Handbook of

Pediatric
Drug Therapy

Handbook of

Pediatric
Drug Therapy

Springhouse Corporation
Springhouse, Pennsylvania

Staff

Executive Director, Editorial
Stanley Loeb

Editorial Director
Helen Klusek Hamilton

Art Director
John Hubbard

Drug Information Editor
George J. Blake, RPh, MS

Copy Editors
Jane V. Cray, Keith de Pinho, Mary Hohenhaus Hardy,
Amy Jirsa, Nancy Papsin, Doris Weinstock

Editorial Assistants
Maree DeRosa, Beverly Lane

Designers
Stephanie Peters (associate art director), Elaine Ezrow

Art Production
Robert Perry (manager), Heather Bernhardt, Anna
Brindisi, Donald Knauss, Robert Wieder

Typography
David Kosten (manager), Diane Paluba (assistant
manager), Elizabeth Bergman, Joyce Rossi Biletz,
Robin Rantz, Valerie Rosenberger

Manufacturing
Deborah Meiris (manager), T.A. Landis, Jennifer Suter

Production Coordination
Aline Miller (manager), Laurie Sander

Indexer
Barbara Hodgson

Library of Congress Cataloging-in-Publication Data
Handbook of pediatric drug therapy.
    p.   cm.

    Includes bibliographical references.
        1. Drugs – Dictionaries.   2. Pediatric pharmacology –
Dictionaries.
I. Springhouse Corporation.
        [DNLM: 1. Drug Therapy – in infancy & childhood –
handbooks.   WS 39 H2355]
RJ560.H29   1990
615.5'8'083 – dc20
DNLM/DLC   89-26164
ISBN 0-87434-217-1   CIP

Contents

Generic drugs for children and adolescents

Appendices and index

Contributors

Edward M. Bednarczyk, RPh, PharmD, Research Fellow, University Hospitals of Cleveland, Division of Cardiology, Cleveland, Ohio: GI drugs, including H_2-receptor antagonists.

Keith A. Burechson, RPh, Assistant Director of Pharmacy, Roxborough Memorial Hospital, Philadelphia, Pa.: topical agents.

James B. Caldwell, RPh, PharmD, Clinical Pharmacist, Anne Arundel General Hospital, Annapolis, Md.: cephalosporins, sulfonamides, and tetracyclines.

Mark A. Campbell, RPh, MS, Pharmacist Specialist, Kaiser Foundation Hospital, San Diego Medical Center, San Diego, Calif.: cancer chemotherapy.

Deborah B. Cooper, RPh, PharmD, Clinical Pharmacist, The Sinai Hospital of Baltimore, Baltimore, Md.: ACE inhibitors, beta-adrenergic blocking agents, and rauwolfia alkaloids.

H. Edward Davidson, RPh, PharmD, Director of Clinical Services, HPI Health Care Services, Atlanta, Ga.: nitrates, cardiac glycosides, and calcium channel blocking agents.

Linda J. Dawson, RPh, PharmD, Fellow in Drug Information, University of Kentucky Medical Center, Lexington, Ky.: tricyclic and MAO inhibitor antidepressants, phenothiazines, and thioxanthines.

Jerri O. Edwards, RPh, PharmD, Clinical Pharmacist, Baker Hospital, Charleston, S.C.: nonsteroidal anti-inflammatory agents and salicylates.

Marcy Portnoff Gever, RPh, MEd, Pharmacist Consultant, West Chester, Pa.: antihistamines.

Joe N. Gibson, RPh, Assistant Director Pharmacy and I.V. Therapy, Nash General Hospital, Rocky Mount, N.C.: systemic and miotic cholinergics and belladonna derivatives.

Margaret R. Glessner, RPh, PharmD, Pharmacy Consultant, Bryn Mawr, Pa.: mydriatic agents.

Edwin L. Gutshall, RPh, PharmD, Director of Pharmacy Services, John Randolph Hospital, Hopewell, Va.: gold salts.

Sarah Johnston-Miller, RPh, MS, PharmD, Advanced Resident in Pharmacy Nutrition Support, Hospital of the University of Pennsylvania, Philadelphia, Pa.: aminoquinolones.

Patricia C. Kienle, RPh, MPA, Assistant Director of Pharmacy, Mercy Hospital, Wilkes-Barre, Pa.: iron supplements, thrombolytic enzymes, and anticoagulants.

Thomas H. Kramer, RPh, PharmD, Research Associate, Department of Pharmacology, College of Medicine, Tucson, Ariz.: hormones.

Michael Lease, RPh, MS, Director of Pharmacy, Montgomery Hospital, Norristown, Pa.: xanthines and pancreatic enzymes.

Robert J. Lipsy, RPh, PharmD, Drug Information Resident, Arizona Poison and Drug Information Center, Tucson, Ariz.: anesthetic agents, barbiturates, and benzodiazepines.

Jan-Elian Markind, RPh, Staff Pharmacist, Graduate Hospital, Philadelphia, Pa.: vitamins and calorics.

Sondra H. McClellan, RPh, PharmD, Clinical Coordinator, Pharmacy Department, Anderson Memorial Hospital, Anderson, S.C.: anticonvulsants and amphetamines.

Barbara L. McHenry, RPh, PharmD, Clinical Pharmacist, Ann Arundel General Hospital, Annapolis, Md.: sulfonamides, tetracyclines, and cephalosporins.

Mary L. Miller, RPh, PharmD, Clinical Pharmacy Fellow in Ambulatory Care, Audie Murphy Memorial V.A. Medical Center, San Antonio, Texas: corticosteroids.

John Ostrosky, RPh, PharmD, Medical College of Virginia Hospital, Richmond, Va.: vaccines and toxins.

Doris M. Sherpinsky, RPh, Staff Pharmacist, Holy Redeemer Hospital and Medical Center, Meadowbrook, Pa.: miscellaneous cardiovascular drugs.

Joanne M. Sica, RPh, MS, Director of Pharmacy, Roxborough Memorial Hospital, Philadelphia, Pa.: adrenergics and several recently approved drugs.

Thomas Simpson, RPh, PharmD, Director of Pharmacy, CPC Santa Ana Psychiatric Hospital, Santa Ana, Calif.: opioids.

Lilliam Sklaver, PharmD, Coordinator of Clinical Research Service, University of Miami School of Medicine, Papanicolaou Comprehensive Cancer Center, Miami, Fla.: diuretics.

Lisa Marie Stevenson, RPh, PharmD, Clinical Pharmacy Resident, University of Kentucky Medical Center, Lexington, Ky.: antidiabetic agents and thyroid hormones.

Paul J. Vitale, RPh, PharmD, Assistant Director Pharmacy/Clinical Services, Anne Arundel General Hospital, Annapolis, Md.: aminoglycosides, penicillins, and other anti-infectives.

Clinical Consultants

John S. Bradley, MD, Assistant Professor of Pediatrics, University of California San Diego, Children's Hospital, San Diego, Calif.

Lawrence W. Brown, MD, ACP, FAAN, FAAP, Associate Professor of Pediatrics and Neurology, Medical College of Pennsylvania, Philadelphia, Pa.

David Burton, MD, Attending Physician, Pediatric Cardiology, St. Christopher's Hospital for Children, Philadelphia, Pa.

Joseph H. Calhoun, MD, Director of Pediatric Ophthalmology, Wills Eye Hospital, Philadelphia, Pa.

Clara Callahan, MD, FAAP, Clinical Assistant Professor of Pediatrics, Jefferson Medical College, Philadelphia, Pa.

Nancy S. Day, MD, Director, Department of Anesthesia, Frankford Hospital, Philadelphia, Pa.

Isaac Djerassi, MD, Director of Research in Oncology and Hematology, Mercy Catholic Medical Center, Philadelphia, Pa.

Stephen C. Duck, MD, Associate Professor of Pediatrics, Medical College of Wisconsin, Milwaukee, Wis.

Bruce Frey, PharmD, Clinical Pharmacist in Pediatrics, Thomas Jefferson University Hospital, Philadelphia, Pa.

Donald P. Goldsmith, MD, Associate Professor of Pediatrics, University of Pennsylvania School of Medicine, Associate Director, Pediatric Rheumatology Center, Philadelphia, Pa.

Susan Jefferies, RN, MSN, Former Pharmacology Research Nurse, National Cancer Institute, Pediatric Branch, Bethesda, Md.

Sheila Jenkins, RN, MSN, Instructor, Bridgeport Hospital School of Nursing, Bridgeport, Conn.

Kathleen A. Kucer, MD, Dermatologist, Chief of Division of Dermatology, Grand View Hospital, Sellersville, Pa.

Linda Sadowski, RN, MSN, Pediatric Critical Care Clinical Specialist, Thomas Jefferson University Hospital, Philadelphia, Pa.

Eileen E. Tyrala, MD, FAAP, Director, Neonatology, Temple University Hospital, Philadelphia, Pa.

Robert H. Wharton, MD, Director of Pediatrics, Spaulding Rehabilitation Hospital, Boston, Mass.

Special thanks to those who assisted with early development of this volume:
Cheryl Conatser, RN, MS, Children's Medical Center of Dallas, Tex.; Valerie D. George, RN, PhD, Cleveland State University, Ohio; Kristin McCarten, RN, BSN, CCRN, Children's Hospital of San Francisco, Calif.; Amy Mikkelson, RN, BSN, CareTeam of Orlando, Winter Park, Fla.; Barbara Pawel, MD, St. Joseph's Hospital and Medical Center, Paterson, N.J.; Patricia A. Rutowski, RN, MSN, Catherine McAuley Health Center, Ann Arbor, Mich.; Cindy Sagady, RN, BSN, Frankford Hospital, Philadelphia, Pa.; Sharon L. Stankoven, RN, BSN, MSA, University of Mich. Medical Center, Ann Arbor, Mich.

How to use this book

The *Handbook of Pediatric Drug Therapy*, the result of the collaboration of pediatricians, pharmacists, and nurse specialists, provides comprehensive, completely updated information on drug therapy in children and adolescents in an easy-to-use encyclopedic format. It covers all aspects of drug information from fundamental pharmacology to specific management of toxicity and overdose. It also includes several unique features – a comprehensive listing of indications that includes clinically approved but unlabeled uses, specific recommendations for use in renal failure, and relevant instructions for administration and monitoring of drug therapy by parents.

An introductory chapter discusses the fundamentals of pharmacotherapeutics in children, provides recommended procedures for correct administration of drugs in all forms and by all routes, and presents a charted summary of emergency drugs.

Generic drug entries

The individual drug entries provide detailed information on virtually all drugs that are considered appropriate for use in children and adolescents, all arranged alphabetically by generic name for easy access. A guideword at the top of each page identifies the generic drug presented on that page. Each entry is complete where it falls alphabetically and does not require cross-referencing to other sections of the book.

In each drug entry, the generic name (with alternate generic names following in parentheses) precedes an alphabetically arranged list of current trade names. An asterisk signals products available only in Canada. To help avoid exposure of sensitive patients to additives that may be hazardous, a graphic symbol identifies products that may contain sulfites (‡), tartrazine (♦), or benzyl alcohol (♦♦). The latter is a preservative that may cause kernicterus in neonates. Drugs available solely as combinations (such as ticarcillin disodium/clavulanate potassium) are listed according to the first generic in the combination. Next, the classification identifies each drug's pharmacologic or chemical category and its major therapeutic uses. When it's appropriate, the next line identifies any drug that the Drug Enforcement Agency (DEA) lists as a controlled substance and specifies the schedule of control as II, III, IV, or V.

How supplied lists the preparations available for each drug (for example, tablets, capsules, solution), specifying available dosage forms and strengths.

Indications, route, and dosage presents all clinically accepted indications for use and includes age- and weight-specific dosage recommendations for infants, children, and adolescents, as appropriate. A preceding dagger signals clinically accepted but unlabeled uses. These dosage instructions reflect current clinical trends in therapeutics as reported by pediatric specialists but should not be considered as absolute and universal recommendations. For individual application, dosage must be considered according to the patient's condition.

Action and kinetics explains the mechanism and effects of the drug's physiologic action.

Kinetics in adults describes absorption, distribution, metabolism, and excretion of the drug; it also specifies onset and duration of action and half-life. It cites information relevant to adults because such information is usually established in adult subjects.

Kinetics in children lists pharmacokinetic information specific to children, if known.

Contraindications and precautions lists conditions associated with special risks in patients who receive the drug and includes the rationale for each warning.

Interactions specifies the clinically significant additive, synergistic, or antagonistic effects that result from combined use of the drug with other drugs.

Effects on diagnostic tests lists significant interference with a diagnostic test or its result by direct effects on the test itself or by systemic drug effects that lead to misleading test results.

Adverse reactions lists the undesirable effects that may follow use of the drug; these effects are arranged by body systems (CNS, CV, DERM, EENT, GI, GU, HEMA, Hepatic, Metabolic, Respiratory, Local, and Other). Local effects occur at the site of drug administration (by application, infusion, or injection); adverse reactions not specific to a single body system (for example, the effects of hypersensitivity) are listed under *Other*. Throughout, adverse reactions that have been reported in children are italicized. At the end of this section, *Note* signals a list of severe and hazardous reactions that mandate discontinuation of the drug.

Overdose and treatment summarizes the clinical manifestations of drug overdose and recommends specific treatment as appropriate. Usually, this segment recommends emesis or gastric lavage, followed by activated charcoal to reduce the amount of drug absorbed and possibly a cathartic to eliminate the toxin. This section specifies antidotes, drug therapy, special care, and the effects of dialysis.

Special considerations offers detailed recommendations for preparation and administration of the drug and for patient care during therapy. A special section unique to this volume, *Information for parents and patient*, lists recommendations for teaching patients and parents correct administration and monitoring, preventing and managing adverse reactions, and teaching the patient self-care, as appropriate.

Appendix

The appendix includes several useful charts and a *Table of equivalents*. The first chart, *Drugs available without prescription*, lists recommendations for using OTC drugs in children. *Calculating body surface area in children* provides an easy-to-use nomogram. *Pediatric recommendations for anesthetic drugs* describes use of inhalant and intravenous anesthetics. *Recommendations for pediatric immunization* includes current CDC and ACIP guidelines, including those for children with HIV infection. *Identifying the unknown poison* correlates common poisons with the signs and symptoms they typically cause. *Antidotes to poisoning or envenomation* lists dosages and other guidelines for use in children.

Index

The index lists trade names of generic drugs and combination products; alternate generic names; and charts, tables, and illustrations.

ABBREVIATIONS

Abbreviation	Meaning
ALT	serum alanine aminotransferase
AST	serum aspartate aminotransferase
ATP	adenosine triphosphate
AV	atrioventricular
b.i.d.	twice a day
BUN	blood urea nitrogen
cAMP	cyclic 3′, 5′ adenosine monophosphate
CHF	congestive heart failure
CNS	central nervous system
CPK	creatinine phosphokinase
CPR	cardiopulmonary resuscitation
CSF	cerebrospinal fluid
CV	cardiovascular
CVP	central venous pressure
DNA	deoxyribonucleic acid
EEG	electroencephalogram
ECG	electrocardiogram
FDA	Food and Drug Administration
g	gram
G	gauge
GI	gastrointestinal
GU	genitourinary
h.s.	at bedtime
I.M.	intramuscular
IU	International Unit
I.V.	intravenous
kg	kilogram
L	liter
m^2	square meter
mm^3	cubic millimeter
MAO	monoamine oxidase
mcg or μg	microgram
mEq	milliequivalent
mg	milligram
MI	myocardial infarction
ml	milliliter
ng	nanogram (millimicrogram)
OTC	over-the-counter
P.O.	by mouth
p.r.n.	as needed
q	every
q.d.	every day
q.i.d.	four times a day
RNA	ribonucleic acid
SA	sinoatrial
S.C.	subcutaneous
SGOT	serum glutamic oxaloacetic transaminase
SGPT	serum glutamic pyruvic transaminase
t.i.d.	three times a day

SELECTED REFERENCES

AMA Drug Evaluations, 6th ed. Chicago: American Medical Association, 1986.

American Hospital Formulary Service. Drug Information 1989. Bethesda, Md.: American Society of Hospital Pharmacists, 1989.

Bhatt, D.R., et al. Neonatal Drug Formulary. Covina, Calif.: California Perinatal Association, 1987.

Billups, N., ed. American Drug Index, 33rd ed. Philadelphia: J.B. Lippincott Co., 1989.

Braunwald, E., et al. Harrison's Principles of Internal Medicine, 11th ed. New York: McGraw-Hill Book Co., 1987.

Briggs, G., et al. Drugs in Pregnancy and Lactation: A Reference Guide to Fetal and Neonatal Risk, 2nd ed. Baltimore: Williams & Wilkins Co., 1986.

Committee on Infectious Diseases, American Academy of Pediatrics. Report of the Committee on Infectious Diseases, 12th ed. Elk Grove Village, Ill.: American Academy of Pediatrics, 1986.

Compendium of Pharmaceuticals and Specialties of 1989, 24th ed. Ottawa, Canada: Canadian Pharamceutical Association, 1989.

Dorland's Illustrated Medical Dictionary, 27th ed. Philadelphia: W.B Saunders Co., 1988.

Drug Interaction Facts. St. Louis: J.B. Lippincott Co. (Facts and Comparisons Division), 1989.

Facts and Comparisons. St. Louis: J.B. Lippincott Co. (Facts and Comparisons Division), 1989.

Ford, D.C., et al. Guidelines for Administration of Intravenous Medications to Pediatric Patients. Bethesda, Md.: American Society of Hospital Pharmacists, 1988.

Gilman, A., et al., eds. Goodman and Gilman's The Pharmacological Basis of Therapeutics, 7th ed. New York: Macmillan Publishing Co., 1985.

Haddad, L.M., and Winchester, J. Clinical Management of Poisoning & Drug Overdose. Philadelphia: W.B. Saunders Co., 1983.

Handbook of Nonprescription Drugs, 8th ed. Washington, D.C.: American Pharmaceutical Association, 1986.

Hansten, P., and Horn, J.R. Drug Interactions, 6th ed. Philadelphia: Lea and Febiger, 1989.

Knobson, J.E., and Anderson, P.O., eds. Handbook of Clinical Drug Data, 6th ed. Hamilton, Ill.: Drug Intelligence Publications, Inc., 1988.

The Merck Manual of Diagnosis and Therapy, 15th ed. Rahway, N.J.: Merck & Co., Inc., 1987.

Pawlack, R., and Herfert, L., eds. Drug administration in the NICU. Petaluma, Calif.: Neonatal Network, 1988.

Physician's Desk Reference, 43rd ed. Oradell, N.J.: Medical Economics Books, 1989.

Physician's Desk Reference for Nonprescription Drugs, 10th ed. Oradell, N.J.: Medical Economics Books, 1989.

Physician's Desk Reference for Ophthalmology, 17th ed. Oradell, N.J.: Medical Economics Books, 1989.

Rowe, P.C., ed. The Harriet Lane Handbook, 11th ed. Chicago: Year Book Medical Publishers, 1987.

Speight, T. Avery's Drug Treatment, 3rd ed. Baltimore: Williams & Wilkins Co., 1987.

Trissel, L. Handbook of Injectable Drugs, 5th ed. Bethesda, Md.: American Society of Hospital Pharmacists, 1988.

United States Pharmacopeia Dispensing Information (USP-DI). Rockville, Md.: United States Pharmacopeial Convention, Inc., 1989.

Foreword

The proliferation of drugs currently available has led to an increased number of drugs prescribed for children, and corresponding increase in the need for accurate and comprehensive information about pediatric drug therapy. According to the National Council on Patient Information and Education (NCPIE), over 6 million children weekly take drugs prescribed or recommended by physicians. However, this report contends that the drug therapy is ultimately incorrect for nearly half of these children. Commonly, the drug is discontinued too soon, the dosage taken is less or more than prescribed, or the drug is not taken at all. Such poor compliance may reflect insufficient instruction by the prescribing practitioner or misunderstanding of instructions by the parents. Improved compliance with drug therapy requires physicians and nurses to possess current accurate information about the drugs and to provide more specific information about drug administration to parents.

Complications of drug therapy may be serious. The NCPIE study notes that drug-related illnesses are responsible for nearly 5% of all hospital admissions, and nearly 50% of these illnesses are serious or fatal.

These worrisome statistics suggest that drug therapy is too often inappropriate or imprecise. The *Handbook of Pediatric Drug Therapy* addresses this need for comprehensive, accurate information about drug therapy in children and adolescents. It is the result of collaboration of pediatricians, pharmacists, and nurse specialists and is designed to provide the practitioner with important and relevant information in an encyclopedic format.

The introductory chapter presents fundamental concepts in pediatric pharmacotherapeutics. It includes recommended procedures for accurate administration of drugs in all forms and by all routes as well as a summary of emergency drugs.

The major portion of the book is devoted to a presentation of drugs, arranged alphabetically by generic name. Individual drug entries offer instant access to current information about the drug, including trade names, all accepted indications for use, age- and weight-specific dosage recommendations, contraindications to use, and precautions. The mechanism of action, pharmacokinetics, interactions, effects on diagnostic tests, and adverse effects are also provided for each drug. Unique to this handbook, the text includes information for treatment of overdose, relevant instructions for administration of the drug by parents, and other special considerations.

The appendices include the latest Centers For Disease Control (CDC) recommendations for immunization of children (with new guidelines for reporting adverse reactions), charts for pediatric use of anesthetics and over-the-counter drugs, a list of signs and symptoms to help identify unknown poisons, and a list of antidotes to poisoning and envenomation. The index lists alternate generic names; all trade names available in the United States and Canada (including selected combination drugs); charts, tables, and illustrations; and introductory pharmacotherapeutic concepts.

The drug information in this reference was reviewed for accuracy and appropriateness for use in children by pediatric specialists. Consequently, the information listed represents current clinical experience and standards of practice that are more comprehensive and clinically relevant than the information available elsewhere. For example, the entries list all clinically approved indications, including unlabeled and selected investigational uses.

This practical reference will be very useful to pediatricians, pediatric nurses, and other health care professionals who manage drug therapy in children and adolescents.

William Banner, MD, PhD
Associate Professor of Pediatrics,
Critical Care Division,
University of Utah/Primary Children's Medical Center
Salt Lake City, Utah

Mary Fran Hazinski, RN, MSN
Clinical Nurse Specialist, Pediatric Critical Care
Nashville, Tenn.

Drug therapy in children

Providing drug therapy to children presents a unique set of challenges. Physiologic differences between children and adults, including variance in vital organ maturity and body composition, greatly influence the action and effectiveness of drugs. However, pharmacokinetic studies, which are usually done in adult subjects, offer little information about specific activity in children. Further complicating pediatric drug therapy is the fact that many drugs currently lack full approval by the U.S. Food and Drug Administration for use in children.

Drug administration routes are essentially the same for children and adults, but injection sites, administration techniques, and, especially, dosages often differ greatly. Moreover, choosing a drug and an administration route, calculating the proper dosage, and administering it correctly are only the first steps. Because drug effects often are less predictable in children than in adults, careful monitoring after administration is necessary to ensure safe and effective therapy.

Factors affecting pharmacokinetics

As they grow, children undergo profound physiologic changes that affect drug absorption, distribution, metabolism, and excretion. Failure to understand these changes and their effects can lead to underestimation or overestimation of drug dosage, with the resultant potential for failure of therapy, severe adverse reactions, or, perhaps, fatal toxicity.

Absorption. In children, various factors influence the rate of drug absorption, including age, physiologic condition, the drug's dosage form and physical properties, and interactions with concurrent drugs and foods.

• *Absorption of oral drugs.* After oral administration, most drug absorption takes place in the small intestine, where the prevalent pH range (4 to 8) favors absorption of the nonionized absorbable form of most drugs. The pH of neonatal gastric fluid is slightly acidic or neutral and becomes more acidic as the infant matures, reaching adult values by age 2. Higher gastric pH affects absorption of some drugs, particularly during the first 2 months of life. For example, high gastric pH increases absorption of nafcillin and penicillin G through decreased acid hydrolysis in the stomach; it decreases absorption of phenytoin and such weak acids as phenobarbital by increasing the ionized form of the drug.

Other physiologic factors also affect oral drug absorption. A neonate's erratic and prolonged gastric emptying time and intestinal transit time can enhance drug absorption. But an older child's faster gastric emptying time and intestinal transit time can decrease drug absorption.

A child's immature biliary function produces a smaller amount of gastric bile salts, resulting in decreased absorption of lipid-soluble drugs, such as vitamin E.

Concurrent administration of various infant formulas or milk products may temporarily raise gastric pH and impede absorption of acidic drugs. Thus, neonates, infants, and young children should receive oral medication on an empty stomach whenever possible.

• *Absorption of parenteral drugs.* Because of their relatively small skeletal muscle mass and variable blood flow, neonates, infants, and young children experience unpredictable and erratic absorption of drugs administered at peripheral sites via intramuscular (I.M.) and subcutaneous injections.

The properties of particular drugs also may influence I.M. absorption in children. For instance, absorption of I.M. phenobarbital is rapid, but absorption of I.M. diazepam is slow.

• *Absorption of topical drugs.* Neonates and infants experience enhanced absorption of topical drugs because of the relative thinness and high water content of their skin and because of their high proportion of body surface area to total body mass. This can lead to systemic, possibly toxic, adverse reactions after use of such common topical agents as rubbing alcohol, hexachlorophene soaps, and steroid and salicyclic acid ointments.

Distribution. Developmental changes in body composition during childhood can significantly affect drug distribution. In a normal neonate, body fluid accounts for 55% to 70% of the total body weight; in a premature infant, this figure may be as high as 85%. In comparison, an adult's proportion of body fluid normally ranges from 50% to 55% of total body weight. The extracellular fluid volume (mostly blood) constitutes 40% of a neonate's weight, compared with 20% of an adult's. Intracellular fluid volume remains fairly constant throughout life and has little effect on drug distribution.

A drug's solubility in lipids or water greatly affects the pediatric dosage. Because most drugs travel through extracellular fluid to reach their receptor sites, the proportion of extracellular fluid volume influences the concentration of a water-soluble drug and subsequently influences its effect. Children have a higher ratio of fluid to solid body weight than adults; thus, their distribution area is proportionately greater for water-soluble drugs. Conversely, because the proportion of fat to lean body mass increases with age, the distribution of fat-soluble drugs is more limited in children than in adults.

Another major factor in the distribution of many drugs is the degree of plasma protein binding. Only unbound, or free, drug can exert its pharmacologic effect, and even a small change in the ratio of protein-bound to unbound active drug can greatly increase drug effect. For instance, a decrease in the percentage of bound drug from 95% to 90% will double the amount of free drug available.

As the result of decreased albumin concentration or weaker intermolecular attraction between the drug and plasma protein, many drugs are less bound to plasma proteins in infants than in adults.

One other physiologic factor affecting drug distribution in neonates is the comparative immaturity of the blood-brain barrier. This allows for greater drug penetration of the cerebrospinal fluid (CSF), particularly by aminoglycoside antibiotics, such as gentamicin and tobramycin.

Metabolism. Most drug metabolism occurs in the liver. In neonates, a large liver (40% of total body mass, as compared with only 2% in adults) provides a markedly greater hepatic surface area available for drug metabolism. Nevertheless, the immaturity of the neonatal liver and hepatic enzyme system may interfere with drug metabolism.

In children, enzymatic functions mature at different rates. These differences influence metabolic mechanisms and, in turn, drug dosages. For example, because glucuronidation (a mechanism that helps eliminate drugs) is insufficiently developed until age 1 month, full pediatric dosages of some drugs may produce adverse or even toxic reactions in a neonate. One such drug is chloramphenicol; administration of a full pediatric dose of chloramphenicol to a neonate may cause the potentially fatal gray baby syndrome. Use of chloramphenicol in neonates, therefore, requires decreased dosages and careful monitoring of blood drug levels.

On the other hand, older infants and children can metabolize some drugs (for example, theophylline) more rapidly than adults. Thus, they may require larger doses of these drugs than those recommended for adults. Failure to recognize such differences may lead to failure of drug therapy.

Other factors that affect a child's ability to metabolize a drug include intrauterine exposure to drugs and the nature of the drug itself. Intrauterine exposure to certain drugs (phenobarbital, for example) may induce precocious development of hepatic enzymes, thereby increasing the neonate's capacity to metabolize drugs or potentially harmful substances, such as bilirubin.

Finally, in children as in adults, concurrent use of certain drugs can produce interactions that stimulate or reduce hepatic enzyme activity. The resultant effect may require a dosage adjustment. For example, concomitant use of phenobarbital can induce metabolism of phenytoin, requiring increased dosage.

Excretion. Because most drugs and their metabolites are excreted in the urine, the maturity of the renal system or the presence of renal disease can profoundly affect a child's dosage requirements. If renal excretion is inadequate, drug accumulation and possible toxicity may result unless the dosage is reduced.

Physiologically, the neonatal renal system differs from an adult's in the following ways:
• a higher resistance to blood flow and a resultant decreased renal fraction of cardiac output
• incomplete glomerular and tubular development and short, incomplete loops of Henle

• a low glomerular filtration rate (GFR), which doesn't reach adult equivalent values until age 2½ to 5 months
• a decreased capacity to concentrate urine or reabsorb various filtered compounds and a reduced ability of the proximal tubule to secrete organic acids. (Tubular secretion and reabsorption rates don't reach adult equivalent values until age 5 to 7 months.)

These physiologic differences can greatly influence drug therapy. For example, a drug that requires a high GFR, such as a thiazide diuretic, produces a diminished response in a neonate, necessitating a higher dosage or substitution of a drug that is less dependent on GFR, such as furosemide.

Calculating pediatric dosages

In the past, drug dosages for children were based on rigid but inexact dosing formulas, such as Young's, Clark's, and Fried's rules. These and other such formulas determine what fraction of an adult dose is appropriate for a child. Such dosage formulas were recently in widespread use, but are now obsolete. Because of individual variations in developmental stage and body composition, following a rigid formula often leads to either underdosage or overdosage, with a resultant drug failure or risk of toxicity.

Today, calculation of pediatric dosages is based on much more exact and individualized parameters: either total body surface area (mg/m^2) or body weight (mg/kg) of the child. Body weight is the most commonly used method because of its ease of calculation. The body surface area method requires both body weight and height, which can then be applied to a nomogram for calculating body surface area (see Appendix), or can be used in the formulas below. Whether you use the surface area method or

---

FORMULAS FOR BODY SURFACE AREA

$S = W^{0.425} \times H^{0.725} \times 71.84$, or
$\log S = \log W \times 0.425 + \log H \times 0.725 + 1.8564$

where S = body surface area in cm^2
W = weight in kg
H = height in cm

---

the body weight method, keep the following general rules in mind:
• Reevaluate all dosages at regular intervals to ensure necessary adjustments as the child develops.
• Ensure that the surface area or body weight dosage recommendation is appropriate for the child's age. A dosage calculation that is appropriate for a neonate may not be so for a premature infant or a toddler.
• When calculating amounts per kilogram of body weight, do not exceed the maximum adult dosage (except with certain drugs, such as theophylline).
• Always double-check all computations before prescribing or administering the dosage.

Administering drugs to children

The best method of drug administration depends on the drug's dosage form and its specific properties, as well as the child's age and physical condition.

Oral administration. To facilitate administration of oral drugs, consider the drug's taste, dosage form, and frequency of administration. If possible, administer oral drugs in the liquid dosage form. To ensure accuracy of dosage, measure and administer the drug in an oral syringe or a calibrated medication cup. Recheck the amount of medication poured into a medication cup by placing the cup at eye level and reading the dose at the base of the meniscus.

If the drug is available only in tablet form, you may crush it and mix it with a compatible syrup or other vehicle, or possibly with food if no alternative is available. However, because crushing some tablets may reduce their effectiveness and because food may interfere with absorption of certain drugs, check with the pharmacist before doing this.

To administer an oral drug to an infant, raise the infant's head to prevent aspiration, gently press down on the chin with your thumb to open his mouth, then give the dose. (Never administer oral drugs to an infant in the prone position unless the infant has been intubated.) If using a syringe to administer the medication, place the tip of the syringe in the pocket between the patient's cheek mucosa and gum. Administer slowly and steadily, to reduce risk of aspiration. As an alternative, you can place the medication in a nipple and allow the infant to suck the contents. However, never mix a drug with the contents of a baby bottle; the child who doesn't finish the entire contents won't receive the correct dose, and some formulas may interfere with drug absorption.

To maximize absorption, administer oral medications on an empty stomach unless otherwise indicated. And, obviously, for safety's sake, never refer to a drug as "candy" or "a treat," even if it has a pleasant taste. Remember to warn parents about this when instructing them about giving medications.

Rectal administration. When administering drugs or fluids through the rectum, keep in mind the special significance children place on this part of the body. Toddlers in particular—especially those for whom toilet-training is or was stressful—likely will resist rectal administration. Older children may perceive the procedure as an invasion of privacy and may react with embarrassment or anger and hostility. To reduce the child's anxiety and increase cooperation, spend some time explaining the procedure and reassure him that it will not hurt.

After administering a suppository, hold the child's buttocks together for a few minutes to prevent expulsion.

Intravenous infusion. Before administering I.V. drugs, check the following points:
• *Compatibility of the solution.* A drug that is compatible with the main I.V. vehicle may be diluted in

---

---

enough fluid to run over 15 to 30 minutes regardless of the concentration. An irritating drug must be diluted in enough fluid to run for over 30 to 60 minutes to offset most irritation. If a drug must be administered using a solution that is incompatible with the main I.V. vehicle or unfavorable to the child's condition or course of treatment, use the minimum amount of solution and infuse it over 15 to 30 minutes regardless of the resulting concentration. To run a second drug through the same I.V. tubing, first flush the tubing with a small amount of solution that is compatible with the second drug.
• *Appropriate dilutions.* In infants, hyperosmolar drugs must be diluted to prevent radical fluid shifts that may induce CNS hemorrhage. Sodium bicarbonate, for example, must be diluted before administration to lower osmolality and reduce the risk of hemorrhage. Diluting irritating drugs in 30 to 60 ml of fluid should substantially reduce any irritation. Generally, however, the minimum amount of compatible fluid should be infused over the shortest recommended time. Remember to include fluids used to administer drugs as part of the child's daily fluid intake.
• *Maximum administration time and infusion rate.* When infusing any routinely scheduled drug, know both the maximum administration time and the maximum infusion rate for that drug. If a drug has

no maximum infusion rate or special concentration requirements, it may be possible to administer via I.V. push. If it has a maximum rate, follow the manufacturer's recommendations.

Intramuscular injection. The optimum site for I.M. injection depends on the patient's age. In children under age 3, the vastus lateralis muscle is the preferred site; in older children, either the gluteus muscle or ventrogluteal area can be used.

The appropriate needle size also depends on the patient's age, as well as the patient's muscle mass (which may be affected by nutritional status) and the drug's viscosity.

Before administering an I.M. injection, explain to the child that, although the injection will hurt slightly, the medication will help him. Clean the injection site with an alcohol swab, using a circular motion and moving from the center outward. If necessary, restrain the child, and always comfort him after the injection.

Subcutaneous injection. The subcutaneous route is used to administer certain medications, including narcotics, insulin, heparin, and some vaccines. The procedure is similar to that for I.M. injection, but shorter needles must be used and the volume of the injection should be limited to 2 ml. Use a ⅜" or ½" needle for an infant or small child and a ⅝" needle for a larger child.

CHOOSING AN I.M. INJECTION SITE

When determining the optimum I.M. injection site for a child, take into account the child's age, weight, and muscle development; the amount of subcutaneous fat over the injection site; the type of drug you're administering; and its absorption rate.

If the child is younger than age 3, you'll generally use the vastus lateralis muscle group for injection. The largest muscle mass in children of this age-group, it has few major blood vessels and nerves. For a child older than age 3, consider the ventrogluteal and dorsogluteal areas as other possible injection sites. These areas also are relatively free of major blood vessels and nerves. Before you select either area, however, make sure that the child has been walking for at least 1 year, to ensure that the muscles are sufficiently developed. If the posterior gluteal muscle is poorly developed, injection carries the risk of injury to the child's sciatic nerve.

If the child is older than age 18 months and if rapid drug absorption is desired, consider using the deltoid muscle. Blood flow is more rapid in the deltoid than in other muscles. But choose this site with caution—the deltoid isn't fully developed until adolescence. In a younger child, it's small and close to the radial nerve, which may be injured during needle insertion.

MAXIMUM I.M. SOLUTION VOLUMES FOR CHILDREN

The amount of drug solution that you can administer safely via I.M. injection depends primarily on the child's age and the selected injection site. The following chart lists the maximum recommended volumes that are appropriate for intramuscular injections in the various muscle groups for children of different ages.

MUSCLE GROUP	AGE				
	BIRTH TO 1½ YEARS	1½ TO 3 YEARS	3 TO 6 YEARS	6 TO 15 YEARS	15 YEARS TO ADULTHOOD
Deltoid	Not recommended	0.5 ml (Not recommended unless other sites aren't available.)	0.5 ml	0.5 ml	1 ml
Gluteus maximus	Not recommended	1 ml (Not recommended unless other sites aren't available.)	1.5 ml	1.5 to 2 ml	2 to 2.5 ml
Ventrogluteal	Not recommended	1 ml (Not recommended unless other sites aren't available.)	1.5 ml	1.5 to 2 ml	2 to 2.5 ml
Vastus lateralis	0.5 to 1 ml	1 ml	1.5 ml	1.5 to 2 ml	2 to 2.5 ml

INTRAMUSCULAR INJECTION SITES FOR INFANTS AND TODDLERS

Dorsogluteal injection site

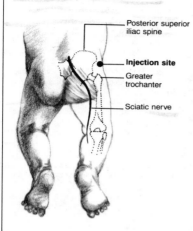

- Posterior superior iliac spine
- **Injection site**
- Greater trochanter
- Sciatic nerve

The dorsogluteal site can be used only after the toddler has been walking for about 1 year.

Vastus lateralis and rectus femoris injection sites

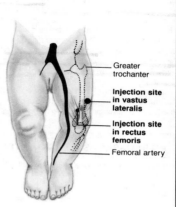

- Greater trochanter
- **Injection site in vastus lateralis**
- **Injection site in rectus femoris**
- Femoral artery

The vastus lateralis and rectus femoris muscles are the recommended sites for I.M. injection in an infant or a toddler.

Ventrogluteal injection site

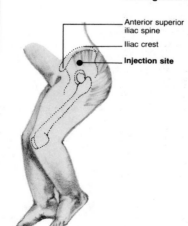

- Anterior superior iliac spine
- Iliac crest
- **Injection site**

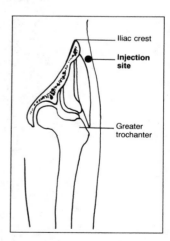

- Iliac crest
- **Injection site**
- Greater trochanter

The ventrogluteal site can be used only after the toddler has been walking for about 1 year.

Intraosseous infusion. The intraosseous route may be indicated in a severe emergency, in which I.V. access is not readily attained for necessary fluid and medication administration. Such emergencies include cardiopulmonary arrest or circulatory collapse, hypokalemia from trauma or dehydration, status epilepticus, status asthmaticus, burns, near drowning, and overwhelming sepsis. The bone marrow serves as a noncollapsible vein; in this situation, fluid infused into the marrow rapidly enters the systemic circulation via an extensive network of venous sinusoids. (See *Lateral view of tibial intraosseous infusion.*) Thus, any substance that can be given I.V. can be given intraosseously, and drug absorption and effectiveness are the same as the I.V. route.

Intraosseous flow rates are determined by both the size of the needle and the flow through the bone marrow. Fluids should flow freely if placement is correct. (When needle placement is correct, the needle stands upright without support.) Normal saline solution has been administered intraosseously at a rate of 600 ml/min and up to 2500 ml/hr when delivered under pressure of 300 mm Hg through a 13 G needle.

With specialized training, insertion of a needle for intraosseous infusion can be accomplished within 3 minutes. It requires the use of a local anesthetic if the patient is awake.

Observe for complications of infusion: extravasation of fluid into subcutaneous tissue from improper needle placement, subperiosteal effusion from failure of fluid to penetrate the marrow cavity, and needle clotting from delay in starting infusion or failure to flush.

Intraosseous infusion is strictly an emergency alternative and should be replaced by I.V. administration as soon as possible.

INTRAOSSEOUS INFUSION SITE

The anteromedial surface of the proximal tibia, approximately 1″ below the tibial tuberosity, is the site of choice for intraosseous infusion.

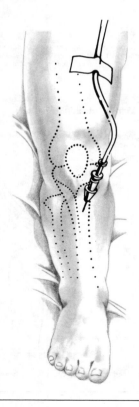

LATERAL VIEW OF TIBIAL INTRAOSSEOUS INFUSION

The tip of the needle lies in the medullary cavity of long bones, where marrow sinusoids drain into large medullary venous channels that provide access to the systemic venous circulation.

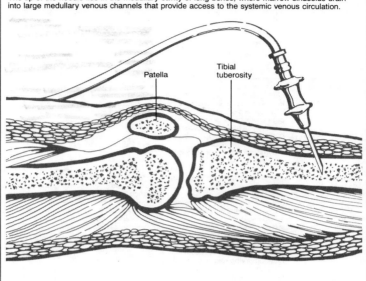

Ear drops. Follow these guidelines for administering ear drops to children.
• Before you begin, warm the drops to room temperature; cold drops can cause pain and vertigo.
• Position the child on his side, with the affected ear up. For a patient younger than age 3, pull the pinna down and back; for a patient age 3 or older, pull the pinna up and back.
• After administering the drops, keep the child in the lateral position for at least 5 minutes.

Nose drops. Follow these guidelines for administering nose drops to children.
• Hyperextend the child's head to visualize the nostrils.
• Minimize bacterial contamination by ensuring that the dropper doesn't touch the nasal mucosa.
• If the drops are for nasal congestion, administer the drops 15 to 30 minutes before mealtime to make feeding easier.

Eye drops and ointments. Follow these guidelines for administering ophthalmic medications.
• Tilt the child's head backward and to one side.
• Hold the lower lid down to expose the conjunctiva, instill the drops or ointment, then release the lid. Gently blot any leakage with a tissue.
• To minimize bacterial contamination of the ophthalmic solution, make sure that the applicator tip doesn't touch the conjunctiva.
• If necessary, restrain an uncooperative child.

Inhalants. Correct administration of an inhalant depends on the patient's full cooperation and therefore requires special instruction. Inhaled agents may have limited usefulness in young children. If you have any doubt about the child's ability to use the medication correctly, consider an alternate route.

When administering medication through a metered-dose inhaler, first explain the equipment and the procedure to the child. Then, instruct the child to hold the device upside down and to close his lips around the mouthpiece. Next, tell him to exhale, to pinch his nostrils shut, and, as inhalation occurs, to release one dose of medication. Instruct him to continue inhaling until his lungs feel full. This same procedure applies if the inhaler is used with an extender.

After use, the inhalation device must be thoroughly cleaned to minimize bacterial contamination.

Emergency drug therapy

Effective management of a pediatric emergency requiring drug therapy requires quick, accurate dosage calculations and proper administration techniques. The accompanying chart, *Pediatric emergency drugs,* summarizes critical dosing and administration information. This chart lists dosages calculated by weight (mg of drug per unit of body weight), according to the latest American Heart Association standards.

PEDIATRIC EMERGENCY DRUGS

DRUG	INDICATION	DOSAGE
Aminophylline	• Bronchial asthma • Bronchospasm	Loading dose: If no prior doses of theophylline have been given, 4 to 6 mg/kg over 15 to 20 minutes; if theophylline has been given previously, 2 to 4 mg over 15 to 20 minutes. Maintenance infusion: 0.9 to 1.25 mg/kg/hour. Therapeutic levels are 10 to 20 mcg/ml.
Atropine sulfate	• Symptomatic bradycardia (or heart rate below 80 beats/minute in a distressed infant younger than age 6 months, with or without hypotension) • Vagally mediated bradycardia during endotracheal intubation • Ventricular asystole • Symptomatic bradycardia with AV block (rare)	0.01 to 0.03 mg/kg/dose by I.V. bolus or endotracheally; if necessary, repeat in 5 minutes. Maximum total dosage is 1 mg for children, 2 mg for adolescents.
Bretylium tosylate	• Ventricular tachycardia or fibrillation	5 to 10 mg/kg I.V. bolus. If still unable to defibrillate, 10 mg/kg I.V. Maintenance dosage: 5 mg/kg q 6 to 8 hours.
Calcium chloride	• Hypocalcemia • Hyperkalemia • Hypermagnesemia • Calcium channel blocker overdose ***Note:*** Calcium is *not* recommended during resuscitation efforts unless hypocalcemia is clearly present.	I.V. bolus of 20 mg/kg/dose; repeat in 10 minutes, if necessary.
Calcium gluceptate	• Acute hypocalcemia	440 mg to 1.1 g I.V. bolus, infused slowly at a rate not to exceed 2 ml/minute. May be given I.M. *only* if I.V. administration is impossible.
Calcium gluconate	• Acute hypocalcemia	200 to 500 mg I.V. bolus infused slowly at a rate not to exceed 5 ml/minute, until tetany is controlled.
Diazepam	• Seizures • Tetanic muscle spasms	Given I.V. Acute anticonvulsant dose: 0.25 mg/kg by slow I.V. bolus at rate not exceeding 5 mg/minute; may repeat q 15 minutes for two doses. Maximum dosage is 5 mg for infants or 15 mg for older children.
Digoxin	• Atrial dysrhythmias	Given I.V. Total digitalizing dose (TDD): Premature infants, 25 to 40 mcg/kg; infants ages 0 to 2 weeks, 35 to 50 mcg/kg; infants ages 2 weeks to 2 years, 40 to 65 mcg/kg; children ages 2 to 10, 35 to 50 mcg/kg. TDD may be divided in equal thirds and given in 8-hour intervals or more. Total daily maintenance: P.O. ⅓ TDD based on original I.V. dosage.
Dobutamine hydrochloride	• Poor myocardial function from diminished cardiac output	I.V. infusion of 5 to 15 mcg/kg/minute.
Dopamine hydrochloride	• Shock • Hypotension or poor peripheral perfusion after resuscitation	Initially, I.V. infusion of 5 to 10 mcg/kg/minute; increase to a maximum of 20 mcg/kg/minute, if necessary, to improve blood pressure, perfusion, and urine output.

(continued)

PEDIATRIC EMERGENCY DRUGS *(continued)*

DRUG	INDICATION	DOSAGE
Epinephrine hydrochloride	• Asystole • Bradydysrhythmias	I.V. bolus, endotracheal, or intracardiac, 0.01 mg/kg (0.1 mg/kg of 1:10,000 solution). Repeat q 5 minutes, as needed.
Furosemide	• Pulmonary edema • Hypercalcemia	As a diuretic, 1 mg/kg I.V. or I.M., then increase dose by an additional 1 mg/kg at 2-hour intervals until desired dose is obtained. For hypercalcemia, 25 to 50 mg I.V or I.M., repeated q 4 hours until desired response is obtained.
Glucose	• Acute hypoglycemia • Adjunctive treatment of shock	*Neonates:* 250 to 500 mg/kg of 25% dextrose per dose. Repeated doses based on serum glucose level. Severe cases or older infants may require 10 to 12 ml of 25% dextrose. I.V. infusion of 10% dextrose may be needed to stabilize blood glucose. *Children:* 50% dextrose for hypoglycemia, 40% to 70% solutions for shock.
Isoproterenol hydrochloride	• Hemodynamically significant bradycardia resistant to atropine • Heart block (rare in children)	I.V. infusion of 0.1 to 1 mcg/kg/minute.
Lidocaine hydrochloride	• Ventricular fibrillation • Ventricular tachycardia • Ventricular ectopy causing hypotension and poor perfusion	I.V. bolus of 1 mg/kg/dose; may be repeated q 5 minutes for three doses and followed by an infusion of 10 to 20 mcg/kg/minute if dysrhythmia continues.
Naloxone	• Opioid-induced respiratory depression	0.01 mg/kg I.V, I.M., or S.C. or via umbilical artery in neonates. Repeat at 2- to 3-minute intervals for one or two additional doses.
Sodium bicarbonate	• Prolonged cardiac arrest or unstable hemodynamic state with documented metabolic acidosis. *Note:* Sodium bicarbonate is not normally indicated during resuscitation efforts.	I.V. bolus of 1 mEq/kg (1 ml/kg or 8.4% solution) in children; for infants, dilute to 0.5 mEq/ml.

SELECTED REFERENCES

Mulhall, A. "Antibiotic Treatment of Neonates... Does Route of Administration Matter?," *Developmental Pharmacology and Therapeutics* 8(1):1-8, 1985.

Prandota, J. "Clinical Pharmacokinetics of Changes in Drug Elimination in Children," *Developmental Pharmacology and Therapeutics* 8(5):311-28, 1985.

Warner, A. "Drug Use in the Neonate: Interrelationships of Pharmacokinetics, Toxicity, and Biochemical Maturity," *Clinical Chemistry* 32(5):721-27, 1986.

acetaminophen
Acephen, Anacin-3, Bromo-Seltzer, Datril, Datril-500, Tempra, Tylenol, Valadol, Valorin

- Classification: nonnarcotic analgesic (antipyretic para-aminophenol derivative)

How supplied
Available without prescription
Tablets: 160 mg, 325 mg, 500 mg, 650 mg
Tablets (chewable): 80 mg
Capsules: 325 mg, 500 mg
Suppositories: 120 mg, 125 mg, 135 mg, 650 mg
Solution: 100 mg/ml
Elixir: 120 mg/5 ml, 160 mg/5 ml, 320 mg/5 ml
Liquid: 160 mg/5 ml; 500 mg/15 ml
Wafers: 120 mg
Effervescent granules: 325 mg/capful

Indications, route, and dosage
Mild pain or fever
Children over age 12 and adults: 325 to 650 mg P.O. or rectally q 4 hours, p.r.n. Maximum dose should not exceed 4 g daily. Patient should not self-medicate for longer than 5 days. Dosage for long-term therapy should not exceed 2.6 g daily.
Children under age 12: 10 mg/kg P.O. per dose, with no more than five doses in any 24-hour period; or 1.5 g/m² P.O. daily in divided doses. Alternatively, give according to age:
Children age 3 months or younger: 40 mg/dose q 4 to 6 hours.
Children age 4 to 11 months: 80 mg/dose q 4 to 6 hours.
Children age 12 to 23 months: 120 mg/dose q 4 to 6 hours.
Children age 2 to 4: 160 mg/dose q 4 to 6 hours.
Children age 4 to 6: 240 mg/dose q 4 to 6 hours.
Children age 6 to 9: 320 mg/dose q 4 to 6 hours.
Children age 9 to 11: 400 mg/dose q 4 to 6 hours.
Children age 11 to 12: 480 mg/dose q 4 to 6 hours.

Action and kinetics
The mechanism and site of action is unclear and may be related to inhibition of prostaglandin synthesis in the CNS.
- *Antipyretic action:* Acetaminophen is believed to exert its antipyretic effect by direct action on the hypothalamic heat-regulating center to block the effects of endogenous pyrogen. This results in increased heat dissipation through sweating and vasodilation.
- *Analgesic action:* Its analgesic effect may be related to an elevation of the pain threshold.
- *Kinetics in adults:* Acetaminophen is absorbed rapidly and completely via the GI tract. Peak plasma

concentrations occur in ½ to 2 hours, slightly faster for liquid preparations. The drug is 25% protein-bound. Plasma concentrations do not correlate well with analgesic effect, but do correlate with toxicity. Approximately 90% to 95% is metabolized in the liver. Acetaminophen is excreted in urine. The average elimination half-life ranges from 1 to 4 hours. In acute overdose, prolongation of elimination half-life is correlated with toxic effects. Half-life over 4 hours is associated with hepatic necrosis; over 12 hours with coma.

Contraindications and precautions
Acetaminophen is contraindicated in patients with known hypersensitivity to this compound. Administer drug cautiously to patients with anemia or hepatic or renal disease because it has been known to induce these disorders; and to patients with a history of GI disease, increased risk of GI bleeding, or decreased renal function. Acetaminophen may mask the signs and symptoms of acute infection (fever, myalgia, erythema); patients with high infection risk (such as those with diabetes) should be carefully evaluated.

Interactions
Concomitant use of acetaminophen may potentiate the effects of anticoagulants and thrombolytic drugs, but this effect appears to be clinically insignificant. Antacids and food delay and decrease the absorption of acetaminophen. Combined caffeine and acetaminophen may enhance the therapeutic effect of acetaminophen. Concomitant use of phenothiazines and acetaminophen in large doses may result in hypothermia.

Effects on diagnostic tests
Acetaminophen may cause a false-positive test result for urinary 5-hydroxyindoleacetic acid (5-HIAA).

Adverse reactions
- CNS: mental changes, stupor, confusion, agitation (with toxic doses), weakness.
- DERM: rash, urticaria, itching, unusual bruising, erythema.
- EENT: unexplained sore throat.
- GI: nausea, vomiting, diarrhea, abdominal cramps, abdominal pain, loss of appetite.
- GU: bloody or cloudy urine, difficult or painful urination, sudden decrease in amount of urine.
- HEMA: unusual bleeding, tiredness or weakness, hemolytic anemia, neutropenia, leukopenia, pancytopenia, thrombocytopenia, methemoglobinemia.
- Hepatic: severe liver damage (toxic doses).
- Other: hypoglycemia, jaundice, unexplained fever.
  Note: Drug should be discontinued if hypersensitivity or signs and symptoms of hepatic toxicity occur.

Overdose and treatment
In acute overdose, plasma levels of 200 mcg/ml 4 hours postinjection or 50 mcg/ml 12 hours postinjection are associated with hepatotoxicity. Clinical manifestations of overdose include cyanosis, anemia, jaundice, skin eruptions, fever, emesis, CNS stimulation, delirium, methemoglobinemia progressing to depression, coma, vascular collapse, convulsions, and death. Acetaminophen poisoning develops in stages:

Stage 1 (12 to 24 hours after ingestion): nausea, vomiting, diaphoresis, anorexia.

Stage 2 (24 to 48 hours after ingestion): clinically improved but elevated liver function tests.

Stage 3 (72 to 96 hours after ingestion): peak hepatotoxicity.

Stage 4 (7 to 8 days after ingestion): recovery.

To treat toxic overdose of acetaminophen, empty stomach immediately by inducing emesis with ipecac syrup if patient is conscious, or by gastric lavage. Administer activated charcoal via nasogastric tube. Oral acetylcysteine (Mucomyst) is a specific antidote for acetaminophen poisoning and is most effective if started within 10 to 12 hours after ingestion, but can help if started within 24 hours after ingestion. Doses vomited within 1 hour of administration must be repeated. Remove charcoal before administering acetylcysteine because it may interfere with this antidote's absorption.

Acetylcysteine minimizes hepatic injury by supplying sulphydryl groups that bind with acetaminophen metabolites. Hemodialysis may be helpful to remove acetaminophen from the body. Monitor laboratory parameters and vital signs closely. Cimetidine has been used investigationally to block acetaminophen's metabolism to toxic intermediates. Provide symptomatic and supportive measures (respiratory support, correction of fluid and electrolyte imbalances). Determine plasma acetaminophen levels at least 4 hours after overdose. If plasma acetaminophen levels indicate hepatotoxicity, perform liver function tests every 24 hours for at least 96 hours.

▶ Special considerations
• Patient should not take more than five doses per day or take the drug for more than 5 days unless specifically prescribed.
• Acetaminophen has no significant anti-inflammatory effect.
• Many nonprescription products contain acetaminophen. Be aware of this when calculating total daily dose.
• Patients unable to tolerate aspirin may be able to tolerate acetaminophen.
• Use this medication cautiously in patients with alcoholism, hepatic disease, viral infection, renal function impairment, or cardiovascular disease.
• When prescribing buffered acetaminophen effervescent granules, consider sodium content for sodium-restricted patients.
• Monitor vital signs, especially temperature, to evaluate drug's effectiveness.
• Assess patient's level of pain and response before and after administration of acetaminophen.
• Store suppository form in refrigerator.

Information for parents and patient
• Teach proper administration of prescribed form.
• Advise parents of patients on chronic high-dose acetaminophen therapy to arrange for monitoring of laboratory parameters, especially BUN and serum creatinine levels, liver function tests, and CBC.
• Warn parents that patient with current or history of rectal bleeding should not use acetaminophen suppositories because they must be retained for at least 1 hour and would cause rectal irritation.
• Explain that high doses or unsupervised chronic use of acetaminophen can cause liver damage. Use of alcoholic beverages increases the risk of liver toxicity.
• Tell parents or patient to avoid unsupervised treatment of a fever above 103.1° F. (39.5° C.), a fever persisting longer than 3 days, or a recurrent fever.
• Warn against taking nonsteroidal anti-inflammatory drugs together with acetaminophen on a regular basis.
• Warn parents to avoid giving tetracycline antibiotics within 1 hour after patient takes buffered acetaminophen effervescent granules.
• Tell parents and patient that this drug should not be used for arthritic or rheumatic conditions without medical approval because it may relieve pain but not other symptoms.
• Tell parents to call if symptoms do not improve or if fever lasts more than 3 days.
• Tell parents of patients on high-dose or long-term therapy that regular follow-up visits are essential.

acetazolamide
acetazolamide sodium
Ak-Zol, Diamox, Diamox Sequels

• Classification: diuretic, antiglaucoma agent, anticonvulsant, agent for preventing and treating acute high-altitude sickness (carbonic anhydrase inhibitor)

How supplied
Available by prescription only
Tablets: 125 mg, 250 mg
Capsules (extended-release): 500 mg
Injection: 500 mg

Indications, route, and dosage
Edema, in congestive heart failure
Children: 5 mg/kg P.O., I.M., or I.V. daily in a.m.
Adults: 250 to 375 mg P.O., I.M., or I.V. daily in a.m.
Myoclonic seizures, refractory generalized tonic-clonic (grand mal) or absence (petit mal) seizures, mixed seizures
Children: 8 to 30 mg/kg P.O., I.M., or I.V. daily, divided t.i.d. or q.i.d. Maximum dosage is 1.5 g daily, or 300 to 900 mg/m² daily.
Adults: 375 mg P.O., I.M., or I.V. daily up to 250 mg q.i.d. Or, Diamox Sequels 250 to 500 mg daily or b.i.d. Initial dosage when used with other anticonvulsants usually is 250 mg daily.

†*Diuresis and alkalization of urine in the treatment of toxicity associated with weakly acidic drugs*
Children: 5 mg/kg I.V. or 150 mg/m² I.V. for 1 to 2 days (in the a.m.).
Adults: 5 mg/kg I.V. p.r.n.
†*Glaucoma*
Neonates: 5 mg/kg P.O. or I.V. q 6 to 8 hours.
†*Hydrocephalus*
Infants: 25 mg/kg/day P.O. or I.V., increased by 25 mg/kg/day to maximum dosage of 100 mg/kg/day divided t.i.d.

Action and kinetics
• *Diuretic action:* Acetazolamide and acetazolamide sodium act by noncompetitive reversible inhibition of the enzyme carbonic anhydrase, which is responsible for formation of hydrogen and bicarbonate ions from carbon dioxide and water. This inhibition results in decreased hydrogen concentration in the renal tubules, promoting excretion of bicarbonate, sodium, potassium, and water; because carbon dioxide is not eliminated as rapidly, systemic acidosis may occur.
• *Antiglaucoma action:* In open-angle glaucoma and perioperatively for acute angle-closure glaucoma, acetazolamide and acetazolamide sodium decrease the formation of aqueous humor, lowering intraocular pressure.
• *Anticonvulsant action:* The mechanism is unknown. Acetazolamide is used with other anticonvulsants in various types of epilepsy, particularly absence seizures.
• *Other actions:* Acetazolamide shortens the period of high-altitude acclimatization; by inhibiting conversion of carbon dioxide to bicarbonate, it may increase carbon dioxide tension in tissues and decrease it in the lungs. The resultant metabolic acidosis may also increase oxygenation during hypoxia.
• *Kinetics in adults:* Acetazolamide is well absorbed from the GI tract after oral administration and distributed throughout body tissues. Acetazolamide is excreted primarily in urine via tubular secretion and passive reabsorption.

Contraindications and precautions
Acetazolamide is contraindicated in patients with hepatic insufficiency because the drug may precipitate hepatic coma; in patients with low potassium or sodium concentration level or hyperchloremic acidosis because it may worsen electrolyte imbalance; and in patients with severe renal impairment because nephrotoxicity has been reported.
　Acetazolamide should be used cautiously in patients with respiratory acidosis or other severe respiratory problems, because the drug may produce acidosis; in patients with diabetes, because it may cause hyperglycemia and glycosuria; in patients taking cardiac glycosides, because they are more susceptible to digitalis toxicity from acetazolamide-induced hypokalemia; and in patients taking diuretics.

Interactions
Acetazolamide alkalizes urine and thus may decrease excretion of amphetamines, procainamide, quinidine,

and flecainide. Acetazolamide may increase excretion of salicylates, phenobarbital, and lithium, lowering plasma levels of these drugs and possibly necessitating dosage adjustments.

Effects on diagnostic tests
Because it alkalizes urine, acetazolamide may cause false-positive proteinuria in Albustix or Albutest. Acetazolamide may also decrease thyroid iodine uptake.

Adverse reactions
• CNS: drowsiness, *decreased alertness in infants,* paresthesias, confusion.
• DERM: rash.
• EENT: transient myopia.
• GI: nausea, vomiting, *anorexia, transient diarrhea, poor oral feeding.*
• GU: crystalluria, renal calculi, hematuria.
• HEMA: aplastic anemia, hemolytic anemia, leukopenia.
• Metabolic: hyperchloremic acidosis, hypokalemia, asymptomatic hyperuricemia, *occasional tachypnea, increased susceptibility to dehydration.*
• Local: pain at injection site, sterile abscesses.
　Note: Drug should be discontinued if blood pH is below 7.2.

Overdose and treatment
Specific recommendations are unavailable. Treatment is supportive and symptomatic. Acetazolamide increases bicarbonate excretion and may cause hypokalemia and hyperchloremic acidosis. Induce emesis or perform gastric lavage. Do not induce catharsis because this may exacerbate electrolyte disturbances. Monitor fluid and electrolyte levels.

▶ Special considerations
• In treating edema, intermittent dosage schedules may minimize tendency to cause metabolic acidosis and permit diuresis.
• Because it alkalizes, drug may cause false-positive results on test for proteinuria.
• Monitor blood pressure and pulse rate; establish baseline values before therapy, and watch for significant changes. Impose safety measures for ambulatory patients until response to the diuretic is known.
• Monitor carefully for electrolyte imbalance, metabolic acidosis, and hematologic changes.
• Establish baseline and periodically review CBC, including WBC count; serum electrolytes, CO_2, BUN, and creatinine levels; and, especially, liver function tests. Patients with liver disease are especially susceptible to diuretic-induced electrolyte imbalance; in extreme cases, stupor, coma, and death can result.
• Administer diuretics in the morning so major diuresis occurs before bedtime. To prevent nocturia, avoid giving diuretics after 6 p.m.
• Consider possible dosage adjustment: reduced dosage for patients with hepatic dysfunction and those taking other antihypertensive agents; increased dosage for patients with renal impairment, oliguria, or decreased diuresis (inadequate urine output may result in circulatory overload, causing water intoxication, pulmonary edema, and congestive heart failure); increased doses of insulin in diabetic patients.

---

*Canada only　　　†Unlabeled clinical use　　　Italicized adverse reactions have been observed in children.

• Monitor for signs of toxicity: postural hypotension; muscle weakness and cardiac dysrhythmia (signs of hypokalemia); leg cramps, nausea, muscle weakness, dry mouth, and dizziness (hyponatremia); lethargy, confusion, stupor, muscle twitching, increased reflexes, and convulsions (water intoxication); severe weakness, headache, abdominal pain, malaise, nausea, and vomiting (metabolic acidosis); sore throat, rash, or jaundice (blood dyscrasias from hypersensitivity); joint swelling, redness, and pain (hyperuricemia).

• Monitor patient for edema. Observe lower extremities of ambulatory children and the sacral area of infants. Check abdominal girth with tape measure to detect ascites. Dosage adjustment may be indicated.

• Patient's weight should be recorded each morning immediately after voiding and before breakfast to provide an index for dosage adjustments.

• Measure head circumference daily during medical management of hydrocephalus.

• Consider possible need for high-potassium diet or supplementation.

• Urinal or commode should be readily available for ambulatory children, as appropriate.

• Suspensions containing 250 mg/5 ml of syrup are the most palatable and can be made by a pharmacist. These will remain stable for about 1 week. Tablets will not dissolve in fruit juice.

• Reconstitute powder by adding at least 5 ml sterile water for injection.

• I.M. injection is painful because of alkalinity of solution. Direct I.V. administration is preferred if drug must be given parenterally.

• Acetazolamide has been used for periodic paralysis in dosages up to 1.5 g daily in divided doses b.i.d. or t.i.d.

• Drug may be given with food to minimize GI discomfort.

Information for parents and patient

• Explain rationale for therapy and diuretic effect of these drugs.

• Teach parents how to observe for signs of adverse effects, especially hypokalemia (weakness, fatigue, muscle cramps, paresthesias, confusion, nausea, vomiting, diarrhea, headache, dizziness, or palpitations), and importance of reporting these symptoms promptly. Advise them to watch closely for signs of chest, back, or leg pain; shortness of breath; or dyspnea, and to report such symptoms immediately.

• Warn parents to supervise the child's activities closely to prevent falls and other injuries that may result from dizziness and incoordination.

• For children who have difficulty swallowing tablets, a single dose may be prepared by softening 1 tablet in 2 teaspoons of warm water and adding 2 teaspoonfuls of honey or syrup (chocolate, cherry) and then having the child take it immediately.

• Advise parents to encourage child to eat potassium-rich foods, such as citrus fruits, potatoes, dates, raisins, and bananas, and to restrict the child's access to salt and high-sodium foods, such as lunch meat, smoked meats, and processed cheeses. Inform them that low-sodium formulas are available for infants.

• Tell parents to avoid giving nonprescription drugs without medical approval; many contain sodium and potassium and can cause electrolyte imbalance.

• Warn parents about photosensitivity reactions. Explain that ultraviolet radiation alters drug structure, causing allergic reactions in some persons; such reactions occur 10 days to 2 weeks after initial sun exposure.

• Emphasize importance of regular follow-up to monitor effectiveness of diuretic therapy.

• Tell parents to report increased edema or excess diuresis (more than 2% weight loss or gain) and to record the child's weight each morning after voiding and before breakfast, on the same scale and wearing the same type of clothing.

acetylcysteine
Airbron*, Mucomyst, Mucosol, Parvolex*

• Classification: mucolytic agent, antidote for acetaminophen overdose (amino acid [L-cysteine] derivative)

How supplied
Available by prescription only
Solution: 10%, 20%
Injection:* 200 mg/ml

Indications, route, and dosage
Acute and chronic bronchopulmonary disease, tracheostomy care, pulmonary complications of surgery, diagnostic bronchial studies
Administer by nebulization, direct application, or intratracheal instillation.
Children and adults: 1 to 2 ml of 10% or 20% solution by direct instillation into trachea as often as every hour; or 3 to 5 ml of 20% solution or 6 to 10 ml of 10% solution administered by nebulizer every 2 to 3 hours. For instillation via percutaneous intratracheal catheter, administer 1 to 2 ml of 20% solution or 2 to 4 ml of 10% solution; via tracheal catheter to treat a specific bronchopulmonary tree segment, administer 2 to 5 ml of 20% solution. For diagnostic bronchial studies (administered before procedure), administer 1 to 2 ml of 20% solution or 2 to 4 ml of 10% solution for two or three doses.
Acetaminophen toxicity
Children and adults: Initially, 140 mg/kg P.O., followed by 70 mg/kg q 4 hours for 17 doses (a total of 1,330 mg/kg) or until acetaminophen assay reveals nontoxic level. Alternatively, may be administered intravenously: Loading dose 150 mg/kg I.V. in 200 ml dextrose 5% in water (D_5W) over 15 minutes, followed by 50 mg/kg I.V. in 500 ml D_5W over 4 hours, followed by 100 mg/kg I.V. in 100 ml D_5W over 16 hours.

Action and kinetics
• *Mucolytic action:* Acetylcysteine produces its mucolytic effect by splitting the disulfide bonds of mucoprotein, the substance responsible for increased viscosity of mucus secretions in the lungs; thus, pul-

monary secretions become less viscous and more liquid.

• *Acetaminophen antidote:* The mechanism by which acetylcysteine reduces acetaminophen toxicity is not fully understood; it is thought that acetylcysteine restores hepatic stores of glutathione or inactivates the toxic metabolite of acetaminophen via a chemical interaction, thereby preventing liver damage.

• *Kinetics in adults:* Most inhaled acetylcysteine acts directly on the mucus in the lungs; the remainder is absorbed by pulmonary epithelium. Action begins within 1 minute after inhalation, and immediately upon direct intratracheal instillation; peak effect occurs in 5 to 10 minutes. After oral administration, acetylcysteine is absorbed from the GI tract. Acetylcysteine is metabolized in the liver.

Contraindications and precautions
Acetylcysteine is contraindicated in patients with known hypersensitivity to the drug; however, it may be given to hypersensitive patients to treat acetaminophen overdose if the allergic symptoms are controlled. It should be used with caution in patients with asthma because bronchospasm may occur; if it does, discontinue acetylcysteine immediately. It also should be used with caution in debilitated patients with respiratory insufficiency, because it may increase airway obstruction; and in all patients who exhibit inadequate cough during therapy, because secretions may occlude airways.

Interactions
Activated charcoal adsorbs orally administered acetylcysteine, preventing its absorption.

Acetylcysteine is incompatible with oxytetracycline, tetracycline, chlortetracycline, erythromycin, lactobionate, amphotericin B, ampicillin, iodized oil, chymotrypsin, trypsin, and hydrogen peroxide; drug should be administered separately.

Effects on diagnostic tests
None reported.

Adverse reactions
• CNS: drowsiness.
• EENT: *rhinorrhea,* hemoptysis.
• GI: *stomatitis, vomiting, nausea, hemoptysis.*
• Other: clammy skin, *bronchospasm, bronchoconstriction,* sensitization (rare), *fever* and chills (rare).
• Long-term use: *transient maculopapular rash.*

Overdose and treatment
No information available.

▶ Special considerations
• Acetylcysteine may be given by tent or Croupette. A sufficient volume (up to 300 ml) of a 10% or 20% solution should be used to maintain a heavy mist in the tent for the time prescribed. Administration may be continuous or intermittent.
• Acetylcysteine solutions release hydrogen sulfide and discolor on contact with rubber and some metals (especially iron, nickel, and copper); drug tarnishes silver (this does not affect drug potency). Solution may turn light purple; this does not affect drug's

safety or efficacy. Use plastic, stainless steel, or other inert metal when administering drug by nebulization. Do not use hand-held bulb nebulizers; output is too small and particle size too large. Do not place directly in the chamber of a heated (hot pot) nebulizer. Dilute with sterile saline solution for inhalation.
• After opening, store in refrigerator or use within 96 hours.
• Monitor cough type and frequency; for maximum effect, instruct patient to clear airway by coughing before aerosol administration. Many clinicians pretreat with bronchodilators before administration of acetylcysteine. Keep suction equipment available; if patient has insufficient cough to clear increased secretions, suction will be needed to maintain open airway.
• When used orally for acetaminophen overdose, dilute with cola, fruit juice, or water to a 5% concentration and administer within 1 hour.
• Mixing with other drugs is not recommended but is often done without apparent loss of effectiveness.
• Monitor blood gases for carbon dioxide retention.

Information for parents and patient
Warn parents and patient of unpleasant odor (rotten egg odor of hydrogen sulfide). Explain that increased amounts of liquefied bronchial secretion plus unpleasant odor may cause nausea and vomiting; have patient rinse mouth with water after nebulizer treatment, because it may leave a sticky coating in the mouth.

_____

acyclovir (acycloguanosine) acyclovir sodium
Zovirax

• Classification: antiviral agent (synthetic purine nucleoside)

_____

How supplied
Available by prescription only
Capsules: 200 mg
Injection: 500 mg/vial
Ointment: 5%

Indications, route, and dosage
Initial and recurrent mucocutaneous herpes simplex virus (HSV-I and HSV-II) or severe initial genital herpes in immunocompromised patient
Neonates: 30 mg/kg I.V. daily in divided doses q 8 hours.
Children age 11 and under: 250 mg/m², given at a constant rate over a period of 1 hour by I.V. infusion q 8 hours for 7 days (5 days for genital herpes).
Children over age 11 and adults: 5 mg/kg, given at a constant rate over a period of 1 hour by I.V. infusion q 8 hours for 7 days (5 days for genital herpes).

Herpes genitalis; non-life-threatening herpes simplex infection in immunocompromised patient

Children and adults: Apply sufficient quantity of ointment to adequately cover all lesions q 3 hours, six times a day for 7 days.

Dosage in renal failure

Oral dose

200 mg q 12 hours if creatinine clearance drops below 10 ml/minute.

I.V. dose

5 mg/kg q 8 hours if creatinine clearance exceeds 50 ml/minute; 5 mg/kg q 12 hours if it ranges from 25 to 50 ml/minute; 5 mg/kg q 24 hours if it ranges from 10 to 25 ml/minute; 2.5 mg/kg q 24 hours if it falls below 10 ml/minute.

Note: In patients undergoing hemodialysis, 5 mg/kg may be given after each dialysis treatment.

Action and kinetics

• *Antiviral action:* Acyclovir is converted by the viral cell into its active form (triphosphate) and inhibits viral DNA polymerase.

In vitro, acyclovir is active against herpes simplex virus Type I, herpes simplex virus Type II, varicella-zoster virus, Epstein-Barr virus, and cytomegalovirus. In vivo, acyclovir may reduce the duration of acute infection and speed lesion healing in initial genital herpes episodes. Patients with frequent herpes recurrences (more than six episodes a year) may receive oral acyclovir prophylactically for 4 to 6 months to prevent recurrences or reduce their frequency.

• *Kinetics in adults:* With oral administration, acyclovir is absorbed slowly and incompletely (15% to 30%). Peak concentrations occur in 1½ to 2 hours. Absorption is not affected by food. With topical administration, absorption is minimal. Acyclovir is distributed widely to organ tissues and body fluids. CSF concentrations equal approximately 50% of serum concentrations. About 9% to 33% of a dose binds to plasma proteins. Acyclovir is metabolized inside the viral cell to its active form. Approximately 10% of a dose is metabolized extracellularly. Up to 92% of systemically absorbed acyclovir is excreted unchanged by the kidneys by glomerular filtration and tubular secretion. In patients with normal renal function, half-life is 2 to 3½ hours. Renal failure may extend half-life to 19 hours.

Contraindications and precautions

Acyclovir is contraindicated in patients with known hypersensitivity to the drug.

Acyclovir should be administered cautiously to patients with dehydration, renal dysfunction, or pre-existing neurologic dysfunction, because it may aggravate these disorders.

The risk of neurologic abnormalities may increase in patients who experience neurologic reactions to interferon or intrathecal methotrexate.

Interactions

Concomitant use with probenecid may result in reduced renal tubular secretion of acyclovir, leading to increased drug half-life, reduced elimination rate, and decreased urinary excretion. This reduced clearance causes more sustained serum drug levels.

Effects on diagnostic tests

Serum creatinine and blood urea nitrogen (BUN) levels may increase during acyclovir therapy.

Adverse reactions

• CNS: headache, encephalopathic signs (lethargy, obtundation, tremors, confusion, hallucinations, agitation, seizures, coma).
• CV: hypotension.
• DERM: rash, transient burning and stinging, pruritus.
• GI: nausea, vomiting, diarrhea.
• GU: hematuria, crystalluria, *reversible renal dysfunction.*
• Local: *inflammation, vesicular eruptions and phlebitis at injection site.*
• Other: arthralgia, resistant viruses (with prolonged or repeated use).

Note: Drug should be discontinued if hypersensitivity or encephalopathic reactions occur.

Overdose and treatment

Overdose has followed I.V. bolus administration in patients with unmonitored fluid status or in patients receiving inappropriately high parenteral dosages. Acute toxicity has not been reported after high oral dosage. Hemodialysis removes acyclovir.

Clinical effects of overdose include signs of nephrotoxicity, including elevated serum creatinine and BUN levels, progressing to renal failure.

▶ Special considerations

• Safety and effectiveness of oral and topical acyclovir in children have not been established. I.V. acyclovir has been used with only a limited number of children. Do not use bacteriostatic water for injection containing benzyl alcohol.
• Drug should not be administered subcutaneously, I.M., by I.V. bolus, or ophthalmically.
• I.V. dose should be infused over at least 1 hour to prevent renal tubular damage.
• Acyclovir's solubility in urine is low. Ensure that patient taking the systemic form of the drug is well hydrated to prevent nephrotoxicity.
• Monitor serum creatinine level. If level does not return to normal within a few days after therapy begins, may increase hydration, adjust dose, or discontinue drug.
• Encephalopathic signs are more likely in patients who have had neurologic reactions to cytotoxic drugs.

Information for parents and patient

• Explain that although drug helps manage the disease, it does not cure it or prevent it from spreading to others.
• For best results, patient should begin taking drug when early symptoms (such as tingling, itching, or pain) occur.
• Teach correct application of ointment: Using a finger cot or rubber glove, apply about a ½" (1 cm) ribbon of ointment for every 4 in² (26 cm²) of surface area

to be covered, thoroughly covering each lesion. Patient should avoid getting ointment in the eye.
• Patient should avoid sexual intercourse during active genital infection.

---

albumin, human (normal serum albumin, human)
Albuminar-5, Albuminar-25, Albutein 5%, Albutein 25%, Buminate 5%, Buminate 25%, Plasbumin-5, Plasbumin-25

• Classification: plasma volume expander (blood derivative)

How supplied
Injection: 5% (50 mg/ml) in vials of 50 ml, 250 ml, 500 ml, 1,000 ml; 25% (250 mg/ml) in vials of 20 ml, 50 ml, 100 ml

Indications, route, and dosage
Shock
Children: 25% to 50% of adult dose in nonemergency. Maximum dose is 6 g/kg/day.
Adults: Initially, 500 ml (5% solution) by I.V. infusion, repeated p.r.n. Dose varies with patient's condition and response. Do not give more than 250 g/48 hours.
Hypoproteinemia
Children: 0.5 to 1 g/kg I.V. Repeat every 24 to 48 hours.
Adults: 1,000 to 1,500 ml 5% solution by I.V. infusion daily, maximum rate 5 to 10 ml/minute; or 25 to 100 g 25% solution by I.V. infusion daily, maximum rate 3 ml/minute. Dose varies with patient's condition and response.
Burns
Dosage varies according to extent of burn and patient's condition. Usually maintain plasma albumin level at 2 to 3 g/dl.
Hyperbilirubinemia
Infants: 1 g albumin (4 ml of 25% solution)/kg before transfusion.

Action and kinetics
• *Plasma volume-expanding action:* Albumin, 5%, supplies colloid to the blood and expands plasma volume. Albumin, 25%, provides intravascular oncotic pressure at 5:1, causing fluid to shift from interstitial space to the circulation and slightly increasing plasma protein concentration.
• *Kinetics in adults:* Albumin is not adequately absorbed from the GI tract. Albumin accounts for approximately 50% of plasma proteins; it is distributed into the intravascular space and extravascular sites, including skin, muscle, and lungs. In patients with reduced circulating blood volume, hemodilution secondary to albumin administration persists for many hours; in patients with normal blood volume, excess fluid and protein are lost. Although albumin is synthesized in the liver, liver is not involved in clearance of albumin from plasma in healthy individuals.
Little is known about excretion in healthy individ-

uals. Administration of albumin decreases hepatic albumin synthesis and increases albumin clearance if plasma oncotic pressure is high. In certain pathologic states, the liver, kidneys, or intestines may provide elimination mechanisms for albumin.

Contraindications and precautions
Albumin is contraindicated in patients with severe anemia and heart failure because of potential for fluid overload.
Administer albumin cautiously to patients without albumin deficiency or to those with low cardiac reserve, severely restricted salt intake, hepatic or renal failure, dehydration, or pulmonary disease, because of potential for hypervolemia.

Interactions
None significant.

Effects on diagnostic tests
Preparations of albumin derived from placental tissue may increase serum alkaline phosphatase level; all products may slightly increase plasma albumin level.

Adverse reactions
• CV: *vascular overload after rapid infusion, hypotension,* tachycardia, flushing, dilutional anemia (with large doses).
• DERM: *urticaria.*
• GI: increased salivation, *nausea, vomiting.*
• Other: *chills, fever,* altered respiration, pulmonary edema with rapid infusions, headache.

Overdose and treatment
Clinical manifestations of overdose include signs of circulatory overload, such as increased venous pressure and distended neck veins, or pulmonary edema; slow flow to a keep-vein-open rate and re-evaluate therapy.

▶ Special considerations
• Premature infants with low serum protein concentrations may receive 1.4 to 1.8 ml of a 25% albumin solution (350 to 450 mg albumin).
• Solution should be a clear amber color; do not use if cloudy or contains sediment. Store at room temperature; freezing may break bottle.
• Use opened solution promptly, discarding unused portion after 4 hours; solution contains no preservatives and becomes unstable.
• One volume of 25% albumin produces the same hemodilution and relative anemia as five volumes of 5% albumin; reference to "1 unit" albumin usually indicates 50 ml of the 25% concentration, containing 12.5 g of albumin.
• Dilute if necessary with normal saline solution or dextrose 5% injection. Use 5-micron or larger filter; do not give through 0.22-micron I.V. filter.
• Be certain patient is properly hydrated before starting infusion; product may be administered without regard to blood typing and crossmatching.
• Avoid rapid I.V. infusion; rate is individualized according to patient's age, condition, and diagnosis. In patients with hypovolemic shock, infuse 5% solution at a rate not exceeding 2 to 4 ml/minute in adults and

---

25% solution (diluted or undiluted) at a rate not exceeding 1 ml/minute in adults; in patients with normal blood volume, infuse 5% solution at a rate not exceeding 5 to 10 ml/minute in adults, and 25% solution (diluted or undiluted), at a rate not exceeding 2 to 3 ml/minute in adults. Do not give more than 250 g in 48 hours.
• Monitor vital signs carefully; observe patient for adverse reactions.
• Monitor intake and output, hemoglobin, hematocrit, and serum protein and electrolyte levels to help determine continuing dosage.
• Each liter contains 130 to 160 mEq of sodium before dilution with any additional I.V. fluids; a 50-ml bottle of solution contains 7 to 8 mEq sodium. This preparation was once known as "salt-poor albumin."

Information for parents and patient
Discuss with parents and patient the benefit of therapy. Explain that drug is derived from donated human blood, but risk of infection (hepatitis, HIV) is low.

---

albuterol sulfate
Proventil, Proventil Syrup, Ventolin, Ventolin Syrup

• Classification: bronchodilator (adrenergic)

How supplied
Available by prescription only
Tablets: 2 mg, 4 mg
Solution: 2 mg/5 ml
Aerosol inhaler: 90 mcg/metered spray

Indications, route, and dosage
To prevent and treat bronchospasm in patients with reversible obstructive airway disease
Children age 2 to 5: Administer 0.1 mg/kg P.O. t.i.d., not to exceed 2 mg t.i.d.
Children age 6 to 11: Administer 2 mg P.O. t.i.d. or q.i.d.
Children age 12 and over and adults: One to two inhalations q 4 to 6 hours. More frequent administration or a greater number of inhalations is not usually recommended. However, because deposition of inhaled medications is variable, higher doses are occasionally used, especially in patients with acute bronchospasm. For tablets, 2 to 4 mg P.O. t.i.d. or q.i.d.; maximum dosage, 8 mg q.i.d.
To prevent exercise-induced bronchospasm
Children age 12 and over and adults: Two inhalations 15 minutes before exercise.

Action and kinetics
• *Bronchodilator action:* Albuterol selectively stimulates beta₂-adrenergic receptors of the lungs, uterus, and vascular smooth muscle. Bronchodilation results from relaxation of bronchial smooth muscles, which relieves bronchospasm and reduces airway resistance.
• *Kinetics in adults:* After oral inhalation, albuterol

appears to be absorbed gradually (over several hours) from the respiratory tract; however, most of the dose is swallowed and absorbed through the GI tract. Onset of action occurs within 5 to 15 minutes, peaks in ½ to 2 hours, and lasts 3 to 6 hours. After oral administration, albuterol is well absorbed through the GI tract. Onset of action occurs within 30 minutes, peaks in 2 to 3 hours, and lasts 4 to 6 hours or longer. Albuterol does not cross the blood-brain barrier. Albuterol is extensively metabolized in the liver to inactive compounds. Albuterol is rapidly excreted in urine and feces. After oral inhalation, 70% of a dose is excreted in urine unchanged and as metabolites within 24 hours; 10% in feces. Elimination half-life is about 4 hours. After oral administration, 75% of a dose is excreted in urine within 72 hours as metabolites; 4% in feces.

Contraindications and precautions
Albuterol is contraindicated in patients with known hypersensitivity to the drug. Administer with caution to patients with hyperthyroidism, diabetes mellitus, cardiovascular disorders (coronary insufficiency or hypertension), or sensitivity to sympathomimetic amines, because drug may worsen these conditions.

Interactions
Concomitant use of orally inhaled albuterol with epinephrine and other orally inhaled sympathomimetic amines may increase sympathomimetic effects and risk of toxicity. Serious cardiovascular effects may follow concomitant use with monoamine oxidase inhibitors and tricyclic antidepressants.
Propranolol and other beta-adrenergic blockers may antagonize the effects of albuterol.

Effects on diagnostic tests
None significant.

Adverse reactions
• CNS: *tremors, nervousness,* sweating, vertigo, central stimulation, hyperactivity, excitement, irritable behavior, insomnia, epistaxis, weakness, dizziness, drowsiness, *headache.*
• CV: *tachycardia,* palpitations, peripheral vasodilation, increased or decreased blood pressure, angina.
• EENT: drying and irritation of nose (inhaled form).
• GI: *nausea, vomiting,* unusual taste, irritation of oropharynx, increased appetite, heartburn.
• Other: difficult urination, cough, dilated pupils, muscle cramps, urticaria, rash, allergic reactions.
Note: Drug should be discontinued if hypersensitivity or paradoxical bronchospasm occurs.

Overdose and treatment
Clinical manifestations of overdose include exaggeration of common adverse reactions, particularly angina, hypertension, hypokalemia, and seizures.
To treat, use selective beta₁-adrenergic blockers (such as metoprolol) with extreme caution; these may induce asthmatic attack. *Dialysis is not appropriate.* Monitor vital signs and electrolyte levels closely.

---

‡May contain sulfites   ◆May contain tartrazine   ◆ ◆ May contain benzyl alcohol

▶ **Special considerations**

• Approved for use in children age 2 and older.

• The preservative sodium bisulfite is present in many adrenergic formulations. Patients with a history of allergy to sulfites should avoid preparations that contain this preservative.

• Therapy should be administered when patient arises in morning and before meals to reduce fatigue by improving lung ventilation.

• Adrenergic inhalation may be alternated with other drug administration (steroids, other adrenergics) if necessary, but should not be administered simultaneously because of danger of excessive tachycardia.

• Do not use discolored or precipitated solutions.

• Protect solutions from light, freezing, and heat. Store at controlled room temperature.

• Systemic absorption can follow applications to nasal and conjunctival membranes, though infrequently. If symptoms of systemic absorption occur, patient should stop the drug.

• Prolonged or too-frequent use may cause tolerance to bronchodilating and cardiac stimulant effect. Rebound bronchospasm may follow end of drug effect.

• Small, transient increases in blood glucose level may occur after oral inhalation.

• Serum potassium levels may decrease after I.V. administration, but potassium supplementation is usually unnecessary.

• Effectiveness of treatment is measured by periodic monitoring of the patient's pulmonary function.

Information for parents and patient

• Treatment should start with first symptoms of bronchospasm.

• Dosage and recommended method of inhaling may vary with type of nebulizer and formulation used. Carefully instruct parents and patient in correct use of nebulizer:

—Administration by metered-dose nebulizers: Shake canister thoroughly to activate; place mouthpiece well into mouth, aimed at back of throat. Close lips and teeth around mouthpiece. Exhale through nose as completely as possible, then inhale through mouth slowly and deeply while actuating the nebulizer to release dose. Hold breath 10 seconds (count "1-100, 2-100, 3-100," until "10-100" is reached); remove mouthpiece, and then exhale slowly.

—Administration by metered powder inhaler: Caution patient not to take forced deep breath, but to breathe with normal force and depth. Observe patient closely for exaggerated systemic drug action.

—Administration by oxygen aerosolization: Administer over 15- to 20-minute period, with oxygen flow rate adjusted to 4 liters/minute. Turn on oxygen supply before patient places nebulizer in mouth. Lips need not be closed tightly around nebulizer opening. Placement of Y tube in rubber tubing permits patient to control administration. Advise patient to rinse mouth immediately after inhalation therapy to help prevent dryness and throat irritation. Rinse mouthpiece thoroughly with warm running water at least once daily to prevent clogging. (It is not dishwasher-safe.) After cleaning, wait until mouthpiece is completely dry before storing. Do not place near artificial heat (dishwasher or oven). Replace reservoir bag every 2 to 3 weeks or as needed; replace mouthpiece every 6 to 9 months or as needed. Replacement of bags or mouthpieces may require a prescription.

• Warn parents and patient to use only as directed, and not to use more than prescribed amount or more often than prescribed. Information and instructions are furnished with the aerosol forms of these drugs. Urge parents and patient to read them carefully and ask questions if necessary.

• Instruct patient to wait 1 full minute after initial one to two inhalations of adrenergic to be sure of necessity for another dose. Drug action should begin immediately and peak within 5 to 15 minutes.

• Teach parents and patient that a single aerosol treatment is usually enough to control an asthma attack and to call promptly if the patient requires more than three aerosol treatments in 24 hours. Explain that overuse of adrenergic bronchodilators may cause tachycardia, palpitations, headache, nausea and dizziness, loss of effectiveness, possible paradoxical reaction, and cardiac arrest.

• Tell parents to call if troubled breathing persists 1 hour after using medication, if symptoms return within 4 hours, if condition worsens, if new (refill) canister is needed within 2 weeks, or if bronchodilator causes dizziness or chest pain.

• Tell parents and patient to wait 15 minutes after using inhalational albuterol before using adrenocorticoids (beclomethasone, dexamethasone, flunisolide, or triamcinolone).

• Tell parents and patient that repeated use may result in paradoxical bronchospasm. If it occurs, they should discontinue drug and report this effect immediately.

• Tell parents and patient that dryness of mouth and throat may occur, and that rinsing with water after each dose may help.

• Patient should avoid other adrenergic medications (for example, decongestants) unless they are prescribed.

• Inform parents and patient that saliva and sputum may appear pink after inhalation treatment.

• Caution patient to keep spray away from eyes.

• Explain that increased fluid intake facilitates clearing of secretions. Teach parents and patient how to accomplish postural drainage, to cough productively, and to clap and vibrate to promote good respiratory hygiene.

• Inform parents and patient about adverse reactions, and advise them to report such reactions promptly.

• Tell parents and patient not to discard drug applicator. Refill units are available.

---

allopurinol
Lopurin, Zyloprim

• Classification: antigout agent (xanthine oxidase inhibitor)

How supplied
Available by prescription only
Tablets (scored): 100 mg, 300 mg

Indications, route, and dosage
Gout, primary or secondary hyperuricemia
Gout may be secondary to diseases such as acute or chronic leukemia, polycythemia vera, multiple myeloma, and psoriasis. Dosage varies with severity of disease; can be given as single dose or divided, but doses larger than 300 mg should be divided.
Adults: Mild gout, 200 to 300 mg P.O. daily; severe gout with large tophi, 400 to 600 mg P.O. daily. Same dose for maintenance in secondary hyperuricemia.
Hyperuricemia secondary to malignancies; to prevent uric acid nephropathy during cancer chemotherapy
Children: 10 mg/kg P.O. q 8 hours to a maximum of 600 mg daily, then titrate dosage according to serum uric acid level; or, 100 to 200 mg/m² divided into four doses.
Adults: 600 to 800 mg P.O. daily for 2 to 3 days, with high fluid intake; or, 350 to 700 mg/m² I.V., as a 24-hour infusion divided into four to six doses.
Dosage in renal failure
Adults: 200 mg P.O. daily if creatinine clearance is 10 to 20 ml/minute; 100 mg P.O. daily if creatinine clearance is less than 10 ml/minute; 100 mg P.O. more than 24 hours apart if creatinine clearance is less than 3 ml/minute.

Action and kinetics
• *Antigout action:* Allopurinol inhibits xanthine oxidase, the enzyme catalyzing the conversion of hypoxanthine to xanthine, and the conversion of xanthine to uric acid. By blocking this enzyme, allopurinol and its metabolite, oxypurinol, prevent the conversion of oxypurines (xanthine and hypoxanthine) to uric acid, thus decreasing serum and urine concentrations of uric acid. The drug has no analgesic, anti-inflammatory, or uricosuric action.
• *Kinetics in adults:* After oral administration, approximately 80% to 90% of a dose of allopurinol is absorbed. Peak concentrations are achieved 2 to 6 hours after a usual dose. Allopurinol is distributed widely throughout the body except in the brain, where concentrations of the drug are 50% of those found in the rest of the body. Allopurinol and oxypurinol are not bound to plasma proteins.
Allopurinol is metabolized to oxypurinol by xanthine oxidase. The half-life of allopurinol is less than 1 hour; of oxypurinol, approximately 13½ hours. Five to seven percent of an allopurinol dose is excreted in urine unchanged within 6 hours of ingestion. After this, it is excreted by the kidneys as oxypurinol, allopurinol, and oxypurinol ribonucleosides. About 70% of the administered daily dose is excreted in urine as oxypurinol and an additional 2% appears in feces as unchanged drug within 48 to 72 hours.

Contraindications and precautions
Allopurinol is contraindicated in patients with hypersensitivity to the drug and in those with idiopathic hemochromatosis. Patients with impaired renal function must be carefully monitored while receiving allopurinol. Dosage adjustments may be necessary in patients with bone marrow depression, lower GI tract disease, and impaired renal function.

Interactions
In patients with decreased renal function, the concomitant use of allopurinol and a thiazide diuretic (captopril or enalapril) may increase the risk of allopurinol-induced hypersensitivity reactions.
Concomitant use with azathioprine and mercaptopurine may increase these drugs' toxic effects, particularly bone marrow depression. Combined use of these drugs requires reduction of initial doses of azathioprine or mercaptopurine to 25% to 33% of the usual dose, with subsequent doses adjusted according to patient response and toxic effects.
Concomitant use of allopurinol with cyclophosphamide may increase the incidence of bone marrow depression through an unknown mechanism. Allopurinol inhibits hepatic microsomal metabolism of dicumarol, thus increasing the half-life of dicumarol; patients receiving the two drugs concomitantly should be observed for increased anticoagulant effects.
Concomitant use of allopurinol with ampicillin or amoxicillin may increase the incidence of skin rash. Concomitant use of allopurinol with iron supplements may increase hepatic iron stores.
Because allopurinol or its metabolites may compete with chlorpropamide for renal tubular secretion, patients who receive these drugs concomitantly should be observed for signs of excessive hypoglycemia.
Concomitant use of co-trimoxazole with allopurinol has been associated with thrombocytopenia.

Effects on diagnostic tests
Increased alkaline phosphatase, AST (SGOT), and ALT (SGPT) levels have been reported in patients on allopurinol therapy.

Adverse reactions
• CNS: headache, peripheral neuropathy, *neuritis,* paresthesia, somnolence.
• DERM: *rash,* Stevens-Johnson syndrome, toxic epidermal necrolysis, alopecia, erythema multiforme, ichthyosis, purpuric lesions, vesicular bullous dermatitis, eczematoid dermatitis, pruritus, urticaria, onycholysis, lichen planus.
• EENT: cataracts, retinopathy, severe furunculosis of nose.
• GI: *nausea, vomiting,* diarrhea, intermittent abdominal pain, gastritis, dyspepsia, metallic taste, loss of taste.
• GU: renal failure, uremia.
• HEMA: agranulocytosis, anemia, aplastic anemia, bone marrow depression, leukopenia, pancytopenia, thrombocytopenia, ecchymosis.
• Hepatic: increased alkaline phosphatase, AST (SGOT), ALT (SGPT) levels; hepatomegaly; hyperbilirubinemia; cholestatic jaundice; granulomatous hepatitis; hepatic necrosis; *hepatotoxicity.*
• Other: acute attacks of gout, fever, myopathy, epistaxis, loss or perversion of taste, hypersensitivity (fever, chills, leukopenia, leukocytosis, eosinophilia, arthralgia, nausea, vomiting), renal failure, uremia.
Note: Drug should be discontinued at first sign of rash, which may precede severe hypersensitivity reaction or any other adverse reaction.

Overdose and treatment
No information available.

▶ Special considerations
• Allopurinol should not be used in children except to treat hyperuricemia secondary to malignancies or Lesch-Neiman syndrome.
• Monitor patient's intake and output. Adequate daily urine output (1 to 2 ml/kg/hour in children) and maintenance of neutral or slightly alkaline urine is desirable.
• If renal insufficiency exists at any time during treatment, allopurinol dose should be reduced.
• Monitor CBC, serum uric acid levels, and hepatic and renal function at start of therapy and periodically thereafter.
• Minimize GI adverse reactions by administering with meals or immediately after. Tablets may be crushed and administered with fluid or food.
• Allopurinol may predispose patient to ampicillin-induced rash.
• Allopurinol-induced rash may occur weeks after discontinuation of drug.
• Skin rash occurs most often in patients taking diuretics and in those with renal disorders.
• Avoid using allopurinol with iron supplements because such use may increase hepatic iron stores.

Information for parents and patient
• Advise parents that they should encourage patient to drink plenty of fluids (10 to 12 8-oz [240 ml] glasses a day) while taking this drug unless otherwise contraindicated.
• Patient should avoid hazardous activities requiring alertness until CNS response to drug is known, because drug may cause drowsiness.
• Patient should avoid alcohol because it decreases effectiveness of allopurinol.
• Tell parents to report all adverse reactions immediately.

---

alprostadil
Prostin VR Pediatric

• Classification: prostaglandin

How supplied
Available by prescription only
Injection: 500 mcg/ml

Indications, route, and dosage
Temporary maintenance of patency of ductus arteriosus until surgery can be performed
Infants: Initial I.V. infusion of 0.05 to 0.1 mcg/kg/minute via infusion pump. After satisfactory response is achieved, reduce infusion rate to the lowest dosage that will maintain response. Maintenance dosage is usually one-hundredth to one-tenth the initial dose. I.V. route is preferred but intraarterial or intraaortic route may be used.

Action and kinetics
• *Ductus arteriosus patency adjunct action:* Alprostadil, also known as prostaglandin E_1 or PGE_1, is a prostaglandin that relaxes or dilates the rings of smooth muscle of the ductus arteriosus and maintains patency in neonates when infused before natural closure.
• *Kinetics in adults:* Alprostadil is administered I.V. and is distributed rapidly throughout the body. Approximately 68% of a dose is metabolized in one pass through the lung, primarily by oxidation; 100% is metabolized within 24 hours. All metabolites are excreted in urine within 24 hours.

Contraindications and precautions
Alprostadil is contraindicated in infants with respiratory distress syndrome because of the potential for adverse cardiovascular effects. It should be used cautiously in infants with bleeding tendencies because it inhibits platelet aggregation.

Interactions
None reported.

Effects on diagnostic tests
None reported.

Adverse reactions
• CNS: *seizures, hyperpyrexia,* cerebral bleeding, *fever, apnea, sedation, lethargy.*
• CV: *flushing, bradycardia, hypotension,* tachycardia, *edema in lower extremities,* damage to the ductus pulmonary artery and aorta (with prolonged infusion).
• GI: *diarrhea,* gastric regurgitation, *nausea, vomiting.*
• HEMA: disseminated intravascular coagulation, anemia, *thrombocytopenia,* bleeding, hyperbilirubinemia, *decreased platelet aggregation.*
• Respiratory: bradypnea, wheezing, hypercapnia, tachypnea, respiratory distress, *bronchospasm.*
• Other: sepsis, hypokalemia, hyperkalemia, *hypocalcemia hypoglycemia, cortical hyperostosis* (with long-term use).

Overdose and treatment
Clinical manifestations are similar to the adverse reactions and include apnea, bradycardia, pyrexia, hypotension, and flushing. Apnea most frequently occurs in neonates weighing less than 2 kg at birth and usually develops during the first hour of drug therapy.
    Treatment of apnea or bradycardia requires discontinuance of the infusion and appropriate supportive therapy, including mechanical ventilation as needed. Pyrexia or hypotension may be treated by reducing the infusion rate. Flushing may be corrected by repositioning the intraarterial catheter.

▶ Special considerations
• Adding a 500-mcg solution to 50 ml of dextrose 5% in water or normal saline solution provides a concentration of 10 mcg/ml. At this concentration, a 0.01 ml/kg/minute infusion rate will deliver 0.1 mcg alprostadil/kg/minute.

• Drug must be diluted before administration. Discard prepared solution after 24 hours.
• Assess all vital functions closely and frequently to prevent adverse effects.
• Monitor arterial pressure by umbilical artery catheter, auscultation, or Doppler transducer. Slow the rate of infusion if arterial pressure falls significantly.
• In infants with restricted pulmonary blood flow, measure drug's effectiveness by monitoring blood oxygenation. In infants with restricted systemic blood flow, measure drug's effectiveness by monitoring systemic blood pressure and blood pH.
• Apnea and bradycardia may reflect drug overdose. Stop the infusion immediately if they occur.
• Monitor respiratory status throughout treatment; have ventilatory assistance immediately available.
• Peripheral arterial vasodilation (flushing) may respond to repositioning of the catheter.
• This drug should be administered only by personnel trained in pediatric intensive care.
• Store alprostadil ampules in refrigerator.

Information for parents and patient
Explain therapy to parents. Advise them to monitor for adverse reactions.

---

aluminum hydroxide
Alagel, ALternaGEL, Alu-Cap, Aluminett, Alu-Tab, Amphojel, Dialume, Hydroxal, Nephrox, Nutrajel

• Classification: antacid, hypophosphatemic agent, adsorbent (aluminum salt)

How supplied
Available without prescription
Tablets: 300 mg, 600 mg
Capsules: 475 mg, 500 mg
Suspension: 320 mg/5 ml, 600 mg/5 ml

Indications, route, and dosage
Hyperphosphatemia in renal failure
Children: 50 to 150 mg/kg/day in divided doses q 4 to 6 hours.

Action and kinetics
• *Antacid action:* Aluminum hydroxide neutralizes gastric acid, reducing the direct acid irritant effect. This increases pH, thereby decreasing pepsin activity.
• *Hypophosphatemic action:* Aluminum hydroxide reduces serum phosphate levels by complexing with phosphate in the gut, resulting in insoluble, nonabsorbable aluminum phosphate, which is then excreted in feces. Calcium absorption increases secondary to decreased phosphate absorption.
• *Kinetics in adults:* Aluminum hydroxide is absorbed minimally; small amounts may be absorbed systemically. Aluminum hydroxide is excreted in feces; some drug may be excreted in breast milk.

Contraindications and precautions
Aluminum hydroxide is contraindicated in patients with hypophosphatemia, appendicitis, impaired renal function, undiagnosed rectal or GI bleeding, constipation, fecal impaction, chronic diarrhea, gastric outlet obstruction, or intestinal obstruction, because the drug may exacerbate these symptoms.

Aluminum hydroxide should be used cautiously in patients with hemorrhoids and in patients with decreased GI motility, such as patients receiving anticholinergics or antidiarrheals, because constipation associated with drug use may be irritating.

Interactions
Aluminum hydroxide may decrease absorption of many drugs, including tetracycline, phenothiazines (especially chlorpromazine), coumarin anticoagulants, chenodiol, antimuscarinics, diazepam, chlordiazepoxide, $histamine_2$ antagonists, isoniazid, vitamin A, digoxin, iron salts, and sodium or potassium phosphate, thereby decreasing their effectiveness; separate drugs by 1 to 2 hours. Drug causes premature release of enterically coated drugs; separate doses by 1 hour.

Effects on diagnostic tests
Aluminum hydroxide therapy may interfere with imaging techniques using sodium pertechnetate Tc 99m and thus impair evaluation of Meckel's diverticulum. It may also interfere with reticuloendothelial imaging of liver, spleen, and bone marrow using technetium Tc 99m sulfur colloid. It may antagonize pentagastrin's effect during gastric acid secretion tests.

Aluminum hydroxide may elevate serum gastrin levels and reduce serum phosphate levels.

Adverse reactions
• GI: *constipation,* appetite loss, decreased bowel motility.
• Metabolic: *hypophosphatemia,* hypokalemia.
• Other: aluminum toxicity.
Note: Drug should be discontinued if anorexia, malaise, muscle weakness, or other signs and symptoms of hypophosphatemia develop.

Overdose and treatment
No specific information available. Patients with impaired renal function are at a higher risk of aluminum toxicity to brain, bone, and parathyroid glands.

▶ Special considerations
• Use with caution in children under age 6.
• Shake suspension well (especially extra-strength suspension) and give with small amounts of water or fruit juice.
• Every 10 ml of drug neutralizes 13 mEq of acid.
• Every 5 ml of drug contains less than 0.3 mEq of sodium.
• After administration through nasogastric tube, tube should be flushed with water to prevent obstruction.
• Constipation may be managed with stool softeners or bulk laxatives. Also, alternate aluminum hydroxide with magnesium-containing antacids (unless patient has renal disease).
• Periodically monitor serum calcium and phosphate levels; decreased serum phosphate levels may lead to

---

increased serum calcium levels. Observe patient for hypophosphatemia signs and symptoms (anorexia, muscle weakness, and malaise).

Information for parents and patient
• Caution parents that patient should take aluminum hydroxide only as directed; should shake suspension well or chew tablets thoroughly; and should follow with sips of water or juice. Patient should not take any other oral medications within 2 hours of antacid dosage.
• Instruct parents to restrict patient's sodium intake, to have patient drink plenty of fluids, and to have patient follow a low-phosphate diet if drug is used for hyperphosphatemia.
• Instruct parents to report black, tarry stools or "coffee ground" vomiting to the physician.
• Advise parents not to switch to another antacid or to give any other medication without medical approval.

---

amantadine hydrochloride
Symmetrel

• Classification: antiviral, antiparkinsonism agent (synthetic cyclic primary amine)

How supplied
Available by prescription only
Capsules: 100 mg
Syrup: 50 mg/5 ml

Indications, route, and dosage
Prophylaxis or symptomatic treatment of influenza type A virus, respiratory tract illnesses in debilitated patients.
Children age 1 to 9: 4.4 to 8.8 mg/kg P.O. daily, divided b.i.d. or t.i.d. Do not exceed 150 mg/day.
Children age 10 and over and adults: 200 mg P.O. daily in a single dose or divided b.i.d.

Treatment should continue for 24 to 48 hours after symptoms disappear. Prophylaxis should start as soon as possible after initial exposure and continue for at least 10 days after exposure. Prophylactic treatment may be continued up to 90 days for repeated or suspected exposures if influenza virus vaccine is unavailable. If used with influenza virus vaccine, continue dose for 2 to 3 weeks until protection from vaccine develops.
Treatment of drug-induced extrapyramidal reactions
Adults: 100 mg P.O. b.i.d., up to 300 mg/day in divided doses. Patient may benefit from as much as 400 mg/day, but doses over 200 mg must be closely supervised.
Dosage in renal failure
Base dosage on creatinine clearance value, as follows:
Creatinine clearance value (ml/minute/1.73 m²) determines maintenance dosage. Thus, if creatinine clearance is > 80 ml/minute, maintenance dosage is 100 mg twice daily; if 60 to 80 ml/minute, 200 mg or 100 mg on alternate days; 40 to 60 ml/minute, 100

mg once daily; 30 to 40 ml/minute, 200 mg twice weekly; 20 to 30 ml/minute, 100 mg three times weekly; 10 to 20 ml/minute, 200 mg or 100 mg alternating every 7 days.

Note: Patients on chronic hemodialysis should receive 200 mg or 100 mg alternating every 7 days.

Action and kinetics
• *Antiviral action:* Amantadine interferes with penetration of influenza A virus into susceptible cells and blocks viral uncoating by ribonucleic acid (RNA). In vitro, amantadine is active only against influenza type A virus. (However, spontaneous resistance frequently occurs.) In vivo, amantadine may protect against influenza type A virus in 70% to 90% of patients; when administered within 24 to 48 hours of onset of illness, it reduces duration of fever and other systemic symptoms.
• *Antiparkinsonism action:* Amantadine is thought to cause the release of dopamine in the substantia nigra.
• *Kinetics in adults:* With oral administration, amantadine is well absorbed from the GI tract. Peak serum levels occur in 1 to 8 hours; usual serum level is 0.2 to 0.9 mcg/ml. (Neurotoxicity may occur at levels exceeding 1.5 mcg/ml.) Amantadine is distributed widely throughout the body and crosses the blood-brain barrier. About 10% of dose is metabolized. About 90% of dose is excreted unchanged in urine, primarily by tubular secretion. Portion of drug may be excreted in breast milk. Excretion rate depends on urine pH (acidic pH enhances excretion). In patients with normal renal function, elimination half-life is approximately 24 hours. In patients with renal dysfunction, elimination half-life may be prolonged to 10 days.

Contraindications and precautions
Amantadine is contraindicated in patients with known hypersensitivity to the drug.

Amantadine should be administered cautiously to patients with a history of hepatic disease, seizures, psychosis, renal disease, recurrent eczematoid dermatitis, epilepsy, cardiovascular disease (especially congestive heart failure), peripheral edema, or orthostatic hypotension, because the drug may exacerbate these disorders. Do not administer to female patients of childbearing age without adequate contraceptive measures because animal studies have demonstrated embryotoxic and teratogenic potential.

Interactions
When used concomitantly, amantadine may potentiate anticholinergic adverse effects of trihexyphenidyl and benztropine (when these drugs are given in high doses), possibly causing confusion and hallucinations. Concomitant use with a combination of hydrochlorothiazide and triamterene may decrease urinary amantadine excretion, resulting in increased serum amantadine levels and possible toxicity.

Concomitant use with CNS stimulants may cause additive stimulation. Concomitant use with alcohol may result in light-headedness, confusion, fainting, and hypotension.

Effects on diagnostic tests
None reported.

Adverse reactions
• CNS: *depression,* fatigue, confusion, dizziness, psychosis, hallucinations, anxiety, irritability, ataxia, insomnia, weakness, headache, light-headedness, difficulty concentrating.
• CV: peripheral edema, *orthostatic hypotension, congestive heart failure.*
• DERM: livedo reticularis (with prolonged use).
• GI: anorexia, nausea, constipation, vomiting, dry mouth.
• GU: *urinary retention.*
Note: Drug should be discontinued if patient develops hypersensitivity reaction.

Overdose and treatment
Clinical effects of overdose include nausea, vomiting, anorexia, hyperexcitability, tremors, slurred speech, blurred vision, lethargy, anticholinergic symptoms, convulsions, and possible ventricular dysrhythmias, including torsade de pointes and ventricular fibrillation.
Note: CNS effects result from increased levels of dopamine in the brain.

Treatment includes immediate gastric lavage or emesis induction along with supportive measures, forced fluids, and, if necessary, I.V. administration of fluids. Urine acidification may be used to increase drug excretion. Physostigmine may be given (1 to 2 mg by slow I.V. infusion at 1- to 2-hour intervals) to counteract CNS toxicity. Seizures or dysrhythmias may be treated with conventional therapy. Patient should be monitored closely.

▶ Special considerations
• Amantadine's safety and effectiveness in children under age 1 have not been established.
• If patient experiences insomnia, administer dose several hours before bedtime.
• Prophylactic drug use is recommended for selected high-risk patients who cannot receive influenza virus vaccine. Manufacturer recommends prophylactic therapy lasting up to 90 days with possible repeated or unknown exposure.

Information for parents and patient
• Warn parents and patient that drug may impair mental alertness.
• Patient should take drug after meals to ensure best absorption.
• Caution parents that patient should avoid abrupt position changes because these may cause light-headedness or dizziness.
• Patient should avoid alcohol while taking drug. Explain that some liquid medications contain alcohol.
• Instruct parents to report adverse reactions promptly, especially dizziness, depression, anxiety, nausea, and urine retention.

ambenonium chloride
Mytelase

• Classification: antimyasthenic agent (cholinesterase inhibitor)

How supplied
Available by prescription only
Tablets: 10 mg

Indications, route, and dosage
Symptomatic treatment of myasthenia gravis
Children: Initially, 0.3 mg/kg/day or 10 mg/m²/day up to 1.5 mg/kg/day or 50 mg/m²/day in three or four doses.
Adults: Dose must be individualized for each patient, but usually ranges from 5 to 25 mg P.O. t.i.d. to q.i.d. Starting dose usually 5 mg P.O. t.i.d. to q.i.d., increased gradually and adjusted at 2-day intervals to avoid drug accumulation and overdose. Maintenance dosage may range from 5 mg to as much as 75 mg per dose.

Action and kinetics
• *Muscle stimulant action:* Ambenonium blocks hydrolysis of acetylcholine by cholinesterase, resulting in acetylcholine accumulation at cholinergic synapses. That leads to increased stimulation of cholinergic receptors at the myoneural junction.

Because of its toxic potential, ambenonium chloride is usually used only in patients who cannot tolerate neostigmine or pyridostigmine (such as those who are hypersensitive to bromides).
• *Kinetics in adults:* Ambenonium is poorly absorbed from the GI tract. Onset of action usually occurs in 20 to 30 minutes. Distribution is largely unknown. The exact metabolic fate is unknown; however, drug is not hydrolyzed by cholinesterases. Duration of effect is usually 3 to 8 hours, depending on patient's physical and emotional status and severity of disease. Excretion is unknown.

Contraindications and precautions
Ambenonium is contraindicated in patients with mechanical obstruction of the intestinal or urinary tract because of its stimulatory effect on smooth muscle and in patients with bradycardia and hypotension because it may exacerbate these conditions.

Administer ambenonium cautiously to patients with epilepsy because of the drug's possible CNS stimulatory effects; to patients with recent coronary occlusion or cardiac dysrhythmias, because the drug stimulates the cardiovascular system; to patients with peptic ulcer, because the drug may stimulate gastric acid secretion; and to patients with bronchial asthma, because the drug may precipitate asthma attacks. Avoid giving large doses to patients with megacolon or decreased GI motility because intoxication may occur after gastric motility has been restored. Other cholinergic drugs should be discontinued before ambenonium administration begins to avoid additive cholinergic effects.

Interactions
Procainamide and quinidine may reverse ambenonium's cholinergic effects on muscle. Use with corticosteroids also may decrease ambenonium's cholinergic effects; however, after corticosteroids are stopped, cholinergic effects may increase, possibly altering muscle strength. Combined use with succinylcholine may cause prolonged respiratory depression from plasma esterase inhibition and resulting delay in succinylcholine hydrolysis. Use with ganglionic blockers, such as mecamylamine, may critically decrease blood pressure; effect is usually preceded by abdominal symptoms. Concomitant use of magnesium may antagonize beneficial effects of anticholinesterase therapy through a direct depressant effect on skeletal muscle.

Effects on diagnostic tests
None reported.

Adverse reactions
• CNS: headache, dizziness, convulsions, confusion, nervousness.
• CV: dysrhythmias (especially bradycardia), decreased cardiac output, hypotension.
• Eye: miosis, lacrimation, diplopia, blurred vision, conjunctival hyperemia.
• GI: nausea, vomiting, diarrhea, increased peristalsis, increased abdominal cramps, increased salivation, increased GI secretions, dysphagia.
• GU: urinary frequency and urgency, incontinence.
• Musculoskeletal: muscle weakness, muscle cramps, fasciculations.
• Respiratory: increased tracheobronchial secretions, laryngospasm, bronchiolar constriction, bronchospasm, respiratory muscle paralysis.
• Other: fever.
   Note: Drug should be discontinued if hypersensitivity, difficulty breathing, incoordination, paralysis, or restlessness or agitation develops.

Overdose and treatment
Clinical signs of overdose include nausea, vomiting, diarrhea, excessive salivation, increased bronchial secretions, excessive sweating, muscle weakness, fasciculations, paralysis, hypotension, and bradycardia.
   Treatment consists mainly of respiratory support and bronchial suctioning. Discontinue drug immediately. Atropine (0.5 to 4 mg I.V.) will block ambenonium's muscarinic effects but will not counter paralytic effects on skeletal muscle. Avoid atropine overdose, because it may cause bronchial plug formation.

▶ Special considerations
• Dosage must be individualized according to severity of disease and patient response.
• Give ambenonium with food or milk to reduce the chance of GI adverse effects.
• Observe and record variations in patient's muscle strength. If muscle weakness is severe, determine if this problem results from drug toxicity or exacerbation of myasthenia gravis. A test dose of edrophonium I.V. will aggravate drug-induced weakness but will temporarily relieve weakness that results from the disease.
• Patients may develop resistance to this drug.

Information for parents and patient
• Tell parents to have patient take drug with food or milk to reduce adverse effects.
• Advise parents to keep daily record of dose and effects during initial phase of therapy to help identify an optimum therapeutic regimen.
• Warn parents to administer drug exactly as prescribed and to give missed dose as soon as possible. If almost time for next dose, patient should skip the missed dose and return to prescribed schedule. Patient should not double the dose.
• Advise parents to store drug away from heat and light and safely out of small children's reach.
• Teach parents how to evaluate muscle strength and to report changes; also advise them to report any skin rash or extreme fatigue.

---

amcinonide
Cyclocort

• Classification: anti-inflammatory agent (adrenocorticoid)

How supplied
Available by prescription only
Cream, lotion, ointment: 0.1%

Indications, route, and dosage
Inflammation of corticosteroid-responsive dermatoses
Children: Apply a light film of cream, lotion, or ointment to affected areas once daily.
Adults: Apply a light film of cream, lotion, or ointment to affected areas b.i.d. or t.i.d. Rub in cream gently and thoroughly until it disappears.

Action and kinetics
• *Anti-inflammatory action:* Amcinonide stimulates the synthesis of enzymes needed to decrease the inflammatory response. Amcinonide is a group II fluorinated corticosteroid with much greater anti-inflammatory activity than hydrocortisone 0.25% to 2.5%. It has vasoconstrictor, antipruritic, and anti-inflammatory actions equal to those of betamethasone dipropionate 0.05% and triamcinolone acetonide 0.5%.
• *Kinetics in adults:* The amount of drug absorbed depends on the amount applied and on the nature of the skin at the application site. It ranges from about 1% in areas with a thick stratum corneum (such as the palms, soles, elbows, and knees) to as high as 36% in areas of the thinnest stratum corneum (face, eyelids, and genitals). Absorption increases in areas of skin damage, inflammation, or occlusion. Some systemic absorption of topical steroids may occur, especially through the oral mucosa.
   After topical application, amcinonide is distributed throughout the local skin and metabolized primarily in the skin. The small amount that is absorbed into

systemic circulation is removed rapidly from the blood and distributed into muscle, liver, skin, intestines, and kidneys and metabolized primarily in the liver to inactive compounds.

Inactive metabolites are excreted by the kidneys, primarily as glucuronides and sulfates, but also as unconjugated products. Small amounts of the metabolites are also excreted in feces.

Contraindications and precautions

Amcinonide is contraindicated in patients who are hypersensitive to any component of the preparation and in patients with viral diseases of the skin, such as varicella or herpes simplex, because it suppresses the patient's immune response.

Amcinonide should be used with extreme caution in patients with impaired circulation because it may increase the risk of skin ulceration.

Interactions

None significant.

Effects on diagnostic tests

None reported.

Adverse reactions

• Local: burning, itching, irritation, dryness, folliculitis, hypertrichosis, acneiform eruptions, hypopigmentation, perioral dermatitis, allergic contact dermatitis, maceration, secondary infection, atrophy, striae, miliaria.

Significant systemic absorption may produce the following reactions.
• CNS: euphoria, insomnia, headache, psychotic behavior, pseudotumor cerebri, mental changes, nervousness, restlessness.
• CV: congestive heart failure, hypertension, edema.
• EENT: cataracts, glaucoma, thrush.
• GI: peptic ulcer, irritation, increased appetite.
• Immune: immunosuppression, increased susceptibility to infection.
• Metabolic: hypokalemia, sodium retention, fluid retention, weight gain, hyperglycemia, osteoporosis, growth suppression in children.
• Musculoskeletal: muscle atrophy.
• Other: withdrawal syndrome (nausea, fatigue, anorexia, dyspnea, hypotension, hypoglycemia, myalgia, arthralgia, fever, dizziness, and fainting).

Note: Drug should be discontinued if local irritation, infection, systemic absorption, or hypersensitivity reaction occurs.

Overdose and treatment

No information available.

▶ Special considerations

• *Children have greater susceptibility to topical corticosteroid-induced HPA axis suppression and Cushing's syndrome than mature patients because of a higher ratio of skin surface area to body weight.* Hypothalamic-pituitary-adrenal (HPA) axis suppression, Cushing's syndrome, and intracranial hypertension have been reported in children receiving topical corticosteroids. Effects of adrenal suppression in children include linear growth retardation, delayed weight gain, low plasma cortisol levels, and absence of response to ACTH stimulation. Signs of intracranial hypertension include bulging fontanelles, headaches, and bilateral papilledema.
• Administration of topical corticosteroids to children should be limited to the least amount compatible with an effective therapeutic regimen. Chronic corticosteroid therapy may interfere with growth and development.
• Monitor patient response. Observe inflamed area and elicit patient comments concerning pruritus. Inspect skin for infection, striae, and atrophy. Skin atrophy is common and may be clinically significant within 3 to 4 weeks of treatment with high-potency preparation; it also occurs more readily at sites where percutaneous absorption is high.
• Do not apply occlusive dressings over topical steroids because this may lead to secondary infection, maceration, atrophy, striae, or miliaria caused by increasing steroid penetration and potency.
• If an occlusive dressing is necessary, minimize adverse reactions by using it intermittently. Do not leave it in place longer than 16 hours each day.
• Stop drug if the patient develops signs of systemic absorption (including Cushing's syndrome, hyperglycemia, or glucosuria), skin irritation or ulceration, hypersensitivity, or infection. (If antifungals or antibiotics are being used with corticosteroids and the infection does not respond immediately, corticosteroids should be stopped until infection is controlled.)

Information for parents and patient

• Instruct parents and patient in application of the drug. Tell them the following:
Method for applying topical preparations
• Wash your hands before and after applying the drug.
• Gently cleanse the area of application. Washing or soaking the area before application may increase drug penetration.
• Apply sparingly in a light film; rub in lightly. Avoid contact with patient's eyes.
• Avoid prolonged application on the face, in skin folds, and in areas near the eyes, genitals, and rectum. High-potency topical corticosteroids are more likely to cause striae in these areas because of their higher rates of absorption.
• Warn patient not to use nonprescription topical preparations other than those specifically recommended.
• Advise parents not to use tight-fitting diapers or plastic pants on a child being treated in the diaper area, since such garments may serve as occlusive dressings.

amikacin sulfate
Amikin

• Classification: antibiotic (aminoglycoside)

How supplied

Available by prescription only
Injection: 50 mg/ml, 250 mg/ml

Indications, route, and dosage
Serious infections caused by susceptible organisms
Neonates with normal renal function: Initially, 10 mg/kg I.M. or I.V. (in dextrose 5% in water administered over 1 to 2 hours); then 7.5 mg/kg q 12 hours I.M. or I.V. infusion.
Neonates age 1 to 7 days, weighing ⩽ *2 kg:* 7.5 mg/kg I.V. or I.M. q 12 hr
Neonates age 1 to 7 days, weighing > *2 kg:* 10 mg/kg I.V. or I.M. q 12 hr
Neonates over age 1 week, weighing ⩽ *2 kg:* 7.5 to 10 mg/kg I.V. or I.M. q 8 hr
Neonates over age 1 week, weighing > *2 kg:* 10 mg/kg I.V. or I.M. q 8 hr
Children and adults with normal renal function: 15 mg/kg/day divided q 8 to 12 hours I.M. or I.V. (in 100 to 200 ml dextrose 5% in water administered over 30 to 60 minutes). May be given by direct I.V. push if necessary.
Meningitis, ventriculitis
Children: Systemic therapy as above; may also use 1 to 2 mg intrathecally daily.
Adults: Systemic therapy as above; may also use up to 20 mg intrathecally or intraventricularly daily.
Dosage in renal failure
Initially, 7.5 mg/kg. Subsequent doses and frequency determined by blood amikacin concentrations and renal function studies. One method is to administer additional 7.5 mg/kg doses and alter dosing interval based upon steady state serum creatinine: creatinine (mg/100 ml) × 9 = dosing interval (in hours). Keep peak serum concentrations between 15 and 35 mcg/ml, and trough serum concentrations between 5 and 10 mcg/ml.

Action and kinetics
• *Antibiotic action:* Amikacin is bactericidal; it binds directly to the 30S ribosomal subunit, thus inhibiting bacterial protein synthesis. Its spectrum of activity includes many aerobic gram-negative organisms (including most strains of *Pseudomonas aeruginosa*) and some aerobic gram-positive organisms. Amikacin may act against some organisms resistant to other aminoglycosides, such as *Proteus, Pseudomonas,* and *Serratia*; some strains of these may be resistant to amikacin. It is ineffective against anerobes.
• *Kinetics in adults:* Amikacin is absorbed poorly after oral administration and is given parenterally; after I.M. administration, peak serum concentrations occur in 45 minutes to 2 hours.
Amikacin is distributed widely after parenteral administration; intraocular penetration is poor. Factors that increase volume of distribution (burns, peritonitis) may increase dosage requirements. CSF penetration is low, even in patients with inflamed meninges. Intraventricular administration produces high concentrations throughout the CNS. Protein binding is minimal. Amikacin crosses the placenta.
Amikacin is excreted primarily in urine by glomerular filtration; small amounts may be excreted in bile and breast milk. Elimination half-life in adults is 2 to 3 hours. In patients with severe renal damage, half-life may extend to 30 to 86 hours. Over time, amikacin accumulates in inner ear and kidneys; urine

concentrations approach 800 mcg/ml 6 hours after a 500-mg I.M. dose.
• *Kinetics in children:* Additional information from studies in neonates show that peak serum levels after I.M. administration occur in 30 minutes. Elimination half life is estimated at 4 to 5 hours in full term infants 7 days of age or older, and 7 to 8 hours in low birth weight infants age 1 to 3 days.

Contraindications and precautions
Amikacin is contraindicated in patients with known hypersensitivity to amikacin or any other aminoglycoside.
Amikacin should be used cautiously in neonates and other infants, patients with decreased renal function; in patients with tinnitus, vertigo, or high-frequency hearing loss, who are susceptible to ototoxicity; in patients with dehydration, because of potential for increased nephrotoxicity with decreased urinary output; in patients with myasthenia gravis, parkinsonism, and hypocalcemia, because the drug may exacerbate symptoms associated with these disorders.

Interactions
Concomitant use with the following drugs may increase the hazard of nephrotoxicity, ototoxicity, and neurotoxicity: amphotericin B, loop diuretics, methoxyflurane, polymyxin B, capreomycin, cisplatin, cephalosporins, and other aminoglycosides; hazard of ototoxicity is also increased during use with ethacrynic acid, furosemide, bumetanide, urea, or mannitol. Dimenhydrinate and other antiemetics and antivertigo drugs may mask amikacin-induced ototoxicity. Amikacin may potentiate neuromuscular blockade from general anesthetics or neuromuscular blocking agents such as succinylcholine and tubocurarine.
Concomitant use with penicillins results in a synergistic bactericidal effect against *Pseudomonas aeruginosa, Escherichia coli, Klebsiella, Citrobacter, Enterobacter, Serratia,* and *Proteus mirabilis.* However, the drugs are physically and chemically incompatible and are inactivated when mixed or given together. In vivo inactivation has also been reported when aminoglycosides and penicillins are used concomitantly.

Effects on diagnostic tests
Amikacin-induced nephrotoxicity may elevate BUN, nonprotein nitrogen, or serum creatinine levels, and increase urinary excretion of casts.

Adverse reactions
• CNS: *headache, lethargy, neuromuscular blockade* with respiratory depression.
• EENT: *ototoxicity (tinnitus, vertigo, hearing loss).*
• GI: *diarrhea.*
• GU: *nephrotoxicity (cells or casts in urine, oliguria, proteinuria, decreased creatinine clearance, increased BUN, serum creatinine, and nonprotein nitrogen levels).*
• HEMA: *blood dyscrasias, purpura* (infants).
• Hepatic: *transient hepatomegaly, elevated hepatic enzymes.*

• Other: hypersensitivity reactions *(eosinophilia, fever, rash, urticaria, pruritus)*, bacterial or fungal superinfections.

Note: Drug should be discontinued if signs of ototoxicity, nephrotoxicity, or hypersensitivity occur.

Overdose and treatment

Clinical signs of overdose include ototoxicity, nephrotoxicity, and neuromuscular toxicity. Drug can be removed by hemodialysis or peritoneal dialysis. Treatment with calcium salts or anticholinesterases reverses neuromuscular blockade.

▶ Special considerations

• Amikacin has been administered intrathecally and intraventricularly. Many clinicians prefer intraventricular administration to ensure adequate CSF levels in the treament of ventriculitis.

• Because amikacin is dialyzable, patients undergoing hemodialysis may need dosage adjustments.

• To prevent emergence of resistance, and because the potential for ototoxicity is unknown, amikacin should only be used in infants when other drugs are ineffective or contraindicated. Patient should be closely monitored during therapy.

• Assess patient's allergic history; do not give an aminoglycoside to patient with a history of hypersensitivity reactions to any aminoglycoside; monitor patient continuously for this and other adverse reactions.

• Obtain results of culture and sensitivity tests before first dose; however, therapy may begin before tests are completed. Repeat tests periodically to assess drug efficacy.

• Monitor vital signs, electrolyte levels, and renal function studies before and during therapy; be sure patient is well hydrated to minimize chemical irritation of renal tubules; watch for signs of declining renal function.

• Keep peak serum levels and trough serum levels at recommended concentrations, especially in patients with decreased renal function. Draw blood for peak level 1 hour after I.M. injection (30 minutes to 1 hour after I.V. infusion); for trough level, draw sample just before the next dose. Time and date all blood samples. Do not use heparinized tube to collect blood samples; it interferes with results.

• Evaluate patient's hearing before and during therapy; monitor for complaints of tinnitus, vertigo, or hearing loss.

• Avoid concomitant use of aminoglycosides with other ototoxic or nephrotoxic drugs.

• Usual duration of therapy is 7 to 10 days; if no response occurs in 3 to 5 days, drug should be discontinued and cultures repeated for reevaluation of therapy.

• Closely monitor patients on long-term therapy—especially debilitated patients and others receiving immunosuppressant or radiation therapy—for possible bacterial or fungal superinfection; monitor especially for fever.

• Do not add or mix other drugs with I.V. infusions—particularly penicillins, which will inactivate aminoglycosides; the two groups are chemically and physically incompatible. If other drugs must be given I.V., temporarily stop infusion of primary drug.

• Aminoglycosides may cause neuromuscular blockade with skeletal weakness and respiratory distress, especially in patients with pre-existing neuromuscular disease or hypocalcemia, in those receiving general anesthetics, and in infants with botulism (through potentiation of botulism toxin).

Parenteral administration

• Consult manufacturer's directions for reconstitution, dilution, and storage of drugs; check expiration dates.

• Administer I.M. dose deep into large muscle mass (gluteal or midlateral thigh); rotate injection sites to minimize tissue injury; do not inject more than 2 g of drug per injection site. Apply ice to injection site for pain.

• Too-rapid I.V. administration may cause neuromuscular blockade. Infuse I.V. drug continuously or intermittently over 30 to 60 minutes for adults, 1 to 2 hours for infants; dilution volume for children is determined individually.

• Solutions should always be clear, colorless to pale yellow (in most cases, darkening indicates deterioration), and free of particles; do not give solutions containing precipitates or other foreign matter.

Information for parents and patient

Teach parents how to recognize signs and symptoms of hypersensitivity; bacterial or fungal superinfections (especially if the child has low resistance from immunosuppressants or irradiation); and other adverse reactions to aminoglycosides. Urge them to report any unusual effects promptly.

---

aminocaproic acid
Amicar

• Classification: fibrinolysis inhibitor (carboxylic acid derivative)

How supplied

Available by prescription only
Tablets: 500 mg
Syrup: 250 mg/ml
Injection: 5 g/20 ml for dilution; 24 g/96 ml for infusion

Indications, route, and dosage
Excessive acute bleeding from hyperfibrinolysis

Adults: 4 to 5 g I.V. or P.O. over first hour, followed with constant infusion of 1 g/hour for about 8 hours or until bleeding is controlled; plasma level should be 130 mcg/ml. Maximum dosage is 30 g/24 hours.

Chronic bleeding tendency

Children: 100 mg/kg I.V., or 3 g/m² I.V. first hour, followed by constant infusion of 33.3 mg/kg/hour or 1 g/m²/hour. Maximum dosage is 18 g/m² for 24 hours.
Adults: 5 to 30 g/day P.O. in divided doses at 3- to 6-hour intervals.

Action and kinetics

• *Hemostatic action:* Aminocaproic acid inhibits plasminogen activators; to a lesser degree, it blocks antiplasmin activity by inhibiting fibrinolysis.

---

‡May contain sulfites   ◆May contain tartrazine   ◆◆May contain benzyl alcohol

• *Kinetics in adults:* Aminocaproic acid is rapidly and completely absorbed from the GI tract. Peak plasma level occurs in 2 hours; sustained plasma levels are achieved by repeated oral doses or continuous I.V. infusion. Aminocaproic acid readily permeates human blood cells and other body cells. It is not protein-bound. Metabolism is insignificant. Duration of action of a single parenteral dose is less than 3 hours; 40% to 60% of a single oral dose is excreted unchanged in urine in 12 hours.

Contraindications and precautions

Aminocaproic acid is contraindicated in patients with active intravascular clotting; do not use in patients with disseminated intravascular coagulation (DIC) without concomitant heparin therapy, because aminocaproic acid may induce thrombus formation.

Administer drug cautiously to patients with thrombophlebitis or cardiac disease because of potential for clotting abnormalities, and to patients with hepatic or renal disease because of potential for drug accumulation.

Interactions

Concomitant use with estrogens and oral contraceptives containing estrogen increases risk of hypercoagulability; use with caution.

Effects on diagnostic tests

Drug may elevate serum potassium level in some patients with decreased renal function; it may increase creatine phosphokinase (CPK), AST (SGOT), and ALT (SGPT) levels.

Adverse reactions

• CNS: dizziness, *malaise*, headache, delirium, hallucinations, seizures, weakness.
• CV: hypotension, bradycardia, dysrhythmias (especially with rapid I.V. infusion).
• DERM: rash.
• EENT: tinnitus, nasal stuffiness, conjunctival suffusion.
• GI: *nausea*, cramps, *diarrhea.*
• GU: diuresis, dysuria, inhibition of ejaculation, prolonged menses, red-brown urine.
• HEMA: generalized thrombosis, thrombophlebitis.
• Other: hepatic failure; skeletal myopathy; elevated CPK, ALT (SGPT), AST (SGOT) levels.
    Note: Drug should be discontinued if signs of allergy or thrombosis appear.

Overdose and treatment

Clinical manifestations of overdose may include nausea, diarrhea, delirium, thrombotic episodes, and cardiac and hepatic necrosis. Discontinue drug immediately. Animal studies have demonstrated subendocardial hemorrhagic lesions after long-term high-dose administration.

▶ Special considerations

• To prepare an I.V. infusion, use normal saline injection, dextrose 5% in water injection, or lactated Ringer's injection for dilution. Dilute doses up to 5 g with 250 ml of solution, doses of 5 g or greater with at least 500 ml.

• Avoid rapid I.V. infusion to minimize risk of CV adverse reactions; use infusion pump to ensure constancy of infusion.
• Monitor coagulation studies, heart rhythm, and blood pressure. Chronic use of this agent requires routine CPK determinations. Be alert for signs of phlebitis.

Information for parents and patient

• Tell parents that patient should change positions slowly to minimize dizziness.
• With long-term use, explain that routine CPK determinations will be necessary.
• Teach parents signs and symptoms of thrombophlebitis, and advise them to report them promptly.

---

aminophylline
Amoline, Phyllocontin, Somophylline, Truphylline

• Classification: bronchodilator (xanthine derivative)

How supplied

Available by prescription only
Tablets: 100 mg, 200 mg
Tablets (controlled-release): 225 mg
Liquid: 105 mg/5 ml
Injection: 250-mg, 500-mg vials and ampules
Rectal suppositories: 250 mg, 500 mg
Rectal solution: 300 mg/5 ml

Indications, route, and dosage
Symptomatic relief of bronchospasm

Patients not currently receiving theophylline or whose serum theophylline level is < 2.5 mcg/ml, and who require rapid relief of symptoms: Loading dose is 6 mg/kg (equivalent to 4.7 mg/kg anhydrous theophylline) I.V. slowly (less than or equal to 25 mg/minute), then maintenance infusion.
Children age 9 to 16: 1 mg/kg/hour for 12 hours; then 0.8 mg/kg/hour.
Children age 6 months to 9 years: 1.2 mg/kg/hour for 12 hours; then 1 mg/kg/hour.
Adults (nonsmokers): 0.7 mg/kg/hour for 12 hours; then 0.5 mg/kg/hour.
Older patients; adults with cor pulmonale: 0.6 mg/kg/hour for 12 hours; then 0.3 mg/kg/hour.
Adults with congestive heart failure (CHF) or liver disease: 0.5 mg/kg/hour for 12 hours; then 0.1 to 0.2 mg/kg/hour.
Otherwise healthy adult smokers: 1 mg/kg/hour for 12 hours; then 0.8 mg/kg/hour.
Patients currently receiving theophylline: Aminophylline infusions of 0.63 mg/kg (0.5 mg/kg anhydrous theophylline) will increase plasma levels of theophylline by 1 mcg/ml. Some clinicians recommend a loading dose of 3.1 mg/kg (2.5 mg/kg anhydrous theophylline) if no obvious signs of theophylline toxicity are present.
Chronic bronchial asthma
Children: 12 mg/kg P.O. daily divided t.i.d. or q.i.d. Alternatively, administer according to age:
Children age 1 to 9: 27.4 mg/kg/day in 4 divided doses.

---

*Canada only   †Unlabeled clinical use   Italicized adverse reactions have been observed in children.

Children age 9 to 12: 22.8 mg/kg/day in 4 divided doses.
Children age 12 to 16: 20.5 mg/kg/day in 4 divided doses.

Monitor serum levels to ensure that theophylline concentrations range from 10 to 20 mcg/ml. However, some patients may respond with adequate bronchodilation at 5 to 10 mcg/ml.
Adults: 600 to 1,600 mg P.O. daily divided t.i.d. or q.i.d.

†*Adjunctive treatment of neonatal apnea*
Loading dose 3 to 6 mg/kg I.V. over at least 20 minutes, followed by maintenance dose of 1 to 2 mg/kg every 8 or 12 hours P.O. or I.V. Peak serum concentrations should be 5 to 12 mcg/ml.

Action and kinetics
• *Bronchodilating action:* Aminophylline acts at the cellular level after it is converted to theophylline. (Aminophylline dihydrate [theophylline ethylenediamine] is 79% theophylline; anhydrous aminophylline is 86% theophylline.) Theophylline acts by either inhibiting phosphodiesterase or blocking adenosine receptors in the bronchi, resulting in relaxation of the smooth muscle. The drug also stimulates the respiratory center in the medulla and prevents diaphragmatic fatigue.
• *Kinetics in adults:* Most dosage forms are absorbed well; absorption of the suppository, however, is unreliable and slow. The rate and onset of action also depend upon the dosage form. Food may alter the rate, but not the extent of absorption, of oral doses. Aminophylline is distributed in all tissues and extracellular fluids. Aminophylline is converted to theophylline, then metabolized to inactive compounds. Aminophylline is excreted in the urine as theophylline (10%).
• *Kinetics in children:* In neonates and infants, aminophylline and theophylline can be converted to caffeine.

Contraindications and precautions
Aminophylline is contraindicated in patients with hypersensitivity to xanthines or ethylenediamine. It should be used cautiously in patients with compromised cardiac or circulatory function, diabetes, glaucoma, hypertension, hyperthyroidism, peptic ulcer, or gastroesophageal reflux, because drug may worsen these conditions.

Interactions
Aminophylline increases the excretion of lithium. Concomitant cimetidine, allopurinol (high dose), propranolol, erythromycin, or troleandomycin may increase serum concentration of aminophylline by decreasing hepatic clearance. Phenobarbital, tobacco, marijuana, and aminoglutethimide decrease effects of aminophylline. Alkali-sensitive drugs reduce activity of aminophylline. Do not add these drugs to I.V. fluids containing aminophylline.

Effects on diagnostic tests
Aminophylline may alter the assay for uric acid, depending on method used, and increases plasma-free fatty acids and urinary catecholamines. Theophylline

levels are falsely elevated in the presence of furosemide, phenylbutazone, probenecid, theobromine, caffeine, tea, chocolate, cola beverages, and acetaminophen, depending on type of assay used.

Adverse reactions
• CNS: *irritability, restlessness, seizures,* headache, insomnia, dizziness, depression, light-headedness, muscle twitching, *sleeplessness.*
• CV: palpitations, marked flushing, hypotension, *sinus tachycardia, ventricular tachycardia and other life-threatening dysrhythmias, extrasystoles, circulatory failure.*
• DERM: urticaria.
• GI: *nausea, vomiting, epigastric pain,* discomfort, dyspepsia, bitter aftertaste, loss of appetite, diarrhea.
• Respiratory: *tachypnea,* respiratory arrest.
• Local: rectal irritation from suppositories.
• Other: fever, urinary retention, *hyperglycemia, diuresis, dehydration.*
Note: Drug should be discontinued if an adverse reaction intensifies; this signals impending overdose.

Overdose and treatment
Clinical manifestations of overdose include nausea, vomiting, insomnia, irritability, tachycardia, extrasystoles, tachypnea, and tonic/clonic seizures. Onset of toxicity may be sudden and severe; dysrhythmias and seizures are the first signs. Induce emesis, except in convulsing patients, then use activated charcoal and cathartics (for example, a mixture of charcoal and sorbitol q 4 hours until serum level declines). Charcoal hemoperfusion may be beneficial. Treat dysrhythmias with lidocaine and seizures with I.V. diazepam; support respiratory and cardiovascular systems.

▶ Special considerations
• Many dosage forms and agents are available; it is important to select the form that offers maximum potential for patient compliance and minimal toxicity to the individual. Controlled-release preparations may not be crushed or chewed.
• Dosage should be calculated from lean body weight, because theophylline does not distribute into fatty tissue, and adjusted according to serum levels.
• Aminophylline releases theophylline in the blood; theophylline blood levels are used to monitor therapy.
• Before giving loading dose, check that patient has not had recent theophylline therapy.
• Do not combine in fluids for I.V. infusion with the following: ascorbic acid, chlorpromazine, codeine phosphate, dimenhydrinate, epinephrine, erythromycine gluceptate, hydralazine, insulin, levorphanol tartrate, meperidine, methadone, methicillin, morphine sulfate, norepinephrine bitartrate, oxytetracycline, penicillin G potassium, phenobarbital, phenytoin, prochlorperazine, promazine, promethazine, tetracycline, vancomycin, vitamin B complex with C.
• I.V. drug administration includes I.V. push at a very slow rate or an infusion with a volume of dextrose 5% or 0.9% sodium chloride to infuse over 15 to 20 minutes.
• GI symptoms may be relieved by taking oral drug

with full glass of water at meals, although food in stomach delays absorption. Enteric-coated tablets may also delay absorption. There is no evidence that antacids reduce GI adverse reactions.

• Suppositories are slowly and erractically absorbed and should be used with caution in children; retention enemas may be absorbed more rapidly. Rectally administered preparations can be given when patient cannot take drug orally. Schedule after evacuation, if possible; may be retained better if given before meal. Advise patient to remain recumbent 15 to 20 minutes after insertion.

• Chronic ingestion of charcoal broiled foods may increase elimination. Caffeinated beverages and chocolate may increase adverse reactions.

• Individuals metabolize xanthines at different rates, and metabolism is influenced by many factors, including age and life-style (smoking). Adjust dose by monitoring response, tolerance, pulmonary function, and theophylline blood levels. Therapeutic level is 10 to 20 mcg/ml, but some patients may respond at lower levels; toxicity occurs at levels over 20 mcg/ml.

• Plasma clearance may be decreased in patients with CHF, hepatic dysfunction, or pulmonary edema. Smokers show accelerated clearance. Dose adjustments necessary.

Information for parents and patient

• Teach parents rationale for therapy and importance of compliance with prescribed regimen; if a dose is missed, patient should take it as soon as possible, but not double up on doses. Advise parents to avoid giving child extra "breathing pills."

• Advise the parents of the adverse effects and possible signs of toxicity.

• Tell parents patient should avoid excessive intake of xanthine-containing foods and beverages.

• Warn that nonprescription remedies may contain ephedrine in combination with theophylline salts; excessive CNS stimulation may result. Tell parents to seek medical approval before giving child *any* other medications.

• Teach parents adjunctive measures to improve respiration: plentiful fluid intake, use of humidifier, chest physiotherapy, postural drainage, and avoidance of exposure to cigarette smoke.

---

amiodarone hydrochloride
Cordarone

• Classification: ventricular and supraventricular antiarrhythmic (benzofuran derivative)

How supplied
Available by prescription only
Tablets: 100 mg*, 200 mg

Indications, route, and dosage
Ventricular and †supraventricular dysrhythmias († recurrent supraventricular tachycardia, atrial fibrillation and flutter, †ventricular tachycardia)

Children: 10 mg/kg P.O. per day or 800 mg/1.72 m² P.O. per day for 10 days or until response is seen. Then 5 mg/kg or 400 mg/1.72 m²; usual maintenance dosage is 2.5 mg/kg or 200 mg/1.72 m² P.O. per day.
Adults: Loading dose of 800 to 1,600 mg P.O. daily for 1 to 3 weeks until initial therapeutic response occurs. Maintenance dosage is 200 to 600 mg P.O. daily. Alternatively, loading dose is 5 to 10 mg/kg by I.V. infusion via central line, followed by I.V. infusion of 10 mg/kg/day for 3 to 5 days.

Note: Intravenous use of amiodarone is investigational.

Action and kinetics
• *Ventricular antiarrhythmic action:* Although it has mixed Class IC and Class III antiarrhythmic effects, amiodarone generally is considered a Class III agent. It widens the action potential duration (repolarization inhibition). With prolonged therapy, the effective refractory period (ERP) increases in the atria, ventricles, AV node, His-Purkinje system, and bypass tracts and conduction slows in the atria, AV node, His-Purkinje system, and ventricles; sinus node automaticity decreases. Amiodarone also noncompetitively blocks beta-adrenergic receptors. Clinically, it has little, if any, negative inotropic effect. Coronary and peripheral vasodilator effects may occur with long-term therapy. Amiodarone is among the most effective antiarrhythmic agents, but its therapeutic applications are somewhat limited by its severe adverse reactions.

• *Kinetics in adults:* Amiodarone has slow, variable absorption. Bioavailability is approximately 35% to 65%. Peak plasma levels occur 3 to 7 hours after oral administration; however, onset of action may be delayed from 2 to 3 days to 2 to 3 months—even with loading doses. Amiodarone is distributed widely because it accumulates in adipose tissue and in organs with marked perfusion, such as the lungs, liver, and spleen. It is also highly protein-bound (96%). The therapeutic serum level is not well-defined but probably ranges from 1 to 2.5 mcg/ml. Amiodarone is metabolized extensively in the liver to a pharmacologically active metabolite, desethyl amiodarone. Amiodarone's main excretory route is hepatic, through the biliary tree (with enterohepatic recirculation). Because no renal excretion occurs, patients with impaired renal function do not require dosage reduction. Terminal elimination half-life—25 to 110 days—is the longest of any antiarrhythmic; in most patients, half-life ranges from 40 to 50 days.

Contraindications and precautions
Amiodarone is contraindicated in patients with pre-existing sinus-node dysfunction and bradycardia causing syncope or second- or third-degree heart block (except if patient has artificial pacemaker) because of its potent effects on the AV conduction system. It should be used with caution in patients with CHF because of the potential for adverse hemodynamic

---

effects; in patients with liver disease, because metabolism may be reduced; and in patients with hypokalemia, because drug may be ineffective.

Interactions

Concomitant use of amiodarone with quinidine, disopyramide, tricyclic antidepressants, or phenothiazines may cause additive effects that lead to a prolonged QT interval, possibly resulting in Torsades de Pointes ventricular tachycardia.

Concomitant use with warfarin may cause prolonged prothrombin time, as a result of enhanced drug displacement from protein-binding sites. Concomitant use with digoxin, quinidine, phenytoin, or procainamide may lead to increased serum levels of these drugs, resulting in enhanced effects.

Effects on diagnostic tests

Amiodarone alters thyroid function test results, causing increased serum thyroxine (T_4) and decreased triiodothyronine (T_3) levels. (However, most patients maintain normal thyroid function during therapy.)

Adverse reactions

• CNS: peripheral neuropathy and extrapyramidal symptoms, headache, malaise, fatigue, *dizziness, paresthesias.*
• CV: *bradycardia,* hypotension, *dysrhythmia.*
• DERM: photosensitivity, blue-gray pigmentation.
• EENT: *corneal microdeposits,* visual disturbances.
• Endocrine: hypothyroidism and hyperthyroidism.
• GI: *nausea, vomiting,* constipation, *anorexia.*
• Hepatic: *altered liver enzyme levels,* hepatic dysfunction.
• Metabolic: electrolyte disturbances.
• Respiratory: *severe pulmonary toxicity* (pneumonitis, alveolitis) with high doses, *pulmonary fibrosis.*
• Other: muscle weakness, *altered thyroid function.*

   Note: Drug should be discontinued if signs or symptoms of pulmonary toxicity or epididymitis occur.

Overdose and treatment

Clinical effects of overdose include bradydysrhythmias. Treatment may involve beta-adrenergic agonists (such as isoproterenol) or artificial pacing to help restore an acceptable heart rate. To treat hypotension, positive inotropic agents (such as dopamine or dobutamine) or vasopressors (such as epinephrine or norepinephrine) may be administered. General supportive measures should be used, as necessary. Amiodarone cannot be removed by dialysis.

▶ Special considerations

• Children receiving amiodarone concomitantly with digoxin may experience more acute effects of interaction. Children may experience faster onset of action and shorter duration of effect than adults.
• Amiodarone has proved effective in treating dysrhythmias resistant to other drug therapy. However, high incidence of adverse effects limits drug's use.
• Divide loading dose into three equal doses, and give with meals to minimize GI intolerance. Maintenance dose may be given once daily but may be divided into two doses taken with meals if GI intolerance occurs.

• Monitor blood pressure and heart rate and rhythm frequently for significant change.
• Periodically monitor hepatic and thyroid function tests. Perform periodic ophthalmologic evaluations to assess corneal microdeposits.
• Monitor for signs and symptoms of pneumonitis, such as exertional dyspnea, nonproductive cough, and pleuritic chest pain. Also check pulmonary function tests and chest X-ray. (Pulmonary toxicity is more common with daily dosages exceeding 600 mg.) Pulmonary complications require discontinuation of amiodarone and, possibly, treatment with corticosteroids.
• Digoxin, quinidine, phenytoin, and procainamide doses should be decreased during amiodarone therapy to avoid toxicity.
• Adverse effects are more prevalent with high doses but usually resolve within about 4 months after drug therapy stops.

Information for parents and patient

• Advise parents that patient should use sunscreen lotion to prevent photosensitivity, which may result in sunburn and blistering.
• Although corneal microdeposits typically appear 1 to 4 months after therapy begins, only 2% to 3% of patients have actual visual disturbances. To minimize this complication, recommend frequent instillation of methylcellulose ophthalmic solution.

---

amitriptyline hydrochloride
Amitril∗, Amitriptylene, Elavil, Emitrip, Endep, Enovil, Levate∗, Mevaril∗, Novotriptyn∗, SK-Amitriptyline

• Classification: tricyclic antidepressant

How supplied

Available by prescription only
Tablets: 10 mg, 25 mg, 50 mg, 75 mg, 100 mg, 150 mg
Injection: 10 mg/ml

Indications, route, and dosage
Depression; †Anorexia or bulimia associated with depression
Adolescents: 30 mg P.O. daily in divided doses; may be increased to 150 mg.
Adults: 50 to 100 mg P.O. daily, divided t.i.d. or may be given at h.s. Increase to 200 mg daily; maximum dosage is 300 mg daily if needed; or 20 to 30 mg I.M. t.i.d. Alternatively, the entire dosage can be given at bedtime.

   Parenteral therapy should be changed to oral route as soon as possible.
†Migraine prophylaxis
Children: 10 mg P.O. h.s., increasing by 10 mg weekly.
†Adjunctive treatment of neurogenic pain
Adults: 25 mg b.i.d. or q.i.d.

Action and kinetics
• *Antidepressant action:* Amitriptyline is thought to exert its antidepressant effects by inhibiting reuptake of norepinephrine and serotonin in CNS nerve ter-

minals (presynaptic neurons), resulting in increased concentrations and enhanced activity of these neurotransmitters in the synaptic cleft. Amitriptyline more actively inhibits reuptake of serotonin than norepinephrine; it carries a high incidence of undesirable sedation, but tolerance to this effect usually develops within a few weeks.

• *Kinetics in adults:* Amitriptyline is absorbed rapidly from the GI tract after oral administration and from muscle tissue after I.M. administration.

Amitriptyline is distributed widely into the body, including the CNS and breast milk. Drug is 96% protein-bound. Peak effect occurs 2 to 12 hours after a given dose, and steady state is achieved within 4 to 10 days; full therapeutic effect usually occurs in 2 to 4 weeks.

Amitriptyline is metabolized by the liver to the active metabolite nortriptyline; a significant first-pass effect may account for variability of serum concentrations in different patients taking the same dosage. Most of drug is excreted in urine.

Contraindications and precautions
Amitriptyline is contraindicated in patients with known hypersensitivity to tricyclic antidepressants, trazodone, and related compounds; in the acute recovery phase of myocardial infarction because of its arrhythmogenic potential; in patients in coma or with severe respiratory depression because of additive depressant effects on CNS; and during or within 14 days of therapy with monoamine oxidase inhibitors.

Amitriptyline should be used with caution in patients with other cardiac disease (dysrhythmias, congestive heart failure [CHF], angina pectoris, valvular disease, or heart block); respiratory disorders; alcoholism, epilepsy and other seizure disorders; scheduled electroconvulsive therapy (ECT); bipolar disease; glaucoma; hyperthyroidism, or in those taking thyroid replacement; Type I and Type II diabetes; prostatic hypertrophy, paralytic ileus, or urinary retention; hepatic or renal dysfunction; Parkinson's disease; and in those undergoing surgery with general anesthesia.

Interactions
Concomitant use of amitriptyline with sympathomimetics, including epinephrine, phenylephrine, phenylpropanolamine, and ephedrine (often found in nasal sprays) may increase blood pressure; use with warfarin may increase prothrombin time and cause bleeding.

Concomitant use with thyroid hormones, pimozide, or antiarrhythmic agents (quinidine, disopyramide, procainamide) may increase incidence of cardiac dysrhythmias and conduction defects.

Amitriptyline may decrease hypotensive effects of centrally acting antihypertensive drugs, such as guanethidine, guanabenz, guanadrel, clonidine, methyldopa, and reserpine. Concomitant use with disulfiram or ethchlorvynol may cause delirium and tachycardia.

Additive effects are likely after concomitant use of amitriptyline with CNS depressants, including alcohol, analgesics, barbiturates, narcotics, tranquilizers, and anesthetics (oversedation); atropine or other anticholinergic drugs, including phenothiazines, antihistamines, meperidine, and antiparkinsonian agents (oversedation, paralytic ileus, visual changes, and severe constipation); or metrizamide (increased risk of convulsions).

Barbiturates and heavy smoking induce amitriptyline metabolism and decrease therapeutic efficacy; phenothiazines and haloperidol decrease its metabolism, decreasing therapeutic efficacy; methylphenidate, cimetidine, oral contraceptives, propoxyphene, and beta blockers may inhibit amitriptyline metabolism, increasing plasma levels and toxicity.

Effects on diagnostic tests
Amitriptyline may prolong conduction time (elongation of Q-T and PR intervals, flattened T waves on ECG); it also may elevate liver function test results, decrease white blood cell counts, and decrease or increase serum glucose levels.

Adverse reactions
• CNS: drowsiness, dizziness, sedation, excitation, tremors, weakness, headache, nervousness, seizures, peripheral neuropathy, extrapyramidal symptoms, anxiety, vivid dreams, decreased libido, confusion (more marked in elderly patients).
• CV: orthostatic hypotension, tachycardia, dysrhythmias, MI, stroke, heart block, CHF, palpitations, hypertension, ECG changes.
• EENT: blurred vision, tinnitus, mydriasis, increased intraocular pressure.
• GI: dry mouth, constipation, abdominal cramping, nausea, vomiting, anorexia, diarrhea, paralytic ileus, jaundice.
• GU: urinary retention.
• Other: sweating, photosensitivity, hypersensitivity (rash, urticaria, drug fever, edema).

After abrupt withdrawal of long-term therapy, nausea, headache, malaise (does not indicate addiction) may occur.

Note: Drug should be discontinued (not abruptly) if signs of hypersensitivity occur. Reevaluate therapy if the following signs and symptoms occur: urine retention, extreme dry mouth, rash, excessive sedation, seizures, tachycardia, sore throat, fever, or jaundice.

Overdose and treatment
The first 12 hours after acute ingestion are a stimulatory phase characterized by excessive anticholinergic activity (agitation, irritation, confusion, hallucinations, hyperthermia, parkinsonian symptoms, seizure, urinary retention, dry mucous membranes, pupillary dilatation, constipation, and ileus). This is followed by CNS depressant effects, including hypothermia, decreased or absent reflexes, sedation, hypotension, cyanosis, and cardiac irregularities, including tachycardia, conduction disturbances, and quinidine-like effects on the ECG.

Severity of overdose is best indicated by widening of the QRS complex and usually represents a serum level in excess of 1,000 mcg/ml; Metabolic acidosis may follow hypotension, hypoventilation, and convulsions. Delayed cardiac anomalies and death may occur.

Treatment is symptomatic and supportive, including maintaining airway, stable body temperature, and fluid and electrolyte balance. Induce emesis with ipe-

---

cac if gag reflex is intact; follow with gastric lavage and repeated doses of activated charcoal to prevent further absorption. Dialysis is of little use. Treatment of seizures may include parenteral diazepam or phenytoin; treatment of dysrhythmias, parenteral phenytoin or lidocaine; and treatment of acidosis, sodium bicarbonate. *Do not give barbiturates;* these may enhance CNS and respiratory depressant effects.

▶ **Special considerations**

• Drug is not recommended for children under age 12.
• Check vital signs regularly for decreased blood pressure or tachycardia; observe patient carefully for other adverse reactions and report changes.
• Check for anticholinergic adverse reactions (urine retention or constipation), which may require dosage reduction.
• Observe patients for mood changes to monitor progress; benefits may not be apparent for several (3 to 6) weeks.
• Do not withdraw full dose of drug abruptly; gradually reduce dosage over period of weeks to avoid rebound effect or other adverse reactions.
• Carefully follow manufacturer's instructions for reconstitution, dilution, and storage of drugs.
• Investigational uses include treating peptic ulcer, migraine and cluster headache prophylaxis, intractable hiccups, post-herpetic neuralgia, and allergy. Potential toxicity has, to date, outweighed most advantages.
• Amitriptyline causes a high incidence of sedative effect. Tolerance to sedative effects usually develops over several weeks.
• The full dose may be given at bedtime to help offset daytime sedation.
• Oral administration should be substituted for the parenteral route as soon as possible.
• Intramuscular administration may result in a more rapid onset of action than oral administration.
• The drug should be discontinued at least 48 hours before surgical procedures.

Information for parents and patient

• Teach parents and patient how and when to administer drug. Warn them not to increase dosage without medical approval and never to discontinue drug abruptly.
• Tell parents that patient should avoid beverages and drugs containing alcohol and should not take any other drug (including nonprescription products) without medical approval.
• Tell patient chewing gum, sugarless hard candy, or ice may alleviate dry mouth. Stress the importance of regular dental hygiene, because dry mouth can increase the incidence of dental caries.
• Advise parents to have patient lie down 30 minutes after first dose and rise slowly to prevent orthostatic hypotension. They should report dizziness that persists.
• Advise taking drug with milk or food to minimize GI distress.
• Urge parents of diabetic children to monitor blood glucose levels because, drug may alter insulin needs.
• Warn parents and patient that excessive exposure

to sunlight, heat lamps, or tanning beds may cause burn and abnormal hyperpigmentation.
• Advise parents and patient that unpleasant side effects (except dry mouth) usually diminish over time.
• The full dose may be taken at bedtime to alleviate daytime sedation. Alternatively, it may be taken in the early evening to avoid morning "hangover."
• Explain that full effects of the drug may not become apparent for up to 4 weeks after initiation of therapy.
• Warn parents that drug may cause drowsiness or dizziness. Patient should avoid hazardous activities that require alertness until the full effects of the drug are known.
• Encourage parents to report troublesome or unusual effects, especially confusion, movement disorders, rapid heartbeat, dizziness, fainting, or difficulty urinating.

---

amobarbital, amobarbital sodium
Amytal

• Classification: sedative-hypnotic, anticonvulsant (barbiturate)
• Controlled substance schedule II

How supplied
Available by prescription only
Tablets: 30 mg, 50 mg, 100 mg
Capsules: 65 mg, 200 mg
Powder for injection: 250 mg, 500 mg/vial
Powder (bulk): 15 g, 30 g

Indications, route, and dosage
Sedation
Children: 3 to 6 mg/kg P.O. daily divided into four equal doses.
Adults: Usually 30 to 50 mg P.O. b.i.d. or t.i.d. but may range from 15 to 120 mg b.i.d. to q.i.d.
Insomnia
Children over age 6: 3 to 5 mg/kg deep I.M. h.s.; I.M. injection not to exceed 5 ml in any one site.
Adults: 65 to 200 mg P.O. or deep I.M. h.s.; I.M. injection not to exceed 5 ml in any one site. Maximum dosage is 500 mg.
Preanesthetic sedation
Children over age 6: 3 to 5 mg/kg P.O. or I.M.
Adults: 200 mg P.O. or I.M. 1 to 2 hours before surgery.
Manic reactions, as an adjunct in psychotherapy; anticonvulsant
Children under age 6: 3 to 5 mg/kg slow I.V. or I.M.
Children over age 6 and adults: 65 to 500 mg slow I.V.; rate not to exceed 100 mg/minute. Maximum dose is 1 g.

Action and kinetics
• *Anticonvulsant action:* The exact cellular site and mechanism(s) of action are unknown. Parenteral amobarbital suppresses the spread of seizure activity produced by epileptogenic foci in the cortex, thalamus, and limbic systems by enhancing the effect of gamma-

---

‡May contain sulfites   ♦May contain tartrazine   ♦♦May contain benzyl alcohol

aminobutyric acid (GABA). Both presynaptic and postsynaptic excitability are decreased.

• *Sedative-hypnotic action:* Amobarbital acts throughout the CNS as a nonselective depressant with an intermediate onset and duration of action. Particularly sensitive to this drug is the mesencephalic reticular activating system, which controls CNS arousal. Amobarbital decreases both presynaptic and postsynaptic membrane excitability by facilitating the action of GABA.

• *Kinetics in adults:* Amobarbital is absorbed well after oral administration. Absorption after I.M. administration is 100%. Onset of action is 45 to 60 minutes. Amobarbital is distributed well throughout body tissues and fluids. Amobarbital is metabolized in the liver by oxidation to a tertiary alcohol. Less than 1% of a dose is excreted unchanged in the urine. The rest is excreted as metabolites. The half-life is biphasic, with a first phase half-life of about 40 minutes and a second phase of about 20 hours. Duration of action is 6 to 8 hours.

Contraindications and precautions

Amobarbital is contraindicated in patients with known hypersensitivity to barbiturates and in patients with bronchopneumonia, status asthmaticus, or other severe respiratory distress because of the potential for respiratory depression.

Amobarbital should not be used in patients who are depressed or have suicidal ideation, because the drug can worsen depression; in patients with uncontrolled acute or chronic pain, because paradoxical excitement can occur; or in patients with porphyria, because this drug can trigger symptoms of this disease.

Amobarbital should be used cautiously in patients who must perform hazardous tasks requiring mental alertness, because the drug causes drowsiness. Administer parenteral amobarbital slowly and with extreme caution to patients with hypotension or severe pulmonary or cardiovascular disease because of potential adverse hemodynamic effects. Because tolerance and physical or psychological dependence may occur, prolonged use of high doses should be avoided.

Use cautiously in patients with renal or hepatic disease, as drug accumulation may occur. CNS depression may be exacerbated in patients with shock or uremia. Use parenteral amobarbital cautiously in patients with cardiovascular disease. Prenatal exposure to barbiturates is associated with an increased incidence of fetal abnormalities, and possibly brain tumors. Use of barbiturates in the third trimester may be associated with physical dependence in neonates.

Interactions

Amobarbital may add to or potentiate CNS and respiratory depressant effects of other sedative-hypnotics, antihistamines, narcotics, antidepressants, monoamine oxidase inhibitors, tranquilizers, and alcohol.

Amobarbital enhances the enzymatic degradation of warfarin and other oral anticoagulants; patients may require increased doses of the anticoagulants. Amobarbital also enhances hepatic metabolism of digitoxin (not digoxin), corticosteroids, theophylline and other xanthines, oral contraceptives and other estrogens, and doxycycline. Amobarbital impairs the effectiveness of griseofulvin by decreasing absorption from the GI tract. Amobarbital may cause unpredictable fluctuations in serum phenytoin levels.

Valproic acid, phenytoin, monoamine oxidase inhibitors, and disulfiram decrease the metabolism of amobarbital and can increase its toxicity.

Rifampin may decrease amobarbital levels by increasing metabolism.

Effects on diagnostic tests

Amobarbital may cause a false-positive phentolamine test. The physiologic effects of amobarbital may impair the absorption of cyanocobalamin ^{57}Co; it may decrease serum bilirubin concentrations in neonates, epileptic patients, and in patients with cogenital nonhemolytic unconjugated hyperbilirubinemia. EEG patterns are altered, with a change in low-voltage, fast activity; changes persist for a time after discontinuation of therapy.

Adverse reactions

• CNS: drowsiness, lethargy, vertigo, headache, CNS depression, mental depression, *paradoxical excitement;* confusion and *agitation.*
• CV: hypotension (after rapid I.V. administration), bradycardia, syncope, circulatory collapse.
• DERM: urticaria, rash, exfoliative dermatitis, Stevens-Johnson syndrome.
• EENT: laryngospasm, bronchospasm, miosis, mydriasis (with severe toxicity).
• GI: nausea, vomiting, diarrhea, constipation, epigastric pain.
• Local: thrombophlebitis, pain and possible tissue damage at extravascular injection site.
• Other: respiratory depression, blood dyscrasias, rebound insomnia, increased dreams or nightmares, possibly seizures (after acute withdrawal or reduction in dosage). Vitamin K deficiency and bleeding have occurred in newborns of mothers treated during pregnancy. *Hyperalgesia* occurs with low doses or in patients with chronic pain.

Note: Drug should be discontinued if hypersensitivity reaction, profound CNS or respiratory depression, or skin eruption occurs.

Overdose and treatment

Clinical manifestations of overdose include unsteady gait, slurred speech, sustained nystagmus, somnolence, confusion, respiratory depression, pulmonary edema, areflexia, and coma. Oliguria, jaundice, hypothermia, fever, and shock with tachycardia and hypotension may occur.

Maintain and support ventilation as necessary; support circulation with vasopressors and I.V. fluids as needed.

Treatment is aimed to maintain and support ventilation and pulmonary function as necessary; support cardiac function and circulation with vasopressors and I.V. fluids as needed. If patient is conscious with a functioning gag reflex and ingestion has been recent, then induce emesis by administering ipecac syrup. Gastric lavage may be performed if a cuffed endotracheal tube is in place to prevent aspi-

---

*Canada only   †Unlabeled clinical use   Italicized adverse reactions have been observed in children.

ration when emesis is inappropriate. Follow with administration of activated charcoal or saline cathartic. Measure fluid intake and output, vital signs, and laboratory parameters. Maintain body temperature.

Alkalinization of urine may be helpful in removing amobarbital from the body; hemodialysis may be useful in severe overdose.

▶ **Special considerations**
• Safe use in children under age 6 has not been established. Use of amobarbital may cause paradoxical excitement in some children.
• Premature infants are more susceptible to the depressant effects of barbiturates because of immature hepatic metabolism. Children receiving barbituates may experience hyperactivity, excitement, or hyperalgesia.
• Dosage of barbiturates must be individualized for each patient, because different rates of metabolism and enzyme induction occur.
• Administer oral amobarbital before meals or on an empty stomach to enhance the rate of absorption.
• Reconstitute powder for injection with sterile water for injection. Roll vial in hands; do not shake. Use 2.5 or 5 ml (for 250 or 500 mg of amobarbital) to make 10% solution. For I.M. use, prepare 20% solution by using 1.25 ml or 2.5 ml of sterile water for injection.
• Administer reconstituted parenteral solution within 30 minutes after opening the vial.
• Do not administer any amobarbital solution that is cloudy or forms a precipitate after 5 minutes of reconstitution.
• Administer I.V. dose at a rate no greater than 100 mg/minute in adults or 60 mg/m²/minute in children to prevent possible hypotension and respiratory depression. Have emergency resuscitative equipment available.
• Administer I.M. dose deep into large muscle mass, giving no more than 5 ml in any one injection site. Sterile abscess or tissue damage may result from inadvertent superficial I.M. or S.C. injection.
• Administering full loading doses over short periods of time to treat status epilepticus may require ventilatory support.
• Assess I.V. site for signs of infiltration or phlebitis.
• May be given rectally if oral or parenteral route is inappropriate.
• Assess level of consciousness before and frequently during therapy to evaluate effectiveness of drug. Monitor seizure character, frequency, and duration for changes. Institute seizure precautions as necessary.
• Vital signs should be checked frequently especially during I.V. administration.
• Assess patient's sleeping pattern before and during therapy to ensure effectiveness of drug.
• Institute safety measures – side rails, assistance when out of bed, call light within reach – to prevent falls and injury.
• Anticipate possible rebound confusion and excitatory reactions in patients.
• Assess cardiopulmonary status frequently for possible alterations. Monitor blood counts for potential adverse reactions.
• Assess renal and hepatic laboratory studies to ensure adequate drug removal.

• Monitor prothrombin times carefully when patient on amobarbital starts or ends anticoagulant therapy. Anticoagulant dosage may need to be adjusted.
• Assess bowel elimination patterns; monitor for complaints of constipation. Advise diet high in fiber, if indicated.
• Observe patient to prevent hoarding or self-dosing, especially in depressed or suicidal patients, or those who are or have a history of being drug-dependent.
• Abrupt discontinuation may cause withdrawal symptoms; discontinue slowly.
• Death is common with an overdose of 2 to 10 g; it may occur at much smaller doses if alcohol is also ingested.
• Avoid administering barbiturates to patients with status asthmaticus.

Information for parents and patient
• Warn parents of possible physical or psychological dependence with prolonged use.
• Warn parents that patient should avoid concurrent use of other drugs with CNS depressant effects, such as antihistamines, analgesics, and alcohol, because they will have additive effects and increase drowsiness. Parents should seek medical approval before giving patient any nonprescription cold or allergy preparations.
• Caution parents and patient not to increase or decrease dose or frequency without medical approval; abrupt discontinuation may trigger rebound insomnia, with increased dreaming, nightmares, or seizures.
• Patient should avoid hazardous tasks that require alertness while taking barbiturates.
• Instruct parents to report any skin eruption or other marked adverse effect.
• Explain that a morning hangover is common after therapeutic use of barbiturates.

---

amoxicillin/clavulanate potassium
Augmentin, Augmentin 125, Augmentin 250, Augmentin 500, Clavulin*

• Classification: antibiotic (aminopenicillin and beta-lactamase inhibitor)

How supplied
Available by prescription only
Oral suspension: 125 mg amoxicillin trihydrate and 31.25 mg clavulanic acid/5 ml (after reconstitution)
Suspension: 250 mg amoxicillin trihydrate and 62.5 mg clavulanic acid/5 ml (after reconstitution)
Chewable tablets: 125 mg amoxicillin trihydrate, 31.25 mg clavulanic acid; 250 mg amoxicillin trihydrate, 62.5 mg clavulanic acid
Film-coated tablets: 250 mg amoxicillin trihydrate, 125 mg clavulanic acid; 500 mg amoxicillin trihydrate, 125 mg clavulanic acid

Indications, route, and dosage
Lower respiratory infections, otitis media, sinusitis, skin and skin structure infections, and urinary tract infections caused by susceptible organisms
Children weighing less than 40 kg: 20 to 40 mg/kg/day (based on the amoxicillin component) given in divided doses q 8 hours.
Adults and children 40 kg or more: 250 mg (based on the amoxicillin component) P.O. q 8 hours. For more severe infections, 500 mg q 8 hours.

Action and kinetics
• *Antibiotic action:* Amoxicillin is bactericidal; it adheres to bacterial penicillin-binding proteins, thus inhibiting bacterial cell wall synthesis.

Clavulanate has only weak antibacterial activity and does not affect mechanism of action of amoxicillin. However, clavulanic acid has a beta-lactam ring and is structurally similar to penicillin and cephalosporins; it binds irreversibly with certain beta-lactamases and prevents them from inactivating amoxicillin, enhancing its bactericidal activity.

This combination acts against penicillinase- and non-penicillinase-producing gram-positive bacteria, *Neisseria gonorrhoeae, N. meningitidis, Hemophilus influenzae, Escherichia coli, Proteus mirabilis, Citrobacter diversus, Klebsiella pneumoniae, P. vulgaris, Salmonella,* and *Shigella.* However, the severity of some infections precludes oral therapy with amoxicillin/potassium clavulanate and requires use of other antibiotics.

• *Kinetics in adults:* Amoxicillin and clavulanate potassium are well absorbed after oral administration; peak serum levels occur at 1 to 2½ hours.

Both amoxicillin and clavulanate potassium distribute into pleural fluid, lungs, and peritoneal fluid; high urine concentrations are attained. Amoxicillin also distributes into synovial fluid, liver, prostate, muscle, and gallbladder; and penetrates into middle ear effusions, maxillary sinus secretions, tonsils, sputum, and bronchial secretions. Amoxicillin and clavulanate cross the placenta and low concentrations occur in breast milk. Amoxicillin and clavulanate potassium have minimal protein-binding of 17% to 20% and 22% to 30%, respectively.

Amoxicillin is metabolized only partially. It is excreted principally in urine by renal tubular secretion and glomerular filtration; the drug is also excreted in breast milk.

Clavulanate potassium appears to undergo extensive metabolism. It is excreted by glomerular filtration. Elimination half-life of amoxicillin in adults is 1 to 1½ hours; it is prolonged to 7½ hours in patients with severe renal impairment. Half-life of clavulanate in adults is about 1 to 1½ hours, prolonged to 4½ hours in patients with severe renal impairment.

Both drugs are removed readily by hemodialysis and minimally removed by peritoneal dialysis.

Contraindications and precautions
Amoxicillin/potassium clavulanate is contraindicated in patients with known hypersensitivity to any other penicillin or to cephalosporins.

Amoxicillin clavulanate potassium should not be used in patients with mononucleosis because many patients develop a rash during therapy.

The combination should be used cautiously in patients with renal impairment because it is excreted in urine; decreased dosage is required in moderate to severe renal failure.

Interactions
Concomitant use with an aminoglycoside antibiotic causes a synergistic bactericidal effect against some strains of enterococci and group B streptococci.

Concomitant use with allopurinol appears to increase incidence of skin rash from both drugs.

Probenecid blocks tubular secretion of amoxicillin, raising its serum concentrations; it has no effect on clavulanate.

Large doses of penicillins may interfere with renal tubular secretion of methotrexate, thus delaying elimination and prolonging elevated serum concentrations of methotrexate.

Effects on diagnostic tests
Amoxicillin/potassium clavulanate alters results of urine glucose tests that use cupric sulfate (Benedict's reagent or Clinitest). Make urine glucose determinations with glucose oxidase methods (Clinistix or Tes-Tape). Positive Coombs' tests have been reported with other clavulanate combinations.

Amoxicillin may falsely decrease serum aminoglycoside concentrations.

Adverse reactions
Adverse reactions to this combination are similar to those occurring with amoxicillin; however, GI reactions may occur more frequently, due to greater absorption of clavulanate.
• GI: nausea, vomiting, diarrhea, pseudomembranous colitis (may be indicated by severe diarrhea).
• GU: acute interstitial nephritis.
• Other: hypersensitivity (*erythematous maculopapular rash, urticaria, anaphylaxis*), bacterial and fungal superinfection.
Note: Drug should be discontinued if immediate hypersensitivity reactions occur, or if bone marrow toxicity or acute interstitial nephritis develops.

Overdose and treatment
Clinical signs of overdose include neuromuscular sensitivity or seizures. After recent ingestion (4 hours or less), empty the stomach by induced emesis or gastric lavage; follow with activated charcoal to reduce absorption. Amoxicillin/potassium clavulanate can be removed by hemodialysis.

▶ Special considerations
• Assess patient's history of allergies; do not give drug to any patient with a history of hypersensitivity reactions to either penicillins or cephalosporins. Try to determine whether previous reactions were true hypersensitivity reactions or another reaction, such as GI distress, which the patient has interpreted as allergy.
• Keep in mind that a negative history for penicillin hypersensitivity does not preclude future allergic re-

actions; monitor patient continuously for possible allergic reactions or other untoward effects.

• More common than allergic rashes is a nonallergic maculopapular rash, usually seen 5 to 9 days into the course of the drug. This rash usually lasts about 3 days. It is not a contraindication to the drug's use in the future.

• In patients with renal impairment, dosage should be reduced if creatinine clearance is below 10 ml/minute.

• Assess level of consciousness, neurologic status, and renal function when high doses are used, because excessive blood levels can cause CNS toxicity.

• Obtain results of cultures and sensitivity tests before first dose; however, therapy may begin before test results are complete. Repeat tests periodically to assess drug efficacy.

• Monitor vital signs, electrolytes, and renal function studies, monitor body weight for fluid retention with extended-spectrum penicillins for possible hypokalemia or hypernatremia.

• Coagulation abnormalities, even frank bleeding, can follow high doses, especially of extended-spectrum penicillins; monitor prothrombin times and platelet counts, and assess patient for signs of occult or frank bleeding.

• Monitor patients on long-term therapy for possible superinfection, especially debilitated patients and others receiving immunosuppressants or radiation therapy; monitor closely, especially for fever.

Oral and parenteral administration

• Give penicillins at least 1 hour before giving bacteriostatic antibiotics (tetracyclines, erythromycins, and chloramphenicol); these drugs inhibit bacterial cell growth, decreasing rate of penicillin uptake by bacterial cell walls.

• Children usually tolerate drug better when taking it with meals.

• Pediatric drops may be placed on child's tongue or added to formula, milk, fruit juice, or soft drink. Be sure child ingests all of prepared dose.

• Suspension and drops are stable for 7 days at room temperature and 14 days in refrigerator after reconstitution.

• When using film-coated tablets, be aware that both dosages contain different amounts of amoxicillin, but the *same amount* of clavulanate; therefore two 250-mg tablets are not the equivalent of one 500-mg tablet.

• Because ampicillin/potassium clavulanate is dialyzable, patients undergoing hemodialysis may need dosage adjustments.

Information for parents and patient

• Tell parents to have patient to chew tablets thoroughly or crush before swallowing and wash down with liquid to ensure adequate absorption of drug; capsule may be emptied and contents swallowed with water.

• Encourage parents to report diarrhea promptly.

• Teach signs and symptoms of hypersensitivity and other adverse reactions, and emphasize need to report any unusual reactions.

• Teach signs and symptoms of bacterial and fungal superinfections to parents and patients; emphasize need to report signs of infection in debilitated patients

and others with low resistance from immunosuppressants or irradiation.

• Be sure parents and patient understand how and when to administer drugs; urge them to complete entire prescribed regimen, to comply with instructions for around-the-clock dosage, and to keep follow-up appointments.

• Counsel parents to check expiration date of drug and to discard unused drug.

████████████████████

amoxicillin trihydrate
Amoxil, Amoxil Pediatric Drops, Polymox, Trimox '125', Trimox '250', Trimox '500', Utimox, Wymox

• Classification: antibiotic (aminopenicillin)

How supplied
Available by prescription only
Capsules: 250 mg, 500 mg
Suspension: 125 mg/5 ml, 250 mg/5 ml, 50 mg/5 ml (after reconstitution, pediatric drops)
Tablets (chewable): 125 mg, 250 mg

Indications, route, and dosage
Systemic infections, upper respiratory tract infections, otitis media, and urinary tract infections caused by susceptible bacteria
Children over age 1 month weighing less than 20 kg: 20 to 40 mg/kg or 500 mg to 1g/m² daily divided q 8 hours.
Children over 20 kg: 750 mg to 1 g. P.O. daily, divided q 8 hours.
Acute, uncomplicated gonorrhea caused by Neisseria gonorrhoeae
Children over age 2 weighing less than 45 kg: 50 mg/kg P.O. as a single dose with probenecid 25 mg/kg (up to 1 g).
Children 45 kg and over and adults: 3 g P.O. as a single dose, with probenecid 1 g. P.O. administered concurrently.
Follow-up therapy with doxycycline or tetracycline is recommended in adult children over 8 years old.
Prophylaxis of bacterial endocarditis in low-risk patients
Children under 27 kg: 50 mg/kg P.O. 1 hour before the procedure, and 25 mg/kg P.O. 6 hours later.
Children 27 kg and over and adults: 3 g P.O. before the procedure, and 1.5 g P.O. 6 hours later.
Dosage in renal failure
Patients who require repeated doses may need adjustment of dosing interval. If creatinine clearance is 10 to 50 ml/min, increase interval to q 12 hours; if creatinine clearance is < 10 ml/min, administer q 12 to 16 hours. Supplemental doses may be necessary after hemodialysis.

Action and kinetics
• *Antibacterial action:* Amoxicillin is bactericidal; it adheres to bacterial penicillin-binding proteins, thus inhibiting bacterial cell wall synthesis.
Amoxicillin's spectrum of action includes

nonpenicillinase-producing gram-positive bacteria, Streptococcus group B, *Neisseria gonorrheae, Proteus mirabilis, Salmonella,* and *H. influenzae.* It is also effective against non-penicillinase producing *S. aureus, S. pyogenes, S. bovis, S. pneumoniae, S. viridans, N. meningitidis, E. coli, S. typhi, B. pertussis, G. vaginalis, Peptococcus,* and *Peptostreptococcus.* However, the severity of some infections precludes oral therapy with amoxicillin and requires use of other antibiotics.

• *Kinetics in adults:* Amoxicillin is approximately 80% absorbed after oral administration; peak serum concentrations occur at 1.0 to 2.5 hours after an oral dose. Amoxicillin distributes into pleural, peritoneal, and synovial fluids, and into the lungs, prostate, muscle, liver, and gallbladder; it also penetrates middle ear, maxillary sinus and bronchial secretions, tonsils, and sputum. Amoxicillin readily crosses the placenta. Amoxicillin is 17% to 20% protein-bound. Amoxicillin is partially metabolized and excreted principally in urine by renal tubular secretion and glomerular filtration; it is also excreted in breast milk. Elimination half-life in adults is 1 to 1½ hours; severe renal impairment increases half-life to 7½ hours.

Contraindications and precautions

Amoxicillin is contraindicated in patients with known hypersensitivity to any other penicillin or to cephalosporins.

Amoxicillin should not be used in patients with infectious mononucleosis, because many patients develop a rash during therapy.

Amoxicillin should be used cautiously in patients with renal impairment because it is excreted by the kidneys; decreased dosage is required in moderate to severe renal failure.

Interactions

Concomitant use with allopurinol appears to increase the incidence of skin rash from both drugs.

Concomitant use with clavulanate potassium enhances effect of amoxicillin against certain beta-lactamase-producing bacteria.

Probenecid blocks renal tubular secretion of amoxicillin, raising its serum concentrations.

Large doses of penicillins may interfere with renal tubular secretion of methotrexate, thus delaying elimination and prolonging elevated serum concentrations of methotrexate.

Concomitant use with an aminoglycoside antibiotic causes a synergistic bactericidal effect against some strains of enterococci and group B streptococci; however, the drugs are physically and chemically incompatible if mixed or given together.

Effects on diagnostic tests

Amoxicillin may alter results of urine glucose tests that use cupric sulfate (Benedict's reagent or Clinitest). Make urine glucose determinations with glucose oxidase methods (Clinistix or Tes-Tape).

Amoxicillin may falsely decrease serum aminoglycoside concentrations.

Adverse reactions

• GI: nausea, vomiting, diarrhea, pseudomembranous colitis.
• GU: acute interstitial nephritis.
• HEMA: anemia, thrombocytopenia, thrombocytopenic purpura, eosinophilia, leukopenia.
• Other: hypersensitivity (erythematous maculopapular rash, urticaria, anaphylaxis), bacterial or fungal superinfection.
   Note: Drug should be discontinued if immediate hypersensitivity reactions occur or if bone marrow toxicity or acute interstitial nephritis develops.

Overdose and treatment

Clinical signs of overdose include neuromuscular sensitivity or seizures. After recent ingestion (4 hours or less), empty the stomach by induced emesis or gastric lavage; follow with activated charcoal to reduce absorption. Amoxicillin can be removed by hemodialysis.

▶ Special considerations

• Assess patient's history of allergies; do not give amoxicillin to any patient with a history of hypersensitivity reactions to either penicillins or cephalosporins. Try to determine whether previous reactions were true hypersensitivity reactions or another reaction, such as GI distress, which the patient has interpreted as allergy.
• Keep in mind that a negative history for penicillin hypersensitivity does not preclude future allergic reactions; monitor patient continuously for possible allergic reactions or other untoward effects.
• More common than allergic rashes is a nonallergic maculopapular rash, usually seen 5 to 9 days into the course of the drug. This rash usually lasts about 3 days. It is not a contraindication to the drug's use in the future.
• In patients with renal impairment, dosage should be reduced if creatinine clearance is below 10ml/minute.
• Assess level of consciousness, neurologic status, and renal function when high doses are used, because excessive blood levels can cause CNS toxicity.
• Obtain results of cultures and sensitivity tests before first dose; however, therapy may begin before test results are complete. Repeat tests periodically to assess drug efficacy.
• Monitor vital signs, electrolytes, and renal function studies, monitor body weight for fluid retention with extended-spectrum penicillins for possible hypokalemia or hypernatremia.
• Coagulation abnormalities, even frank bleeding, can follow high doses, especially of extended-spectrum penicillins; monitor prothrombin times and platelet counts, and assess patient for signs of occult or frank bleeding.
• Monitor patients on long-term therapy for possible superinfection, especially debilitated patients and others receiving immunosuppressants or radiation therapy; monitor closely, especially for fever.

Oral administration

• Give penicillins at least 1 hour before giving bacteriostatic antibiotics (tetracyclines, erythromycins, and chloramphenicol); these drugs inhibit bacterial

cell growth, decreasing rate of penicillin uptake by bacterial cell walls.
• Give oral penicillin at least 1 hour before or 2 hours after meals to enhance gastric absorption; food may or may not decrease absorption.

Information for parents and patient
• Tell parents to have patients chew tablets thoroughly or crush before swallowing and wash down with liquid to ensure adequate absorption of drug; capsule may be emptied and contents swallowed with water; suspension should be shaken well to ensure correct dosage.
• Encourage parents to report diarrhea promptly.
• Teach signs and symptoms of hypersensitivity and other adverse reactions, and emphasize need to report any unusual reactions.
• Teach signs and symptoms of bacterial and fungal superinfections to parents and patients; emphasize need to report signs of infection in debilitated patients and others with low resistance from immunosuppressants or irradiation.
• Be sure parents understand how and when to administer drugs; urge them to complete entire prescribed regimen, to comply with instructions for around-the-clock dosage, and to keep follow-up appointments.
• Counsel parents to check expiration date of drug and to discard unused drug.

amphetamine sulfate

• Classification: CNS stimulant, short-term adjunctive anorexigenic agent, sympathomimetic amine (amphetamine)
• Controlled substance schedule II

How supplied
Available by prescription only
Tablets: 5 mg, 10 mg
Capsules: 5 mg, 10 mg

Indications, route, and dosage
Attention deficit disorder with hyperactivity
Children age 3 to 5: 2.5 mg P.O. daily, with 2.5-mg increments weekly, as needed.
Children age 6 and older: 5 mg P.O. daily, with 5-mg increments weekly, as needed.
Narcolepsy
Children under age 6: Dosage seldom exceeds 40 mg daily.
Children age 6 to 12: 5 mg P.O. daily, with 5-mg increments weekly, as needed.
Children over age 12: 10 mg P.O. daily, with 10-mg increments weekly, as needed.
Adults: 5 to 60 mg P.O. daily in divided doses.

Action in kinetics
• *CNS stimulant action:* Amphetamines are sympathomimetic amines with CNS stimulant activity; in hyperactive children, they have a paradoxical calming effect. The cerebral cortex and reticular activating system appear to be their primary sites of activity; amphetamines release nerve terminal stores of norepinephrine, promoting nerve impulse transmission. At high dosages, effects are mediated by dopamine.
• *Anorexigenic action:* Anorexigenic effects are thought to occur in the hypothalamus, where decreased smell and taste acuity decreases the appetite.

Amphetamines are used to treat narcolepsy and as adjuncts to psychosocial measures in attention deficit disorder in children. Their precise mechanisms of action in these conditions are unknown.
• *Kinetics in adults:* Amphetamine sulfate is absorbed completely within 3 hours after oral administration; therapeutic effects persist for 4 to 24 hours. Drug is distributed widely throughout the body, with high concentrations in the brain. It is metabolized by hydroxylation and deamination in the liver and is excreted in urine.

Contraindications and precautions
Amphetamines are contraindicated in children with hypersensitivity or idiosyncratic reaction to sympathomimetic amines; in those with symptomatic cardiovascular disease, hyperthyroidism, nephritis, angina pectoris, hypertension, glaucoma, or agitated states; and in patients with a history of drug or alcohol abuse. They also are contraindicated for concomitant use with monoamine oxidase (MAO) inhibitors or within 14 days of discontinuing MAO inhibitors.

Amphetamines should be used with caution in patients with diabetes mellitus; in debilitated or hyperexcitable patients; and in children with Gilles de la Tourette's syndrome. Avoid long-term therapy, when possible, because of the risk of psychic or physical dependence.

Interactions
Concomitant use with MAO inhibitors (or drugs with MAO-inhibiting effects such as furazolidone) or within 14 days of such therapy may cause hypertensive crisis; concomitant use with antihypertensives may antagonize their hypertensive effects.

Concomitant use with antacids, sodium bicarbonate, or acetazolamide may enhance reabsorption of amphetamine and prolong its duration of action, whereas concomitant use with ammonium chloride or ascorbic acid enhances amphetamine excretion or shortens duration of action. Use with phenothiazines or haloperidol decreases amphetamine effects; barbiturates counteract amphetamine by CNS depression, whereas caffeine or other CNS stimulants produce additive effects.

Amphetamines may alter insulin requirements.

Effects on diagnostic tests
Amphetamines may elevate plasma corticosteroid levels and also may interfere with urinary steroid determinations.

Adverse reactions
• CNS: restlessness, tremor, agitation, talkativeness, insomnia, irritability, dizziness, headache, chills, overstimulation, dysphoria.
• CV: tachycardia, palpitations, hypertension, hypotension.

• GI: nausea, vomiting, cramps, dry mouth, diarrhea, constipation, metallic taste, anorexia, weight loss.
• Other: urticaria, impotence, changes in libido.
Note: Drug should be discontinued if signs of hypersensitivity or idiosyncrasy occur.

Overdose and treatment
Symptoms of acute overdose include increasing restlessness, irritability, insomnia, tremor, hyperreflexia, diaphoresis, mydriasis, flushing, confusion, hypertension, tachypnea, fever, delirium, self-injury, dysrhythmias, convulsions, coma, circulatory collapse, and death.

Treat overdose symptomatically and supportively: if ingestion is recent (within 4 hours) use gastric lavage or emesis; activated charcoal, saline catharsis, and urinary acidification may enhance excretion. Forced fluid diuresis may help. In massive ingestion, hemodialysis or peritoneal dialysis may be needed. Keep patient in a cool room, monitor his temperature, and minimize external stimulation. Haloperidol may be used for psychotic symptoms; diazepam, for hyperactivity.

▶ Special considerations
Amphetamines should be used cautiously in children who are debilitated or hyperexcitable or in children with diabetes mellitus or Gilles de la Tourette's syndrome. Avoid long-term therapy when possible because of the risk of psychic dependence or habituation.
• Children should receive lowest effective dose with dosage adjusted individually according to response; after long-term use, dosage should be lowered gradually to prevent acute rebound depression.
• Amphetamines may impair ability to perform tasks requiring mental alertness, such as schoolwork or driving a car.
• Vital signs should be checked regularly for increased blood pressure or other signs of excessive stimulation; avoid late-day or evening dosing, especially of long-acting dosage forms, to minimize insomnia.
• Amphetamine use for analeptic effect is discouraged; CNS stimulation superimposed on CNS depression may cause neuronal instability and seizures.
• Carefully follow manufacturer's directions for reconstitution, dilution, storage, and administration of all preparations. Prolonged administration of CNS stimulants to children with attention deficit disorders may be associated with temporarily decreased growth.
• Amphetamines are not recommended for weight reduction in children under age 12 and are contraindicated for agitation in children under age 3.
• Temporary suppression of normal bone growth has followed long-term use of amphetamines. Monitor use carefully.
• Amphetamines have a high potential for abuse; they are not recommended to combat the fatigue of exhaustion or the need for sleep but are often abused illegally for this purpose by students, athletes, and truck drivers.
• In the event of overdose, protect patient from excessive noise or stimulation.

Information for parents and patient
• Explain rationale for therapy and the potential risks and benefits.
• Warn patient not to use drug to mask fatigue.
• Encourage patient to get adequate rest; unusual, compensatory fatigue may result as drug wears off.
• Tell parent that patient should avoid drinks containing caffeine to prevent added CNS stimulation and should not increase dosage.
• Advise narcoleptic patients to take first dose on awakening.
• Tell patient not to chew or crush sustained-release dosage forms.
• Advise diabetic patients to monitor blood glucose levels carefully because drug may alter insulin needs.
• Advise patient to avoid hazardous tasks that require mental alertness until CNS effects are known.

---

amphotericin B
Fungizone

• Classification: antifungal (polyene macrolide)

How supplied
Available by prescription only
Injection: 50-mg lyophilized cake
Cream: 3%
Lotion: 3%
Ointment: 3%

Indications, route, and dosage
Systemic (potentially fatal) fungal infections caused by susceptible organisms; †fungal endocarditis; fungal septicemia
Children: Some clinicians recommend an initial test dose of 0.05 to 0.1 mg infused (some may give up to 1 mg) over 20 to 30 minutes. Maintenance dose is 0.25 to 0.5 mg/kg/day. Initially, dose should be administered over 2 to 6 hours. Dosage may be increased as tolerated by increments of 0.25 to 0.5 mg/kg/day to a maximum of 1 mg/kg/day (30 mg/m²/day) or 1.5 mg/kg every other day.
Adults: Some clinicians recommend an initial test dose of 1 mg in 250 ml dextrose 5% in water (D_5W) infused over 2 to 4 hours. If this test dose is tolerated, 5 mg in 500 ml of D_5W is given on the next day, followed by 10 mg in 1 liter D_5W on day 3. Additional increases of 5 to 10 mg per day are administered as tolerated. Duration of therapy depends on nature and severity of the infection.
Cutaneous or mucocutaneous candidal infection
Children and adults: Apply topical product b.i.d., t.i.d., or q.i.d. for 1 to 3 weeks. Apply up to several months for interdigital or paronychial lesions.

Action and kinetics
• *Antifungal action:* Amphotericin B is fungistatic. It binds to sterols in the fungal cell membrane, increasing membrane permeability of fungal cells causing subsequent leakage of intracellular components; it

also may interfere with some human cell membranes that contain sterols.

The spectrum of activity includes *Histoplasma capsulatum*, *Coccidioides immitis*, *Blastomyces dermatitidis*, *Cryptococcus neoformans*, *Candida* species, *Aspergillus fumigatus*, *Mucor* species, *Rhizopus* species, *Absidia* species, *Entomophthora* species, *Basidiobolus* species, *Paracoccidioides brasiliensis*, *Sporothrix schenckii*, and *Rhodotorula* species.

• *Kinetics in adults:* Amphotericin B is absorbed poorly from the GI tract. Amphotericin B distributes well into inflamed pleural cavities and joints; in low concentrations into aqueous humor, bronchial secretions, pancreas, bone, muscle, and parotids. CSF concentrations reach about 3% of serum concentrations. The drug is 90% to 95% bound to plasma proteins. It reportedly crosses the placenta. The metabolic fate of amphotericin B is not well defined. Amphotericin B's elimination is biphasic; second phase half-life is about 15 days. About 2% to 5% of the drug is excreted unchanged in urine. Amphotericin B is not readily removed by hemodialysis.

Contraindications and precautions
Amphotericin B is contraindicated in patients with known hypersensitivity to the drug, unless no other therapy is effective. It should be used with caution in patients taking other nephrotoxic drugs.

Interactions
Concomitant use with aminoglycosides, cisplatin, and other nephrotoxic drugs should be avoided, when possible, because of added nephrotoxic effects.

Because amphotericin B induces hypokalemia, concomitant use with digoxin increases the risk of digitalis toxicity. Because of added potassium depletion, concomitant use with corticosteroids requires careful monitoring of serum electrolyte levels and cardiac function. Amphotericin B-induced hypokalemia may enhance effects of skeletal muscle relaxants. It potentiates the effects of flucytosine and other antibiotics, presumably by increasing cell membrane permeability.

Effects on diagnostic tests
Amphotericin B therapy may increase BUN, serum creatinine, alkaline phosphatase, and bilirubin levels.

Amphotericin B may cause hypokalemia and hypomagnesemia and may decrease white blood cell, red blood cell, and platelet counts.

Adverse reactions
• CNS: headache, peripheral neuropathy; with intrathecal administration – peripheral nerve pain, paresthesias.
• CV: hypotension, dysrhythmias.
• DERM: with topical application – possible dryness, erythema, burning pruritus, contact dermatitis.
• GI: anorexia, weight loss, *nausea, vomiting*, dyspepsia, diarrhea, epigastric cramps.
• GU: abnormal renal function with hypokalemia, azotemia, hyposthenuria, renal tubular acidosis, nephrocalcinosis; with large doses – permanent renal impairment, anuria, oliguria.
• HEMA: normochromic, normocytic anemia.

• Local: burning, stinging, irritation, tissue damage with extravasation, thrombophlebitis, pain at injection site.
• Other: arthralgia, myalgia, muscle weakness secondary to hypokalemia, *fever, chills*, anaphylactoid reactions, hypomagnesemia, malaise, generalized pain.

Overdose and treatment
Overdose may affect cardiovascular and respiratory function. Treatment is largely supportive.

▶ Special considerations
• Cultures and histologic and sensitivity testing must be completed and diagnosis confirmed before starting therapy in nonimmunocompromised patient.
• Prepare infusion as manufacturer directs, with strict aseptic technique, using *only* 10 ml of sterile water to reconstitute. To avoid precipitation, do not mix with solutions containing sodium chloride, other electrolytes, or bacteriostatic agents, such as benzyl alcohol.
• Lyophilized cake contains no preservatives. Do not use if solution contains a precipitate or other foreign particles. Store cake at 35.6° to 46.4° F. (2° to 8° C.). Protect drug from light, and check expiration date.
• For I.V. infusion, use an in-line membrane with a mean pore diameter larger than 1 micron.
• Infuse slowly; rapid infusion may cause cardiovascular collapse.
• Do not mix or piggyback antibiotics with amphotericin B infusion; the I.V. solution appears compatible with small amounts of heparin sodium, hydrocortisone sodium succinate, and methylprednisolone sodium succinate.
• Give in distal veins, and monitor site for discomfort or thrombosis; if thrombosis occurs, alternate-day therapy may be considered.
• Vital signs should be checked every 30 minutes for at least 4 hours after start of I.V. infusion; fever may appear in 1 to 2 hours but should subside within 4 hours of discontinuing drug.
• Monitor intake and output, and check for changes in urine appearance or volume; renal damage may be reversible if drug is stopped at earliest sign of dysfunction.
• Monitor potassium and magnesium levels closely; monitor calcium and magnesium levels twice weekly; perform liver and renal function studies and CBCs weekly.
• Severity of some adverse reactions can be reduced by premedication with aspirin, acetaminophen, antihistamines, antiemetics, meperidine, or small doses of corticosteroids; by addition of phosphate buffer to the solution; and by alternate-day dosing. If reactions are severe, drug may have to be discontinued for varying periods.
• Use topical products for folds of groin, neck, or armpit; avoid occlusive dressing with ointment, and discontinue if signs of hypersensitivity develop.
• Topical products may stain skin or clothes.
• Store at room temperature. Solution is stable at room temperature and in indoor light for 24 hours or in refrigerator for 1 week.
• For bladder irrigation, mix with sterile water for injection.

‡May contain sulfites   ♦May contain tartrazine   ♦ ♦May contain benzyl alcohol

Information for parents and patient
• Teach parents and patient signs and symptoms of hypersensitivity and other adverse reactions, especially those associated with I.V. therapy. Warn them that patient is likely to have fever and chills, which can be quite severe when therapy is initiated. These symptoms usually subside with repeated doses. Encourage patient feedback during infusion.
• Warn that therapy may take several months; teach personal hygiene and other measures to prevent spread and recurrence of lesions.
• Urge compliance and appropriate follow-up.
• Tell parents and patient that topical products may stain skin and clothing; cream or lotion may be removed from clothing with soap and water.

---

ampicillin
Amcill, Apo-Ampi*, Novoampicillin*, Omnipen, Omnipen Pediatric Drops, Penbritin*, Polycillin, Principen, Roampicillin, Super Totacillin

ampicillin sodium
Ampicin*, Ampilean*, NaMPICIL, Omnipen-N, Pen A/N, Penbritin*, Polycillin-N, Totacillin-N

ampicillin trihydrate
D-Amp, Polycillin, Principen (capsules and suspension), Totacillin (capsules and suspension)

• Classification: antibiotic (aminopenicillin)

How supplied
Available by prescription only
Capsules: 250 mg, 500 mg
Suspension: 100 mg/ml (pediatric drops), 125 mg/5 ml, 250 mg/5 ml, 500 mg/5 ml (after reconstitution)
Parenteral: 125 mg, 250 mg, 500 mg, 1 g, 2 g
Pharmacy bulk package: 10 g vial
Infusion: 500 mg, 1 g, 2 g

Indications, route, and dosage
Meningitis
Neonates age 0 to 7 days weighing < 2 kg: 50 to 75 mg/kg I.M. or I.V. q 12 hours.
Neonates age 0 to 7 days weighing > 2 kg: 50 to 75 mg/kg I.M. or I.V. q 8 hours.
Neonates over 7 days weighing < 2 kg: 50 mg/kg I.M. or I.V. q 8 hours.
Neonates over 7 days weighing > 2 kg: 50 mg/kg I.M. or I.V. q 6 hours.
Children age 2 months to 12 years: 200 to 400 mg/kg I.V. daily in divided doses q 4 to 6 hours. Usually administered with chloraamphenicol I.V.
Adults: 8 to 14 g, or 150 to 200 mg/kg I.V. or I.M. daily in equally divided doses every 3 to 4 hours
Septicemia
Neonates age 0 to 7 days weighing < 2 kg: 25 mg/kg I.M. or I.V. q 12 hours

Neonates age 0 to 7 days weighing > 2 kg: 25 mg/kg I.M. or I.V. q 8 hours.
Neonates over 7 days weighing < 2 kg: 25 mg/kg I.M. or I.V. q 8 hours.
Neonates over 7 days weighing > 2 kg: 25 mg/kg I.M. or I.V. q 6 hours
Children age 2 months to 12 years: 100 to 200 mg/kg I.V. daily, divided q 3 to 4 hours.
Adults: 8 to 14 g or 150 to 200 mg/kg I.V. or I.M. daily in equally divided doses q 3 to 4 hours
Treatment of mild to moderate infections caused by susceptible gram negative and gram positive bacteria
Children older than 1 month: 50 to 100 mg/kg P.O. I.M. or I.V. divided q 6 to 8 hours
Treatment of severe infections caused by susceptible gram negative and gram positive bacteria
Children older than 1 month: 200 to 400 mg/kg I.M. or I.V. daily divided q 4 to 6 hours
Acute, uncomplicated gonorrhea caused by Neisseria gonorrhoeae
Children weighing 45 kg or more and adults: 3.5 g P.O. as a single dose. Administer with probenecid 1 g P.O.
   Follow-up therapy with doxycycline or tetracycline is recommended in adults and children over 8 years old.
Prophylaxis of bacterial endocarditis in patients receiving dental surgery
Children weighing over 27 kg and adults: 1 to 2 g I.M. or I.V. 30 minutes to 1 hour prior to the procedure and 8 hours later. Should be administered with gentamycin 1.5 mg/kg I.M. or I.V. Alternatively, penicillin V 1 g P.O. may be used as the follow-up medication.
Children weighing 27 kg and less: 50 mg/kg I.M. or I.V. 30 minutes to 1 hour prior to the procedure and 8 hours later. Should be administered with gentamycin 2 mg/kg I.M. or I.V. Alternatively, penicillin V 500 mg may be used as the follow-up medication.
Prophylaxis of bacterial endocarditis in patients receiving GI, GU, or biliary tract surgery
Children weighing over 27 kg and adults: 2 g I.M. or I.V. 30 minutes to 1 hour prior to the procedure and 8 hours later. Should be administered with gentamycin 1.5 mg/kg I.M. or I.V.
Children weighing 27 kg and less: 50 mg/kg I.M. or I.V. 30 minutes to 1 hour prior to the procedure and 8 hours later. Should be administered with gentamycin 2 mg/kg I.M. or I.V.
Dosage in renal failure
Dosing interval should be increased to q 12 hours in patients with severe renal impairment (creatinine clearance ≤ 10 ml/min).

Action and kinetics
• *Antibiotic action:* Ampicillin is bactericidal; it adheres to bacterial penicillin-binding proteins, thus inhibiting bacterial cell wall synthesis.
   Ampicillin's spectrum of action includes nonpenicillinase-producing gram-positive bacteria. It is also effective against many gram-negative organisms, including: *Neisseria gonorrhoeae, N. meningitidis, Hemophilus influenzae, Escherichia coli, Proteus*

---

mirabilis, Salmonella, and *Shigella.* Ampicillin should be used in gram-negative systemic infections only when organism sensitivity is known.

• *Kinetics in adults:* Approximately 42% of ampicillin is absorbed after an oral dose; peak serum concentrations occur at 1 to 2 hours. After I.M. administration, peak serum concentrations occur at 1 hour. Peak serum levels are higher and more prolonged in premature or full-term neonates younger than 6 days old. Ampicillin distributes into pleural, peritoneal, and synovial fluids, lungs, prostate, liver, and gallbladder; it also penetrates middle ear effusions, maxillary sinus and bronchial secretions, tonsils, and sputum. Ampicillin readily crosses the placenta; it is minimally protein-bound at 15% to 25%. Neonates with meningitis can experience CSF concentrations ranging from 11% to 65% of serum levels. Ampicillin is metabolized only partially. Ampicillin is excreted in urine by renal tubular secretion and glomerular filtration. It is also excreted in breast milk. Elimination half-life is about 1 hour to 1½ hours; in patients with extensive renal impairment, half-life is extended to 10 to 24 hours.

Contraindications and precautions

Ampicillin is contraindicated in patients with known hypersensitivity to any other penicillin or to cephalosporins.

Ampicillin should not be used in patients with infectious mononucleosis because many patients develop a rash during therapy.

Ampicillin should be used cautiously in patients with renal impairment because it is excreted in urine; decreased dosage is required in moderate to severe renal failure.

Interactions

Concomitant use with an aminoglycoside antibiotic causes a synergistic bactericidal effect against some strains of enterococci and group B streptococci. However, the drugs are physically and chemically incompatible and are inactivated if mixed or given together.

Concomitant use with allopurinol appears to increase incidence of skin rash from both drugs.

Concomitant use with clavulanate results in increased bactericidal effects, because clavulanic acid is a beta-lactamase inhibitor.

Probenecid inhibits renal tubular secretion of ampicillin, raising its serum concentrations.

Large doses of penicillins may interfere with renal tubular secretion of methotrexate, thus delaying elimination and elevating serum concentrations of methotrexate.

Effects on diagnostic tests

Ampicillin alters results of urine glucose tests that use cupric sulfate (Benedict's reagent or Clinitest). Make urine glucose determinations with glucose oxidase methods (Clinistix or Tes-Tape).

Ampicillin may falsely decrease serum aminoglycoside concentrations.

Adverse reactions

• GI: nausea, vomiting, diarrhea, glossitis, stomatitis, pseudomembranous colitis.

• GU: acute interstitial nephritis.

• HEMA: anemia, thrombocytopenia, thrombocytopenic purpura, eosinophilia, leukopenia.

• Local: pain at injection site, vein irritation, thrombophlebitis.

• Other: *metabolic alkalosis,* hypersensitivity (erythematous maculopapular rash, urticaria, anaphylaxis), bacterial and fungal superinfection.

Note: Drug should be discontinued if immediate hypersensitivity reaction occurs or if bone marrow toxicity, pseudomembranous colitis, or acute interstitial nephritis develops.

Overdose and treatment

Clinical signs of overdose include neuromuscular sensitivity or seizures. After recent ingestion (within 4 hours), empty the stomach by induced emesis or gastric lavage; follow with activated charcoal to reduce absorption. Ampicillin can be removed by hemodialysis.

▶ Special considerations

• Administer I.M. or I.V. only for severe infections or if patient is unable to take oral drug.

• Assess patient's history of allergies; do not give a penicillin to any patient with a history of hypersensitivity reactions to either penicillins or cephalosporins. Try to determine whether previous reactions were true hypersensitivity reactions or another reaction, such as GI distress, which the patient has interpreted as allergy.

• Keep in mind that a negative history for penicillin hypersensitivity does not preclude future allergic reactions; monitor patient continuously for possible allergic reactions or other untoward effects.

• More common than allergic rashes is a nonallergic maculopapular rash, usually seen 5 to 9 days into the course of the drug. This rash usually lasts about 3 days. It is not a contraindication to the drug's use in the future.

• In patients with renal impairment, dosage should be reduced if creatinine clearance is below 10ml/minute.

• Assess level of consciousness, neurologic status, and renal function when high doses are used, because excessive blood levels can cause CNS toxicity.

• Obtain results of cultures and sensitivity tests before first dose; however, therapy may begin before test results are complete. Repeat tests periodically to assess drug efficacy.

• Monitor vital signs, electrolytes, and renal function studies, monitor body weight for fluid retention with extended-spectrum penicillins for possible hypokalemia or hypernatremia.

• Coagulation abnormalities, even frank bleeding, can follow high doses, especially of extended-spectrum penicillins; monitor prothrombin times and platelet counts, and assess patient for signs of occult or frank bleeding.

• Monitor patients on long-term therapy for possible superinfection, especially debilitated patients and others receiving immunosuppressants or radiation therapy; monitor closely, especially for fever.

---

‡May contain sulfites   ◆May contain tartrazine   ◆◆May contain benzyl alcohol

Oral and parenteral administration
• Give penicillins at least 1 hour before giving bacteriostatic antibiotics (tetracyclines, erythromycins, and chloramphenicol); these drugs inhibit bacterial cell growth, decreasing rate of penicillin uptake by bacterial cell walls.
• Always consult manufacturer's directions for reconstitution, dilution, and storage of drugs, check expiration dates.
• Give oral penicillin at least 1 hour before or 2 hours after meals to enhance gastric absorption; food may or may not decrease absorption.
• Refrigerate oral suspensions (stable for 14 days); shake well before administering, to assure correct dosage.
• Administer I.M. dose deep into large muscle mass (gluteal or midlateral thigh); rotate injection sites to minimize tissue injury; do not inject more than 2 g of drug per injection site. Apply ice to injection site for pain.
• Do not add or mix other drugs with I.V. infusions — particularly aminoglycosides, which will be inactivated if mixed with penicillins; they are chemically and physically incompatible. If other drugs must be given I.V., temporarily stop infusion of primary drug.
• Infuse I.V. drug continuously or intermittently (over 30 minutes) and assess I.V. site frequently to prevent infiltration or phlebitis; rotate infusion site q 48 hours; intermittent I.V. infusion may be diluted in 50 to 100 ml sterile water, 0.9% sodium chloride, dextrose 5% in water, dextrose 5% in water and half normal saline, or lactated Ringer's solution.
• Solutions should always be clear, colorless to pale yellow, and free of particles, do not give solutions containing precipitates or other foreign matters.

Information for parents and patient
• Explain that drug should not be taken with acidic beverages such as fruit juices.
• Teach signs and symptoms of hypersensitivity and other adverse reactions, and emphasize need to report any unusual reactions. Explain that a rash is fairly common. Teach how to differentiate it from allergic reaction.
• Encourage parents to report diarrhea promptly.
• Teach signs and symptoms of bacterial and fungal superinfections to parents and patients; emphasize need to report signs of infection in debilitated patients and others with low resistance from immunosuppressants or irradiation.
• Be sure parents and patient understand how and when to administer drugs; urge them to complete entire prescribed regimen, to comply with instructions for around-the-clock dosage, and to keep follow-up appointments.
• Counsel parents to check expiration date of drug and to discard unused drug.

---

amyl nitrite

• Classification: vasodilator, cyanide poisoning adjunct (nitrate)

How supplied
Available by prescription only
Nasal inhalant: 0.18 ml, 0.3 ml

Indications, route, and dosage
Angina pectoris
Adults: 0.18 to 0.3 ml by inhalation (one glass ampule inhaler), p.r.n.
†*Adjunct treatment of cyanide poisoning*
Children and adults: 0.3 ml by inhalation for 15 to 30 seconds; repeat every 60 seconds until I.V. sodium nitrite infusion and I.V. sodium thiosulfate infusion are available.

Action and kinetics
• *Vasodilating action:* Amyl nitrite reduces myocardial oxygen demand by decreasing left ventricular end-diastolic pressure (preload) and systemic vascular resistance and arterial pressure (afterload). It also increases collateral coronary blood flow. By relaxing vascular smooth muscle, it produces generalized vasodilation. Amyl nitrite also relaxes all other smooth muscle, including bronchial and biliary smooth muscle. In cyanide poisoning, it converts hemoglobin to methemoglobin, which reacts with cyanide to form cyanmet-hemoglobin.
• *Kinetics in adults:* Inhaled amyl nitrite is absorbed readily through the respiratory tract; action begins in 30 seconds and lasts 3 to 5 minutes. Amyl nitrite, an organic nitrite, is metabolized by the liver to form inorganic nitrites, which are much less potent vasodilators than the parent drug. One third of the inhaled dose is excreted in urine.

Contraindications and precautions
Amyl nitrite is contraindicated in patients with severe anemia or hypersensitivity, head trauma, or cerebral hemorrhage because it dilates the meningeal vessels. Use cautiously in patients with hypotension or glaucoma. Because it reduces maternal blood pressure and blood flow to the placenta, amyl nitrite could harm the fetus if administered to a pregnant woman.

Interactions
Concomitant use of alcohol, phenothiazines, beta blockers, or antihypertensives may cause excessive hypotension.

Effects on diagnostic tests
Amyl nitrite therapy alters the Zlatkis-Zak color reaction, causing a false decrease in serum cholesterol levels.

Adverse reactions
• CNS: severe, persistent (sometimes throbbing) headache; dizziness; weakness; muscle twitching.

• CV: orthostatic hypotension, tachycardia, palpitations, fainting.
• DERM: cutaneous vasodilation, visible flushing on face and neck; perspiration; cold sweats.
• GI: nausea, vomiting.
• HEMA: methemoglobinemia.
   Note: Drug should be discontinued if a severe drop in blood pressure occurs or if patient faints.

Overdose and treatment
Clinical signs of overdose include methemoglobinemia, characterized by blue skin and mucous membranes, hypotension, tachycardia, palpatations, skin changes, diaphoresis, dizziness, syncope, vertigo, headache, nausea, vomiting, anorexia, increased intracranial pressure, confusion, moderate fever, and paralysis. Hypoxia may lead to metabolic acidosis, cyanosis, convulsions, coma, and cardiac collapse. Treat with high-flow oxygen and methylene blue. Usual dose of methylene blue for adults and children is 1 to 2 mg/kg I.V. given slowly over several minutes. In severe cases, this dose may be repeated only once; doses exceeding 4 mg/kg may produce methemoglobinemia.

▶ Special considerations
• Keep patient sitting or lying down during and immediately after inhalation. Crush ampule (has a woven gauze covering) between fingers, and hold to nose for inhalation.
• Monitor for orthostatic hypotension; do not allow patient to make rapid postural changes while inhaling drug.
• Amyl nitrite is highly flammable; keep away from open flame and extinguish all cigarettes before use.
• Amyl nitrite is used illegally to enhance sexual pleasure, chiefly by homosexuals. Street names include "Amy" and "poppers."

Information for parents and patient
• Explain that ampule must be crushed to release drug.
• Warn parents that patient should use drug only when seated or lying down.

---

anthralin
Anthra-Derm, Drithocreme,
Drithocreme HP 1%

• Classification: topical antipsoriatic (germicide)

How supplied
Available by prescription only
Ointment: 0.1%, 0.25%, 0.5%, 1%
Cream: 0.1%, 0.25%, 0.5%, 1%

Indications, route, and dosage
Quiescent or chronic psoriasis
Children and adults: Apply thinly daily or as directed. Start with lowest concentration and increase, p.r.n.

Action and kinetics
• *Antipsoriatic action:* Although the mechanism of action is not fully known, it is thought that anthralin decreases the mitotic rate and reduces the proliferation of epidermal cells in psoriasis by inhibiting the synthesis of nucleic protein in psoriatic cell tissue.
• *Kinetics in adults:* Limited absorption with topical use.

Contraindications and precautions
Anthralin is contraindicated in patients with hypersensitivity to the drug. Drug should not be used on acute or inflammatory eruptions or applied to the face or genitalia. Avoid contact with the eyes or mucous membranes. Use cautiously in patients with renal disease because renal abnormalities may occur.

Interactions
None reported.

Effects on diagnostic tests
None reported.

Adverse reactions
• DERM: contact dermatitis, irritation, erythema.
   Note: Drug should be discontinued if sensitization develops.

Overdose and treatment
If accidental oral ingestion occurs, force fluids and contact local or regional poison information center.

▶ Special considerations
• Avoid use on eyes and mucous membranes.
• Drug may stain skin, hair, and fabrics.
• Patients with renal disease and those having extensive or prolonged applications should have periodic urine tests for albuminuria.

Information for parents and patient
• Advise parents or patient how to apply drug. At the end of the treatment period, patient should bathe or shower to remove any excess cream.
• Because anthralin may stain skin, clothing, or bed linens a red-brown to purple-brown color, use protective dressings.
• Parents or patient should avoid applying to normal skin by coating area surrounding lesion with petrolatum and should avoid applying cream to uninvolved scalp areas. They should wash hands thoroughly after use.
• Advise parents or patient to decrease the frequency of application if redness develops on adjacent normal skin.

---

antihemophilic factor (AHF)
Factorate, Hemofil T, Humafac, Koāte-HT, Profilate

- Classification: antihemophilic agent (blood derivative)

How supplied
Available by prescription only
Injection: Vials, with diluent. Number of units on label. A new porcine product is now available for patients with congenital hemophilia A who have antibodies to human Factor VIII:C.

Indications, route, and dosage
Hemophilia A (Factor VIII deficiency)
Children and adults: 10 to 20 units/kg I.V. push or infusion q 8 to 24 hours. Maintenance doses may be less. Administer solutions containing less than 34 AHF units/ml at a rate of 10 to 20 ml over 3 minutes; administer solutions containing 34 or more AHF units/ml at a maximum of 2 ml/minute. Dosage varies with individual needs.

One AHF unit is equal to the activity present in 1 ml normal pooled human plasma less than 1 hour old.

Do not confuse commercial product with blood bank-produced cryoprecipitated Factor VIII from individual human donors.

AHF is designed for I.V. use only; use plastic syringe, because solution adheres to glass surfaces.

Action and kinetics
- *Antihemophilic action:* AHF replaces deficient clotting factor that converts prothrombin to thrombin.
- *Kinetics in adults:* AHF must be given parenterally for systemic effect. AHF equilibrates intravascular and extravascular compartments; it does not readily cross placenta. Drug is cleared rapidly from plasma and consumed during blood clotting. Half-life ranges from 4 to 24 hours (average 12 hours).

Contraindications and precautions
Administer AHF cautiously to patients with hepatic disease and to neonates and infants because of susceptibility to hepatitis, which it may transmit.

The risk potential for viral transmission has been considerably reduced by heat treatment of all available AHF products, using a newer method similar to pasteurization.

Interactions
None significant.

Effects on diagnostic tests
None reported.

Adverse reactions
- CNS: headache, paresthesia, clouding or loss of consciousness.
- CV: tachycardia; hypotension; possible intravascular hemolysis in patients with blood type A, B, or AB.
- DERM: erythema, urticaria.
- EENT: disturbed vision.
- GI: nausea, vomiting, viral hepatitis.
- Other: chills, fever, backache, flushing, cough, chest pain, hypersensitivity reactions (erythema, urticaria, bronchospasm), stinging at infusion site.
    Note: Drug should be discontinued if signs of allergic reaction occur.

Overdose and treatment
Large or frequently repeated doses of AHF in patients with blood group A, B, or AB may cause intravascular hemolysis; monitor complete blood count and direct Coombs' test, and if intravascular hemolysis occurs, give serologically compatible type O red blood cells.

▶ Special considerations
- Administer cautiously to neonates and older infants because of susceptibility to hepatitis.
- Refrigerate concentrate until needed; before reconstituting, warm concentrate and diluent bottles to room temperature. To mix, gently roll vial between your hands; do not shake or mix with other I.V. solutions. Keep product away from heat (but do not refrigerate because that may cause precipitation of active ingredient), and use within 3 hours.
- Take baseline pulse rate before I.V. administration. If pulse rate increases significantly during administration, flow rate should be reduced or drug discontinued. Adverse reactions are usually related to too-rapid infusion.
- Monitor coagulation studies before and during therapy; monitor vital signs regularly, and be alert for allergic reactions.
- Prophylactic oral diphenhydramine may be prescribed if patient has history of transient allergic reactions to AHF.
- All products are now heat-treated by special method similar to pasteurization to decrease risk of transmitting hepatitis. Patient should be immunized with hepatitis B vaccine to decrease the risk of transmission of hepatitis.

Information for parents and patient
- Teach parents how to use, inject, and store prescribed product.
- Patient should not take salicylates or other drugs that inhibit platelet formation.

ascorbic acid (vitamin C)
Arco-Cee, Ascorbicap, Cebid Timecelles, Cecon Solution, Cemill-500, Cemill-1000, Cetane, Cevalin, Cevi-Bid, Ce-Vi-Sol, Cevita, C-Long, C-Span, Dull-C, Flavorcee, Vitacee

- Classification: nutritional supplement (water-soluble vitamin)

How supplied
Available by prescription only
Injection: 100 mg/ml in 2-ml and 10-ml ampules; 250 mg/ml in 10-ml ampules and 10-ml, 30-ml, and 50-

ml vials; 500 mg/ml in 2-ml and 5-ml ampules and 50-ml vials; 500 mg/ml (with monothioglycerol) in 1-ml ampules

Available without prescription, as appropriate
Tablets: 25 mg, 50 mg, 100 mg, 250 mg, 500 mg, 1,000 mg, 1,500 mg; effervescent — 1,000 mg sugar-free; chewable — 100 mg, 250 mg, 500 mg; timed-release — 500 mg, 750 mg, 1,000 mg, 1,500 mg
Capsules (timed-release): 500 mg
Crystals: 100 g (4 g/tsp), 1,000 g (4 g/tsp, sugar-free)
Powder: 100 g (4 g/tsp), 500 g (4 g/tsp), 1,000 g (4 g/tsp, sugar-free)
Liquid: 50 ml (35 mg/0.6 ml)
Solution: 50 ml (100 mg/ml)
Syrup: 20 mg/ml in 120 ml and 480 ml; 500 mg/5ml in 5 ml, 10 ml, 120 ml, and 473 ml

Indications, route, and dosage
Frank and subclinical scurvy
Infants: 50 to 100 mg P.O., I.M., I.V., or S.C. daily.
Children: 100 to 300 mg, depending on severity, P.O., S.C., I.M., or I.V. daily, then at least 35 mg/day for maintenance.
Adults: 100 mg to 2 g, depending on severity, P.O., S.C., I.M., or I.V. daily, then at least 50 mg/day for maintenance.
Extensive burns, delayed fracture or wound healing, postoperative wound healing, severe febrile or chronic disease states
Children: 100 to 200 mg P.O., S.C., I.M., or I.V. daily.
Adults: 200 to 500 mg P.O., S.C., I.M., or I.V. daily.
Prevention of ascorbic acid deficiency in those with poor nutritional habits or increased requirements
Infants: At least 35 mg P.O., S.C., I.M., or I.V. daily.
Children: At least 40 mg P.O., S.C., I.M., or I.V. daily.
Adults: 45 to 50 mg P.O., S.C., I.M., or I.V. daily.

Action and kinetics
• *Nutritional action:* Ascorbic acid, an essential vitamin, is involved with the biological oxidations and reductions used in cellular respiration. It is essential for the formation and maintenance of intracellular ground substance and collagen. In the body, ascorbic acid is reversibly oxidized to dehydroascorbic acid and influences tyrosine metabolism, conversion of folic acid to folinic acid, carbohydrate metabolism, resistance to infections, and cellular respiration. Ascorbic acid deficiency causes scurvy, a condition marked by degenerative changes in the capillaries, bone, and connective tissues. Restoring adequate ascorbic acid intake completely reverses symptoms of ascorbic acid deficiency. Data regarding the use of ascorbic acid as a urinary acidifier are conflicting.
• *Kinetics in adults:* After oral administration, ascorbic acid is absorbed readily. After very large doses, absorption may be limited because absorption is an active process. Absorption also may be reduced in patients with diarrhea or GI diseases. Normal plasma concentrations of ascorbic acid are about 10 to 20 mcg/ml. Plasma concentrations below 1.5 mcg/ml are associated with scurvy. However, leukocyte concentrations (although not usually measured) may better

reflect ascorbic acid tissue saturation. Approximately 1.5 g of ascorbic acid is stored in the body. Within 3 to 5 months of ascorbic acid deficiency, clinical signs of scurvy become evident.

Ascorbic acid is distributed widely in the body, with large concentrations found in the liver, leukocytes, platelets, glandular tissues, and lens of the eye. Ascorbic acid crosses the placenta; cord blood concentrations are usually two to four times the maternal blood concentrations. Ascorbic acid is distributed into breast milk and is metabolized in the liver. It is reversibly oxidized to dehydroascorbic acid. Some is metabolized to inactive compounds that are excreted in urine. The renal threshold is approximately 14 mcg/ml. When the body is saturated and blood concentrations exceed the threshold, unchanged ascorbic acid is excreted in urine. Renal excretion is directly proportional to blood concentrations. Ascorbic acid is also removed by hemodialysis.

Contraindications and precautions
Ascorbic acid products containing tartrazine can cause allergic reactions, including bronchial asthma, in susceptible individuals (many are also allergic to aspirin). Prolonged use of large doses of ascorbic acid may increase its metabolism. If intake is then reduced to normal levels, rebound scurvy may occur. Ingestion of large doses of this vitamin during pregnancy has caused scurvy in neonates.

Patients on sodium-restricted diets must consider that each gram of sodium ascorbate contains approximately 5 mEq of sodium.

Interactions
Concomitant use of ascorbic acid with acidic drugs in large doses (more than 2 g/day) may lower urine pH, causing renal tubular reabsorption of acidic drugs. Conversely, concomitant use with basic drugs (for example, amphetamines or tricyclic antidepressants) may cause decreased reabsorption and therapeutic effect.

Concurrent use of ascorbic acid with sulfonamides may cause crystallization. A combination of 30 mg of iron with 200 mg of ascorbic acid is sometimes recommended. Concomitant use with iron maintains it in the ferrous state and increases iron absorption in the GI tract, but this increase may not be significant.

Concomitant use of ascorbic acid with dicumarol influences the intensity and duration of the anticoagulant effect; use with warfarin may inhibit the anticoagulant effect; use with ethinyl estradiol may increase plasma levels of ethinyl estradiol.

Smoking may decrease serum ascorbic acid levels, thus increasing dosage requirements of this vitamin.

Salicylates inhibit ascorbic acid uptake by leukocytes and platelets. Although no evidence exists that salicylates precipitate ascorbic acid deficiency, patients receiving high doses of salicylates with ascorbic acid supplements must be observed for symptoms of ascorbic acid deficiency.

Effects on diagnostic tests
Ascorbic acid is a strong reducing agent; it alters results of tests that are based on oxidation-reduction reactions.

---

‡May contain sulfites   ◆ May contain tartrazine   ◆ ◆ May contain benzyl alcohol

Large doses of ascorbic acid (more than 500 mg) may cause false-negative glucose determinations using the glucose oxidase method, or false-positive results using the copper reduction method or Benedict's reagent.

Ascorbic acid should not be used for 48 to 72 hours before an amine-dependent test for occult blood in the stool is conducted. A false-negative result may occur.

Depending on the reagents used, ascorbic acid may also cause interactions with other diagnostic tests.

Adverse reactions
• CNS: faintness or dizziness with rapid I.V. administration.
• DERM: discomfort at injection site.
• GI: diarrhea, epigastric burning.
• GU: oxalate or urate renal calculi.
• Other: *dental erosion after prolonged use of chewable tablets.*

Overdose and treatment
Excessively high doses of parenteral ascorbic acid are excreted renally after tissue saturation and rarely accumulate. Serious adverse effects or toxicity is very uncommon. Severe effects require discontinuation of therapy.

▶ Special considerations
• Administer large doses of ascorbic acid (1,000 mg/day) in divided amounts because the body uses only a limited amount and excretes the rest in urine. Large doses may increase small-intestine pH and impair vitamin B_{12} absorption. The recommended daily allowance of ascorbic acid is 35 to 45 mg in children and 50 to 60 mg in adults.
• Administer oral solutions of ascorbic acid directly into the mouth or mix with food. Effervescent tablets should be dissolved in a glass of water immediately before ingestion.
• Administer the I.V. solution slowly.
• Conditions that raise the metabolic rate (hyperthyroidism, fever, infection, burns and other severe trauma, postoperative states, neoplastic disease, and chronic alcoholism) significantly raise ascorbic acid requirements.
• Reportedly, patients taking oral contraceptives require ascorbic acid supplements.
• Use ascorbic acid cautiously in patients with renal insufficiency because the vitamin is normally excreted in urine.
• Persons whose diets are deficient in fruits and vegetables can develop subclinical ascorbic acid deficiency. Observe for such deficiency in patients on restricted diets and those receiving long-term treatment with I.V. fluids or hemodialysis.
• Overt symptoms of ascorbic acid deficiency include irritability; emotional disturbances; general debility; pallor; anorexia; sensitivity to touch; limb and joint pain; follicular hyperkeratosis (particularly on thighs and buttocks); easy bruising; petechiae; bloody diarrhea; delayed healing; loosening of teeth; sensitive, swollen, and bleeding gums; and anemia.
• Protect ascorbic acid solutions from light.

Information for parents and patient
• Infants fed on cow's milk alone require supplemental ascorbic acid.
• Teach parents and patient about good dietary sources of ascorbic acid, such as citrus fruits, leafy vegetables, tomatoes, green peppers, and potatoes.
• Replacement dosage of ascorbic acid is higher if the patient smokes.
• Tell parents of patients who are prone to renal calculi, who have diabetes, who are undergoing tests for occult blood in stools, or who are on sodium-restricted diets or anticoagulant therapy to avoid high doses of ascorbic acid.

---

asparaginase
Elspar, Kidrolase

• Classification: antineoplastic (enzyme [L-asparagine amidohydrolase, cell cycle-phase specific, G_1 phase])

How supplied
Available by prescription only
Injection: 10,000-IU vials

Indications, route, and dosage
Dosage and indications may vary. Check current literature for recommended protocol.
Acute lymphocytic leukemia
Children: 6,000 IU/m² three times a week. Usually administered with vincristine and prednisone.
Adults: When used alone, 200 IU/kg daily I.V. for 28 days. When used in combination with other chemotherapeutic agents, dosage is highly individualized.

Action and kinetics
• *Antineoplastic action:* Asparaginase exerts its cytotoxic activity by inactivating the amino acid, asparagine, which is required by tumor cells to synthesize proteins. Because the tumor cells cannot synthesize their own asparagine, protein synthesis and eventually synthesis of DNA and RNA are inhibited.
• *Kinetics in adults:* Asparaginase is not absorbed across the GI tract after oral administration; therefore the drug must be given I.V. or I.M. Asparaginase distributes primarily within the intravascular space, with detectable concentrations in the thoracic and cervical lymph. The drug crosses the blood-brain barrier to a minimal extent. The metabolic fate of asparaginase is unclear; hepatic sequestration by the reticuloendothelial system may occur. The plasma elimination half-life, which is not related to dose, sex, age, or hepatic or renal function, ranges from 8 to 30 hours.

Contraindications and precautions
Asparaginase is contraindicated in patients with a history of anaphylactoid reactions to the drug or in patients with pancreatitis or a history of pancreatitis.

Drug should be used cautiously in patients with impaired liver function, infections, or recent therapy with antineoplastics or radiation because of risk of increased adverse effects.

Interactions

Concomitant use of asparaginase with methotrexate decreases the effectiveness of methotrexate, because asparaginase destroys the actively replicating cells that methotrexate requires for its cytotoxic action. Concomitant use of asparaginase and vincristine can cause additive neuropathy and disturbances of erythropoiesis. When asparaginase is used with prednisone, hyperglycemia may result from an additive effect on the pancreas.

Effects on diagnostic tests

Asparaginase therapy alters the results of thyroid function tests by decreasing concentrations of serum thyroxine-binding globulin.

Adverse reactions

• CNS: lethargy, somnolence, *headache*, confusion, agitation, tremor, *CNS depression and hyperexcitability.*
• DERM: rash, urticaria.
• GI: *vomiting* (may last up to 24 hours), anorexia, *abdominal pain, nausea*, cramps, weight loss, stomatitis.
• GU: azotemia, *renal failure*, uric acid nephropathy, glycosuria, polyuria.
• HEMA: *hypofibrinogenemia and depression of other clotting factors*, thrombocytopenia, leukopenia, depression of serum albumin, elevated bilirubin, jaundice.
• Hepatic: elevated ALT (SGPT) and AST (SGOT) levels; hepatotoxicity.
• Metabolic: elevated alkaline phosphatase and bilirubin (direct and indirect) levels; increase or decrease in total lipids; *hyperglycemia;* increased blood ammonia.
• Other: *hemorrhagic pancreatitis, anaphylaxis* (relatively common), *fever, chills, hypersensitivity.*
   Note: Drug should be discontinued at the first sign of renal failure or pancreatitis.

Overdose and treatment

Clinical manifestations of overdose include nausea and diarrhea.
   Treatment is generally supportive and includes antiemetics and antidiarrheals.

▶ Special considerations

• Asparaginase toxicity appears to be less severe in children than in adults.
• Reconstitute drug for I.M. administration with 2 ml unpreserved normal saline or sterile water for injection. Do not shake the solution; this can break down the protein and decrease potency. Do not use if precipate forms.
• I.M. injections should not contain more than 2 ml per injection. They are usually given in the thigh, alternating injection sites (left thigh/right thigh). Applying ice to the site before and after injection helps minimize discomfort and bleeding. I.M. administration requires adequate platelet count.
• For I.V. administration: Reconstitute with 5 ml of sterile water for injection or sodium chloride injection.

Solution will be clear or slightly cloudy. May further dilute with sodium chloride injection or dextrose 5% in water and administer I.V. over 30 minutes. Filtration through a 5-micron in-line filter during administration will remove particulate matter that may develop on standing; filtration through a 0.22-micron filter will result in a loss of potency. Do not use if precipitate forms.
• Refrigerate unopened dry powder. Reconstituted solution is stable 6 hours at room temperature, 24 hours refrigerated.
• Don't use as sole agent to induce remission unless combination therapy is inappropriate. May be used alone for consolidation of remission in children and adults with acute lymphocytic leukemia. Not recommended for maintenance therapy.
• Should be administered in hospital setting with close supervision. Monitor patient for 30 to 60 minutes after administration.
• I.V. administration of asparaginase with or immediately before vincristine or prednisone may increase toxicity reactions.
• Conduct skin test before initial dose. Observe site for 1 hour. Erythema and wheal formation indicate a positive reaction.
• Hypersensitivity reactions may not occur after first dose, but may develop later during therapy.
• Risk of hypersensitivity increases with repeated doses. Patient may be desensitized, but this doesn't rule out risk of allergic reactions. Routine administration of 2-unit I.V. test dose may identify high-risk patients.
• L-asparaginase may be derived from *Escherichia coli* (commercial preparation) or from *Erwinia caratovora*. A patient who reacts to one type may not react to the other. Both types should be tried before discontinuing drug because of hypersensitivity. *Erwinia* asparaginase is available from the National Cancer Institute for patients who are allergic to the commercial form.
• Because of vomiting, patient may need parenteral fluids for 24 hours or until oral fluids are tolerated.
• Monitor CBC and bone marrow function. Bone marrow regeneration may take 5 to 6 weeks.
• Obtain frequent serum amylase determinations to check pancreatic status. If elevated, asparaginase should be discontinued.
• Tumor lysis can result in uric acid nephropathy. Prevent occurrence by increasing fluid intake. Allopurinol should be started before therapy begins.
• Watch for signs of bleeding, such as petechiae and melena.
• Monitor blood glucose and test urine before and during therapy. Watch for signs of hyperglycemia, such as glycosuria and polyuria. Patient may need short-term insulin therapy.
• Keep epinephrine, diphenhydramine, and I.V. corticosteroids available for treatment of anaphylaxis.
• Follow institutional policy for safe handling of antineoplastics.

Information for parents and patient

• Advise the parents to encourage the patient to drink plenty of fluids to increase urine output and facilitate excretion of uric acid.

• Teach parents and patient to observe for signs of bleeding (easy bruising, bleeding gums, petechiae).
• Explain that drowsiness may occur during therapy or for several weeks after treatment has ended. Patient should avoid hazardous activities requiring mental alertness. CNS toxicities occur mainly in adults.

---

aspirin
A.S.A., A.S.A. Enseals, Aspergum, Bayer Timed-Release, Buffinol, Easprin, Ecotrin, Empirin, Encaprin, Entrophen, Measurin, Novasen*, Sal-Adult*, Sal-Infant*, Supasa*, Zorprin

• Classification: nonnarcotic analgesic, antipyretic, anti-inflammatory, antiplatelet (salicylate)

How supplied
Available without prescription
Tablets: 65 mg, 81 mg, 325 mg (5 grains), 500 mg, 600 mg, 650 mg
Tablets (enteric-coated): 325 mg, 500 mg, 650 mg
Tablets (extended-release): 650 mg
Capsules: 325 mg, 500 mg
Chewing gum: 227.5 mg
Suppositories: 60 to 120 mg

Available by prescription only
Tablets (enteric-coated): 975 mg
Tablets (extended-release): 800 mg

Indications, route, and dosage
Arthritis
Children: 90 to 130 mg/kg/day P.O., divided q 4 to 6 hours.
Adults: 2.6 to 5.2 g P.O. daily in divided doses.
Mild pain
Children: 40 to 60 mg/kg/day, P.O. or rectally, divided q 4 to 6 hours, p.r.n.
Severe pain
Children: 65 to 100 mg/kg P.O. or rectally daily, divided q 4 to 6 hours, p.r.n.
Kawasaki syndrome
Children: 90 to 130 mg/kg/day P.O., divided q 4 to 6 hours.

Action and kinetics
• *Analgesic action:* Aspirin produces analgesia by an ill-defined effect on the hypothalamus (central action) and by blocking generation of pain impulses (peripheral action). The peripheral action may involve blocking of prostaglandin synthesis via inhibition of cyclo-oxygenase enzyme.
• *Anti-inflammatory effects:* Although the exact mechanism is unknown, aspirin is believed to inhibit prostaglandin synthesis; it may also inhibit the synthesis or action of other mediators of inflammation.
• *Antipyretic effect:* Aspirin relieves fever by acting on the hypothalamic heat-regulating center to produce peripheral vasodilation. This increases peripheral blood supply and promotes sweating, which leads to loss of heat and to cooling by evaporation.

• *Anticoagulant effects:* Aspirin appears to impede clotting by blocking prostaglandin synthetase action, which prevents formation of the platelet-aggregating substance thromboxane A_2. This interference with platelet activity is irreversible and can prolong bleeding time.
• *Kinetics in adults:* Aspirin is absorbed rapidly and completely from the GI tract. Therapeutic blood salicylate concentrations for analgesia and anti-inflammatory effect are 15 to 50 mg/100 ml; responses vary with the patient.
Aspirin is distributed widely into most body tissues and fluids. Protein-binding to albumin is concentration dependent, ranges from 75% to 90%, and decreases as serum concentration increases. Severe toxic side effects may occur at serum concentrations greater than 400 mcg/ml.
Aspirin is hydrolyzed partially in the GI tract to salicylic acid with almost complete metabolism in the liver.
Aspirin is excreted in urine as salicylate and its metabolites. Elimination half-life ranges from 15 to 20 minutes.

Contraindications and precautions
Children or teenagers who have chicken pox or flu symptoms should avoid aspirin and other salicylates because they have been associated with Reye's syndrome, a rare but life-threatening condition. Aspirin is contraindicated in patients with known hypersensitivity to aspirin or other nonsteroidal anti-inflammatory drugs (NSAIDs). Aspirin-induced bronchospasm is commonly associated with asthma, nasal polyps, and chronic urticaria. Patients sensitive to yellow tartrazine dye should avoid aspirin.
Aspirin is also contraindicated in patients with GI ulcer or GI bleeding because the drug's irritant effects may worsen these conditions.
Administer cautiously to patients with hypoprothrombinemia, vitamin K deficiency, bleeding disorders, renal impairment, or liver disease, because the drug may cause bleeding. Patients should avoid aspirin during pregnancy, especially during the third trimester, because of potential adverse maternal and fetal effects.

Interactions
When used concomitantly, anticoagulants and thrombolytic drugs may to some degree potentiate the platelet-inhibiting effects of aspirin. Concomitant use of aspirin with drugs that are highly protein-bound (phenytoin, sulfonylureas, warfarin) may cause displacement of either drug and adverse effects. Monitor therapy closely for both drugs. Concomitant use with other GI-irritant drugs such as alcohol, steroids, antibiotics, and other NSAIDs may potentiate the aspirin's adverse GI effects. Use together with caution. Concomitant use with other ototoxic drugs, such as aminoglycosides, bumetanide, capreomycin, ethacrynic acid, furosemide, cisplatin, vancomycin, or erythromycin, may potentiate ototoxic effects. Aspirin decreases renal clearance of lithium carbonate, thus increasing serum lithium levels and the risk of adverse effects. Aspirin is antagonistic to the urico-

---

suric effect of phenylbutazone, probenecid, and sulfinpyrazone.

Ammonium chloride and other urine acidifiers increase aspirin blood levels; monitor for aspirin toxicity. Furosemide may impair aspirin excretion. Antacids in high doses, and other urine alkalizers, decrease aspirin blood levels; monitor for decreased salicylate effect. Corticosteroids enhance aspirin elimination. Food and antacids delay and decrease absorption of aspirin.

Effects on diagnostic tests
Aspirin interferes with urinary glucose analysis performed with Clinistix, Tes-Tape, Clinitest, and Benedict's solution, and with urinary 5-Hydroxyindoleacetic acid (5-HIAA) and vanillylmandelic acid (VMA) tests. Serum uric acid levels may be falsely increased. Aspirin may interfere with the Gerhardt test for urine acetoacetic acid.

Adverse reactions
• DERM: rash, bruising.
• EENT: tinnitus, hearing loss.
• GI: nausea, vomiting, *GI distress,* anorexia, dyspepsia, heartburn, occult bleeding.
• GU: reduced creatinine clearance, albuminuria, proteinuria.
• Hepatic: elevated liver enzyme levels, hepatitis, *hepatoxicity.*
• Other: *hypersensitivity manifested by anaphylaxis or asthma,* prolonged bleeding time.
   Note: Drug should be discontinued if the following occur: hypersensitivity, salicylism, tinnitus, headache, dizziness, confusion, impaired vision.

Overdose and treatment
Clinical manifestations of overdose include respiratory alkalosis, hyperpnea, and tachypnea, because of increased CO_2 production and direct stimulation of the respiratory center.

   To treat aspirin overdose, empty the patient's stomach immediately by inducing emesis with ipecac syrup if patient is conscious, or by gastric lavage. Administer repeated doses of activated charcoal via nasogastric tube. Provide symptomatic and supportive measures (respiratory support and correction of fluid and electrolyte imbalances). Closely monitor laboratory parameters and vital signs. Enhance renal excretion by administering sodium bicarbonate to alkalinize urine. Use cooling blanket or sponging if patient's rectal temperature is above 104° F. (40° C.). Hemodialysis is effective in removing aspirin but is only used in severely poisoned individuals or those at risk for pulmonary edema.

▶ Special considerations
• Because of epidemiologic association with Reye's syndrome, the Centers for Disease Control recommend that children with chicken pox or flulike symptoms not be given aspirin or other salicylates.
• Do not use long-term salicylate therapy in children under age 14; safety of this use has not been established.
• Children may be more susceptible to toxic effects of aspirin. Use with caution.

• Children usually should not take aspirin more than five times a day or for more than 5 days.
• Use aspirin with caution in patients with a history of GI disease, increased risk of GI bleeding, or decreased renal function.
• Administer non-enteric-coated tablets with food or after meals to minimize gastric upset.
• Tablets may be chewed, broken, or crumbled and administered with food or fluids to aid swallowing.
• Do not crush enteric-coated tablets.
• Patient should take a full glass of water or milk with aspirin to ensure passage into stomach. Patient should sit up for 15 to 30 minutes after taking drug to prevent lodging of drug in esophagus.
• Administer antacids, if prescribed, with aspirin, except enteric-coated forms. Separate doses of antacids and enteric-coated aspirin by 1 to 2 hours to ensure adequate absorption.
• Monitor vital signs frequently, especially temperature.
• Aspirin may mask the signs and symptoms of acute infection (fever, myalgia, erythema); carefully evaluate patients at risk for infections, such as those with diabetes.
• Monitor CBC, platelet count, prothrombin time; and BUN, serum creatinine, and liver function studies periodically during therapy to detect abnormalities.
• Assess hearing function before and periodically during therapy to prevent ototoxicity.
• Assess level of pain and inflammation before initiation of therapy. Evaluate effectiveness of therapy as evidenced by relief of these symptoms.
• Assess for signs and symptoms of potential hemorrhage, such as petechiae, bruising, coffee ground vomitus, and black tarry stools.
• If fever or illness causes fluid depletion, dosage should be reduced.
• Enteric-coated products are absorbed slowly and are not suitable for acute therapy. They are better suited for long-term therapy such as for arthritis.
• Avoid giving effervescent aspirin preparations to sodium-restricted patients.
• Stop aspirin therapy 1 week before elective surgery, if possible.
• Moisture may cause aspirin to lose potency. Store in a cool, dry place, and avoid using if tablets smell like vinegar.
• Avoid administering aspirin to patient who is allergic to tartrazine dye.

Information for parents and patient
• Tell parents to have child take tablet or capsule forms of medication with 8 oz of water and not lie down for 15 to 30 minutes after swallowing the drug.
• Tell parents to have patient take the medication 30 minutes before or 2 hours after meals, or with food or milk if gastric irritation occurs.
• Advise parents of patients on chronic therapy to arrange for monitoring of laboratory parameters, especially BUN and serum creatinine levels, liver function test, CBC, and prothrombin times.
• Warn parents of patients with current or history of rectal bleeding to avoid using salicylate suppositories. The latter must be retained in the rectum for at least 1 hour and could cause irritation and bleeding.

‡May contain sulfites   ◆May contain tartrazine   ◆◆May contain benzyl alcohol

• Warn against patient taking aspirin-containing medications without medical approval.
• Warn parents or patient that use of alcoholic beverages with aspirin may cause increased GI irritation and possibly GI bleeding.
• Patient should take a missed dose as soon as he remembers, unless it is almost time for next dose; in that case, he should skip the missed dose and return to regular schedule.
• Tell parents or patient not to take aspirin for more than 5 consecutive days unless otherwise directed.
• Tell parents to keep aspirin out of children's reach; encourage use of child-resistant closures because aspirin is a leading cause of poisoning.
• Advise parents of patients receiving high-dose, long-term aspirin therapy to watch for petechiae, bleeding gums, and signs of GI bleeding.

---

atropine sulfate

• Classification: antiarrhythmic, vagolytic (belladonna alkaloid)

How supplied
Available by prescription only
Injection: 0.05 mg/ml, 0.1 mg/ml, 0.3 mg/ml, 0.4 mg/ml, 0.5 mg/ml, 0.6 mg/ml, 0.8 mg/ml, 1 mg/ml, and 1.2 mg/ml
Tablets: 0.4 mg

Indications, route, and dosage
Symptomatic bradycardia, bradydysrhythmia (junctional or escape rhythm) and heart block
Children: 0.01 mg/kg up to maximum 0.4 mg; or 0.3 mg/m^2; may repeat q 4 to 6 hours. Minimum dose is 0.1 mg to prevent paradoxical bradycardia.
Adults: Usually 0.5 to 1 mg by I.V. push; repeat q 5 minutes, to a maximum of 2 mg. Lower doses (less than 0.5 mg) may cause bradycardia.
Preoperatively for diminishing secretions and blocking cardiac vagal reflexes
Children: 0.01 mg/kg I.M. up to a maximum dose of 0.4 mg 45 to 60 minutes before anesthesia.
Adults: 0.4 to 0.6 mg I.M. 45 to 60 minutes before anesthesia.
Antidote for anticholinesterase insecticide poisoning
Children: 0.05 mg/kg I.M. or I.V., repeated q 10 to 30 minutes as needed. Maintenance dosage, 0.01 mg/kg (maximum, 0.25 mg).
Adults: 2 mg I.M. or I.V. repeated every 20 to 30 minutes until muscarinic symptoms disappear. Severe cases may require up to 6 mg I.M. or I.V q 1 hour.

Action and kinetics
• *Antiarrhythmic action:* An anticholinergic (parasympatholytic) agent with many uses, atropine remains the mainstay of pharmacologic treatment for bradydysrhythmias. It blocks acetylcholine's effects on the SA and AV nodes, thereby increasing SA and AV node conduction velocity. It also increases sinus

node discharge rate and decreases the AV node's effective refractory period. These changes result in an increased heart rate (both atrial and ventricular).
Atropine has variable – and clinically negligible – effects on the His-Purkinje system. Small doses (< 0.5 mg) and occasionally larger doses may lead to a paradoxical slowing of the heart rate, which may be followed by a more rapid rate.
As a cholinergic blocking agent, atropine decreases the action of the parasympathetic nervous system on certain glands (bronchial, salivary, and sweat), resulting in decreased secretions. It also decreases cholinergic effects on the iris, ciliary body, and intestinal and bronchial smooth muscle.
As an antidote for cholinesterase poisoning, atropine blocks the cholinomimetic effects of these pesticides.
• *Kinetics in adults:* I.V. administration is the most common route for bradydysrhythmia treatment. With endotracheal administration, atropine is well absorbed from the bronchial tree (drug has been used in 1-mg doses in acute bradydysrhythmia when an I.V. line has not been established). Atropine is well absorbed after oral and I.M. administration.
Atropine is well distributed throughout the body, including the CNS. Atropine is metabolized in the liver to several metabolites.
Drug is excreted primarily through the kidneys; however, small amounts may be excreted in the feces and in expired air.

Contraindications and precautions
Atropine should be used with caution in children with acute myocardial infarction because it may promote dysrhythmias, including ventricular fibrillation and tachycardia as well as atrial fibrillation; the resulting increase in heart rate may increase mycocardial oxygen consumption and worsen myocardial ischemia.
Atropine should be used cautiously in those children with narrow-angle glaucoma, obstructive uropathy, obstructive gastrointestinal tract disease, myasthenia gravis, paralytic ileus, intestinal atony, unstable cardiovascular status from acute hemorrhage, and toxic megacolon, because the drug may worsen these symptoms or disorders.

Interactions
Concomitant use of atropine and other anticholinergics or drugs with anticholinergic effects produce additive effects.

Effects on diagnostic tests
None reported.

Adverse reactions
• CNS: headache; restlessness; ataxia; disorientation; hallucinations; delirium; coma; insomnia; dizziness; excitement, agitation, confusion.
• CV: tachycardia (possibly extreme), palpitations, angina.
• DERM: hot, flushed skin.
• EENT: mydriasis, photophobia (with 1-mg dose); blurred vision, mydriasis (with 2-mg dose).
• GI: dry mouth, thirst, constipation, nausea, vomiting.

---

*Canada only   †Unlabeled clinical use   Italicized adverse reactions have been observed in children.

- GU: urinary retention.
- HEMA: leukocytosis.
- Other: hyperpyrexia.

Overdose and treatment

Clinical signs of overdose reflect excessive anticholinergic activity, especially cardiovascular and CNS stimulation.

Treatment includes physostigmine administration, to reverse excessive anticholinergic activity, and general supportive measures, as necessary.

▶ Special considerations

- Monitor patient's vital signs, urine output, visual changes, and check for signs of impending toxicity.
- Give ice chips, cool drinks, or sugarless hard candy to relieve dry mouth.
- Constipation may be relieved by stool softeners or bulk laxatives.
- Observe for tachycardia if patient has cardiac disorder.
- With I.V. administration, drug may cause paradoxical initial bradycardia, which usually disappears within 2 minutes.
- Monitor patient's fluid intake and output; drug causes urinary retention and hesitancy. If possible, patient should void before taking drug.
- High doses may cause hyperpyrexia, urinary retention, and CNS effects, including hallucinations and confusion (anticholinergic delirium). Other anticholinergic drugs may increase vagal blockage.
- Adverse reactions very considerably with dose.
- Observe for tachycardia if patient has cardiac disorder.

Information for parents and patient

- Warn patient to avoid alcoholic beverages, because they may cause additive CNS effects.
- Advise patient to consume plenty of fluids and dietary fiber to help avoid constipation.
- Tell parents or patient to promptly report dry mouth, blurred vision, skin rash, eye pain, any significant change in urine volume, or pain or difficulty on urination.
- Warn parents or patient that drug may cause increased sensitivity or intolerance to high temperatures, resulting in dizziness.
- Instruct parents to watch for signs of confusion and to check child for rapid or pounding heartbeat and to report these effects promptly.

---

auranofin
Ridaura

- Classification: antiarthritic (gold salt)

How supplied

Available by prescription only
Capsules: 3 mg

Indications, route, and dosage
Rheumatoid arthritis

†*Children:* Initially, 0.1 mg/kg daily. Increase dosage as needed. Usual maintenance dosage is 0.15 mg/kg daily. Maximum dosage is 0.2 mg/kg daily.

Adults: 6 mg P.O. daily, administered either as 3 mg b.i.d. or 6 mg once daily. After 4 to 6 months, may be increased to 9 mg daily. If response remains inadequate after 3 months at 9 mg daily, discontinue the drug.

Action and kinetics

- *Antiarthritic action:* Auranofin suppresses or prevents, but does not cure, adult or juvenile arthritis and synovitis. It is anti-inflammatory in active arthritis. This drug is thought to reduce inflammation by altering the immune system. Auranofin has been shown to decrease high serum concentrations of immunoglobulins and rheumatoid factors in patients with arthritis. However, the exact mechanism of action remains unknown.
- *Kinetics in adults:* When administered P.O., 25% of auranofin is absorbed through the GI tract. Time to peak plasma concentration is 1 to 2 hours. The drug is 60% protein-bound and is distributed widely in body tissues. Synovial fluid levels are approximately 50% of blood concentrations. No correlation between blood-gold concentrations and safety or efficacy has been determined. The metabolic fate of auranofin is not known. Sixty percent of the absorbed auranofin (15% of the administered dose) is excreted in the urine and the remainder in the feces. The average plasma half-life is 26 days, compared with about 6 days for gold sodium thiomalate.

Contraindications and precautions

Auranofin is contraindicated in patients with a known hypersensitivity to gold or other heavy metals or with a history of blood dyscrasias, because the drug may induce blood dyscrasias; in patients with severe diabetes, CHF, hemorrhagic conditions, systemic lupus erythematosus, tuberculosis, or exfoliative dermatitis, because it may exacerbate these conditions; in patients with colitis, because the drug can precipitate GI distress; and in patients with impaired renal or hepatic function.

Auranofin should be used cautiously in patients with decreased cerebral or cardiovascular circulation, a history of drug rash, a history of hepatic or renal disease, or severe hypertension.

Interactions

Concomitant use of auranofin with other drugs that may cause blood dyscrasias can produce additive hematologic toxicity.

Effects on diagnostic tests

Serum protein-bound iodine test, especially when done by the chloric acid digestion method, gives false readings during and for several weeks after gold therapy.

Adverse reactions

- GI: abdominal pain, *diarrhea,* nausea, vomiting, stomatitis, enterocolitis, anorexia, metallic taste, dyspepsia, flatulence.

• GU: transient proteinuria, hematuria, nephrotic syndrome.
• HEMA: thrombocytopenia (with or without purpura), aplastic anemia, agranulocytosis, leukopenia, eosinophilia.
• Hepatic: jaundice, elevated liver enzymes.
• Other: hypersensitivity (syncope [rarely], bradycardia, *anaphylactic shock*), interstitial pneumonitis, sore throat, sensory change in the hands and feet (with long-term use).

Overdose and treatment

When severe reactions to gold occur, corticosteroids, dimercaprol (a chelating agent), or penicillamine may be given to aid recovery. Prednisone 40 to 100 mg daily in divided doses is recommended to manage severe renal, hematologic, pulmonary, or enterocolitic reactions to gold. Dimercaprol may be used concurrently with steroids to facilitate the removal of the gold when steroid treatment alone is ineffective. Use of chelating agents is controversial, and caution is recommended.

▶ Special considerations

• Safe dosage in children has not been established; use in children under age 6 is not recommended.
• Auranofin should be discontinued if the platelet count falls below 100,000/mm³.
• Carefully monitor for toxic reactions (pruritus, rash, metallic taste, sore mouth, or GI reactions).
• Gold therapy is contraindicated in patients with a history of necrotizing enterocolitis, pulmonary fibrosis, exfoliative dermatitis, bone marrow aplasia, or severe hematologic disorders; and in patients receiving other drugs that have the potential to cause blood dyscrasias.
• CBC and platelet count should be monitored at least monthly.
• Moderately severe skin reactions and mucous membrane reactions often benefit from a topical steroid cream, an oral antihistamine, and soothing lotions.
• Do not restart gold therapy after a severe reaction.
• Gold therapy may alter liver function tests.

Information for parents and patient

• Emphasize the importance of monthly follow-up blood tests to monitor patient's platelet count.
• Explain that beneficial drug effect may be delayed for 3 months. However, if response is inadequate after 6 to 9 months, auranofin will probably be discontinued.
• Patient should take the drug as prescribed and not alter the dosage schedule.
• Diarrhea is the most common adverse reaction. Tell parents that patient should continue taking the drug if he experiences mild diarrhea; increasing his intake of dietary fiber can minimize watery diarrhea; however, if stool contains blood, parents should call physician immediately.
• Tell parents that patient can continue taking concomitant drug therapy, such as nonsteroidal anti-inflammatory drugs, if prescribed.
• Dermatitis is a common adverse reaction. Advise parents to report any rashes or other skin problems immediately.
• Stomatitis is also common. It is often preceded by

a metallic taste. Advise parents to report this symptom immediately.
• Advise parents to minimize patient's exposure to sunlight or artificial ultraviolet light because skin rash may develop or be aggravated by such exposure.
• Tell parents and patient that good oral hygiene is important.

---

aurothioglucose
Solganal

• Classification: antiarthritic (gold salt)

How supplied

Available by prescription only
Injection: 50 mg/ml suspension in sesame oil with aluminum monosterate 2% and propylparaben 0.1% in a 10-ml container

Indications, route, and dosage
Rheumatoid arthritis

Children age 6 to 12: One-quarter usual adult dose. Alternatively, 1 mg/kg I.M. (not to exceed 25 mg per dose) once weekly for 20 weeks.
Adults: Initially, 10 mg I.M., followed by 25 mg for second and third doses at weekly intervals. Then, 50 mg weekly until 1 g has been given. If improvement occurs without toxicity, continue 25 to 50 mg at 3- to 4-week intervals indefinitely as maintenance therapy.

Action and kinetics

• *Antiarthritic action:* Aurothioglucose is thought to be effective against rheumatoid arthritis by altering the immune system to reduce inflammation. Although the exact mechanism of action remains unknown, these compounds have reduced serum concentrations of immunoglobulins and rheumatoid factors in patients with arthritis.
• *Kinetics in adults:* Absorption of aurothioglucose is slow and erratic because it is in oil suspension. Higher tissue concentrations occur with parenteral gold salts, with a mean steady-state plasma level of 1 to 5 mcg/ml. Drug is distributed widely throughout the body in lymph nodes, bone marrow, kidneys, liver, spleen, and tissues. About 85% to 90% is protein-bound. Aurothioglucose is not broken down into its elemental form. The half-life with cumulative dosing is 14 to 40 days. About 70% of the drug is excreted in the urine, 30% in the feces.

Contraindications and precautions

Gold compounds are contraindicated in patients with uncontrolled diabetes mellitus, systemic lupus erythematosus, Sjögren's syndrome, agranulocytosis, or blood dyscrasias; in patients who recently received radiation therapy; in breast-feeding patients, because the drug distributes into breast milk; and in patients with a history of sensitivity to gold compounds. They should be administered cautiously to patients with marked hypertension, compromised cerebral or cardiovascular function, or renal or hepatic dysfunction,

---

may be increased by 0.5 mg/kg daily (up to a maximum of 2.5 mg/kg daily) at 4-week intervals.

Action and kinetics
• *Immunosuppressant action:* The mechanism of azathioprine's immunosuppressive activity is unknown; however, the drug may inhibit RNA and DNA synthesis, mitosis, or (in patients undergoing renal transplantation) coenzyme formation and functioning. Azathioprine suppresses cell-mediated hypersensitivity and alters antibody production.
• *Kinetics in adults:* Azathioprine is well absorbed orally. Azathioprine and its major metabolite, mercaptopurine, are distributed throughout the body; both are 30% protein-bound. Azathioprine and its metabolites cross the placenta. Azathioprine is metabolized primarily to mercaptopurine. Small amounts of azathioprine and mercaptopurine are excreted in urine intact; most of a given dose is excreted in urine as secondary metabolites.

Contraindications and precautions
Azathioprine is contraindicated in patients with known hypersensitivity to the drug and in pregnant patients. It should be used cautiously in patients with hepatic or renal dysfunction; in patients receiving cadaveric kidneys, who may have decreased elimination; and in rheumatoid arthritis patients previously treated with alkylating agents — cyclophosphamide, chlorambucil, or melphalan — who are at increased risk of neoplasia.

Interactions
Azathioprine's major metabolic pathway is inhibited by allopurinol, which competes for the oxidative enzyme xanthine oxidase; during concomitant use with allopurinol, azathioprine dosage should be reduced to 25% to 33% of the usual amount.

Azathioprine may reverse neuromuscular blockade resulting from use of the nondepolarizing muscle relaxants tubocurarine and pancuronium.

Effects on diagnostic tests
Azathioprine alters CBC and differential blood counts, decreases serum uric acid levels, and elevates liver enzymes test results.

Adverse reactions
• GI: nausea, vomiting, anorexia, diarrhea, oral mucous membrane ulceration, esophagitis with possible ulceration.
• HEMA: leukopenia, macrocytic anemia, pancytopenia, thrombocytopenia, bone marrow depression.
• Hepatic: jaundice, biliary stasis, hepatic venoocclusive disease.
• Other: skin rash, hair loss, drug fever, arthralgias, increased risk of infection and malignancy.
Note: Drug should be discontinued or dosage reduced if patient develops signs of hypersensitivity, leukopenia, pancytopenia, or thrombocytopenia, jaundice, or hepatic veno-occlusive disease; or if WBC falls below 3,000/mm³, to prevent progression to irreversible bone marrow depression.

Overdose and treatment
Clinical signs of overdose include nausea, vomiting, diarrhea, and extension of hematologic effects. Supportive treatment may include treatment with blood products if necessary.

▶ Special considerations
• Monitor patient for signs of hepatic damage: clay-colored stools, dark urine, jaundice, pruritus, and elevated liver enzyme levels.
• If infection occurs, drug dosage should be reduced and infection treated.
• If nausea and vomiting occur, divide dose and/or give with or after meals.
• Monitor for unusual bleeding or bruising, fever, or sore throat.
• Maximum effectiveness occurs when azathioprine is administered during the antibody response induction period, starting either at the time of or within 2 days after antigenic stimulation.
• If used to treat rheumatoid arthritis, nonsteroidal anti-inflammatory agents should be continued when azathioprine therapy is initiated.
• Hematologic status should be monitored while patient is receiving azathioprine. CBCs, including platelet counts, should be taken at least weekly during the 1st month, twice monthly for the 2nd and 3rd months, then monthly.
• Chronic immunosuppression with azathioprine is associated with an increased risk of neoplasia.

Information for parents and patient
• Teach parents and patient about disease and rationale for therapy; explain possible side effects and importance of reporting them, especially any unusual bleeding or bruising, fever, sore throat, mouth sores, abdominal pain, pale stools, or dark urine.
• Encourage compliance with therapy and follow-up visits.
• Advise parents and adolescent females that patient should avoid pregnancy during therapy and for 4 months after stopping therapy.
• Tell parents and patient with rheumatoid arthritis that clinical response may not be apparent for up to 12 weeks.
• Suggest taking drug with or after meals or in divided doses to prevent nausea.

azlocillin sodium
Azlin

• Classification: antibiotic (extended-spectrum penicillin, acylaminopenicillin)

How supplied
Available by prescription only
Injection: 2 g, 3 g, 4 g per vial

Indications, route, and dosage
Serious infections caused by susceptible organisms
Premature neonates < 7 days old: 50 mg/kg I.V. or I.M. q 12 hours

Full-term neonates < 7 days old: 100 mg/kg I.V. or I.M. q 12 hours

Infants and children: 240 to 350 mg/kg/ I.V. daily, divided q 4 to 6 hours.

Children with acute exacerbation of cystic fibrosis: 75 mg/kg I.V. q 4 hours (450 mg/kg daily). Maximum daily dosage is 24 g. Some clinicians recommend 100 to 200 mg/kg I.V. q 8 hours.

Adults: 200 to 350 mg/kg I.V. daily given in four to six divided doses. Usual dose is 3 g q 4 hours (18 g/day). Maximum daily dosage is 24 g. May be administered by I.V. intermittent infusion or by direct slow I.V. injection.

Dosage in renal failure
Reduced dosage is required in patients with creatinine clearance below 30 ml/minute. Measurement of serum level may be necessary.

Action and kinetics
• *Antibiotic action:* Azlocillin is bactericidal; it adheres to bacterial penicillin-binding proteins, thus inhibiting bacterial cell wall synthesis. Extended-spectrum penicillins are more resistant to inactivation by certain beta-lactamases, especially those produced by gram-negative organisms, but are still liable to inactivation by certain others.

Azlocillin's spectrum of activity includes many gram-negative aerobic and anaerobic bacilli; many gram-positive and gram-negative aerobic cocci; and some gram-positive aerobic and anaerobic bacilli. Azlocillin may be effective against some strains of carbenicillin-resistant and ticarcillin-resistant gram-negative bacilli. Azlocillin is less active against *Enterobacteriaceae* than other members of this class, such as mezlocillin and piperacillin, but it is more effective against *Pseudomonas aeruginosa.*

• *Kinetics in adults:* No appreciable absorption occurs after oral administration. After an I.M. dose, peak plasma concentrations occur at ½ to 2 hours.

Azlocillin is distributed widely after parenteral administration, with good penetration into various organs, tissues, and secretions. It penetrates minimally into uninflamed meninges and slightly into bone and sputum. Volume of distribution is between 0.14 and 0.3 L/kg. Azlocillin is 20% to 46% protein-bound; it crosses the placenta.

Azlocillin is metabolized partially; 15% of a dose is metabolized to inactive metabolites.

Azlocillin is excreted primarily (50% to 70%) in urine by glomerular filtration and tubular secretion. It is also excreted in bile and in breast milk. Elimination half-life in adults is about 1 to 1½ hours; in patients with extensive renal impairment, half-life is extended to 4 to 8½ hours.

• *Kinetics in children:* Half life is inversely proportional to age, and is 2.6 to 4.4 hours in premature neonates, 2.5 to 3.4 hours in full-term neonates, 1.9 hours in children 1 to 3 months old, and 0.93 to 0.97 hours in children older than 30 months. *The serum half-life may be shorter in children with cystic fibro-*

sis, which may result in lower than expected serum concentrations. Azlocillin is removed by hemodialysis but not by peritoneal dialysis.

Contraindications and precautions
Azlocillin is contraindicated in patients with known hypersensitivity to any other penicillin or to cephalosporins.

Azlocillin should be used with caution in patients with renal impairment because it is excreted in urine; decreased dosage is required in moderate to severe renal failure.

Interactions
Concomitant use with aminoglycoside antibiotics results in synergistic bactericidal effect against *P. aeruginosa, Escherichia coli, Klebsiella, Citrobacter, Enterobacter, Serratia,* and *Proteus mirabilis.* However, the drugs are physically and chemically incompatible and are inactivated if mixed or given together. In vivo inactivation of aminoglycosides has also been reported when aminoglycosides and extended spectrum penicillins are used concomitantly.

Concomitant use of azlocillin (and other extended-spectrum penicillins) with clavulanic acid also produces a synergistic bactericidal effect against certain beta-lactamase-producing bacteria.

Probenecid blocks tubular secretion of azlocillin, raising its serum concentration levels.

Large doses of penicillins may interfere with renal tubular secretion of methotrexate, delaying elimination and elevating serum concentrations of methotrexate.

Effects on diagnostic tests
Azlocillin alters results of tests for urinary or serum proteins; it interferes with turbidimetric methods that use sulfosalicylic acid, trichloracetic acid, acetic acid, or nitric acid. Azlocillin does not interfere with tests using bromphenal blue (Albustix, Albutest, Multi-Stix).

Azlocillin may falsely decrease serum aminoglycoside concentrations. Systemic effects of azlocillin may cause hypokalemia and hypernatremia and may prolong prothrombin times; azlocillin may also cause transient elevations in liver function study results and transient reductions in red blood cell, white blood cell, and platelet counts.

Adverse reactions
• CNS: neuromuscular irritability, headache, dizziness.
• GI: nausea, diarrhea, vomiting.
• HEMA: bleeding with high doses, neutropenia, eosinophilia, leukopenia, thrombocytopenia.
• Metabolic: hypokalemia.
• Local: pain at injection site, vein irritation, phlebitis.
• Other: hypersensitivity (edema, fever, chills, rash, pruritus, urticaria, anaphylaxis), overgrowth of non-susceptible organisms.

Note: Drug should be discontinued if immediate hypersensitivity reactions or bleeding complications occur and if severe diarrhea occurs, because that may indicate pseudomembranous colitis.

Overdose and treatment
Clinical signs of overdose include neuromuscular hypersensitivity or seizures resulting from CNS irritations by high drug concentrations: A 4- to 6-hour hemodialysis will remove 6% to 50% of azlocillin.

▶ Special considerations
• Azlocillin may be more suitable than carbenicillin or ticarcillin for patients on salt-free diets; azlocillin contains only 2.17 mEq of sodium per gram.
• Elimination half-life is prolonged in neonates; safety of azlocillin in neonates has not been established.
• Assess patient's history of allergies; do not give a penicillin to any patient with a history of hypersensitivity reactions to either penicillins or cephalosporins. Try to determine whether previous reactions were true hypersensitivity reactions or another reaction, such as GI distress, which the patient has interpreted as allergy.
• Keep in mind that a negative history for penicillin hypersensitivity does not preclude future allergic reactions; monitor patient continuously for possible allergic reactions or other untoward effects.
• More common than allergic rashes is a nonallergic maculopapular rash, usually seen 5 to 9 days into the course of the drug. This rash usually lasts about 3 days. It is not a contraindication to the drug's use in the future.
• In patients with renal impairment, dosage should be reduced if creatinine clearance is below 10ml/minute.
• Assess level of consciousness, neurologic status, and renal function when high doses are used, because excessive blood levels can cause CNS toxicity.
• Obtain results of cultures and sensitivity tests before first dose; however, therapy may begin before test results are complete. Repeat tests periodically to assess drug efficacy.
• Monitor vital signs, electrolytes, and renal function studies, monitor body weight for fluid retention with extended-spectrum penicillins for possible hypokalemia or hypernatremia.
• Coagulation abnormalities, even frank bleeding, can follow high doses, especially of extended-spectrum penicillins; monitor prothrombin times and platelet counts, and assess patient for signs of occult or frank bleeding.
• Monitor patients on long-term therapy for possible superinfection, especially debilitated patients and others receiving immunosuppressants or radiation therapy; monitor closely, especially for fever.

Parenteral administration
• Give penicillins at least 1 hour before giving bacteriostatic antibiotics (tetracyclines, erythromycins, and chloramphenicol); these drugs inhibit bacterial cell growth, decreasing rate of penicillin uptake by bacterial cell walls.
• Always consult manufacturer's directions for reconstitution, dilution, and storage of drugs, check expiration dates.
• Do not add or mix other drugs with I.V. infusions—particularly aminoglycosides, which will be inactivated if mixed with penicillins; they are chemically and physically incompatible. If other drugs must be given I.V., temporarily stop infusion of primary drug.

• Infuse I.V. drug continuously or intermittently (over 30 minutes) and assess I.V. site frequently to prevent infiltration or phlebitis; rotate infusion site q 48 hours; intermittent I.V. infusion may be diluted in 50 to 100 ml sterile water, 0.9% sodium chloride, dextrose 5% in water, dextrose 5% in water and half normal saline or lactated Ringer's solution. May infuse in smaller volume or give I.V. push.
• Solutions should always be clear, colorless to pale yellow, and free of particles; do not give solutions containing precipitates or other foreign matter.

Information for parents and patient
• Encourage parents to report diarrhea promptly.
• Teach signs and symptoms of hypersensitivity and other adverse reactions, and emphasize need to report any unusual reactions.
• Teach signs and symptoms of bacterial and fungal superinfections; emphasize need to report signs of infection in debilitated patients and others with low resistance from immunosuppressants or irradiation.
• Be sure parents and patient understand how and when to administer drugs; urge them to complete entire prescribed regimen, to comply with instructions for around-the-clock dosage, and to keep follow-up appointments.
• Counsel parents to check expiration date of drug and to discard unused drug.
• Azlocillin is almost always used with another antibiotic, such as an aminoglycoside, in life-threatening situations.
• Monitor serum electrolyte levels to avoid adverse effects.
• Because azlocillin is partially dialyzable, patients undergoing hemodialysis may need dosage adjustments. Some clinicians administer 3 g I.V. after each dialysis treatment, then every 12 hours.

‡May contain sulfites   ◆May contain tartrazine   ◆ ◆May contain benzyl alcohol

B

bacampicillin hydrochloride
Spectrobid

• Classification: antibiotic (aminopenicillin)

How supplied
Available by prescription only
Suspension: 125 mg/5 ml (after reconstitution)
Tablets: 400 mg

Indications, route, and dosage
Upper and lower respiratory tract, urinary tract, and skin infections caused by susceptible organisms
Children weighing less than 25 kg: 25 mg/kg P.O. q 12 hours.
Children and adults weighing more than 25 kg: 400 to 800 mg P.O. q 12 hours.
Gonorrhea
Children and adults weighing more than 25 kg: Usual dosage is 1.6 g plus 1 g probenecid given as a single dose.

Action and kinetics
• *Antibiotic action:* Bacampicillin is precursor of ampicillin with no innate bactericidal activity; ampicillin is the active metabolite. Ampicillin is bactericidal; it adheres to bacterial penicillin-binding proteins, thus inhibiting bacterial cell wall synthesis. Each milligram of bacampicillin yields 623 to 727 mcg of ampicillin.

Ampicillin's spectrum of activity includes nonpenicillinase-producing gram-positive bacteria, *Neisseria gonorrhoeae, N. meningitidis, Hemophilus influenzae, Escherichia coli, Proteus mirabilis, Salmonella,* and *Shigella.* However, severity of some infections precludes oral therapy with bacampicillin.
• *Kinetics in adults:* Bacampicillin is hydrolyzed rapidly to ampicillin after oral administration, both in GI tract and plasma; peak plasma concentrations occur 30 to 90 minutes after an oral dose.

No unchanged bacampicillin is found in serum after oral administration; ampicillin distributes into pleural, peritoneal, and synovial fluids; lungs, prostate, muscle, liver, and gallbladder; it also penetrates middle ear effusions, maxillary sinus and bronchial secretions, tonsils, and sputum. Ampicillin crosses the placenta; it is 15% to 25% protein-bound.

Bacampicillin is hydrolyzed to ampicillin; ampicillin is metabolized partially.

Ampicillin and metabolites are excreted in urine by renal tubular secretion and glomerular filtration; they are also excreted in breast milk. Elimination half-life in adults is 1 to 1½ hours, extended to 7½ hours in patients with severe renal impairment.

Contraindications and precautions
Bacampicillin is contraindicated in patients with known hypersensitivity to any other penicillin or to cephalosporins.

Bacampicillin should not be used in patients with infectious mononucleosis because many patients develop a rash during therapy.

Bacampicillin should be used cautiously in patients with renal impairment, because it is excreted in urine; decreased dosage is required in moderate to severe renal failure.

Interactions
Concomitant use with an aminoglycoside antibiotic causes a synergistic bactericidal effect against some strains of enterococci and group B streptococci.

Concomitant use with allopurinol may increase incidence of rash from either drug.

Probenecid inhibits renal tubular secretion of ampicillin, increasing its serum concentrations. Large doses of penicillins may interfere with renal tubular secretion of methotrexate, delaying elimination and elevating serum concentrations of methotrexate.

Effects on diagnostic tests
Bacampicillin alters results of urine glucose tests that use cupric sulfate (Benedict's reagent or Clinitest). Make urine glucose determinations with glucose oxidase methods (Clinistix or Tes-Tape).

Bacampicillin may falsely decrease serum aminoglycoside concentrations.

Adverse reactions
• GI: nausea, vomiting, diarrhea, glossitis, stomatitis, pseudomembranous colitis.
• GU: acute interstitial nephritis.
• HEMA: anemia, thrombocytopenia, thrombocytopenic purpura, eosinophilia, leukopenia.
• Other: hypersensitivity (erythematous maculopapular rash, urticaria, anaphylaxis), bacterial or fungal superinfection.
Note: Drug should be discontinued if immediate hypersensitivity reaction, bone marrow toxicity, acute interstitial nephritis, or pseudomembranous colitis occurs.

Overdose and treatment
Clinical signs of overdose include neuromuscular sensitivity or seizures. After recent ingestion (4 hours or less), empty the stomach by induced emesis or gastric lavage; follow with activated charcoal to reduce absorption. Bacampicillin and ampicillin can be removed by hemodialysis.

▶ Special considerations
• Assess patient's history of allergies; do not give a penicillin to any patient with a history of hypersensitivity reactions to either penicillins or cephalosporins. Try to determine whether previous reactions

were true hypersensitivity reactions or another re-action, such as GI distress, which the patient has interpreted as allergy.

• Keep in mind that a negative history for penicillin hypersensitivity does not preclude future allergic re-actions; monitor patient continuously for possible al-lergic reactions or other untoward effects.

• More common than allergic rashes is a nonallergic maculopapular rash, usually seen 5 to 9 days into the course of the drug. This rash usually lasts about 3 days. It is not a contraindication to the drug's use in the future.

• In patients with renal impairment, dosage should be reduced if creatinine clearance is below 10 ml/minute.

• Assess level of consciousness, neurologic status, and renal function when high doses are used, because excessive blood levels can cause CNS toxicity.

• Obtain results of cultures and sensitivity tests before first dose; however, therapy may begin before test results are complete. Repeat tests periodically to as-sess drug efficacy.

• Monitor vital signs, electrolytes, and renal function studies; monitor body weight for fluid retention with extended-spectrum penicillins for possible hypoka-lemia or hypernatremia.

• Coagulation abnormalities, even frank bleeding, can follow high doses, especially of extended-spectrum penicillins; monitor prothrombin times and platelet counts, and assess patient for signs of occult or frank bleeding.

• Monitor patients on long-term therapy for possible superinfection, especially debilitated patients and others receiving immunosuppressants or radiation therapy; monitor closely for fever.

Oral administration

• Give penicillins at least 1 hour before giving bac-teriostatic antibiotics (tetracyclines, erythromycins, and chloramphenicol); these drugs inhibit bacterial cell growth, decreasing rate of penicillin uptake by bacterial cell walls.

• Give oral penicillin at least 1 hour before or 2 hours after meals to enhance gastric absorption; food may or may not decrease absorption. Oral dosage is max-imally absorbed from an empty stomach, but food does not cause significant loss of potency of bacampicillin tablets; food impairs absorption of bacampicillin sus-pension.

• Refrigerate oral suspensions (stable for 14 days); shake well before administering to ensure correct dos-age.

• Because the active metabolite of bacampicillin (am-picillin) is dialyzable, patients undergoing hemodi-alysis may need dosage adjustments.

Information for parents and patient

• Teach signs and symptoms of hypersensitivity and other adverse rections, and emphasize need to report any unusual reactions.

• Teach signs and symptoms of bacterial and fungal superinfection; emphasize need to report signs of in-fection in debilitated patients and others with low resistance from immunosuppressants or irradiation.

• Be sure parents and patient understand how and when to administer drug; urge them to complete entire prescribed regimen, to comply with instructions for around-the-clock dosage, and to keep follow-up ap-pointments.

• Counsel parents to check expiration date of drug and to discard unused drug.

• Tell parents to call if rash, fever, or chills develop, and to report diarrhea promptly. A rash is the most common allergic reaction. However, non-allergic rash may also occur.

bacitracin
Ak-tracin, Baciguent, Baci-IM

• Classification: antibiotic (polypeptide)

How supplied
Available by prescription
Injection: 10,000-unit and 50,000-unit vials
Ophthalmic ointment: 500 units/g
Topical ointment: 500 units/g
Available without prescription in topical ointment combination products containing neomycin, poly-myxin B, and bacitracin

Indications, route, and dosage
†*Antibiotic-associated* Clostridium difficile *diarrhea and colitis*
Adults: 20,000 to 25,000 units P.O. q 6 hours for 7 to 10 days.
Pneumonia or empyema caused by suscepti-ble staphylococci
Infants over 2.5 kg: 1,000 units/kg I.M. daily, divided q 8 to 12 hours. Do not give for more than 12 days.
Infants under 2.5 kg: 900 units/kg I.M. daily, divided q 8 to 12 hours. Do not give for more than 12 days.

Although current labeling indicates bacitracin is only used in infants, adults with susceptible staphy-lococcal infections may receive 10,000 to 25,000 units I.M. q 6 hours (maximum 25,000 units/dose, 100,000 units daily).

Note: Although commercially available bacitracin specifies parenteral pediatric dosage, *pediatric spe-cialists reserve such use for therapy of last resort.*
Topical infections, impetigo, abrasions, cuts, and minor wounds
Children and adults: Apply thin film b.i.d., t.i.d., or more often, depending on severity of condition.

Action and kinetics
• *Antibacterial action:* Bacitracin impairs bacterial cell-wall synthesis, damaging the bacterial plasma membrane and making the cell more vulnerable to osmotic pressure. Drug is effective against many gram-positive organisms, including *Clostridium difficile.* In most cases, however, parenteral bacitracin has been replaced by penicillin and penicillinase-resistant pen-icillins, by cephalosporins for most penicillinase-pro-ducing staphylococci, and by vancomycin for resistant strains. Drug is only minimally active against gram-negative organisms.
• *Kinetics in adults:* With I.M. administration, baci-tracin is absorbed rapidly and completely; serum con-

centrations range from 0.2 to 2 mcg/ml. Bacitracin is not absorbed from the GI tract and not significantly absorbed from intact or denuded skin wounds or mucous membranes. Bacitracin is distributed widely throughout all body organs and fluids except CSF (unless meninges are inflamed). Bacitracin binds to plasma protein only minimally and is not significantly metabolized. When administered I.M., 10% to 40% of dose is excreted by the kidneys.

Contraindications and precautions
Bacitracin is contraindicated in patients with known hypersensitivity or previous toxic reactions to the agent. Bacitracin should be administered cautiously (if at all) to patients with preexisting renal dysfunction because it is nephrotoxic. Topical ointment is contraindicated for application in external ear canal if eardrum is perforated.

Interactions
Systemically administered bacitracin may induce additive damage when given concomitantly with other nephrotoxic drugs. It also may prolong or increase neuromuscular blockade induced by anesthetics or neuromuscular blocking agents.

Effects on diagnostic tests
Urinary sediment tests may show increased protein and cast excretion. Serum creatinine and BUN levels may increase during bacitracin therapy.

Adverse reactions
• DERM: urticaria; rash; stinging and other allergic reactions, such as itching, burning, and swelling of lips or face (with topical application).
• EENT: *ototoxicity.*
• GI: nausea, vomiting, anorexia, diarrhea, rectal itching or burning.
• GU: nephrotoxicity (albuminuria, cylindruria, oliguria, anuria, increased BUN level, tubular and glomerular necrosis).
• HEMA: blood dyscrasias, eosinophilia.
• Local: pain at injection site.
• Other: superinfection, fever, anaphylaxis, neuromuscular blockade, allergic reactions, chest tightness, hypotension, overgrowth of nonsusceptible organisms.
   Note: Drug should be discontinued if renal toxicity occurs or if patient develops hypersensitivity reaction.

Overdose and treatment
With parenteral administration over several days, bacitracin may cause nephrotoxicity. Acute oral overdose may cause nausea, vomiting, and minor GI upset.
   Treatment is supportive.

▶ Special considerations
• Culture and sensitivity tests should be done before treatment starts.
• Obtain baseline renal function studies before starting therapy, and monitor results daily for signs of deterioration.
• Patients allergic to neomycin may also be allergic to bacitracin.

• Injectable forms of the drug may be used for I.M. administration only. I.V. administration may cause severe thrombophlebitis. Dilute injectable drug in solution containing sodium chloride and 2% procaine hydrochloride (if hospital policy permits). After reconstitution, bacitracin concentration should range from 5,000 to 10,000 units/ml. Inject deeply into upper outer quadrant of buttocks (may be painful). Do not give if patient is sensitive to procaine or para-aminobenzoic acid (PABA) derivatives.
• Ensure adequate fluid intake and monitor output closely.
• Monitor patient's urine pH. It should be kept above 6 with good hydration and alkalinizing agents (such as sodium bicarbonate), if necessary, to limit nephrotoxicity.
• Drug may be used orally with neomycin as bowel preparation or in solution as wound irrigating agent.

Information for parents and patient
• Advise parents to discontinue topical use of the drug and to call physician promptly if patient's condition worsens or does not respond to the drug.
• Patient with a skin infection should avoid sharing washcloths and towels with family members and should wash hands before and after applying ointment.
• Advise parents administering ophthalmic ointment to cleanse eye area of excess exudate before applying ointment. Warn them not to touch tip of tube to any part of eye or surrounding tissue.
• Warn parents and patient that ophthalmic ointment may cause blurred vision. Tell them to stop drug immediately and report signs of sensitivity, such as itchy eyelids or constant burning.
• Instruct parents to store ophthalmic ointment in tightly closed, light-resistant container.
• Patient should not share eye medications with others.

---

beclomethasone dipropionate

Nasal inhalants
Beconase, Vancenase

Oral inhalants
Beclovent, Becotide*, Vanceril

• Classification: anti-inflammatory, antiasthmatic agent (glucocorticoid)

How supplied
Available by prescription only
Nasal aerosol: 42 mcg/metered spray
Oral inhalation aerosol: 42 mcg/metered spray

Indications, route, and dosage
Steroid-dependent asthma
Oral inhalation
Children age 6 to 12: One to two inhalations t.i.d. or q.i.d. Maximum of 10 inhalations daily.
Adults: Two to four inhalations t.i.d. or q.i.d. Maximum of 20 inhalations daily.

Perennial or seasonal rhinitis; prevention of recurrence of nasal polyps after surgical removal

Nasal inhalation

Children age 6 to 12: One spray in each nostril t.i.d. (252 mcg daily).

Children and adults over age 12: One spray (42 mcg) in each nostril b.i.d. to q.i.d. Usual total dosage is 168 to 336 mcg daily.

Action and kinetics

• *Anti-inflammatory action:* Beclomethasone stimulates the synthesis of enzymes needed to decrease the inflammatory response. The anti-inflammatory and vasoconstrictor potency of topically applied beclomethasone is, on a weight basis, about 5,000 times greater than that of hydrocortisone, 500 times greater than that of betamethasone or dexamethasone, and about five times greater than that of fluocinolone or triamcinolone.

• *Antiasthmatic action:* Beclomethasone is used as a nasal inhalant to treat symptoms of seasonal or perennial rhinitis and to prevent the recurrence of nasal polyps after surgical removal, and as an oral inhalant to treat bronchial asthma in patients who require chronic administration of corticosteroids to control symptoms.

• *Kinetics in adults:* After nasal inhalation, the drug is absorbed primarily through the nasal mucosa, with minimal systemic absorption. After oral inhalation, the drug is absorbed rapidly from the lungs and GI tract. Greater systemic absorption is associated with oral inhalation, but systemic effects do not occur at usual doses because of rapid metabolism in the liver and local metabolism of drug that reaches the lungs. Onset of action usually occurs in a few days but may take as long as 3 weeks in some patients.

Distribution after intranasal administration has not been described. There is no evidence of tissue storage of beclomethasone or its metabolites. About 10% to 25% of a nasal spray or orally inhaled dose is deposited in the respiratory tract. The remainder, deposited in the mouth and oropharynx, is swallowed. When absorbed, it is 87% bound to plasma proteins.

Beclomethasone that is swallowed undergoes rapid metabolism in the liver or GI tract to a variety of metabolites, some of which have minor glucocorticoid activity. The portion that is inhaled into the respiratory tract is partially metabolized before absorption into systemic circulation. Most of the drug is metabolized in the liver.

Excretion of beclomethasone administered by inhalation has not been described; however, when the drug is administered systemically, its metabolites are excreted mainly in feces via biliary elimination and to a lesser extent in urine. The biological half-life of beclomethasone averages 15 hours.

Contraindications and precautions

Beclomethasone is contraindicated in patients with acute status asthmaticus and in patients who are hypersensitive to any component of the preparation.

Drug should be used with caution in patients receiving systemic corticosteroids, because of increased risk of hypothalamic-pituitary-adrenal axis suppression; when substituting inhalation for oral systemic administration, because withdrawal symptoms may occur; and in patients with tuberculosis, healing nasal septal ulcers, oral or nasal surgery or trauma, or bacterial, fungal, or viral respiratory infection.

Interactions

None reported.

Effects on diagnostic tests

None reported.

Adverse reactions

• EENT: (after oral inhalation) flushing, rash, dry mouth, hoarseness, irritation of the tongue or throat, and impaired sense of taste; (after nasal inhalation) itchy nose, dryness, burning, irritation and sneezing, infrequent epistaxis, bloody mucus.

• Immune: immunosuppression (may allow fungal overgrowth and infections of the nose, mouth, or throat).

Note: Drug should be discontinued if no improvement is evident after 3 weeks, or if nasal or oral infections develop.

Overdose and treatment

No information available.

▶ Special considerations

• In children, systemic corticosteroid therapy may be successfully substituted with nasal or oral inhalant corticosteroid therapy, thus reducing the risk of adverse systemic effects. However, the risk of HPA axis suppression and Cushing's syndrome still exists, particularly if excessive dosages are used. Manifestations of adrenal suppression in children include retardation of linear growth, delayed weight gain, low plasma cortisol concentrations, and lack of response to corticotropin stimulation.

• Beclomethasone is not recommended for children under age 6.

• The therapeutic effects of intranasal inhalants, unlike those of sympathomimetic decongestants, are not immediate. Full therapeutic benefit requires regular use and is usually evident within a few days, although a few patients may require up to 3 weeks of therapy for maximum benefit.

• Use of nasal or oral inhalation therapy may occasionally allow a patient to discontinue systemic corticosteroid therapy. Systemic corticosteroid therapy should be discontinued by gradually tapering the dosage while carefully observing the patient for signs of adrenal insufficiency (joint pain, lassitude, depression).

• After the desired clinical effect is obtained, maintenance dose should be reduced to the smallest amount necessary to control symptoms.

• The drug should be discontinued if the patient develops signs of systemic absorption (including Cushing's syndrome, hyperglycemia, or glucosuria), mucosal irritation or ulceration, hypersensitivity, or infection. (If antifungals or antibiotics are being used with corticosteroids and the infection does not respond immediately, discontinue corticosteroids until the infection is controlled.)

Information for parents and patient

For patients using a *nasal* inhaler

• Instruct patient to use only as directed. Inform him that full therapeutic effect is not immediate but requires regular use of inhaler.

• Encourage patient with blocked nasal passages to use an oral decongestant ½ hour before intranasal corticosteroid administration to ensure adequate penetration. Advise patient to clear nasal pasages of secretions before using the inhaler.

• Ask parents and patient to read manufacturer's instructions and demonstrate use of inhaler. Assist patient until proper use of inhaler is demonstrated.

• Instruct parents and patient to clean inhaler according to manufacturer's instructions.

For patients using an *oral* inhaler

• Instruct parents and patient to use only as directed.

• Advise patient to use the bronchodilator before the corticosteroid inhalant to enhance penetration of the corticosteroid into the bronchial tree. Patient should wait several minutes to allow time for the bronchodilator to relax the smooth muscle.

• Ask parents and patient to read manufacturer's instructions and demonstrate use on inhaler. Assist patient until proper use of inhaler is demonstrated.

• Instruct patient to hold breath for a few seconds to enhance placement and action of the drug and to wait 1 minute before taking subsequent puffs of medication.

• Patient should rinse mouth with water after using the inhaler to decrease the chance of oral fungal infections. Tell parents to check patient's nasal and oral mucous membranes frequently for signs of fungal infection.

• Instruct parents and patient to clean inhaler according to manufacturer's instructions.

• Asthma patients should not increase use of corticosteroid inhaler during a severe asthma attack. Instead, parents should call for adjustment of therapy possibly by adding a systemic steroid.

For patients using *either* type of inhaler

• Tell parents and patient to report decreased response; an adjustment in dosage or discontinuation of the drug may be necessary.

• Instruct parents to observe for adverse effects, and if fever or local irritation develops, to discontinue use and report the effect promptly.

---

bendroflumethiazide
Naturetin

• Classification: diuretic, antihypertensive (thiazide)

How supplied
Available by prescription only
Tablets: 2.5 mg, 5 mg, 10 mg

Indications, route, and dosage
Edema, hypertension
Children: Initially, 0.1 to 0.4 mg/kg or 3 to 12 mg/m^2 daily in one or two doses. Maintenance dosage is 0.05 to 0.1 mg/kg or 9 mg/m^2 daily in one or two doses.

Adults: 2.5 to 20 mg P.O. daily or b.i.d. in divided doses.

Action and kinetics
• *Diuretic action:* Bendroflumethiazide increases urinary excretion of sodium and water by inhibiting sodium reabsorption in the cortical diluting tubule of the nephron, thus relieving edema.

• *Antihypertensive action:* The exact mechanism of bendroflumethiazide's antihypertensive effect is unknown; its effect may partially result from direct arteriolar vasodilation and a decrease in total peripheral resistance.

• *Kinetics in adults:* Bendroflumethiazide is well absorbed from the GI tract. Extent of distribution is unknown. Bendroflumethiazide is excreted unchanged in urine.

Contraindications and precautions
Bendroflumethiazide is contraindicated in patients with anuria and in those with known sensitivity to the drug or to other sulfonamide derivatives. Bendroflumethiazide should be used cautiously in patients with severe renal disease, because it may decrease glomerular filtration rate and precipitate azotemia; in patients with impaired hepatic function or liver disease, because electrolyte changes may precipitate coma; and in patients taking digoxin, because hypokalemia may predispose patients to digitalis toxicity.

Naturetin contains tartrazine, which may cause such allergic reactions as bronchospasm in asthmatic and aspirin-sensitive patients.

Interactions
Bendroflumethiazide potentiates the hypotensive effects of most other antihypertensive drugs; this may be used to therapeutic advantage.

Bendroflumethiazide may potentiate hyperglycemic, hypotensive, and hyperuricemic effects of diazoxide, and its hyperglycemic effect may increase insulin requirements in diabetic patients.

Bendroflumethiazide may reduce renal clearance of lithium, elevating serum lithium levels, and may necessitate a 50% reduction in lithium dosage.

Bendroflumethiazide turns urine slightly more alkaline and may decrease urinary excretion of some amines, such as amphetamine and quinidine; alkaline urine may also decrease therapeutic efficacy of methenamine compounds, such as methenamine mandelate.

Cholestyramine and colestipol may bind bendroflumethiazide, preventing its absorption; administer drugs 1 hour apart.

Effects on diagnostic tests
Bendroflumethiazide therapy may alter serum electrolyte levels and may increase serum urate, glucose, cholesterol, and triglyceride levels.

Bendroflumethiazide may interfere with tests for parathyroid function and should be discontinued before such tests.

Adverse reactions
• CV: volume depletion and dehydration, orthostatic hypotension, hypercholesterolemia, hypertriglyceridemia.
• DERM: dermatitis, photosensitivity, rash.
• GI: anorexia, nausea, pancreatitis.
• HEMA: aplastic anemia, agranulocytosis, leukopenia, thrombocytopenia.
• Hepatic: hepatic encephalopathy.
• Metabolic: asymptomatic hyperuricemia; gout; hyperglycemia and impairment of glucose tolerance; fluid and electrolyte imbalances, including hypokalemia, dilutional hyponatremia and hypochloremia, and hypercalcemia; metabolic acidosis.
• Other: hypersensitivity reactions, such as pneumonitis and vasculitis.
   Note: Drug should be discontinued if rising BUN and serum creatinine levels indicate renal impairment or if patient shows signs of impending coma.

Overdose and treatment
Clinical signs of overdose include GI irritation and hypermotility, diuresis, and lethargy, which may progress to coma.
   Treatment is mainly supportive; monitor and assist respiratory, cardiovascular, and renal function as indicated. Monitor fluid and electrolyte balance. Induce vomiting with ipecac syrup in conscious patient; otherwise, use gastric lavage to avoid aspiration. Do not give cathartics; these promote additional loss of fluids and electrolytes.

▶ Special considerations
• Diuretic effect lasts more than 18 hours, permitting longer dosage intervals.
• Monitor weight and serum electrolyte levels regularly.
• Monitor serum potassium levels; encourage high-potassium diet. Foods rich in potassium include citrus fruits, tomatoes, bananas, dates, and apricots. Watch for signs of hypokalemia (for example, muscle weakness or cramps). Patients also taking digitalis have an increased risk of digitalis toxicity from the potassium-depleting effect of this drug.
• Bendroflumethiazide may be used with potassium-sparing diuretics to attenuate potassium loss.
• Check insulin requirements in patients with diabetes.
• Monitor serum creatinine and BUN levels regularly. Drug is not as effective if these levels are more than twice normal.
• Monitor blood uric acid levels.
• A.M. administration is recommended to prevent nocturia.
• Antihypertensive effects persist for approximately 1 week after discontinuation of the drug.
• Instruct parents to observe for and to report any joint swelling, pain, or redness; these signs may indicate hyperuricemia.

Information for parents and patient
• Explain rationale of therapy and diuretic effects of these drugs.
• Advise parents to watch for and promptly report signs of electrolyte imbalance: weakness, fatigue, muscle cramps, paresthesias, confusion, nausea, vomiting, diarrhea, headache, dizziness, and palpitations.
• Tell parents to report any increased edema or excess diuresis (more than a 2% weight loss or gain) and to record child's weight each morning after voiding and before breakfast on the same scale and wearing the same type of clothing.
• Advise parents to give drug with food to minimize gastric irritation; to encourage child to eat potassium-rich foods, such as citrus fruits, potatoes, dates, raisins, and bananas; and to restrict child's access to salt and high-sodium foods, such as lunch meat, smoked meats, and processed cheeses.
• Tell parents to seek medical approval before giving the patient nonprescription drugs; many contain sodium and potassium and can cause electrolyte imbalances.
• Explain photosensitivity reactions. In thiazide-related photosensitivity, ultraviolet radiation alters drug structure, causing allergic reactions in some persons; such reactions occurs 10 days to 2 weeks after initial sun exposure.
• Warn parents to supervise the child's activities closely to prevent falls and other injuries that may result from dizziness, especially at beginning of therapy.
• Caution patient to change position slowly, especially when rising to upright position, to prevent dizziness from orthostatic hypotension.
• Advise parents to watch patient closely for signs of chest, back, or leg pain, or shortness of breath, and to call immediately if they occur.
• Advise parents to administer drug only as prescribed and at the same time each day, to prevent nighttime diuresis and interrupted sleep.
• Emphasize importance of regular medical follow-up to monitor effectiveness of diuretic therapy.

bentiromide
Chymex

• Classification: pancreatic function test (para-aminobenzoic acid derivative)

How supplied
Available by prescription only
Solution: 500 mg/17.5 ml

Indications, route, and dosage
Screening test for pancreatic exocrine insufficiency
Children age 6 to 12: 14 mg/kg followed with an 8-oz glass of water. Maximum dose is 500 mg.
Children over age 12 and adults: After overnight fast and morning void, administer a single 500-mg dose P.O. and follow with an 8-oz glass of water.
   Give patient another glass of water 2 hours after dose. An additional two glasses of water are recommended during postdosing hours 2 to 6.

Action and kinetics
• *Pancreatic function testing action:* After oral administration, bentiromide is cleaved by the pancreatic enzyme chymotrypsin, causing the release of para-aminobenzoic acid (PABA). This test is not conclusive, because a negative result does not rule out pancreatic disease and a positive result is only a strong indicator of a problem. Confirmatory tests are required.
• *Kinetics in adults:* The absorption process depends on the presence of chymotrypsin in the small intestine. PABA is absorbed after hydrolysis of bentiromide by chymotrypsin; the extent of absorption may be altered by other conditions, including gastric stasis, maldigestion, and malabsorption. The mean peak plasma level in healthy adults is about 6 mcg/ml and occurs in 2 to 3 hours. In patients with chronic pancreatitis, mean peak plasma levels are reduced to 3 mcg/ml and occur in 2 to 6 hours. The distribution into body tissues and fluids has not been determined for bentiromide or PABA. Bentiromide is hydrolyzed in the small intestine, and the metabolites are further broken down in the liver. PABA and its metabolites are excreted in urine.

Contraindications and precautions
Bentiromide is contraindicated in patients with hypersensitivity to bentiromide or PABA; such patients may have an anaphylactic reaction. Drug should be used with caution in pregnancy and breast-feeding, because safety of such use has not been established.

Interactions
When used concomitantly, bentiromide may displace methotrexate from PABA binding sites. Pancreatic enzyme preparations may yield a false-negative result; they should be discontinued 5 days before testing with bentiromide.

Effects on diagnostic tests
Bentiromide therapy alters no other tests, but several factors may invalidate bentiromide test results. Various drugs, including acetaminophen, benzocaine, chloramphenicol, thiazides, lidocaine, PABA preparations, procainamide, procaine, and sulfonamides, are metabolized into arylamines, which increase the PABA content in urine. Foods such as apples, plums, prunes, and cranberries have a similar effect. All of these drugs and foods should be discontinued at least 3 days before testing with bentiromide.

Adverse reactions
• CNS: headache.
• GI: diarrhea, gas, nausea, vomiting.
• Respiratory: shortness of breath (rare).
• Other: weakness.
   Note: Drug should be discontinued if shortness of breath occurs.

Overdose and treatment
No information available.

▶ Special considerations
• A pre-test urine sample may help determine dietary PABA levels.
• Hydrate the patient after administration of benti-

romide by giving 250 ml of water immediately and 250 to 750 ml during the next 6 hours.
• Patient's urine should be collected for exactly 6 hours after administration for analysis.
• Monitor blood glucose levels for possible adjustment of insulin in diabetic patients during fast.

Information for parents and patient
• Tell parents that patient should avoid the medications and foods listed in "Interactions" and "Effects on diagnostic tests" sections for the specified times and should fast after midnight the night before test.
• Have patient void just prior to testing to ensure accurate results.

benzonatate
Tessalon

• Classification: nonnarcotic antitussive agent (local anesthetic [ester])

How supplied
Available by prescription only
Capsules: 100 mg

Indications, route, and dosage
Cough suppression
Children under age 10: 8 mg/kg P.O. in three to six divided doses.
Children over age 10 and adults: 100 mg P.O. t.i.d.; up to 600 mg daily.

Action and kinetics
• *Antitussive action:* Benzonatate suppresses the cough reflex at its source by anesthetizing peripheral stretch receptors located in the respiratory passages, lungs, and pleura.
• *Kinetics in adults:* Action begins within 15 to 20 minutes and lasts for 3 to 8 hours. Distribution, metabolism, and excretion have not been established.

Contraindications and precautions
Benzonatate is contraindicated in patients with a known hypersensitivity to the drug or to related compounds, such as tetracaine.

Interactions
None significant.

Effects on diagnostic tests
None reported.

Adverse reactions
• CNS: dizziness, headache, sedation.
• DERM: rash, eruptions, pruritus.
• EENT: nasal congestion, sensation of burning in eyes.
• GI: nausea, constipation, GI upset.
• Other: chills, chest numbness, hypersensitivity.

Overdose and treatment
CNS stimulation from overdose of drug may cause restlessness and tremors, which may lead to chronic convulsions followed by profound CNS depression.

Empty stomach by gastric lavage and follow with activated charcoal. Treat convulsions with a short-acting barbiturate given I.V; do not use CNS stimulants. Mechanical respiratory support may be necessary in severe cases.

▶ Special considerations
Monitor cough type and frequency and volume and quality of sputum. Encourage fluid intake to help liquefy sputum.

Information for parents and patient
• Instruct parents and patient never to chew or dissolve capsules in the mouth, because local anesthesia will result.
• Teach parents comfort measures for a nonproductive cough: Patient should limit talking; use a cold mist or steam vaporizer; and use sugarless hard candy to increase saliva flow.

---

benzthiazide
Aquatag, Exna, Hydrex, Marazide, Proaqua

• Classification: diuretic, antihypertensive (thiazide)

How supplied
Available by prescription only
Tablets: 25 mg, 50 mg

Indications, route, and dosage
Edema
Children: 1 to 4 mg/kg P.O. or 30 to 120 mg/m^2 daily in three divided doses.
Adults: 50 to 200 mg P.O. daily or in divided doses.

Action and kinetics
• *Diuretic action:* Benzthiazide increases urinary excretion of sodium and water by inhibiting sodium reabsorption in the cortical diluting tubule of the nephron, thereby relieving edema.
• *Antihypertensive action:* The exact mechanism of benzthiazide's antihypertensive effect is unknown; it may be partially because of direct arteriolar vasodilation and a decrease in total peripheral resistance.
• *Kinetics in adults:* Benzthiazide is well absorbed from the GI tract. Diuresis begins within 2 hours. Like other thiazide diuretics, it is thought to enter extracellular space. Peak effect occurs in 3 to 6 hours. Benzthiazide is excreted unchanged in urine.

Contraindications and precautions
Benzthiazide is contraindicated in anuria and in patients with known sensitivity to the drug or other sulfonamide derivatives. Benzthiazide should be used cautiously in patients with severe renal disease, because it may decrease glomerular filtration rate and precipitate azotemia; in patients with impaired hepatic function or liver disease, because electrolyte changes may precipitate coma; and in patients taking digoxin, because hypokalemia may predispose patients to digitalis toxicity.

Aquatag and Exna contain tartrazine, which may cause such allergic reactions as bronchospasm in asthmatic and aspirin-sensitive patients.

Interactions
Benzthiazide potentiates the hypotensive effects of most other antihypertensive drugs; this may be used to therapeutic advantage.

Benzthiazide may potentiate hyperglycemic, hypotensive, and hyperuricemic effects of diazoxide, and its hyperglycemic effect may increase insulin requirements in diabetic patients.

Benzthiazide may reduce renal clearance of lithium, elevating serum lithium levels, and may necessitate reduction in lithium dosage by 50%.

Benzthiazide turns urine slightly more alkaline and may decrease urinary excretion of some amines, such as amphetamine and quinidine; alkaline urine may also decrease therapeutic efficacy of methenamine compounds, such as methenamine mandelate.

Cholestyramine and colestipol may bind benzthiazide, preventing its absorption; give drugs 1 hour apart.

Effects on diagnostic tests
Benzthiazide therapy may alter serum electrolyte levels and may increase serum urate, glucose, cholesterol, and triglyceride levels.

Benzthiazide may interfere with tests for parathyroid function and should be discontinued before such tests.

Adverse reactions
• CV: volume depletion and dehydration, orthostatic hypotension, hypercholesterolemia, hypertriglyceridemia.
• DERM: dermatitis, photosensitivity, rash.
• GI: anorexia, nausea, pancreatitis.
• HEMA: aplastic anemia, agranulocytosis, leukopenia, thrombocytopenia.
• Hepatic: hepatic encephalopathy.
• Metabolic: asymptomatic hyperuricemia; gout; hyperglycemia and impairment of glucose tolerance; fluid and electrolyte imbalances, including hypokalemia, dilutional hyponatremia and hypochloremia, and hypercalcemia; metabolic alkalosis.
• Other: hypersensitivity reactions, such as pneumonitis and vasculitis.

Note: Drug should be discontinued if rising BUN and serum creatinine levels indicate renal impairment or if patient shows signs of hypersensitivity reaction or impending coma.

Overdose and treatment
Clinical signs of overdose include GI irritation and hypermotility, diuresis, and lethargy, which may progress to coma.

Treatment is mainly supportive; monitor and assist respiratory, cardiovascular, and renal function as indicated. Monitor fluid and electrolyte balance. Induce vomiting with ipecac in conscious patient; otherwise,

---

use gastric lavage to avoid aspiration. Do not give cathartics; these promote additional loss of fluids and electrolytes.

▶ **Special considerations**
• Monitor weight and serum electrolyte levels regularly.
• Monitor serum potassium levels; encourage high-potassium diet. Foods rich in potassium include citrus fruits, tomatoes, bananas, dates, and apricots. Watch for signs of hypokalemia (for example, muscle weakness or cramps). Patients also taking digitalis have an increased risk of digitalis toxicity from the potassium-depleting effect of this drug.
• Benzthiazide may be used with potassium-sparing diuretics to attenuate potassium loss.
• Check insulin requirements in patients with diabetes.
• Monitor serum creatinine and BUN levels regularly. Drug is not as effective if these levels are more than twice normal.
• Monitor blood uric acid levels.
• A.M. administration is recommended to prevent nocturia.
• Antihypertensive effects persist for approximately 1 week after discontinuation of the drug.
• Instruct parents to observe for and to report any joint swelling, pain, or redness; these signs may indicate hyperuricemia.

Information for parents and patient
• Explain rationale of therapy and diuretic effects of drug.
• Advise parents to watch for and promptly report signs of electrolyte imbalance: weakness, fatigue, muscle cramps, paresthesias, confusion, nausea, vomiting, diarrhea, headache, dizziness, and palpitations.
• Tell parents to report any increased edema or excess diuresis (more than a 2% weight loss or gain), and to record child's weight each morning after voiding and before breakfast on the same scale and wearing the same type of clothing.
• Advise parents to give drug with food to minimize gastric irritation; to encourage child to eat potassium-rich foods, such as citrus fruits, potatoes, dates, raisins, and bananas; and to restrict child's access to salt and high-sodium foods, such as lunch meat, smoked meats, and processed cheeses.
• Tell parents to seek medical approval before giving the patient nonprescription drugs; many contain sodium and potassium and can cause electrolyte imbalances.
• Explain photosensitivity reactions. In thiazide-related photosensitivity, ultraviolet radiation alters drug structure, causing allergic reactions in some persons; such reactions occurs 10 days to 2 weeks after initial sun exposure.
• Warn parents to supervise the child's activities closely to prevent falls and other injuries that may result from dizziness, especially at beginning of therapy.
• Caution patient to change position slowly, especially when rising to upright position, to prevent dizziness from orthostatic hypotension.
• Advise parents to watch patient closely for signs of

chest, back, or leg pain, or shortness of breath, and to call immediately if they occur.
• Advise parents to administer drug only as prescribed and at the same time each day, to prevent nighttime diuresis and interrupted sleep.
• Emphasize importance of regular medical follow-up to monitor effectiveness of diuretic therapy.

betamethasone
Systemic: Betnelan★, Celestone

betamethasone benzoate
Topical: Beben★, Benisone, Uticort

betamethasone dipropionate
Topical: Alphatrex, Diprolene Ointment, Diprosone

betamethasone sodium phosphate
Systemic: Betnesol★, BSP, Celestone Phosphate, Prelestone, Selestoject

betamethasone sodium phosphate and betamethasone acetate
Systemic: Celestone Soluspan

betamethasone valerate
Topical: Betacort★, Betaderm★, Betatrex, Beta-Val, Betnovate★, Celestoderm-V★ Ectosone★, Metaderm★, Novobetamet★, Valisone★

• Classification: anti-inflammatory (glucocorticoid)

How supplied
Available by prescription only
Betamethasone
Syrup: 600 mcg/5 ml
Tablets: 600 mcg
Tablets (extended-release): 1 mg
Betamethasone benzoate
Lotion, ointment, gel, cream: 0.025%
Betamethasone dipropionate
Lotion, ointment, cream: 0.05%
Aerosol: 0.1%
Betamethasone sodium phosphate
Effervescent tablets★: 500 mcg
Injection: 4 mg (3 mg base)/ml in 5-ml vials
Enema★: 5 mg (base)
Betamethasone sodium phosphate and betamethasone acetate suspension
Injection: betamethasone acetate 3 mg and betamethasone sodium phosphate (equivalent to 3 mg base) per ml
Betamethasone valerate
Lotion, ointment: 0.1%;
Cream: 0.01%, 0.1%
Aerosol solution: 0.1%

Indications, route, and dosage

Severe inflammation or immunosuppression

Adults: 0.6 to 7.2 mg or 2 to 6 mg (extended-release) P.O. daily.

Betamethasone sodium phosphate

Adults: 0.5 to 9 mg I.M., I.V., or into joint or soft tissue daily.

Betamethasone sodium phosphate and betamethasone acetate suspension

Children: 0.0625 to 0.25 mg/kg P.O. divided t.i.d. or q.i.d.; or 21 to 125 mcg/kg I.M. or 625 mcg to 3.75 mg/m² q 12 to 24 hours.

Adults: 1.5 to 12 mg into joint or soft tissue q 1 to 2 weeks, p.r.n.

Adrenocortical insufficiency

Children: 17.5 mcg/kg P.O. daily or 500 mcg/m² P.O. daily in three or four divided doses; or 17.5 mcg/kg or 500 mg/m² I.M. q 3 days.

Adults: 0.6 to 7.2 mg P.O. daily, or up to 9 mg I.M. or I.V. daily.

Inflammation of corticosteroid-responsive dermatoses

Betamethasone

Children: Apply sparingly to affected areas once a day.

Adults: Apply sparingly to affected areas two or three times daily.

Betamethasone benzoate

Children: Apply cream, gel, lotion, or ointment sparingly to affected areas once a day.

Adults: Apply cream, gel, lotion, or ointment sparing to affected areas two or three times daily.

Betamethasone dipropionate

Children: Apply cream, lotion, ointment or aerosol spray sparingly to affected areas once a day.

Adults: Apply cream, or ointment sparingly to affected areas once or twice daily. Apply topical aerosol as a 3-second spray three times a day. Apply lotion to affected areas twice a day.

Betamethasone valerate

Children: Apply 0.01% cream to affected areas once or twice a day. Apply 0.1% cream, lotion, or ointment to affected areas once a day.

Adults: Apply cream or ointment to affected areas one to three times a day. Apply lotion to affected areas once or twice a day.

Action and kinetics

• *Anti-inflammatory action:* Betamethasone stimulates the synthesis of enzymes needed to decrease the inflammatory response. Betamethasone is a long-acting steroid with an anti-inflammatory potency 25 times that of an equal weight of hydrocortisone. It has essentially no mineralocorticoid activity. Betamethasone tablets and syrup are used as oral anti-inflammatory agents. Betamethasone sodium phosphate is highly soluble, has a prompt onset of action, and may be given I.V. Betamethasone sodium phosphate and betamethasone acetate (Celestone Soluspan) combines the rapid-acting phosphate salt and the slightly soluble, slowly released acetate salt to provide rapid anti-inflammatory effects with a sustained duration of action. It is a suspension and should not be given I.V. It is particularly useful as an anti-inflammatory agent in intra-articular, intradermal, and intralesional injections.

• *Kinetics in adults:* Betamethasone is absorbed readily after oral administration. After oral and I.V. administration, peak effects occur in 1 to 2 hours. Onset and duration of action of the suspensions for injection vary, depending on whether they are injected into an intra-articular space or a muscle, and on the local blood supply. Systemic absorption occurs slowly following intra-articular injections.

The amount absorbed after topical use depends on the potency of the preparation, the amount applied, and the skin at the application site. It ranges from about 1% in areas with a thick stratum corneum (such as the palms, soles, elbows, and knees) to as high as 36% in areas with a thin stratum corneum (face, eyelids, and genitals). Absorption increases in areas of skin damage, inflammation, or occlusion. Some systemic absorption of topical steroids occurs, especially through the oral mucosa.

After topical application, betamethasone is distributed throughout the local skin and metabolized primarily in the skin. Any drug absorbed is removed rapidly from the blood, distributed into various tissues (muscle, liver, skin, intestines, and kidneys), and metabolized primarily in the liver to inactive glucuronide and sulfate metabolites. The inactive metabolites and small amounts of unmetabolized drug are excreted by the kidneys. Insignificant quantities of drug are also excreted in feces. The biological half-life of betamethasone is 36 to 54 hours.

Contraindications and precautions

Betamethasone is contraindicated in patients with hypersensitivity to ingredients of adrenocorticoid preparations or with systemic fungal infections. Patients who are receiving betamethasone should not be given live virus vaccines because betamethasone suppresses the immune response.

Betamethasone should be used with extreme caution in patients with GI ulceration, renal disease, hypertension, osteoporosis, diabetes mellitus, thromboembolic disorders, idiopathic thrombocytopenic purpura, seizures, myasthenia gravis, congestive heart failure (CHF), tuberculosis, hypoalbuminemia, hypothyroidism, cirrhosis of the liver, emotional instability, psychotic tendencies, hyperlipidemias, glaucoma, or cataracts, because the drug may exacerbate these conditions.

Because adrenocorticoids increase susceptibility to and mask symptoms of infection, betamethasone should not be used (except in life-threatening situations) in patients with viral or bacterial infections not controlled by anti-infective agents.

Topical use of betamethasone is contraindicated in patients who are hypersensitive to any component of the preparation and in patients with viral, fungal, or tubercular skin lesions. It should be used with extreme caution in patients with impaired circulation, because it may increase the risk of skin ulceration.

Interactions

When used concomitantly, betamethasone may decrease the effects of oral anticoagulants (rarely); increase the metabolism of isoniazid and salicylates;

and cause hyperglycemia, requiring dosage adjustment of insulin in diabetic patients. Use with barbiturates, phenytoin, and rifampin may cause decreased corticosteroid effects because of increased hepatic metabolism. Use with cholestyramine, colestipol, and antacids decreases betamethasone's effect by adsorbing the corticosteroid, decreasing the amount absorbed.

Betamethasone may enhance hypokalemia associated with diuretic or amphotericin B therapy. The hypokalemia may increase the risk of toxicity in patients concurrently receiving digitalis glycosides.

Concomitant use with estrogens may reduce the metabolism of corticosteroids by increasing the concentrations of transcortin. The half-life of the corticosteroid is then prolonged because of increased protein binding. Concomitant administration of ulcerogenic drugs such as nonsteroidal anti-inflammatory agents may increase the risk of GI ulceration.

Effects on diagnostic tests

Adrenocorticoid therapy suppresses reactions to skin tests, causes false-negative results in the nitroblue tetrazolium tests for systemic bacterial infections, and decreases ^{131}I uptake and protein-bound iodine concentrations in thyroid function tests.

It may increase glucose and cholesterol levels; decrease serum potassium, calcium, thyroxine, and triiodothyronine levels; and increase urine glucose and calcium levels.

Adverse reactions

When administered in high doses or for prolonged therapy, betamethasone suppresses release of adrenocorticotropic hormone (ACTH) from the pituitary gland; the adrenal cortex then stops secreting endogenous corticosteroids. The degree and duration of hypothalamic-pituitary-adrenal (HPA) axis suppression produced is highly variable among patients and depends on the dose, time, and frequency of administration, and duration of glucocorticoid therapy. In children, it may cause premature closure of the epiphyseal growth plates.

• CNS: euphoria, insomnia, headache, psychotic behavior, pseudotumor cerebri, mental changes, nervousness, restlessness, *psychoses*.
• CV: CHF, *hypertension*, edema.
• DERM: delayed healing, *acne*, skin eruptions, striae.
• EENT: *cataracts*, glaucoma, thrush.
• GI: *peptic ulcer*, irritation, increased appetite.
• Immune: immunosuppression, *increased susceptibility to infection*.
• Metabolic: *hypokalemia*, sodium retention, fluid retention, weight gain, hyperglycemia, *osteoporosis*, growth suppression in children, *glycosuria*.
• Musculoskeletal: muscle atrophy, weakness, *myopathy*.
• Other: pancreatitis, *hirsutism, cushingoid symptoms*, withdrawal syndrome (nausea, fatigue, anorexia, dyspnea, hypotension, hypoglycemia, myalgia, arthralgia, fever, dizziness, and fainting), ecchymoses. Sudden withdrawal may be fatal or may exacerbate the underlying disease. Acute adrenal insufficiency may follow increased stress (infection,

surgery, trauma) or abrupt withdrawal after long-term therapy.

Note: Topical should be discontinued if local irritation, infection, systemic absorption, or hypersensitivity reaction occurs.

Overdose and treatment

Acute ingestion, even in massive doses, is rarely a clinical problem. Toxic signs and symptoms rarely occur if drug is used for less than 3 weeks, even at large doses. However, chronic use causes adverse physiologic effects, including suppression of the HPA axis, cushingoid appearance, muscle weakness, and osteoporosis.

▶ Special considerations

• Investigational use includes prevention of respiratory distress syndrome in premature infants (hyaline membrane disease). Give 6 mg (2 ml) of Celestone Soluspan I.M. once daily 24 to 36 hours before induced delivery.
• Chronic use of betamethasone in children and adolescents may delay growth and maturation.
• If possible, avoid long-term administration of pharmacologic dosages of glucocorticoids in children because these drugs may retard bone growth. Manifestations of adrenal suppression in children include retardation of linear growth, delayed weight gain, low plasma cortisol concentrations, and lack of response to corticotropin stimulation. In children who require prolonged therapy, closely monitor growth and development. Alternate-day therapy is recommended to minimize growth suppression.
• Establish baseline blood pressure, fluid intake and output, weight, and electrolyte status. Watch for any sudden patient weight gain, edema, change in blood pressure, or change in electrolyte status.
• During times of physiologic stress (trauma, surgery, infection), the patient may require additional steroids and may experience signs of steroid withdrawal; patients who were previously steroid-dependent may need systemic corticosteroids to prevent adrenal insufficiency.
• After long-term therapy, the drug should be reduced gradually. Rapid reduction may cause withdrawal symptoms.
• Be aware of the patient's psychological history and watch for any behavioral changes.
• Observe for signs of infection or delayed wound healing.
• Acute withdrawal of drug may result in fever, myalgia, arthralgia, malaise, hypotension, hypoglycemia, and shock.

Topical use

• Diprolene Ointment may suppress the HPA axis at doses as low as 7 g per day. Patient should not use more than 45 g per week and should not use occlusive dressings. Treatment with Diprolene Ointment is not recommended in children under age 12.
• *Pediatric patients may demonstrate greater susceptibility to topical corticosteroid-induced HPA axis suppression and Cushing's syndrome than mature patients because of a higher ratio of skin surface area to body weight.* HPA axis suppression, Cushing's syndrome, and intracranial hypertension have been re-

ported in children receiving topical corticosteroids. Signs of adrenal suppression in children include linear growth retardation, delayed weight gain, low plasma cortisol levels, and absence of response to ACTH stimulation. Signs of intracranial hypertension include bulging fontanelles, headaches, and bilateral papilledema.

• Administration of topical corticosteroids to children should be limited to the least effective amount. Chronic corticosteroid therapy may interfere with growth and development.

• Stop drug if the patient develops signs of systemic absorption (including Cushing's syndrome, hyperglycemia, or glucosuria), skin irritation or ulceration, hypersensitivity, or infection. (If antifungals or antibiotics are being used with betamethasone and the infection does not respond immediately, betamethasone should be discontinued until infection is controlled.)

Information for parents and patient
• Be sure that the parents and patient understand that patient must use betamethasone exactly as prescribed. Give the patient instructions on what to do if a dose is inadvertently missed.

• Warn the parents and patient not to discontinue the drug abruptly.

• Inform the parents and patient of the possible therapeutic and adverse effects of the drug, so that they may report any complications as soon as possible.

• Advise the parents that the patient should wear a Medic Alert bracelet or necklace indicating the need for supplemental adrenocorticoids during times of stress.

• Instruct parents and patient in application of the drug. Tell them the following:

Method for applying topical preparations
• Wash your hands before and after applying the drug.
• Gently cleanse the area of application. Washing or soaking the area before application may increase drug penetration.

• Apply sparingly in a light film; rub in lightly. Avoid contact with patient's eyes.

• Avoid prolonged application on the face, in skin folds, and in areas near the eyes, genitals, and rectum. High-potency topical corticosteroids are more likely to cause striae in these areas because of their higher rates of absorption.

• Monitor patient response. Observe area of inflammation and elicit patient comments concerning pruritus. Inspect skin for infection, striae, and atrophy. Skin atrophy is common and may be clinically significant within 3 to 4 weeks of treatment with high-potency preparations; it also occurs more readily at sites where percutaneous absorption is high.

• Do not apply occlusive dressings over topical steroids because this may lead to secondary infection, maceration, atrophy, striae, or miliaria caused by increasing steroid penetration and potency.

• If an occlusive dressing is necessary, minimize adverse reactions by using it intermittently. Do not leave it in place longer than 16 hours each day.

• Warn patient not to use nonprescription topical preparations other than those specifically recommended.

• Advise parents to avoid exposing treated areas to

sunlight. Tell them not to use tight-fitting diapers or plastic pants on a child being treated in the diaper area, since such garments may serve as occlusive dressings.

---

bethanechol chloride
Duvoid, Myotonachol, Urabeth, Urecholine

• Classification: urinary tract and GI tract stimulant (cholinergic agonist)

How supplied
Available by prescription only
Tablets: 5 mg, 10 mg, 25 mg, 50 mg
Injection: 5 mg/ml

Indications, route, and dosage
Acute postoperative nonobstructive (functional) urinary retention, neurogenic atony of urinary bladder with retention, abdominal distention, megacolon
Children over age 8: 0.6 mg/kg/day P.O. or 0.15 to 0.20 mg/kg S.C. t.i.d. or q.i.d.
Adults: 10 to 50 mg P.O. b.i.d., t.i.d., or q.i.d. Or 2.5 to 10 mg S.C. *Never give I.M. or I.V.* When used for urinary retention, some patients may require 50 to 100 mg P.O. per dose. Use such doses with extreme caution. Test dose: 2.5 mg S.C. repeated at 15- to 30-minute intervals to total of four doses to determine the minimal effective dose; then use minimal effective dose q 6 to 8 hours. Adjust dosage to meet individual requirements.

Action and kinetics
• *Urinary tract stimulant action:* Bethanechol directly binds to and stimulates muscarinic receptors of the parasympathetic nervous system. That increases tone of the bladder's detrusor muscle, usually resulting in contraction, decreased bladder capacity, and subsequent urination.

• *GI stimulant action:* Bethanechol directly stimulates cholinergic receptors, leading to increased gastric tone and motility and peristalsis restoration in patients with abdominal distention or megacolon. Bethanechol improves lower esophageal sphincter tone by directly stimulating cholinergic receptors, thereby alleviating gastric reflux.

• *Kinetics in adults:* Bethanechol is poorly absorbed from the GI tract (absorption varies considerably among patients). After oral administration, action usually begins in 30 to 90 minutes; after S.C. administration, in 5 to 15 minutes. Distribution is largely unknown; however, therapeutic doses do not penetrate the blood-brain barrier. Metabolism is unknown. Usual duration of effect after oral administration is 1 hour; after S.C. administration, up to 2 hours. Excretion is unknown.

Contraindications and precautions
Bethanechol is contraindicated in patients with uncertain bladder wall strength or integrity; in patients

---

for whom increased muscular activity of the GI or urinary tract poses a risk; in patients with mechanical obstruction of the GI or urinary tract because of drug's stimulatory effect on smooth muscle; in patients with bradycardia, vagotonia, hyperthyroidism, hypotension, or Parkinson's disease, because the drug may exacerbate these conditions; in patients with epilepsy because of the drug's possible CNS stimulatory effects; in patients with cardiac or coronary artery disease because of stimulatory effects on the cardiovascular system; in patients with peptic ulcer, because drug may stimulate gastric acid secretion; and in patients with asthma, because the drug may precipitate asthma attacks.

Administer bethanechol cautiously to patients with hypertension and vasomotor instability, because of its stimulatory effects, and to patients with peritonitis or other acute GI inflammatory conditions, because the drug may aggravate these conditions.

Interactions
Concomitant use with procainamide and quinidine may reverse bethanechol's cholinergic effect on muscle. Concomitant use with ganglionic blockers, such as mecamylamine, may cause a critical blood pressure decrease; this effect is usually preceded by abdominal symptoms.

Effects on diagnostic tests
Bethanechol increases serum levels of amylase, lipase, bilirubin, and AST (SGOT), and increases sulfobromophthalein retention time.

Adverse reactions
• CNS: headache, malaise.
• CV: bradycardia, *orthostatic hypotension,* cardiac arrest, reflex tachycardia, transient syncope, complete heart block, and decreased diastolic blood pressure.
• DERM: *flushing,* sweating.
• EENT: lacrimation, miosis.
• GI: abdominal cramps, diarrhea, *salivation, nausea,* vomiting, belching, borborygmus, involuntary defecation, colicky pain.
• GU: urinary retention, urinary urgency.
• Other: *bronchospasm,* increased bronchial secretions, asthma attack, substernal pressure or pain from bronchoconstriction or esophageal spasm.
   Note: Drug should be discontinued if difficulty breathing, restlessness or agitation, incoordination, blood pressure changes, hypersensitivity, or skin rash occurs.

Overdose and treatment
Clinical signs of overdose include nausea, vomiting, abdominal cramps, diarrhea, involuntary defecation, urinary urgency, excessive salivation, miosis, excessive tearing, bronchospasm, increased bronchial secretions, hypotension, excessive sweating, bradycardia or reflex tachycardia, and substernal pain.

Treatment requires discontinuation of the drug and administration of atropine by S.C., I.M., or I.V. route. (Atropine must be administered cautiously; an overdose could cause bronchial plug formation.)

▶ **Special considerations**
• Regularly monitor patient's vital signs, especially heart rate and respirations, and fluid intake and output; evaluate for changes in muscle strength and observe closely for adverse drug reactions or signs of acute toxicity.
• Impose safety precautions. Patient may become restless or have hallucinations and may need assistance with ambulation.
• Never give bethanechol I.M. or I.V., because that could cause circulatory collapse, hypotension, severe abdominal cramps, bloody diarrhea, shock, or cardiac arrest. Give only by subcutaneous route when giving parenterally.
• For administration to treat urinary retention, bedpan should be readily available.
• For administration to prevent abdominal distention and GI distress, insertion of a rectal tube will facilitate passage of gas.
• Give bethanechol on an empty stomach; eating soon after drug administration may cause nausea and vomiting.
• Patients with hypertension receiving bethanechol may experience a precipitous drop in blood pressure.

Information for parents and patient
• Instruct parents to have patient take medication exactly as ordered; patient may take drug with food and milk to reduce gastric irritation, if appropriate.
• Advise parents to report dyspnea, irregular pulse rate, increased salivation, nausea, vomiting, diarrhea, severe abdominal pain, muscle weakness, or sweating.

---

bitolterol mesylate
Tornalate

• Classification: bronchodilator (adrenergic, beta₂ agonist)

How supplied
Available by prescription only
Aerosol inhaler: 370 mcg/metered spray

Indications, route, and dosage
To prevent and treat bronchial asthma and bronchospasm
Children age 12 and older and adults: For symptomatic relief of bronchospasm, two inhalations at an interval of at least 1 to 3 minutes followed by a third inhalation, if needed; to prevent bronchospasm, two inhalations q 8 hours. Usually, dose should not exceed three inhalations q 6 hours or two inhalations q 4 hours. However, because deposition of inhaled medications is variable, higher doses are occasionally used, especially in patients with acute bronchospasm.

Action and kinetics
• *Bronchodilator action:* Bitolterol selectively stimulates beta₂-adrenergic receptors of the lungs. Bronchodilation results from relaxation of bronchial smooth muscles, which relieves bronchospasm and reduces

airway resistance. Some cardiovascular stimulation may occur as a result of beta$_1$-adrenergic stimulation, including mild tachycardia, palpitations, and changes in blood pressure or heart rate.

• *Kinetics in adults:* After oral inhalation, bronchodilation results from local action on the bronchial tree, with most of the inhaled dose being swallowed. Onset of action occurs within 3 to 5 minutes, peaks in ½ to 2 hours, and lasts 4 to 8 hours. Bitolterol is widely distributed throughout the body. Bitolterol is hydrolyzed by esterases to active metabolites. After oral administration, bitolterol and its metabolites are excreted primarily in urine.

Contraindications and precautions
Bitolterol is contraindicated in patients with known hypersensitivity to drug. Administer cautiously to patients with cardiovascular disorders (ischemic heart disease, hypertension, or cardiac dysrhythmias), hyperthyroidism, diabetes, seizure disorders, or sensitivity to other sympathomimetic amines.

Interactions
Concomitant use with other orally inhaled beta-adrenergic agonists may produce additive sympathomimetic effects. Evidence suggests that cardiotoxic effects may be increased when bitolterol is used with a theophylline salt, such as aminophylline.

Propranolol and other beta blockers may antagonize the effects of bitolterol.

Effects on diagnostic tests
Bitolterol therapy may increase AST (SGOT) levels and decrease platelet or leukocyte count. Proteinuria may also occur.

Adverse reactions
• CNS: tremors, nervousness, dizziness, headache, insomnia, light-headedness, hyperkinesia.
• CV: palpitations, tachycardia, chest discomfort, premature ventricular contractions, flushing, changes in blood pressure.
• EENT: throat irritation.
• GI: nausea, vomiting, unusual taste, irritation of oropharynx, increased appetite, heartburn.
• Other: dyspnea, cough, dyspepsia, bronchospasm.
   Note: Drug should be discontinued if hypersensitivity or bronchoconstriction occurs.

Overdose and treatment
Clinical manifestations of overdose include exaggeration of common adverse reactions, especially dysrhythmias, extreme tremors, nausea, and vomiting.

Treatment requires supportive measures. To reverse effects, use selective beta$_1$-adrenergic blockers (acebutolol, atenolol, metaprolol) with extreme caution (may induce asthmatic attack). Monitor vital signs and ECG closely.

▶ Special considerations
• The preservative sodium bisulfite is present in many adrenergic formulations. Patients with a history of allergy to sulfites should avoid preparations that contain this preservative.
• Therapy should be administered when patient arises

in morning and before meals to reduce fatigue by improving lung ventilation.
• Adrenergic inhalation may be alternated with other adrenergics if necessary, but should not be administered simultaneously because of danger of excessive tachycardia.
• Do not use discolored or precipitated solutions.
• Protect solutions from light, freezing, and heat. Store at controlled room temperature.
• Systemic absorption can follow applications to nasal and conjunctival membranes, though infrequently. If symptoms of systemic absorption occur, patient should stop using the drug.
• Prolonged or too-frequent use may cause tolerance to bronchodilating and cardiac stimulant effect. Rebound bronchospasm may follow end of drug effect.
• Repeated use may result in paradoxical bronchospasm. Discontinue immediately if this occurs.

Information for parents and patient
• Treatment should start with first symptoms of bronchospasm.
• Dosage and recommended method of inhaling may vary with type of nebulizer and formulation used. Tell parents and patient to use only as directed and not to use more than prescribed amount or more often than prescribed. Information and instructions are furnished with the aerosol forms of these drugs. Urge parents and patient to read them carefully and ask questions if necessary.
• Give parents and patient instructions on proper use of inhaler:
  — Administration by metered-dose nebulizers: Shake canister to activate; place mouthpiece well into mouth, aimed at back of throat. Close lips and teeth around mouthpiece. Exhale through nose, then inhale through mouth slowly and deeply while actuating the nebulizer to release dose. Breath hold 10 seconds (count "1-100, 2-100, 3-100" to "10-100"); remove mouthpiece, then exhale slowly.
  — Administration by metered powder inhaler: Caution patient not to take forced deep breaths, but to breathe normally. Observe patient closely for exaggerated systemic drug action.
  — Patients requiring more than three aerosol treatments within 24 hours should be under close medical supervision.
  — Administration by oxygen aerosolization: Administer over 15 to 20 minutes, with oxygen flow rate adjusted to 4 liters/minute. Turn on oxygen supply before patient places nebulizer in mouth. (Patient need not close lips tightly around nebulizer opening.) Placement of Y tube in rubber tubing permits patient to control administration. Advise patient to rinse mouth immediately after inhalation therapy to help prevent dryness and throat irritation. Rinse mouthpiece with warm running water at least once daily to prevent clogging. (It is not dishwasher-safe.) Wait until mouthpiece is dry before storing. Do not place near artificial heat (dishwasher or oven). Replace reservoir bag every 2 to 3 weeks or as needed; replace mouthpiece every 6 to 9 months or as needed. Replacement of bags or mouthpieces may require a prescription.
• Instruct patient to wait 1 full minute after initial one or two inhalations to be sure of necessity for

another dose. Drug action should begin immediately and peak within 5 to 15 minutes.

• Teach parents and patient that a single aerosol treatment is usually enough to control an asthma attack and to call promptly if the patient requires more than three aerosol treatments in 24 hours. Explain that overuse of adrenergic bronchodilators may cause tachycardia, palpitations, headache, nausea and dizziness, loss of effectiveness, possible paradoxical reaction, and cardiac arrest.

• To ensure proper delivery of dose, plastic mouthpiece should be cleaned with warm tap water and dried thoroughly at least once daily. Tell patient that dryness of mouth and throat may occur, but that rinsing with water after each dose may help.

• Tell parents to call promptly if troubled breathing persists 1 hour after using drug, if symptoms return within 4 hours, if condition worsens, if new (refill) canister is needed within 2 weeks, or if bronchodilator causes dizziness or chest pain.

• Tell parents and patient to wait 15 minutes after use of bitolterol before using adrenocorticoid inhaler.

• Tell parents that patient should avoid other adrenergic medications unless they are prescribed.

• Inform parents and patient that saliva and sputum may appear pink after inhalation treatment.

• Caution patient to keep spray away from eyes.

• Explain that increased fluid intake facilitates clearing of secretions. Teach parents and patient how to accomplish postural drainage, to cough productively, and to clap and vibrate to promote good respiratory hygiene.

• Inform parents and patient taking repeated doses about adverse reactions, and advise them to report such reactions promptly.

• Tell parents and patient not to discard drug applicator. Refill units are available.

---

bleomycin sulfate
Blenoxane

• Classification: antineoplastic (antibiotic [cell cycle-phase specific, G_2 and M phase])

How supplied
Available by prescription only
Injection: 15-unit ampules (1 unit = 1 mg)

Indications, route, and dosage
Dosage and indications may vary. Check literature for current protocol.
Hodgkin's disease, squamous cell carcinoma, osteosarcoma, non-Hodgkin's lymphoma, or testicular carcinoma
Children and adults: 10 to 20 units/m² (0.25 to 0.5 units/kg) I.V., I.M., or S.C., one or two times weekly. After 50% reduction in tumor size, maintenance dose of 1 unit daily or 5 units weekly. Reduce dosage when used in combination with other agents.

Action and kinetics
• *Antineoplastic action:* The exact mechanism of bleomycin's cytotoxicity is unknown. Its action may be through scission of single- and double-stranded DNA and inhibition of DNA, RNA, and protein synthesis. Bleomycin also appears to inhibit cell progression out of the G_2 phase.

• *Kinetics in adults:* Bleomycin is poorly absorbed across the GI tract following oral administration. I.M. administration results in lower serum levels than those occurring after equivalent I.V. doses. Bleomycin distributes widely into total body water, mainly in the skin, lungs, kidneys, peritoneum, and lymphatic tissue. Its metabolic fate is unknown; however, extensive tissue inactivation occurs in the liver and kidney and much less in the skin and lungs. Bleomycin and its metabolites are excreted primarily in urine. The terminal plasma elimination phase half-life is reported at 2 hours.

Contraindications and precautions
Bleomycin is contraindicated in patients with a history of hypersensitivity or idiosyncratic reaction to the drug. Use with caution in patients with renal impairment because drug accumulation may occur; also use cautiously in patients with pulmonary impairment and monitor the patient carefully for signs of pulmonary toxicity, because pulmonary fibrosis may occur. Patient should have chest X-rays every 1 to 2 weeks during therapy, and evaluation of pulmonary diffusion capacity for carbon dioxide every month.

Interactions
Concomitant use with vincristine increases the effectiveness of bleomycin. The proposed mechanism is that vincristine arrests cells in mitosis, making them more susceptible to bleomycin. Bleomycin may decrease oral bioavailability of diagoxin and phenytoin.

Effects on diagnostic tests
Bleomycin therapy may increase blood and urine concentrations of uric acid.

Adverse reactions
• CNS: hyperesthesia of scalp and fingers, headache.
• DERM: *rash,* erythema, vesiculation, and hardening and discoloration of palmar and plantar skin in 8% of patients; desquamation of hands, feet, and pressure areas; hyperpigmentation; acne.
• GI: *stomatitis,* prolonged anorexia in 13% of patients, *nausea, vomiting,* diarrhea.
• Respiratory: fine crackles, fever, dyspnea, nonproductive cough; *dose-limiting pulmonary fibrosis* in 10% of patients, *pneumonitis.*
• Other: reversible alopecia, swelling of interphalangeal joints, leukocytosis, *allergic reaction* (fever up to 106° F. [41.1° C.] with chills up to 5 hours after injection; *anaphylaxis* in 1% to 6% of patients), *Raynaud's phenomenon.*
   Note: Drug should be discontinued if patient develops signs of pulmonary fibrosis or mucocutaneous toxicity.

Overdose and treatment
Clinical manifestations of overdose include pulmonary fibrosis, fever, chills, vesiculation, and hyperpigmentation.

Treatment is usually supportive and includes antipyretics for fever.

▶ Special considerations
• Vital signs and patency of catheter or I.V. line should be monitored throughout administration.
• Carefully follow all established procedures for the safe and proper handling, administration, and disposal of chemotherapy.
• Treat extravasation promptly.
• Attempt to ease anxiety in patient and family before treatment.
• Monitor BUN, hematocrit, platelet count, ALT (SGPT), AST (SGOT), LDH, serum bilirubin, serum creatinine, uric acid, and total and differential leukocytes.
• To prepare solution for I.M. administration, reconstitute the drug with 1 to 5 ml of normal saline solution, sterile water for injection, or dextrose 5% in water.
• For I.V. administration, dilute with a minimum of 5 ml of diluent and administer over 10 minutes as I.V. push injection.
• Prepare infusions of bleomycin in glass bottles, as absorption of drug to plastic occurs with time. However, plastic syringes do not interfere with bleomycin activity.
• Use precautions in preparing and handling drug; wear gloves and wash hands after preparing and administering.
• Drug can be administered by intracavitary, intraarterial, or intratumoral injection. It can also be instilled into bladder for bladder tumors.
• Cumulative lifetime dosage should not exceed 400 units.
• Response to therapy may take 2 to 3 weeks.
• Administer a 1-unit test dose before therapy to assess hypersensitivity to bleomycin. For patients with lymphoma, first two doses should be 2 units or less, and patient should be monitored for any allergic reaction. If no reaction occurs, then follow the dosing schedule. The test dose can be incorporated as part of the total dose for the regimen.
• Have epinephrine, diphenhydramine, I.V. corticosteroids, and oxygen available in case of anaphylactic reaction.
• Premedication with aspirin, steroids, and diphenhydramine may reduce drug fever and risk of anaphylaxis.
• Dosage should be reduced in patients with renal or pulmonary impairment.
• Drug concentrates in keratin of squamous epithelium. To prevent linear streaking, don't use adhesive dressings on skin.
• Allergic reactions may be delayed especially in patients with lymphoma.
• Pulmonary function tests should be performed to establish a baseline and then monitored periodically.
• Monitor chest X-rays and auscultate the lungs.
• Bleomycin is stable for 24 hours at room temperature

and 48 hours under refrigeration. Refrigerate unopened vials containing dry powder.

Information for parents and patient
• Advise parents and the patient that hair should grow back after treatment is discontinued.
• Urge parents to avoid patient's exposure to persons with bacterial or viral infections as chemotherapy can make the patient more susceptible to infection, and to report infection immediately.
• Advise parents to have child use proper hygiene and caution when using toothbrush and dental floss. Chemotherapy can increase incidence of microbial infection, delayed healing, and bleeding gums.
• Tell parents that patient's dental work should be completed before initiation of therapy whenever possible, or delayed until blood counts are normal.
• Explain that easy bruising may occur because of drug's effects on blood count.
• Tell parents and patient to immediately report redness, pain, or swelling at injection site. Local tissue injury and scarring may result if I.V. infiltrates.
• Advise parents that patient and others in the same household should not receive live-virus immunizations during therapy and for several weeks after therapy.

boric acid
Borofax, Collyrium, Ear-Dry, Neo-Flo, Ocu-Bath, Swim Ear, Ting

• Classification: topical anti-infective (acid)

How supplied
Available without prescription
Ophthalmic ointment: 5%, 10%
Otic ointment: 2.75% boric acid in isopropyl alcohol
Topical ointment: 5%, 10% ointment

Indications, route, and dosage
External ear canal infection
Children and adults: Fill ear canal with solution and plug with cotton. Repeat t.i.d. or q.i.d.
Relief of abrasions, dry skin, minor burns, insect bites, and other skin irritations
Children over age 2 and adults: Apply 5% or 10% ointment to affected area t.i.d. or q.i.d.
Eyelid inflammation and irritation
Children and adults: Apply 5% or 10% ophthalmic ointment to inner surface of lower eyelid b.i.d. or t.i.d.

Action and kinetics
• *Local anti-infection action:* Boric acid destroys or inhibits the growth of microorganisms. It is indicated to treat irritated and inflamed eyelids and to inhibit or destroy bacteria present in the ear canal.
• *Kinetics in adults:* Unknown.

Contraindications and precautions
Boric acid is contraindicated in patients with hypersensitivity to any components of the preparations. Otic preparation is contraindicated in patients with perforated eardrum or excoriated membranes in the ear.

---

‡May contain sulfites   ♦May contain tartrazine   ♦♦May contain benzyl alcohol

Ophthalmic preparation is contraindicated in patients with eye lacerations or abraded cornea. Topical form is contraindicated for children under age 2 and for patients with abraded skin or granulating wounds, because significant absorption may occur and cause systemic symptoms.

Interactions
Do not use with eye drops or contact lens wetting solutions containing polyvinyl alcohol; concomitant use with boric acid for ophthalmic use may form insoluble complexes with polyvinyl alcohol.

Effects on diagnostic tests
None reported.

Adverse reactions
- CNS: restlessness, delirium, convulsions, headache.
- CV: circulatory collapse, tachycardia.
- DERM: urticaria.
- Ear: irritation or itching.
- GI: nausea, vomiting, diarrhea, irritation.
- GU: renal damage, hypothermia.
- Other: overgrowth of nonsusceptible organisms.

Note: Drug should be discontinued if ophthalmic use causes eye pain, changes in vision, continued redness or irritation of the eye; if the condition worsens or persists; or if signs of hypersensitivity or systemic toxicity occur.

Overdose and treatment
Clinical manifestations of overdose include hypotension, shock, restlessness, weakness, seizures, nausea, vomiting, diarrhea, oliguria, hypothermia, hyperthermia, and erythematous rash.

To treat accidental substantial ingestion, induce emesis, then administer a cathartic unless the patient is comatose or obtunded. Treat hypotension with fluids. Treat seizures with I.V. diazepam.

▶ Special considerations
- Use with caution in children, who are at increased risk for systemic absorption.
- When used topically, drug is a mild antiseptic and astringent. Drug is a weak bacteriostatic, fungistatic agent.
- Avoid long-term use.
- Ophthalmic use is not recommended when soft contact lenses are in place.
- Boric acid ointments for topical use are not recommended for ophthalmic use.
- During otic use, watch for signs of superinfection (continual pain, inflammation, fever).

Information for parents and patient
- Teach correct otic administration: To place ear drops correctly for a child under age 3 years, pull the pinna down and straight back; for a child age 3 and over, pull the pinna up and back.
- Advise parents administering boric acid as an otic agent to moisten cotton plug with medication when using cotton plug in ear and not to touch dropper to ear.
- Advise patient not to use ophthalmic preparation when contact lenses are in place.

- Advise parents and patient to avoid long-term topical use or use on abraded skin.
- Drug should be stored out of small children's reach to prevent accidental ingestion.

---

bretylium tosylate
Bretylate*, Bretylol

- Classification: ventricular antiarrhythmic (adrenergic blocking agent)

How supplied
Available by prescription only
Injection: 50 mg/ml

Indications, route, and dosage
Ventricular fibrillation
†*Children and adults:* 5 mg/kg undiluted by rapid I.V. injection. If necessary, increase dose to 10 mg/kg and repeat q 15 to 30 minutes until 30 mg/kg has been given.
Unstable ventricular tachycardia and other ventricular dysrhythmias
Children and adults: Initially, 500 mg diluted to 50 ml with dextrose 5% in water or normal saline solution and infused I.V. over more than 8 minutes at 5 to 10 mg/kg. Dosage may be repeated in 1 to 2 hours. Thereafter, give q 6 to 8 hours. Infused in diluted solution of 500 ml dextrose 5% in water or normal saline solution at 1 to 2 mg/minute. For I.M. injection, administer 5 to 10 mg/kg undiluted. Repeat in 1 to 2 hours if needed. Thereafter, repeat q 6 to 8 hours.

Action and kinetics
- *Ventricular antiarrhythmic action:* Bretylium is a Class III antiarrhythmic used to treat ventricular fibrillation and tachycardia. Like other Class III antiarrhythmics, it widens the action potential duration (repolarization inhibition) and increases the effective refractory period (ERP); it does not affect conduction velocity. These actions follow a transient increase in conduction velocity and shortening of the action potential duration and ERP.

Initial effects stem from norepinephrine release from sympathetic ganglia and postganglionic adrenergic neurons immediately after drug administration. Norepinephrine release also accounts for an increased threshold for successful defibrillation, increased blood pressure, and increased heart rate. This initial phase of drug's action is brief (up to 1 hour).

Bretylium also alters the disparity in action potential duration between ischemic and nonischemic myocardial tissue; its antiarrhythmic action may result from this activity.

Hemodynamic drug effects include increased blood pressure, heart rate, and possible cardiac irritability (all resulting from initial norepinephrine release). The drug-induced adrenergic blockade ultimately predominates, leading to vasodilation and a subsequent blood pressure drop (primarily orthostatic). This effect has been referred to as chemical sympathectomy.
- *Kinetics in adults:* Bretylium is incompletely and

---

erratically absorbed from the GI tract; it is well absorbed after I.M. administration. With I.M. administration, the drug's antiarrhythmic (ventricular tachycardia and ectopy) action begins within about 20 to 60 minutes but may not reach maximal level for 6 to 9 hours when given by this route (for this reason, I.M. administration is not recommended for treating life-threatening ventricular fibrillation).

With I.V. administration, antifibrillatory action begins within a few minutes. However, suppression of ventricular tachycardia and other ventricular dysrhythmias occurs more slowly—usually within 20 minutes to 2 hours; peak antiarrhythmic effects may not occur for 6 to 9 hours. Bretylium is distributed widely throughout the body. It does not cross the blood-brain barrier. Only about 1% to 10% is plasma protein-bound. No metabolites have been identified. Bretylium is excreted in the urine mostly as unchanged drug; half-life ranges from 5 to 10 hours (longer in patients with renal impairment). Duration of effect ranges from 6 to 24 hours and may increase with continued dosage increases. (Patients with ventricular fibrillation may require continuous infusion to maintain desired effect.)

Contraindications and precautions
Bretylium is contraindicated in patients with digitalis-induced dysrhythmias, because the resulting release of norepinephrine may aggravate digitalis toxicity.

Bretylium should be used with extreme caution in patients with aortic stenosis and/or pulmonary hypertension, because these patients may be unable to compensate for the fall in blood pressure; and in patients with fixed cardiac output, aortic stenosis, and pulmonary hypertension, because the drug may cause sudden severe hypotension.

Interactions
Concomitant use of bretylium with other antiarrhythmic agents may cause additive toxic effects and additive or antagonistic cardiac effects. Concomitant use with digitalis may exacerbate ventricular tachycardia associated with digitalis toxicity. When used concomitantly with pressor amines (sympathomimetics), bretylium may potentiate the action of these drugs.

Effects on diagnostic tests
None reported.

Adverse reactions
• CNS: vertigo, dizziness, light-headedness, syncope (usually secondary to hypotension).
• CV: *severe hypotension* (especially orthostatic), bradycardia, anginal pain, *premature ventricular contractions*.
• GI: severe nausea, vomiting (with rapid infusion).

Overdose and treatment
Clinical effects of overdose primarily involve severe hypotension.

Treatment includes administration of vasopressors (such as dopamine or norepinephrine), to support blood pressure, and general supportive measures, as necessary. Volume expanders and positional changes also may be effective.

▶ Special considerations
• Drug is not a first-line agent, according to American Heart Association advanced cardiac life-support guidelines. With ventricular fibrillation, drug should follow lidocaine; with ventricular tachycardia, drug should follow lidocaine and/or procainamide.
• Ventricular tachycardia and other ventricular dysrhythmias respond to drug less rapidly than ventricular fibrillation.
• Drug is ineffective against atrial dysrhythmias.
• Drug has been used investigationally to treat hypertension. Usual dosage is 100 to 400 mg P.O. t.i.d.
• Administer I.V. infusion at appropriate rate to avoid or minimize adverse reactions.
• For I.M. injection, do not exceed 5-ml volume in any one site (1 ml per site for children; 0.5 ml per site for infants) and rotate sites.
• Patient should remain supine and avoid sudden postural changes until tolerance to hypotension develops.
• Simultaneous initiation of therapy with digitalis and bretylium should be avoided.
• Monitor ECG and blood pressure throughout therapy for any significant change. If supine systolic pressure falls below 75 mm Hg, norepinephrine, dopamine, or volume expanders may be prescribed to raise blood pressure.
• Closely monitor patient who is receiving pressor amines (sympathomimetics) to correct hypotension; bretylium potentiates these drugs' effects.
• Observe for increased anginal pain in susceptible patients.
• Because bretylium is excreted exclusively by the kidneys, patients with renal impairment require dosage modification. Dosage interval should be increased because renal impairment prolongs the elimination half-life increases threefold to sixfold.
• Subtherapeutic doses (less than 5 mg/kg) may cause hypotension.

---

brompheniramine maleate
Bromamine, Brombay, Bromphen, Chlorphed, Dehist, Dimetane, Histaject Modified, Nasahist B, N-D Stat Revised, Oraminic II, Veltrane

• Classification: antihistamine H_1-receptor antagonist (alkylamine)

How supplied
Available with or without prescription
Tablets: 4 mg
Tablets (timed-release): 8 mg, 12 mg
Elixir: 2 mg/5 ml
Injection: 10 mg/ml, 100 mg/ml

Indications, route, and dosage
Rhinitis, allergy symptoms
Children under age 12: 0.125 mg/kg or 3.75 mg/m² I.M., I.V., or S.C. three or four times a day; or 0.5 mg/kg or 15 mg/m² P.O. daily in three or four divided doses. Alternatively, adjust dosage according to age: *Children age 2 to 6:* 1 mg q 4 to 6 hours.

---

‡May contain sulfites ◆May contain tartrazine ◆◆May contain benzyl alcohol

Children age 6 to 12: 2 mg q 4 to 6 hours.
Alternatively, children age 6 and older may receive timed-release tablets: one 8- or 12-mg tablet q 12 hours.
Children age 12 and over and adults: 4 to 8 mg P.O. t.i.d. or q.i.d.; or (timed-release) 8 to 12 mg P.O. every 8 or 12 hours (maximum timed-release dosage is 24 mg daily); or 5 to 20 mg q 6 to 12 hours I.M., I.V., or S.C. Maximum dosage is 40 mg daily.

Action and kinetics
Antihistamine action: Antihistamines compete with histamine for histamine H_1-receptor sites on the smooth muscle of the bronchi, GI tract, uterus, and large blood vessels; by binding to cellular receptors, they prevent access of histamine and suppress histamine-induced allergic symptoms, even though they do not prevent its release.
• *Kinetics in adults:* Brompheniramine is absorbed readily from the GI tract and is distributed widely into the body. Approximately 90% to 95% of brompheniramine is metabolized by the liver. Brompheniramine and its metabolites are excreted primarily in urine; a small amount is excreted in feces.

Contraindications and precautions
Brompheniramine is contraindicated in patients with known hypersensitivity to this drug and in those taking antihistamines with similar chemical structures (chlorpheniramine, dexchlorpheniramine, and triprolidine); in patients experiencing asthmatic attacks, because brompheniramine thickens bronchial secretions; and in patients who have taken MAO inhibitors within the previous 2 weeks. (See Interactions.)

Brompheniramine should be used with caution in patients with narrow-angle glaucoma; in those with pyloroduodenal obstruction or urinary bladder obstruction from prostatic hypertrophy or narrowing of the bladder neck, because of their marked anticholinergic effects; in patients with cardiovascular disease, hypertension, or hyperthyroidism, because of the risk of palpitations and tachycardia; and in patients with renal disease, diabetes, bronchial asthma, urinary retention, or stenosing peptic ulcers.

Interactions
MAO inhibitors interfere with the metabolism of brompheniramine and thus prolong and intensify their central depressant and anticholinergic effects; additive CNS depression may occur when brompheniramine is given concomitantly with other CNS depressants, such as alcohol, barbiturates, tranquilizers, sleeping aids, and antianxiety agents.

Brompheniramine may diminish the effects of sulfonylureas and partially may counteract the anticoagulant effects of heparin.

Effects on diagnostic tests
Brompheniramine should be discontinued 4 days before performing diagnostic skin tests; it can prevent, reduce, or mask positive skin test response.

Adverse reactions
• CNS: dizziness, tremors, irritability, insomnia, drowsiness, stimulation, impaired coordination.
• CV: hypotension, palpitations.
• DERM: urticaria, rash.
• EENT: blurred vision.
• GI: anorexia, nausea, vomiting, dry mouth and throat, constipation.
• GU: urinary retention.
• HEMA: thrombocytopenia, agranulocytosis.
• Respiratory: thickened bronchial secretions.
   Note: Drug should be discontinued if signs of acute hypersensitivity in the form of severe agranulocytosis occur: high fever, chills, and, possibly, gangrenous mouth and throat ulcers, pneumonia, and exhaustion.

Overdose and treatment
Clinical manifestations of overdose may include either those of CNS depression (sedation, reduced mental alertness, apnea, and cardiovascular collapse) or of CNS stimulation (insomnia, hallucinations, tremors, or convulsions). Anticholinergic symptoms, such as dry mouth, flushed skin, fixed and dilated pupils, and GI symptoms, are common, especially in children.

Treat overdose by inducing emesis with ipecac syrup (in conscious patients), followed by activated charcoal to reduce further drug absorption. Use gastric lavage if patient is unconscious or ipecac fails. Treat hypotension with vasopressors, and control seizures with diazepam or phenytoin I.V. *Do not give stimulants.*

▶ Special considerations
• Drug is contraindicated during an acute asthma attack because it may not alleviate the symptoms; also, antimuscarinic effects can cause thickening of secretions.
• Children, especially those under age 6, may experience paradoxical hyperexcitabilty with restlessness, insomnia, nervousness, euphoria, tremors, and seizures.
• Note that liquid form may contain alcohol.
• Brompheniramine is not indicated for use in neonates. Timed-release tablets are not recommended for children under age 11.
• Monitor blood counts during therapy; watch for signs of blood dyscrasias.
• Reduce GI distress by giving antihistamines with food; give sugarless gum, appropriate hard candy, or ice chips to relieve dry mouth. Increase fluid intake (if allowed) or humidify air to decrease adverse effect of thickened secretions.
• If tolerance develops, another antihistamine may be substituted.
• Some antihistamines may mask ototoxicity from high doses of aspirin and other salicylates.
• Drug causes less drowsiness than some antihistamines.
• Store parenteral solutions and elixirs away from light and freezing temperatures; solution may crystallize if stored below 32° F. (0° C.). Crystals will dissolve when warmed to 86° F. (30° C.).

Information for parents and patient
• Advise patient to take drug with meals or snack to prevent gastric upset and to use any of the following

measures to relieve dry mouth: warm water rinses, artificial saliva, ice chips, or sugarless gum or candy. Patient should avoid overusing mouthwash, which may add to dryness (alcohol content) and destroy normal flora.

• Warn parents that child should avoid hazardous activities that require balance or alertness until extent of CNS effects are known. Urge them to seek medical approval before administering tranquilizers, sedatives, pain relievers, or sleeping medications.

• Warn parents and patient to stop administration of drug 4 days before diagnostic skin tests, to preserve accuracy of tests.

• Instruct parents not to administer more than 24 mg/day (for children age 12 and older) or 12 mg/day (for children age 6 to 11).

bumetanide
Bumex

• Classification: loop diuretic

How supplied
Available by prescription only
Tablets: 0.5 mg, 1 mg, 2 mg
Injection: 0.25 mg/ml

Indications, route, and dosage
Edema (CHF, hepatic and renal disease)
†*Children:* 0.02 to 0.1 mg/kg P.O., I.M., or I.V. q 12 hours.

Note: The injectable form is not recommended for use in neonates because it contains benzyl alcohol.
Adults: 0.5 to 2 mg P.O. once daily. If diuretic response is not adequate, give a second or third dose at 4- to 5-hour intervals. Maximum dosage is 10 mg/day. Give parenterally when oral route is not feasible. Usual initial dose is 0.5 to 1 mg I.V. or I.M. If response is not adequate, give a second or third dose at 2- to 3-hour intervals. Maximum dosage is 10 mg/day.

Action and kinetics
• *Diuretic action:* This loop diuretic inhibits sodium and chloride reabsorption in the proximal part of the ascending loop of Henle, promoting the excretion of sodium, water, chloride, and potassium. Bumetanide produces renal and peripheral vasodilation and may temporarily increase glomerular filtration rate and decrease peripheral vascular resistance.
• *Kinetics in adults:* After oral administration, 85% to 95% of a dose of bumetanide is absorbed; food delays oral absorption. I.M. bumetanide is completely absorbed. Diuresis usually begins 30 to 60 minutes after oral and 40 minutes after I.M. administration; peak diuresis occurs 1 to 2 hours after either. Diuresis begins a few minutes after I.V. administration and peaks in 15 to 30 minutes. Bumetanide is approximately 92% to 96% protein-bound; it is unknown whether the drug enters CSF or breast milk or crosses the placenta. Bumetanide is metabolized by the liver to at least five metabolites; it is excreted in urine

(80%) and feces (10% to 20%). Half-life ranges from 1 to 1½ hours; duration of effect is about 2 to 4 hours.

Contraindications and precautions
Bumetanide is contraindicated in patients with known hypersensitivity, anuria, hepatic coma, or electrolyte depletion, and in patients with increasing BUN and creatinine levels or oliguria, despite its use as a diuretic in patients with renal impairment.

Bumetanide should be used cautiously in patients allergic to sulfonamides, including furosemide, because cross-sensitivity may occur; in patients with hepatic cirrhosis and ascites, because electrolyte alterations may precipitate hepatic encephalopathy; and in patients receiving cardiac glycosides (digoxin, digitoxin), because bumetanide-induced hypokalemia may predispose them to digitalis toxicity. Rapid I.V. administration increases hazard of ototoxicity.

Interactions
Bumetanide potentiates the hypotensive effect of most other antihypertensive agents and of other diuretics; both actions are used to therapeutic advantage.

Concomitant use of bumetanide with potassium-sparing diuretics (spironolactone, triamterene, amiloride) may decrease bumetanide-induced potassium loss; use with other potassium-depleting drugs, such as steroids and amphotericin B, may cause severe potassium loss.

Bumetanide may reduce renal clearance of lithium and increase lithium levels; lithium dosage may require adjustment.

Indomethacin and probenecid may reduce bumetanide's diuretic effect, and their combined use is not recommended; however, if there is no therapeutic alternative, an increased dose of bumetanide may be required.

Concomitant administration of bumetanide with ototoxic or nephrotoxic drugs may result in enhanced toxicity.

Bumetanide could prolong neuromuscular blockade by tubocurarine or gallamine, although this has not been reported.

Effects on diagnostic tests
Bumetanide therapy alters electrolyte balance and liver and renal function tests.

Adverse reactions
• CNS: dizziness, headache.
• CV: volume depletion and dehydration, orthostatic hypotension, ECG changes.
• DERM: rash.
• EENT: transient deafness.
• GI: nausea.
• HEMA: transient thrombocytopenia and leukopenia.
• Metabolic: hypochloremic alkalosis; asymptomatic hyperuricemia; fluid and electrolyte imbalances, including dilutional hyponatremia, hypokalemia, hypocalcemia, and hypomagnesemia; hyperglycemia and impairment of glucose tolerance.
• Other: muscle pain and tenderness.
Note: Drug should be discontinued if dehydration or hypotension occurs or if BUN and serum creatinine levels rise.

Overdose and treatment
Clinical manifestations of overdose include profound electrolyte and volume depletion, which may cause circulatory collapse.

Treatment of bumetanide overdose is primarily supportive; replace fluid and electrolytes as needed.

▶ **Special considerations**
• Safety and efficacy of bumetanide in children have not been established.
• Use this loop diuretic with caution in neonates. The usual pediatric dose can be used, but dosage intervals should be extended.
• Monitor blood pressure and pulse rate (especially during rapid diuresis) to establish baseline values before therapy, and watch for significant changes.
• Advise safety measures for all ambulatory patients until response to the diuretic is known.
• Establish baseline and periodically review CBC, including WBC count; serum electrolytes, CO_2, BUN, and creatinine levels; and results of liver function test.
• Administer drug in the morning so major diuresis occurs before bedtime. To prevent nocturia, do not prescribe diuretics for use after 6 p.m.
• Consider possible dosage adjustment in the following circumstances: reduced dosage for patients with hepatic dysfunction; increased dosage in patients with renal impairment, oliguria, or decreased diuresis (inadequate urine output may result in circulatory overload, causing water intoxication, pulmonary edema, and CHF); increased doses of insulin in diabetic patients; and reduced dosages of other antihypertensive agents.
• Monitor patient for edema and ascites. Observe lower extremities of ambulatory children and the sacral area of those on bed rest.
• Patient should be weighed each morning immediately after voiding and before breakfast wearing the same type of clothing and on the same scale. Weight provides guide for clinical response to diuretic therapy.
• Consult dietitian on possible need for dietary potassium supplementation.
• Patients taking digitalis are at increased risk of digitalis toxicity from potassium depletion.
• Ototoxicity may follow prolonged use or administration of large doses.
• Patients with liver disease are especially susceptible to diuretic-induced electrolyte imbalance; in extreme cases, stupor, coma, and death can result.
• Patient should have urinal or commode readily available.
• Give I.V. bumetanide slowly, over 1 or 2 minutes. For I.V. infusion, dilute bumetanide in dextrose 5% in water, normal saline solution, or lactated Ringer's solution and use within 24 hours.

Information for parents and patient
• Explain to the parents and patient the rationale for therapy and the diuretic effect of these drugs.
• Advise parents to have patient eat potassium-rich foods, such as citrus fruits, potatoes, dates, raisins, and bananas; to avoid high-sodium foods, such as lunch meat, smoked meats, and processed cheeses;

and not to add salt to other foods. Recommend salt substitutes.
• With initial doses, caution patient to change position slowly, especially when rising to upright position, to prevent dizziness form orthostatic hypotension.
• Teach parents signs of adverse effects, especially hypokalemia (weakness, fatigue, muscle cramps, paresthesias, confusion, nausea, vomiting, diarrhea, headache, dizziness, or palpitations), and importance of reporting such symptoms promptly.
• Tell parents to report if patient experiences increased edema or excess diuresis (more than 2% weight loss or gain).
• Instruct parents to call at once if patient shows signs of chest, back, or leg pain; dyspnea; or shortness of breath.
• Emphasize importance of regular medical follow-up to monitor effectiveness of diuretic therapy.

⬛

busulfan
Myleran

• Classification: antineoplastic (alkylating agent [cell cycle-phase nonspecific])

How supplied
Available by prescription only
Tablets: 2 mg

Indications, route, and dosage
Dosage and indications may vary. Check current literature for recommended protocol.
Chronic myelogenous leukemia
Children: 0.06 to 0.12 mg/kg or 1.8 to 4.6 mg/m² P.O. daily.
Adults: 4 to 8 mg P.O. daily but may range from 1 to 12 mg P.O. daily (0.06 mg/kg or 1.8 mg/m²).

Action and kinetics
• *Antineoplastic action:* Busulfan is an alkylating agent that exerts its cytotoxic activity by interfering with DNA replication and RNA transcription, causing a disruption of nucleic acid function.
• *Kinetics in adults:* Busulfan is well absorbed from the GI tract and is cleared rapidly from the plasma. Distribution into the brain and CSF is unknown. Busulfan is metabolized in the liver. Busulfan and its metabolites are excreted in urine.

Contraindications and precautions
Busulfan is contraindicated in patients with a history of resistance to therapy with busulfan.

Busulfan should be used with caution in patients of childbearing age because it can impair fertility, in those with a history of gout from hyperuricemic effects of the drug, and in patients whose immune system is compromised because of potential for additive toxicity. The drug can cause further myelosuppression, increasing the patient's risk of infection.

Interactions
None reported.

Effects on diagnostic tests

Drug-induced cellular dysplasia may interfere with interpretation of cytologic studies.

Busulfan therapy may increase blood and urine levels of uric acid as a result of increased purine catabolism that accompanies cell destruction.

Adverse reactions

• DERM: transient hyperpigmentation, anhidrosis.
• GI: *nausea, vomiting, diarrhea,* cheilosis, glossitis, stomatitis.
• GU: amenorrhea, testicular atrophy, renal calculi, uric acid nephropathy, cholestatic jaundice, impotence.
• HEMA: *bone marrow depression* (dose-limiting); WBC count falling after about 10 days and continuing to fall for 2 weeks after stopping drug; thrombocytopenia, leukopenia, anemia, *leukemia.*
• Metabolic: Addison-like wasting syndrome, profound hyperuricemia from increased cell lysis.
• Other: gynecomastia, alopecia, *irreversible pulmonary fibrosis (commonly termed "busulfan lung"),* pulmonary infiltrates, hyperpigmentation, gynecomastia, ovarian failure, cellular dysplasia.

Note: Drug should be discontinued if the leukocyte count decreases to approximately 15,000/mm³, or if patient's clinical symptoms and changes on chest X-ray support pulmonary fibrosis.

Overdose and treatment

Clinical manifestations of overdose include hematologic manifestations such as leukopenia and thrombocytopenia.

Treatment is supportive and includes transfusion of blood components and antibiotics for infections that may develop.

▶ Special considerations

• Avoid all I.M. injections, if possible, when platelets are below 100,000/mm³.
• Patient response usually begins 1 to 2 weeks (increased appetite, sense of well-being, decreased total leukocyte count, reduction in size of spleen) after discontinuing the drug.
• Encourage high fluid intake to aid drug excretions by the kidneys and to help prevent hyperuricemia. Patients with large tumor loads may receive allopurinol concurrently to avoid uric acid deposition during tumor lysis.
• Use cautiously in patients recently given other myelosuppressive drugs or radiation treatment and in those with depressed neutrophil or platelet count.
• Watch for signs of infection (fever, sore throat).
• Pulmonary fibrosis may be delayed for 4 to 6 months.
• Monitor BUN, hematocrit, platelet count, ALT (SGPT), AST (SGOT), LDH, serum bilirubin, serum creatinine, uric acid total and differential leukocyte, CDBC, and kidney function.
• Follow all established procedures for safe handling, administration, and disposal of chemotherapy.

Information for parents and patient

• Persistent cough and progressive dyspnea with alveolar exudate may result from drug toxicity, not pneumonia. Instruct parents and patient to report respiratory symptoms so dose adjustments can be made.
• Advise parents to administer aspirin-containing products cautiously and to watch closely for signs of bleeding. Advise them to report bleeding promptly .
• Emphasize the importance of taking the drug as prescribed and of continuing to take it despite nausea and vomiting.
• Advise parents to avoid patient's exposure to persons with bacterial or viral infections because chemotherapy can increase susceptibility to infection, and to report any signs of infection promptly.
• Teach oral hygiene including caution when using dental floss and toothbrush.
• Advise parents that patient's dental work should be completed before initiation of therapy whenever possible, or delayed until blood counts are normal.
• Advise parents that immunizations should be avoided during busulfan therapy if possible.
• Explain potential reproductive side effects (amenorrhea, gynecomastia in males).
• Inform patient that alopecia may occur.
• Instruct parents and patient to report exposure to chicken pox promptly so that zoster immune globulin may be given as soon as possible to patient without immunity to this infection.

butabarbital

Barbased, Butalan, Butatran, Buticaps, Butisol, Day-Barb*, Neo-Barb*, Sarisol No. 2

• Classification: sedative-hypnotic (barbiturate)
• Controlled substance schedule III

How supplied

Available by prescription only
Tablets: 15 mg, 30 mg, 50 mg, 100 mg
Capsules: 15 mg, 30 mg
Elixir: 30 mg/5 ml, 33.3 mg/5 ml

Indications, route, and dosage
Sedation

Children: 2 mg/kg P.O. t.i.d. or 60 mg/m² t.i.d.
Adults: 15 to 30 mg P.O. t.i.d. or q.i.d.
Preoperative sedation

Children: 2 to 6 mg/kg; up to a maximum of 100 mg/dose.
Adults: 50 to 100 mg P.O. 60 to 90 minutes before surgery.
Insomnia

Children: Dosage must be individualized.
Adults: 50 to 100 mg P.O. h.s.

Action and kinetics

• *Sedative-hypnotic action:* The exact cellular site and mechanism(s) of action are unknown. Butabarbital acts throughout the CNS as a nonselective depressant with an intermediate onset and duration of action. Particularly sensitive to the drug is the reticular activating system, which controls CNS arousal. Butabarbital decreases both presynaptic and postsynaptic

membrane excitability by facilitating the action of gamma-aminobutyric acid (GABA).
• *Kinetics in adults:* Butabarbital is absorbed well after oral administration, with peak concentrations occurring in 3 to 4 hours. Onset of action occurs in 45 to 60 minutes. Serum concentrations needed for sedation and hypnosis are 2 to 3 mcg/ml and 25 mcg/ml, respectively.

Butabarbital is distributed well throughout body tissues and fluids.

Butabarbital is metabolized extensively in the liver by oxidation. Its duration of action is 6 to 8 hours.

Inactive metabolites of butabarbital are excreted in urine. Only 1% to 2% of an oral dose is excreted in urine unchanged. The terminal half-life ranges from 30 to 40 hours.

Contraindications and precautions

Butabarbital is contraindicated in patients with known hypersensitivity to barbiturates and in patients with bronchopneumonia, status asthmaticus, or other severe respiratory distress because of the potential for respiratory depression. Butabarbital should not be used in patients who are depressed or have suicidal ideation, because the drug can worsen depression; in patients with uncontrolled acute or chronic pain, because exacerbation of pain or paradoxical excitement can occur; or in patients with porphyria, because this drug can trigger symptoms of this disease. Some butabarbital preparations contain tartrazine, which may precipitate an allergic reaction. Do not administer butabarbital to patients with a tartrazine sensitivity.

Butabarbital should be used cautiously in patients who must perform hazardous tasks requiring mental alertness, because the drug causes drowsiness. Prolonged use of high doses should be avoided because tolerance and physical or psychological dependence may occur.

Use cautiously in patients with renal or hepatic dysfunction because of the risk of drug accumulation.

Interactions

Butabarbital may add to or potentiate the CNS and respiratory depressant effects of other sedative-hypnotics, antihistamines, narcotics, antidepressants, tranquilizers, and alcohol. Butabarbital enhances the enzymatic degradation of warfarin and other oral anticoagulants; patients may require increased doses of the anticoagulants. Drug also enhances hepatic metabolism of some drugs, including digitoxin (not digoxin), corticosteroids, oral contraceptives and other estrogens, theophylline and other xanthines, and doxycycline. Butabarbital impairs the effectiveness of griseofulvin by decreasing absorption from the GI tract.

Valproic acid, phenytoin, disulfiram, and monoamine oxidase inhibitors decrease the metabolism of butabarbital and can increase its toxicity. Rifampin may decrease butabarbital levels by increasing hepatic metabolism.

Effects on diagnostic tests

Butabarbital may cause a false-positive phentolamine test. The physiologic effects of the drug may impair the absorption of cyanocobalamin ^{57}Co; it may decrease serum bilirubin concentrations in neonates, epileptic patients, and patients with congenital nonhemolytic unconjugated hyperbilirubinemia. EEG patterns are altered, with a change in low-voltage, fast activity; changes persist for a time after discontinuation of therapy. Barbiturates may increase sulfobromophthalein retention.

Adverse reactions

• CNS: drowsiness, lethargy, vertigo, headache, CNS depression, *paradoxical excitement*, confusion and agitation, rebound insomnia, increased dreams, nightmares, possibly seizures (after acute withdrawal or reduction in dosage).
• CV: hypotension, bradycardia, syncope, circulatory collapse.
• DERM: urticaria, rash, exfoliative dermatitis, Stevens-Johnson syndrome.
• EENT: miosis.
• GI: epigastric pain, nausea, vomiting, diarrhea, constipation.
• Other: laryngospasm, bronchospasm, blood dyscrasias. Vitamin K deficiency and bleeding have been reported in newborns of mothers treated during pregnancy. Hyperalgesia occurs with low doses or in patients with chronic pain.
Note: Drug should be discontinued if hypersensitivity reaction, profound CNS or respiratory depression, or skin eruption occurs.

Overdose and treatment

Clinical manifestations of overdose include unsteady gait, slurred speech, sustained nystagmus, somnolence, confusion, respiratory depression, pulmonary edema, areflexia, and coma. Jaundice, hypothermia followed by fever, oliguria, and typical shock syndrome with tachycardia and hypotension may occur.

To treat, maintain and support ventilation and pulmonary function, as necessary; support cardiac function and circulation with vasopressors and I.V. fluids, as needed. If patient is conscious with a functioning gag reflex and ingestion was recent, induce emesis by administering ipecac syrup. If emesis is contraindicated, perform gastric lavage while a cuffed endotracheal tube is in place, to prevent aspiration. Follow by administering repeated doses of activated charcoal or saline cathartic. Measure intake and output, vital signs, and laboratory parameters. Maintain body temperature. Alkalinization of urine may be helpful in removing drug from the body; hemodialysis may be useful in severe overdose.

▶ Special considerations

• Butabarbital may cause paradoxical excitement in children. Dosage depends on age and weight of child and degree of sedation required. Use with caution.
• Premature infants are more susceptible to the depressant effects of barbiturates because of immature hepatic metabolism. Children receiving barbiturates may experience hyperactivity, excitement, or hyperalgia.
• Dosage must be individualized for each patient, because different rates of metabolism and enzyme induction occur.
• May be given rectally if oral route is inappropriate.

• Assess level of consciousness before and frequently during therapy to evaluate effectiveness of drug. Monitor neurologic status for possible alterations or deteriorations. Monitor seizure character, frequency, and duration for changes. Institute seizure precautions, as necessary.

• Assess patient's sleeping patterns before and during therapy to ensure effectiveness of drug.

• Institute safety measures — side rails, assistance when out of bed, call light within reach — to prevent falls and injury.

• Anticipate possible rebound confusion and excitatory reactions in patient.

• Assess bowel elimination patterns and monitor for complaints of constipation. Advise diet high in fiber, if indicated.

• Observe patient to prevent hoarding or self-dosing, especially in depressed or suicidal patients, or those who are or have a history of being drug-dependent.

• Abrupt discontinuation may cause withdrawal symptoms; discontinue slowly.

• Death is common with an overdose of 2 to 10 g; it may occur at much smaller doses if alcohol is also ingested.

• Avoid administering barbiturates to patients with status asthmaticus.

• Tablet may be crushed and mixed with food or fluid if patient has difficulty swallowing. Capsule may be opened and contents mixed with food or fluids to aid in swallowing.

• Assess cardiopulmonary status frequently; monitor vital signs for significant changes.

• Monitor patients for possible allergic reaction resulting from tartrazine sensitivity.

• Periodically evaluate blood counts and renal and hepatic studies for abnormalities and adverse effects.

• Monitor prothrombin times carefully when patient on butabarbital starts or ends anticoagulant therapy. Anticoagulant dosage may need to be adjusted.

• Watch for signs of barbiturate toxicity (coma, pupillary constriction, cyanosis, clammy skin, hypotension). Overdose can be fatal.

• Prolonged administration is not recommended; drug has not been shown to be effective after 14 days. A drug-free interval of at least 1 week is advised between dosing periods.

Information for parents and patient

• Warn parents or patient to avoid concurrent use of other drugs with CNS depressant effects, such as antihistamines, analgesics, and alcohol, because they will have additive effects and result in increased drowsiness. Instruct parents to seek medical approval before giving patient any nonprescription cold or allergy preparations.

• Caution parents and patient not to increase or decrease dose or frequency without medical approval; abrupt discontinuation of medication may trigger rebound insomnia, with increased dreaming, nightmares, or seizures.

• Patient should avoid hazardous tasks that require alertness while taking barbiturates.

• Be sure parents and patient understand that barbiturates can cause physical or psychological dependence (addiction).

• Instruct parents to report any skin eruption or other marked adverse reaction.

• Explain that a morning hangover is common after therapeutic use of barbiturates.

caffeine
NōDōz, Tirend, Vivarin

- Classification: CNS stimulant, analeptic, respiratory stimulant (methylxanthine)

How supplied
Available by prescription only
Injection: caffeine (125 mg/ml) with sodium benzoate (125 mg/ml)

Available without prescription
Tablets: 100 mg, 150 mg, 200 mg
Capsules (timed-release): 200 mg, 250 mg

Indications, route, and dosage
CNS depression
Infants and children: 8 mg/kg I.M., I.V., or S.C. q 4 hours, p.r.n.
Adults: 100 to 200 mg P.O. q 4 hours, p.r.n.; timed-release, 200 or 250 mg q 4 to 6 hours. For emergencies—500 mg I.M. or I.V.; maximum single dose 1 g.
Note: This use is strongly discouraged by many clinicians.
†Neonatal apnea
Neonates: 5 to 10 mg/kg caffeine and sodium benzoate (about 4 mg/kg caffeine) or 250 mg/m² (about 125 mg/m² caffeine). Maximum single dose is 500 mg. I.V., I.M., or P.O. as a loading dose, followed by 2.5 to 5 mg/kg I.V., I.M., or P.O. daily, according to patient tolerance and plasma caffeine levels. Alternatively, if caffeine citrate is used, 10 to 20 mg/kg as a loading dose, followed by 5 to 10mg/kg/day for maintenance.

Action and kinetics
- *CNS stimulant action:* Caffeine, like theophylline, is a xanthine derivative; it increases levels of cyclic 3':5'-adenosine monophosphate by inhibiting phosphodiesterase. Caffeine stimulates all levels of the CNS; it hastens and clarifies thinking and improves arousal and psychomotor coordination.
- *Respiratory stimulant action:* In respiratory depression and in neonatal apnea (unlabeled use), larger doses of caffeine increase respiratory rate. Caffeine increases contractile force and decreases fatigue of skeletal muscle.
- *Kinetics in adults:* Caffeine is well absorbed from the GI tract; absorption after I.M. injection may be slower. Caffeine is distributed rapidly throughout the body; it crosses the blood-brain barrier and placenta. Approximately 17% protein-bound, caffeine's plasma half-life is 3 to 4 hours in adults. Caffeine is metabolized by the liver; in neonates, liver metabolism is

much less evident and half-life may approach 80 hours. Drug is excreted in urine.

Contraindications and precautions
Caffeine is contraindicated in patients with known hypersensitivity to caffeine; in patients with symptomatic cardiac dysrhythmias or palpitations; and for 6 weeks after acute myocardial infarction because of its arrhythmogenic potential. It also is contraindicated in patients with a history of peptic ulcer disease; large amounts of caffeine may reactivate ulcers by stimulating gastric acid secretion. Use injectable form with caution in neonates: sodium benzoate content reportedly causes kernicterus.

Caffeine does not reverse alcohol intoxication or its depressant effects; excessive use of caffeine in patients with such conditions may deepen CNS depression. Withdrawal of caffeine may cause acute abstinence syndrome from physical tolerance.

Interactions
Concomitant use of caffeine with oral contraceptives, cimetidine, or disulfiram inhibits caffeine metabolism and increases its effects; use with other xanthine derivatives (theophylline) may increase incidence of stimulant-induced adverse reactions, such as tremor, tachycardia, insomnia, and nervousness. Concomitant use of beta agonists (terbutaline, albuterol, metaproterenol) increases incidence of cardiac effects and tremors.

Effects on diagnostic tests
Caffeine may increase blood glucose levels and cause false-positive urate levels; it also may cause false-positive test results for pheochromocytoma or neuroblastoma by increasing certain urinary catecholamines.

Adverse reactions
- CNS: *irritability, agitation, insomnia, restlessness,* nervousness, mild delirium, headache, excitement, agitation, *muscle tremors, twitches,* tinnitus, lightheadedness, *seizures* (with toxic doses).
- CV: *tachycardia, bradycardia, decreased blood pressure,* palpitations.
- DERM: hyperesthesia.
- GI: *nausea, vomiting,* diarrhea, abdominal pain, *gastric irritation.*
- GU: *diuresis.*
- Other: *flushing, tachypnea, respiratory depression.*
Note: Drug should be discontinued if signs of hypersensitivity, tachycardia, palpitations, or dizziness occur.

Overdose and treatment
Clinical manifestations of overdose in adults may include insomnia, dyspnea, altered states of consciousness, muscle twitching, seizure, diuresis, dysrhythmias, and fever. In infants, symptoms may

include alternating hypotonicity and hypertonicity, opisthotonoid posture, tremors, bradycardia, hypotension, and severe acidosis.

Treat overdose symptomatically and supportively; lavage and charcoal may help. Carefully monitor vital signs, ECG, and fluid and electrolyte balance. Seizures may be treated with diazepam or phenobarbital; diazepam can exacerbate respiratory depression.

▶ Special considerations
• For control of neonatal apnea, maintain plasma caffeine level at 5 to 20 mcg/ml.
• Adverse CNS effects are usually more severe in children.
• In neonates, avoid using caffeine products containing sodium benzoate because they may cause kernicterus.
• Restrict caffeine-containing beverages in patients with dysrhythmic symptoms or those who are taking aminophylline or theophylline.
• Caffeine content in beverages (mg/180 ml) is the following: cola drinks, 17 to 55; tea, 40 to 100; instant coffee, 60 to 180; brewed coffee, 100 to 150; decaffeinated coffee, 1 to 6.
• Many nonprescription pain relievers contain caffeine, but evidence concerning its analgesic effects conflicts. Caffeine (30%) may be used in a hydrophilic base or hydrocortisone cream to treat atopic dermatitis.
• Caffeine has been used to relieve headache after lumbar puncture and, in topical creams, to treat atopic dermatitis.

Information for parents and patient
• Advise parents to have patient avoid excessive caffeine consumption and therefore CNS stimulation by learning caffeine content of beverages and foods.
• Warn parents not to exceed recommended dosage, not to substitute caffeine for needed sleep, and to discontinue drug if dizziness or tachycardia occurs.

calcitriol
Rocaltrol

• Classification: antihypocalcemic (vitamin D analog)

How supplied
Available by prescription only
Capsules: 0.25 mcg, 0.5 mcg

Indications, route, and dosage
Hypocalcemia in chronic dialysis
Children: Initially, 0.25 mcg P.O. daily. Increase dosage at 2- to 4-week intervals to 0.25 to 2 mcg daily. Maintenance dose is 0.25 mcg every other day up to 0.5 to 1.25 mcg daily.
Adults: Initially, 0.25 mcg P.O. daily. Increase dosage at 2- to 4-week intervals to 0.5 to 3 mcg daily.
Hypoparathyroidism
Children: Initially, 0.25 mcg P.O. daily. Increase dosage at 2- to 4-week intervals to 0.04 to 0.08 mcg daily

Adults: Initially, 0.25 mcg P.O. daily. Increase dosage at 2- to 4-week intervals to 0.25 to 2.7 mcg daily.
Renal osteodystrophy
Children: Initially, 0.25 mcg P.O. daily. Increase dosage at 2- to 4-week intervals to 0.014 to 0.041 mcg/kg daily.
Adults: Initially, 0.25 mcg P.O. daily. Adjust dosage at 2- to 4-week intervals to 0.25 every other day up to 3 mcg or more daily.

Action and kinetics
• *Antihypocalcemic action:* Calcitriol is a vitamin D analog (1,25 dihydroxycholecalciterol), or activated cholecalciferol. It promotes absorption of calcium from the intestine by forming a calcium-binding protein. It reverses the signs of rickets and osteomalacia in patients who cannot activate or utilize ergocalciferol or cholecalciferol. In patients with renal failure it reduces bone pain, muscle weakness, and parathyroid serum levels.
• *Kinetics in adults:* Calcitriol is absorbed readily after oral administration. Calcitriol is distributed widely and protein-bound. Calcitriol is metabolized in the liver and kidney, with a half-life of 3 to 8 hours. No activation step is required. Calcitriol is excreted primarily in the feces.

Contraindications and precautions
Calcitriol is contraindicated in patients with hypercalcemia or sensitivity to vitamin D. Use cautiously in patients taking digitalis, because dyshypercalcemia may precipitate cardiac dysrhythmias.

Interactions
Antacids may alter calcitriol absorption. Barbiturates, phenytoin, and primidone may increase metabolism of calcitriol and reduce activity. The increases in calcium may potentiate the effects of digitalis glycosides.

Effects on diagnostic tests
Calcitriol therapy may falsely elevate cholesterol determinations made using the Zlatkis-Zak reaction. It also alters serum alkaline phosphatase concentrations and may alter electrolytes, such as magnesium, phosphate, and calcium in serum and urine.

Adverse reactions
• CNS: headache, somnolence, irritability.
• EENT: conjunctivitis, photophobia, rhinorrhea.
• GI: nausea, vomiting, constipation, metallic aftertaste, dry mouth, anorexia.
• GU: polyuria.
• Other: weakness, bone and muscle pain, hyperthermia, hypertension, weight loss.
  Note: Drug should be discontinued if adverse reactions become severe.

Overdose and treatment
Clinical manifestation of overdose is hypercalcemia. Treatment requires discontinuation of drug, institution of a low-calcium diet, increased fluid intake, and supportive measures. Calcitonin administration may help reverse hypercalcemia. In severe cases, death has followed cardiovascular and renal failure.

---

‡May contain sulfites   ◆May contain tartrazine   ◆◆May contain benzyl alcohol

▶ **Special considerations**
• Some infants may be hyperreactive to drug.
• Monitor serum calcium levels several times weekly after initiating therapy.
• Protect drug from heat and light.

Information for parents and patient
• Instruct parents on the importance of a diet rich in calcium.
• Advise parents to report any adverse reactions immediately.
• Tell parents to avoid administering to patients magnesium-containing antacids and other self-prescribed drugs.

---

calcium salts

calcium chloride
calcium citrate
Citracal

calcium glubionate
Neo-Calglucon

calcium gluceptate
calcium gluconate
Kalcinate

calcium glycerophosphate
calcium lactate
calcium phosphate, dibasic
calcium phosphate, tribasic
Posture

• Classification: therapeutic agent for electrolyte balance, cardiotonic (calcium supplement)

How supplied
Available by prescription only
Calcium chloride
Injection: 10% solution (1 g/10 ml) in 10-ml ampules, vials, and syringes (contains 270 mg [13.5 mEq] of elemental calcium/g)
Calcium gluceptate
Injection: 22% solution (1.1 g/5 ml) in 5-ml ampules or 50-ml vials (contains 82 mg [4.1 mEq] of elemental calcium/g)
Calcium gluconate
Injection: 10% solution (1 g/10 ml) in 10-ml ampules and vials, 10-ml or 20-ml vials (contains 90 mg [4.5 mEq] of elemental calcium/g)

Available without prescription
Calcium citrate
Tablets: 950 mg (contains 211 mg [10.6 mEq] of elemental calcium/g)
Calcium glubionate
Syrup: 1.8 g/5 ml (contains 64 mg [3.2 mEq] of elemental calcium/g)
Calcium gluconate
Tablets: 500 mg, 650 mg, 975 mg, 1 g (contains 90 mg [4.5 mEq] of elemental calcium/g)

Calcium lactate
Tablets: 325 mg, 650 mg (contains 130 mg [6.5 mEq] of elemental calcium/g)
Calcium phosphate, dibasic
Tablets: 468 mg (contains 230 mg [11.5 mEq] of elemental calcium/g)
Calcium phosphate, tribasic
Tablets: 300 mg, 600 mg (contains 400 mg [20 mEq] of elemental calcium/g)

Indications, route, and dosage
Cardiotonic use during cardiopulmonary resuscitation
Children: 0.27 mEq/kg I.V. using calcium chloride. Repeat dose in 10 minutes if necessary. Additional doses should be based upon documented calcium deficit.
Adults: 2.7 mEq I.V. using calcium chloride, repeated PRN; or 4.5 to 6.3 mEq I.V. using calcium gluceptate, repeated PRN; or 2.3 to 3.7 mEq I.V. using calcium gluconate, repeated PRN. Some clinicians routinely employ doses of 7 to 14 mEq calcium chloride. When given by intracardiac injection (into the ventricular cavity) the usual adult dose is 2.7 to 5.4 mEq using calcium chloride.
Emergency elevation of serum calcium
Infants: Up to 1 mEq I.V. daily; repeat every 1 to 3 days.
Children: 1 to 7 mEq I.V. daily; repeat every 1 to 3 days.
Adults: 7 to 14 mEq I.V.; repeat P.R.N.
Hypocalcemic tetany
Neonates: 2.4 mEq I.V. daily in divided doses.
Children: 0.5 to 0.7 mEq/kg I.V. t.i.d. or q.i.d.
Adults: 4.5 to 16 mEq I.V.; repeat P.R.N.

Action and kinetics
• *Calcium replacement:* Calcium is essential for maintaining the functional integrity of the nervous, muscular, and skeletal systems, and for cell-membrane and capillary permeability. Calcium salts are used as a source of calcium cation to treat or prevent calcium depletion in patients in whom dietary measures are inadequate. Conditions associated with hypocalcemia are chronic diarrhea, vitamin D deficiency, steatorrhea, sprue, pregnancy and lactation, menopause, pancreatitis, renal failure, alkalosis, hyperphosphatemia, and hypoparathyroidism.
• *Kinetics in adults:* The I.M. and I.V. calcium salts are absorbed directly into the bloodstream. I.V. injection gives an immediate blood level, which will decrease to previous levels in about 30 to 120 minutes. The oral dose is absorbed actively in the duodenum and proximal jejunum and, to a lesser extent, in the distal part of the small intestine. Calcium is absorbed only in the ionized form. Pregnancy and reduction of calcium intake may increase the efficiency of absorption. Vitamin D in its active form is required for calcium absorption.

Calcium enters the extracellular fluid and then is incorporated rapidly into skeletal tissue. Bone contains 99% of the total calcium; 1% is distributed equally between the intracellular and extracellular fluids. CSF concentrations are about 50% of serum calcium concentrations. No significant metabolism

---

ocurrs. Calcium is excreted mainly in feces as unabsorbed calcium that was secreted via bile and pancreatic juice into the lumen of the GI tract. Most calcium entering the kidney is reabsorbed in the loop of Henle and the proximal and distal convoluted tubules. Only small amounts of calcium are excreted in the urine.

Contraindications and precautions
Calcium chloride is contraindicated in ventricular fibrillation during cardiac resuscitation; in patients with hypercalcemia; in patients with a history of cardiac or renal insufficiency, respiratory acidosis and failure, metastatic bone disease, or hypercalcemia; and in patients with digitalis toxicity.

I.M. administration of calcium gluconate and calcium gluceptate may be tolerated, but the I.V. route is preferred in all cases except emergencies. Do not give S.C.

Interactions
Concomitant use of calcium salts with cardiac glycosides increases digitalis toxicity; administer calcium very cautiously, if at all, to digitalized patients.

Calcium may antagonize the therapeutic effects of calcium channel blocker drugs (verapamil).

Calcium should not be physically mixed with phosphates, carbonates, sulfates, or tartrates, especially at high concentrations. Calcium competes with magnesium and may compete for absorption, thus decreasing the amount of bioavailable magnesium. Concurrent administration of calcium decreases the therapeutic effect of tetracycline as a result of chelation.

Effects on diagnostic tests
I.V. calcium may produce transient elevation of plasma 11-hydroxycorticosteroid concentrations (Glen-Nelson technique) and false-negative values for serum and urine magnesium as measured by the Titan yellow method.

Adverse reactions
• CNS: hypercalcemia may cause dizziness and a change in mental status; somnolence, headache, confusion, psychosis; from I.V. use, tingling sensation, sense of oppression or "heat waves."
• CV: *mild fall in blood pressure;* with rapid I.V. injection, vasodilation, *bradycardia, cardiac dysrhythmias,* cardiac arrest.
• GI: with oral administration, *ingestion,* constipation, *irritation,* hemorrhage, gastric distention, nausea, vomiting; with I.V. administration, chalky taste, GI hemorrhage, nausea, vomiting, thirst, abdominal pain.
• GU: polyuria, *renal calculi,* nocturia, azotemia.
• Metabolic: hypercalcemia, hypophosphatemia.
• Local: with S.C. or I.M. injection, possible pain and irritation, burning, necrosis, sloughing of skin, cellulitis, soft-tissue calcification; with I.V. administration, *venous irritation, phlebitis, extravasation,* muscle pain, *cellulitis, soft-tissue necrosis* and calcification, requiring skin grafting (especially after I.V. push).

Overdose and treatment
Acute hypercalcemia syndrome is characterized by a markedly elevated plasma calcium level, lethargy, weakness, nausea and vomiting, and coma, and may lead to sudden death.

In case of overdose, calcium should be discontinued immediately. After oral ingestion of calcium overdose, treatment includes removal by emesis or gastric lavage followed by supportive therapy, as needed.

▶ Special considerations
• Monitor ECG when giving calcium I.V. Such injections should not exceed 0.7 and 1.5 mEq/minute in adults. Stop injection if patient complains of discomfort.
• Calcium chloride should be given I.V. only.
• I.V. calcium should be administered slowly through a small-bore needle into a large vein to avoid extravasation and necrosis.
• I.V. route is recommended in children, but not by scalp vein because calcium salts can cause tissue necrosis.
• Drug precipitates with bicarbonate. When giving drug I.V., avoid mixing with sodium bicarbonate; be sure I.V. tubing has been flushed.
• After I.V. injection, patient should be recumbent for 15 minutes to prevent orthostasis.
• If perivascular infiltration occurs, discontinue I.V. immediately. Venospasm may be reduced by administering 1% procaine hydrochloride and hyaluronidase to the affected area.
• Never give calcium chloride I.M.
• Monitor serum calcium levels frequently, especially in patients with renal impairment.
• Hypercalcemia may result when large doses are given to patients with chronic renal failure.
• Severe necrosis and sloughing of tissue may occur after extravasation. Calcium gluconate is less irritating to veins and tissue than calcium chloride.
• Assess Chvostek's and Trousseau's signs periodically to check for tetany.
• Crash carts usually contain both gluconate and chloride. Be sure to specify form to be administered.
• If GI upset occurs with oral calcium, give 2 to 3 hours after meals.
• Oxalic acid (found in rhubarb and spinach), phytic acid (in bran and whole-grain cereals), and phosphorus (in milk and dairy products) may interfere with absorption of calcium.
• With oral product, patient may need laxatives or stool softeners to manage constipation.
• Monitor for symptoms of hypercalcemia (nausea, vomiting, headache, mental confusion, anorexia), and report them immediately. Calcium absorption of an oral dose is decreased in patients with certain disease states such as achlorhydria, renal osteodystrophy, steatorrhea, or uremia.

Information for parents and patient
• Tell parents and patient not to exceed the manufacturer's recommended dosage of calcium.
• Warn parents and patient not to use bonemeal or dolomite as a source of calcium; they may contain lead.
• Patient should avoid tobacco and limit intake of alcohol and caffeine-containing beverages.

---

‡May contain sulfites   ♦May contain tartrazine   ♦♦May contain benzyl alcohol

cantharidin
Cantharone, Verr-Canth

• Classification: keratolytic (cantharide derivative)

How supplied
Available by prescription only
Liquid: 0.7%

Indications, route, and dosage
Removal of ordinary and periungual warts
Children and adults: Apply directly to lesion and cover completely. Allow to dry, then cover with nonporous adhesive tape. Remove tape in 24 hours (or less if it causes extreme pain) and replace with loose bandage. Reapply, if necessary.
Removal of moluscum contagiosum
Children and. adults: Coat each lesion. Repeat in a week on new or remaining lesions, this time covering with occlusive tape. Remove tape in 4 to 6 hours.
Removal of plantar warts
Children and adults: Pare away keratin. Apply drug to wart and 1 to 3 mm around the wart. Allow to dry; then cover with nonporous tape. Debride 1 to 3 weeks after treatment. Repeat 3 times, if necessary, on large lesions.

Action and kinetics
• *Keratolytic action:* Cantharidin causes exfoliation of benign epithelial growths as a consequence of acantholytic action. This action does not go beyond the epidermal cells; the basal layer remains intact.
• *Kinetics in adults:* Absorption is limited with topical use.

Contraindications and precautions
Cantharidin is contraindicated in patients with hypersensitivity to the drug. Avoid use near eyes or mucous membranes. Do not use on sensitive areas, such as the face or genitalia, or on moles, birthmarks, or hair-growing warts. Drug should be used with caution in patients with diabetes or impaired peripheral circulation.

Interactions
None reported.

Effects on diagnostic tests
None reported.

Adverse reactions
• Local: irritation, burning, tingling, tenderness at site; may cause annular warts.
  Note: Drug should be discontinued if sensitization develops.

Overdose and treatment
Cantharidin is a strong vesicant. If spilled on skin, wipe off at once with acetone, alcohol, or tape remover and wash with soap and water.

▶ Special considerations
• Apply directly to lesion and cover with nonporous tape. Avoid applying to normal skin tissue. Use only on affected area. Be sure to wash hands well after using drug.
• Use of mild antibacterial is recommended until tissue re-epithelializes.
• Cantharidin should never be dispensed for application by parents or patient.

Information for parents and patient
Advise parents or patient that cantharidin may cause tingling, itching, or burning a few hours after application. The application site may be extremely tender for a week after application.

captopril
Capoten

• Classification: antihypertensive, adjunctive treatment of CHF (ACE inhibitor)

How supplied
Available by prescription only
Tablets: 12.5 mg, 25 mg, 37.5 mg, 50 mg, 100 mg

Indications, route, and dosage
Mild to severe hypertension
Neonates: 0.01 mg/kg P.O. q 6 to 12 hours.
Infants and children: Initially, 0.3 mg/kg P.O. t.i.d. Increase dosage at intervals of 8 to 24 hours by 0.3 mg/kg. Children who are receiving diuretics, have renal function impairment, or are sodium- or water-depleted should be started at 0.15 mg/kg P.O. t.i.d.
Children over age 12 and adults: Initially, 25 mg P.O. b.i.d. or t.i.d.; if necessary, dosage may be increased to 50 mg t.i.d. after 1 to 2 weeks; if control is still inadequate after 1 to 2 weeks more, a diuretic may be added. Dosage may be raised to a maximum of 150 mg t.i.d. (450 mg/day) while continuing the diuretic. Daily dose may be given b.i.d.
Congestive heart failure
Neonates: 0.1 to 0.4 mg/kg P.O. q 6 to 24 hours.
Infants: 0.5 to 0.6 mg/kg/day P.O. divided q 6 to 12 hours.
Children to age 12: 25 mg/day divided q 12 hours.
Children over age 12 and adults: Initially, 25 mg P.O. t.i.d.; may be increased to 50 mg t.i.d., with maximum of 450 mg/day. In patients taking diuretics, initial dosage is 6.25 to 12.5 mg t.i.d.

Action and kinetics
• *Antihypertensive action:* Captopril inhibits ACE, preventing pulmonary conversion of angiotensin I to angiotensin II, a potent vasoconstrictor. Reduced formation of angiotensin II decreases peripheral arterial resistance, which results in decreased aldosterone secretion, thus reducing sodium and water retention and lowering blood pressure.
• *Cardiac load-reducing action:* Captopril decreases systemic vascular resistance (afterload) and pulmo-

nary capillary wedge pressure (preload), thus increasing cardiac output in patients with CHF.
• *Kinetics in adults:* Captopril is absorbed through the GI tract; food may reduce absorption by up to 40%. Antihypertensive effect begins in 15 minutes; peak blood levels occur at 1 hour. Maximum therapeutic effect may require several weeks. Captopril is distributed into most body tissues except the CNS; drug is approximately 25% to 30% protein-bound. About 50% of captopril is metabolized in the liver. Drug and its metabolites are excreted primarily in urine; small amounts are excreted in feces. Duration of effect is usually 2 to 6 hours; this increases with higher doses. Elimination half-life is less than 3 hours. Duration of action may be increased in patients with renal dysfunction.

Contraindications and precautions
Captopril is contraindicated in patients with known hypersensitivity to captopril or other ACE inhibitors.
  Captopril should be used cautiously in patients with impaired renal function or collagen vascular disease and in patients taking drugs known to depress leukocytes or immune response; such patients are at increased risk of developing neutropenia, especially if they have impaired renal function.

Interactions
Indomethacin, aspirin, and other nonsteroidal antiinflammatory drugs may decrease captopril's antihypertensive effect; antacids also decrease captopril's effects and should be given at different dose intervals.
  Captopril may increase antihypertensive effects of diuretics or other antihypertensive drugs.
  Patients with impaired renal function or CHF and patients concomitantly receiving drugs that can increase serum potassium levels – for example, potassium-sparing diuretics, potassium supplements, or salt substitutes – may develop hyperkalemia during captopril therapy.

Effects on diagnostic tests
Captopril may cause false-positive results for urinary acetone; it also may cause hyperkalemia and may transiently elevate liver enzyme levels.

Adverse reactions
• CNS: dizziness, fainting.
• CV: tachycardia, *hypotension,* angina pectoris, CHF, pericarditis.
• DERM: *urticarial or maculopapular rash,* pruritus.
• EENT: *loss of taste (dysgeusia).*
• GI: anorexia.
• GU: *proteinuria,* nephrotic syndrome, membranous glomerulopathy, renal failure, urinary frequency.
• HEMA: leukopenia, *neutropenia,* agranulocytosis, pancytopenia.
• Metabolic: hyperkalemia.
• Other: fever, angioedema of face and extremities, cough.
  Note: Drug should be discontinued if neutropenia or renal failure occurs.

Overdose and treatment
Overdose is manifested primarily by severe hypotension. After acute ingestion, empty stomach by induced emesis or gastric lavage. Follow with activated charcoal to reduce absorption. Subsequent treatment is usually symptomatic and supportive. In severe cases, hemodialysis may be considered.

▶ **Special considerations**
• Safety and efficacy of captopril in children have not been established; use only if potential benefit outweighs risk.
• Diuretic therapy is usually discontinued 2 to 3 days before beginning captopril therapy, to reduce risk of hypotension; if drug does not adequately control blood pressure, diuretics may be reinstated.
• Perform WBC and differential counts before treatment, every 2 weeks for 3 months, and periodically thereafter. Monitor serum potassium levels because potassium retention has been noted.
• Lower dosage or reduced dosing frequency is necessary in patients with impaired renal function. Titrate patient to effective levels over a 1- to 2-week interval, then reduce dosage to lowest effective level.
• Give drug 1 hour before meals; food reduces absorption.
• Several weeks of therapy may be required before the beneficial effects of captopril are seen.
• Proteinuria and nephrotic syndrome may occur in patients who are on captopril therapy.
• If patient is receiving antacids, give them at different dose intervals (1 to 2 hours) because they may decrease captopril's effects.

Information for parents and patient
• Tell parents to watch for and report signs of lightheadedness, especially in first few days, so dosage can be adjusted; signs of infection, such as sore throat or fever, because drug may decrease WBC count; facial swelling or difficulty breathing, because drug may cause angioedema; and loss of taste, which may necessitate discontinuing drug.
• Advise parents that patient should avoid sudden position changes, to minimize orthostatic hypotension.
• Warn parents to seek medical approval before giving patient OTC cold preparations.
• Patient should take drug 1 hour before meals.

carbamazepine
Epitol, Mazepine, Tegretol

• Classification: anticonvulsant, analgesic (iminostilbene derivative; chemically related to tricyclic antidepressants)

How supplied
Available by prescription only
Tablets: 200 mg
Tablets (chewable): 100 mg
Suspension: 100 mg/5 ml

Indications, route, and dosage
Generalized tonic-clonic (grand mal), complex-partial (psychomotor), mixed seizure patterns

†*Children age 5 and under:* Initially, 5 mg/kg P.O. daily in four divided doses. Increase at 5- to 7-day intervals, initially to 10 mg/kg daily, then higher (up to 20 mg/kg daily).

Children age 6 to 12: Initially, 100 mg P.O. b.i.d., increasing by 100 mg/day at 6- to 8-hour intervals. Do not exceed 1,000 mg/day. Alternatively, give 20 mg/kg P.O. daily divided t.i.d. to q.i.d.

Children over age 12 and adults: 200 mg P.O. b.i.d. on day 1. May increase by 200 mg P.O. per day, in divided doses at 6- to 8-hour intervals. Adjust to minimum effective level when control is achieved; do not exceed 1,000 mg/day in children age 12 to 15, or 1,200 mg/day in those over age 15. In rare instances, higher doses have been used.

Trigeminal neuralgia

Adults: 100 mg P.O. b.i.d. with meals on day 1. Increase by 100 mg q 12 hours until pain is relieved. Don't exceed 1.2 g daily. Maintenance dose is 200 to 400 mg P.O. b.i.d.

Action and kinetics

• *Anticonvulsant action:* Carbamazepine is chemically unrelated to other anticonvulsants and its mechanism of action is unknown. It appears to limit seizure propagation by reducing polysynaptic responses.

Many clinicians consider carbamazepine the drug of choice for initial anticonvulsant therapy, especially in children; it is increasingly preferred to phenobarbital in children because it has less effect on alertness and behavior. In seizure disorders, carbamazepine can be used alone or with other anticonvulsants.

• *Analgesic action:* In trigeminal neuralgia, carbamazepine is a specific analgesic through its reduction of synaptic neurotransmission.

• *Kinetics in adults:* Carbamazepine is absorbed slowly from the GI tract; peak plasma concentrations occur at 2 to 8 hours.

Carbamazepine is distributed widely throughout the body; it crosses the placenta and accumulates in fetal tissue. The drug is approximately 75% protein-bound. Therapeutic serum levels are 3 to 14 mcg/ml; nystagmus can occur above 4 mcg/ml and ataxia, dizziness, and anorexia at or above 10 mcg/ml. Serum levels may be misleading because an unmeasured active metabolite also can cause toxicity.

Carbamazepine is metabolized by the liver to an active metabolite. It may also induce its own metabolism; over time, higher doses are needed to maintain plasma levels.

Carbamazepine is excreted in urine (70%) and feces (30%); carbamazepine levels in breast milk approach 60% of serum levels.

Contraindications and precautions

Carbamazepine is contraindicated in patients with known hypersensitivity to carbamazepine and tricyclic antidepressants and in patients with past or present bone marrow depression; it also is contraindicated for use with monoamine oxidase (MAO) inhibitors or within 14 days of such use.

Use carbamazepine with caution in patients with cardiovascular, renal, or hepatic damage; increased intraocular pressure; or atypical absence seizures.

Interactions

Concomitant use of carbamazepine with MAO inhibitors may cause hypertensive crisis; use with calcium channel blockers (verapamil and possibly diltiazem) may increase serum levels of carbamazepine significantly (therefore, carbamazepine dosage should be decreased by 40% to 50% when given with verapamil); concomitant use with erythromycin, cimetidine, isoniazid, or propoxyphene also may increase serum carbamazepine levels.

Concomitant use with phenobarbital, phenytoin, or primidone lowers serum carbamazepine levels. When used with warfarin, phenytoin, haloperidol, ethosuximide, or valproic acid, carbamazepine may increase the metabolism of these drugs; it may decrease the effectiveness of theophylline and oral contraceptives.

Effects on diagnostic tests

Carbamazepine may elevate liver enzyme levels; it also may decrease values of thyroid function tests.

Adverse reactions

• CNS: *dizziness,* vertigo, *drowsiness,* fatigue, ataxia, worsening of seizures, hallucinations, speech disturbances, *neuritis.*

• CV: congestive heart failure, hypertension, hypotension, aggravation of coronary artery disease, thrombophlebitis, dysrhythmias (deaths have occurred).

• DERM: rash, urticaria, erythema multiforme, Stevens-Johnson syndrome.

• EENT: conjunctivitis, dry mouth and pharynx, blurred vision, *diplopia,* nystagmus.

• GI: *nausea,* vomiting, abdominal pain, diarrhea, anorexia, stomatitis, glossitis, dry mouth.

• GU: *urinary frequency or retention,* impotence, albuminuria, glycosuria, elevated blood urea nitrogen levels.

• HEMA: aplastic anemia, agranulocytosis, eosinophilia, leukocytosis, thrombocytopenia.

• Hepatic: abnormal liver function tests, hepatitis.

• Metabolic: water intoxication, hypocalcemia.

• Other: diaphoresis, fever, chills, pulmonary hypersensitivity, paralysis, abnormal movements, leg cramps, joint pain, *tinnitus.*

Note: Drug should be discontinued if signs of hypersensitivity, significant elevation of liver function tests, or hematologic abnormalities occur; or if any of the following signs of bone marrow depression appear: fever, sore throat, mouth ulcers, easy bruising, or petechial or purpuric hemorrhage.

Overdose and treatment

Symptoms of overdose may include irregular breathing, respiratory depression, tachycardia, blood pressure changes, shock, dysrhythmias, impaired consciousness (ranging to deep coma), convulsions, restlessness, drowsiness, psychomotor disturbances, nausea, vomiting, anuria, or oliguria.

Treat overdose with repeated gastric lavage, especially if the patient ingested alcohol concurrently.

---

*Canada only   †Unlabeled clinical use   Italicized adverse reactions have been observed in children.

Oral charcoal and laxatives may hasten excretion. Carefully monitor vital signs, ECG, and fluid and electrolyte balance. Diazepam may control convulsions but can exacerbate respiratory depression.

▶ **Special considerations**
• Safety and efficacy have not been established for children under age 2.
• Carbamazepine dosage should be adjusted according to individual response.
• Drug is structurally similar to tricyclic antidepressants.
• Hematologic toxicity is rare but serious.
• Chewable tablets and suspension are available for children.
• Unlabeled uses of carbamazepine include neurogenic diabetes insipidus, certain psychiatric disorders, and management of alcohol withdrawal.
• Consider that poor response or low serum levels may result from auto-induction of metabolism, not non-confidence.

Information for parents and patient
• Tell parents that carbamazepine may cause GI distress. Advise parents that patient should take drug with food at equally spaced intervals.
• Warn parents that patient should not stop drug abruptly.
• Encourage parents to promptly report unusual bleeding, bruising, jaundice, dark urine, pale stools, abdominal pain, impotence, fever, chills, sore throat, mouth ulcers, edema, or disturbances in mood, alertness, or coordination.
• Emphasize importance of follow-up laboratory tests and continued medical supervision. Periodic eye examinations are recommended.
• Warn parents and patient that drug may cause drowsiness, dizziness, and blurred vision. Advise parents that patient should avoid hazardous activities that require alertness, especially during first week of therapy and when dosage is increased.

---

carbarsone
Carbarsone Pulvules

• Classification: amebicide (organic arsenical)

How supplied
Available by prescription only
Capsules: 250 mg

Indications, route, and dosage
Intestinal amebiasis
Children: Average total dosage is 75 mg/kg P.O. given in three divided doses daily over a 10-day period. Recommended total varies according to age—age 2 to 4: 2 g total (66 mg t.i.d.); age 5 to 8: 3 g total (100 mg t.i.d.); age 9 to 12: 4 g total (133 mg t.i.d.); and over age 12: 5 g total (167 mg t.i.d.).
Adults: 250 mg P.O. b.i.d. or t.i.d. for 10 days. Rectal (as retention enema): 2 g dissolved in 200 ml of warm 2% sodium bicarbonate solution, every other night for

five doses. Discontinue oral therapy when enema is given.

Action and kinetics
• *Amebicidal action:* Carbarsone is amebicidal against protozoa, especially *Entamoeba histolytica,* and acts primarily in the intestinal lumen, probably by combining with sulfhydryl groups of enzymes in the parasite. Because of its toxic potential, carbarsone is not considered a first-line drug.
• *Kinetics in adults:* Carbarsone is absorbed readily from the GI tract after oral and rectal administration. Carbarsone may be partially converted to methylated products in the liver. It is excreted slowly by the kidney; it is unknown whether it is excreted in breast milk.

Contraindications and precautions
Carbarsone is contraindicated in patients with hepatic or renal disease because it is metabolized in the liver and excreted by the kidneys; in patients with contracted visual or color fields because of its adverse ocular effects; and in patients with a history of hypersensitivity to topically or systemically administered arsenic agents.
Because carbarsone is excreted slowly, this drug accumulates over time; therefore, the total daily dosage should not exceed the maximum recommended daily dosage, and duration of treatment should not exceed 10 days.

Interactions
No interactions with carbarsone have been well documented.

Effects on diagnostic tests
Proteinuria and abnormal results of liver function tests may occur as adverse effects of carbarsone therapy.

Adverse reactions
• CNS: neuritis, seizures, hemorrhagic encephalitis.
• DERM: *rash,* eruptions, exfoliative dermatitis, pruritus.
• EENT: sore throat, retinal edema, visual disturbances.
• GI: epigastric pain and burning, irritation, *nausea, vomiting, diarrhea,* abdominal pain or cramps, anorexia, constipation, increased motility.
• GU: polyuria, albuminuria, kidney dysfunction.
• HEMA: agranulocytosis.
• Hepatic: hepatomegaly, jaundice, hepatitis, liver necrosis.
• Other: edema of wrists, ankles, and knees; weight loss; splenomegaly; pulmonary congestion; fever.
Note: Drug should be discontinued if signs of hypersensitivity or toxicity occur.

Overdose and treatment
Clinical manifestations of overdose are from arsenic toxicity and include nausea, vomiting, abdominal pain, diarrhea, shock, coma, seizures, kidney dysfunction, and ulceration of the skin and mucous membranes.
The antidote for carbarsone toxicity is dimercaprol (British anti-Lewisite, or BAL) 3 to 4 mg/kg every 6 hours for 2 days, then every 12 hours for 8 more days.

Dimercaprol may be ineffective if aplastic anemia, hemorrhagic encephalitis, or jaundice has developed. Supportive treatment includes gastric lavage, oxygen therapy, I.V. fluid therapy, and stabilization of body temperature. Hemodialysis may be helpful in severe cases.

▶ **Special considerations**
• Skin rashes may occur but are usually mild; GI complaints (nausea, vomiting, diarrhea) may occur.
• Divide carbarsone capsule to obtain required dose. Give in a 4-oz (120-ml) glass of orange juice or milk, in a small amount of 1% sodium bicarbonate solution, or in jelly or other food.
• Low-residue diet may alleviate GI upset.
• Tell the patient to report any unusual symptoms, even after the drug is discontinued.
• Liver function tests should precede therapy. During therapy, regularly repeat careful inspection of the skin, vision testing, and palpation of liver and spleen for possible adverse reactions.
• Monitor intake and output and bowel function.
• Enema to obtain stool specimen should use isotonic saline solution or tap water; hypertonic solutions may alter appearance of amebae. Send stool specimens to laboratory promptly; movements of parasites are seen only in warm stool. Amebic cysts in stool indicate need for additional therapy. Stool specimen should be checked 1 week after stopping therapy and monthly thereafter, for 1 year.
• Rest periods of 10 to 14 days must follow each 10-day course of treatment because slow excretion of carbarsone allows drug accumulation and therefore potential toxicity. Be prepared for arsenic toxicity and have antidote at hand.

Information for parents and patient
• Patient should limit physical activities during treatment.
• Teach parents about symptoms and adverse reactions that should be reported.
• To help prevent reinfection, teach parents and patient proper hygiene, including disposal of feces and hand washing after defecation and before handling, preparing, or eating food. Emphasize the control of contamination by flies and the risks of eating raw food.
• Advise parents that isolation is not required but that patient must refrain from preparing, processing, or serving food until treatment is complete.
• Advise use of liquid soap or reserved bar of soap to prevent cross-contamination.

---

carbenicillin disodium
Geopen, Pyopen

• Classification: antibiotic (extended-spectrum penicillin, alpha-carboxypenicillin)

How supplied
Available by prescription only
Injection: 1 g, 2 g, 5 g per vial

Pharmacy bulk package: 10 g, 20 g, 30 g per vial
I.V. infusion piggyback: 2 g, 5 g, 10 g

Indications, route, and dosage
Serious infections caused by Pseudomonas aeruginosa *or anaerobes*
Children age 1 month and over: 400 to 500 mg/kg I.V. daily by continuous or intermittent infusion (not to exceed 40 g daily)
Adults: 400 to 500 mg/kg (30 to 40 g) I.V. by continuous infusion or divided q 4 hours
Serious infections caused by Escherichia coli *or* Proteus
Children age 1 month or older: 250 to 400 mg/kg/day I.V. by continuous infusion or in divided doses
Adults: 1 to 2 g I.M. or I.V. q 6 hours
Severe infections caused by susceptible strains of E. coli, Hemophilus influenzae, Proteus, Pseudomonas, Streptococcus pneumoniae, *and anaerobes*
Neonates weighing < 2 kg: Initially, give a loading dose of 100 mg I.V. followed by 75 mg/kg I.V. q 8 hours, increasing to 100 mg/kg I.V. q 6 hours after the infant reaches 1 week of age.
Neonates weighing > 2 kg: Initially, 100 mg/kg I.V. followed by 75 mg/kg I.V. q 6 hours during the first 3 days. Dosage may be increased to 100 mg I.V. q 6 hours when the infant is over 3 days old.
Urinary tract infections
Children: 50 to 200 mg/kg daily I.M. or I.V. infusion, divided into doses given q 4 to 6 hours.
Adults: 200 mg/kg daily I.M. or I.V. infusion, divided into doses given q 4 to 6 hours.
  The maximum daily dosage of carbenicillin disodium in an adult is 40 g.
Dosage in renal failure (creatinine clearance < 10 ml/min)
Adults: 2 g I.V. q 8 to 12 hours. Alternatively, give the usual dose q 24 to 48 hours.
Adults undergoing hemodialysis: 2 g I.V. q 4 hours for serious infections. Alternatively, administer as above with supplemental 750 mg to 2 g I.V. after each treatment.
Adults undergoing peritoneal dialysis: 2 g I.V. q 6 to 12 hours.

Action and kinetics
• *Antibiotic action:* Carbenicillin is bactericidal; it adheres to bacterial penicillin-binding proteins, thus inhibiting bacterial cell wall synthesis.
  Extended-spectrum penicillins are more resistant to inactivation by certain beta-lactamases, especially those produced by gram-negative organisms, but are still liable to inactivation by certain others.
  Carbenicillin's spectrum of activity includes many gram-negative aerobic and anaerobic bacilli, many gram-positive and gram-negative aerobic cocci, and some gram-positive aerobic and anaerobic bacilli.
• *Kinetics in adults:* No appreciable absorption occurs after oral administration. After an I.M. dose, peak plasma concentrations occur at 0.5 to 2.0 hours.
  Carbenicillin disodium is distributed widely after parenteral administration; it penetrates minimally into uninflamed meninges and only slightly into bone and sputum. Carbenicillin disodium crosses the placenta

---

and is 30% to 60% protein-bound. It may concentrate in biliary fluid.

Carbenicillin disodium is metabolized partially.

Drug and its metabolites are excreted primarily (79% to 99%) in urine by glomerular filtration and tubular secretion; some drug is excreted in breast milk. Elimination half-life in adults is about 1 hour; in patients with extensive renal impairment, half-life is extended to 9½ to 23 hours. Carbenicillin disodium is removed by hemodialysis but not by peritoneal dialysis.

• *Kinetics in children:* Serum half-life is prolonged in neonates. Excretion may be enhanced in children with cystic fibrosis.

Contraindications and precautions

Carbenicillin disodium is contraindicated in patients with known hypersensitivity to any other penicillin or to cephalosporins.

Carbenicillin disodium should be used with caution in patients with renal impairment, because it is excreted in urine; decreased dosage is required in moderate to severe renal failure.

Interactions

Concomitant use of carbenicillin with aminoglycoside antibiotics results in synergistic bactericidal effects against *Pseudomonas aeruginosa, E. coli, Klebsiella, Citrobacter, Enterobacter, Serratia,* and *Proteus mirabilis.* However, the drugs are physically and chemically incompatible and are inactivated if mixed or given together. Concomitant use of carbenicillin disodium (and other extended-spectrum penicillins) with clavulanic acid produces synergistic bactericidal effects against certain beta-lactamase-producing bacteria.

Probenecid blocks tubular secretion of carbenicillin, raising its serum concentrations.

Large doses of penicillins may interfere with renal tubular secretion of methotrexate, delaying elimination and elevating serum concentrations of methotrexate.

Effects on diagnostic tests

Carbenicillin disodium alters results of urine glucose tests that use cupric sulfate (Benedict's reagent or Clinitest). Make urine glucose determinations with glucose oxidase methods (Clinistix or Tes-Tape). Carbenicillin disodium causes increased serum uric acid values (cupric sulfate method) and false elevations of urine specific gravity in dehydrated patients with low urine output; positive Coombs' tests have been reported.

Carbenicillin may falsely decrease serum aminoglycoside concentrations.

Carbenicillin intefemes with some human leukocyte antigen (HLA) tests and could cause inaccurate HLA typing. This drug's systemic effects may cause hypokalemia and hypernatremia and may prolong prothrombin times; it may also cause transient elevations in liver function study results and transient reductions in red blood cell, white blood cell, and platelet counts.

Adverse reactions

• CNS: neuromuscular irritability seizures.
• GI: nausea, vomiting.
• GU: acute interstitial nephritis.
• HEMA: bleeding with high doses, neutropenia, eosinophilia, leukopenia, *thrombocytopenia,* anemia.
• Local: pain at injection site, vein irritation, phlebitis.
• Metabolic: hypokalemia, *hypernatremia.*
• Other: hypersensitivity (edema, fever, chills, rash, pruritus, urticaria, anaphylaxis), bacterial and fungal superinfection.

Note: Drug should be discontinued if immediate hypersensitivity reactions or bleeding complications occur; and if severe diarrhea occurs, because that may indicate pseudomembranous colitis.

Overdose and treatment

Clinical signs of overdose include neuromuscular hypersensitivity or seizures resulting from CNS irritation by high drug concentrations. Carbenicillin disodium can be removed by hemodialysis; about 45% to 70% of a given dose is removed after 4 to 6 hours of hemodialysis.

▶ Special considerations

• Assess patient's history of allergies; do not give carbenicillin to any patient with a history of hypersensitivity reactions to either penicillins or cephalosporins. Try to determine whether previous reactions were true hypersensitivity reactions or another reaction, such as GI distress, which the patient has interpreted as allergy.

• Keep in mind that a negative history for penicillin hypersensitivity does not preclude future allergic reactions; monitor patient continuously for possible allergic reactions or other untoward effects.

• In patients with renal impairment, dosage should be reduced if creatinine clearance is below 10 ml/minute.

• Assess level of consciousness, neurologic status, and renal function when high doses are used, because excessive blood levels can cause CNS toxicity.

• Obtain results of cultures and sensitivity tests before test results are complete. Repeat test periodically to assess drug efficacy.

• Monitor vital signs, electrolytes, and renal function studies; monitor body weight for fluid retention with extended-spectrum penicillins for possible hypokalemia or hypernatremia.

• Coagulation abnormalities, even frank bleeding, can follow high doses, especially of extended-spectrum penicllins; monitor prothrombin times and platelet counts, and assess patient for signs of occult or frank bleeding.

• Monitor patients on long-term therapy for possible superinfection, especially debilitated patients and others receiving immunosuppressants or radiation therapy; monitor closely, especially for fever.

Parenteral administration

• Use this drug cautiously in patients on sodium-restricted diets; sodium content is high (4.7 to 6.5 mEq/g).

• Give penicillins at least 1 hour before giving bacteriostatic antibiotics (tetracyclines, erythromycins, and chloramphenicol); these drugs inhibit bacterial cell growth, decreasing rate of penicillin uptake by bacterial cell walls.

• Consult manufacturer's directions for reconstitution, dilution, and storage of drugs; check expiration dates.

• Administer I.M. dose deep into large muscle mass (gluteal or midlateral thigh); rotate injection sites to minimize tissue injury; do not inject more than 2 g or drug per injection site. Apply ice to injection site for pain.

• Do not add or mix other drugs with I.V. infusions — particularly aminoglycosides, which will be inactivated if mixed with penicillins; they are chemically and physically incompatible. If other drugs must be given I.V., temporarily stop infusion of primary drug.

• Do not reconstitute with sterile water containing benzyl alcohol.

• Infuse I.V. drug continuously or intermittently (over 30 minutes) and assess I.V. site frequently to prevent infiltration or phlebitis; rotate infusion site q 48 hours; intermittent I.V. infusion may be diluted in 50 to 100 ml sterile water, 0.9% sodium chloride, dextrose 5% in water, dextrose 5% in water and half normal saline, or lactated Ringer's solution.

• Solutions should always be clear, colorless to pale yellow, and free of particles; do not give solutions containing precipitates or other foreign matter.

• Carbenicillin is almost always used with another antibiotic, such as an aminoglycoside, in life-threatening situations.

• Dosage reduction is not required unless the patient's creatinine clearance is below 10 ml/minute.

• Check complete blood count, differential, and platelet count frequently. Drug may cause thrombocytopenia. Observe carefully for signs of overt or occult bleeding.

• High blood concentrations of this drug may cause seizures.

• Because carbenicillin is dialyzable, patients undergoing hemodialysis may need dosage adjustments.

• Pharmacy bulk packages (10 g, 20 g, 30 g) are not intended for direct I.V. infusion.

Information for parents and patient

• Teach signs and symptoms of hypersensitivity and other adverse reactions, and emphasize need to report any unusual reactions.

• Teach signs and symptoms of bacterial and fungal superinfection to parents and patients, especially debilitated patients and others with low resistance from immunosuppressants or irradiation; emphasize need to report signs of infection.

carbinoxamine maleate
Clistin

• Classification: antihistamine, H_1-receptor antagonist (ethanolamine derivative)

How supplied
Available by prescription only
Tablets: 4 mg

Indications, route, and dosage
Rhinitis, allergy symptoms
Children age 1 to 3: 2 mg P.O. t.i.d. or q.i.d.
Children age 3 to 6: 2 to 4 mg P.O. t.i.d. or q.i.d.
Children over age 6: 4 to 6 mg P.O. t.i.d. or q.i.d.
Adults: 4 to 8 mg P.O. t.i.d. or q.i.d.

Action and kinetics
• *Antihistamine action:* Antihistamines compete with histamine for histamine H_1-receptor sites on the smooth muscle of the bronchi, GI tract, uterus, and large blood vessels; by binding to cellular receptors, they prevent access of histamine and suppress histamine-induced allergic symptoms, even though they do not prevent its release.

• *Kinetics in adults:* Carbinoxamine apparently is metabolized primarily in the liver; it is apparently excreted primarily in urine.

Contraindications and precautions
Carbinoxamine is contraindicated in patients with known hypersensitivity to this drug or other antihistamines with similar chemical structures (diphenhydramine and clemastine); in patients experiencing asthmatic attacks, because carbinoxamine thickens bronchial secretions; and in patients who have taken MAO inhibitors within the preceding 2 weeks.

Carbinoxamine should be used with caution in patients with narrow-angle glaucoma; in those with pyloroduodenal obstruction or urinary bladder obstruction from narrowing of the bladder neck, because of their marked anticholinergic effects; in patients with cardiovascular disease, hypertension, or hyperthyroidism, because of the risk of palpitations and tachycardia; and in patients with renal disease, diabetes, bronchial asthma, urinary retention, or stenosing peptic ulcer.

Interactions
MAO inhibitors interfere with the detoxification of antihistamines and thus prolong and intensify their central depressant and anticholinergic effects. Concomitant use of carbinoxamine with other CNS depressants, such as alcohol, barbiturates, tranquilizers, sleeping aids, and antianxiety agents, produces additive sedative effects.

Carbinoxamine may diminish the effects of sulfonylureas and may partially counteract the anticoagulant action of heparin.

Effects on diagnostic tests
Discontinue carbinoxamine 4 days before diagnostic skin tests; antihistamines can prevent, reduce, or mask positive skin test response.

Adverse reactions
• CNS: drowsiness, dizziness, stimulation.
• GI: anorexia, constipation, nausea, vomiting, dry mouth.
• GU: urinary retention.

Overdose and treatment
Clinical manifestations of overdose may include either CNS depression (sedation, reduced mental alertness,

apnea, and cardiovascular collapse) or CNS stimulation (insomnia, hallucinations, tremors, and convulsions). Atropine-like symptoms, such as dry mouth, flushed skin, fixed and dilated pupils, and GI symptoms, are common, especially in children.

Treat overdose by inducing emesis with ipecac syrup (in conscious patient), followed by activated charcoal to reduce further drug absorption. Use gastric lavage if patient is unconscious or ipecac fails. Treat hypotension with vasopressors, and control seizures with diazepam or phenytoin. *Do not give stimulants.*

▶ Special considerations
• Neonates, especially premature infants, may experience paradoxical excitability with restlessness, insomnia, nervousness, euphoria, tremors, and seizures.
• Antihistamines are contraindicated in acute asthma attack because they may not alleviate the symptoms and because antimuscarinic effects can cause thickening of secretions.
• Reduce GI distress by giving drug with food; give sugarless gum or candy or ice chips to relieve dry mouth; increase fluid intake (if allowed) or humidify air to decrease adverse effect of thickened secretions.

Information for parents and patient
• Advise patient to report use of salicylates; this drug may mask ototoxic effects of other drugs.
• Advise patient to take drug with meals or snack to prevent gastric upset and to use any of the following measures to relieve dry mouth: warm water rinses, artificial saliva, ice chips, or sugarless gum or appropriate candy. Patient should avoid overusing mouthwash, which may add to dryness (alcohol content) and destroy normal flora.
• Warn parents that child should avoid hazardous activities that require alertness until extent of CNS effects are known. Tell them to seek medical approval before administering tranquilizers, sedatives, pain relievers, or sleeping medications.
• Warn parents to discontinue drug 4 days before diagnostic skin tests, to preserve accuracy of tests.

---

carisoprodol
Rela, Sodol, Soma, Soprodol

• Classification: skeletal muscle relaxant (carbamate derivative)

How supplied
Available by prescription only
Tablets: 350 mg

Indications, route, and dosage
Adjunct for relief of discomfort in acute, painful musculoskeletal conditions
Children over age 12 and adults: Administer 350 mg P.O. t.i.d. and h.s.

Action and kinetics
• *Skeletal muscle relaxant action:* Carisoprodol does not relax skeletal muscle directly, but apparently as a result of its sedative effects. However, the exact mechanism of action is unknown. Animal studies suggest that the drug modifies central perception of pain without eliminating peripheral pain reflexes, and has slight antipyretic activity.
• *Kinetics in adults:* With usual therapeutic doses, onset of action occurs within 30 minutes and persists 4 to 6 hours. Carisoprodol is widely distributed throughout the body. Carisoprodol is metabolized in the liver. The drug may induce microsomal enzymes in the liver. The drug is excreted in urine mainly as its metabolites; less than 1% of a dose is excreted unchanged. The drug may be removed by hemodialysis or peritoneal dialysis.

Contraindications and precautions
Carisoprodol is contraindicated in patients with acute intermittent porphyria, because the drug may exacerbate the condition, and in those who have demonstrated allergic or idiosyncratic reactions to the drug or its related compounds (meprobamate).

Administer cautiously to patients with impaired renal or hepatic function. Patients allergic or sensitive to the dye tartrazine should avoid taking Rela tablets. Although tartrazine sensitivity is rare, it frequently occurs in patients sensitive to aspirin.

Administer cautiously to patients with CNS depression, because effects may be additive. Psychological dependence and abuse have been reported in those with a history of drug abuse or dependence. Avoid use in patients with head injury or coma.

Interactions
Concomitant use with other CNS depressants, including alcohol, produces additive CNS depression. When used with other depressant drugs (general anesthetics, opioid analgesics, antipsychotics, tricyclic antidepressants, or anxiolytics), exercise care to avoid overdose. Concurrent use with monoamine oxidase inhibitors or tricyclic antidepressants may increase CNS depression, respiratory depression, and hypotensive effects. Dosage adjustments (reduction of one or both) are required.

Effects on diagnostic tests
None significant.

Adverse reactions
• CNS: drowsiness, dizziness, vertigo, ataxia, tremor, insomnia, agitation, irritability, headache, depression, syncope.
• CV: tachycardia, postural hypotension (orthostatic), facial flushing.
• DERM: rash, erythema, urticaria, pruritus, fixed drug eruption.
• GI: nausea, vomiting, hiccups, increased bowel activity, epigastric distress.
• HEMA: eosinophilia.
• Other: asthmatic episodes, fever, angioneurotic edema, weakness, stinging or burning eyes, anaphylaxis.
Note: Drug should be discontinued if allergic or idiosyncratic reactions occur during therapy. May be treated with epinephrine, antihistamines, or corti-

---

‡May contain sulfites   ◆May contain tartrazine   ◆◆May contain benzyl alcohol

costeroids as needed. Hypersensitivity possible to drug or to tartrazine in formulation.

Overdose and treatment
Clinical manifestations of overdose include exaggerated CNS depression, stupor, coma, shock, and respiratory depression.

Treatment of a conscious patient requires emptying the stomach by emesis or gastric lavage; activated charcoal may be used after gastric lavage to adsorb any remaining drug. If patient is comatose, secure endotracheal tube with cuff inflated before gastric lavage. Provide supportive therapy by maintaining adequate airway and assisted ventilation. CNS stimulants and pressor agents should be used cautiously. Monitor vital signs, fluid and electrolyte levels, and neurologic status closely.

Monitor urine output, and avoid overhydration. Forced diuresis using mannitol, peritoneal dialysis, or hemodialysis may be beneficial. Continue to monitor patient for relapse from incomplete gastric emptying and delayed absorption. Contact local or regional poison control center for more information.

▶ Special considerations
• Safety and efficacy have not been established in children under age 12. However, some clinicians suggest a dosage of 25 mg/kg or 750 mg/m² divided q.i.d. for children age 5 and older.
• Use with caution with other CNS depressants, because effects may be cumulative.
• Initially, allergic or idiosyncratic reactions may occur (first to the fourth dose). Symptoms usually subside after several hours; treat with supportive and symptomatic measures.
• Psychological dependence may follow long-term use.
• Withdrawal symptoms (abdominal cramps, insomnia, chilliness, headache, and nausea) may occur with abrupt termination of drug after prolonged use of higher-than-recommended doses.
• Rela contains tartrazine, which may cause allergic reactions, including bronchial asthma, in susceptible individuals. Such patients also may be sensitive to aspirin.

Information for parents and patient
• Patient may take drug with food to avoid GI upset.
• Inform parents that carisoprodol may cause dizziness and faintness in some patients. Symptoms may be controlled by making position changes slowly and in stages. Parents should report persistent symptoms.
• Tell parents that patient should avoid alcoholic beverages and use cough or cold preparations containing alcohol cautiously while taking this medication. He should also avoid other CNS depressants (effects may be additive) unless prescribed.
• Warn parents and patient that drug may cause drowsiness. Patient should avoid hazardous activities that require alertness until CNS depressant effects can be determined.
• Advise parents to discontinue drug immediately and to call if rash, diplopia, dizziness, or other unusual signs or symptoms appear.
• Tell parents to store drug away from direct heat, light, and moisture (not in bathroom medicine cabinet).
• Instruct parents to have child take missed dose only if remembered within 1 hour. If remembered later, patient should skip that dose and go back to regular schedule. Patient should not double the dose.

---

carmustine (BCNU)
BiCNU

• Classification: antineoplastic (alkylating agent; nitrosourea [cell cycle-phase nonspecific])

How supplied
Available by prescription only
Injection: 100-mg vial (lyophilized), with a 3-ml vial of absolute alcohol supplied as a diluent

Indications, route, and dosage
Dosage and indications may vary. Check current literature for recommended protocol.
†*Brain, colon, and stomach cancer; Hodgkin's disease; non-Hodgkin's lymphomas; melanomas; multiple myeloma; hepatoma*
Children and adults: 75 to 100 mg/m² I.V. by slow infusion daily for 2 consecutive days, repeated q 6 weeks if platelet count is above 100,000/mm³ and WBC count is above 4,000/mm³. Reduce dosage by 50% when WBC count is below 2,000/mm³ and platelet count is below 25,000/mm³.
Alternate therapy: 200 mg/m² I.V. slow infusion as a single dose, repeated q 6 to 8 weeks; or 40 mg/m² I.V. slow infusion for 5 consecutive days, repeated q 6 weeks.

Action and kinetics
• *Antineoplastic action:* The cytotoxic action of carmustine is mediated through its metabolites, which inhibit several enzymes involved with DNA formation. This agent can also cause cross-linking of DNA. Cross-linking interferes with DNA, RNA, and protein synthesis. Cross-resistance between carmustine and lomustine has been shown to occur.
• *Kinetics in adults:* Carmustine is not absorbed across the GI tract. Carmustine is cleared rapidly from the plasma. After I.V. administration, carmustine and its metabolites distribute rapidly into the CSF. Carmustine also is distributed in breast milk. Carmustine is metabolized extensively in the liver. Approximately 60% to 70% of carmustine and its metabolites are excreted in urine within 96 hours, 6% to 10% is excreted as carbon dioxide by the lungs, and 1% is excreted in feces. Enterohepatic circulation and storage of the drug in adipose tissue can occur and may cause delayed hematologic toxicity.

Contraindications and precautions
Carmustine is contraindicated in patients with a history of hypersensitivity to the drug.

Drug should be withheld or dosage reduced in the presence of hepatic or renal insufficiency because drug accumulation may occur; in patients with compro-

---

mised hematologic status because of the drug's adverse hematologic effects; and in patients with recent exposure to cytotoxic medications or radiation therapy.

Interactions
Concomitant use with cimetidine increases the bone marrow toxicity of carmustine. The mechanism of this interaction is unknown. Avoid concomitant use of these drugs.

Effects on diagnostic tests
Carmustine therapy may increase BUN, serum alkaline phosphatase, AST (SGOT), and bilirubin concentrations.

Adverse reactions
• DERM: hyperpigmentation upon accidental contact of drug with skin; alopecia.
• GI: *nausea,* possibly severe, lasting 2 to 6 hours after dose; *vomiting.*
• GU: nephrotoxicity.
• HEMA: bone marrow depression (dose-limiting, usually occurring 4 to 6 weeks after a dose), *leukopenia, thrombocytopenia.*
• Hepatic: *reversible liver damage.*
• Metabolic: possible hyperuricemia in lymphoma patients when rapid cell lysis occurs.
• Local: *intense pain at infusion site.*
• Other: *pulmonary fibrosis, delayed renal damage.*

Overdose and treatment
Clinical manifestations of overdose include leukopenia, thrombocytopenia, nausea, and vomiting.

Treatment consists of supportive measures, including transfusion of blood components, antibiotics for infections that may develop, and antiemetics.

▶ Special considerations
• Reconstitute the 100-mg vial with the 3 ml of absolute alcohol provided by the manufacturer, then dilute further with 27 ml sterile water for injection. Resultant solution contains 3.3 mg carmustine/ml in 10% ethanol. Dilute in normal saline or dextrose 5% in water for I.V. infusion. Give over 1 to 2 hours. Discard excess drug.
• Follow all established procedures for the safe and proper handling, administration, and disposal of chemotherapy.
• Vital signs and patency of catheter or I.V. line throughout administration should be monitored.
• Wear gloves to administer carmustine infusion and when changing I.V. tubing. Avoid contact with skin because carmustine will cause a brown stain. If drug comes into contact with skin, wash off thoroughly.
• Solution is unstable in plastic I.V. bags. Administer only in glass containers.
• Carmustine may decompose at temperatures above 80° F. (26.6° C.).
• If powder liquefies or appears oily, it is a sign of decomposition. Discard.
• Reconstituted solution may be stored in refrigerator for 24 hours.
• Don't mix with other drugs during administration.
• Avoid all I.M. injections, if possible, when platelets

are below 100,000/mm³. If necessary, transfuse with platelets before I.M. injection.
• To reduce pain on infusion, dilute further, slow infusion rate, and apply warm packs to cause vasodilatation.
• Intense flushing of the skin may occur during an I.V. infusion, but usually disappears within 2 to 4 hours.
• To reduce nausea, give antiemetic before administering.
• Monitor BUN, CBC, hematocrit, platelet count, ALT (SGPT), AST (SGOT), LDH, serum bilirubin, serum creatinine, uric acid, total and differential leukocyte, and others as required per specific agent.
• At first sign of extravasation, infusion should be discontinued and area infiltrated with liberal injections of 0.5 mEq/ml sodium bicarbonate solution.
• Carmustine has been applied topically in concentrations of 0.5% to 2% to treat mycosis fungoides.
• Because carmustine crosses the blood-brain barrier, it may be used to treat primary brain tumors.

Information for parents and patient
• Advise parents that immunizations should be avoided during carmustine therapy if possible.
• Warn parents to watch patient for signs of infection (fever, sore throat) and bone marrow toxicity (anemia, fatigue, easy bruising, nose or gum bleeds, melena). Advise them to take neutropenic patient's temperature every 4 hours and to report fever promptly.
• Remind parents to have child return for follow-up blood work weekly, or as needed.
• Advise parents to avoid patient's exposure to persons with bacterial or viral infections because chemotherapy can increase susceptibility to infection. They should watch for and report any signs of infection promptly. Urge them to report exposure to chicken pox immediately so that zoster immune globulin may be given as soon as possible to a child without immunity to this infection.
• Advise parents to avoid administering over-the-counter products containing aspirin to the patient because they may precipitate bleeding. Advise them to report any signs of bleeding promptly.
• Instruct parents and patient in proper oral hygiene including caution when using toothbrush and dental floss.
• Advise parents that patient's dental work should be completed before initiation of therapy whenever possible, or delayed until blood counts are normal.
• Warn parents that patient may bruise easily because of drug's effect on blood count. Patient should avoid dangerous activities such as contact sports when platelets are low.

‡May contain sulfites   ◆May contain tartrazine   ◆◆May contain benzyl alcohol

cefaclor
Ceclor

• Classification: antibiotic (second-generation cephalosporin)

How supplied
Available by prescription only
Capsules: 250 mg, 500 mg
Suspension: 125 mg/5 ml, 250 mg/5 ml

Indications, route, and dosage
Infections of respiratory or urinary tracts, skin, and soft tissue; and otitis media caused by susceptible organisms
Children: 20 mg/kg P.O. daily in divided doses q 8 hours. In more serious infections, 40 mg/kg daily are recommended, not to exceed 1 g/day.
Adults: 250 to 500 mg P.O. q 8 hours. Total daily dosage should not exceed 4 g.

Action and kinetics
• *Antibacterial action:* Cefaclor is primarily bactericidal; however, it may be bacteriostatic. Activity depends on the organism, tissue penetration, drug dosage, and rate of organism multiplication. It acts by adhering to penicillin-binding enzymes, thereby inhibiting bacterial protein synthesis.

Cefaclor has the same bactericidal spectrum as second-generation cephalosporins, except that it has increased activity against ampicillin- or amoxicillin-resistant *Hemophilus influenzae.*
• *Kinetics in adults:* Cefaclor is well absorbed from the GI tract; peak serum levels occur 30 to 60 minutes after an oral dose. Food will delay but not prevent complete GI tract absorption. Cefaclor is distributed widely into most body tissues and fluids; CSF penetration is poor. Cefaclor crosses the placenta; it is 25% protein-bound. Cefaclor is not metabolized. It is excreted primarily in urine by renal tubular secretion and glomerular filtration; small amounts of drug are excreted in breast milk. Elimination half-life is ½ to 1 hour in patients with normal renal function; endstage renal disease prolongs half-life to 3 to 5½ hours. Hemodialysis removes cefaclor.

Contraindications and precautions
Cefaclor is contraindicated in patients with known hypersensitivity to any cephalosporin; it should be used cautiously in patients with penicillin allergy, who usually are more susceptible to such reactions.

Interactions
Probenecid competitively inhibits renal tubular secretion of cefaclor, resulting in higher, prolonged serum levels of these drugs.

Concomitant use with nephrotoxic agents (vancomycin, colistin, polymyxin B, or aminoglycosides) or loop diuretics increases the risk of nephrotoxicity.

Concomitant use of cefaclor with bacteriostatic agents (tetracyclines, erythromycin, or chloramphenicol) may impair its bactericidal activity.

Effects on diagnostic tests
Cefaclor may cause false-positive Coombs' test results. Cefaclor also causes false-positive results in urine glucose tests utilizing cupric sulfate (Benedict's reagent or Clinitest); use glucose oxidase tests (Clinistix or Tes-Tape) instead.

Cefaclor causes false elevations in serum or urine creatinine levels in tests using Jaffé's reaction.

Adverse reactions
• CNS: dizziness, headache, somnolence, paresthesias, and seizures.
• DERM: maculopapular rash, dermatitis.
• GI: nausea, vomiting, diarrhea, anorexia, *pseudomembranous colitis,* heartburn, glossitis, dyspepsia, abdominal cramping, tenesmus, anal pruritus.
• GU: red and white cells in urine, nephrotoxicity.
• HEMA: transient leukopenia, *lymphocytosis,* anemia, eosinophilia.
• Other: *hypersensitivity (serum sickness [erythema multiforme, rashes, urticaria, polyarthritis, fever]),* bacterial and fungal superinfection.
Note: Drug should be discontinued if signs of toxicity, immediate hypersensitivity reaction, or serum sickness occur or if severe diarrhea indicates pseudomembranous colitis; consider alternative therapy if the following symptoms occur: fever, eosinophilia, hematuria, neutropenia, or unexplained elevations in BUN or serum creatinine levels.

Overdose and treatment
Clinical signs of overdose include neuromuscular hypersensitivity; seizure may follow high CNS concentrations. Remove cefaclor by hemodialysis or peritoneal dialysis.

▶ Special considerations
• Safety and effectiveness have not been established for infants younger than age 1 month.
• To prevent toxic accumulation, reduced dosage may be required if patient's creatinine clearance is below 40 ml/minute.
• Review patient's history of allergies; do not give cefaclor to any patient with a history of hypersensitivity reactions to cephalosporins; administer cautiously to patients with penicillin allergy.
• Hypersensitivity reactions have been reported more frequently in children than in adults. Such reactions may occur after the first or second exposure to the drug.
• Administer cephalosporins at least 1 hour before bacteriostatic antibiotics (tetracyclines, erythromycins and chloramphenicol); these drugs inhibit bacterial cell growth, decreasing cephalosporin uptake by bacterial cell walls.
• For treatment of B hemolytic streptococcal infections, cefaclor should be administered for at least 10 days.
• Cefaclor may be given with food to minimize GI distress.
• Total daily dosage may be administered b.i.d. rather than t.i.d. with similar therapeutic effect.
• Refrigerate oral suspensions (stable for 14 days); shake well before administering to ensure correct dosage.

---

*Canada only   †Unlabeled clinical use   Italicized adverse reactions have been observed in children.

• Stock oral suspension is stable for 14 days if refrigerated.

• Because cefaclor is dialyzable, patients who are receiving treatment with hemodialysis or peritoneal dialysis may require drug dosage adjustment.

• Try to determine whether previous reactions were true hypersensitivity reactions and not another reaction, such as GI distress, that patient has interpreted as allergy.

• Monitor continuously for possible hypersensitivity or other untoward effects.

• Obtain results of cultures and sensitivity tests before first dose, but do not delay therapy; check test results periodically to assess drug efficacy.

• Monitor renal function studies; dosages of certain cephalosporins must be lowered in patients with severe renal impairment. In decreased renal function, monitor BUN levels, serum creatinine levels, and urine output for significant changes.

• Monitor patients on long-term therapy for possible superinfection, especially debilitated patients and others receiving immunosuppressants or radiation therapy.

• Cephalosporins cause false-positive results in urine glucose tests utilizing cupric sulfate solutions (Benedict's reagent or Clinitest); glucose oxidase tests (Clinistix or Tes-Tape) are not affected.

Information for parents and patient

• Teach parents signs and symptoms of hypersensitivity, bacterial and fungal superinfection, and other adverse reactions; urge them to report any unusual reactions.

• Warn parents that patient should not ingest alcohol in any form within 72 hours of cephalosporin dose. Emphasize that some liquid forms of acetaminophen contain alcohol.

• Advise adding live-culture yogurt or buttermilk to patient's diet to prevent intestinal superinfection resulting from suppression of normal intestinal flora.

• Advise parents of diabetic child to monitor urine glucose level with Clinistix or Tes-Tape and not to use Clinitest.

• Patient should take drug with food if GI irritation occurs.

• Advise parents of infants of potential for yeast infections, especially in diaper area. Instruct them to keep diaper area clean and dry and to avoid use of plastic pants.

• Be sure parents understand how and when to give drug; urge them to complete entire prescribed regimen, to comply with instructions for around-the-clock dosage, and to keep follow-up appointments. Advise them to check expiration date of drug and to discard unused drug.

cefadroxil monohydrate
Duricef, Ultracef

• Classification: antibiotic (first-generation cephalosporin)

How supplied
Available by prescription only
Capsules: 500 mg
Tablets: 1 g
Suspension: 125 mg/5 ml, 250 mg/5 ml, 500 mg/5 ml

Indications, route, and dosage
Urinary tract, skin, and soft tissue infections caused by susceptible organisms
Children: 30 mg/kg P.O. daily in two divided doses.
Adults: 500 mg to 2 g P.O. daily, depending on the infection treated. Usually given in once-daily or b.i.d. doses.
Dosage in renal failure
In patients with a creatinine clearance of 10 to 50 ml/minute, extend dosing interval to every 24 hours. If creatinine clearance is less than 10 ml/minute, administer every 48 hours.

Action and kinetics
• *Antibacterial action:* Cefadroxil is primarily bactericidal; however, it may be bacteriostatic. Activity depends on the organism, tissue penetration, drug dosage, and rate of organism multiplication. It acts by adhering to penicillin-binding enzymes, thereby inhibiting bacterial protein synthesis.

Cefadroxil is active against many gram-positive cocci, including penicillinase-producing *Staphylococcus aureus* and *epidermidis; Streptococcus pneumoniae,* group B streptococci, and group A beta-hemolytic streptococci; and susceptible gram-negative organisms including *Klebsiella pneumoniae, Escherichia coli, Proteus mirabilis,* and *Shigella.*

• *Kinetics in adults:* Cefadroxil is absorbed rapidly and completely from the GI tract after oral administration; peak serum levels occur at 1 to 2 hours.

It is distributed widely into most body tissues and fluids, including the gallbladder, liver, kidneys, bone, bile, sputum, and pleural and synovial fluids; CSF penetration is poor. Cefadroxil crosses the placenta; it is 20% protein-bound.

Cefadroxil is not metabolized. It is excreted primarily unchanged in the urine via glomerular filtration and renal tubular secretion; small amounts of drug may be excreted in breast milk. Elimination half-life is about 1 to 2 hours in patients with normal renal function; end-stage renal disease prolongs half-life to 25 hours. Cefadroxil can be removed by hemodialysis.

• *Kinetics in children:* Serum half-life is prolonged in neonates and infants younger than age 1.

Contraindications and precautions
Cefadroxil is contraindicated in patients with known hypersensitivity to any cephalosporin; it should be used cautiously in patients with penicillin allergy, who usually are more susceptible to such reactions.

---

‡May contain sulfites   ◆May contain tartrazine   ◆◆May contain benzyl alcohol

Interactions

Probenecid competitively inhibits renal tubular secretion of cephalosporins, resulting in higher, prolonged serum levels of these drugs.

Concomitant use with nephrotoxic agents (vancomycin, colistin, polymyxin B, or aminoglycosides) or loop diuretics increases the risk of nephrotoxicity.

Concomitant use with bacteriostatic agents (tetracyclines, erythromycin, or chloramphenicol) may interfere with bactericidal activity.

Effects on diagnostic tests

Cefadroxil causes false-positive results in urine glucose tests utilizing cupric sulfate (Benedict's reagent or Clinitest); use glucose oxidase test (Clinistix or Tes-Tape) instead. Cefadroxil causes false elevations in serum or urine creatinine levels in tests using Jaffé's reaction.

Positive Coombs' test results occur in about 3% of patients taking cephalosporins.

Adverse reactions

• CNS: dizziness, headache, malaise, paresthesias, seizures.
• DERM: maculopapular and erythematous rashes, urticaria.
• GI: *pseudomembranous colitis*, nausea, anorexia, vomiting, diarrhea, glossitis, dyspepsia, abdominal cramps, anal pruritus, tenesmus.
• GU: genital pruritus, moniliasis.
• HEMA: transient neutropenia, eosinophilia, leukopenia, anemia.
• Other: dyspnea, bacterial and fungal superinfection.

   Note: Drug should be discontinued if signs of toxicity or immediate hypersensitivity reaction occur or if severe diarrhea indicates pseudomembranous colitis; alternative therapy should be considered if the following symptoms occur: fever, eosinophilia, hematuria, neutropenia, or unexplained elevations in BUN or serum creatinine levels.

Overdose and treatment

Clinical signs of overdose include neuromuscular hypersensitivity; seizure may follow high CNS concentrations. Remove cefadroxil by hemodialysis. Other treatment is supportive.

▶ Special considerations

• Longer half-life permits once- or twice-daily dosing.
• Because cefadroxil is dialyzable, patients who are receiving treatment with hemodialysis may require dosage adjustment.
• Review patient's history of allergies; do not give cefadroxil to any patient with a history of hypersensitivity reactions to cephalosporins; administer cautiously to patients with penicillin allergy.
• Try to determine whether previous reactions were true hypersensitivity reactions and not another reaction, such as GI distress, that the patient has interpreted as allergy.
• Monitor continuously for possible hypersensitivity or other untoward effects.
• Obtain results of cultures and sensitivity tests before first dose, but do not delay therapy; check test results periodically to assess drug efficacy.

• Monitor patients on long-term therapy for possible superinfection, especially debilitated patients and others receiving immunosuppressants or radiation therapy.

Oral administration

• Administer cephalosporins at least 1 hour before bacteriostatic antibiotics (tetracyclines, erythromycins, and chloramphenicol); these drugs inhibit bacterial cell growth, decreasing cephalosporin uptake by bacterial cell walls.
• Administer cephalosporin at least 1 hour before or 2 hours after meals for maximum absorption.
• Refrigerate oral suspensions (stable for 14 days); shake well before administering to ensure correct dosage.

Information for parents and patient

• Teach parents signs and symptoms of hypersensitivity, bacterial and fungal superinfection, and other adverse reactions; urge them to report any unusual reactions.
• Warn parents that patient should not ingest alcohol in any form within 72 hours of cephalosporin dose. Emphasize that some liquid forms of acetaminophen contain alcohol.
• Advise adding live-culture yogurt or buttermilk to patient's diet to prevent intestinal superinfection resulting from suppression of normal intestinal flora.
• Advise parents of diabetic child to monitor urine glucose level with Clinistix or Tes-Tape and not to use Clinitest.
• Patient should take oral drug with food if GI irritation occurs.
• Advise parents of infants of potential for yeast infections, especially in diaper area. Instruct them to keep diaper area clean and dry and to avoid use of plastic pants.
• Be sure parents understand how and when to give drug; urge them to complete entire prescribed regimen, to comply with instructions for around-the-clock dosage, and to keep follow-up appointments.
• Advise them to check expiration date of drug and to discard unused drug.

---

cefamandole nafate
Mandol

• Classification: antibiotic (second-generation cephalosporin)

How supplied

Available by prescription only
Injectable solution: 500 mg, 1 g, 2 g, 10 g
Pharmacy bulk package: 10 g

Indications, route, and dosage

Serious respiratory, genitourinary, skin and soft-tissue, and bone and joint infections; septicemia; peritonitis from susceptible organisms
Infants and children: 50 to 100 mg/kg I.M. or I.V. daily in equally divided doses q 4 to 8 hours. May be

---

*Canada only   †Unlabeled clinical use   Italicized adverse reactions have been observed in children.

increased to total daily dosage of 150 mg/kg (not to exceed maximum adult dose) for severe infections.

Adults: 500 mg to 1 g I.M. or I.V. q 4 to 8 hours. In life-threatening infections, up to 2 g q 4 hours may be needed.

Total daily dosage is same for I.M. or I.V. administration and depends on susceptibility of organism and severity of infection. Cefamandole should be injected deep I.M. into a large muscle mass, such as the gluteus or the lateral aspect of the thigh.

Dosage in renal failure

In patients with impaired renal function, doses or frequency of administration must be modified according to degree of renal impairment, severity of infection, and susceptibility of organism.

DOSAGE IN ADULTS		
Creatinine clearance (ml/min/ 1.73 m²)	Severe infections	Life-threatening infections (maximum)
>80	1 to 2 g q 6 hours	2 g q 4 hours
50 to 80	750 mg to 1.5 g q 6 hours	1.5 g q 4 hours; or 2 g q 6 hours
25 to 50	750 mg to 1.5 g q 8 hours	1.5 g q 6 hours; or 2 g q 8 hours
10 to 25	500 mg to 1 g q 8 hours	1 g q 6 hours; or 1.25 g q 8 hours
2 to 10	500 to 750 mg q 12 hours	670 mg q 8 hours; or 1 g q 12 hours
<2	250 to 500 mg q 12 hours	500 mg q 8 hours; or 750 mg q 12 hours

Action and kinetics

• *Antibacterial action:* Cefamandole is primarily bactericidal; however, it may be bacteriostatic. Activity depends on the organism, tissue penetration, drug dosage, and rate of organism multiplication. It acts by adhering to penicillin-binding enzymes, thereby inhibiting bacterial protein synthesis.

Cefamandole is active against *Escherichia coli* and other coliform bacteria, *Staphylococcus aureus* (penicillinase- and nonpenicillinase-producing), *Staphylococcus epidermidis*, group A beta hemolytic streptococci, *Klebsiella, Hemophilus influenzae, proteus mirabilis,* and *Enterobacter* as the second-generation drugs. *Bacteroides fragilis* and *Acinetobacter* are resistant.

• *Kinetics in adults:* Cefamandole is not absorbed from the GI tract and must be given parenterally; peak serum levels occur ½ to 2 hours after an I.M. dose.

Cefamandole is distributed widely into most body tissues and fluids, including the gallbladder, liver, kidneys, bone, sputum, bile, and pleural and synovial fluids; *CSF penetration is poor.* Cefamandole crosses the placenta; it is 65% to 75% protein-bound.

Cefamandole is not metabolized. It is excreted primarily in urine by renal secretion and glomerular filtration; small amounts of drug are excreted in breast milk. Elimination half-life is about ½ to 2 hours in patients with normal renal function; severe renal disease prolongs half-life to 12 to 18 hours. Hemodialysis removes some cefamandole.

Contraindications and precautions

Cefamandole is contraindicated in patients with known hypersensitivity to any cephalosporin. It should be used with caution in patients with penicillin allergy, who usually are more susceptible to such reactions; in patients with coagulopathy; and in severely debilitated and malnourished patients, who are at greater risk of bleeding complications.

Interactions

Probenecid competitively inhibits renal tubular secretion of cephalosporins, resulting in higher, prolonged serum levels of these drugs.

Concomitant use with nephrotoxic agents (vancomycin, colistin, polymixin B, or aminoglycosides) or loop diuretics increases the risk of nephrotoxicity.

Concomitant use of cefamandole with bacteriostatic agents (tetracyclines, erythromycin, or chloramphenicol) may impair its bactericidal activity.

Concomitant use with alcohol may cause severe disulfiram-like reactions.

Effects on diagnostic tests

Cefamandole causes false-positive results in urine glucose tests utilizing cupric sulfate (Benedict's reagent or Clinitest); use glucose oxidase tests (Clinistix or Tes-Tape) instead. Cefamandole also causes false elevations in serum or urine creatinine levels in tests using Jaffé's reaction.

Cefamandole may cause positive Coombs' test results, and may elevate liver function test results or prothrombin times.

Adverse reactions

• CNS: headache, malaise, paresthesias, dizziness, seizures.
• DERM: maculopapular and erythematous rashes, urticaria.
• GI: *pseudomembranous colitis,* nausea, anorexia, vomiting, diarrhea, glossitis, dyspepsia, abdominal cramps, tenesmus, anal pruritus.
• GU: nephrotoxicity, vaginitis.
• HEMA: transient neutropenia, eosinophilia, hemolytic anemia, *hypoprothrombinemia,* bleeding.
• Local: at injection site — pain, induration, sterile abscesses, temperature elevation, tissue sloughing; phlebitis and thrombophlebitis with I.V. injection.
• Other: hypersensitivity (serum sickness [erythema multiforme, rashes, polyarthritis, fever]), dyspnea, bacterial and fungal superinfection.

Note: Drug should be discontinued if signs of toxicity, immediate hypersensitivity reaction, serum sickness, or hypoprothrombinemia occur or if severe diarrhea indicates pseudomembranous colitis; consider alternative therapy if the following symptoms occur: fever, eosinophilia, hematuria, neutropenia, hypoprothrombinemia, or unexplained elevations in BUN or serum creatinine levels.

Overdose and treatment
Clinical signs of overdose include neuromuscular hypersensitivity. Seizure may follow high CNS concentrations. Hypoprothrombinemia and bleeding may occur; they may be treated with vitamin K or blood products. Some cefamandole may be removed by hemodialysis.

▶ Special considerations
• Cefamandole injection contains 3.3 mEq of sodium per gram of drug.
• Safe use in infants younger than age 1 month has not been established.
• For most cephalosporin-sensitive organisms, cefamandole offers little advantage over other cephalosporins; it is less effective than cefoxitin against anaerobic infections.
• Consult manufacturer's directions for reconstitution, dilution, and storage of drugs; check expiration dates.
• For I.V. use, reconstitute 1 g with 10 ml of sterile water for injection, dextrose 5%, or 0.9% sodium chloride for injection. Administer slowly, over 3 to 5 minutes, or by intermittent infusion or continuous infusion in compatible solutions. Check package insert.
• Don't mix with I.V. infusions containing magnesium or calcium ions, which are chemically incompatible and may cause irreversible effects.
• Do not add or mix other drugs with I.V. infusions — particularly aminoglycosides, which will be inactivated if mixed with cephalosporins; if other drugs must be given I.V., temporarily stop infusion of primary drug.
• Adequate dilution of I.V. infusion, adequate flushing of I.V. after administration of drug, and rotation of the site every 48 hours help minimize local vein irritation; use of small-gauge needle in larger available vein may be helpful.
• For I.M. use, dilute 1 g of cefamandole in 3 ml of sterile water for injection, bacteriostatic water for injection, 0.9% sodium chloride for injection, or 0.9% bacteriostatic sodium chloride for injection. Do not administer more than 2 ml per injection site.
• Administer deeply into large muscle mass (gluteal or midlateral thigh) to ensure maximum absorption. Rotate injection sites to minimize tissue injury.
• I.M. cefamandole is less painful than cefoxitin injection; it does not require addition of lidocaine.
• After reconstitution, solution remains stable for 24 hours at room temperature or 96 hours under refrigeration. Solution should be light yellow to amber. Do not use solution if it is discolored or contains a precipitate.
• Administer cephalosporins at least 1 hour before bacteriostatic antibiotics (tetracyclines, erythromycins, and chloramphenicol); these drugs inhibit bacterial cell growth, decreasing cephalosporin uptake by bacterial cell walls.
• Monitor for signs or symptoms of bleeding. Monitor patient's prothrombin times and platelet levels. Patient may require prophylactic use of vitamin K to prevent bleeding.
• Bleeding can be reversed by administering vitamin K or blood products.
• Review patient's history of allergies; do not give cefamandole to any patient with a history of hypersensitivity reactions to cephalosporins; administer cautiously to patients with penicillin allergy.
• Try to determine whether previous reactions were true hypersensitivity reactions and not another reaction, such as GI distress, that the patient has interpreted as allergy.
• Monitor continuously for possible hypersensitivity or other untoward effects.
• Obtain results of cultures and sensitivity tests before first dose, but do not delay therapy; check test results periodically to assess drug efficacy.
• Monitor patients on long-term therapy for possible superinfection, especially debilitated patients and others receiving immunosuppressants or radiation therapy.

Information for parents and patient
• Teach parents signs and symptoms of hypersensitivity, bacterial and fungal superinfection, and other adverse reactions; urge them to report any unusual reactions.
• Warn parents that patient should not ingest alcohol in any form within 72 hours of cephalosporin dose. Emphasize that some liquid forms of acetaminophen contain alcohol.
• Advise adding live-culture yogurt or buttermilk to patient's diet to prevent intestinal superinfection resulting from suppression of normal intestinal flora.
• Explain that drug may cause hypoprothrombinemia. Parents may need to restrict patient's activities to prevent injury and bleeding.
• Advise parents of diabetic child to monitor urine glucose level with Clinistix or Tes-Tape and not to use Clinitest.
• Advise parents of infants of potential for yeast infections, especially in diaper area. Instruct them to keep diaper area clean and dry and to avoid use of plastic pants.

---

cefazolin sodium
Ancef, Kefzol

• Classification: antibiotic (first-generation cephalosporin)

How supplied
Available by prescription only
Injection (parenteral): 250 mg, 500 mg, 1 g, 5 g, 10 g
Infusion: 500 mg/100 ml vial, 500-mg or 1-g Redi Vials, Faspaks, or ADD-Vantage vials

Indications, route, and dosage
Serious respiratory, genitourinary, skin and soft-tissue, and bone and joint infections; septicemia, endocarditis from susceptible organisms
Children over age 1 month: 8 to 16 mg/kg I.M. or I.V. q 8 hours, or 6 to 12 mg/kg q 6 hours. For severe infections, 25 to 33 mg/kg, divided q 6 to 8 hours.
Adults: 250 mg I.M. or I.V. q 8 hours to 1 g q 6 hours. Maximum dosage is 12 g/day in life-threatening situations.

★Canada only   †Unlabeled clinical use   Italicized adverse reactions have been observed in children.

Total daily dosage is same for I.M. or I.V. administration and depends on the susceptibility of organism and severity of infection. Cefazolin should be injected deep I.M. into a large muscle mass, such as the gluteus or the lateral aspect of the thigh.

Dosage in renal failure

Doses or frequency of administration must be modified according to the degree of renal impairment, severity of infection, and susceptibility of organism.

Creatinine clearance (ml/min/1.73 m²)	Dosage in adults
≥ 55	Usual adult dose
35 to 54	Full dose q 8 hours or less frequently
11 to 34	½ usual dose q 12 hours
≤ 10	½ usual dose q 18 to 24 hours

Creatinine clearance (ml/min/1.73 m²)	Dosage in children
> 70	Usual pediatric dose
40 to 70	7.5 to 30 mg per kg of body weight q 12 hours
20 to 40	3.125 to 12.5 mg per kg of body weight q 12 hours
5 to 20	2.5 to 10 mg per kg of body weight q 24 hours

Action and kinetics

• *Antibacterial action:* Cefazolin is primarily bactericidal; however, it may be bacteriostatic. Activity depends on the organism, tissue penetration, drug dosage, and rate of organism multiplication. It acts by adhering to penicillin-binding enzymes, thereby inhibiting bacterial protein synthesis.

Cefazolin is active against *Escherichia coli, Enterobacteriaceae, gonococci, Klebsiella, Proteus mirabilis, Staphylococcus aureus, Streptococcus pneumoniae,* and group A beta-hemolytic streptococcus.

• *Kinetics in adults:* Cefazolin is not well absorbed from the GI tract and must be given parenterally; peak serum levels occur 1 to 2 hours after an I.M. dose.

Cefazolin is distributed widely into most body tissues and fluids, including the gallbladder, liver, kidneys, bone, sputum, bile, and pleural and synovial fluids; CSF penetration is poor. It crosses the placenta; it is 74% to 86% protein-bound.

Cefazolin is not metabolized. It is excreted primarily unchanged in urine by renal tubular secretion and glomerular filtration; small amounts of drug are excreted in breast milk. Elimination half-life is about 1 to 2 hours in patients with normal renal function; end-stage renal disease prolongs half-life to 12 to 50 hours. Hemodialysis or peritoneal dialysis removes cefazolin.

• *Kinetics in children:* Serum half-life is prolonged in neonates and in infants up to age 1.

Contraindications and precautions

Cefazolin is contraindicated in patients with known hypersensitivity to any cephalosporin; it should be used with caution in patients with penicillin allergy, who usually are more susceptible to such reactions.

Interactions

Probenecid competitively inhibits renal tubular secretion of cephalosporins, resulting in higher, prolonged serum levels of these drugs.

Concomitant use with nephrotoxic agents (vancomycin, colistin, polymixin B, or aminoglycosides) or loop diuretics increases the risk of nephrotoxicity.

Concomitant use with bacteriostatic agents (tetracyclines, erythromycin, or chloramphenicol) may interfere with bactericidal activity.

Effects on diagnostic tests

Cephalosporins cause false-positive results in urine glucose tests utilizing cupric sulfate (Benedict's reagent or Clinitest); use glucose oxidase tests (Clinistix or Tes-Tape) instead. Cefazolin causes false elevations in serum or urine creatinine levels in tests using Jaffé's reaction.

Cefazolin also causes positive Coombs' test results and may elevate liver function test results.

Adverse reactions

• CNS: dizziness, headache, malaise, paresthesias, seizures.
• DERM: maculopapular and erythematous rashes, urticaria.
• GI: *pseudomembranous colitis,* nausea, anorexia, vomiting, diarrhea, glossitis, dyspepsia, abdominal cramps, anal pruritus, tenesmus.
• GU: genital pruritus, vaginitis, nephrotoxicity.
• HEMA: *transient neutropenia, leukopenia, eosinophilia, anemia.*
• Local: at injection site — pain, induration, sterile abscesses, tissue sloughing; *phlebitis* and thrombophlebitis with I.V. injection.
• Other: hypersensitivity, dyspnea, fever, bacterial and fungal superinfection.

Note: Drug should be discontinued if signs of toxicity or immediate hypersensitivity reaction occur or if severe diarrhea indicates pseudomembranous colitis; consider alternative therapy if the following symptoms occur: fever, eosinophilia, hematuria, neutropenia, or unexplained elevations in BUN or serum creatinine levels.

Overdose and treatment

Clinical signs of overdose include neuromuscular hypersensitivity; seizure may follow high CNS concentrations. Remove cefazolin by hemodialysis.

▶ Special considerations

• For patients on sodium restrictions note that cefazolin injection contains 2 mEq of sodium per gram of drug.
• Safety of using cefazolin in infants younger than age 1 month has not been established.

---

‡May contain sulfites   ◆May contain tartrazine   ◆ ◆ May contain benzyl alcohol

• Because of the long duration of effect, most infections can be treated with a single dose every 8 hours.
• For I.M. use, reconstitute with sterile water, bacteriostatic water, or 0.9% sodium chloride solution: 2 ml to a 250-mg vial, 2 ml to a 500-mg vial, and 2.5 ml to a 1-g vial produces concentrations of 125 mg/ml, 225 mg/ml, and 330 mg/ml respectively.
• Reconstituted solution is stable for 24 hours at room temperature; for 96 hours if refrigerated.
• I.M. cefazolin injection is less painful than that of other cephalosporins.
• Because hemodialysis removes cefazolin, patients who are undergoing hemodialysis may require dosage adjustment.
• Review patient's history of allergies; do not give cefazolin to any patient with a history of hypersensitivity reactions to cephalosporins; administer cautiously to patients with penicillin allergy.
• Try to determine whether previous reactions were true hypersensitivity reactions and not another reaction, such as GI distress, that the patient has interpreted as allergy.
• Monitor continuously for possible hypersensitivity or other untoward effects.
• Obtain results of cultures and sensitivity tests before first dose, but do not delay therapy; check test results periodically to assess drug efficacy.
• Monitor patients on long-term therapy for possible superinfection, especially debilitated patients and others receiving immunosuppressants or radiation therapy.

Administration
• Administer cephalosporins at least 1 hour before bacteriostatic antibiotics (tetracyclines, erythromycins, and chloramphenicol); these drugs inhibit bacterial cell growth, decreasing cephalosporin uptake by bacterial cell walls.
• Consult manufacturer's directions for reconstitution, dilution, and storage of drugs; check expiration dates.
• Administer I.M. dose deep into large muscle mass (gluteal or midlateral thigh); rotate injection sites to minimize tissue injury.
• Do not add or mix other drugs with I.V. infusions—particularly aminoglycosides, which will be inactivated if mixed with cephalosporins; if other drugs must be given I.V., temporarily stop infusion of primary drug.
• Adequate dilution of I.V. infusion and rotation of the site every 48 hours help minimize local vein irritation; use of small-gauge needle in larger available vein may be helpful.

Information for parents and patient
• Teach parents signs and symptoms of hypersensitivity, bacterial and fungal superinfection, and other adverse reactions; urge them to report any unusual reactions.
• Warn parents that patient should not ingest alcohol in any form within 72 hours of cephalosporin dose. Emphasize that some liquid forms of acetaminophen contain alcohol.
• Advise parents to add live-culture yogurt or buttermilk to child's diet to prevent intestinal superinfection resulting from suppression of normal intestinal flora.
• Advise parents of diabetic child to monitor urine glucose level with Clinistix or Tes-Tape and not to use Clinitest.

cefoperazone sodium
Cefobid

• Classification: antibiotic (third-generation cephalosporin)

How supplied
Available by prescription only
Parenteral: 1 g, 2 g
Infusion: 1 g, 2 g piggyback

Indications, route, and dosage
Serious respiratory tract, intraabdominal, gynecologic, and skin infections; bacteremia; and septicemia caused by susceptible organisms
Children: 25 to 100 mg/kg/day q 12 hours I.M. or I.V.
Adults: Usual dosage is 1 to 2 g q 12 hours I.M. or I.V. In severe infections or infections caused by less sensitive organisms, the total daily dosage or frequency may be increased up to 16 g/day in certain situations.
Dosage in renal failure
No dosage adjustment is usually necessary in patients with renal impairment. However, dosages of 4 g/day should be given cautiously to patients with hepatic disease. Adults with combined hepatic and renal function impairment should not receive more than 1 g (base) daily without serum determinations. In patients who are receiving hemodialysis treatments, a dose should be scheduled to follow hemodialysis.

Action and kinetics
• *Antibacterial action:* Cefoperazone is primarily bactericidal; however, it may be bacteriostatic. Activity depends on the organism, tissue penetration, drug dosage, and rate of organism multiplication. It acts by adhering to penicillin-binding enzymes, thereby inhibiting bacterial protein synthesis. Third-generation cephalosporins appear more active against some beta-lactamase-producing gram-negative organisms.

Cefoperazone is active against some gram-positive organisms and many enteric gram-negative bacilli, including *Streptococcus pneumoniae* and *Streptococcus pyogenes, Staphylococcus aureus* (penicillinase- and nonpenicillinase-producing), *Staphylococcus epidermidis,* enterococcus, *Escherichia coli, Klebsiella, Hemophilus influenzae, Enterobacter, Citrobacter, Proteus,* some *Pseudomonas* species (including *Pseudomonas aeruginosa*), and *Bacteroides fragilis. Acinetobacter* and *Listeria* usually are resistant. Cefoperazone is less effective than moxalactam, cefotaxime, or ceftizoxime against Enterobacteriaceae but is slightly more active than those drugs against *Pseudomonas aeruginosa.*
• *Kinetics in adults:* Cefoperazone is not absorbed from the GI tract and must be given parenterally; peak serum levels occur 1 to 2 hours after an I.M. dose.

Cefoperazone is distributed widely into most body tissues and fluids, including the gallbladder, liver, kidneys, bone, sputum, bile, and pleural and synovial fluids; CSF penetration is achieved in patients with inflamed meninges. Cefoperazone crosses the placenta. Protein binding is dose-dependent and decreases as serum levels rise; average is 82% to 93%.

Cefoperazone is not substantially metabolized. It is excreted primarily in bile; some drug is excreted in urine by renal tubular secretion and glomerular filtration; and small amounts, in breast milk. Elimination half-life is about 1½ to 2½ hours in patients with normal hepatorenal function; biliary obstruction or cirrhosis prolongs half-life to about 3½ to 7 hours. Hemodialysis removes cefoperazone.

• *Kinetics in children:* Serum half-life is prolonged in neonates and in infants up to age 1.

Contraindications and precautions

Cefoperazone is contraindicated in patients with known hypersensitivity to any cephalosporin. It should be used with caution in patients with penicillin allergy, who usually are more susceptible to such reactions; in patients with coagulopathy; and in debilitated or malnourished patients, who are at greater risk of bleeding complications.

Interactions

Concomitant use with aminoglycosides results in synergistic activity against *Pseudomonas aeruginosa* and *Serratia marcescens;* such combined use slightly increases the risk of nephrotoxicity.

Concomitant use with clavulanic acid results in synergistic activity against many Enterobacteriaceae, *Bacteroides fragilis, P. aeruginosa,* and *S. aureus.*

Concomitant use with alcohol may cause disulfiram-like reactions (flushing, sweating, tachycardia, headache, and abdominal cramping).

Probenecid competitively inhibits renal tubular secretions of cephalosporins, causing prolonged serum levels of these drugs.

Effects on diagnostic tests

Cephalosporins cause false-positive results in urine glucose tests utilizing cupric sulfate (Benedict's reagent or Clinitest); use glucose oxidase (Clinistix or Tes-Tape) instead.

Cefoperazone may cause positive Coombs' test results, and elevated liver function test results and prothrombin times.

Adverse reactions

• CNS: headache, malaise, paresthesias, dizziness, seizures.
• DERM: maculopapular and erythematous rashes, urticaria.
• GI: pseudomembranous colitis, nausea, anorexia, vomiting, diarrhea, glossitis, dyspepsia, abdominal cramps, tenesmus, anal pruritus.
• GU: genital pruritus.
• HEMA: transient neutropenia, eosinophilia, hemolytic anemia, hypoprothrombinemia, bleeding.
• Hepatic: mildly elevated liver enzyme levels.
• Local: at injection site—pain, induration, sterile abscesses, temperature elevation, tissue sloughing; phlebitis and thrombophlebitis with I.V. injection.
• Other: hypersensitivity (serum sickness [erythema multiforme, rashes, polyarthritis, fever]), bacterial and fungal superinfection.

Note: Drug should be discontinued if signs of toxicity, immediate hypersensitivity reaction, serum sickness, or hypoprothrombinema occur or if severe diarrhea indicates pseudomembranous colitis; alternative therapy should be considered if the patient develops fever, eosinophilia, hematuria, or neutropenia.

Overdose and treatment

Clinical signs of overdose include neuromuscular hypersensitivity. Seizure may follow high CNS concentrations. Hypoprothrombinemia and bleeding may occur and may require treatment with vitamin K or blood products. Hemodialysis will remove cefoperazone.

▶ Special considerations

• Safety and effectiveness in children under age 12 have not been established.
• Diarrhea may be more common with cefoperazone than with other cephalosporins because of the high degree of biliary excretion.
• Patients with biliary disease may need lower doses.
• For patients on sodium-restricted diets, note that cefoperazone injection contains 1.5 mEq of sodium per gram of drug.
• Give drug at least 1 hour before giving bacteriostatic antibiotics (tetracyclines, erythromycins, and chloramphenicol); these drugs decrease cefoperazone uptake by bacterial cell walls.
• Do not add or mix other drugs with I.V. infusions—particularly aminoglycosides, which will be inactivated if mixed with cefoperazone; if other drugs must be given I.V., temporarily stop infusion of primary drug.
• Adequate dilution of I.V. infusion and rotation of the site every 48 hours help minimize local vein irritation; use of small-gauge needle in large available vein may be helpful.
• To prepare I.M. injection, use the appropriate diluent, including sterile water for injection or bacteriostatic water for injection. Follow manufacturer's recommendations for mixing drug with sterile water for injection and lidocaine 2% injection. Final solution for I.M. injection will contain 0.5% lidocaine and will be less painful upon administration (recommended for concentrations of 250 mg/ml or greater). Cefoperazone should be injected deep I.M. into a large muscle mass, such as the gluteus or the lateral aspect of the thigh.
• Store drug in refrigerator and away from light before reconstituting.
• Shake solution vigorously to ensure complete drug dissolution. Allow solution to stand after reconstituting to allow foam to dissipate and solution to clear.
• After reconstitution, solution is stable for 24 hours at a controlled room temperature or 5 days if refrigerated. Protecting drug from light is unnecessary.
• Because cefoperazone is dialyzable, patients undergoing treatment with hemodialysis may require dosage adjustment.

‡May contain sulfites   ◆May contain tartrazine   ◆◆May contain benzyl alcohol

• Review patient's history of allergies; do not give cefoperazone to any patient with a history of hypersensitivity reactions to cephalosporins; administer cautiously to patients with penicillin allergy, because they are more susceptible to such reactions.
• Try to determine whether previous reactions were true hypersensitivity reactions and not merely an adverse reaction that patient perceived as allergy.
• Monitor continuously for possible hypersensitivity reactions or other untoward effects.
• Obtain results of cultures and sensitivity tests before first dose, but do not delay therapy; check test results periodically to assess drug efficacy.
• Monitor renal and hepatic function; dosage of cefoperazone must be adjusted in patients with renal and hepatic impairment.
• Monitor prothrombin times and platelet counts and assess patient for signs of hypoprothrombinemia, which may occur, with or without bleeding, during therapy—usually in debilitated or malnourished patients.
• Monitor patients on long-term therapy for possible bacterial and fungal superinfection, especially debilitated patients and others receiving immunosuppressants or radiation therapy.

Information for parents and patient
• Teach signs and symptoms of hypersensitivity and other adverse reactions, and emphasize need to report any unusual effects.
• Teach signs and symptoms of bacterial and fungal superinfection to parents and patients, especially those with low resistance from immunosuppressants or irradiation; emphasize need to report infections promptly.
• Warn parents that patient should not ingest alcohol in any form within 72 hours of cefoperazone dose. Emphasize that some liquid medications contain alcohol.
• Advise adding live-culture yogurt or buttermilk to patient's diet to prevent intestinal superinfection resulting from suppression of normal intestinal flora.
• Advise parents of diabetic children to monitor urine glucose level with Clinistix or Tes-Tape and not to use Clinitest.
• Counsel parents to check drug's expiration date and to discard outdated or unused drug.

ceforanide
Precef

• Classification: antibiotic (second-generation cephalosporin)

How supplied
Available by prescription only
Injection: 500 mg, 1 g
Infusion: 500 mg, 1 g piggyback

Indications, route, and dosage
Serious lower respiratory, urinary, skin, and bone and joint infections; endocarditis; and septicemia from susceptible organisms
Children: 20 to 40 mg/kg/day in equally divided doses q 12 hours.
Adults: 0.5 to 1 g I.V. or I.M. q 12 hours.
Prophylaxis of surgical infections
Adults: 0.5 to 1 g I.M. or I.V. 1 hour before surgery.
Total daily dosage is the same for I.M. or I.V. administration and depends on susceptibility of organism and severity of infection. Ceforanide should be injected deep I.M. into a large muscle mass, such as the gluteus or lateral aspect of the thigh.
Dosage in renal failure
In patients with impaired renal function, doses or frequency of administration must be modified according to the degree of renal impairment, severity of infection, and susceptibility of organism. To prevent toxic accumulation, reduced dosage may be required in patients with creatinine clearance below 60 ml/minute.

Creatinine clearance (ml/min/1.73 m²)	Dosage in adults
≥60	Usual adult dose
20 to 59	500 mg to 1 g q 24 hr
5 to 19	500 mg to 1 g q 48 hr
<5	500 mg to 1 g q 48 to 72 hr

Action and kinetics
• *Antibacterial action:* Ceforanide is primarily bactericidal; however, it may be bacteriostatic. Activity depends on the organism, tissue penetration, drug dosage, and rate of organism multiplication. It acts by adhering to penicillin-binding enzymes, thereby inhibiting bacterial protein synthesis.
Ceforanide is active against many gram-positive organisms and enteric gram-negative bacilli, including *Streptococcus pneumoniae, Klebsiella pneumoniae, Escherichia coli, Hemophilus influenzae, Proteus mirabilis, Staphylococcus aureus* and *epidermidis,* and *Streptococcus pyogenes; Bacteroides fragilis, Pseudomonas,* and *Acinetobacter* are resistant. Ceforanide is less effective than cefamandole or cefuroxime against *S. aureus* or *H. influenzae.*
• *Kinetics in adults:* Ceforanide is not absorbed from the GI tract and must be given parenterally; peak serum levels occur 1 hour after an I.M. dose.
Ceforanide is distributed widely into most body tissues and fluids, including the gallbladder, liver, kidneys, bone, skeletal muscle, uterus, jejunum, myocardium, and bile. CSF penetration is poor. It is unknown if ceforanide crosses the placenta. Ceforanide is about 80% protein-bound.
Ceforanide is not metabolized. It is excreted primarily in urine by renal tubular secretion and glomerular filtration; elimination half-life is 2½ to 3½ hours in patients with normal renal function; 5½ to 25 hours in patients with end-stage renal disease. Hemodialysis removes ceforanide.

• *Kinetics in children:* Serum half-life is prolonged in neonates and in infants up to age 1.

Contraindications and precautions

Ceforanide is contraindicated in patients with known hypersensitivity to any cephalosporin. It should be used with caution in patients with penicillin allergy, who usually are more susceptible to such reactions.

Interactions

Probenecid competitively inhibits renal tubular secretion of cephalosporins, resulting in higher, prolonged serum levels of these drugs.

Concomitant use of ceforanide with nephrotoxic agents (vancomycin, colistin, polymixin B, or aminoglycosides) or loop diuretics increases the risk of nephrotoxicity. Concomitant use with bacteriostatic agents (tetracyclines, erythromycin, or chloramphenicol) may impair its bactericidal activity.

Effects on diagnostic tests

Cephalosporins cause false-positive results in urine glucose tests utilizing cupric sulfate (Benedict's reagent or Clinitest); use glucose oxidase tests (Clinistix or Tes-Tape) instead. Ceforanide causes false elevations in serum or urine creatinine levels in tests using Jaffé's reaction.

Ceforanide may elevate results of liver function tests and may cause positive Coombs' test results.

Adverse reactions

• CNS: confusion, headache, lethargy, seizures.
• DERM: maculopapular and erythematous rashes, urticaria.
• GI: *pseudomembranous colitis,* nausea, anorexia, vomiting, diarrhea, glossitis, dyspepsia, abdominal cramps.
• GU: genital pruritus, hematuria, nephrotoxicity.
• HEMA: transient neutropenia, leukopenia, eosinophilia, thrombocytopenia, anemia.
• Hepatic: transient elevation in liver enzymes.
• Local: at injection site—pain, induration, sterile abscesses, tissue sloughing; phlebitis and thrombophlebitis with I.V. injection.
• Other: hypersensitivity (dyspnea, serum sickness [erythema multiforme, rashes, polyarthritis, fever]), bacterial and fungal superinfection.
Note: Drug should be discontinued if signs of toxicity, immediate hypersensitivity reaction, or serum sickness occur or if severe diarrhea indicates pseudomembranous colitis; alternative therapy should be considered if patient develops fever, eosinophilia, hematuria, neutropenia, or unexplained elevations in BUN or serum creatinine levels.

Overdose and treatment

Clinical signs of overdose include neuromuscular hypersensitivity. Seizure may follow high CNS concentrations. Hemodialysis removes ceforanide.

▶ Special considerations

• Use in infants younger than age 1 is not recommended.
• Review patient's history of allergies; do not give a cephalosporin to any patient with a history of hy-

persensitivity reactions to cephalosporins; administer cautiously to patients with penicillin allergy.
• Try to determine whether previous reactions were true hypersensitivity reactions and not another reaction, such as GI distress, that the patient has interpreted as allergy.
• Obtain results of cultures and sensitivity tests before first dose, but do not delay therapy; check test results periodically to assess drug efficacy.
• Administer cephalosporins at least 1 hour before bacteriostatic antibiotics (tetracyclines, erythromycins, and chloramphenicol); these drugs inhibit bacterial cell growth, decreasing cephalosporin uptake by bacterial cell walls.
• Consult manufacturer's directions for reconstitution, dilution, and storage of drugs; check expiration dates.
• Upon reconstitution, ceforanide injection may appear cloudy. Let it stand briefly to allow solution to deaerate and clarify. Check package insert for compatible diluents.
• Administer I.M. dose deep into large muscle mass (gluteal or midlateral thigh); rotate injection sites to minimize tissue injury.
• Do not add or mix other drugs with I.V. infusions—particularly aminoglycosides, which will be inactivated if mixed with cephalosporins; if other drugs must be given I.V., temporarily stop infusion of primary drug.
• Administer I.V. dose slowly with compatible solution.
• Adequate dilution of I.V. infusion and rotation of the site every 48 hours help minimize local vein irritation; use of small-gauge needle in larger available vein may be helpful.
• Monitor continuously for possible hypersensitivity or other untoward effects.
• Because ceforanide is hemodializable, patients undergoing treatment with hemodialysis may require dosage adjustments.
• Monitor patients on long-term therapy for possible superinfection, especially debilitated patients and others receiving immunosuppressants or radiation therapy.

Information for parents and patient

• Teach parents signs and symptoms of hypersensitivity, bacterial and fungal superinfection, and other adverse reactions; urge them to report any unusual reactions.
• Warn parents that patient should not ingest alcohol in any form within 72 hours of cephalosporin dose. Emphasize that some liquid forms of acetaminophen contain alcohol.
• Advise adding live-culture yogurt or buttermilk to patient's diet to prevent intestinal superinfection resulting from suppression of normal intestinal flora.
• Advise parents of diabetic child to monitor urine glucose level with Clinistix or Tes-Tape and not to use Clinitest.
• Advise parents of infants of potential for yeast infections, especially in diaper area. Instruct them to keep diaper area clean and dry and to avoid use of plastic pants.

cefotaxime sodium
Claforan

- Classification: antibiotic (third-generation cephalosporin)

How supplied
Available by prescription only
Injection: 500 mg, 1 g, 2 g
Pharmacy bulk package: 10-g vial
Infusion: 1 g, 2 g

Indications, route, and dosage
Serious lower respiratory, urinary, CNS, gynecologic, and skin infections; bacteremia; septicemia caused by susceptible organisms
Neonates age 0 to 7 days: 50 mg/kg daily q 12 hours
Neonates age 8 days to 4 weeks: 50 mg/kg daily q 8 hours
Children over age 1 month: 50 to 180 mg/kg I.M. or I.V. divided q 4 to 6 hours. If body weight exceeds 50 kg, adult dosage should be used. Maximum daily dosage should not exceed 12 g.
Adults: Usual dosage is 1 g I.V. or I.M. q 6 to 8 hours. Up to 12 g daily can be administered in life-threatening infections.

Total daily dosage is same for I.M. or I.V. administration and depends on susceptibility of organism and severity of infection. Cefotaxime should be injected deep I.M. into a large muscle mass, such as the gluteus or the lateral aspect of the thigh.
Dosage in renal failure
In patients with impaired renal function, doses or frequency of administration must be modified according to the degree of renal impairment, severity of infection, and susceptibility of organism. To prevent toxic accumulation, increased dosage interval may be required in patients with creatinine clearance below 50 ml/minute.

Action and kinetics
- *Antibacterial action:* Cefotaxime is primarily bactericidal; however, it may be bacteriostatic. Activity depends on the organism, tissue penetration, drug dosage, and rate of organism multiplication. It acts by adhering to penicillin-binding enzymes, thereby inhibiting bacterial protein synthesis. Third-generation cephalosporins appear more active against some beta-lactamase-producing gram-negative organisms.

Cefotaxime is active against some gram-positive organisms and many enteric gram-negative bacilli, including streptococci (*Streptococcus pneumoniae* and *pyogenes*), *Staphylococcus aureus* (penicillinase- and nonpenicillinase-producing); *Staphylococcus epidermidis*; *Escherichia coli*; *Klebsiella* species; *Hemophilus influenzae*; *Enterobacter* species; *Proteus* species; and *Peptostreptococcus* species; and some strains of *Pseudomonas aeruginosa*. *Listeria* and *Acinetobacter* are often resistant. The active metabolite of cefotaxime, desacetylcefotaxime, may act synergistically with the parent drug against some bacterial strains.

- *Kinetics in adults:* Cefotaxime is not absorbed from the GI tract and must be given parenterally; peak serum levels occur 30 minutes after an I.M. dose.

Cefotaxime is distributed widely into most body tissues and fluids, including the gallbladder, liver, kidneys, bone, sputum, bile, and pleural and synovial fluids. *Unlike most other cephalosporins, cefotaxime has good CSF penetration;* it crosses the placenta. Cefotaxime is 13% to 38% protein-bound.

Cefotaxime is metabolized partially to an active metabolite, desacetylcefotaxime. Cefotaxime and its metabolites are excreted primarily in urine by renal tubular secretion; some drug may be excreted in breast milk. About 25% of cefotaxime is excreted in urine as the active metabolite; elimination half-life in normal adults is about 1 to 1½ hours for cefotaxime and about 1½ to 2 for desacetylcefotaxime; severe renal impairment prolongs cefotaxime's half-life to 11½ hours and that of the metabolite to as much as 56 hours. Hemodialysis removes both the drug and its metabolites.
- *Kinetics in children:* Serum half-life is prolonged in neonates and infants up to age 1.

Contraindications and precautions
Cefotaxime is contraindicated in patients with known hypersensitivity to any cephalosporin. It should be used with caution in patients with penicillin allergy, who usually are more susceptible to such reactions.

Interactions
Concomitant use with aminoglycosides results in apparent synergistic activity against Enterobacteriaceae and some strains of *Pseudomonas aeruginosa* and *Serratia marcescens;* such combined use may increase the risk of nephrotoxicity slightly.

Probenecid may block renal tubular secretion of cefotaxime and prolong its half-life.

Effects on diagnostic tests
Cephalosporins cause false-positive results in urine glucose tests utilizing cupric sulfate (Benedict's reagent or Clinitest); use glucose oxidase (Clinistix or Tes-Tape) instead. Cefotaxime also causes false elevations in urine creatinine levels in tests using Jaffé's reaction.

Cefotaxime may cause positive Coombs' tests results and elevations of liver function test results.

Adverse reactions
- CNS: headache, malaise, paresthesias, dizziness, seizures.
- DERM: maculopapular and erythematous rashes, urticaria.
- GI: *pseudomembranous colitis,* nausea, anorexia, vomiting, *diarrhea,* glossitis, dyspepsia, abdominal cramps, tenesmus, anal pruritus.
- GU: genital pruritus.
- HEMA: transient neutropenia, eosinophilia, hemolytic anemia.
- Local: at injection site—pain, induration, sterile abscesses, temperature elevation, tissue sloughing; phlebitis and thrombophlebitis with I.V. injection.
- Other: hypersensitivity (serum sickness [erythema

multiforme, rashes, urticaria, polyarthritis, fever]), dyspnea, bacterial and fungal superinfection.

Note: Drug should be discontinued if signs of toxicity, immediate hypersensitivity reaction, or serum sickness occur or if severe diarrhea indicates pseudomembranous colitis; alternative therapy should be considered if patient develops fever, eosinophilia, hematuria, or neutropenia.

Overdose and treatment
Clinical signs of overdose include neuromuscular hypersensitivity. Seizure may follow high CNS concentrations. Cefotaxime may be removed by hemodialysis.

▶ Special considerations
• For patients on sodium restriction, note that cefotaxime contains 2.2 mEq of sodium per gram of drug.
• Review patient's history of allergies; do not give a cephalosporin to any patient with a history of hypersensitivity reactions to cephalosporins; administer cautiously to patients with penicillin allergy.
• Try to determine whether previous reactions were true hypersensitivity reactions and not another reaction, such as GI distress, that the patient has interpreted as allergy.
• Monitor continuously for possible hypersensitivity or other untoward effects.
• Obtain results of cultures and sensitivity tests before first dose, but do not delay therapy; check test results periodically to assess drug efficacy.
• For I.M. injection, add 2 ml, 3 ml, or 5 ml of sterile or bacteriostatic water for injection to each 500-mg, 1-g, or 2-g vial. Shake well to dissolve drug completely. Check solution for particles and discoloration. Color ranges from light yellow to amber.
• Do not inject more than 1 g or more than 2 ml into a single I.M. site to prevent pain and tissue reaction.
• Administer I.M. dose deep into large muscle mass (gluteal or midlateral thigh); rotate injection sites to minimize tissue injury.
• Do not mix with any aminoglycoside or with sodium bicarbonate or any fluid with a pH above 7.5.
• For I.V. use, reconstitute all strengths of an I.V. dose with 10 ml of sterile water for injection. For infusion bottles, add 50 to 100 ml of 0.9% NaCl injection or 5% dextrose injection. May be further reconstituted to 50 to 1,000 ml with fluids recommended by manufacturer.
• Do not add or mix other drugs with I.V. infusions— particularly aminoglycosides, which will be inactivated if mixed with cephalosporins; if other drugs must be given I.V., temporarily stop infusion of primary drug.
• Adequate dilution of I.V. infusion, flushing with compatible solution after administration of drug, and rotation of the site every 48 hours help minimize local vein irritation; use of small-gauge needle in larger available vein may be helpful.
• Administer cefotaxime by direct intermittent I.V. over 3 to 5 minutes. Cefotaxime also may be given more slowly into a flowing I.V. line of compatible solution.
• Solution is stable for 24 hours at room temperature or at least 5 days under refrigeration. Cefotaxime may be stored in disposable glass or plastic syringes.

• Because cefotaxime is hemodialyzable, patients undergoing treatment with hemodialysis may require dosage adjustment.
• Monitor patients on long-term therapy for possible superinfection, especially debilitated patients and others receiving immunosuppressants or radiation therapy.
• Administer cephalosporins at least 1 hour before bacteriostatic antibiotics (tetracyclines, erythromycins, and chloramphenicol); these drugs inhibit bacterial cell growth, decreasing cephalosporin uptake by bacterial cell walls.

Information for parents and patient
• Teach parents signs and symptoms of hypersensitivity, bacterial and fungal superinfection, and other adverse reactions; urge them to report any unusual reactions.
• Warn parents that patient should not ingest alcohol in any form within 72 hours of cephalosporin dose. Emphasize that some liquid forms of acetaminophen contain alcohol.
• Advise adding live-culture yogurt or buttermilk to patient's diet to prevent intestinal superinfection resulting from suppression of normal intestinal flora.
• Advise parents of diabetic child to monitor urine glucose level with Clinistix or Tes-Tape and not to use Clinitest.
• Advise parents of infants of potential for yeast infections, especially in diaper area. Instruct them to keep diaper area clean and dry and to avoid use of plastic pants.

cefoxitin sodium
Mefoxin

• Classification: antibiotic (second-generation cephalosporin, cephamycin)

How supplied
Available by prescription only
Injection: 1 g, 2 g
Pharmacy bulk package: 10 g
Infusion: 1 g, 2 g in 50-ml or 100-ml container

Indications, route, and dosage
Serious respiratory, genitourinary, skin, soft-tissue, bone and joint, blood, and intraabdominal infections caused by susceptible organisms
Children: 80 to 160 mg/kg daily given in four to six equally divided doses.
Adults: 1 to 2 g q 6 to 8 hours for uncomplicated forms of infection. Up to 12 g daily in life-threatening infections.
Surgical prophylaxis
Children over age 3 months: 30 to 40 mg/kg I.M. or I.V. just before surgery (½ to 1 hour before initial incision), and q 6 hours after the first dose for no more than 24 hours.

Total daily dosage is same for I.M. or I.V. administration and depends on susceptibility of organism and severity of infection. Cefoxitin should be injected deep I.M. into a large muscle mass, such as the gluteus or lateral aspect of the thigh.

Dosage in renal failure

In patients with impaired renal function, doses or frequency of administration must be modified according to the degree of renal impairment, severity of infection, and susceptibility of organism. To prevent toxic accumulation, reduced dosage may be required in patients with creatinine clearance below 50 ml/minute.

Creatinine clearance (ml/min/1.73 m²)	Dosage in adults
>50	Usual adult dose
30 to 50	1 to 2 g q 8 to 12 hours
10 to 29	1 to 2 g q 12 to 24 hours
5 to 9	500 mg to 1 g q 12 to 24 hours
<5	500 mg to 1 g q 24 to 48 hours

Action and kinetics

• *Antibacterial action:* Cefoxitin is primarily bactericidal; however, it may be bacteriostatic. Activity depends on the organism, tissue penetration, drug dosage, and rate of organism multiplication. It acts by adhering to penicillin-binding enzymes, thereby inhibiting bacterial protein synthesis.

Cefoxitin is active against many gram-positive organisms and enteric gram-negative bacilli, including *Escherichia coli* and other coliform bacteria, *Staphylococcus aureus* (penicillinase- and nonpenicillinase-producing), *Staphylococcus epidermidis*, streptococci, *Klebsiella*, and Bacteroides species, (including *fragilis*). *Enterobacter, Pseudomonas,* and *Acinetobacter* are resistant to cefoxitin.

• *Kinetics in adults:* Cefoxitin is not absorbed from the GI tract and must be given parenterally; peak serum levels occur 20 to 30 minutes after an I.M. dose.

Cefoxitin is distributed widely into most body tissues and fluids, including the gallbladder, liver, kidneys, bone, sputum, bile, and pleural and synovial fluids; *CSF penetration is poor.* Cefoxitin crosses the placenta; it is 50% to 80% protein-bound.

About 2% of a cefoxitin dose is metabolized. Cefoxitin is excreted primarily in urine by renal tubular secretion and glomerular filtration; small amounts of drug are excreted in breast milk. Elimination half-life is about ½ to 1 hour in patients with normal renal function; half-life is prolonged in patients with severe renal dysfunction to 6½ to 21½ hours. Cefoxitin can be removed by hemodialysis but not by peritoneal dialysis.

• *Kinetics in children:* Serum half-life is prolonged in neonates and infants up to age 1.

Contraindications and precautions

Cefoxitin is contraindicated in patients with known hypersensitivity to any cephalosporin. It should be used with caution in patients with penicillin allergy.

Interactions

Probenecid competitively inhibits renal tubular secretion of cephalosporins, resulting in higher, prolonged serum levels of these drugs.

Concomitant use of cefoxitin with nephrotoxic agents (vancomycin, colistin, polymyxin B, or aminoglycosides) or loop diuretics increases the risk of nephrotoxicity. Concomitant use with bacteriostatic agents (tetracyclines, erythromycin, or chloramphenicol) may impair cefoxitin's bactericidal activity.

Effects on diagnostic tests

Cefoxitin causes false-positive results in urine glucose tests utilizing cupric sulfate (Benedict's reagent or Clinitest); use glucose oxidase tests (Clinistix or Tes-Tape) instead. Cefoxitin also causes false elevations in serum or urine creatinine levels in tests using Jaffé's reaction.

Cefoxitin may elevate liver function test results and may cause positive Coombs' test results.

Adverse reactions

• CNS: headache, malaise, paresthesias, dizziness, seizures.
• DERM: maculopapular and erythematous rashes, urticaria.
• GI: *pseudomembranous colitis,* nausea, anorexia, vomiting, diarrhea, glossitis, dyspepsia, abdominal cramps, tenesmus, anal pruritus.
• GU: genital pruritus, vaginitis, hematuria, nephrotoxicity.
• HEMA: transient neutropenia, eosinophilia, hemolytic anemia.
• Local: at injection site – pain, induration, sterile abscesses, tissue sloughing; phlebitis and thrombophlebitis with I.V. injection.
• Other: hypersensitivity, (serum sickness [erythema multiforme, rashes, polyarthritis, fever]); bacterial and fungal superinfection.

Note: Drug should be discontinued if signs of toxicity, immediate hypersensitivity reaction, or serum sickness occur or if severe diarrhea indicates pseudomembranous colitis; alternative therapy should be considered if the patient develops fever, eosinophilia, hematuria, neutropenia, or unexplained elevations in BUN or serum creatinine levels.

Overdose and treatment

Clinical signs of overdose include neuromuscular hypersensitivity. Seizure may follow high CNS concentrations. Cefoxitin may be removed by hemodialysis.

▶ Special considerations

• Cefoxitin injection contains 2.3 mEq of sodium per gram of drug.
• Reduced dosage may be indicated in infants younger than age 3 months. Safety has not been established.
• Review patient's history of allergies; do not give cefoxitin to any patient with a history of hypersen-

sitivity reactions to cephalosporins; administer cautiously to patients with penicillin allergy.
• Try to determine whether previous reactions were true hypersensitivity reactions and not another reaction, such as GI distress, that the patient has interpreted as allergy.
• Obtain results of cultures and sensitivity tests before first dose, but do not delay therapy; check test results periodically to assess drug efficacy.
• Consult manufacturer's directions for reconstitution, dilution, and storage of drugs; check expiration dates.
• After reconstituting, shake vial and then let stand until clear to ensure complete drug dissolution. Solution is stable for 24 hours at room temperature or for 1 week if refrigerated or 26 weeks if frozen.
• Solution may range from colorless to light amber and may darken during storage. Slight color change does not indicate loss of potency.
• Administer cephalosporins at least 1 hour before bacteriostatic antibiotics (tetracyclines, erythromycins, and chloramphenicol); these drugs inhibit bacterial cell growth, decreasing cephalosporin uptake by bacterial cell walls.
• For I.M. injection, reconstitute with 0.5% to 1% lidocaine hydrochloride (without epinephrine) to minimize pain at injection site; or with sterile water for injection, as ordered.
• Administer I.M. dose deep into large muscle mass (gluteal or midlateral thigh); rotate injection sites to minimize tissue injury.
• For I.V. use, reconstitute 1 g of cefoxitin with at least 10 ml of sterile water for injection, or 2 g of cefoxitin with 10 to 20 ml. Solutions of dextrose 5% and 0.9% NaCl for injection can also be used.
• Do not add or mix other drugs with I.V. infusions—particularly aminoglycosides, which will be inactivated if mixed with cephalosporins; if other drugs must be given I.V., temporarily stop infusion of primary drug.
• Adequate dilution of I.V. infusion and rotation of the site every 48 hours help minimize local vein irritation; use of small-gauge needle in larger available vein may be helpful.
• Cefoxitin has been associated with thrombophlebitis. Assess I.V. site frequently for signs of infiltration or phlebitis. Change I.V. site every 48 to 72 hours.
• Monitor continuously for possible hypersensitivity or other untoward effects.
• Monitor patients on long-term therapy for possible superinfection, especially debilitated patients and others receiving immunosuppressants or radiation therapy.
• Because cefoxitin is hemodialyzable, patients undergoing treatment with hemodialysis may require dosage adjustments.

Information for parents and patient
• Teach parents signs and symptoms of hypersensitivity, bacterial and fungal superinfection, and other adverse reactions; urge them to report any unusual reactions.
• Warn parents that patient should not ingest alcohol in any form within 72 hours of cephalosporin dose. Emphasize that some liquid forms of acetaminophen contain alcohol.

• Advise adding live-culture yogurt or buttermilk to patient's diet to prevent intestinal superinfection resulting from suppression of normal intestinal flora.
• Advise parents of diabetic child to monitor urine glucose level with Clinistix or Tes-Tape and not to use Clinitest.
• Advise parents of infants of potential for yeast infections, especially in diaper area. Instruct them to keep diaper area clean and dry and to avoid use of plastic pants.

▬▬▬▬▬▬▬▬▬▬▬▬▬▬▬

ceftazidime
Fortaz, Tazicef

• Classification: antibiotic (third-generation cephalosporin)

How supplied
Available by prescription only
Injection: 500 mg, 1 g, 2 g
Pharmacy bulk package: 6 g
Infusion: 1 g, 2 g in 100-ml vials and bags

Indications, route, and dosage
Bacteremia, septicemia, and serious respiratory, urinary, gynecologic, intraabdominal, CNS, and skin infections from susceptible organisms
Neonates age 0 to 4 weeks: 30 mg/kg I.V. q 12 hours.
Children age 1 month to 12 years: 30 to 50 mg/kg I.V. q 8 hours.
Children with cystic fibrosis: 150 to 300 mg/kg/day divided q 6 hours. Do not exceed 6 g daily.
Adults: 1 g I.V. or I.M. q 8 to 12 hours; up to 6 g daily in life-threatening infections.
    Total daily dosage is same for I.M. or I.V. administration and depends on susceptibility of organism and severity of infection. Ceftazidime should be injected deep I.M. into a large muscle mass, such as the gluteus or lateral aspect of the thigh.
Dosage in renal failure
In patients with impaired renal function, doses or frequency of administration must be modified according to the degree of renal impairment, severity of infection, and susceptibility of organism. To prevent toxic accumulation, reduced dosage may be required in patients with creatinine clearance below 50 ml/minute.

Creatinine clearance (ml/min/1.73 m²)	Dosage in adults
> 50	Usual adult dose
31 to 50	1 g q 12 hours
16 to 30	1 g q 24 hours
6 to 15	500 mg q 24 hours
< 5	500 mg q 48 hours
Hemodialysis patients	1 g after each hemodialysis period
Peritoneal dialysis patients	500 mg q 24 hours

Action and kinetics

• *Antibacterial action:* Ceftazidime is primarily bactericidal; however, it may be bacteriostatic. Activity depends on the organism, tissue penetration, drug dosage, and rate of organism multiplication. It acts by adhering to penicillin-binding enzymes, thereby inhibiting bacterial protein synthesis. Third-generation cephalosporins appear more active against some beta-lactamase-producing gram-negative organisms.

Ceftazidime is active against some gram-positive organisms and many enteric gram-negative bacilli, including streptococci (*Streptococcus pneumoniae* and *S. pyogenes*); *Staphylococcus aureus* (penicillinase- and nonpenicillinase-producing); *Escherichia coli; Klebsiella; Proteus; Enterobacter; Hemophilus influenzae; Pseudomonas;* and some strains of *Bacteroides.* It is more effective than any cephalosporin or penicillin derivative against *Pseudomonas.* Some other third-generation cephalosporins are more active against gram-positive organisms and anaerobes.

• *Kinetics in adults:* Ceftazidime is not absorbed from the GI tract and must be given parenterally; peak serum levels occur 1 hour after an I.M. dose.

Ceftazidime is distributed widely into most body tissues and fluids, including the gallbladder, liver, kidneys, bone, sputum, bile, and pleural and synovial fluids; unlike most other cephalosporins, ceftazidime has good CSF penetration; it crosses the placenta. Ceftazidime is 5% to 24% protein-bound.

Ceftazidime is not metabolized. It is excreted primarily in urine by glomerular filtration; small amounts of drug are excreted in breast milk. Elimination half-life is about 1½ to 2 hours in patients with normal renal function; up to 35 hours in patients with severe renal disease. Hemodialysis or peritoneal dialysis removes ceftazidime.

• *Kinetics in children:* Serum half-life is prolonged in neonates and infants up to age 1.

Contraindications and precautions

Ceftazidime is contraindicated in patients with known hypersensitivity to any cephalosporin. It should be used with caution in patients with penicillin allergy, who usually are more susceptible to such reactions.

Interactions

Concomitant use with aminoglycosides results in synergistic activity against *Pseudomonas aeruginosa* and some strains of *Enterobacteriaceae;* such combined use may slightly increase the risk of nephrotoxicity.

Concomitant use with clavulanic acid results in synergistic activity against some strains of *Bacteroides fragilis.*

Effects on diagnostic tests

Ceftazidime causes false-positive results in urine glucose tests utilizing cupric sulfate (Benedict's reagent or Clinitest); use glucose oxidase (Clinistix or Tes-Tape) instead. Ceftazidime also causes false elevations in urine creatinine levels in tests using Jaffé's reaction.

Ceftazidime may cause positive Coombs' test results and elevated liver function test results.

Adverse reactions

• CNS: headache, dizziness, seizures.
• DERM: maculopapular and erythematous rashes, urticaria.
• GI: *pseudomembranous enterocolitis,* nausea, vomiting, diarrhea, dysgeusia, abdominal cramps.
• GU: hematuria, genital pruritus.
• HEMA: *eosinophilia, thrombocytosis, neutropenia,* leukopenia, anemia.
• Hepatic: transient elevation in liver enzymes.
• Local: at injection site – pain, induration, sterile abscesses, tissue sloughing; phlebitis and thrombophlebitis with I.V. injection.
• Other: hypersensitivity, (dyspnea, serum sickness [erythema multiforme, rashes, polyarthritis, fever]), bacterial and fungal superinfection.

Note: Drug should be discontinued if signs of toxicity, immediate hypersensitivity reaction, or serum sickness occur or if severe diarrhea indicates pseudomembranous colitis; alternative therapy should be considered if patient develops fever, eosinophilia, hematuria, or neutropenia.

Overdose and treatment

Clinical signs of overdose include neuromuscular hypersensitivity. Seizure may follow high CNS concentrations. Ceftazidime may be removed by hemodialysis or peritoneal dialysis.

▶ Special considerations

• For patients on sodium restriction, note that ceftazidime contains 2.3 mEq of sodium per gram of drug.
• Ceftazidime powders for injection contain 118 mg sodium carbonate per gram of drug; ceftazidime sodium is more water-soluble and is formed in situ upon reconstitution.
• Ceftazidime vials are supplied under reduced pressure. When the antibiotic is dissolved, carbon dioxide is released and a positive pressure develops. Each brand of ceftazidime includes specific instructions for reconstitution. Read and follow these instructions carefully.
• Because ceftazidime is hemodialyzable, patients undergoing treatments with hemodialysis or peritoneal dialysis may require dosage adjustment.
• Review patient's history of allergies; do not give ceftazidime to any patient with a history of hypersensitivity reactions to cephalosporins; administer cautiously to patients with penicillin allergy.

• Try to determine whether previous reactions were true hypersensitivity reactions and not another reaction, such as GI distress, that patient has interpreted as allergy.
• Obtain results of cultures and sensitivity tests before first dose, but do not delay therapy; check test results periodically to assess drug efficacy.
• Monitor continuously for possible hypersensitivity or other untoward effects.
• Monitor patients on long-term therapy for possible superinfection, especially debilitated patients and others receiving immunosuppressants or radiation therapy.
• Consult manufacturer's directions for reconstitution, dilution, and storage of drugs; check expiration dates.
• Administer cephalosporins at least 1 hour before bacteriostatic antibiotics (tetracyclines, erythromycins, and chloramphenicol); these drugs inhibit bacterial cell growth, decreasing cephalosporin uptake by bacterial cell walls.
• Administer I.M. dose deep into large muscle mass (gluteal or midlateral thigh); rotate injection sites to minimize tissue injury.
• Do not add or mix other drugs with I.V. infusions—particularly aminoglycosides, which will be inactivated if mixed with cephalosporins; if other drugs must be given I.V., temporarily stop infusion of primary drug.
• Adequate dilution of I.V. infusion and rotation of the site every 48 hours help minimize local vein irritation; use of small-gauge needle in larger available vein may be helpful.

Information for parents and patient

• Teach parents signs and symptoms of hypersensitivity, bacterial and fungal superinfection, and other adverse reactions; urge them to report any unusual reactions.
• Warn parents that patient should not ingest alcohol in any form within 72 hours of cephalosporin dose. Emphasize that some liquid forms of acetaminophen contain alcohol.
• Advise parents to add live-culture yogurt or buttermilk to child's diet to prevent intestinal superinfection resulting from suppression of normal intestinal flora.
• Advise parents of diabetic child to monitor urine glucose level with Clinistix or Tes-Tape and not to use Clinitest.
• Be sure parents understand how and when to give drug; urge them to complete entire prescribed regimen, to comply with instructions for around-the-clock dosage, and to keep follow-up appointments.
• Advise them to check expiration date of drug and to discard unused drug.

ceftizoxime sodium
Cefizox

• Classification: antibiotic (third-generation cephalosporin)

How supplied
Available by prescription only
Injection: 1 g, 2 g
Infusion: 1 g, 2 g in 100-mg vials

Indications, route, and dosage
Bacteremia, septicemia, meningitis, and serious respiratory, urinary, gynecologic, intraabdominal, bone and joint and skin infections from susceptible organisms
Children and infants age 6 months and older: 150 to 200 mg/kg/day I.V. or I.M. divided q 6 to 8 hours.
Adults: Usual dosage is 1 to 2 g I.V. or I.M. q 8 to 12 hours. In life-threatening infections, up to 2 g q 4 hours.

Total daily dosage is same for I.M. or I.V. administration and depends on susceptibility of organism and severity of infection. Ceftizoxime should be injected deep I.M. into a large muscle mass, such as the gluteus or lateral aspect of the thigh.
Mild to moderate infections caused by susceptible organisms
Children and infants over 6 months and older: 100 to 150 mg/kg/day I.V. or I.M., divided q 8 hours.
Dosage in renal failure
In patients with impaired renal function, doses or frequency of administration must be modified according to the degree of renal impairment, severity of infection, and susceptibility of organism. To prevent toxic accumulation, reduced dosage may be required in patients with creatinine clearance below 80 ml/minute.

DOSAGE IN ADULTS		
Creatinine clearance (ml/min/ 1.73 m²)	**Less severe infections**	**Life-threatening infections**
> 80	Usual adult dose	Usual adult dose
50 to 79	500 mg q 8 hours	750 mg to 1.5 g q 8 hours
5 to 49	250 to 500 mg q 12 hours	500 mg to 1 g q 12 hours
0 to 4	500 mg q 48 hours; or 250 mg q 24 hours	500 mg to 1 g q 48 hours; or 500 mg q 24 hours

Action and kinetics
• *Antibacterial action:* Ceftizoxime is primarily bactericidal; however, it may be bacteriostatic. Activity depends on the organism, tissue penetration, drug dosage, and rate of organism multiplication. It acts

‡May contain sulfites   ◆May contain tartrazine   ◆◆May contain benzyl alcohol

by adhering to penicillin-binding enzymes, thereby inhibiting bacterial protein synthesis. Third-generation cephalosporins appear more active against some beta-lactamase-producing gram-negative organisms.

Ceftizoxime is active against some gram-positive organisms and many enteric gram-negative bacilli, including streptococci (*Streptococcus pneumoniae* and *pyogenes*; *Staphylococcus aureus* (penicillinase- and nonpenicillinase-producing); *Staphylococcus epidermidis*; *Escherichia coli*; *Klebsiella*; *Hemophilus influenzae*; *Enterobacter*; *Proteus*; *Peptostreptococcus*; some strains of *Pseudomonas* and *Acinetobacter*. Cefotaxime and moxalactam are slightly more active than ceftizoxime against gram-positive organisms but are less active against gram-negative organisms.

• *Kinetics in adults:* Ceftizoxime is not absorbed from the GI tract and must be given parenterally; peak serum levels occur at ½ to 1½ hours after an I.M. dose.

Ceftizoxime is distributed widely into most body tissues and fluids, including the gallbladder, liver, kidneys, bone, sputum, bile, and pleural and synovial fluids; unlike most other cephalosporins, ceftizoxime has good CSF penetration and achieves adequate concentration in inflamed meninges; ceftizoxime crosses the placenta. Ceftizoxime is 28% to 31% protein-bound.

Ceftizoxime is excreted unmetabolized, primarily in urine by renal tubular secretion and glomerular filtration; small amounts of drug are excreted in breast milk. Elimination half-life is about 1½ to 2 hours in patients with normal renal function; severe renal disease prolongs half-life up to 30 hours. Hemodialysis or peritoneal dialysis removes minimal amounts of ceftizoxime.

• *Kinetics in children:* Serum half-life is prolonged in neonates and infants up to age 1.

Contraindications and precautions
Ceftizoxime is contraindicated in patients with known hypersensitivity to any cephalosporin. It should be used with caution in patients with penicillin allergy, who usually are more susceptible to such reactions.

Interactions
Probenecid competitively inhibits renal tubular secretion of cephalosporins, causing higher, prolonged serum levels.

Concomitant use of ceftizoxime with bacteriostatic agents (tetracyclines, erythromycin, or chloramphenicol) may impair its bactericidal effects. Concomitant use with aminoglycosides may slightly increase the risk of nephrotoxicity.

Effects on diagnostic tests
Ceftizoxime causes false-positive results in urine glucose tests utilizing cupric sulfate (Benedict's reagent or Clinitest); use glucose oxidase (Clinistix or Tes-Tape) instead. Ceftizoxime also causes false elevations in urine creatinine levels using Jaffé's reaction.

Ceftizoxime may cause positive Coombs' test results and elevated liver function test results.

Adverse reactions
• CNS: headache, malaise, paresthesias, dizziness, seizures.
• DERM: maculopapular and erythematous rashes, urticaria.
• GI: *pseudomembranous colitis,* nausea, anorexia, vomiting, diarrhea, glossitis, dyspepsia, abdominal cramps, tenesmus, anal pruritus, altered taste.
• GU: genital pruritus, nephrotoxicity, vaginitis, hematuria.
• HEMA: transient neutropenia, eosinophilia, hemolytic anemia.
• Local: at injection site – pain, induration, sterile abscesses, tissue sloughing; phlebitis and thrombophlebitis with I.V. injection.
• Other: hypersensitivity, (serum sickness [erythema multiforme, rashes, polyarthritis, fever]), bacterial and fungal superinfection.

Note: Drug should be discontinued if signs of toxicity, immediate hypersensitivity reaction, or serum sickness occur or if severe diarrhea indicates pseudomembranous colitis; alternative therapy should be considered if patient develops fever, eosinophilia, hematuria, or neutropenia.

Overdose and treatment
Clinical signs of overdose include neuromuscular hypersensitivity. Seizure may follow high CNS concentrations. Ceftizoxime may be removed by hemodialysis.

▶ Special considerations
• For patients on sodium restriction, note that ceftizoxime contains 2.6 mEq of sodium per gram of drug.
• Administer cephalosporins at least 1 hour before bacteriostatic antibiotics (tetracyclines, erythromycins, and chloramphenicol); these drugs inhibit bacterial cell growth, decreasing cephalosporin uptake by bacterial cell walls.
• Drug may be supplied as frozen, sterile solution in plastic containers. Thaw at room temperature. Thawed solution is stable for 24 hours at room temperature, or for 10 days if refrigerated. Do not refreeze.
• For I.M. use, reconstitute with sterile water for injection. Shake vial well to ensure complete dissolution of drug. To administer a dose that exceeds 1 g, divide the dose and inject it into separate sites to prevent tissue injury.
• Administer I.M. dose deep into large muscle mass (gluteal or midlateral thigh); rotate injection sites to minimize tissue injury.
• For I.V. use, reconstitute I.V. dose with sterile water for injection. Solution should clear after shaking well and range in color from yellow to amber. If particles are visible, discard solution. Reconstituted solution is stable for 8 hours at room temperature or 48 hours if refrigerated.
• Do not add or mix other drugs with I.V. infusions – particularly aminoglycosides, which will be inactivated if mixed with cephalosporins; if other drugs must be given I.V., temporarily stop infusion of primary drug.
• Adequate dilution of I.V. infusion and rotation of the site every 48 hours help minimize local vein irritation; use of small-gauge needle in larger available vein may be helpful.

• Administer I.V. as a direct injection slowly over 3 to 5 minutes directly or through tubing of compatible infusion fluid. If given as intermittent infusion, dilute reconstituted drug in 50 to 100 ml of compatible fluid. Check package insert.

• Review patient's history of allergies; do not give ceftizoxime to any patient with a history of hypersensitivity reactions to cephalosporins; administer cautiously to patients with penicillin allergy.

• Try to determine whether previous reactions were true hypersensitivity reactions and not another reaction, such as GI distress, that the patient has interpreted as allergy.

• Obtain results of cultures and sensitivity tests before first dose, but do not delay therapy; check test results periodically to assess drug efficacy.

• Monitor continuously for possible hypersensitivity or other untoward effects.

• Monitor patients on long-term therapy for possible superinfection, especially debilitated patients and others receiving immunosuppressants or radiation therapy.

Information for parents and patient

• Teach parents signs and symptoms of hypersensitivity, bacterial and fungal superinfection, and other adverse reactions; urge parents to report any unusual reactions.

• Warn parents that patient should not ingest alcohol in any form within 72 hours of cephalosporin dose.

• Advise adding live-culture yogurt or buttermilk to child's diet to prevent intestinal superinfection resulting from suppression of normal intestinal flora.

• Advise parents of diabetic child to monitor urine glucose level with Clinistix or Tes-Tape and not to use Clinitest.

• Tell parents to have patient take oral drug with food if GI irritation occurs.

ceftriaxone sodium
Rocephin

• Classification: antibiotic (third-generation cephalosporin)

How supplied
Available by prescription only
Injection: 250 mg, 500 mg, 1 g, 2 g
Pharmacy bulk package: 10 g
Infusion: 1 g, 2 g

Indications, route, and dosage
Bacteremia, septicemia, and serious respiratory, urinary, gynecologic, intraabdominal, and skin infections from susceptible organisms
Neonates: 50 to 75 mg/kg/day I.V. or I.M., divided q 12 to 24 hours, not to exceed 2 g.
Children: 50 to 75 mg/kg/day divided q 12 hours; usual duration 4 to 14 days.
Adults: 1 to 2 g I.M. or I.V. once daily or in equally divided doses twice daily. Total daily dosage should not exceed 4 g.

Meningitis
Neonates: 75 mg/kg I.V. as single dose, then 100 mg/kg/day I.V. divided q 12 hours.
Children and adults: 100 mg/kg/day given divided q 12 hours; not to exceed 4 g.

Uncomplicated gonococcal infection
Neonates: 150 mg as single dose.
Children and adults: 250 mg I.M. as a single dose.

May give loading dose of 75 mg/kg. Total daily dosage is same for I.M. or I.V. administration and depends on susceptibility of organism and severity of infection. Ceftriaxone should be injected deep I.M. into a large muscle mass, such as the gluteus or lateral aspect of the thigh.

Action and kinetics
• *Antibacterial action:* Ceftriaxone is primarily bactericidal; however, it may be bacteriostatic. Activity depends on the organism, tissue penetration, and drug dosage and on the rate of organism multiplication. It acts by adhering to penicillin-binding enzymes, thereby inhibiting bacterial protein synthesis. Third-generation cephalosporins appear more active against some beta-lactamase-producing gram-negative organisms.

Ceftriaxone is active against some gram-positive organisms and many enteric gram-negative bacilli, including streptococci; *Streptococcus pneumoniae* and *pyogenes; Staphylococcus aureus* (penicillinase and nonpenicillinase producing); *Staphylococcus epidermis; Escherichia coli; Klebsiella; Hemophilus influenzae, Enterobacter; Proteus;* some strains of *Pseudomonas* and *Peptostreptococcus.* Most strains of *Listeria, Pseudomonas,* and *Acinetobacter* are resistant. Ceftriaxone's activity is most like that of cefotaxime and ceftizoxime.

• *Kinetics in adults:* Ceftriaxone is not absorbed from the GI tract and must be given parenterally; peak serum levels occur at 1½ to 4 hours after an I.M. dose.

Ceftriaxone is distributed widely into most body tissues and fluids, including the gallbladder, liver, kidneys, bone, sputum, bile, and pleural and synovial fluids; unlike most other cephalosporins, ceftriaxone has good CSF penetration. Ceftriaxone crosses the placenta. Protein binding is dose-dependent and decreases as serum levels rise; average is 58% to 96%.

Ceftriaxone is partially metabolized and excreted principally in urine; some drug is excreted in bile by biliary mechanisms, and small amounts are excreted in breast milk. Elimination half-life is 5½ to 11 hours in adults with normal renal function; severe renal disease prolongs half-life only moderately. Neither hemodialysis nor peritoneal dialysis will remove ceftriaxone.

• *Kinetics in children:* Serum half-life is prolonged in neonates and infants up to age 1.

Contraindications and precautions
Ceftriaxone is contraindicated in patients with known hypersensitivity to any cephalosporin. It should be used with caution in patients with penicillin allergy, who usually are more susceptible to such reactions; in hyperbilirubinemic neonates, especially prema-

---

‡May contain sulfites   ♦May contain tartrazine   ♦♦May contain benzyl alcohol

tures; and in patients with history of colitis or other GI disease.

Interactions
Concomitant use with aminoglycosides produces synergistic antimicrobial activity against *Pseudomonas aeruginosa* and some strains of *Enterobacteriaceae.*

Effects on diagnostic tests
Ceftriaxone causes false-positive results in urine glucose tests utilizing cupric sulfate (Benedict's reagent or Clinitest); use glucose oxidase (Clinistix or Tes-Tape) instead. Ceftriaxone also causes false elevations in urine creatinine levels in tests using Jaffé's reaction.

Ceftriaxone may cause positive Coombs' test results, and elevations in liver function test results.

Adverse reactions
• CNS: headache, dizziness, seizures.
• DERM: maculopapular and erythematous rashes, urticaria.
• GI: pseudomembranous enterocolitis, *nausea, vomiting, diarrhea,* dysgeusia, *abdominal cramps.*
• GU: genital pruritus, hematuria, casts.
• HEMA: eosinophilia, neutropenia, thrombocytosis, *leukopenia,* anemia, *thrombocytopenia.*
• Hepatic: transient elevation in liver enzymes.
• Local: at injection site — *pain,* induration, sterile abscesses, tissue sloughing; *phlebitis* and thrombophlebitis with I.V. injection.
• Other: *hypersensitivity,* (dyspnea, *fever, chills, pruritus,* serum sickness [erythema multiforme, rashes, polyarthritis, fever]).
    Note: Drug should be discontinued if signs of toxicity, immediate hypersensitivity reaction, or serum sickness occur or if severe diarrhea indicates pseudomembranous colitis; alternative therapy should be considered if patient develops fever, eosinophilia, hematuria, or neutropenia.

Overdose and treatment
Clinical signs of overdose include neuromuscular hypersensitivity. Seizure may follow high CNS concentrations. Treatment is supportive.

▶ Special considerations
• For patients on sodium restriction, note that ceftriaxone injection contains 3.6 mEq of sodium per gram of drug.
• Long serum half-life allows once a day administration.
• Ceftriaxone is used commonly in home care programs for management of serious infections, such as osteomyelitis.
• Dosage adjustment usually is not necessary in patients with renal insufficiency because of partial biliary excretion. In patients with impaired hepatic and renal function, dosage should not exceed 2 g/day without monitoring of serum levels.
• For infections caused by *Streptococcus pyogenes*, treatment should continue for at least 10 days.
• Review patient's history of allergies; do not give ceftriaxone to any patient with a history of hyper-

sensitivity reactions to cephalosporins; administer cautiously to patients with penicillin allergy.
• Try to determine whether previous reactions were true hypersensitivity reactions and not another reaction, such as GI distress, that the patient has interpreted as allergy.
• Monitor continuously for possible hypersensitivity or other untoward effects.
• Obtain results of cultures and sensitivity tests before first dose, but do not delay therapy; check test results periodically to assess drug efficacy.
• Monitor patients on long-term therapy for possible superinfection, especially debilitated patients and others receiving immunosuppressants or radiation therapy.
• Administer cephalosporins at least 1 hour before bacteriostatic antibiotics (tetracyclines, erythromycins, and chloramphenicol); these drugs inhibit bacterial cell growth, decreasing cephalosporin uptake by bacterial cell walls.
• Consult manufacturer's directions for reconstitution, dilution, and storage of drugs; check expiration dates.
• Administer I.M. dose deep into large muscle mass (gluteal or midlateral thigh); rotate injection sites to minimize tissue injury.
• Do not add or mix other drugs with I.V. infusions — particularly aminoglycosides, which will be inactivated if mixed with cephalosporins; if other drugs must be given I.V., temporarily stop infusion of primary drug.
• Adequate dilution of I.V. infusion and rotation of the site every 48 hours help minimize local vein irritation; use of small-gauge needle in larger available vein may be helpful.

Information for parents and patient
• Teach parents signs and symptoms of hypersensitivity, bacterial and fungal superinfection, and other adverse reactions; urge them to report any unusual reactions.
• Warn parents that patient should not ingest alcohol in any form within 72 hours of cephalosporin dose. Emphasize that some liquid forms of acetaminophen contain alcohol.
• Advise adding live-culture yogurt or buttermilk to patient's diet to prevent intestinal superinfection resulting from suppression of normal intestinal flora.
• Advise parents of diabetic child to monitor urine glucose level with Clinistix or Tes-Tape and not to use Clinitest.
• Advise parents of infants of potential for yeast infections, especially in diaper area. Instruct them to keep diaper area clean and dry and to avoid use of plastic pants.

---

cefuroxime sodium
Kefurox, Zinacef

• Classification: antibiotic (second-generation cephalosporin)

How supplied
Available by prescription only
Injection: 750 mg, 1.5 g
Infusion: 750 mg, 1.5-g Infusion Packets

Indications, route, and dosage
Serious lower respiratory, urinary tract, skin and skin structure infections; septicemia; meningitis caused by susceptible organisms
Neonates: 10 mg/kg/day I.M. or I.V. divided q 12 hours.
Children and infants over age 3 months: 50 to 100 mg/kg I.M. or I.V. daily. Higher dosages (in equally divided doses every 6 to 8 hours) are administered when treating meningitis.
Adults: Usual dosage is 750 mg to 1.5 g I.M. or I.V. q 8 hours, usually for 5 to 10 days. For life-threatening infections and infections caused by less susceptible organisms, 1.5 g I.M. or I.V. q 6 hours; for bacterial meningitis, up to 3 g I.V. q 8 hours.
Meningitis caused by **Streptococcus pneumoniae, Hemophilus influenzae, Neisseria meningitidis,** *and* **S. aureus.**
Children and infants over age 3 months: 200 to 240 mg/kg/day I.V. divided q 6 to 8 hours. Dosage should not exceed 3 g per 8 hour period.

Total daily dosage is same for I.M. or I.V. administration and depends on susceptibility of organism and severity of infection. Cefuroxime should be injected deep I.M. into a large muscle mass, such as the gluteus or lateral aspect of the thigh.

Dosage in renal failure
In patients with impaired renal function, doses or frequency of administration must be modified according to the degree of renal impairment, severity of infection, and susceptibility of organism. To prevent toxic accumulation, reduced dosage may be required in patients with creatinine clearance below 20 ml/minute.

Creatinine clearance (ml/min/1.73 m²)	Dosage in adults
>20	750 mg to 1.5 g q 8 hours
10 to 20	750 mg q 12 hours
<10	750 mg q 24 hours
Hemodialysis patients	750 mg at the end of each dialysis period

Action and kinetics
• *Antibacterial action:* Cefuroxime is primarily bactericidal; however, it may be bacteriostatic. Activity depends on the organism, tissue penetration, drug dosage, and rate of organism multiplication. It acts by adhering to penicillin-binding enzymes, thereby inhibiting bacterial protein synthesis.

Cefuroxime is active against many gram-positive organisms and enteric gram-negative bacilli, including *Streptococcus pneumoniae* and *pyogenes, Hemophilus influenzae, Klebsiella* species, *Staphylococcus aureus, Escherichia coli, Enterobacter,* and *Neisseria gonorrhoea;* its spectrum is similar to that of cefamandole, but it is more stable against beta-lactamases. *Bacteroides fragilis, Pseudomonas,* and *Acinetobacter* are resistant to cefuroxime.

• *Kinetics in adults:* Cefuroxime is not well absorbed from the GI tract and must be given parenterally; peak serum levels occur 15 to 60 minutes after an I.M. dose.

Cefuroxime is distributed widely into most body tissues and fluids, including the gallbladder, liver, kidneys, bone, bile, and pleural and synovial fluids; CSF penetration is greater than that of most first- and second-generation cephalosporins and achieves adequate therapeutic levels in inflamed meninges. Cefuroxime crosses the placenta; it is 33% to 50% protein-bound.

Cefuroxime is not metabolized. It is primarily excreted in urine by renal tubular secretion and glomerular filtration; elimination half-life is 1 to 2 hours in patients with normal renal function; end-stage renal disease prolongs half-life 15 to 22 hours. Some of the drug is excreted in breast milk. Hemodialysis removes cefuroxime.

• *Kinetics in children:* Serum half-life is prolonged in neonates and infants up to age 1.

Contraindications and precautions
Cefuroxime is contraindicated in patients with known hypersensitivity to any cephalosporin. It should be used with caution in patients with penicillin allergy, who usually are more susceptible to such reactions.

Interactions
Probenecid competitively inhibits renal tubular secretion of cephalosporins, resulting in higher, prolonged serum levels of these drugs.

Concomitant use of cefuroxime with nephrotoxic agents (vancomycin, colistin, polymyxin B, or aminoglycosides) or loop diuretics increases the risk of nephrotoxicity. Concomitant use with bacteriostatic agents (tetracyclines, erythromycin, or chloramphenicol) may impair its bactericidal activity.

Effects on diagnostic tests
Cefuroxime causes false-positive results in urine glucose tests utilizing cupric sulfate (Benedict's reagent or Clinitest); use glucose oxidase tests (Clinistix or Tes-Tape) instead. Cefuroxime also causes false elevations in serum or urine creatinine levels in tests using Jaffé's reaction.

Cefuroxime may elevate liver function test results and may cause positive Coombs' test results.

Adverse reactions
• CNS: headache, malaise, paresthesias, dizziness, seizures.
• DERM: maculopapular and erythematous rashes, urticaria.

• GI: *pseudomembranous colitis,* nausea, anorexia, vomiting, diarrhea, glossitis, dyspepsia, abdominal cramps, tenesmus, anal pruritus.
• GU: genital pruritus, hematuria, nephrotixicity.
• HEMA: transient neutropenia, eosinophilia, hemolytic anemia, decrease in hemoglobin and hematocrit levels.
• Local: at injection site — pain, induration, sterile abscesses, temperature elevation, tissue sloughing; phlebitis and thrombophlebitis with I.V. injection.
• Other: hypersensitivity, (dyspnea, serum sickness [erythema multiforme, rashes, polyarthritis, and fever]), bacterial and fungal superinfection.
   Note: Drug should be discontinued if signs of toxicity, immediate hypersensitivity reaction, or serum sickness occur or if severe diarrhea indicates pseudomembranous colitis; alternative therapy should be considered if the following symptoms occur: fever, eosinophilia, hematuria, neutropenia, or unexplained elevations in BUN or serum creatinine levels.

Overdose and treatment
Clinical signs of overdose include neuromuscular hypersensitivity. Seizure may follow high CNS concentrations. Hemodialysis or peritoneal dialysis will remove cefuroxime.

▶ Special considerations
• For patients on sodium restriction, note that cefuroxime contains 2.4 mEq of sodium per gram of drug.
• Cefuroxime is a second-generation cephalosporin similar to cefamandole. However, cefuroxime has not been associated with prothrombin deficiency and bleeding. It offers the advantage of effectiveness in treating meningitis.
• Check solutions for particulate matter and discoloration. Solution may range in color from light yellow to amber without affecting potency.
• Shake I.M. solution gently before administration to ensure complete drug dissolution. Administer deep I.M. in a large muscle mass, preferably the gluteus. Aspirate before injecting to prevent inadvertent injection into a blood vessel. Rotate injection sites to prevent tissue damage. Apply ice to injection site to relieve pain.
• Do not add or mix other drugs with I.V. infusions — particularly aminoglycosides, which will be inactivated if mixed with cephalosporins; if other drugs must be given I.V., temporarily stop infusion of primary drug.
• Adequate dilution of I.V. infusion and rotation of the site every 48 hours help minimize local vein irritation; use of small-gauge needle in larger available vein may be helpful.
• For direct intermittent I.V., inject solution slowly into vein over 3 to 5 minutes or slowly through tubing of free-running, compatible I.V. solution.
• Reconstituted solution retains potency for 24 hours at room temperature or for 48 hours if refrigerated.
• Because cefuroxime is hemodialyzable, patients undergoing treatment with hemodialysis or peritoneal dialysis may require dosage adjustments.
• Review patient's history of allergies; do not give cefuroxime to any patient with a history of hyper-

sensitivity reactions to cephalosporins; administer cautiously to patients with penicillin allergy.
• Try to determine whether previous reactions were true hypersensitivity reactions and not another reaction, such as GI distress, that the patient has interpreted as allergy.
• Obtain results of cultures and sensitivity tests before first dose, but do not delay therapy; check test results periodically to assess drug efficacy.
• Monitor continuously for possible hypersensitivity or other untoward effects.
• Monitor patients on long-term therapy for possible superinfection, especially debilitated patients and others receiving immunosuppressants or radiation therapy.
• Administer cephalosporins at least 1 hour before bacteriostatic antibiotics (tetracyclines, erythromycins, and chloramphenicol); these drugs inhibit bacterial cell growth, decreasing cephalosporin uptake by bacterial cell walls.

Information for parents and patient
• Teach parents signs and symptoms of hypersensitivity, bacterial and fungal superinfection, and other adverse reactions; urge them to report any unusual reactions.
• Warn parents that patient should not ingest alcohol in any form within 72 hours of cephalosporin dose. Emphasize that some liquid forms of acetaminophen contain alcohol.
• Advise adding live-culture yogurt or buttermilk to patient's diet to prevent intestinal superinfection resulting from suppression of normal intestinal flora.
• Advise parents of diabetic child to monitor urine glucose level with Clinistix or Tes-Tape and not to use Clinitest.
• Advise parents of infants of potential for yeast infections, especially in diaper area. Instruct them to keep diaper area clean and dry and to avoid use of plastic pants.

■

cephalexin monohydrate
Ceporex*, Keflex, Novolexin*

• Classification: antibiotic (first-generation cephalosporin)

How supplied
Available by prescription only
Tablets: 250 mg, 500 mg, 1 g
Capsules: 500 mg, 1,250 mg
Suspension: 100 mg/5 ml, 125 mg/5 ml, and 250 mg/5 ml

Indications, route, and dosage
Respiratory, genitourinary, skin and soft-tissue or bone and joint infections, and otitis media caused by susceptible organisms
Children: 25 to 50 mg/kg P.O. q 6 hours. Maximum 25 mg/kg q 6 hours.
Adults: 250 mg to 1 g P.O. q 6 hours.

Streptococcal pharyngitis
Children over age 1 year: 25 to 50 mg/kg P.O. divided q 12 hours.

Otitis media
Children: 75 to 100 mg/kg/day divided q 6 hours.

Dosage in renal failure
To prevent toxic accumulation in patients with impaired renal function, those with creatinine clearance below 40 ml/minute should receive reduced dosage.

Action and kinetics

• *Antibacterial action:* Cephalexin is primarily bactericidal; however, it may be bacteriostatic. Activity depends on the organism, tissue penetration, drug dosage, and rate of organism multiplication. It acts by adhering to penicillin-binding enzymes, thereby inhibiting bacterial protein synthesis.

Cephalexin is active against many gram-positive organisms, including penicillinase-producing *Staphylococcus aureus* and *epidermidis, Streptococcus pneumoniae,* group B streptococci, and group A beta-hemolytic streptococci; susceptible gram-negative organisms include *Klebsiella pneumoniae, Escherichia coli, Proteus mirabilis,* and *Shigella.*

• *Kinetics in adults:* Cephalexin is absorbed rapidly and completely from the GI tract after oral administration; peak serum levels occur within 1 hour. Food delays but does not prevent complete absorption.

Cephalexin is distributed widely into most body tissues and fluids, including the gallbladder, liver, kidneys, bone, sputum, bile, and pleural and synovial fluids; CSF penetration is poor. Cephalexin crosses the placenta; it is 6% to 15% protein-bound.

Cephalexin is not metabolized. It is excreted primarily unchanged in urine by glomerular filtration and renal tubular secretion; small amounts of drug may be excreted in breast milk. Elimination half-life is about ½ to 1 hour in patients with normal renal function; 7½ to 14 hours in patients with severe renal impairment. Hemodialysis or peritoneal dialysis removes cephalexin.

• *Kinetics in children:* The serum half-life is prolonged in neonates and in infants younger than age 1.

Contraindications and precautions

Cephalexin is contraindicated in patients with known hypersensitivity to any cephalosporin. It should be used with caution in patients with penicillin allergy, who usually are more susceptible to such reactions, and in patients with renal impairment.

Interactions

Probenecid competitively inhibits renal tubular secretion of cephalosporins, resulting in higher, prolonged serum levels of these drugs.

Concomitant use with nephrotoxic agents (vancomycin, colistin, polymyxin B, or aminoglycosides) or loop diuretics increases the risk of nephrotoxicity.

Concomitant use with bacteriostatic agents (tetracyclines, erythromycin, or chloramphenicol) may interfere with bactericidal activity.

Effects on diagnostic tests

Cephalexin causes false-positive results in urine glucose tests utilizing cupric sulfate (Benedict's reagent

or Clinitest); use glucose oxidase test (Clinistix or Tes-Tape) instead. Cephalexin also causes false elevations in serum or urine creatinine levels in tests using Jaffé's reaction.

Positive Coombs' test results occur in about 3% of patients taking cephalexin.

Adverse reactions

• CNS: dizziness, headache, malaise, paresthesias, seizures.
• DERM: maculopapular and erythematous rashes, urticaria.
• GI: *pseudomembranous colitis, nausea, anorexia, vomiting,* diarrhea, *glossitis, dyspepsia, abdominal cramps,* anal pruritus, tenesmus.
• GU: genital pruritus, vaginitis, hematuria, nephrotoxicity.
• HEMA: transient neutropenia, eosinophilia, anemia, neutropenia.
• Other: hypersensitivity, (dyspnea, serum sickness [erythema, multiforme, rashes, polyarthritis, and fever]), bacterial and fungal superinfection.

Note: Drug should be discontinued if signs of toxicity or immediate hypersensitivity reaction occur or if severe diarrhea indicates pseudomembranous colitis; alternative therapy should be considered if the following symptoms occur: fever, eosinophilia, hematuria, neutropenia, or unexplained elevations in BUN or serum creatinine levels.

Overdose and treatment

Clinical signs of overdose include neuromuscular hypersensitivity; seizure may follow high CNS concentrations. Remove cephalexin by hemodialysis or peritoneal dialysis. Other treatment is supportive.

▶ Special considerations

• To prepare the oral suspension, add the required amount of water to the powder in two portions. Shake well after each addition. After mixing, store in refrigerator. Suspension is stable for 14 days without significant loss of potency. Store mixture in tightly closed container. Shake well before using.
• Administer oral cephalosporin at least 1 hour before or 2 hours after meals for maximum absorption.
• Refrigerate oral suspensions (stable for 14 days); shake well before administering to ensure correct dosage.
• Because cephalexin is dialyzable, patients undergoing treatment with hemodialysis or peritoneal dialysis may require dosage adjustment.
• Although cephalexin can eradicate group A Streptococcus from the nasopharynx, it has not been shown to be effective prophylaxis for rheumatic fever and rheumatic heart disease.
• Review patient's history of allergies; do not give cephalexin to any patient with a history of hypersensitivity reactions to cephalosporins; administer cautiously to patients with penicillin allergy.
• Try to determine whether previous reactions were true hypersensitivity reactions and not another reaction, such as GI distress, that the patient has interpreted as allergy.
• Obtain results of cultures and sensitivity tests before

first dose, but do not delay therapy; check test results periodically to assess drug efficacy.
• Monitor continuously for possible hypersensitivity or other untoward effects.
• Monitor renal function studies; dosages of certain cephalosporins must be lowered in patients with severe renal impairment. In decreased renal function, monitor BUN levels, serum creatinine levels, and urine output for significant changes.
• Monitor patients on long-term therapy for possible superinfection, especially debilitated patients and others receiving immunosuppressants or radiation therapy.

Information for parents and patient

• Teach parents signs and symptoms of hypersensitivity, bacterial and fungal superinfection, and other adverse reactions; urge them to report any unusual reactions.
• Warn parents that patient should not ingest alcohol in any form within 72 hours of cephalosporin dose. Emphasize that some liquid forms of acetaminophen contain alcohol.
• Advise adding live-culture yogurt or buttermilk to child's diet to prevent intestinal superinfection resulting from suppression of normal intestinal flora.
• Advise parents of diabetic child to monitor urine glucose level with Clinistix or Tes-Tape and not to use Clinitest.
• Patient should take drug with food if GI irritation occurs.
• Advise parents of infants of potential for yeast infections, especially in diaper area. Instruct them to keep diaper area clean and dry and to avoid use of plastic pants.
• Be sure parents understand how and when to give drug; urge them to complete entire prescribed regimen, to comply with instructions for around-the-clock dosage, and to keep follow-up appointments.
• Advise them to check expiration date of drug and to discard unused drug.

---

cephalothin sodium
Keflin, Seffin

• Classification: antibiotic (first-generation cephalosporin)

How supplied
Available by prescription only
Injection: 1 g, 2 g, 4 g
Infusion: 1 g/50 ml, 2 g/50 ml, 1 g/dl, 2 g/dl
Pharmacy bulk package: 10 g, 20 g

Indications, route, and dosage
Serious respiratory, genitourinary, GI, skin and soft-tissue, bone and joint infections; septicemia; endocarditis; meningitis
Children: 14 to 27 mg/kg I.V. q 4 hours, or 20 to 40 mg/kg q 6 hours; dosage should be proportionately less in accordance with age, weight, and severity of infection.

Adults: 500 mg to 1 g I.M. or I.V. (or intraperitoneally) q 4 to 6 hours; in life-threatening infections, up to 2 g q 4 hours.

Mild to moderate infections caused by susceptible organisms
Infants over age 3 months: 80 to 100 mg/kg I.V. or I.M. divided q 6 hours.
Cephalothin should be injected deep I.M. into a large muscle mass, such as the gluteus or lateral aspect of the thigh. I.V. route is preferable in severe or life-threatening infections.

Dosage in renal failure
Dosage schedule is determined by the degree of renal impairment, severity of infection, and susceptibility of causative organism. To prevent toxic accumulation, reduced dosage may be required in patients with creatinine clearance below 50 ml/minute.

Creatinine clearance (ml/min/1.73 m^2)	Dosage in adults
>80	Usual adult dose
50 to 80	Up to 2 g q 6 hours
25 to 50	Up to 1.5 g q 6 hours
10 to 25	Up to 1 g q 6 hours
2 to 10	Up to 500 mg q 6 hours
<2	Up to 500 mg q 8 hours

Action and kinetics
• *Antibacterial action:* Cephalothin is primarily bactericidal; however, it may be bacteriostatic. Activity depends on the organism, tissue penetration, drug dosage, and rate of organism multiplication. It acts by adhering to penicillin-binding enzymes, thereby inhibiting bacterial protein synthesis.
Like other first-generation cephalosporins, cephalothin is active mainly against gram-positive organisms and some gram-negative organisms. Susceptible organisms include *Escherichia coli* and other coliform bacteria, Enterobacteriaceae, enterococci, gonococci, group A beta-hemolytic streptococci, *Klebsiella, Proteus mirabilis, Salmonella, Staphylococcus aureus, Shigella, Streptococcus pneumoniae,* staphylococci, and *Streptococcus viridans.*
• *Kinetics in adults:* Cephalothin is not absorbed from the GI tract and must be given parenterally; peak serum levels occur 30 minutes after an I.M. dose.
Cephalothin is distributed widely into most body tissues and fluids, including the gallbladder, liver, kidneys, bone, sputum, bile, and pleural and synovial fluids; CSF penetration is poor. Cephalothin crosses the placenta; it is 65% to 79% protein-bound.
Cephalothin is metabolized partially by the liver and kidneys. It is excreted primarily in urine by renal tubular secretion and glomerular filtration. Small amounts of drug are excreted in breast milk. Elimination half-life is ½ to 1 hour in patients with normal renal function; 19 hours in patients with severe renal disease. Hemodialysis or peritoneal dialysis removes cephalothin.
• *Kinetics in children:* Serum half-life is prolonged in neonates and infants up to age 1.

Contraindications and precautions

Cephalothin is contraindicated in patients with known hypersensitivity to any cephalosporin; it should be used with caution in patients with penicillin allergy, who usually are more susceptible to such reactions.

Interactions

Probenecid competitively inhibits renal tubular secretion of cephalosporins, resulting in higher, prolonged serum levels of these drugs.

Concomitant use with nephrotoxic agents (vancomycin, colistin, polymyxin B, or aminoglycosides) or loop diuretics increases the risk of nephrotoxicity.

Concomitant use with bacteriostatic agents (tetracyclines, erythromycin, or chloramphenicol) may impair cephalothin's bactericidal activity.

Effects on diagnostic tests

Cephalothin causes false-positive results in urine glucose tests utilizing cupric sulfate (Benedict's reagent or Clinitest); use glucose oxidase tests (Clinistix or Tes-Tape) instead. Cephalothin also causes false elevations in serum or urine creatinine levels in tests using Jaffé's reaction.

Cephalothin may cause positive Coombs' test results or elevate liver function test results.

Adverse reactions

• CNS: headache, malaise, paresthesias, dizziness, seizures.

• DERM: maculopapular and erythematous rashes, urticaria.

• GI: *pseudomembranous colitis,* nausea, anorexia, vomiting, diarrhea, glossitis, dyspepsia, abdominal cramps, tenesmus, anal pruritus.

• GU: *nephrotoxicity,* genital pruritus, hematuria.

• HEMA: transient neutropenia, eosinophilia, hemolytic anemia.

• Local: at injection site – pain, induration, sterile abscesses, tissue sloughing; *phlebitis* and thrombophlebitis with I.V. injection.

• Other: hypersensitivity, dyspnea, fever, bacterial and fungal superinfection.

    Note: Drug should be discontinued if signs of toxicity or immediate hypersensitivity reaction occur or if severe diarrhea indicates pseudomembranous colitis; alternative therapy should be considered if the following symptoms occur: fever, eosinophilia, hematuria, neutropenia, or unexplained elevations in BUN or serum creatinine levels.

Overdose and treatment

Clinical signs of overdose include neuromuscular hypersensitivity; seizure may follow high CNS concentrations. Remove cephalothin by hemodialysis or peritoneal dialysis.

▶ Special considerations

• For patients on sodium restriction, consider that cephalothin contains approximately 2.8 mEq per gram of drug.

• Review patient's history of allergies; do not give cephalothin to any patient with a history of hypersensitivity reactions to cephalosporins; administer cautiously to patients with penicillin allergy.

• Try to determine whether previous reactions were true hypersensitivity reactions and not another reaction, such as GI distress, that the patient has interpreted as allergy.

• Obtain results of cultures and sensitivity tests before first dose, but do not delay therapy; check test results periodically to assess drug efficacy.

• I.M. injection is painful; avoid this route if possible. If necessary, inject I.M. dose deeply into a large muscle mass to reduce pain. Apply ice to injection site. Rotate injection sites to prevent tissue irritation.

• For I.M. administration, reconstitute each gram of cephalothin with 4 ml of sterile water for injection, providing 500 mg in each 2.2 ml. If contents do not dissolve completely, add an addition 0.2 to 0.4 ml of diluent, and warm contents slightly.

• For I.V. administration, dilute contents of a 4-g vial with at least 20 ml of sterile water for injection, dextrose 5% for injection, or 0.9% sodium chloride for injection and add to one of the following I.V. solutions: lactated Ringer's injection, dextrose 5% injection, dextrose 5% in lactated Ringer's injection, Ionosol B in dextrose 5% in water, lactated Ringer's injection, Normosol-R in dextrose 5% in water, Ringer's injection, or 0.9% sodium chloride injection. Choose solution and fluid volume according to patient's size and fluid and electrolyte status.

• Do not add or mix other drugs with I.V. infusions – particularly aminoglycosides, which will be inactivated if mixed with cephalosporins; if other drugs must be given I.V., temporarily stop infusion of primary drug.

• Adequate dilution of I.V. infusion and rotation of the site every 48 hours help minimize local vein irritation; use of small-gauge needle in larger available vein may be helpful.

• Administer reconstituted I.M. and I.V. solutions within 12 hours. Solutions for continuous infusion should start within 12 hours and be completed within 24 hours.

• Reconstituted solutions are stable for 96 hours under refrigeration. Low temperature may cause solution to precipitate. Warm to room temperature with gentle agitation before using.

• Discoloration in solution stored at room temperature does not indicate loss of potency.

• Do not freeze drug in plastic syringes.

• Solutions reconstituted in original container and frozen immediately are stable for as long as 12 weeks at $-20°$ C. Do not thaw solution until ready to use. Do not heat to thaw or refreeze once thawed.

• Because cephalothin is dialyzable, patients undergoing treatment with hemodialysis or peritoneal dialysis may require dosage adjustments.

• Monitor continuously for possible hypersensitivity or other untoward effects.

• Monitor patients on long-term therapy for possible superinfection, especially debilitated patients and others receiving immunosuppressants or radiation therapy.

• Administer cephalosporins at least 1 hour before bacteriostatic antibiotics (tetracyclines, erythromycins, and chloramphenicol); these drugs inhibit bacterial cell growth, decreasing cephalosporin uptake by bacterial cell walls.

---

‡May contain sulfites   ◆May contain tartrazine   ◆◆May contain benzyl alcohol

Information for parents and patient
• Teach parents signs and symptoms of hypersensitivity, bacterial and fungal superinfection, and other adverse reactions; urge them to report any unusual reactions.
• Warn parents that patient should not ingest alcohol in any form within 72 hours of cephalosporin dose. Emphasize that some liquid forms of acetaminophen contain alcohol.
• Advise adding live-culture yogurt or buttermilk to patient's diet to prevent intestinal superinfection resulting from suppression of normal intestinal flora.
• Advise parents of diabetic child to monitor urine glucose level with Clinistix or Tes-Tape and not to use Clinitest.
• Advise parents of infants of potential for yeast infections, especially in diaper area. Instruct them to keep diaper area clean and dry and to avoid use of plastic pants.

cephapirin sodium
Cefadyl

• Classification: antibiotic (first-generation cephalosporin)

How supplied
Available by prescription only
Injection: 500 mg, 1 g, 2 g
Infusion: 1 g, 2 g, and 4 g piggyback
Pharmacy bulk package: 20 g

Indications, route, and dosage
Serious respiratory, genitourinary, GI, skin and soft-tissue, bone and joint infections (including osteomyelitis); septicemia; endocarditis
Children over age 3 months: 10 to 20 mg/kg I.V. or I.M. q 6 hours; dosage depends on age, weight, and severity of infection. Consistency: 50 to 80 mg/kg/day divided q 6 hours.
Adults: 500 mg to 1 g I.V. or I.M. q 4 to 6 hours up to 12 g daily.

Cephapirin should be injected deep I.M. into a large muscle mass, such as the gluteus or lateral aspect of the thigh.
Dosage in renal failure
Depending on the causative organism and severity of infection, patients with reduced renal function may be treated adequately with a lower dosage (7.5 to 15 mg/kg q 12 hours). Patients with severely reduced renal function and who are to be dialyzed should receive the same dosage just before dialysis and every 12 hours thereafter. To prevent toxic accumulation, reduced dosage may be required in patients with creatinine clearance below 10 ml/minute.

Action and kinetics
• *Antibacterial action:* Cephapirin is primarily bactericidal; however, it may be bacteriostatic. Activity depends on the organism, tissue penetration, drug dosage, and rate of organism multiplication. It acts by adhering to penicillin-binding enzymes, thereby inhibiting bacterial protein synthesis.

Like other first-generation cephalosporins, cephapirin is active mainly against gram-positive organisms and some gram-negative organisms. Susceptible organisms include *Streptococcus pneumoniae, Escherichia coli,* group A beta-hemolytic streptococci, *Hemophilus influenzae, Klebsiella, Proteus mirabilis, Staphylococcus aureus,* and *Streptococcus viridans.*
• *Kinetics in adults:* Cephapirin is not absorbed from the GI tract and must be given parenterally; peak serum levels occur 30 minutes after an I.M. dose.

It is distributed widely into most body tissues and fluids, including the gallbladder, liver, kidneys, bone, sputum, bile, and pleural and synovial fluids; CSF penetration is poor. Cephapirin crosses the placenta; it is 44% to 50% protein-bound.

Cephapirin is metabolized partially. Cephapirin and metabolites are excreted primarily in urine by renal tubular secretion and glomerular filtration; small amounts of drug are excreted in breast milk. Elimination half-life is about ½ to 1 hour in patients with normal renal function; severe renal dysfunction prolongs half-life to 1 to 1½ hours. Hemodialysis removes cephapirin.
• *Kinetics in children:* Serum half-life is prolonged in neonates and infants up to age 1.

Contraindications and precautions
Cephapirin is contraindicated in patients with known hypersensitivity to any cephalosporin. It should be used with caution in patients with penicillin allergy, who usually are more susceptible to such reactions.

Interactions
Probenecid competitively inhibits renal tubular secretion of cephalosporins, resulting in higher, prolonged serum levels of these drugs.

Concomitant use with nephrotoxic agents (vancomycin, colistin, polymyxin B, or aminoglycosides) or loop diuretics increases the risk of nephrotoxicity.

Concomitant use with bacteriostatic agents (tetracyclines, erythromycin, or chloramphenicol) may impair bactericidal activity.

Effects on diagnostic tests
Cephapirin causes false-positive results in urine glucose tests utilizing cupric sulfate (Benedict's reagent or Clinitest); use glucose oxidase tests (Clinistix or Tes-Tape) instead. Cephapirin also causes false elevations in serum or urine creatinine levels in tests using Jaffé's reaction.

Cephapirin may cause positive Coombs' test results and may elevate liver function test results.

Adverse reactions
• CNS: dizziness, headache, malaise, paresthesias, seizures.
• DERM: maculopapular and erythematous rashes, urticaria.
• GI: *pseudomembranous colitis,* nausea, anorexia, vomiting, diarrhea, glossitis, dyspepsia, abdominal cramps, tenesmus, anal pruritus.
• GU: genital pruritus, vaginitis, *nephrotoxicity,* hematuria.

★Canada only   †Unlabeled clinical use   Italicized adverse reactions have been observed in children.

- HEMA: transient neutropenia, eosinophilia, anemia.
- Local: pain, induration, sterile abscesses, tissue sloughing; phlebitis and thrombophlebitis with I.V. injection.
- Other: hypersensitivity, dyspnea, bacterial and fungal superinfection.

Note: Drug should be discontinued if signs of toxicity or immediate hypersensitivity reaction occur or if severe diarrhea indicates pseudomembranous colitis; alternative therapy should be considered if the following symptoms occur: fever, eosinophilia, hematuria, neutropenia, or unexplained elevations in BUN or serum creatinine levels.

Overdose and treatment
Clinical signs of overdose include neuromuscular hypersensitivity; seizure may follow high CNS concentrations. Remove cephapirin by hemodialysis.

▶ **Special considerations**
- For patients on sodium restriction, consider that cephapirin contains approximately 2.4 mEq sodium per gram of drug.
- Safe use has not been established in infants younger than age 3 months.
- Administer cephalosporins at least 1 hour before bacteriostatic antibiotics (tetracyclines, erythromycins, and chloramphenicol); these drugs inhibit bacterial cell growth, decreasing cephalosporin uptake by bacterial cell walls.
- Review patient's history of allergies; do not give cephapirin to any patient with a history of hypersensitivity reactions to cephalosporins; administer cautiously to patients with penicillin allergy.
- Try to determine whether previous reactions were true hypersensitivity reactions and not another reaction, such as GI distress, that the patient has interpreted as allergy.
- Obtain results of cultures and sensitivity tests before first dose, but do not delay therapy; check test results periodically to assess drug efficacy.
- For I.M. administration, reconstitute 1-g or 2-g vial with 1 to 2 ml respectively of sterile or bacteriostatic water for injection, so that 1.2 ml contains 500 mg of cephapirin.
- Inform patient that I.M. injection is painful. Administer deep into large muscle mass; apply ice to reduce pain. Rotate injection sites.
- For I.V. use, reconstitute 1-g or 2-g vial with 10 ml or more of 0.9% NaCl injection, bacteriostatic water for injection or dextrose injection as diluent.
- Do not add or mix other drugs with I.V. infusions—particularly aminoglycosides, which will be inactivated if mixed with cephalosporins; if other drugs must be given I.V., temporarily stop infusion of primary drug.
- Adequate dilution of I.V. infusion and rotation of the site every 48 hours help minimize local vein irritation; use of small-gauge needle in larger available vein may be helpful.
- Administer direct I.V. infusion over 4 to 5 minutes. For intermittent infusion, use Y-tube administration set. Dilute 4-g vial with 40 ml of bacteriostatic water, dextrose, or NaCl for injection. Stop primary infusion during cephapirin infusion.

- Reconstituted cephapirin is stable for 10 days under refrigeration and for 12 to 48 hours at room temperature. Solution may become slightly yellow, which does not indicate loss of potency.
- Because cephapirin is dialyzable, patients undergoing treatment with hemo- or peritoneal dialysis may require dosage adjustments.
- Monitor continuously for possible hypersensitivity or other untoward effects.
- Monitor patients on long-term therapy for possible superinfection, especially debilitated patients and others receiving immunosuppressants or radiation therapy.

Information for parents and patient
- Teach parents signs and symptoms of hypersensitivity, bacterial and fungal superinfection, and other adverse reactions; urge them to report any unusual reactions.
- Warn parents that patient should not ingest alcohol in any form within 72 hours of cephalosporin dose. Emphasize that some liquid forms of acetaminophen contain alcohol.
- Advise adding live-culture yogurt or buttermilk to parent's diet to prevent intestinal superinfection resulting from suppression of normal intestinal flora.
- Advise parents of diabetic child to monitor urine glucose level with Clinistix or Tes-Tape and not to use Clinitest.
- Advise parents of infants of potential for yeast infections, especially in diaper area. Instruct them to keep diaper area clean and dry and to avoid use of plastic pants.

---

cephradine
Anspor, Velosef

- Classification: antibiotic (first-generation cephalosporin)

How supplied
Available by prescription only
Capsules: 250 mg, 500 mg
Suspension: 125 mg/5 ml, 250 mg/5 ml
Injection: 250 mg, 500 mg, 1 g, 2 g, 4 g
Infusion: 2 g

Indications, route, and dosage
Serious respiratory, genitourinary, GI, skin and soft-tissue, bone and joint infections; septicemia; endocarditis; and otitis media
Children over age 1: 12 to 25 mg/kg/day P.O., I.M., or I.V., divided q 6 hours. Do not exceed 4 g/day. Consider alternate: 50 to 100 mg/kg/day I.M. or I.V. divided q 6 hours.
Adults: 500 mg to 1 g I.M. or I.V. b.i.d. to q.i.d.; do not exceed 8 g daily. Or 250 to 500 mg P.O. q 6 hours. Severe or chronic infections may require larger and/or more frequent doses (up to 1 g P.O. q 6 hours).
Otitis media caused by H. influenzae
Children over age 9 months: 75 to 100 mg/kg/day divided q 6 to 12 hours.

Larger doses (up to 1 g q.i.d.) may be given for severe or chronic infections in all patients regardless of age and weight. Parenteral therapy may be followed by oral therapy. Injections should be given deep I.M. in a large muscle mass, such as the gluteus or lateral aspect of the thigh. Maximum dose should not exceed 4 g/day.

Dosage in renal failure

To prevent toxic accumulation, reduced dosage may be required in patients with creatinine clearance below 20 ml/minute.

After an initial loading dose of 750 mg, adults with impaired renal function may require a reduction in dose as follows:

Creatinine clearance (ml/min/1.73 m²)	Dosage in adults
> 20	500 mg q 6 hours
5 to 20	250 mg q 6 hours
< 5	250 mg q 12 hours

Action and kinetics

• *Antibacterial action:* Cephradine is primarily bactericidal; however, it may be bacteriostatic. Activity depends on the organism, tissue penetration, drug dosage, and rate of organism multiplication. It acts by adhering to penicillin-binding enzymes, thereby inhibiting bacterial cell synthesis.

Like other first-generation cephalosporins, cephradine is active against many gram-positive organisms and some gram-negative organisms. Susceptible organisms include *Escherichia coli* and other coliform bacteria, group A beta-hemolytic streptococci, *Hemophilus influenzae, Klebsiella, Proteus mirabilis, Staphylococcus aureus, Streptococcus pneumoniae,* staphylococci, and *Streptococcus viridans.*

• *Kinetics in adults:* Cephradine is well absorbed from the GI tract; peak serum levels occur within 1 hour after an oral dose and between 1 and 2 hours after an I.M. dose.

Cephradine is distributed widely into most body tissues and fluids, including the gallbladder, liver, kidneys, bone, sputum, bile, and pleural and synovial fluids; CSF penetration is poor. Cephradine crosses the placenta; it is 6% to 20% protein-bound.

Cephradine is not metabolized. It is excreted primarily in urine by renal tubular and glomerular filtration; small amounts are excreted in breast milk. Elimination half-life is about ½ to 2 hours in normal renal function; end-stage renal disease prolongs half-life to 8 to 15 hours. Hemodialysis or peritoneal dialysis removes cephradine.

• *Kinetics in children:* Serum half-life is prolonged in neonates and infants under age 1.

Contraindications and precautions

Cephradine is contraindicated in patients with known hypersensitivity to any cephalosporin. It should be used with caution in patients with penicillin allergy, who usually are more susceptible to such reactions.

Interactions

Probenecid competitively inhibits renal tubular secretion of cephalosporins, resulting in higher, prolonged serum levels of these drugs.

Concomitant use with nephrotoxic agents (vancomycin, colistin, polymyxin B, or aminoglycosides) or loop diuretics increases the risk of nephrotoxicity.

Concomitant use with bacteriostatic agents (tetracyclines, erythromycin, or chloramphenicol) may interfere with bactericidal activity.

Effects on diagnostic tests

Cephradine causes false-positive results in urine glucose tests utilizing cupric sulfate (Benedict's reagent or Clinitest); use glucose oxidase tests (Clinistix or Tes-Tape) instead. Cephradine also causes false elevations in serum or urine creatinine levels in tests using Jaffe's reaction.

Cephradine may cause positive Coombs' test results or elevate liver function test results.

Adverse reactions

• CNS: dizziness, headache, malaise, paresthesias, seizures.
• DERM: maculopapular and erythematous rashes, urticaria.
• GI: *pseudomembranous colitis,* nausea, anorexia, vomiting, heartburn, glossitis, dyspepsia, abdominal cramping, diarrhea, tenesmus, anal pruritus.
• GU: genital pruritus, vaginitis, nephrotoxicity, hematuria.
• HEMA: transient neutropenia, eosinophilia.
• Local: at injection site—pain, induration, sterile abscesses, tissue sloughing; phlebitis and thrombophlebitis with I.V. injection.
• Other: hypersensitivity, dyspnea, fever, bacterial and fungal superinfection.

Note: Drug should be discontinued if signs of toxicity or immediate hypersensitivity reaction occur or if severe diarrhea indicates pseudomembranous colitis; alternative therapy should be considered if the following symptoms occur: fever, eosinophilia, hematuria, neutropenia, or unexplained elevations in BUN or serum creatinine levels.

Overdose and treatment

Clinical signs of overdose include neuromuscular hypersensitivity; seizure may follow high CNS concentrations. Remove cephradine by hemodialysis.

▶ Special considerations

• For patients on sodium restriction, note that cephradine injection contains 6 mEq of sodium per gram of drug.
• Cephradine is the only cephalosporin available in both oral and injectable forms.
• Administer cephalosporins at least 1 hour before bacteriostatic antibiotics (tetracyclines, erythromycins, and chloramphenicol); these drugs inhibit bacterial cell growth, decreasing cephalosporin uptake by bacterial cell walls.
• Review patient's history of allergies; do not give a cephalosporin to any patient with a history of hypersensitivity reactions to cephalosporins; administer cautiously to patients with penicillin allergy.

• Try to determine whether previous reactions were true hypersensitivity reactions and not another reaction, such as GI distress, that the patient has interpreted as allergy.

• Obtain results of cultures and sensitivity tests before first dose, but do not delay therapy; check test results periodically to assess drug efficacy.

• Reconstituted oral suspension may be stored for 7 days at room temperature or for 14 days in refrigerator.

• Refrigerate oral suspensions (stable for 14 days); shake well before administering to ensure correct dosage.

• For I.M. administration, reconstitute with sterile water for injection or with bacteriostatic water for injection as follows: 1.2 ml to 250-mg vial; 2 ml to 500-mg vial; 4 ml to 1 g-vial. I.M. solutions stored at room temperature must be used within 2 hours; if refrigerated, within 24 hours. Solutions may vary in color from light straw to yellow without affecting potency.

• A solution containing 30 mg (anhydrous base) per milliliter is approximately isotonic.

• I.M. injection is painful. Inject deeply into a large muscle mass; apply ice to injection site to reduce pain. Rotate injection sites to prevent tissue irritation.

• Do not add or mix other drugs with I.V. infusions — particularly aminoglycosides, which wll be inactivated if mixed with cephalosporins; if other drugs must be given I.V., temporarily stop infusion of primary drug.

• Adequate dilution of I.V. infusion and rotation of the site every 48 hours help minimize local vein irritation; use of small-gauge needle in larger available vein may be helpful.

• When preparing cephradine for I.V. administration, use preparation specifically supplied for infusion, when available.

• If administration time is prolonged, infusions should be replaced every 10 hours with freshly prepared solution.

• Monitor continuously for possible hypersensitivity or other untoward effects.

• Because cephradine is dialyzable, patients undergoing treatment with hemodialysis may require dosage adjustments.

• Monitor patients on long-term therapy for possible superinfection, especially debilitated patients and others receiving immunosuppressants or radiation therapy.

Information for parents and patient

• Teach parents signs and symptoms of hypersensitivity, bacterial and fungal superinfection, and other adverse reactions; urge them to report any unusual reactions.

• Warn parents that patient should not ingest alcohol in any form within 72 hours of cephalosporin dose. Emphasize that some liquid forms of acetominophen contain alcohol.

• Advise adding live-culture yogurt or buttermilk to patient's diet to prevent intestinal superinfection resulting from suppression of normal intestinal flora.

• Advise parents of diabetic child to monitor urine glucose level with Clinistix or Tes-Tape and not to use Clinitest.

• Patient should take oral drug with food if GI irritation occurs.

• Advise parents of infants of potential for yeast infections, especially in diaper area. Instruct them to keep diaper area clean and dry and to avoid use of plastic pants.

• Be sure parents understand how and when to give drug; urge them to complete entire prescribed regimen, to comply with instructions for around-the-clock dosage, and to keep follow-up appointments.

• Advise them to check expiration date of drug and to discard unused drug.

---

chloral hydrate
Aquachloral, Noctec, Novochlorhydrate

• Classification: sedative-hypnotic (general CNS depressant)
• Controlled substance schedule IV

How supplied
Available by prescription only
Capsules: 250 mg, 500 mg
Syrup: 250 mg/5 ml, 500 mg/5 ml
Suppositories: 325 mg, 500 mg, 650 mg

Indications, route, and dosage
Sedation
Children: 8 mg/kg P.O. t.i.d. Maximum dosage is 500 mg t.i.d.
Adults: 250 mg P.O. or rectally t.i.d. after meals.
Insomnia
Children: 50 mg/kg single dose. Maximum dosage is 1 g.
Adults: 500 mg to 1 g P.O. or rectally 15 to 30 minutes before bedtime.
Premedication
Children: 50 to 75 mg/kg P.O. or rectally. Selected patients may receive 100 mg/kg.

Action and kinetics
• *Sedative-hypnotic action:* Chloral hydrate has CNS depressant activities similar to those of the barbiturates. Nonspecific CNS depression occurs at hypnotic doses; however, respiratory drive is only slightly affected. The drug's primary site of action is the reticular activating system, which controls arousal. The cellular site(s) of action are not known.

• *Kinetics in adults:* Chloral hydrate is absorbed well after oral and rectal administration. Sleep occurs 30 to 60 minutes after a 500-mg to 1-g dose.

Chloral hydrate and its active metabolite trichloroethanol are distributed throughout the body tissue and fluids. Trichloroethanol is 35% to 41% protein-bound.

Chloral hydrate is metabolized rapidly and nearly completely in the liver and erythrocytes to the active metabolite trichloroethanol. It is further metabolized in the liver and kidneys to trichloroacetic acid and other inactive metabolites.

The inactive metabolites of chloral hydrate are excreted primarily in urine. Minor amounts are excreted

---

in bile. The half-life of trichloroethanol is 8 to 10 hours.

Contraindications and precautions

Chloral hydrate is contraindicated in patients with known hypersensitivity to chloral derivatives; in patients with severe cardiac disease; and in patients with marked renal or hepatic failure because elimination of the drug will decrease.

Chloral hydrate should be used cautiously in patients with signs and symptoms of depression, suicidal ideation, or history of drug abuse or addiction, because the drug depresses CNS function; and in patients who need to perform hazardous tasks requiring mental alertness or physical coordination. Do not administer oral forms of chloral hydrate to patients with esophagitis, gastritis, or gastric or duodenal ulcers, because the drug is irritating to the GI tract. Rectal chloral hydrate may exacerbate proctitis or ulcerative colitis.

Interactions

Concomitant use with alcohol, sedative-hypnotics, narcotics, antihistamines, tranquilizers, tricyclic antidepressants, or other CNS depressants will add to or potentiate their effects. Concomitant use with alcohol may cause vasodilation, tachycardia, sweating, and flushing in some patients.

Administration of chloral hydrate followed by I.V. furosemide may cause a hypermetabolic state by displacing thyroid hormone from binding sites, resulting in sweating, hot flashes, tachycardia, and variable blood pressure.

Chloral hydrate may displace oral anticoagulants such as warfarin from protein-binding sites, causing increased hypoprothrombinemic effects.

Effects on diagnostic tests

Chloral hydrate therapy may produce false-positive results for urine glucose with tests using cupric sulfate, such as Benedict's reagent and possibly Clinitest. It does not interfere with Clinistix or Tes-Tape results. It will interfere with fluorometric tests for urine catecholamines; do not use drug for 48 hours before the test. Drug may also interfere with Reddy-Jenkins-Thorn test for urinary 17-hydroxycorticosteroids. It also may cause a false-positive phentolamine test.

Adverse reactions

• CNS: hangover, headache, ataxia, confusion, hallucinations, disorientation, excitement, nightmares, paranoia.
• DERM: rash, urticaria, erythema, eczematoid dermatitis, scarlatiniform exanthema.
• GI: gastric irritation, nausea, vomiting, diarrhea, flatulence, altered taste.
• GU: ketonuria.
• HEMA: leukopenia, eosinophilia.
  Note: Drug should be discontinued if hypersensitivity occurs, if patient becomes incoherent or disoriented, or if patient exhibits paranoid behavior.

Overdose and treatment

Clinical manifestations of overdose include stupor, coma, respiratory depression, pinpoint pupils, hypotension, and hypothermia. Esophageal stricture may follow gastric necrosis and perforation. GI hemorrhage has also been reported. Hepatic damage and jaundice may occur.

Treatment is supportive of respiration (including mechanical ventilation if needed), blood pressure, and body temperature. If the patient is conscious, empty stomach by emesis or gastric lavage. Hemodialysis will remove chloral hydrate and its metabolite, trichloroethanol. Peritoneal dialysis is ineffective.

▶ Special considerations

• Chloral hydrate is safe and effective as a premedication for EEG and other procedures.
• Not a first-line drug because of potential for adverse or toxic side effects.
• Withdrawal phenomenon can follow use for sedation.
• Assess level of consciousness before administering drug to ensure appropriate baseline level.
• Give chloral hydrate capsules with a full glass of water to lessen GI upset; dilute syrup in a half glass of water or juice before administration to improve taste.
• Monitor vital signs frequently.
• Store drug in dark container away from heat and moisture to prevent deterioration. Store suppositories in refrigerator.

Information for parents and patient

• Advise parents that patient should take with a full glass of water and should dilute syrup with juice or water before taking.
• Instruct parents and patient in proper administration of drug form prescribed.
• Warn parents that patient should not attempt tasks that require mental alertness or physical coordination until the CNS effects of the drug are known.
• Tell parents that patient should avoid alcohol and other CNS depressants.
• Instruct parents to call for medical approval before using any nonprescription allergy or cold preparations.
• Warn parents and patient not to increase the dose or discontinue the drug except as prescribed.

chlorambucil
Leukeran

• Classification: antineoplastic (alkylating agent [cell cycle-phase nonspecific])

How supplied

Available by prescription only
Tablets: 2 mg

Indications, route, and dosage

Dosage and indications may vary. Check current literature for recommended protocol.

†*Minimal-change nephrotic syndrome*

Children: 100 to 200 mg/kg daily. Usually given for 8 to 12 weeks with prednisone. Additional courses of therapy may be necessary.

---

†*Chronic lymphocytic leukemia, diffuse lymphocytic lymphoma, Hodgkin's disease, autoimmune hemolytic anemias, lupus glomerulonephritis, macroglobulinemia*
Children: 100 to 200 mg/kg or 4.5 mg/m² as a single daily dose.
Adults: 0.1 to 0.2 mg/kg P.O. daily or 3 to 6 mg/m² P.O. daily as a single dose or in divided doses; for 3 to 6 weeks. Usual dose is 4 to 10 mg daily. Reduce dose if within 4 weeks of a full course of radiation therapy.

Chronic lymphocytic leukemia (alternative schedule)
Adults: Initially 400 mcg once every 2 weeks. Increase dosage by 100 mcg until response or toxicity occurs. Usually given with prednisone.

Action and kinetics
• *Antineoplastic action:* Chlorambucil exerts its cytotoxic activity by cross-linking strands of cellular DNA and RNA, disrupting normal nucleic acid function.
• *Kinetics in adults:* Chlorambucil is well absorbed from the GI tract. The distribution of chlorambucil is not well understood. However, the drug and its metabolites have been shown to be highly bound to plasma and tissue proteins. Chlorambucil is metabolized in the liver. The primary metabolite, phenylacetic acid mustard, also possesses cytotoxic activity. The metabolites of chlorambucil are excreted in urine. The half-life of the parent compound is 2 hours and that of the phenylacetic acid metabolite 2½ hours. Chlorambucil is probably not dialyzable.

Contraindications and precautions
Chlorambucil is contraindicated in patients with a history of hypersensitivity to the drug or of resistance to previous therapy with the drug. Cross-sensitivity, which manifests as a rash, may occur between chlorambucil and other alkylating agents.

Dosage adjustments must be considered in patients with hematologic impairment because of the drug's hematologic toxicity.

Patients should not receive a full dose of chlorambucil if a full course of radiation therapy or other myelosuppressive drugs were administered within the preceding 4 weeks because of the potential for additive toxicity. When used to treat non-malignant disease, the risk of inducing a malignancy with chlorambucil must be considered.

Interactions
Chlorambucil toxicity is potentiated by barbiturates, possibly by inducing hepatic activation of chlorambucil. Dosage of chlorambucil should be reduced or the barbiturate discontinued during chlorambucil therapy.

Effects on diagnostic tests
Chlorambucil therapy may increase concentrations of serum alkaline phosphatase, AST (SGOT), and blood and urine uric acid.

Adverse reactions
• CNS: seizures (with high doses), *hallucinations.*
• DERM: rash, pruritus, peripheral neuropathy (rare).
• GI: nausea, vomiting, anorexia, abdominal pain, diarrhea.
• GU: sterile cystitis.
• HEMA: pancytopenia (dose-limiting), *bone marrow depression, leukemia.*
• Metabolic: hyperuricemia.
• Other: *pulmonary infiltrates and fibrosis;* drug fever; alopecia (rare); hepatotoxicity; increased risk of secondary malignancy with prolonged, high-dose therapy; possible sterility.

Overdose and treatment
Clinical manifestations of overdose include vomiting, ataxia, abdominal pain, muscle twitching, and major motor seizures in children and reversible pancytopenia in adults. Treatment is usually supportive with transfusion of blood components if necessary and appropriate anticonvulsant therapy if seizures occur. Induction of emesis, activated charcoal, and gastric lavage may be useful in removing unabsorbed drug.

▶ Special considerations
• Oral suspension can be prepared in the pharmacy by crushing tablets and mixing powder with a suspending agent and simple syrup.
• Avoid all I.M. injections when platelets are below 100,000/mm³.
• Anticoagulants and aspirin products should be used cautiously. Watch closely for signs of bleeding.
• Severe pancytopenia may last for 10 days. It is reversible up to a cumulative dose of 6.5 mg/kg in a single course.
• To prevent hyperuricemia with resulting uric acid nephropathy, allopurinol may be used with adequate hydration. Monitor uric acid. I.V. sodium bicarbonate solution may be needed to alkalinize urine.
• Store tablets in a tightly closed, light-resistant container.
• Attempt to alleviate or reduce anxiety in parents and patient family before treatment.
• Monitor BUN, hematocrit, platelet count, ALT (SGPT), AST (SGOT), LDH, serum bilirubin, serum creatinine, uric acid total and differential leukocyte.

Information for parents and patient
• Emphasize to the parents and patient importance of continuing medication despite nausea and vomiting, and of keeping appointments for periodic blood work. Administering drug before breakfast or at bedtime, and encouraging small, frequent meals may minimize nausea.
• Advise parents to call if vomiting occurs shortly after the child takes the dose or if symptoms of infection or bleeding are present.
• Advise parents to avoid giving the patient nonprescription products containing aspirin.
• Advise parents to avoid patient's exposure to persons with bacterial or viral infections because chemotherapy can increase susceptibility to infection. Parents should promptly report any signs of infection and any exposure to chicken pox if the patient has no immunity to it.

• Advise parents that patient's dental work should be completed before therapy whenever possible, or should be deferred until blood counts are normal.
• Warn parents that patient may bruise easily because of the drug's effect on blood count. Patient should avoid contact sports when platelets are low.
• Advise parents that immunizations should be avoided if possible.

chloramphenicol
Antibiopto, Chloromycetin, Chloroptic, Econochlor, Fenicol*, Isopto-Fenicol, Novochlorocap*, Ophthochlor, Pentamycetin*

chloramphenicol palmitate
Chloromycetin Palmitate

chloroamphenicol sodium succinate
Chloromycetin Sodium Succinate, Mychel S, Pentamycetin*

• Classification: antibiotic (dichloroacetic acid derivative)

How supplied
Available by prescription only
Capsules: 250 mg, 500 mg
Suspension: 150 mg/5 ml
Injection: 1-g, 10-g vial
Ophthalmic solution: 0.5%
Ophthalmic ointment: 1%
Topical cream: 1%
Otic solution: 0.5%

Indications, route, and dosage
Meningitis, bacteremia, or other severe infections when other antibiotics are contraindicated or ineffective
Premature and full-term infants up to age 2 weeks: 6.25 mg/kg (base) I.V. or P.O., q 6 hours.
Infants age 2 weeks and over: 12.5 mg/kg (base) I.V. or P.O. q 6 hours or 25 mg/kg I.V. or P.O. q 12 hours.
    In severe infections, up to 75 mg/kg/day P.O. or 100 mg/kg/day I.V. may be given.
Adults: 12.5 mg/kg (base) I.V. or P.O. q 6 hours. Do not exceed 4 g (base) daily.
External ear canal infection
Adults and children: 2 to 3 drops into ear canal t.i.d or q.i.d.
Surface bacterial infection involving conjunctiva or cornea
Adults and children: Instill 2 drops of solution in eye every hour until condition improves, or instill q.i.d., depending on severity of infection. Apply small amount of ointment to lower conjunctival sac at bedtime as supplement to drops. To use ointment alone, apply small amount to lower conjunctival sac q 3 to 6 hours or more frequently if necessary. Continue until condition improves.

Action and kinetics
• *Antibacterial action:* Chloramphenicol palmitate and chloramphenicol sodium succinate must be hydrolyzed to chloramphenicol before antimicrobial activity can take place. The active compound then inhibits bacterial protein synthesis by binding to the ribosome's 50S subunit, thus inhibiting peptide bond formation.
    Chloramphenicol usually produces bacteriostatic effects on susceptible bacteria, including *Rickettsia, Chlamydia,* and *Mycoplasma* and certain *Salmonella* strains, as well as most gram-positive and gram-negative organisms. It is used to treat *Hemophilus influenzae,* Rocky Mountain spotted fever, meningitis, lymphogranuloma, psittacosis, severe meningitis, and bacteremia.
• *Kinetics in adults:* After oral administration, chloramphenicol is well absorbed from the GI tract. Palmitate and sodium succinate salts are hydrolyzed quickly to chloramphenicol. Peak serum concentrations occur in 1 to 3 hours. In patients receiving chloramphenicol palmitate, mean serum concentrations resemble those achieved by the base. Recommended therapeutic range is 10 to 20 mcg/ml for peak levels and 5 to 10 mcg/ml for trough levels.
    With I.V. administration, serum concentrations vary greatly, depending on patient's metabolism. Chloramphenicol is distributed widely to most body tissues and fluids, including CSF, liver, and kidneys; it readily crosses the placenta. Approximately 50% to 60% of the drug binds to plasma proteins.
    Parent drug is metabolized primarily by hepatic glucuronyl transferase to inactive metabolites.
    About 8% to 12% of dose is excreted by the kidneys as unchanged drug; the remainder is excreted as inactive metabolites. (However, some drug may be excreted in breast milk.) Plasma half-life ranges from about 1½ to 4½ hours in adults with normal hepatic and renal function. Plasma half-life of parent drug is prolonged in patients with hepatic dysfunction. Peritoneal hemodialysis does not remove significant drug amounts. Plasma chloramphenicol levels may be elevated in patients with renal impairment after I.V. chloramphenicol administration.
• *Kinetics in children:* Because hepatic enzymes necessary for the conjugation of chloramphenicol are lacking in the fetus and neonate, they risk toxic accumulation of the active drug. The half-life of chloramphenicol in neonates up to 2 days old may be 24 hours or more, and it may be variable (especially in low birth weight infants). The half-life decreases to about 10 hours in infants 10 to 16 days old. Frequent serum determinations should be made in neonates and infants.

Contraindications and precautions
Chloramphenicol is contraindicated in patients with minor infections (such as influenza, throat infections, and colds) or as prophylaxis against infection, because potential toxicity may outweigh therapeutic benefit; it is also contraindicated in patients with known hypersensitivity or history of toxic reaction to the drug.
    Chloramphenicol should be administered cautiously to infants and to patients with renal or hepatic dysfunction, acute intermittent porphyria, or glucose-6-phosphate dehydrogenase (G6PD) deficiency because

---

*Canada only   †Unlabeled clinical use   Italicized adverse reactions have been observed in children

of potential for adverse effects (including gray-baby syndrome). Drug should be used cautiously with other drugs that can cause bone marrow suppression.

Interactions

When used concomitantly, chloramphenicol inhibits hepatic metabolism of phenytoin, dicumarol, tolbutamide, chlorpropamide, phenobarbital, and cyclophosphamide (by inhibiting microsomal enzyme activity); that leads to prolonged plasma half-life of these drugs and possible toxicity from increased serum drug concentrations. When used concomitantly, chloramphenicol may antagonize penicillin's bactericidal activity.

Concomitant use with acetaminophen causes an elevated serum chloramphenicol level (by an unknown mechanism), possibly resulting in an enhanced pharmacologic effect. Concomitant use with iron salts, folic acid, and vitamin B_{12} reduces the hematologic response to these substances.

Effects on diagnostic tests

False elevation of urinary para-aminobenzoic acid (PABA) levels will result if chloramphenicol is administered during a bentiromide test for pancreatic function. Treatment with chloramphenicol will cause false-positive results on tests for urine glucose level using cupric sulfate (Clinitest). Erythrocyte, platelet, and leukocyte counts in the blood and possibly the bone marrow may decrease during chloramphenicol therapy (from reversible or irreversible bone marrow depression). Hemoglobinuria or lactic acidosis may also occur.

Adverse reactions

• CNS: headache, mild depression, confusion, delirium, peripheral neuropathy (with prolonged therapy).
• DERM: possible contact sensitivity; itching, burning, urticaria, angioneurotic edema in patients hypersensitive to any drug components (topical application).
• EENT: itching or burning ears (with otic application); optic neuritis in patients with cystic fibrosis; glossitis; decreased visual acuity; optic atrophy in children; stinging, burning, or itching eyes (ophthalmic); urticaria; vesicular or maculopapular dermatitis (otic).
• GI: nausea, vomiting, stomatitis, diarrhea, enterocolitis, jaundice.
• HEMA: granulocytopenia, *aplastic anemia* (not related to dose or route of administration, irreversible, and idiopathic), hypoplastic anemia, granulocytopenia, thrombocytopenia (dose-related, reversible).
• Other: infection by nonsusceptible organisms (with topical or systemic administration); hypersensitivity reaction (fever, rash, urticaria, anaphylaxis); sore throat; angioedema; gray syndrome in premature and newborn infants (abdominal distention, gray cyanosis, vasomotor collapse, respiratory distress, and possible death within a few hours of symptom onset).
Note: Drug should be discontinued if patient develops hypersensitivity reaction, optic or peripheral neuritis, or blood dyscrasias.

Overdose and treatment

Clinical effects of parenterally administered overdose include anemia and metabolic acidosis followed by hypotension, hypothermia, abdominal distention, and possible death. Clinical effects of acute oral overdose include nausea, vomiting, and diarrhea.

Initial treatment is symptomatic and supportive. Chloramphenicol may be removed by charcoal hemoperfusion.

▶ Special considerations

• Use drug cautiously in children under age 2 because of risk of gray syndrome (although most cases occur in first 48 hours after birth). Drug has prolonged half-life in neonates, necessitating special dose.
• Children may be at increased risk for bone marrow suppression, which may be irreversible. Monitor closely for signs of adverse bone marrow effects (fever, fatigue, petechiae). Because bone marrow reaction may be delayed, continue to monitor CBC after therapy ends.
• Culture and sensitivity tests may be done concurrently with first dose and then as needed.
• Use drug only when clearly indicated for severe infection. Because of potential for severe toxicity, it should be reserved for potentially life-threatening infections.
• If administering drug concomitantly with penicillin, give penicillin 1 hour or more before chloramphenicol to avoid reduction in penicillin's bactericidal activity.
• For I.V. administration, reconstitute 1-g vial of powder for injection with 10 ml of sterile water for injection; concentration will be 100 mg/ml. Solution remains stable for 30 days at room temperature; however, refrigeration is recommended. Do not use cloudy solutions. Administer I.V. infusion slowly, over at least 1 minute. Check injection site daily for phlebitis and irritation.
• Monitor complete blood count, platelet count, reticulocyte count, and serum iron level before therapy begins and every 2 days during therapy. Discontinue immediately if test results indicate anemia, leukopenia, or thrombocytopenia.
• Observe patient for signs and symptoms of superinfection by nonsusceptible organisms.

Information for parents and patient

• Patient should take oral drug forms on an empty stomach 1 hour before or 2 hours after meals. (Advise patient who develops adverse GI effects to take drug with food.)
• Instruct parents to report adverse reactions, especially nausea, vomiting, diarrhea, bleeding, fever, confusion, sore throat, or mouth sores.
• Tell parents that patient should take medication for prescribed period and to take it exactly as directed, even after he feels better.
• Instruct parents and patient to wash hands before and after applying topical ointment or solution.
• For use of otic solution, warn against touching ear with dropper; during use of topical cream, warn against sharing washcloths and towels with family members.
• For use of ophthalmic form, teach correct method of applying drug after cleansing eye area of excess ex-

udate. Warn patient not to touch applicator tip to eye or surrounding tissue. Instruct parents to observe for signs and symptoms of sensitivity, such as itchy eyelids or constant burning, and if they occur, to report them immediately and to discontinue use of the drug.
• To prevent yeast infections, advise parents of infants and toddlers to keep the child's diaper area clean and dry and to avoid tight-fitting or plastic pants.
• Chloramphenicol solutions lose potency at temperatures above body temperature. Advise storage away from excessive heat.

---

chlordiazepoxide
Libritabs

chlordiazepoxide hydrochloride
Apo-Chlordiazepoxide*, Librium, Lipoxide, SK-Lygen, Medilium*, Murcil, Novopoxide*, Reposans-10, Sereen, Solium*

• Classification: antianxiety agent; anticonvulsant; sedative-hypnotic (benzodiazepine)
• Controlled substance schedule IV

How supplied
Available by prescription only
Tablets: 5 mg, 10 mg, 25 mg
Capsules: 5 mg, 10 mg, 25 mg
Powder for injection: 100 mg/ampule

Indications, route, and dosage
Mild to moderate anxiety and tension
Children over age 6: 5 mg P.O. b.i.d. to q.i.d.; or 0.5 mg/kg/day, divided b.i.d. to q.i.d.
Maximum dosage is 10 mg P.O. b.i.d. to t.i.d.
Adults: 5 to 10 mg t.i.d. or q.i.d.
Note: Parenteral form is not recommended in children under age 12.

Action and kinetics
• *Anxiolytic action:* Chlordiazepoxide depresses the CNS at the limbic and subcortical levels of the brain. It produces an antianxiety effect by influencing the effect of the neurotransmitter gamma-aminobutyric acid (GABA) on its receptor in the ascending reticular activating system, which increases inhibition and blocks both cortical and limbic arousal after stimulation of the reticular formation.
• *Anticonvulsant action:* Chlordiazepoxide suppresses the spread of seizure activity produced by the epileptogenic foci in the cortex, thalamus, and limbic structures by enhancing presynaptic inhibition.
• *Kinetics in adults:* When given orally, chlordiazepoxide is absorbed well through the GI tract. Action begins in 30 to 45 minutes, with peak action in 1 to 3 hours. I.M. administration results in erratic absorption of the drug; onset of action usually occurs in 15 to 30 minutes. After I.V. administration, rapid onset of action occurs in 1 to 5 minutes.
Chlordiazepoxide is distributed widely throughout the body. Drug is 80% to 90% protein-bound.

Chlordiazepoxide is metabolized in the liver to several active metabolites; most metabolites are excreted in urine as glucuronide conjugates. The half-life of chlordiazepoxide is 5 to 30 hours.

Contraindications and precautions
Chlordiazepoxide is contraindicated in patients with known hypersensitivity to the drug; in patients with acute narrow-angle glaucoma or untreated open-angle glaucoma, because of the drug's possible anticholinergic effect; in patients in shock or coma, because the drug's hypnotic or hypotensive effect may be prolonged or intensified; in patients with acute alcohol intoxication who have depressed vital signs, because the drug will worsen CNS depression; and in infants younger than age 30 days, in whom slow metabolism causes the drug to accumulate.

Chlordiazepoxide should be used cautiously in patients with psychoses, because it is rarely beneficial in such patients and may induce paradoxical reactions; in patients with myasthenia gravis or Parkinson's disease, because drug may exacerbate the disorder; in patients with impaired renal or hepatic function, which prolongs elimination of the drug; in elderly or debilitated patients, who are usually more sensitive to the drug's CNS effects; and in individuals prone to addiction or drug abuse.

Interactions
Chlordiazepoxide potentiates the CNS depressant effects of phenothiazines, narcotics, barbiturates, alcohol, antihistamines, monoamine oxidase inhibitors, general anesthetics, and antidepressants. Concomitant use with cimetidine and possibly disulfiram diminishes hepatic metabolism of chlordiazepoxide, which increases its plasma concentration. Heavy smoking accelerates chlordiazepoxide's metabolism, thus lowering clinical effectiveness. Oral contraceptives may impair the metabolism of chlordiazepoxide. Antacids may delay the absorption of chlordiazepoxide. Concomitant use with levodopa may decrease the therapeutic effects of levodopa. Benzodiazepines may decrease serum levels of haloperidol.

Effects on diagnostic tests
Chlordiazepoxide therapy may elevate results of liver function tests. Minor changes in EEG patterns, usually low-voltage, fast activity, may occur during and after chlordiazepoxide therapy. Chlordiazepoxide may cause a false-positive pregnancy test, depending on method used. It may also alter urinary 17-ketosteroids (Zimmerman reaction), urine alkaloid determination (Frings thin layer chromatography method), and urinary glucose determinations (with Clinistix and Diastix, but not Tes-Tape).

Adverse reactions
• CNS: confusion, depression, drowsiness, lethargy, hangover effect, ataxia, dizziness, syncope, nightmares, fatigue, slurred speech, tremors, vertigo, paradoxical reactions (such as hyperaggressiveness, rage).
• CV: cardiovascular collapse, transient hypotension, palpitations, bradycardia.
• DERM: rash, urticaria, hair loss.

• EENT: diplopia, blurred vision, nystagmus.
• GI: constipation, dry mouth, nausea, vomiting, difficulty swallowing, anorexia, abdominal discomfort.
• GU: urinary incontinence or retention.
• Local: pain, phlebitis, and desquamation at injection site.
• Other: respiratory depression, dysarthria, headache, hepatic dysfunction, changes in libido, active intermittent porphyria.

Note: Drug should be discontinued if hypersensitivity or the following paradoxical reactions occur: acute hyperexcited state, anxiety, hallucinations, increased muscle spasticity, insomnia, or rage.

Overdose and treatment

Clinical manifestations of overdose include somnolence, confusion, coma, hypoactive reflexes, dyspnea, labored breathing, hypotension, bradycardia, slurred speech, and unsteady gait or impaired coordination.

Support blood pressure and respiration until drug effects subside; monitor vital signs. Mechanical ventilatory assistance via endotracheal tube may be required to maintain a patent airway and support adequate oxygenation. Use I.V. fluids and vasopressors like dopamine and phenylephrine to treat hypotension as needed. Use gastric lavage if ingestion was recent, but only if an endotracheal tube is in place to prevent aspiration. Induce emesis if the patient is conscious. After emesis or lavage, administer activated charcoal with a cathartic as a single dose. Do not administer barbiturates if excitation occurs. Dialysis is of limited value.

▶ Special considerations

• Safety of oral use has not been established in children under age 6. Safety of parenteral use has not been established in children under age 12.
• Because children, particularly very young ones, are sensitive to the CNS depressant effects of benzodiazepines, caution must be exercised. A neonate whose mother took a benzodiazepine during pregnancy may exhibit withdrawal symptoms.
• Administer with milk or immediately after meals to prevent GI upset. Give antacid, if needed, at least 1 hour before or after dose to prevent interaction and ensure maximum drug absorption and effectiveness.
• Crush tablet or empty capsule and mix with food if patient has difficulty swallowing.
• Assess level of consciousness and neurologic status before and frequently during therapy for changes. Monitor for paradoxical reactions, especially early in therapy.
• Assess sleep patterns and quality. Institute seizure precautions. Assess for changes in seizure character, frequency, or duration.
• Assess vital signs frequently during therapy. Significant changes in blood pressure and heart rate may indicate impending toxicity.
• Comfort measures — such as back rubs and relaxation techniques — may enhance drug effectiveness.
• As needed, institute safety measures — raised side rails and ambulatory assistance — to prevent injury. Anticipate possible rebound excitement reactions.
• Patient should be observed to prevent drug hoarding or self-dosing, especially in depressed or suicidal patients or those who are, or who have a history of being, drug-dependent. Patient's mouth should be checked to be sure tablet or capsule was swallowed.
• After prolonged use, abrupt discontinuation may cause withdrawal symptoms; discontinue gradually.
• I.M. administration is not recommended because of erratic and slow absorption. However, if I.M. route is used, reconstitute with special diluent only. Do not use diluent if hazy. Inject I.M. deep into large muscle mass.
• For I.V. administration, drug should be reconstituted with sterile water or normal saline solution and infused slowly, directly into a large vein, at a rate not exceeding 50 mg/minute for adults. Do not infuse chlordiazepoxide into small veins. Avoid extravasation into subcutaneous tissue. Observe the infusion site for phlebitis. Keep resuscitation equipment nearby in case of an emergency.
• Prepare solutions for I.V. or I.M. use immediately before administration. Discard any unused portions.
• Patients should remain in bed under observation for at least 3 hours after parenteral administration of chlordiazepoxide.
• Lower doses are effective in patients with renal or hepatic dysfunction. Closely monitor renal and hepatic studies for signs of dysfunction.

Information for parents and patient

• Warn parents and patient that sudden changes in position may cause dizziness. Advise parents to have child dangle legs a few minutes before getting out of bed to prevent falls and injury.
• Warn parents that patient should avoid use of alcohol or other CNS depressants, such an antihistamines, analgesics, monoamine oxidase inhibitors, antidepressants, and barbiturates, while taking benzodiazepines to prevent additive depressant effects.
• Caution parents that patient should take the drug exactly as prescribed and should not give medication to others. Tell parents not to increase the dose or frequency and to call before giving patient any nonprescription cold or allergy preparations that may potentiate CNS depressant effects.
• Warn parents that patient should avoid activities requiring alertness and good psychomotor coordination until the CNS response to the drug is determined. Instruct patient in safety measures to prevent injury.
• Patient should avoid using antacids, which may delay drug absorption, unless prescribed.
• Be sure parents and patient understand that benzodiazepines can cause physical and psychological dependence with prolonged use.
• Warn parents that patient should not stop taking the drug abruptly to prevent withdrawal symptoms after prolonged use.
• Tell parents and patient that smoking decreases the drug's effectiveness. Encourage patient to stop smoking during therapy.
• Tell parents to report any adverse effects. These are often dose-related and can be relieved by dosage adjustments.
• Explain to adolescent patient and her parents the importance of reporting suspected pregnancy immediately.

---

‡May contain sulfites   ◆May contain tartrazine   ◆ ◆May contain benzyl alcohol

chloroquine hydrochloride
Aralen Hydrochloride

chloroquine phosphate
Aralen Phosphate

• Classification: antimalarial, amebicide, anti-inflammatory (4-aminoquinoline)

How supplied
Available by prescription only
Chloroquine hydrochloride
Injection: 50 mg/ml (40 mg/ml base)
Chloroquine phosphate
Tablets: 250 mg (150-mg base), 500 mg (300-mg base)

Indications, route, and dosage
Suppressive prophylaxis and treatment of acute attacks of malaria
Children: Initially, 10 mg (base)/kg P.O., then 5 mg (base)/kg P.O. at 6, 24, and 48 hours (do not exceed adult dosage). Or 5 mg (base)/kg I.M. initially; repeat in 6 hours if needed. Switch to oral therapy as soon as possible.
Adults: Initially, 600 mg (base) P.O., then 300 mg P.O. at 6, 24, and 48 hours. Or 160 to 200 mg (base) I.M. initially; repeat in 6 hours if needed. Switch to oral therapy as soon as possible. Continue oral therapy for 3 days until approximately 1.5 g of base has been administered.
Suppressive treatment of malaria
Children and adults: 5 mg (base)/kg P.O. (not to exceed 300 mg) weekly on same day of the week (begin 2 weeks before entering endemic area and continue for 8 weeks after leaving). If treatment begins after exposure, double the initial dose (600 mg for adults, 10 mg/kg for children) in two divided doses P.O. 6 hours apart.
Extraintestinal amebiasis
Children: 10 mg/kg of chloroquine (hydrochloride) base for 2 to 3 weeks. Maximum dose, 300 mg daily.
Adults: 600 mg of chloroquine (1 g of chloroquine phosphate) once daily for 2 days, then 300 mg chloroquine (500 mg chloroquine phosphate) once daily for 2 to 3 weeks.
†Rheumatoid arthritis
Adults: 250 mg of chloroquine phosphate daily with evening meal.

Action and kinetics
• *Antimalarial action:* Chloroquine binds to DNA, interfering with protein synthesis. It also inhibits both DNA and RNA polymerases.
• *Amebicidal action:* Mechanism of action is unknown.
• *Anti-inflammatory action:* Mechanism of action is unknown. Chloroquine may antagonize histamine and serotonin and inhibit prostaglandin effects by inhibiting conversion of arachidonic acid to prostaglandin F_2; it also may inhibit chemotaxis of polymorphonuclear leukocytes, macrophages, and eosinophils.
Chloroquine's spectrum of activity includes the a-sexual erythrocytic forms of *Plasmodium malariae,*

P. ovale, P. vivax, many strains of *P. falciparum,* and *Entamoeba histolytica.*
• *Kinetics in adults:* Chloroquine is absorbed readily and almost completely, with peak plasma concentrations occurring at 1 to 2 hours. Chloroquine is 55% bound to plasma proteins. It concentrates in the liver, spleen, kidneys, heart, and brain and is strongly bound in melanin-containing cells. About 30% of an administered dose of chloroquine is metabolized by the liver to monodesethylchloroquine and bidesethylchloroquine. About 70% of an administered dose is excreted unchanged in urine; unabsorbed drug is excreted in feces. Small amounts of the drug may be present in urine for months after the drug is discontinued. It is excreted in breast milk.

Contraindications and precautions
Chloroquine is contraindicated in patients who have experienced retinal or visual field changes or hypersensitivity reactions to 4-aminoquinoline compounds unless these compounds are the only agents to which the malarial strain is sensitive.
Chloroquine should be used cautiously in patients with psoriasis, porphyria, or glucose-6-phosphate dehydrogenase deficiency, because the drug may exacerbate these conditions. Because chloroquine concentrates in the liver and may cause adverse hepatic effects, it should be used cautiously in patients with hepatic disease or alcoholism and in patients receiving other hepatotoxic drugs.

Interactions
Concomitant administration of kaolin or magnesium trisilicate may decrease absorption of chloroquine.

Effects on diagnostic tests
Chloroquine may cause inversion or depression of the T wave or widening of the QRS complex on ECG. Rarely, it may cause decreased WBC, RBC, or platelet counts.

Adverse reactions
• CNS: mild and transient headache, neuromyopathy, psychic stimulation, fatigue, irritability, nightmares, seizures, dizziness, toxic psychosis, apathy, confusion, depression.
• CV: hypotension, ECG changes, cardiomyopathy.
• DERM: pruritus, lichen planus-like eruptions, skin and mucosal pigmentary changes, pleomorphic skin eruptions.
• EENT: visual disturbances (blurred vision; difficulty in focusing; reversible corneal changes; generally irreversible, sometimes progressive or delayed, retinal changes, such as narrowing of arterioles; macular lesions; pallor of optic disk; optic atrophy; patchy retinal pigmentation, often leading to blindness); ototoxicity (nerve deafness, vertigo, tinnitus).
• GI: anorexia, abdominal cramps, diarrhea, nausea, vomiting, stomatitis.
• HEMA: agranulocytosis, hemolytic anemia, aplastic anemia, thrombocytopenia.
• Other: bleaching of hair.
Note: Drug should be discontinued at the first sign of visual changes not explainable by difficulties of accommodation or corneal opacities or of hematologic

---

*Canada only   †Unlabeled clinical use   Italicized adverse reactions have been observed in children.

abnormalities not attributable to the disease being treated, or if muscular weakness occurs during therapy.

Overdose and treatment

Symptoms of chloroquine overdose may appear within 30 minutes after ingestion and may include headache, drowsiness, visual changes, cardiovascular collapse, and convulsions followed by respiratory and cardiac arrest.

Treatment is symptomatic. The stomach should be emptied by emesis or lavage. After lavage, activated charcoal in an amount at least five times the estimated amount of drug ingested may be helpful if given within 30 minutes of ingestion.

Ultra-short-acting barbiturates may help control seizures. Intubation may become necessary. Peritoneal dialysis and exchange transfusions also may be useful. Forced fluids and acidification of the urine are helpful after the acute phase.

▶ Special considerations

• Children are extremely susceptible to toxicity; monitor closely for adverse effects.
• If chloroquine hydrochloride is given intravenously, it should be diluted and administered very slowly.
• Be aware that chloroquine-resistant malaria is endemic in certain parts of the world. It may require treatment with sulfadoxine/pyrimethamine (Fansidar).
• Give drug immediately before or after meals to minimize GI side effects.
• If patient experiences intolerable GI effects, half of weekly dose can be given on 2 separate days.
• Obtain a baseline ECG, blood counts, and an ophthalmologic examination, and check periodically for changes.
• Monitor patient for signs and symptoms of cumulative effects, such as blurred vision, increased sensitivity to light, muscle weakness, impaired hearing, tinnitus, fever, sore throat, unusual bleeding or bruising, unusual pigmentation of the oral mucous membranes, and jaundice. Maximal effects may not occur for 6 months.
• Muscle weakness and alterations of deep tendon reflexes may require discontinuing the drug.

Information for parents and patient

• Tell parents to report any vision or hearing changes, muscle weakness, or darkening of urine immediately.
• Tell parents that patient should take drug after meals to help prevent GI distress. Tell parents to report any pronounced GI distress and to separate use of magnesium or kaolin compounds from drug by at least 4 hours.
• Advise parents that patient should wear sunglasses in bright light or sunlight to reduce risk of ocular damage and should avoid prolonged exposure to sunlight to avoid exacerbation of drug-induced dermatoses.
• Counsel parents to have patient complete the entire prescribed course of therapy and comply with follow-up blood tests and examinations.
• Warn parents to store drug out of small children's reach.

---

chlorothiazide
Diachlor, Diuril, Ro-Chlorozide, SK-Chlorothiazide

• Classification: diuretic, antihypertensive (thiazide)

How supplied

Available by prescription only
Tablets: 250 mg, 500 mg
Suspension: 250 mg/5 ml
Injection: 500-mg vial

Indications, route, and dosage
Diuresis

Children under age 6 months: May require up to 33 mg/kg P.O. daily in two divided doses. Experience with I.V. chlorothiazide in children is limited. Parenteral use is generally not recommended for infants.
Children age 6 months or over: 20 to 22 mg/kg or 600 mg/m^2 P.O. daily in two divided doses. Total daily dosage may range from 375 mg to 1 g for children age 2 to 12 and 175 to 375 mg for children under age 2.
Adults: 500 mg to 2 g P.O. or I.V. daily or in two divided doses.

Action and kinetics

• *Diuretic action:* Chlorothiazide increases urinary excretion of sodium and water by inhibiting sodium reabsorption in the cortical diluting tubule of the nephron, thus relieving edema.
• *Antihypertensive action:* The exact mechanism of chlorothiazide's antihypertensive effect is unknown. It may partially result from direct arteriolar vasodilation and a decrease in total peripheral resistance.
• *Kinetics in adults:* Chlorothiazide is absorbed incompletely and variably from the GI tract. After P.O administration, onset of action is ½ to 2 hours; duration of action, 6 to 12 hours. Chlorothiazide is excreted unchanged in urine.

Contraindications and precautions

Chlorothiazide is contraindicated in patients with anuria and in those with known sensitivity to the drug or to other sulfonamide derivatives; it should be avoided in jaundiced neonates. Chlorothiazide should be used with caution in patients with severe renal disease, because it may decrease glomerular filtration rate and precipitate azotemia; in patients with impaired hepatic function or liver disease, because electrolyte changes may precipitate coma; and in patients taking digoxin, because hypokalemia may predispose them to digitalis toxicity.

Interactions

Chlorothiazide potentiates the hypotensive effects of most other antihypertensive drugs; this may be used to therapeutic advantage.

Chlorothiazide may potentiate hyperglycemic, hypotensive, and hyperuricemic effects of diazoxide, and its hyperglycemic effect may increase insulin requirements in diabetic patients.

---

‡May contain sulfites   ♦May contain tartrazine   ♦ ♦May contain benzyl alcohol

Chlorothiazide may reduce renal clearance of lithium, elevating serum lithium levels, and may necessitate reduction in lithium dosage by 50%.

Chlorothiazide turns urine slightly more alkaline and may decrease urinary excretion of some amines, such as amphetamine and quinidine; alkaline urine may also decrease therapeutic efficacy of methenamine compounds, such as methenamine mandelate.

Cholestyramine and colestipol may bind chlorothiazide, preventing its absorption; give drugs 1 hour apart.

Effects on diagnostic tests

Chlorothiazide therapy may alter serum electrolyte levels and may increase serum urate, glucose, cholesterol, and triglyceride levels. It may also interfere with tests for parathyroid function and should be discontinued before such tests.

Adverse reactions

- CV: volume depletion and dehydration, orthostatic hypotension, hypercholesteremia, hypertriglyceridemia.
- DERM: dermatitis, photosensitivity, rash.
- GI: anorexia, nausea, pancreatitis.
- HEMA: aplastic anemia, agranulocytosis, leukopenia, thrombocytopenia.
- Hepatic: hepatic encephalopathy, *hyperbilirubinemia.*
- Metabolic: *symptomatic hyperuricemia;* gout; *hyperglycemia* and impairment of glucose tolerance; *glycosuria; fluid and electrolyte imbalances,* including *hypokalemia,* dilutional hyponatremia, hypochloremia, and *hypercalcemia; metabolic alkalosis; dehydration;* and *vitamin K depletion.*
- Other: *hypersensitivity reactions* (pneumonitis and vasculitis, skin reactions, photosensitivity, respiratory distress, fever).

Note: Drug should be discontinued if rising BUN and serum creatinine levels indicate renal impairment, if patient exhibits symptoms of hypersensitivity, or if patient shows signs of impending coma.

Overdose and treatment

Clinical signs of overdose include GI irritation and hypermotility, diuresis, and lethargy, which may progress to coma.

Treatment is mainly supportive; monitor and assist respiratory, cardiovascular, and renal function as indicated. Monitor fluid and electrolyte balance. Induce vomiting with ipecac in conscious patient; otherwise, use gastric lavage to avoid aspiration. Do not give cathartics; these promote additional loss of fluids and electrolytes.

▶ Special considerations

- Chlorothiazide is the only thiazide available in liquid form.
- Give chlorothiazide sodium for I.V. injection only (never I.M. or S.C.), because it is extremely irritating to tissues; do not administer with whole blood or blood products.
- Inspect skin and mucous membranes of patients on prolonged therapy for petechiae, which require reduced dosage or discontinuation of drug.

- Monitor weight and serum electrolyte levels regularly.
- Monitor serum potassium levels; encourage high-potassium diet. Foods rich in potassium include citrus fruits, tomatoes, bananas, dates, and apricots. Watch for signs of hypokalemia (for example, muscle weakness or cramps). Patients also taking digitalis have an increased risk of digitalis toxicity from the potassium-depleting effect of chlorothiazide.
- This thiazide may be used with potassium-sparing diuretics to attenuate potassium loss.
- Check insulin requirements in patients with diabetes.
- Monitor serum creatinine and BUN levels regularly. Drug is not as effective if these levels are more than twice normal.
- Monitor blood uric acid levels.
- A.M. administration is recommended to prevent nocturia.
- Antihypertensive effects persist for approximately 1 week after discontinuation of the drug.
- Instruct parents to watch for and report any joint swelling, pain, or redness; these signs may indicate hyperuricemia.

Information for parents and patient

- Explain rationale of therapy and diuretic effects of drug.
- Advise parents to watch for and promptly report signs of electrolyte imbalance: weakness, fatigue, muscle cramps, paresthesias, confusion, nausea, vomiting, diarrhea, headache, dizziness, and palpitations.
- Tell parents to report any increased edema or excess diuresis (more than a 2% weight loss or gain) and to record the child's weight each morning after voiding and before breakfast, on the same scale wearing the same type of clothing.
- Advise parents to give drug with food to minimize gastric irritation; to encourage child to eat potassium-rich foods, such as citrus fruits, potatoes, dates, raisins, and bananas; and to restrict child's access to salts and high-sodium foods, such as lunch meat, smoked meats, and processed cheeses. Inform parents that low-sodium formulas are available for infants.
- Tell parents to seek medical approval before giving the patient nonprescription drugs; many contain sodium and potassium and can cause electrolyte imbalances.
- Explain photosensitivity reactions. In thiazide-related photosensitivity, ultraviolet radiation alters drug structure, causing allergic reactions in some persons; such reactions occur 10 days to 2 weeks after initial sun exposure.
- Caution patient to change position slowly, especially when rising to upright position, to prevent dizziness from orthostatic hypotension.
- Warn parents to supervise the child's activities closely to prevent falls and other injuries that may result from dizziness, especially at beginning of therapy.
- Advise parents to watch the patient closely for signs of chest, back, leg pain, or shortness of breath, and to call immediately if they occur.
- Advise parents to administer the drug only as pre-

---

scribed and at the same time each day, to prevent nighttime diuresis and interrupted sleep.
• Emphasize importance of regular medical follow-up to monitor effectiveness of diuretic therapy.

---

chlorpheniramine maleate
Alermine, Aller-Chlor, Allerid O.D., Chlo-Amine, Chlor-100, Chlor-Mal, Chlor-Niramine, Chlorphen∗, Chlor-Pro, Chlorspan, Chlortab, Chlor-Trimeton, Chlor-Tripolon∗, Hal-Chlor, Histray, Novopheniram∗, Phenetron, T.D. Alermine, Teldrin, Trymegen

• Classification: antihistamine
(H$_1$-receptor antagonist) (propylamine-derivative antihistamine)

How supplied
Available with or without prescription
Tablets (chewable): 2 mg
Tablets: 4 mg
Tablets (timed-release): 8 mg, 12 mg
Capsules (timed-release): 8 mg, 12 mg
Syrup: 2 mg/5 ml
Injection: 10 mg/ml, 100 mg/ml

Indications, route, and dosage
Rhinitis, allergy symptoms
Children age 2 to 5: 1 mg of syrup q 4 to 6 hours. Maximum dosage is 4 mg/day.
Children age 6 to 11: 2 mg of tablets or syrup q 4 to 6 hours; or one 8-mg timed-release tablet in 24 hours. Maximum dosage is 12 mg/day.
Children age 12 and older and adults: 4 mg of tablets or syrup q 4 to 6 hours; or 8 to 12 mg of timed-release tablets b.i.d. or t.i.d. Maximum dosage is 24 mg/day.

Action and kinetics
• *Antihistamine action:* Antihistamines compete with histamine for histamine H$_1$-receptor sites on smooth muscle of the bronchi, GI tract, uterus, and large blood vessels; they bind to cellular receptors, preventing access of histamine, thereby suppressing histamine-induced allergic symptoms. They do not directly alter histamine or its release.
• *Kinetics in adults:* Chlorpheniramine is well absorbed from the GI tract; action begins within 30 to 60 minutes and peaks in 2 to 6 hours. Food in the stomach delays absorption but does not affect bioavailability. Chlorpheniramine is distributed extensively into the body. Drug is metabolized largely in GI mucosal cells and liver (first-pass effect). Chlorpheniramine's half-life is 12 to 43 hours in adults; drug and metabolites are excreted in urine.
• *Kinetics in children:* Half-life is 10 to 13 hours.

Contraindications and precautions
Chlorpheniramine is contraindicated in children with known hypersensitivity to this medication or antihistamines with similar chemical structures, such as dexchlorpheniramine, brompheniramine, or triproli-

dine; during an acute asthmatic attack, because it thickens bronchial secretions; and in patients who have taken MAO inhibitors within the preceding 2 weeks.

Antihistamines should be used with caution in patients with narrow-angle glaucoma; in those with pyloroduodenal obstruction or urinary bladder obstruction from narrowing of the bladder neck, because of their marked anticholinergic effects; in patients with cardiovascular disease, hypertension, or hyperthyroidism, because of the risk of palpitations and tachycardia; and in patients with renal disease, diabetes, bronchial asthma, urinary retention, or stenosing peptic ulcers.

Not indicated for use in premature or newborn infants. Such use causes seizures and other severe reactions.

Interactions
MAO inhibitors interfere with the detoxification of chlorpheniramine and thus prolong and intensify its central depressant and anticholinergic effects; additive sedation may occur when antihistamines are given concomitantly with other CNS depressants, such as alcohol, barbiturates, tranquilizers, sleeping aids, or antianxiety agents.

Chlorpheniramine enhances the effects of epinephrine and may diminish the effects of sulfonylureas and partially counteract the anticoagulant action of heparin.

Effects on diagnostic tests
Discontinue chlorpheniramine 4 days before diagnostic skin tests; antihistamines can prevent, reduce, or mask positive skin test response.

Adverse reactions
• CNS: stimulation, sedation, drowsiness, dizziness, vertigo, disturbed coordination, excitability.
• CV: hypotension, palpitations.
• DERM: urticaria, rash.
• GI: anorexia, nausea, constipation, epigastric distress, vomiting, dry mouth and throat.
• GU: urinary retention.
• Respiratory: thick bronchial secretions.

Overdose and treatment
Clinical manifestations of overdose may include either CNS depression (sedation, reduced mental alertness, apnea, and cardiovascular collapse) or CNS stimulation (insomnia, hallucinations, tremors, and convulsions). Atropine-like symptoms, such as dry mouth, flushed skin, fixed and dilated pupils, and GI symptoms are common, especially in children.

Treat overdose by inducing emesis with ipecac syrup (in conscious patient), followed by activated charcoal to reduce further drug absorption. Use gastric lavage if patient is unconscious or ipecac fails. Treat hypotension with vasopressors, and control seizures with diazepam or phenytoin. *Do not give stimulants.* Administering ammonium chloride or vitamin C to acidify urine will promote drug excretion.

---

‡May contain sulfites　　　◆May contain tartrazine　　　◆◆May contain benzyl alcohol

▶ **Special considerations**
• Give 100 mg/ml of injectable form S.C. or I.M. *only.*
Not recommended for I.V. use; I.V. preparation contains preservatives.
• Do not use parenteral solutions intradermally.
• Administer I.V. solution slowly, over 1 minute.
• Children, especially those under age 6, may experience paradoxical hyperexcitability with restlessness, insomnia, nervousness, euphoria, tremors, and seizures.
• Reduce GI distress by giving chlorpheniramine with food; give sugarless gum, appropriate hard candy, or ice chips to relieve dry mouth; increase fluid intake (if allowed) or humidify air to decrease adverse effect of thickened secretions.
• Sustained-release tablets should be swallowed whole; do not crush or permit patient to chew tablet.
• Store syrup and parenteral solution away from light.

Information for parents and patient
• Advise patient to take drug with meals or snack to prevent gastric upset and to use any of the following measures to relieve dry mouth: warm water rinses, artificial saliva, ice chips, or sugarless gum or lollipop. Patient should avoid overusing mouthwash, which may add to dryness (alcohol content) and destroy normal flora.
• Warn parents that child should avoid hazardous activities that require balance or alertness until extent of CNS effects are known. Tell them to seek medical approval before administering tranquilizers, sedatives, pain relievers, or sleeping medications.
• Warn parents to discontinue drug 4 days before diagnostic skin tests, to preserve accuracy of tests.

---

chlorpromazine hydrochloride
Chlor-Promanyl★, Chlorzine, Largactil★, Novo-chlorpromazine★, Ormazine, Promapar, Promaz, Sonazine, Thorazine, Thor-Prom

• Classification: antipsychotic, antiemetic (aliphatic phenothiazine)

How supplied
Available by prescription only
Tablets: 10 mg, 25 mg, 50 mg, 100 mg, 200 mg
Capsules (sustained-release): 30 mg, 75 mg, 150 mg, 200 mg, 300 mg
Syrup: 10 mg/5ml
Oral concentrate: 30 mg/ml, 100 mg/ml
Suppositories: 25 mg, 100 mg
Injection: 25 mg/ml

Indications, route, and dosage
Psychosis
Children over age 6 months: 0.25 mg/kg P.O. q 4 to 6 hours; or 0.25 mg/kg I.M. q 6 to 8 hours; or 0.5 mg/kg rectally q 6 to 8 hours. Maximum dosage is 40 mg in children under age 5, and 75 mg in children age 5 to 12.
Adults: 30 to 75 mg P.O. daily in two to four divided

doses. Dosage may be increased twice weekly by 20 to 50 mg until symptoms are controlled. Most patients respond to 200 mg daily, but doses up to 800 mg may be necessary.
Nausea and vomiting
Infants over age 6 months and children: 0.55 mg/kg P.O. or I.M. q 6 to 8 hours; alternatively give 1.1 mg/kg rectally q 6 to 8 hours p.r.n.
Adults: 10 to 225 mg P.O. or I.M. q 4 to 6 hours, p.r.n.; or 50 to 100 mg rectally q 6 to 8 hours, p.r.n.
Acute nausea and vomiting during surgery
Children 6 months and older: 0.275 mg/kg I.M.; repeat in 30 minutes p.r.n. or give fractional 1-mg doses q 2 minutes to a maximum of 0.275 mg/kg; repeat fractional regimen in 30 minutes p.r.n.
Tetanus
Children age 6 months and older: 0.55 mg/kg I.M. or I.V. q 6 to 8 hours.
Note: Maximum I.M. dosage is 40 mg daily in children < age 5 and < 22.7 kg, and 75 mg daily in children age 5 to 12 weighing 22.7 to 45.5 kg.

Action and kinetics
• *Antipsychotic action:* Chlorpromazine is thought to exert its antipsychotic effects by postsynaptic blockade of CNS dopamine receptors, thereby inhibiting dopamine-mediated effects; antiemetic effects are attributed to dopamine receptor blockade in the medullary chemoreceptor trigger zone (CTZ). Chlorpromazine has many other central and peripheral effects; it produces both alpha and ganglionic blockade and counteracts histamine- and serotonin-mediated activity. Its most prominent adverse reactions are antimuscarinic and sedative; it causes fewer extrapyramidal effects than other antipsychotics.
• *Kinetics in adults:* Rate and extent of absorption vary with route of administration. Oral tablet absorption is erratic and variable, with onset ranging from ½ to 1 hour; peak effects occur at 2 to 4 hours and duration of action is 4 to 6 hours. Sustained-release preparations have similar absorption, but action lasts for 10 to 12 hours. Suppositories act in 60 minutes and last 3 to 4 hours. Oral concentrates and syrups are much more predictable; I.M. drug is absorbed rapidly.
Chlorpromazine is distributed widely into the body, including breast milk; concentration is usually higher in CNS than plasma. Steady-state serum level is achieved within 4 to 7 days. Drug is 91% to 99% protein-bound.
Chlorpromazine is metabolized extensively by the liver and forms 10 to 12 metabolites; some are pharmacologically active.
Most of drug is excreted as metabolites in urine; some is excreted in feces via the biliary tract. It may undergo enterohepatic circulation.

Contraindications and precautions
Antipsychotics are contraindicated in patients with known hypersensitivity to phenothiazines and related compounds, including allergic reactions involving hepatic function; in patients with blood dyscrasias and bone marrow depression because chlorpromazine may induce agranulocytosis; in patients with disorders accompanied by coma, brain damage, or CNS depres-

sion because of additive CNS depressant effects; in patients with circulatory collapse or cerebrovascular disease because of the potential for hypotensive or adverse cardiac effects; and for use with adrenergic blocking agents or spinal or epidural anesthetics because of the alpha-blocking potential of chlorpromazine.

Chlorpromazine should be used cautiously in patients with cardiac disease (dysrhythmias, congestive heart failure, angina pectoris, valvular disease, or heart block), encephalitis, Reye's syndrome, head injury, respiratory disease, epilepsy and other seizure disorders, glaucoma, prostatic hypertrophy, urinary retention, hepatic or renal dysfunction, Parkinson's disease, pheochromocytoma, or hypocalcemia. Drug therapy for nausea and vomiting in children is discouraged to avoid masking serious underlying illness such as Reye's syndrome.

Interactions

Concomitant use of chlorpromazine with sympathomimetics, including epinephrine, phenylephrine, phenylpropanolamine, and ephedrine (often found in nasal sprays), and appetite suppressants may decrease their stimulatory and pressor effects. Chlorpromazine may cause epinephrine reversal: the beta-adrenergic agonist activity of epinephrine is evident while its alpha effects are blocked, leading to decreased diastolic and increased systolic pressures and tachycardia.

Chlorpromazine may inhibit blood pressure response to centrally acting antihypertensive drugs such as guanethidine, guanabenz, guanadrel, clonidine, methyldopa, and reserpine. Additive effects are likely after concomitant use of chlorpromazine and CNS depressants (including alcohol, analgesics, barbiturates, narcotics, tranquilizers, and general, spinal, or epidural anesthetics), or parenteral magnesium sulfate (oversedation, respiratory depression, and hypotension); antiarrhythmic agents, quinidine, disopyramide, and procainamide (increased incidence of cardiac dysrhythmias and conduction defects); atropine and other anticholinergic drugs, including antidepressants, monoamine oxidase inhibitors, phenothiazines, antihistamines, meperidine, and antiparkinsonian agents (oversedation, paralytic ileus, visual changes, and severe constipation); nitrates (hypotension); and metrizamide (increased risk of seizures).

Beta-blocking agents may inhibit chlorpromazine metabolism, increasing plasma levels and toxicity.

Concomitant use with propylthiouracil increases risk of agranulocytosis; concomitant use with lithium may cause severe neurologic toxicity with an encephalitis-like syndrome, and a decreased therapeutic response to chlorpromazine.

Pharmacokinetic alterations and subsequent decreased therapeutic response to chlorpromazine may follow concomitant use with phenobarbital (enhanced renal excretion), aluminum- and magnesium-containing antacids and antidiarrheals (decreased absorption), caffeine, and with heavy smoking (increased metabolism).

Chlorpromazine may antagonize therapeutic effect of bromocriptine on prolactin secretion; it also may decrease the vasoconstricting effects of high-dose dopamine and may decrease effectiveness and increase toxicity of levodopa (by dopamine blockade). Chlorpromazine may inhibit metabolism and increase toxicity of phenytoin.

Effects on diagnostic tests

Chlorpromazine causes false-positive test results for urinary porphyrins, urobilinogen, amylase, and 5-hydroxyindoleacetic acid (5-HIAA), because of darkening of urine by metabolites; it also causes false-positive results in urine pregnancy tests using human chorionic gonadotropin (HCG).

Chlorpromazine elevates tests for liver function and protein-bound iodine and causes quinidine-like ECG effects.

Adverse reactions

• CNS: extrapyramidal symptoms—dystonia, akathisia, torticollis, tardive dyskinesia (dose-related, with long-term therapy), sedation, pseudoparkinsonism, drowsiness (frequent); neuroleptic malignant syndrome (dose-related; if untreated, fatal respiratory failure in over 10% of patients); dizziness, headache, insomnia, exacerbation of psychotic symptoms.
• CV: asystole, orthostatic hypotension, tachycardia, dizziness, fainting, dysrhythmias, ECG changes, increased anginal pain (after I.M. injection).
• EENT: blurred vision, tinnitus, mydriasis, increased intraocular pressure, ocular changes (retinal pigmentary change with long-term use).
• GI: dry mouth, constipation, nausea, vomiting, anorexia, diarrhea.
• GU: urinary retention, gynecomastia, hypermenorrhea, inhibited ejaculation.
• HEMA: transient leukopenia, agranulocytosis, thrombocytopenia, anemia (within 30 to 90 days).
• Local: contact dermatitis from concentrate or injectable, muscle necrosis from I.M. injection.
• Other: hyperprolactinemia, photosensitivity, increased appetite or weight gain, hypersensitivity (rash, urticaria, drug fever, edema, cholestatic jaundice [in 2% to 4% of patients within first 30 days]).

After abrupt withdrawal of long-term therapy, gastritis, nausea, vomiting, dizziness, tremors, feeling of heat or cold, sweating, tachycardia, headache, or insomnia may occur.

Note: Drug should be discontinued immediately if the following reactions occur: hypersensitivity, jaundice, agranulocytosis; neuroleptic malignant syndrome (marked hyperthermia, extrapyramidal effects, autonomic dysfunction); and severe extrapyramidal symptoms even after dose is lowered. Chlorpromazine should be discontinued 48 hours before and 24 hours after myelography using metrizamide, because of the risk of convulsions. When feasible, withdraw drug slowly and gradually; many drug effects persist after withdrawal.

Overdose and treatment

CNS depression is characterized by deep, unarousable sleep and possible coma, hypotension or hypertension, extrapyramidal symptoms, abnormal involuntary muscle movements, agitation, seizures, dysrhythmias, ECG changes, hypothermia or hyperthermia, and autonomic nervous system dysfunction.

---

‡May contain sulfites   ♦May contain tartrazine   ♦♦May contain benzyl alcohol

Treatment is symptomatic and supportive, including maintaining vital signs, airway, stable body temperature, and fluid and electrolyte balance.

Do not induce vomiting: Drug inhibits cough reflex, and aspiration may occur. Use gastric lavage, then activated charcoal and saline cathartics; dialysis does not help. Regulate body temperature as needed. Treat hypotension with I.V. fluids: *Do not give epinephrine.* Treat seizures with parenteral diazepam or barbiturates; dysrhythmias with parenteral phenytoin (1 mg/kg with rate titrated to blood pressure); extrapyramidal reactions with barbiturates, benztropine, or parenteral diphenhydramine 2 mg/kg/minute.

▶ Special considerations

• Chlorpromazine is not recommended for patients under age 6 months. Sudden infant death syndrome has been reported in children under age 1 receiving the drug.

• Chlorpromazine has also been used to treat high fever in malignant hyperthermia syndrome.

• Unless otherwise specified, antipsychotics are not recommended for children under age 12; be very careful when using phenothiazines for nausea and vomiting, because acutely ill children (chicken pox, measles, CNS infections, dehydration) are at greatly increased risk of dystonic reactions.

• Check vital signs regularly for decreased blood pressure (especially before and after parenteral therapy) or tachycardia; observe patient carefully for other adverse reactions.

• Check intake and output for urinary retention or constipation, which may require dosage reduction.

• Monitor bilirubin levels weekly for first 4 weeks; monitor complete blood count, ECG (for quinidine-like effects), liver and renal function studies, electrolyte levels (especially potassium), and eye examinations at baseline and periodically thereafter, especially in patients on long-term therapy.

• Observe patient for mood changes to monitor progress; benefits may not be apparent for several weeks.

• Monitor for involuntary movements. Check patient receiving prolonged treatment at least once every 6 months.

• Do not withdraw drug abruptly; although physical dependence does not occur with antipsychotic drugs, rebound exacerbation of psychotic symptoms may occur, and drug effects may persist.

• Carefully follow manufacturer's instructions for reconstitution, dilution, administration, and storage; slightly discolored liquids may or may not be all right to use. Check with pharmacist.

• Drug may cause a pink-brown discoloration of urine.

• Chlorpromazine has a high incidence of sedation, orthostatic hypotension, and photosensitivity reactions (3%). Patient should avoid exposure to sunlight or heat lamps.

• Sustained-release preparations should not be crushed or opened, but swallowed whole.

• Oral formulations may cause stomach upset and may be administered with food or fluid.

• Dilute the concentrate in 2 to 4 oz of liquid, preferably water, carbonated drinks, fruit juice, tomato juice, milk, puddings, or applesauce.

• Store the suppository form in a cool place.

• If tissue irritation occurs, chlorpromazine injection may be diluted with normal saline solution or 2% procaine.

• Dilute the injection to 1 mg/ml with normal saline solution and administer at a rate of 1 mg/2 minutes for children and 1 mg/minute for adults.

• The I.M. injection should be given deep in the upper outer quadrant of the buttocks. Massaging the area after administration may prevent abscess formation. Do not extravasate because skin necrosis can occur.

• The liquid and injectable formulations may cause a rash if skin contact occurs.

• Solution for injection may be slightly discolored. Do not use if drug is excessively discolored or if a precipitate is evident. Monitor blood pressure before and after parenteral administration.

• Shake the syrup before administration.

Information for parents and patient

• Explain rationale and anticipated risks and benefits of therapy, and that full therapeutic effect may not occur for several weeks.

• Teach signs and symptoms of adverse reactions and importance of reporting any unusual effects, especially involuntary movements.

• Tell parents that patient should avoid beverages and drugs containing alcohol and should not take any other drug (especially CNS depressants), including nonprescription products, without medical approval.

• Instruct parents of diabetic children to monitor blood glucose levels because drug may alter insulin needs.

• Teach parents or patient how and when to take drug, not to increase dose without medical approval, and never to discontinue drug abruptly; suggest taking full dose at bedtime if daytime sedation is troublesome.

• Advise parents to have patient lie down for 30 minutes after first dose (1 hour if I.M.) and to rise slowly from sitting or supine position to prevent orthostatic hypotension.

• Patient should avoid hazardous activities that require alertness and psychomotor coordination until full effects of drug are established. Excessive sedative effects tend to subside after several weeks.

• Drugs are locally irritating; advise taking with milk of food to minimize GI distress. Warn that oral concentrates and solutions will irritate skin. Patient should not crush or open sustained-released products but swallow them whole.

• Warn parents that excessive exposure to sunlight, heat lamps, or tanning beds may cause photosensitivity reactions (burn and abnormal hyperpigmentation).

• Tell parents that patient should avoid exposure to extremes of heat or cold because of risk of hypothermia or hyperthermia induced by altered thermoregulatory function.

• Recommend sugarless gum, hard candy, or ice chips to relieve dry mouth.

• Explain that drug may cause pink to brown discoloration of urine.

• Explain the risks of dystonic reactions and tardive dyskinesia, and tell the parents or patient to report abnormal body movements.

• Advise parents that if liquid preparation spills on the skin, rash and irritation may result.
• Encourage parents to call if patient has difficulty urinating, sore throat, dizziness, or fainting.
• Explain what fluids are appropriate for diluting the concentrate and the dropper technique for measuring dose. Teach parents and patient how to use the suppository form.
• Tell parents to shake syrup before administration.

chlortetracycline hydrochloride
Aureomycin, Aureomycin Ophthalmic

• Classification: antibiotic, anti-infective (tetracycline)

How supplied
Available by prescription only
Ophthalmic ointment: 10 mg/g in 3.75-g tube
Suspension: 1%

Available without prescription
Topical ointment: 3% in 14.2-g and 30-g tubes

Indications, route, and dosage
Superficial infections of the skin caused by susceptible bacteria
Children and adults: Rub into affected area b.i.d.
Superficial ophthalmic bacterial infections
Children and adults: Small amount of ophthalmic ointment placed in conjunctival sac every 2 to 12 hours or 1 to 2 drops of ophthalmic suspension b.i.d., t.i.d., or q.i.d.
Ophthalmic chlamydial infections
Children and adults: Small amount of ophthalmic ointment placed in conjunctival sac or 2 drops of ophthalmic suspension in each eye b.i.d., t.i.d., or q.i.d.
Ophthalmia neonatorum prophylaxis
Newborn: 1- to 2-cm ribbon of ophthalmic ointment or 1 to 2 drops of ophthalmic suspension applied to neonate's conjunctival sac shortly after birth.

Action and kinetics
• *Antibacterial and anti-infective action:* Inhibits binding of transfer RNA to the messenger RNA complex at the 30S subunit, inhibiting bacterial protein synthesis. Chlortetracycline is a broad-spectrum bacteriostatic agent.
• *Kinetics in adults:* Unknown.

Contraindications and precautions
Chlortetracycline is contraindicated in patients with hypersensitivity to any of the tetracyclines and in pregnant patients in the second and third trimesters. Use with caution to avoid overgrowth of nonsusceptible organisms during long-term use.

Interactions
None significant.

Effects on diagnostic tests
Although the oral administration of chlortetracycline has been reported to decrease serum cholesterol levels, no such effect has been reported with the topical or ophthalmic administration of chlortetracycline.

Adverse reactions
• DERM: dermatitis, drying.
• Eye: foreign body sensation, transient stinging or burning sensation, increased tearing.

Overdose and treatment
Chlortetracycline content of an entire tube of ophthalmic ointment is insufficient to cause toxicity when accidently ingested orally. Nausea, vomiting, abdominal discomfort, or headache may occur, but severe toxicity is unlikely; induced emesis is indicated only after substantial ingestion. Antacids may be used to treat gastric irritation. Treat patient symptomatically.

▶ Special considerations
• Avoid having topical ointment come in contact with eyes.
• Drug has lanolin base; do not use in patients allergic to wool.
• Prolonged use may result in overgrowth of nonsusceptible organisms.
• Treated skin fluoresces under ultraviolet light.
• Patients with chlamydial ophthalmic infections should also receive an oral anti-infective for at least 3 weeks.
• Mild infections usually respond in 48 hours. If no improvement is seen or if condition worsens, discontinue drug. Therapy should continue for 48 hours after eye appears normal.
• When ointment is used for prophylaxis of ophthalmia neonatorum, the neonate's eyelids should be massaged gently to spread the ointment.
• After application, the ointment or suspension should *not* be flushed from the eye.

Information for parents and patient
Topical ointment
• Tell parents and patient to clean infected area of skin before application and to cover with sterile dressing if necessary.
• Tell parents to call if rash or fever develops or if condition worsens.
• Warn parents and patient that ointment may stain clothing.
• Explain that drug may cause photosensitivity, and advise patient to avoid prolonged sun exposure during use.
• Long-term use of topical ointment may cause tooth discoloration in children under age 8.
Ophthalmic ointment
• Tell parents and patient to remove excess exudate before each new application to enhance comfort.
• Patient should use ointment for full period prescribed.

■■■■■■■■

chlorthalidone
Hygroton, Hylidone, Novothalidone*, Thalitone, Uridone*

• Classification: diuretic, antihypertensive (thiazide-like diuretic)

How supplied
Available by prescription only
Tablets: 25 mg, 50 mg, 100 mg

Indications, route, and dosage
Edema, hypertension
Children: 2 mg/kg or 60 mg/m² P.O. three times weekly.
Adults: 25 to 100 mg P.O. daily.

Action and kinetics
• *Diuretic action:* Chlorthalidone increases urinary excretion of sodium and water by inhibiting sodium reabsorption in the cortical diluting tubule of the nephron, thus relieving edema.
• *Antihypertensive action:* The exact mechanism of chlorthalidone's hypotensive effect is unknown. This effect may partially result from direct arteriolar vasodilation and a decrease in total peripheral resistance.
• *Kinetics in adults:* Chlorthalidone is absorbed from the GI tract; extent of absorption is unknown. Chlorthalidone is 90% bound to erythrocytes. Between 30% and 60% of a given dose of chlorthalidone is excreted unchanged in urine; half-life is 54 hours.

Contraindications and precautions
Chlorthalidone is contraindicated in patients with anuria and in those with known sensitivity to the drug or to other sulfonamide derivatives. Chlorthalidone should be used cautiously in patients with severe renal disease, because it may decrease glomerular filtration rate and precipitate azotemia; in patients with impaired hepatic function or liver disease, because electrolyte changes may precipitate coma; and in patients taking digoxin, because hypokalemia may predispose them to digitalis toxicity.

Interactions
Chlorthalidone potentiates the hypotensive effects of most other antihypertensive drugs; this may be used to therapeutic advantage.

Chlorthalidone may potentiate hyperglycemic, hypotensive, and hyperuricemic effects of diazoxide, and its hyperglycemic effect may increase insulin requirements in diabetic patients. Chlorthalidone may reduce renal clearance of lithium, elevating serum lithium levels, and may necessitate reduction in lithium dosage by 50%.

Chlorthalidone turns urine slightly more alkaline and may decrease urinary excretion of some amines, such as amphetamine and quinidine; alkaline urine also may decrease therapeutic efficacy of methenamine compounds, such as methenamine mandelate.

Cholestyramine and colestipol may bind chlorthalidone, preventing its absorption; give drugs 1 hour apart.

Effects on diagnostic tests
Chlorthalidone therapy may alter serum electrolyte levels and may increase serum urate, glucose, cholesterol, and triglyceride levels.

Chlorthalidone may interfere with tests for parathyroid function and should be discontinued before such tests.

Adverse reactions
• CV: volume depletion and dehydration, orthostatic hypotension, hypercholesterolemia, hypertriglyceridemia.
• DERM: dermatitis, photosensitivity, rash.
• GI: anorexia, nausea, pancreatitis.
• HEMA: aplastic anemia, agranulocytosis, leukopenia, thrombocytopenia.
• Hepatic: hepatic encephalopathy.
• Metabolic: asymptomatic hyperuricemia; gout; hyperglycemia and impairment of glucose tolerance; fluid and electrolyte imbalances, including hypokalemia (may be profound), dilutional hyponatremia, hypochloremia, and hypercalcemia; metabolic alkalosis.
• Other: hypersensitivity reactions, such as pneumonitis and vasculitis.
Note: Drug should be discontinued if rising BUN and serum creatinine levels indicate renal impairment or if patient shows signs of impending coma.

Overdose and treatment
Clinical signs of overdose include GI irritation and hypermotility, diuresis, and lethargy, which may progress to coma.

Treatment is mainly supportive; monitor and assist respiratory, cardiovascular, and renal function as indicated. Monitor fluid and electrolyte balance. Induce vomiting with ipecac in conscious patient; otherwise, use gastric lavage to avoid aspiration. Do not give cathartics; these promote additional loss of fluids and electrolytes.

▶ Special considerations
• Monitor weight and serum electrolyte levels regularly.
• Monitor serum potassium levels; encourage high-potassium diet. Foods rich in potassium include citrus fruits, tomatoes, bananas, dates, and apricots. Watch for signs of hypokalemia (for example, muscle weakness or cramps). Patients also taking digitalis have an increased risk of digitalis toxicity from the potassium-depleting effect of chlorthalidone.
• Drug may be used with potassium-sparing diuretics to attenuate potassium loss.
• Check insulin requirements in patients with diabetes.
• Monitor serum creatinine and BUN levels regularly. Drug is not as effective if these levels are more than twice normal.
• Monitor blood uric acid levels.
• A.M. administration is recommended to prevent nocturia.
• Antihypertensive effects persist for approximately 1 week after discontinuation of the drug.

• Instruct parents to watch for and report any joint swelling, pain, or redness; these signs may indicate hyperuricemia.

Information for parents and patient
• Explain rationale of therapy and diuretic effects of drug.
• Advise parents to watch for and promptly report signs of electrolyte imbalance: weakness, fatigue, muscle cramps, paresthesias, confusion, nausea, vomiting, diarrhea, headache, dizziness, and palpitations.
• Tell parents to report any increased edema or excess diuresis (more than a 2% weight loss or gain) and to record the child's weight each morning after voiding and before breakfast, on the same scale wearing the same type of clothing.
• Advise parents to give drug with food to minimize gastric irritation; to encourage child to eat potassium-rich foods, such as citrus fruits, potatoes, dates, raisins, and bananas; and to restrict child's access to salts and high-sodium foods, such as lunch meat, smoked meats, and processed cheeses.
• Tell parents to seek medical approval before giving the patient nonprescription drugs; many contain sodium and potassium and can cause electrolyte imbalances.
• Explain photosensitivity reactions. In thiazide-related photosensitivity, ultraviolet radiation alters drug structure, causing allergic reactions in some persons; such reactions occur 10 days to 2 weeks after initial sun exposure.
• Caution patient to change position slowly, especially when rising to upright position, to prevent dizziness from orthostatic hypotension.
• Warn parents to supervise the child's activities closely to prevent falls and other injuries that may result from dizziness, especially at beginning of therapy.
• Advise parents to watch the patient closely for signs of chest, back, or leg pain, or shortness of breath, and to call immediately if they occur.
• Advise parents to administer the drug only as prescribed and at the same time each day, to prevent nighttime diuresis and interrupted sleep.
• Emphasize importance of regular medical follow-up to monitor effectiveness of diuretic therapy.

chlorzoxazone
Paraflex, Parafon Forte DSC

• Classification: skeletal muscle relaxant (benzoxazole derivative)

How supplied
Available by prescription only.
Tablets (scored): 250 mg, 500 mg

Indications, route, and dosage
Adjunct in acute, painful musculoskeletal conditions
Children: 20 mg/kg or 600 mg/m^2 daily divided t.i.d. or q.i.d., or 125 to 500 mg t.i.d. or q.i.d., depending on age and weight.
Adults: 250, 500, or 750 mg P.O. t.i.d. or q.i.d.

Action and kinetics
• *Skeletal muscle relaxant action:* Chlorzoxazone does not relax skeletal muscle directly, but apparently as a result of its sedative effects. However, the exact mechanism of action is unknown.
  Animal studies suggest that the drug modifies central perception of pain without eliminating peripheral pain reflexes.
• *Kinetics in adults:* Chlorzoxazone is rapidly and completely absorbed from the GI tract. Onset of action occurs within 1 hour; duration of action is 3 to 4 hours. Chlorzoxazone is widely distributed in the body. Chlorzoxazone is metabolized in the liver to inactive metabolites. Drug is excreted in urine as glucuronide metabolite.

Contraindications and precautions
Chlorzoxazone is contraindicated in patients with known sensitivity to the drug or impaired hepatic function, because the drug is metabolized by the liver. Use with caution in patients with allergies or a history of allergic reactions to drugs.

Interactions
Concomitant use with other CNS depressants, including alcohol, produces further CNS depression. When used with other depressant drugs (general anesthetics, opioid analgesics, antipsychotics, anxiolytics, or tricyclic antidepressants), exercise care to avoid overdose. Concurrent use with monoamine oxidase inhibitors or tricyclic antidepressants may result in increased CNS depression, respiratory depression, and hypotensive effects. Reduce dosage of one or both agents.

Effects on diagnostic tests
None reported.

Adverse reactions
• CNS: drowsiness, dizziness, tremor, insomnia, agitation, irritability, headache, depression.
• DERM: rash, pruritus, urticaria.
• GI: nausea, vomiting, constipation, diarrhea, epigastric distress.
  Note: Drug should be discontinued if signs or symptoms of hepatic dysfunction or hypersensitivity occur.

Overdose and treatment
Clinical manifestations of overdose include nausea, vomiting, diarrhea, drowsiness, dizziness, lightheadedness, headache, malaise, or sluggishness, followed by loss of muscle tone, decreased or absent deep tendon reflexes, respiratory depression, and hypotension.
  To treat overdose, induce emesis or perform gastric lavage followed by activated charcoal. Closely monitor vital signs and neurologic status. Provide supportive

measures, including maintenance of adequate airway and assisted ventilation. Use caution if administering pressor agents.

▶ Special considerations
• Tablets may be crushed and mixed with food, milk, or fruit juice to aid dosing in children and to minimize GI upset.
• Chlorzoxazone may cause drowsiness.
• Drug may turn urine orange or reddish purple.
• Be aware of other CNS depressant drugs patient is taking, because effects are cumulative.

Information for parents and patient
• Caution parents that patient should avoid hazardous activities that require alertness or physical coordination until CNS depression is determined.
• Warn parents that child should avoid alcoholic beverages and that cough and cold preparations may contain alcohol.
• Tell parents to store drug away from direct heat or light (not in bathroom medicine cabinet, where heat and humidity cause deterioriation of drug).
• Tell parent that child should take missed dose only if remembered within 1 hour of scheduled time. If beyond 1 hour, patient should skip dose and go back to regular schedule. Patient should not double the dose.
• Tell parents that patient should not to stop taking this drug without specific medical instructions.
• Explain that patient's urine may turn orange or reddish purple, but this is a harmless effect.
• Tell parents that tablets may be crushed and mixed with food, milk, or fruit juice to aid administration.

---

cholestyramine
Questran

• Classification: antilipemic, bile acid sequestrant (anion exchange resin)

How supplied
Available by prescription only
Powder: 378-g cans, 9-g single-dose packets. Each scoop of powder or single-dose packet contains 4 g of cholestyramine resin.

Indications, route, and dosage
Hyperlipidemia, hypercholesterolemia
Drug is indicated in primary hyperlipidemia, pruritus, and diarrhea caused by excess bile acid; as adjunctive therapy to reduce elevated serum cholesterol levels; in patients with primary hypercholesterolemia; and to reduce the risks of atherosclerotic coronary artery disease and myocardial infarction.
Children age 6 to 12: 80 mg/kg, or 2.35 g/m^2 P.O. t.i.d.
Adults: 4 g before meals and h.s., not to exceed 32 g daily.

Action and kinetics
• *Antilipemic action:* Bile is normally excreted into the intestine to facilitate absorption of fat and other lipid materials. Cholestyramine binds with bile acid, forming an insoluble compound that is excreted in feces. With less bile available in the digestive system, less fat and lipid materials in food are absorbed, more cholesterol is used by the liver to replace its supply of bile acids, and the serum cholesterol level decreases. In partial biliary obstruction, excess bile acids accumulate in dermal tissue, resulting in pruritus; by reducing levels of dermal bile acids, cholestyramine combats pruritus.
Cholestyramine can also act as an antidiarrheal in postoperative diarrhea caused by bile acids in the colon.
• *Kinetics in adults:* Cholestyramine is not absorbed. Cholesterol levels may begin to decrease 24 to 48 hours after the start of therapy and may continue to fall for up 12 months. In some patients, the initial decrease is followed by a return to or above baseline cholesterol levels on continued therapy. Relief of pruritus associated with cholestasis occurs 1 to 3 weeks after initiation of therapy. Diarrhea associated with bile acids may cease in 24 hours. Insoluble cholestyramine with bile acid complex is excreted in feces.

Contraindications and precautions
Cholestyramine is contraindicated in patients with complete biliary obstruction and in patients hypersensitive to any of its components. Cholestyramine powder contains tartrazine (FD&C Yellow No. 5), which may cause allergic reactions in susceptible individuals.
Use resin cautiously in patients with constipation because of the risk of fecal impaction; in patients with malabsorption, whose condition may deteriorate from further decreased absorption of fats and fat-soluble vitamins E, A, D, and K; and in pregnant patients, because impaired maternal absorption of vitamins and other nutrients is a potential threat to the fetus.

Interactions
Cholestyramine may reduce absorption of other oral medications, such as acetaminophen, corticosteroids, thiazide diuretics, thyroid preparations, and cardiac glycosides, thus decreasing their therapeutic effects. Its binding potential may also decrease anticoagulant effects of warfarin; concurrent depletion of vitamin K may either negate this effect or increase anticoagulant activity; careful monitoring of prothrombin time is mandatory.
Dosage of any oral medication may require adjustment to compensate for possible binding with cholestyramine; give other drugs at least 1 hour before or 4 to 6 hours after cholestyramine (longer if possible); readjustment must also be made when cholestyramine is withdrawn, to prevent high-dose toxicity.

Effects on diagnostic tests
Cholestyramine therapy alters serum concentrations of alkaline phosphatase, aspartate aminotransferase, chloride, phosphorus, potassium, calcium, and sodium. Impaired calcium absorption may lead to osteoporosis.

Cholecystography using iopanoic acid will yield abnormal results because iopanoic acid is also bound by cholestyramine.

Adverse reactions
• DERM: rash; irritation of skin, tongue, and perianal area.
• GI: *constipation, diarrhea,* fecal impaction, aggravation of hemorrhoids, abdominal discomfort, flatulence, nausea, *vomiting,* steatorrhea.
• Other: *vitamin A, D, and K deficiency from decreased absorption;* hyperchloremic acidosis with long-term use or very high dosage.

Note: Drug should be discontinued if constipation continues even after reduction in dosage; if a paradoxical increase in serum cholesterol level occurs; or if clinical response is inadequate after 3 months of therapy.

Overdose and treatment
Overdose of cholestyramine has not been reported. Chief potential risk is intestinal obstruction; treatment would depend on location and degree of obstruction and on amount of gut motility.

▶ Special considerations
• Safe dosage has not been established for children under age 6.
• Children may be at greater risk for hyperchloremic acidosis during cholestyramine therapy.
• To mix, sprinkle powder on surface of preferred beverage or wet food, let stand a few minutes, and stir to obtain uniform suspension; avoid excess foaming by using large glass and mixing slowly. Use at least 90 ml of water or other fluid (if carbonated fluid is used, minimize excess foaming by mixing the powder slowly in a large glass), soups, milk, or pulpy fruit; rinse container and have patient drink this to be sure he ingests entire dose.
• Monitor levels of cardiac glycosides and other drugs to ensure appropriate dosage during and after therapy with cholestyramine.
• Determine serum cholesterol level frequently during first few months of therapy and periodically thereafter.
• Monitor bowel function. Treat constipation promptly by decreasing dosage, adding a stool softener, or discontinuing drug.
• Monitor for signs of vitamin A, D, or K deficiency.

Information for parents and patient
• Explain disease process and rationale for therapy, and encourage compliance with continued blood testing and special diet; although therapy is not curative, it helps control serum cholesterol level.
• Attempt to increase awareness of other cardiac risk factors; encourage patient to control weight, take regular exercise, and not to smoke.
• Tell patient to mix drug with fluids or pulpy fruits. Patient should not take the powder in dry form

choline magnesium trisalicylates
Trilisate

choline salicylate
Arthropan

• Classification: nonnarcotic analgesic, antipyretic, anti-inflammatory (salicylate)

How supplied
Available by prescription only
Tablets: 500 mg, 750 mg, 1,000 mg of salicylate (as choline and magnesium salicylate)
Solution: 500 mg of salicylate/5 ml (as choline and magnesium salicylate); 870 mg/5 ml (as choline salicylate)

Indications, route, and dosage
Arthritis, mild
Adults: 1 to 2 teaspoonfuls (5 to 10 ml) or 1 to 2 tablets b.i.d. Total daily dose can also be given at one time.
Rheumatoid arthritis and osteoarthritis
Adults: 2 to 3 teaspoonfuls (10 to 15 ml) or 2 to 3 tablets b.i.d. Total daily dose can also be given at one time.

Each 500-mg tablet or 5 ml of liquid choline and magnesium salicylate or 870 mg of choline salicylate is equal in salicylate content to 650 mg of aspirin.
Juvenile rheumatoid arthritis
Children: 107 to 133 mg/kg/day of choline salicylate in divided doses.
Mild-to-moderate pain
Children: 2 g/m²/day in 4 to 6 divided doses or as shown below.
Children age 2 to 4: 217.5 mg (1.3 ml) q 4 hours, p.r.n.
Children age 4 to 6: 326.5 mg (1.9 ml) q 4 hours, p.r.n.
Children age 6 to 9: 435 mg (2.5 ml) q 4 hours, p.r.n.
Children age 9 to 11: 543.8 mg (3.1 ml) q 4 hours, p.r.n.
Children age 11 to 12: 652.5 mg (3.8 ml) q 4 hours, p.r.n.
Adults: 2 to 3 g P.O. daily in divided doses.

Action and kinetics
• *Analgesic action:* Choline salicylates produce analgesia by an ill-defined effect on the hypothalamus (central action) and by blocking generation of pain impulses (peripheral action). The peripheral action may involve inhibition of prostaglandin synthesis.
• *Anti-inflammatory action:* These drugs exert their anti-inflammatory effect by inhibiting prostaglandin synthesis; they may also inhibit the synthesis or action of other inflammation mediators.
• *Antipyretic action:* Choline salicylates relieve fever by acting on the hypothalamic heat-regulating center to produce peripheral vasodilation. This increases peripheral blood supply and promotes sweating, which leads to loss of heat and to cooling by evaporation.

These drugs do not affect platelet aggregation and should not be used to prevent thrombosis.

• *Kinetics in adults:* These salicylate salts are absorbed rapidly and completely from the GI tract. Peak therapeutic effect occurs in 2 hours. Protein binding depends on concentration and ranges from 75% to 90%, decreasing as serum concentration increases. Severe toxic side effects may occur at serum concentrations greater than 400 mcg/ml. Drugs are hydrolyzed to salicylate in the liver. Metabolites are excreted in urine.

Contraindications and precautions

These drugs are contraindicated in patients with known hypersensitivity to salicylates or other nonsteroidal anti-inflammatory drugs (NSAIDs) and when GI ulcer or GI bleeding are present.

Choline salicylates should be used cautiously in patients with a history of GI disease and increased risk of GI bleeding because the drug may worsen these conditions; and in patients with decreased renal or hepatic function because of potential for drug accumulation (especially magnesium salicylate).

Salicylates may mask the signs and symptoms of acute infection (fever, myalgia, erythema); carefully evaluate patients with high risk (for example, those with diabetes). Choline salicylates are usually well tolerated by patients with "triad" symptoms, as compared with aspirin or other NSAIDs. Use of choline salicylates should be avoided in the third trimester of pregnancy.

Interactions

Concomitant use of choline salicylates with drugs that are highly protein-bound (phenytoin, sulfonylureas, warfarin) may cause displacement of either drug, and adverse effects. Monitor therapy closely for both drugs. The adverse GI effects of choline salicylates may be potentiated by concomitant use of other GI-irritant drugs (such as steroids, antibiotics, and other NSAIDs). Use together with caution. Choline salicylates decrease renal clearance of lithium carbonate, thus increasing serum lithium levels and the risk of adverse effects. Ammonium chloride and other urine acidifiers increase choline salicylate blood levels; monitor for choline salicylate blood levels and thus toxicity. Antacids in high doses, and other urine alkalizers, decrease choline salicylate blood levels; monitor for decreased salicylate effect. Corticosteroids enhance salicylate elimination; monitor for decreased effect. Food and antacids delay and decrease absorption of choline salicylates.

Effects on diagnostic tests

Choline salicylates may interfere with urinary glucose analysis performed via Clinistix, Tes-Tape, Clinitest, and Benedict's solution. These drugs also interfere with urinary 5-hydroxyindole acetic acid (5-HIAA) and vanillylmandelic acid (VMA).

Adverse reactions

• DERM: rash, bruising.
• EENT: tinnitus, hearing loss.
• GI: nausea, vomiting, GI distress, occult bleeding.

• Other: hypersensitivity manifested by anaphylaxis or asthma, abnormal liver function tests, hepatitis.

Note: Drug should be discontinued if the following occur: hypersensitivity (aspirin-induced bronchospasm) reaction, severe hepatic dysfunction, or signs and symptoms of salicylism.

Overdose and treatment

Clinical manifestations of overdose include respiratory alkalosis, hyperpnea, and tachypnea from increased CO_2 production and direct stimulation of the respiratory center.

To treat overdose of choline salicylates, empty stomach immediately by inducing emesis with ipecac syrup, if patient is conscious, or by gastric lavage. Administer activated charcoal via nasogastric tube. Provide symptomatic and supportive measures (respiratory support and correction of fluid and electrolyte imbalances). Monitor laboratory parameters and vital signs closely. Hemodialysis is effective in removing choline salicylates but is used only in severe poisoning.

▶ Special considerations

• The safety of long-term choline salicylate use in children under age 14 has not been established.
• Because of epidemiologic association with Reye's syndrome, the Centers for Disease Control recommend that children with chicken pox or flulike symptoms should not be given salicylates.
• Febrile, dehydrated children can develop toxicity rapidly. Ordinarily, they should not receive more than five doses in 24 hours.
• Children may be more susceptible to toxic effects of salicylates. Use with caution.
• Use salicylates with caution in patients with a history of GI disease, increased risk of GI bleeding, or decreased renal function.
• Administer non-enteric-coated tablets with food or after meals to minimize gastric upset.
• Tablets may be chewed, broken, or crumbled and administered with food or fluids to aid swallowing.
• Do not crush enteric-coated tablets.
• Patient should take drug with enough water or milk to ensure passage into stomach. Patient should sit up for 15 to 30 minutes after taking it to prevent lodging in esophagus.
• Monitor vital signs frequently, especially temperature.
• Salicylates may mask the signs and symptoms of acute infection (fever, myalgia, erythema); carefully evaluate patients at risk for infections, such as those with diabetes.
• Monitor CBC; platelets; prothrombin times; and BUN, serum creatinine, and liver function studies periodically during salicylate therapy to detect abnormalities.
• Assess hearing function before and periodically during therapy to prevent ototoxicity.
• Assess level of pain and inflammation before initiation of therapy. Evaluate effectiveness of therapy as evidenced by relief of these symptoms.
• Assess signs and symptoms of potential hemorrhage, such as petechiae, bruising, coffee ground vomitus, and black tarry stools.

• If fever or illness causes fluid depletion, dosage should be reduced.

• Do not mix choline salicylates with antacids.

• Administer oral solution of choline salicylate mixed with fruit juice. Follow with sufficient water to ensure passage into stomach.

• Monitor serum magnesium levels to prevent possible magnesium toxicity.

Information for parents and patient
• Tell parents to have child take tablet with 8 oz of water and not to lie down for 15 to 30 minutes after swallowing the drug.

• Tell parent to have patient take the medication 30 minutes before or 2 hours after meals, or with food or milk if gastric irritation occurs.

• Explain that taking the drug as directed is necessary to achieve the desired effect; 1 to 4 weeks of treatment may be needed before benefit is seen.

• Advise parents that patient on chronic salicylate therapy may need follow-up tests.

• Advise parents to avoid giving patient aspirin-containing medication without medical approval.

• Explain that use of alcoholic beverages with salicylates may cause increased GI irritation and possibly GI bleeding.

• Patient should take missed dose as soon as he remembers, unless it is almost time for next dose; then skip the missed dose and return to regular schedule.

• Patient should not take this drug for more than 10 consecutive days unless otherwise directed.

chorionic gonadotropin, human (HCG)
A.P.L., Chorex 5, Chorex 10, Chorigon, Choron 10, Corgonject-5, Follutein Gonic, Pregnyl, Profasi HP

• Classification: spermatogenesis stimulant (gonadotropin)

How supplied
Available by prescription only
Injection: 200 USP units/ml, 500 USP units/ml, 1,000 USP units/ml, 2,000 USP units/ml

Indications, route, and dosage
Nonobstructive prepubertal cryptorchidism
Children age 4 to 9: 5,000 USP units I.M. every other day for 4 doses or 4,000 USP units I.M. three times a week for 3 weeks or 15 doses of 500 to 1,000 USP units I.M. given over 6 weeks.

Action and kinetics
• *Spermatogenesis stimulant action:* HCG stimulates androgen production in Leydig's cells of the testis and causes maturation of the cells lining the seminiferous tubules of the testes.

• *Kinetics in adults:* HCG must be administered I.M. Peak blood concentrations occur within 6 hours. HCG is distributed primarily into the testes and the ovaries. Metabolism is unknown. HCG is excreted in urine.

Contraindications and precautions
HCG is contraindicated in patients with precocious puberty or androgen-responsive cancer (prostatic, testicular, male breast), because it stimulates androgen production; and in patients with known hypersensitivity to HCG. HCG should be used cautiously in patients with asthma, seizure disorders, migraines, or cardiac or renal diseases, because it may exacerbate these conditions.

Interactions
None reported.

Effects on diagnostic tests
None reported.

Adverse reactions
• CNS: headache, fatigue, irritability, restlessness, depression.

• GU: early puberty (growth of testes, penis, pubic and axillary hair; voice change, down on upper lip; growth of body hair).

• Local: pain at injection site.

• Other: gynecomastia, edema.

▶ Special considerations
• Treating prepubertal cryptorchidism with HCG can help predict future need for orchidopexy. Induction of androgen secretion may induce precocious puberty in patient treated for cryptorchidism.

• Young male patients receiving HCG must be observed carefully for the development of precocious puberty.

• Carefully monitor patients with disorders that may be aggravated by fluid retention.

Information for parents and patient
• Teach parents how to assess for edema and to report it promptly.

• Advise parents to report signs of precocious puberty promptly. Instruct them to report the following: axillary, facial, or pubic hair; penile growth; acne; and deepening of voice.

cimetidine
Tagamet

• Classification: antiulcer agent (histamine₂-receptor antagonist)

How supplied
Available by prescription only
Tablets: 200 mg, 300 mg, 400 mg, 800 mg
Injection: 150 mg/ml
Liquid: 300 mg/5 ml

Indications, route, and dosage
Active duodenal or benign gastric ulcer
†*Neonates:* 10 to 20 mg/kg/day P.O., divided q 6 to 12 hours.

†*Infants and children:* 20 to 40 mg/kg/day to maximum of 1.2 g, divided q 6 hours.

Adults: 800 mg P.O. h.s. for 4 to 6 weeks. Alternatively, some clinicians give 300 mg P.O. q.i.d. (with meals and h.s.) or 400 mg P.O. b.i.d. (in the morning and h.s.). Some patients may require 1,600 mg P.O. h.s.

Maintenance therapy for duodenal ulcer
Adults: 400 mg P.O. h.s.

Duodenal ulcers and hypersecretory conditions; prophylaxis of stress ulcers, †gastroesophageal reflux, gastric ulcers; †preoperative use to prevent aspiration pneumonitis
†*Children:* 20 to 40 mg/kg/day given in divided doses q 6 hours.

Symptomatic relief of gastroesophageal reflux
Adults: 300 mg P.O. q.i.d., before meals and h.s.

Upper GI bleeding, peptic esophagitis, stress ulcer
Children: 20 to 40 mg/kg daily in divided doses.
Adults: 1 to 2 g I.V. or P.O. daily, in four divided doses.

Action and kinetics

• *Antiulcer action:* Cimetidine competitively inhibits histamine's action at histamine$_2$ (H$_2$) receptors in gastric parietal cells, inhibiting basal and nocturnal gastric acid secretion (such as from stimulation by food, caffeine, insulin, histamine, betazole, or pentagastrin). Cimetidine may also enhance gastromucosal defense and healing.

A 300-mg oral or parenteral dose inhibits about 80% of gastric acid secretion for 4 to 5 hours.

• *Kinetics in adults:* Approximately 60% to 75% of oral dose is absorbed. Absorption rate (but not extent) may be affected by food. Cimetidine is distributed to many body tissues. About 15% to 20% of drug is protein-bound. Cimetidine apparently crosses the placenta and is distributed in breast milk. Approximately 30% to 40% of dose is metabolized in the liver. Drug has a half-life of 2 hours in patients with normal renal function. Cimetidine is excreted primarily in urine (48% of oral dose, 75% of parenteral dose); 10% of oral dose is excreted in feces. Some drug is also excreted in breast milk.

Contraindications and precautions

Cimetidine is contraindicated in patients with cimetidine allergy or cross-sensitivity to other H$_2$-receptor antagonists.

Use caution when administering large parenteral doses to patients with asthma, because the drug may exacerbate the symptoms of the disease.

Use caution when administering cimetidine to patients with cirrhosis, severely impaired hepatic function, and moderately to severely impaired renal function, because drug accumulation may occur.

Interactions

Cimetidine decreases the metabolism of the following drugs, thus increasing potential toxicity and possibly necessitating dosage reduction: beta-adrenergic blockers (such as propranolol), phenytoin, lidocaine, procainamide, quinidine, benzodiazepines, disulfiram, metronidazole, theophylline, aminophylline, tricyclic antidepressants, oral contraceptives, isoniazid, warfarin, and carmustine.

The ability of cimetidine to inhibit drug metabolism is currently being evaluated as a potential treatment of acetaminophen overdose. (It may decrease the formation of hepatotoxic metabolites.)

Effects on diagnostic tests

Cimetidine may antagonize pentagastrin's effect during gastric acid secretion tests; it may cause false-negative results in skin tests using allergen extracts.

Cimetidine therapy increases prolactin levels, serum alkaline phosphatase levels, and serum creatinine levels.

FD and C blue dye #2 used in Tagamet tablets may impair interpretation of Hemoccult and Gastroccult tests on gastric content aspirate. Be sure to wait at least 15 minutes after tablet administration before drawing the sample, and follow test manufacturer's instructions closely.

Adverse reactions

• CNS: *dizziness*, confusion (particularly in critically ill patients), headache, depression, *agitation, restlessness.*
• CV: *bradycardia, hypotension.*
• GI: jaundice, *diarrhea, GI upset.*
• GU: interstitial nephritis, reversible impotence, urinary retention, mild *gynecomastia* with prolonged use.
• HEMA: agranulocytosis (rare), *neutropenia* (rare), thrombocytopenia, aplastic anemia.
• Other: *rash,* allergic reaction, pain at I.M. injection site, fever (rare), *urticaria, myalgia.*

Overdose and treatment

Clinical effects of overdose include respiratory failure and tachycardia. Overdose is rare; intake of up to 10 g has caused no untoward effects.

Support respiration and maintain a patent airway. Induce emesis or use gastric lavage; follow with activated charcoal to prevent further absorption. Treat tachycardia with propranolol if necessary.

▶ Special considerations

• Safe use in children under age 16 has not been determined.
• Neonatal use remains experimental.
• Give single daily dose at bedtime, b.i.d. doses morning and evening, and multiple doses with meals and at bedtime.
• When administering drug I.V., do not exceed recommended infusion rates (I.V. push, 2 to 5 minutes; intermittent infusion, 15 to 30 minutes) because this may increase the risk of adverse cardiovascular effects.
• Antacids may decrease drug absorption; give antacids at least 1 hour apart from cimetidine.
• Patients with renal disease may require a modified dosage schedule.
• Avoid discontinuing drug abruptly.
• For I.V. use, cimetidine must not be diluted before administration. Do not dilute drug with sterile water for injection; use normal saline solution, dextrose 5% or 10% injection, lactated Ringer's solution, or 5% sodium bicarbonate injection to a total volume of 20 ml.

• After administration of the liquid via nasogastric tube, tube should be flushed afterward to clear it and ensure drug's passage to stomach.
• Hemodialysis removes cimetidine; schedule dose after dialysis session.
• Other unlabeled uses include pancreatic insufficiency, hives, heartburn, psoriasis, and hirsutism.

Information for parents and patient
• Patient should take drug as directed, preferably with or after meals and at bedtime, and continue taking it even after pain subsides, to allow for adequate healing. Patient should avoid smoking, caffeine, and alcohol, which may increase gastric acid secretion and worsen disease.
• Inform parents about adverse reactions that should be reported.
• Warn parents and patient not to change dosage or discontinue drug without medical approval.

---

cisplatin (cis-platinum)
Platinol

• Classification: antineoplastic (cell cycle-phase nonspecific)

How supplied
Available by prescription only
Injection: 10-mg and 50-mg vials (lyophilized)

Indications, route, and dosage
Dosage and indications may vary. Check current literature for recommended protocol.
†*Neuroblastoma,* †*osteogenic sarcoma*
Children: 90 mg/m² I.V. once every 3 weeks; or 30 mg/m² I.V. once weekly.
†*Recurrent brain tumors*
Children: 60 mg/m² I.V. once daily for 2 consecutive days every 3 to 4 weeks.
Note: Prehydration and mannitol diuresis may significantly reduce renal toxicity and ototoxicity.

Action and kinetics
• *Antineoplastic action:* Cisplatin exerts its cytotoxic effects by binding with DNA and inhibiting DNA synthesis and, to a lesser extent, by inhibition of protein and RNA synthesis. Cisplatin also acts as a bifunctional alkylating agent, causing intrastrand and interstrand cross-links of DNA. Interstrand cross-linking appears to correlate well with the cytotoxicity of the drug.
• *Kinetics in adults:* Cisplatin is not administered orally or intramuscularly. Cisplatin distributes widely into tissues, with the highest concentrations found in the kidneys, liver, and prostate. Cisplatin can accumulate in body tissues; drug can be detected up to 6 months after the last dose. It does not readily cross the blood-brain barrier. The drug is extensively and irreversibly bound to plasma proteins and tissue proteins. Its metabolic fate is unclear. Cisplatin is excreted primarily unchanged in urine. In patients with normal renal function, the half-life of the initial elimination phase

is 25 to 79 minutes and the terminal phase 58 to 78 hours. The terminal half-life of total cisplatin is up to 10 days.

Contraindications and precautions
Cisplatin is contraindicated in patients with a history of hypersensitivity to cisplatin or other platinum-containing compounds. Patients who have been previously exposed to these agents should undergo skin testing before cisplatin therapy because of potential for allergic reaction. The drug is also contraindicated in patients with myelosuppression or hearing impairment because drug may worsen these conditions.
Cisplatin should be used with caution or dosage adjusted in patients with impaired renal function because of the drug's nephrotoxic effects. It is usually not used in patients with a creatinine clearance below 50 ml/minute. Perform baseline audiometry before therapy begins. Cisplatin can impair fertility. Aspermia has been reported after cisplatin therapy.

Interactions
Concomitant use with aminoglycosides potentiates the cumulative nephrotoxicity caused by cisplatin. Additive toxicity is the mechanism for this interaction. Therefore, aminoglycosides should not be used within 2 weeks of cisplatin therapy. Concomitant use with loop diuretics increases the risk of ototoxicity. Closely monitor the patient's audiologic status.

Effects on diagnostic tests
Cisplatin therapy may increase BUN, serum creatinine, and serum uric acid levels. It may decrease creatinine clearance, serum calcium, magnesium, phosphate, and potassium levels, indicating nephrotoxicity.

Adverse reactions
• CNS: *peripheral neuritis,* loss of taste, seizures, headache.
• EENT: tinnitus, high-frequency hearing loss may occur in both ears. *Ototoxicity* may be more severe in children.
• GI: *nausea and vomiting,* beginning 1 to 4 hours after dose and lasting 24 hours; diarrhea; metallic taste; stomatitis.
• GU: more prolonged and severe renal toxicity with repeated courses of therapy (dose-limiting), *renal damage.*
• HEMA: mild myelosuppression in 25% to 30% of patients; *bone marrow depression, hemolysis,* leukopenia; thrombocytopenia; anemia; nadirs in circulating platelets and leukocytes on days 18 to 23, with recovery by day 39, *hemolytic uremic syndrome.*
• Other: anaphylactoid reaction, hyperuricemia, *fever, Raynaud's syndrome, hypomagnesemia, hypocalcemia, hypokalemia.*
Note: Drug should be discontinued if signs of neurotoxicity appear.

Overdose and treatment
Clinical manifestations of overdose include leukopenia, thrombocytopenia, nausea, and vomiting.
Treatment is generally supportive and includes transfusion of blood components, antibiotics for pos-

sible infections, and antiemetics. Cisplatin can be removed by dialysis, but only within 3 hours after administration.

▶ **Special considerations**
• Pediatric dosage of cisplastin has not been fully established. Unlabeled uses of cisplatin include osteogenic sarcoma and neuroblastoma.
• Follow all established procedures for the safe and proper handling, administration, and disposal of chemotherapy.
• Vital signs and patency of catheter or I.V. line throughout administration should be monitored.
• Attempt to alleviate or reduce anxiety in parents and patient family before treatment.
• Review hematologic status and creatinine clearance before therapy.
• Reconstitute 10-mg vial with 10 ml and 50-mg vial with 50 ml of sterile water for injection to yield a concentration of 1 mg/ml. The drug may be diluted further in a saline-containing solution for I.V. infusion.
• I.V. infusion is given over 6 to 8 hours. Administration by I.V. push increases risk of nephrotoxicity.
• Do not use aluminum needles for reconstitution or administration of cisplatin; a black precipitate may form. Use stainless steel needles.
• Drug is stable for 24 hours in normal saline solutions at room temperature. Do not refrigerate because precipitation may occur. Discard any solution containing precipitate.
• Infusions are most stable in chloride-containing solutions, such as normal saline, 0.5 normal saline, or 0.25 normal saline.
• Mannitol may be given as a 12.5-g I.V. bolus before starting cisplatin infusion. Follow by infusion of mannitol at rate up to 10 g/hour, as necessary, to maintain urine output during cisplatin infusion and for 6 to 24 hours after infusion.
• Hydrate patient with normal saline solution before giving drug. Maintain urine output of 100 ml/hour for 4 consecutive hours before and for 24 hours after infusion. Weigh all diapers to determine urine output.
• Hydrate patient by encouraging oral fluids intake when possible.
• Avoid all I.M. injections when platelets are low.
• Determine baseline weight.
• Nausea and vomiting may be severe and protracted (up to 24 hours). Antiemetics can be started 24 hours before therapy. Monitor fluid intake and output. Continue I.V. hydration until patient can tolerate adequate oral intake.
• High-dose metoclopramide (2 mg/kg I.V.) has been used to prevent and treat nausea and vomiting. Dexamethasome 10 to 20 mg has been given intravenously with metoclopramide to help alleviate nausea and vomiting. Some clinicians recommend a combination of diphenhydramine and metoclopramide
• Monitor CBC, platelet count, and renal function studies before initial and subsequent doses. Do not repeat dose unless platelet count is over 100,000/mm³, WBC count is over 4,000/mm³, serum creatinine level is under 1.5 mg/dl, or BUN level is under 25 mg/dl.
• Renal toxicity becomes more severe with repeated doses. Renal function should return to normal before

next dose can be given, but drug can be given if it doesn't.
• Monitor electrolytes extensively; aggressive supplementation is often required after a course of therapy. Hypomagnesemia is common and often requires magnesium supplementation.
• Anaphylactoid reaction usually responds to immediate treatment with epinephrine, corticosteroids, or antihistamines.
• Drug is given with Adriamycin for osteosarcoma.
• Avoid contact with skin. If contact occurs, wash drug off immediately with soap and water.

Information for parents and patient
• Advise parents to encourage the child to drink plenty of fluids to facilitate uric acid excretion.
• Advise parents and patient to report numbness and tingling (peripheral neuropathy) and tremors or weakness (hypomagnesemia).
• Tell parents and patient to report tinnitus immediately, to prevent permanent hearing loss. Patient should have audiometric tests before initial and subsequent courses.
• Emphasize the importance of continuing drug despite nausea and vomiting, and of keeping appointments for periodic blood work.
• Advise parents to call promptly if symptoms of infection or bleeding are present.
• Advise parents to prevent patient's exposure to persons with bacterial or viral infections because chemotherapy can increase susceptibility to infection. Parents should report any signs of infection promptly. They should promptly report exposure to chicken pox in susceptible patients.
• Instruct parents and patient in proper oral hygiene including caution when using toothbrush and dental floss.
• Advise parents that dental work should be completed before initiation of therapy whenever possible, or should be delayed until blood counts are normal.
• Advise parents that immunizations should be avoided during cisplatin therapy if possible.
• Patient should avoid contact sports when platelets are low.

clemastine fumarate
Tavist, Tavist-1

• Classification: antihistamine, H_1-receptor antagonist (ethanolamine-derivative)

How supplied
Available by prescription only
Tablets: 1.34 mg, 2.68 mg
Syrup: 0.7 mg/5 ml

Indications, route, and dosage
Rhinitis, allergy symptoms
Children age 6 to 11: 0.67 mg b.i.d.; not to exceed 4.02 mg/day.
Children age 12 and older and adults: 1.34 to 2.68

mg P.O. b.i.d. or t.i.d. Maximum recommended daily dosage is 8.04 mg.

Allergic skin manifestation of urticaria and angioedema

Children age 6 to 11: 1.34 mg b.i.d.; not to exceed 4.02 mg/day.

Children age 12 and older and adults: 2.68 mg up to t.i.d. maximum.

Action and kinetics

• *Antihistamine action:* Antihistamines compete with histamine for histamine H_1-receptor sites on the smooth muscle of the bronchi, GI tract, uterus, and large blood vessels; by binding to cellular receptors, they prevent access of histamine and suppress histamine-induced allergic symptoms, even though they do not prevent its release.

• *Kinetics in adults:* Clemastine is absorbed readily from the GI tract; action begins in 15 to 30 minutes and peaks in 2 to 7 hours. Clemastine is excreted in urine.

Contraindications and precautions

Clemastine is contraindicated in children with known hypersensitivity to this drug or other antihistamines with similar chemical structures (carbinoxamine and diphenhydramine); during an acute asthmatic attack, because it thickens bronchial secretions; and in patients who have taken MAO inhibitors within the preceding 2 weeks.

Clemastine should be used with caution in patients with narrow-angle glaucoma; in those with pyloro-duodenal obstruction or urinary bladder obstruction from narrowing of the bladder neck, because of their marked anticholinergic effects; in patients with cardiovascular disease, hypertension, or hyperthyroidism, because of the risk of palpitations and tachycardia; and in patients with renal disease, diabetes, bronchial asthma, urinary retention, or stenosing peptic ulcers.

Clemastine is not indicated for use in premature infants or neonates, because such use has caused seizures and other severe reactions. Children, especially those under age 6, may experience paradoxical hyperexcitability.

Interactions

MAO inhibitors interfere with the detoxification of clemastine and thus prolong and intensify their central depressant and anticholinergic effects. Additive CNS depression may occur when clemastine is given concomitantly with other CNS depressants, such as alcohol, barbiturates, tranquilizers, sleeping aids, or antianxiety agents.

Clemastine may diminish the effects of sulfonyl-ureas and may partially counteract the anticoagulant effects of heparin.

Effects on diagnostic tests

Discontinue clemastine 4 days before diagnostic skin tests; antihistamines can prevent, reduce, or mask positive skin test response.

Adverse reactions

• CNS: sedation, drowsiness.
• CV: hypotension, palpitations, tachycardia.
• DERM: rash, urticaria.
• GI: epigastric distress, anorexia, nausea, vomiting, constipation, dry mouth.
• GU: urinary retention.
• HEMA: hemolytic anemia, thrombocytopenia, agranulocytosis.
• Respiratory: thick bronchial secretions.

Overdose and treatment

Clinical manifestations of overdose may include either CNS depression (sedation, reduced mental alertness, apnea, and cardiovascular collapse) or CNS stimulation (insomnia, hallucinations, tremors, and seizures). *Anticholinergic symptoms, such as dry mouth, flushed skin, fixed and dilated pupils, and GI symptoms, are common, especially in children.*

Treat overdose by inducing emesis with ipecac syrup (in conscious patient), followed by activated charcoal to reduce further drug absorption. Use gastric lavage if patient is unconscious or ipecac fails. Treat hypotension with vasopressors, and control seizures with diazepam or phenytoin. *Do not give stimulants.*

▶ Special considerations

• Children, especially those under age 6, may experience paradoxical hyperexcitability with restlessness, insomnia, nervousness, euphoria, tremors, and seizures.

• Drug is contraindicated during an acute asthma attack because it may not alleviate the symptoms and because antimuscarinic effects can cause thickening of secretions.

• Reduce GI distress by giving drug with food; give sugarless gum, lollipops, or ice chips to relieve dry mouth; increase fluid intake (if allowed) or humidify air to decrease adverse effect of thickened secretions.

• Clemastine is indicated for treatment of urticaria only at dosages of 2.68 mg up to t.i.d.

Information for parents and patient

• Advise patient to take drug with meals or snack to prevent gastric upset and to use any of the following measures to relieve dry mouth: warm water rinses, artificial saliva, ice chips, or sugarless gum or candy. Patient should avoid overusing mouthwash, which may add to dryness (alcohol content) and destroy normal flora.

• Warn parents that child should avoid hazardous activities that require balance or alertness until extent of CNS effects are known. Tell them to seek medical approval before administering tranquilizers, sedatives, pain relievers, or sleeping medications.

• Warn parents to discontinue drug 4 days before diagnostic skin tests, to preserve accuracy of tests.

---

‡May contain sulfites ◆May contain tartrazine ◆◆May contain benzyl alcohol

■■■■■■■■■■

clindamycin hydrochloride
Cleocin HCl

clindamycin palmitate hydrochloride
Cleocin Pediatric

clindamycin phosphate
Cleocin Phosphate, Cleocin T

• Classification: antibiotic (lincomycin derivative)

How supplied
Available by prescription only
Capsules: 75 mg, 150 mg
Solution: 75 mg/5 ml
Injection: 150 mg/ml
Topical solution: 10 mg/ml

Indications, route, and dosage
Infections caused by sensitive organisms
Neonates: 15 to 30 mg/kg/day, divided q 6 to 8 hours.
Children over age 1 month: 8 to 25 mg/kg P.O. daily, divided q 6 to 8 hours; or 15 to 40 mg/kg I.M. or I.V. daily, divided q 6 hours.
Adults: 150 to 450 mg P.O. q 6 hours; or 300 mg I.M. or I.V. q 6, 8, or 12 hours. Up to 2,700 mg I.M. or I.V. daily, divided q 6, 8, or 12 hours. May be used for severe infections.
Acne vulgaris
Adolescents and adults: Apply thin film of topical solution to affected areas b.i.d.

Action and kinetics
• *Antibacterial action:* Clindamycin inhibits bacterial protein synthesis by binding to ribosome's 50S subunit. Clindamycin may produce bacteriostatic or bactericidal effects on susceptible bacteria, including most aerobic gram-positive cocci and several anaerobic gram-negative and gram-positive organisms. It is considered a first-line drug in the treatment of *Bacteroides fragilis* and most other gram-positive and gram-negative anaerobes. It is also effective against *Mycoplasma pneumoniae, Leptotrichia buccalis,* and some gram-positive cocci and bacilli.
• *Kinetics in adults:* When administered orally, clindamycin is absorbed rapidly and almost completely from the GI tract, regardless of formulation. Peak concentrations of 1.9 to 3.9 mcg/ml occur in 45 to 60 minutes. Drug may also be given I.M. with good absorption. Peak concentrations occur in about 3 hours. With 300-mg dose, peak concentrations are about 6 mcg/ml; with 600-mg dose, about 10 mcg/ml.
Clindamycin is distributed widely to most body tissues and fluids (except CSF) and crosses the placenta. Approximately 93% of drug is bound to plasma proteins.
Partially metablized to inactive metabolites, about 10% dose is excreted unchanged in urine; the remainder as inactive metabolites (with some drug excreted in breast milk). Plasma half-life is 2½ to 3 hours in patients with normal renal function; 3½ to 5 hours in anephric patients; and 7 to 14 hours in patients with hepatic disease. Peritoneal dialysis and hemodialysis do not remove drug.

Contraindications and precautions
Clindamycin is contraindicated in patients hypersensitive to the drug or to lincomycin, and those with a history of inflammatory bowel disease or antibiotic-induced colitis.
Clindamycin should be administered cautiously to patients with renal or hepatic dysfunction because it may exacerbate these conditions; to patients with asthma or significant allergies; to newborns; and to patients with tartrazine sensitivity. Topical solution should be administered cautiously to atopic patients because of potential for contact dermatitis.

Interactions
When used concomitantly, clindamycin may potentiate the action of neuromuscular blocking agents (such as tubocurarine and pancuronium). Concomitant use with kaolin products may reduce GI absorption of clindamycin. Concomitant use with such antidiarrheals as diphenoxylate and opiates may prolong or worsen clindamycin-induced diarrhea by reducing excretion of bacterial toxins. When used concomitantly, erythromycin may act as an antagonist, blocking clindamycin from reaching its site of action. When used concurrently with other acne preparations (such as benzoyl peroxide or tretinoin), topical clindamycin may cause a cumulative irritant or drying effect. Reportedly, clindamycin inactivates aminoglycosides in vitro.

Effects on diagnostic tests
Liver function test results may become abnormal in some patients during clindamycin therapy.

Adverse reactions
• DERM: maculopapular rash, urticaria, erythema multiforme, contact dermatitis and dryness (with topical solution).
• EENT: stinging in eyes (with topical solution).
• GI: nausea; vomiting; abdominal pain; diarrhea; pseudomembranous enterocolitis (usually from *Clostridium difficile*); esophagitis; flatulence; anorexia; bloody or tarry stools; dysphagia; *elevated serum glutamic-oxaloacetic transaminase (SGOT), alkaline phosphatase, and bilirubin levels, jaundice.*
• HEMA: *transient leukopenia, eosinophilia, thrombocytopenia.*
• Local: pain, induration, sterile abscess (with I.M. injection); *thrombophlebitis, pain (with I.V. administration).*
• Other: unpleasant or bitter taste, anaphylaxis, sensitization and systemic adverse effects (with topical solution), *hypersensitivity reaction; hypotension with rapid I.V. administration, superinfection.*
    Note: Drug should be discontinued if patient develops persistent diarrhea or hypersensitivity reaction.

Overdose and treatment
No information available.

▶ Special considerations
• Administer drug cautiously, if at all, to neonates and infants. Monitor closely, especially for diarrhea. Drug is not recommended for use in infants younger than 1 month.
• Clindamycin is not indicated for the treatment of meningitis because of poor CNS penetration.
• Culture and sensitivity tests should be done before treatment starts and should be repeated as needed.
• Do not refrigerate reconstituted oral solution, because it will thicken. Drug remains stable for 2 weeks at room temperature.
• I.M. preparation should be given deep I.M. Rotate sites. Doses exceeding 600 mg are not recommended.
• I.M. injection may increase creatinine phosphokinase levels because of muscle irritation.
• For I.V. infusion, dilute each 300 mg in 50 ml of dextrose 5%, normal saline, or lactated Ringer's solution and give no faster than 30 mg/minute. Do not administer more than 1.2 g/hour. Monitor I.V. site; applying warm packs may ease discomfort at I.V. site.
• Give oral forms with food to decrease GI upset. Absorption may only be slightly delayed.
• Do not physically mix with any other medications such as aminophylline, ampicillin, barbiturates, calcium, gluconate, magnesium sulfate, phenytoin.
• Topical form may produce adverse systemic effects.
• Monitor renal, hepatic, and hematopoietic functions during prolonged therapy.
• Do not administer diphenoxylate compound (Lomotil) to treat drug-induced diarrhea because this may worsen and prolong diarrhea. Monitor patient's output. Check for melena.

Information for the parents and patient
• Warn patient that I.M. injection may be painful.
• Instruct parents to report adverse effects – especially diarrhea. Warn them not to treat diarrhea themselves.
• Advise parents and patient to take capsules with full glass of water to prevent dysphagia.
• Instruct parents and patient using topical solution to wash, rinse, and dry affected areas before application. Warn them not to use topical solution near eyes, nose, mouth, or other mucous membranes, and caution them to avoid sharing washcloths and towels with family members.

clonazepam
Klonopin, Rivotril

• Classification: anticonvulsant (benzodiazepine)
• Controlled substance schedule IV

How supplied
Available by prescription only
Tablets: 0.5 mg, 1 mg, 2 mg

Indications, route, and dosage
Absence (petit mal) and atypical absence seizures; akinetic and myoclonic seizures
Children up to age 10 or weighing 30 kg or less: 0.01 to 0.03 mg/kg P.O. daily (not to exceed 0.05 mg/kg daily), divided q 8 hours. Increase dosage by 0.25 to 0.5 mg q 3rd day to a maximum maintenance dosage of 0.1 to 0.2 mg/kg daily.
Adults: Initial dosage should not exceed 1.5 mg P.O. daily, divided into three doses. May be increased by 0.5 to 1 mg q 3 days until seizures are controlled. Maximum recommended daily dosage is 20 mg.
Nocturnal myoclonus
Adults: 0.5 mg t.i.d. or 1.5 mg at bedtime.

Action and kinetics
• *Anticonvulsant action:* Mechanism of anticonvulsant activity is unknown; clonazepam appears to act in the limbic system, thalamus, and hypothalamus.
   Clonazepam is used to treat myoclonic, atonic, and absence seizures resistant to other anticonvulsants and to suppress or eliminate attacks of sleep-related nocturnal myoclonus (restless legs syndrome).
• *Kinetics in adults:* Clonazepam is well absorbed from the GI tract; action begins in 20 to 60 minutes and persists for 6 to 8 hours in infants and children and up to 12 hours in adults. Clonazepam is distributed widely throughout the body; it is approximately 47% protein-bound. Clonazepam is metabolized by the liver to several metabolites. Clonazepam is excreted in urine.

Contraindications and precautions
Clonazepam is contraindicated in patients with known hypersensitivity to clonazepam and other benzodiazepines and in patients with significant hepatic disease, chronic respiratory disease, and untreated open-angle glaucoma or narrow-angle glaucoma. It should be used with caution (and at lower doses) in patients with decreased renal function.

Interactions
Concomitant use of clonazepam with other CNS depressants (alcohol, narcotics, tranquilizers, anxiolytics, barbiturates) and other anticonvulsants will produce additive CNS depressant effects. Concomitant use with valproic acid may induce absence seizures.

Effects on diagnostic tests
Clonazepam may elevate liver function test values.

Adverse reactions
• CNS: *drowsiness, ataxia, behavioral disturbances,* slurred speech, tremor, confusion, headache, *CNS depression.*
• CV: thrombophlebitis, dysrhythmias (deaths have occurred).
• DERM: rash.
• EENT: *increased salivation,* diplopia, nystagmus, abnormal eye movements, rhinorrhea.
• GI: constipation, gastritis, change in appetite, nausea, abnormal thirst, sore gums.
• GU: dysuria, enuresis, nocturia, urinary retention.
• HEMA: leukopenia, thrombocytopenia, eosinophilia.

---

‡May contain sulfites   ◆May contain tartrazine   ◆ ◆May contain benzyl alcohol

• Metabolic: hypocalcemia.
• Respiratory: respiratory depression, chest congestion, shortness of breath, *increased bronchial secretions.*
   Note: Drug should be discontinued if signs of hypersensitivity occur or if liver function or hematologic tests show significant abnormalities.

Overdose and treatment

Symptoms of overdose may include ataxia, confusion, coma, decreased reflexes, and hypotension. Treat overdose with gastric lavage and supportive therapy. Vasopressors should be used to treat hypotension. Carefully monitor vital signs, ECG, and fluid and electrolyte balance. Clonazepam is not dialyzable.

▶ Special considerations

• Long-term safety in children has not been established.
• Because children, particularly young ones, are sensitive to the CNS depressant effects of benzodiazepines, caution must be exercised. A neonate whose mother took a benzodiazepine during pregnancy may exhibit withdrawal symptoms.
• Administer with milk or immediately after meals to prevent GI upset. Give antacid, if needed, at least 1 hour before or after dose to prevent interaction and ensure maximum drug absorption and effectiveness.
• Crush tablet or empty capsule and mix with food if patient has difficulty swallowing.
• Assess level of consciousness and neurologic status before and frequently during therapy for changes. Monitor for paradoxical reactions, especially early in therapy.
• Assess sleep patterns and quality. Institute seizure precautions. Assess for changes in seizure character, frequency, or duration.
• Assess vital signs frequently during therapy. Significant changes in blood pressure and heart rate may indicate impending toxicity.
• Monitor renal and hepatic function periodically to ensure adequate drug removal and prevent cumulative effects.
• Comfort measures—such as back rubs and relaxation techniques—may enhance drug effectiveness.
• As needed, institute safety measures—raised side rails and ambulatory assistance—to prevent injury. Anticipate possible rebound excitement reactions.
• Patient should be observed to prevent drug hoarding or self-dosing, especially in depressed or suicidal patients or those who are, or who have a history of being, drug-dependent. Patient's mouth should be checked to be sure tablet or capsule was swallowed.
• After prolonged use, abrupt discontinuation may precipitate status epilepticus; after long-term use, lower dosage gradually.
• Concomitant use with barbiturates or other CNS depressants may impair ability to perform tasks requiring mental alertness, such as driving a car. Warn patient to avoid such combined use.
• Neurologically impaired children may experience excessive salivation.

Information for parents and patient

• Warn parents that patient should avoid use of alcohol or other CNS depressants, such an antihistamines, analgesics, monoamine oxidase inhibitors, antidepressants, and barbiturates, while taking benzodiazepines to prevent additive depressant effects.
• Caution parents and patient that patient should not take the drug except as prescribed and should not give medication to others. Tell them not to increase the dose or frequency and to call before taking any nonprescription cold or allergy preparations that may potentiate CNS depressant effects.
• Warn parents that patient should avoid activities requiring alertness and good psychomotor coordination until the CNS response to the drug is determined. Instruct patient in safety measures to prevent injury.
• Tell parents that patient should avoid using antacids, which may delay drug absorption, unless prescribed.
• Be sure parents and patient understand that clonazepam may cause physical and psychological dependence with prolonged use.
• Warn parents that patient should not to stop taking the drug abruptly to prevent severe withdrawal symptoms after prolonged therapy.
• Tell parents and patient that smoking decreases the drug's effectiveness. Encourage patient to stop smoking during therapy.
• Teach parents signs and symptoms of adverse reactions and need to report them promptly. These are often dose-related and can be relieved by dosage adjustments.
• Explain to adolescent patient and her parents the importance of reporting suspected pregnancy immediately.

clonidine hydrochloride
Catapres, Catapres-TTS, Dixarit*

• Classification: antihypertensive (centrally acting antiadrenergic agent)

How supplied

Available by prescription only
Tablets: 0.1 mg, 0.2 mg, 0.3 mg
Transdermal: TTS-1 (releases 0.1 mg/24 hours), TTS-2 (releases 0.2 mg/24 hours), TTS-3 (releases 0.3 mg/24 hours)

Indications, route, and dosage
Hypertension

Children age 6 years and older: Initially, 0.05 mg P.O. b.i.d.; increase by 0.05 mg daily until desired response is achieved.
Adults: Initially, 0.1 mg P.O. b.i.d.; then increased by 0.1 to 0.2 mg daily or every few days until desired response is achieved. Usual dosage range is 0.2 to 1.2 mg daily in divided doses. Maximum effective dosage is 2.4 mg/day. If transdermal patch is used, apply to area of intact skin once every 7 days.
†*Prophylaxis for vascular headache*
Adults: 0.05 mg P.O. t.i.d.

---

*Canada only   †Unlabeled clinical use   Italicized adverse reactions have been observed in children.

†Adjunctive therapy in opiate withdrawal

Adults: 5 to 17 mcg/kg P.O. daily in divided doses for up to 10 days. Adjust dosage to avoid hypotension and excessive sedation, and slowly withdraw drug.

Action and kinetics

• *Antihypertensive action:* Clonidine decreases peripheral vascular resistance by stimulating central alpha-adrenergic receptors, thus decreasing cerebral sympathetic outflow; drug may also inhibit renin release. Initially, clonidine may stimulate peripheral alpha-adrenergic receptors, producing transient vasoconstriction.

• *Kinetics in adults:* Clonidine is absorbed well from the GI tract when administered orally; after oral administration, blood pressure begins to decline in 30 to 60 minutes, with maximal effect occurring in 2 to 4 hours. Clonidine is absorbed well percutaneously after transdermal topical administration; transdermal therapeutic plasma levels are achieved 2 to 3 days after initial application. Clonidine is distributed widely into the body and is metabolized in the liver, where nearly 50% is transformed to inactive metabolites. Approximately 65% of a given dose is excreted in urine; 20% is excreted in feces. Half-life of clonidine ranges from 6 to 20 hours in patients with normal renal function. After oral administration, the antihypertensive effect lasts up to 8 hours; after transdermal application, the antihypertensive effect persists for up to 7 days.

Contraindications and precautions

Clonidine is contraindicated in patients with known hypersensitivity to the drug.

Clonidine should be used cautiously in patients with severe coronary insufficiency, diabetes mellitus, myocardial infarction, cerebrovascular disease, chronic renal failure, a history of depression, or those taking other antihypertensives.

Interactions

Clonidine may increase CNS depressant effects of alcohol, barbiturates, and other sedatives.

Tricyclic antidepressants, MAO inhibitors, and tolazoline may inhibit the antihypertensive effects of clonidine; use with propranolol or other beta blockers may cause a paradoxical hypertensive response.

Effects on diagnostic tests

Clonidine may decrease urinary excretion of vanillylmandelic acid and catecholamines; it may slightly increase blood or serum glucose levels and may cause a weakly positive Coombs' test.

Adverse reactions

• CNS: drowsiness, dizziness, fatigue, sedation, nervousness, headache.
• CV: orthostatic hypotension, bradycardia, severe rebound hypertension.
• DERM: pruritus, contact dermatitis from transdermal patch.
• EENT: dry mouth.
• GI: constipation.
• GU: impotence, urinary retention.
• Metabolic: glucose intolerance.

Overdose and treatment

Clinical signs of overdose include bradycardia, CNS depression, respiratory depression, hypothermia, apnea, seizures, lethargy, agitation, irritability, diarrhea, and hypotension; hypertension has also been reported. After overdose with oral clonidine, *do not induce emesis,* because rapid onset of CNS depression can lead to aspiration. After adequate airway is ensured, empty stomach by gastric lavage followed by administration of activated charcoal. If overdose occurs in patients receiving transdermal therapy, remove transdermal patch. Further treatment is usually symptomatic and supportive.

▶ Special considerations

• Efficacy and safety in children have not been established; use drug only if potential benefit outweighs risk.
• Monitor pulse and blood pressure frequently; dosage is usually adjusted to patient's response and tolerance.
• Do not discontinue abruptly; reduce dosage gradually over 2 to 4 days to prevent severe rebound hypertension.
• Patients with renal impairment may respond to smaller doses of the drug.
• Give 4 to 6 hours before scheduled surgery.
• Clonidine may be used to lower blood pressure quickly in some hypertensive emergencies.
• Monitor weight daily during initiation of therapy, to monitor fluid retention.
• Clonidine has been used investigationally to prevent migraine, to treat severe dysmenorrhea and menopausal flushing, as an adjunct to smoking cessation therapy, and to aid rapid detoxification in the management of opiate withdrawal in opiate-dependent patients.
• Therapeutic plasma levels are achieved 2 or 3 days after applying transdermal form. Patient may need oral antihypertensive therapy during this interim period.

Information for parents and patient

• Explain disease and rationale for therapy; emphasize importance of regular medical follow-up.
• Teach parents signs and symptoms of adverse effects and need to report them; patient should also report excessive weight gain (more than 2% per week).
• Warn parents that patient should avoid hazardous activities that require mental alertness until tolerance develops to sedation, drowsiness, and other CNS effects.
• Advise parents that patient should avoid sudden position changes to minimize orthostatic hypotension.
• Advise parents and patient that ice chips, hard candy, or gum will relieve dry mouth.
• Warn parents to call for specific instructions before giving patient nonprescription cold preparations.
• Advise taking last dose at bedtime to ensure nighttime blood pressure control.
• Advise parents that patient should not discontinue drug suddenly; rebound hypertension may develop.

clorazepate dipotassium
Novoclopate*, Tranxene*, Tranxene-SD
Half Strength, Tranxene-SD

- Classification: antianxiety agent; anticonvulsant; sedative-hypnotic (benzodiazepine)
- Controlled substance schedule IV

How supplied
Available by prescription only
Capsules: 3.75 mg, 7.5 mg, 15 mg
Tablets: 3.75 mg, 7.5 mg, 11.25 mg, 15 mg, 22.5 mg

Indications, route, and dosage
As an adjunct in epilepsy
Children between age 9 and 12: Maximum recommended initial dosage is 7.5 mg P.O. b.i.d. Dosage increases should be no greater than 7.5 mg/week. Maximum daily dosage should not exceed 60 mg/day. Safety and efficacy have not been established in children younger than age 9.
Children over age 12 and adults: Maximum recommended initial dosage is 7.5 mg P.O. t.i.d. Dosage increases should be no greater than 7.5 mg/week. Maximum daily dosage should not exceed 90 mg.

Action and kinetics
- *Anxiolytic and sedative actions:* Clorazepate depresses the CNS at the limbic and subcortical levels of the brain. It produces an antianxiety effect by enhancing the effect of the neurotransmitter gamma-aminobutyric acid (GABA) on its receptor in the ascending reticular activating system, which increases inhibition and blocks both cortical and limbic arousal.
- *Anticonvulsant action:* Clorazepate suppresses the spread of seizure activity produced by epileptogenic foci in the cortex, thalamus, and limbic structures by enhancing presynaptic inhibition.
- *Kinetics in adults:* After oral administration, clorazepate is hydrolyzed in the stomach to desmethyldiazepam, which is absorbed completely and rapidly. Peak serum levels occur at 1 to 2 hours.

Clorazepate is distributed widely throughout the body. Approximately 80% to 95% of an administered dose is bound to plasma protein.

Desmethyldiazepam is metabolized in the liver to oxazepam.

Inactive glucuronide metabolites are excreted in urine. The half-life of desmethyldiazepam ranges from 30 to 200 hours.

Contraindications and precautions
Clorazepate is contraindicated in infants younger than age 30 days, in whom slow metabolism of the drug causes it to accumulate; in patients with known hypersensitivity to the drug; in patients with acute narrow-angle glaucoma or untreated open-angle glaucoma, because of the drug's possible anticholinergic effect; in patients in shock or coma, because the drug's hypnotic or hypotensive effect may be prolonged or intensified and in patients with acute alcohol intoxication who have depressed vital signs, because the drug will worsen CNS depression.

Clorazepate should be used cautiously in patients with psychoses, because the drug is rarely beneficial in such patients and may induce paradoxical reactions; in patients with myasthenia gravis or Parkinson's disease, because it may exacerbate the disorder; in patients with impaired renal or hepatic function, which prolongs elimination of the drug; in debilitated patients, who are usually more sensitive to the drug's CNS effects; and in individuals prone to addiction or drug abuse.

Interactions
Clorazepate potentiates the CNS depressant effects of phenothiazines, narcotics, barbiturates, alcohol, antihistamines, monoamine oxidase inhibitors, general anesthetics, and antidepressants. Concomitant use with cimetidine and possibly disulfiram causes diminished hepatic metabolism of clorazepate, which increases its plasma concentration.

Heavy smoking accelerates clorazepate's metabolism, thus lowering clinical effectiveness. Antacids delay the drug's absorption and reduce the total amount absorbed.

Benzodiazepines may reduce serum levels of haloperidol. Clorazepate may decrease the therapeutic effectiveness of levodopa.

Effects on diagnostic tests
Clorazepate therapy may elevate liver function test results. Minor changes in EEG patterns, usually low-voltage, fast activity, may occur during and after clorazepate therapy.

Adverse reactions
- CNS: confusion, depression, drowsiness, lethargy, hangover effect, ataxia, dizziness, syncope, nightmares, fatigue, slurred speech, tremors, vertigo, headache, paradoxical reactions.
- CV: bradycardia, palpitations, cardiovascular collapse, transient hypotension.
- DERM: rash, urticaria.
- EENT: diplopia, blurred vision, nystagmus.
- GI: constipation, dry mouth, nausea, vomiting, anorexia, dysphagia, abdominal discomfort.
- GU: urinary incontinence or retention.
- Other: respiratory depression, dysarthria, behavior problems, hepatic dysfunction, changes in libido.

Note: Drug should be discontinued if hypersensitivity or the following paradoxical reactions occur: acute hyperexcited state, anxiety, hallucinations, increased muscle spasticity, insomnia, or rage.

Overdose and treatment
Clinical manifestations of overdose include somnolence, confusion, coma, hypoactive reflexes, dyspnea, labored breathing, hypotension, bradycardia, slurred speech, and unsteady gait or impaired coordination.

Support blood pressure and respiration until drug effects subside; monitor vital signs. Mechanical ventilatory assistance via endotracheal tube may be required to maintain a patent airway and support adequate oxygenation. Treat hypotension with I.V. fluids and vasopressors such as dopamine and phen-

---

ylephrine as needed. Induce emesis if patient is conscious. Use gastric lavage if ingestion was recent, but only if an endotracheal tube is present to prevent aspiration. After emesis or lavage, administer activated charcoal with a cathartic as a single dose. Dialysis is of limited value. Do not use barbiturates if excitation occurs; they may exacerbate excitation or CNS depression.

▶ **Special considerations**
• Safety has not been established in children under age 9.
• Clorazepate produces a milder sedative effect than the other benzodiazepines.
• Because children, particularly young onges, are sensitive to the CNS depressant effects of benzodiazepines, caution must be exercised. A neonate whose mother took a benzodiazepine during pregnancy may exhibit withdrawal symptoms.
• Administer with milk or immediately after meals to prevent GI upset. Give antacid, if needed, at least 1 hour before or after dose to prevent interaction and ensure maximum drug absorption and effectiveness.
• Crush tablet or empty capsule and mix with food if patient has difficulty swallowing.
• Assess level of consciousness and neurologic status before and frequently during therapy for changes. Monitor for paradoxical reactions, especially early in therapy.
• Assess sleep patterns and quality. Institute seizure precautions. Assess for changes in seizure character, frequency, or duration.
• Assess vital signs frequently during therapy. Significant changes in blood pressure and heart rate may indicate impending toxicity.
• Monitor renal and hepatic function periodically to ensure adequate drug removal and prevent cumulative effects.
• Comfort measures – such as back rubs and relaxation techniques – may enhance drug effectiveness.
• As needed, institute safety measures – raised side rails and ambulatory assistance – to prevent injury. Anticipate possible rebound excitement reactions.
• Patient should be observed to prevent drug hoarding or self-dosing, especially in depressed or suicidal patients or those who are, or who have a history of being, drug-dependent. Patient's mouth should be checked to be sure tablet or capsule was swallowed.
• After prolonged use, abrupt discontinuation may cause withdrawal symptoms; discontinue gradually.
• Lower doses are effective in elderly patients and patients with renal or hepatic dysfunction.
• Store in a cool, dry place away from direct light.

Information for parents and patient
• Warn parents that patient should avoid use of alcohol or other CNS depressants, such an antihistamines, analgesics, monoamine oxidase (MAO) inhibitors, antidepressants, and barbiturates, while taking benzodiazepines to prevent additive depressant effects.
• Caution parents and patient that patient should not take the drug except as prescribed and should not give medication to others. Tell them not to increase the dose or frequency and to seek medical approval

before taking any nonprescription cold or allergy preparations.
• Warn parents that patient should avoid activities requiring alertness and good psychomotor coordination until the CNS response to the drug is determined. Instruct patient in safety measures to prevent injury.
• Patient should avoid using antacids, which may delay drug absorption, unless prescribed.
• Be sure parents and patient understand that clorazepate can cause physical and psychological dependence with prolonged use.
• Warn parents that patient should not to stop taking the drug abruptly to prevent withdrawal symptoms after prolonged therapy.
• Tell parents and patient that smoking decreases the drug's effectiveness. Encourage patient to stop smoking during therapy.
• Tell parents to report any adverse effects. These are often dose-related and can be relieved by dosage adjustments.
• Explain to adolescent patient and her parents the importance of reporting suspected pregnancy immediately.
• Warn parents and patient that sudden position changes may cause dizziness. Patient should dangle legs for a few minutes before getting out of bed to prevent falls and injury.
• Patient who needs to take an antacid should take it 1 hour before or after clorazepate.

clotrimazole
Gyne-Lotrimin, Lotrimin, Mycelex, Mycelex-G

• Classification: topical antifungal (synthetic imidazole derivative)

How supplied
Available by prescription only
Vaginal tablets: 100 mg, 500 mg
Vaginal cream: 1%
Topical cream: 1%
Topical lotion: 1%
Topical solution: 1%
Lozenges: 10 mg

Indications, route, and dosage
Tinea pedis, tinea cruris, tinea versicolor, tinea corporis, cutaneous candidiasis
Children and adults: Apply thinly and massage into cleansed affected and surrounding area, morning and evening, for prescribed period (usually 1 to 4 weeks; however, therapy may take up to 8 weeks).
Vulvovaginal candidiasis
Adults: Insert one 100-mg tablet intravaginally daily at bedtime for 7 consecutive days. Alternatively, nonpregnant women may insert two 100-mg tablets once daily for 3 consecutive days or one 500-mg tablet one time only at bedtime. If vaginal cream is used, insert one applicatorful intravaginally, once daily at bedtime for 7 to 14 consecutive days.

Oropharyngeal candidiasis
Children and adults: Administer orally and dissolve slowly (15 to 30 minutes) in mouth; usual dosage is one lozenge 5 times daily for 14 consecutive days.

Action and kinetics
• *Antifungal action:* Clotrimazole alters cell membrane permeability by binding with phospholipids in the fungal cell membrane. Clotrimazole inhibits or kills many fungi, including yeast and dermatophytes, and also is active against some gram-positive bacteria.
• *Kinetics in adults:* Absorption is limited with topical administration. Distribution is minimal with local application.

Contraindications and precautions
Clotrimazole is contraindicated in patients with hypersensitivity to the drug. Clotrimazole lozenges should be used cautiously in patients with hepatic impairment because abnormal liver function test results have been reported. It should be used with caution intravaginally during first trimester of pregnancy because of possible adverse effects on the fetus.

Interactions
None reported.

Effects on diagnostic tests
Abnormal liver function test results have been reported in patients receiving clotrimazole lozenges.

Adverse reactions
• GI: lower abdominal cramps.
• GU: vaginal burning, urinary frequency.
• Local: blistering, erythema, pruritus, burning, stinging, irritation.
  Note: Drug should be discontinued if hypersensitivity occurs.

Overdose and treatment
Discontinue therapy.

▶ Special considerations
• Clotrimazole is not recommended for use in children under age 3.
• Patients treated with clotrimazole lozenges, especially those who have preexisting liver dysfunction, should have periodic liver function tests.

Information for parents and patient
• Emphasize that clotrimazole lozenges must dissolve slowly in the mouth to achieve maximum effect. Patient should not chew lozenges.
• Intravaginal medication should be inserted high into the vagina. Patient should use a sanitary napkin to prevent staining of clothing and to absorb discharge.
• Patient should complete the full course of therapy. Improvement usually will be noted within a week. Parents or patient should call if no improvement occurs in 4 weeks or if condition worsens.
• Advise parents or patient to watch for and report irritation or sensitivity and, if either occurs, to discontinue use.

cloxacillin sodium
Cloxapen, Tegopen

• Classification: antibiotic (penicillinase-resistant penicillin)

How supplied
Available by prescription only
Capsules: 250 mg, 500 mg
Oral solution: 125 mg/5 ml (after reconstitution)

Indications, route, and dosage
Systemic infections caused by susceptible organisms
Children over 1 month of age and less than 20 kg: 50 to 100 mg/kg P.O. daily, divided into doses given q 6 hours. Maximum dose is 4 g daily.
Adults and children 20 kg and over: 2 to 4 g P.O. daily, divided into doses given q 6 hours.

Action and kinetics
• *Antibiotic action:* Cloxacillin is bactericidal; it adheres to bacterial penicillin-binding proteins, thereby inhibiting bacterial cell wall synthesis.
  Cloxacillin resists the effects of penicillinases — enzymes that inactivate penicillin — and therefore is active against many strains of penicillinase-producing bacteria; this activity is most pronounced against penicillinase-producing staphylococci; some strains may remain resistant. Cloxacillin is also active against gram-positive aerobic and anaerobic bacilli but has no significant effect on gram-negative bacilli.
• *Kinetics in adults:* Cloxacillin is absorbed rapidly but incompletely (37% to 60%) from the GI tract; it is relatively acid stable. Peak plasma concentrations occur ½ to 2 hours after an oral dose. Food may decrease both rate and extent of absorption. Cloxacillin is distributed widely. CSF penetration is poor but enhanced in meningeal inflammation. Cloxacillin crosses the placenta; it is 90% to 96% protein-bound. Partially metabolized drug and metabolites are excreted in urine by renal tubular secretion and glomerular filtration; they are also excreted in breast milk. Elimination half-life in adults is ½ to 1 hour, extended minimally to 2½ hours in patients with renal impairment.
• *Kinetics in children:* Plasma levels are generally higher and serum half-life is longer in neonates as compared with older children. Serum half-life in infants age 1 to 2 weeks is 0.8 to 1.5 hours.

Contraindications and precautions
Cloxacillin is contraindicated in patients with known hypersensitivity to any other penicillin or to cephalosporins.
  Cloxacillin should be administered with caution to patients with renal impairment, because it is excreted in urine; decreased dosage is required in moderate to severe renal failure.

Interactions

Concomitant use with aminoglycosides produces synergistic bactericidal effects against *Staphylococcus aureus*. However, the drugs are physically and chemically incompatible and are inactivated when mixed or given together. In vivo inactivation has been reported when aminoglycosides and penicillins are used concomitantly.

Probenecid blocks renal tubular secretion of carbenicillin, raising its serum concentrations.

Effects on diagnostic tests

Cloxacillin alters test results for urine and serum proteins; it produces false-positive or elevated results in turbidimetric urine and serum protein tests using sulfosalicylic acid or trichloroacetic acid; it also reportedly produces false results on the Bradshaw screening test for Bence Jones protein.

Cloxacillin may cause transient elevations in liver function study results and transient reductions in red blood cell, white blood cell, and platelet counts.

Elevated liver function test results may indicate drug-induced cholestasis or hepatitis.

Cloxacillin may falsely decrease serum aminoglycoside concentrations.

Adverse reactions

• GI: nausea, vomiting, epigastric distress, diarrhea, pseudomembranous colitis, intrahepatic cholestasis.
• GU: acute interstitial nephritis.
• HEMA: eosinophilia, leukopenia, granulocytopenia, thrombocytopenia, agranulocytosis.
• Other: hypersensitivity (rash, urticaria, chills, fever, sneezing, wheezing, anaphylaxis), bacterial and fungal superinfection.

Note: Drug should be discontinued if immediate hypersensitivity reactions occur or if signs of acute interstitial nephritis or pseudomembranous colitis occur. Alternate therapy should be considered if any of the following occurs: drug fever, eosinophilia, hematuria, neutropenia, or unexplained elevations in serum creatinine or BUN levels, or in liver function studies.

Overdose and treatment

Clinical signs of overdose include neuromuscular irritability or seizures. No specific recommendation is available. Treatment is symptomatic. After recent ingestion (within 4 hours), empty the stomach by induced emesis or gastric lavage; follow with activated charcoal to reduce absorption. Cloxacillin is not appreciably removed by hemodialysis or peritoneal dialysis.

▶ Special considerations

• Elimination of cloxacillin is reduced in neonates; safe use of drug in neonates has not been established.
• Assess patient's history of allergies; do not give cloxacillin to any patient with a history of hypersensitivity reactions to either penicillins or cephalosporins. Try to determine if previous reactions were true hypersensitivity reactions or another reaction, such as GI distress, which the patient has interpreted as allergy.
• Keep in mind that a negative history for penicillin hypersensitivity does not preclude future allergic reactions; monitor patient continuously for possible allergic reactions or other untoward effects.
• In patients with renal impairment, dosage should be reduced if creatinine clearance is below 10 ml/minute.
• Assess level of consciousness, neurologic status, and renal function when high doses are used, because excessive blood levels can cause CNS toxicity.
• Obtain results of cultures and sensitivity tests before test results are complete. Repeat test periodically to assess drug efficacy.
• Monitor vital signs, electrolytes, and renal function studies; monitor body weight for fluid retention with extended-spectrum penicillins for possible hypokalemia or hypernatremia.
• Coagulation abnormalities, even frank bleeding, can follow high doses, especially of extended-spectrum penicllins; monitor prothrombin times and platelet counts, and asseess patient for signs of occult or frank bleeding.
• Monitor patients on long-term therapy for possible superinfection, especially debilitated patients and others receiving immunosuppressants or radiation therapy; monitor closely, especially for fever.
• Give drug at least 1 hour before giving bacteriostatic antibiotics (tetracyclines, erythromycins, and chloramphenicol); these drugs inhibit bacterial cell growth, decreasing rate of drug uptake by bacterial cell walls.
• Give cloxacillin at least 1 hour before or 2 hours after meals to enhance gastric absorption; food may or may not decrease absorption. Give drug with water only; acid in fruit juice or carbonated beverage may inactivate drug.

Information for parents and patient

• Tell patients to refrigerate oral solution, and to shake it well before giving to ensure correct dosage.
• Teach signs and symptoms of hypersensitivity and other adverse reactions, and emphasize need to report any unusual reactions.
• Teach signs and symptoms of bacterial and fungal superinfection to parents and patient, especially debilitated patients and others with low resistance from immunosuppressants or irradiation; emphasize need to report signs of infection. To help prevent yeast infection, advise parents to keep child's diaper area clean and dry and to avoid use of plastic pants.
• Be sure parents understand how and when to give drug; urge them to complete entire prescribed regimen, to comply with instructions for around-the-clock dosage, and to keep follow-up appointments.
• Counsel parents to check expiration date of drug and to discard unused drug.

codeine phosphate
codeine sulfate

- Classification: analgesic, antitussive (opioid)
- Controlled substance schedule II

How supplied
Available by prescription only
Tablets: 15-mg, 30-mg, 60-mg; 15-mg, 30-mg, 60-mg (soluble)
Oral solution: 15 mg/5 ml codeine phosphate
Injection: 25 mg/5 ml, 30 mg/ml, 60 mg/ml codeine phosphate

Indications, route, and dosage
Mild to moderate pain
Children: 0.5 mg/kg (or 15 mg/m²) I.V. or P.O. every 4 to 6 hours.
Adults: 15 to 60 mg P.O. or 15 to 60 mg (phosphate) S.C. or I.M. q 4 hours, p.r.n. or around the clock.
Nonproductive cough
Children: 0.25 to 0.5 mg/kg P.O. q 4 hours. Maximum dialy dose is 30 mg. Alternatively, adjust dosage according to child's age.
Children age 2 to 6: 1 mg/kg daily divided into 4 equal doses, administered q 4 to 6 hours.
Children age 6 to 11: 5 to 10 mg q 4 to 6 hours, not to exceed 60 mg daily.
Adults: 10 to 20 mg P.O. q 4 to 6 hours. Maximum dosage: 120 mg/24 hours.

Action and kinetics
- *Analgesic action:* Codeine (methylmorphine) has analgesic properties that result from its agonist activity at the opiate receptors.
- *Antitussive action:* Codeine has a direct suppressant action on the cough reflex center.
- *Kinetics in adults:* Codeine is well absorbed after oral or parenteral administration. It is about two thirds as potent orally as parenterally. After oral or subcutaneous administration, action occurs in less than 30 minutes. Peak analgesic effect is seen at ½ to 1 hour, and the duration of action is 4 to 6 hours.

Codeine is distributed widely throughout the body; it crosses the placenta and enters breast milk.

Codeine is metabolized mainly in the liver, by demethylation, or conjugation with glucuronic acid. Codeine is excreted mainly in the urine as norcodeine and free and conjugated morphine.

Contraindications and precautions
Codeine is contraindicated in patients with known hypersensitivity to the drug or phenanthrene opioids (hydrocodone, hydromorphene, morphine, oxycodone, or oxymorphone).

Administer codeine with extreme caution to patients with supraventricular dysrhythmias; avoid, or administer drug with extreme caution to patients with head injury or increased intracranial pressure, because drug obscures neurologic parameters; and during pregnancy and labor, because drug readily crosses placenta (premature infants are especially sensitive to respiratory and CNS depressant effects of opioids).

Administer codeine cautiously to patients with renal or hepatic dysfunction, because drug accumulation or prolonged duration of action may occur; to patients with pulmonary disease (asthma, chronic obstructive pulmonary disease), because drug depresses respiration and suppresses cough reflex; to patients undergoing biliary tract surgery, because drug may cause biliary spasm; to patients with convulsive disorders, because drug may precipitate seizures; to elderly or debilitated patients, who are more sensitive to both therapeutic and adverse drug effects; and to patients prone to physical or psychic addiction, because of the high risk of addiction to this drug.

Interactions
Concomitant use with other CNS depressants (narcotic analgesics, general anesthetics, antihistamines, phenothiazines, barbiturates, benzodiazepines, sedative-hypnotics tricyclic antidepressants, monoamine oxidase inhibitors, alcohol, and muscle relaxants) potentiates drug's respiratory and CNS depression, sedation, and hypotensive effects. Concomitant use with cimetidine may also increase respiratory and CNS depression, causing confusion, disorientation, apnea, or seizures.

Drug accumulation and enhanced effects may result from concomitant use with other drugs that are extensively metabolized in the liver (rifampin, phenytoin, digitoxin); combined use with anticholinergics may cause paralytic ileus.

Patients who become physically dependent on this drug may experience acute withdrawal syndrome if given a narcotic antagonist.

Severe cardiovascular depression may result from concomitant use with general anesthetics.

Effects on diagnostic tests
Codeine may increase plasma amylase and lipase levels, delay gastric emptying, increase biliary tract pressure resulting from contraction of the sphincter of Oddi, and may interfere with hepatobiliary imaging studies.

Adverse reactions
- CNS: sedation, drowsiness, dysphoria, dizziness, euphoria, insomnia, agitation, confusion, headache, tremor, miosis, seizures, psychic dependence, *CNS depression.*
- CV: tachycardia, bradycardia, palpitations, chest wall rigidity, hypertension, hypotension, syncope, edema, shock, cardiopulmonary arrest.
- DERM: flushing, rashes, pruritus, pain at injection site.
- GI: dry mouth, anorexia, *biliary spasms* (colic), ileus, nausea, vomiting, *constipation.*
- GU: urinary retention or hesitancy, decreased libido.
- Other: apnea, *respiratory depression.*

Note: Drug should be discontinued if hypersensitivity, seizures, or life-threatening cardiac dysrhythmias occur.

Overdose and treatment

The most common signs and symptoms of overdose are CNS depression, respiratory depression, and miosis (pinpoint pupils). Other acute toxic effects include hypotension, bradycardia, hypothermia, shock, apnea, cardiopulmonary arrest, circulatory collapse, pulmonary edema, and convulsions.

To treat acute overdose, first establish adequate respiratory exchange via a patent airway and ventilation as needed; administer narcotic antagonist (naloxone) to reverse respiratory depression. (Because the duration of action of codeine is longer than that of naloxone, repeated naloxone dosing is necessary.) Naloxone should not be given unless the patient has clinically significant respiratory or cardiovascular depression. Monitor vital signs closely.

If the patient presents within 2 hours of ingestion of an oral overdose, empty the stomach immediately by inducing emesis (ipecac syrup) or using gastric lavage. Use caution to avoid any risk of aspiration. Administer activated charcoal via nasogastric tube for further removal of the drug in an oral overdose.

Provide symptomatic and supportive treatment (continued respiratory support, correction of fluid or electrolyte imbalance). Monitor laboratory parameters, vital signs, and neurologic status closely.

▶ Special considerations

• Administer with extreme caution to patients with head injury, increased intracranial pressure, seizures, asthma, chronic obstructive pulmonary disease, alcoholism, severe hepatic or renal disease, acute abdominal conditions, cardiac dysrhythmias, hypovolemia, or psychiatric disorders, and to debilitated patients. Reduced doses may be necessary.
• Consider possible interactions with other drugs the patient is taking.
• Keep resuscitative equipment and a narcotic antagonist (naloxone) available. Be prepared to provide support of ventilation and gastric lavage.
• Parenteral administration provides better analgesia than oral administration. Intravenous administration should be given by slow injection, preferably in diluted solution. Rapid I.V. injection increases the incidence of adverse effects.
• Injections by I.M. or S.C. route should be given cautiously to patients who are chilled, hypovolemic, or in shock, because decreased perfusion may lead to accumulation of the drug and toxic effects. Rotate I.M. or S.C. injection sites to avoid induration.
• Before administration, visually inspect all parenteral products for particulate matter and discoloration.
• Oral solutions of varying concentrations are available. Carefully note the strength of the solution.
• Especially in children, regular dosage schedule (rather than "p.r.n. pain") is preferred to alleviate the symptoms and anxiety that accompany pain.
• The duration of respiratory depression may be longer than the analgesic effect. Monitor the patient closely with repeated dosing.
• With chronic administration, evaluate the patient's respiratory status before each dose. Because severe respiratory depression may occur (especially with accumulation from chronic dosing), watch for respiratory

rate below the patient's baseline level. Evaluate the patient for restlessness, which may be a sign of compensatory response for hypoxia.
• Opiates or agonist-antagonists may cause orthostatic hypotension in ambulatory patients. Have the patient sit or lie down to relieve dizziness or fainting.
• Since opiates depress respiration, when they are used postoperatively encourage patient turning, coughing, and deep-breathing to avoid atelectases.
• If patient's condition allows, instruct patient to breathe deeply, cough, and change position every 2 hours to avoid respiratory complications.
• If gastric irritation occurs, give oral products with food; food delays absorption and onset of analgesia.
• Opiates may obscure the signs and symptoms of an acute abdominal condition or worsen gallbladder pain.
• The antitussive activity of codeine is used to control persistent, exhausting cough or dry, non-productive cough.
• The first sign of tolerance to the therapeutic effect is usually a shortened duration of effect.
• Codeine and aspirin have additive analgesic effects. Give together for maximum pain relief.
• Codeine has much less abuse potential than morphine.
• Monitor for bowel sounds, firm abdomen, and constipation.

Information for parents and patients

• Warn patients that codeine-containing cough preparations may be hazardous in young children. Advise them to use a calibrated device for measuring each dose and not to exceed the recommended daily dose.
• Warn parents that drug may produce drowsiness and sedation. Patient should avoid hazardous activities that require full alertness and coordination.
• Tell parents that patient should avoid ingestion of beverages or elixirs that contain alcohol when taking drug, because this will cause additive CNS depression.
• Explain that constipation may result from taking drug. Suggest measures to increase dietary fiber content, or recommend a stool softener.
• Patient should void at least every 4 hours to prevent urinary retention.
• Tell the parents to have the patient take the medication as prescribed and to call the physician if significant adverse effects occur.
• Tell parents not to increase dosage if patient is not experiencing the desired effect, but to call the physician for prescribed dosage adjustment.
• Instruct the parents not to double the dose. Tell them that patient may take a missed dose as soon as he remembers unless it's almost time for the next dose. If this is so, the patient should skip the missed dose and go back to the regular dosage schedule.
• Explain the signs of overdose to the parents and patient.
• Tell parents to call immediately for emergency help if they think the patient has taken an overdose.

██████████████

colchicine

• Classification: antigout agent *(Colchicum autumnale* alkaloid)

How supplied
Available by prescription only
Injection: 1 mg (1/60 g)/2 ml ampule
Tablets: 0.6 mg (1/100 grain), 0.5 mg (1/120 grain) as sugar-coated granules

Indications, route, and dosage
†*Familial Mediterranean fever*
Colchicine has been used effectively to treat familial Mediterranean fever (hereditary disorder characterized by acute episodes of fever, peritonitis, and pleuritis).
Children less than 30 kg: 0.02 mg/kg/day P.O.
Children from 30 to 50 kg: 0.6 mg/kg/day P.O.
Adults: 1 to 2 mg/day in divided doses.

Action and kinetics
• *Antigout action:* Colchicine's exact mechanism of action is unknown, but it is involved in leukocyte migration inhibition; reduction of lactic acid production by leukocytes, resulting in decreased deposits of uric acid; and interference with kinin formation.
• *Anti-inflammatory action:* Colchicine reduces the inflammatory response to deposited uric acid crystals and diminishes phagocytosis.
• *Kinetics in adults:* When administered P.O., colchicine is absorbed from the GI tract. Unchanged drug may be reabsorbed from the intestine by biliary processes. Colchicine is distributed rapidly into various tissues after reabsorption from the intestine. It is concentrated in leukocytes and distributed into the kidneys, liver, spleen, and intestinal tract but is absent in the heart, skeletal muscle, and brain. Colchicine is metabolized partially in the liver and also slowly metabolized in other tissues. Colchicine and its metabolites are excreted primarily in the feces, with lesser amounts excreted in urine.

Contraindications and precautions
Colchicine is contraindicated in patients with serious GI, renal, or cardiac disorders and should be used cautiously in patients who may have early signs of these disorders, because the drug may exacerbate these conditions. Colchicine is also contraindicated in patients with blood dyscrasias or hypersensitivity to colchicine. Use with caution in debilitated patients.

Interactions
When used concomitantly, colchicine and sulfinpyrazone may lead to leukemia in some patients. However, a cause-and-effect relationship has not been established. Colchicine induces reversible malabsorption of vitamin B_{12}, may increase sensitivity to CNS depressants, and may enhance the response to sympathomimetic agents. Colchicine is inhibited by acidifying agents and by alcohol consumption; its actions are increased by alkalinizing agents.

Effects on diagnostic tests
Colchicine therapy may increase alkaline phosphatase, AST (SGOT), and ALT (SGPT) levels and may decrease serum carotene, cholesterol, and thrombocyte values.
Colchicine may cause false-positive results of urine tests for red blood cells or hemoglobin.

Adverse reactions
• CNS: peripheral neuritis, purpura, myopathy, mental confusion, loss of deep tendon reflexes.
• GI: vomiting, diarrhea, abdominal pain, nausea, hepatotoxicity, pancreatitis, ileus.
• GU: dysuria, urinary frequency.
• HEMA: bone marrow depression with aplastic anemia, agranulocytosis, thrombocytopenia.
• Other: alopecia, azoospermia, dermatosis, hypersensitivity, pain and erythema at I.V. infusion site.

Overdose and treatment
Clinical manifestations of overdose include nausea, vomiting, abdominal pain, and diarrhea. Diarrhea may be severe and bloody from hemorrhagic gastroenteritis. Burning sensations in the throat, stomach, and skin also may occur. Extensive vascular damage may result in shock, hematuria, and oliguria, indicating kidney damage. Patient develops severe dehydration, hypotension, muscle weakness, and ascending paralysis of the CNS. Patient usually remains conscious, but delirium and convulsions may occur. Death may result from respiratory depression.
There is no known specific antidote. Treatment begins with gastric lavage and preventive measures for shock. Recent studies support the use of hemodialysis and peritoneal dialysis; atropine and morphine may relieve abdominal pain; paregoric usually is administered to control diarrhea and cramps. Respiratory assistance may be needed.

▶ Special considerations
• To avoid cumulative toxicity, a course of oral colchicine should not be repeated for at least 3 days; a course of I.V. colchicine should not be repeated for several weeks.
• Do not administer I.M. or subcutaneously; severe local irritation occurs.
• Obtain baseline laboratory studies, including CBC, before initiating therapy and periodically thereafter.
• Give I.V. colchicine by slow I.V. push over 2 to 5 minutes by direct I.V. injection or into tubing of a free-flowing I.V. line with compatible I.V. fluid. Avoid extravasation. Do not dilute colchicine injection with normal saline solution, dextrose 5% injection, or any other fluid that might change pH of colchicine solution. If lower concentration of colchicine injection is needed, dilute with sterile water for injection. However, if diluted solution becomes turbid, do not inject.
• Discontinue drug if weakness, anorexia, nausea, vomiting, or diarrhea occurs. First sign of acute overdosage may be GI symptoms, followed by vascular damage, muscle weakness, and ascending paralysis. Delirium and convulsions may occur without loss of consciousness.
• Store the drug in a tightly closed, light-resistant container, away from moisture and high temperatures.

---

*Canada only   †Unlabeled clinical use   Italicized adverse reactions have been observed in children.

• Colchicine has been used to relieve symptoms of leukemia, but it does not alter the disease state.

Information for parents and patient
• Advise parents to report rash, sore throat, fever, unusual bleeding, bruising, tiredness, weakness, numbness, or tingling.
• Tell parents that patient should discontinue colchicine at the first sign of nausea, vomiting, stomach pain, or diarrhea. Advise parents to report persistent symptoms.
• Patient should avoid alcohol during colchicine therapy because alcohol may inhibit drug action.

---

colestipol hydrochloride
Colestid

• Classification: antilipemic (anion exchange resin)

How supplied
Available by prescription only
Granules: 500-mg bottles, 5-g packets

Indications, route, and dosage
Primary hypercholesterolemia and xanthomas
Children: 10 to 20 g or 500 mg/kg daily in two to four divided doses (lower dosages of 125 to 250 mg/kg used when serum cholesterol levels are 15% to 20% above normal after only dietary management).
Adults: 15 to 30 g P.O. daily in two to four divided doses.

Action and kinetics
• *Antilipemic action:* Bile is normally excreted into the intestine to facilitate absorption of fat and other lipid materials. Colestipol binds with bile acid, forming an insoluble compound that is excreted in feces. With less bile available in the digestive system, less fat and lipid materials in food are absorbed, more cholesterol is used by the liver to replace its supply of bile acids, and the serum cholesterol level decreases.
• *Kinetics in adults:* Colestipol is not absorbed. Cholesterol levels may decrease in 24 to 48 hours, with peak effect occurring at 1 month. In some patients, the initial decrease is followed by a return to or above baseline cholesterol levels on continued therapy. Colestipol is excreted in feces; cholesterol levels return to baseline within 1 month after therapy stops.

Contraindications and precautions
Colestipol is contraindicated in patients with complete biliary obstruction or complete atresia, because bile is not secreted into the intestine; in patients with primary biliary cirrhosis, because cholesterol levels may be further increased in these cases; and in patients with known hypersensitivity to the drug.

Use colestipol cautiously in patients with constipation because of the risk of fecal impaction; in patients with malabsorption, because the condition may deteriorate from further decreased absorption of fats and fat-soluble vitamins A, D, E, and K; and in preg-

nant patients, because impaired maternal absorption of vitamins and other nutrients is a potential threat to the fetus.

Interactions
Colestipol impairs absorption of digitalis glycosides (including digoxin and digitoxin), tetracycline, penicillin G, chenodril, and thiazide diuretics, thus decreasing their therapeutic effect.

Dosage of any oral medication may require adjustment to compensate for possible binding with colestipol; give other drugs at least 1 hour before or 4 to 6 hours after colestipol (longer if possible); readjustment must also be made when colestipol is withdrawn, to prevent high-dose toxicity.

Effects on diagnostic tests
Colestipol alters serum levels of alkaline phosphatase, aspartate aminotransferase, chloride, phosphorus, potassium, and sodium.

Adverse reactions
• DERM: rashes; sore skin, tongue, and perianal skin.
• GI: constipation, fecal impaction, aggravation of hemorrhoids, abdominal discomfort, flatulence, nausea, vomiting, steatorrhea.
• Other: vitamin A, D, and K deficiency from decreased absorption; hyperchloremic acidosis with long-term use or very high dosage.
Note: Drug should be discontinued if constipation worsens even after reduction in dosage; if a paradoxical increase in serum cholesterol level occurs; or if inadequate clinical response occurs after 1 to 3 months of treatment except when treating xanthoma tuberosum, which may require up to 12 months of treatment.

Overdose and treatment
Overdose of colestipol has not been reported. Chief potential risk is intestinal obstruction; treatment would depend on location and degree of obstruction and on amount of gut motility.

▶ Special considerations
• Safety in children has not been established. Drug is not usually recommended for use in children; however, it has been used in a few children with hypercholesteremia.
• To mix, sprinkle granules on surface of preferred beverage or wet food, let stand a few minutes, and stir to obtain uniform suspension; avoid excess foaming by using large glass and mixing slowly. Use at least 90 ml of water or other fluid, soups, milk, or pulpy fruit; rinse container and have patient drink this to be sure he ingests entire dose.
• Monitor levels of cardiac glycosides and other drugs to ensure appropriate dosage during and after therapy with colestipol.
• Determine serum cholesterol level frequently during first few months of therapy and periodically thereafter.
• Monitor bowel function; treat constipation promptly by decreasing dosage, increasing fluid intake, adding a stool softener, or discontinuing drug.
• Monitor for signs of vitamin A, D, or K deficiency.

---

‡May contain sulfites   ◆May contain tartrazine   ◆◆May contain benzyl alcohol

Information for parents and patient
• Explain disease process and rationale for therapy. Although therapy is not curative, it helps control serum cholesterol level. Encourage parents and patient to comply with continued blood testing and special diet.
• Teach parents how to administer drug.

collagenase
Biozyme-C, Santyl

• Classification: topical proteolytic enzyme preparation (derived from *Clostridium histolytica*)

How supplied
Available by prescription only
Ointment: 250 units/g

Indications, route, and dosage
To promote debridement of necrotic tissue in dermal ulcers and severe burns
Children and adults: Apply ointment to lesion daily or every other day.

Action and kinetics
• *Enzymatic debriding agent:* Collagenase liquefies necrotic tissue without damaging granulation tissue. It hydrolyzes peptide bonds of undenatured and denatured collagen.
• *Kinetics in adults:* Absorption is limited with topical use.

Contraindications and precautions
Collagenase is contraindicated in patients with hypersensitivity to the drug. It should be used with caution near the eyes.

Interactions
When used concomitantly, the enzyme activity of collagenase is adversely affected by detergents, benzalkonium chloride, hexachlorophene, nitrofurazone, tincture of iodine, and any medication or material containing heavy metal ions.

Effects on diagnostic tests
None reported.

Adverse reactions
• Local: pain, burning, erythema.
Note: Drug should be discontinued if sensitization occurs.

Overdose and treatment
Action of enzyme can be stopped by applying aluminum acetate solution to the lesion as soon as possible.

▶ Special considerations
• Store drug at temperature not exceeding 98.6° F. (37° C.).
• Avoid local skin irritation by covering the skin surrounding the lesion with a protectant.

• Observe patient for sensitivity reaction with prolonged use.
• Monitor debilitated patients for systemic infections; debriding enzymes may increase risk of bacteremia.
• Use strict aseptic technique when applying collagenase. Cleanse lesion with hydrogen peroxide or 0.9% sodium chloride buffer solution.
• Discontinue therapy when debridement of tissue has been achieved and granulation tissue has developed.
• When infection is present, use an appropriate topical antibacterial. Neosporin is compatible with collagenase and should be applied before applying collagenase.

Information for parents and patient
Teach parents or patient to cover surrounding area with a protectant (zinc oxide paste) to decrease possibility of irritation, to cleanse lesion with hydrogen peroxide or 0.9% sodium chloride buffer solution, and to maintain strict aseptic conditions when changing dressings.

corticotropin (adrenocorticotropic hormone, ACTH)
ACTH, Acthar, ACTHGel, Cortigel-40, Cortigel-80, Cortrophin Gel, Cortrophin-Zinc, HP Acthar Gel

• Classification: diagnostic aid, replacement hormone, treatment for multiple sclerosis and nonsuppurative thyroiditis (anterior pituitary hormone)

How supplied
Available by prescription only
Injection: 25 units/vial, 40 units/vial
Repository injection: 40 units/ml, 80 units/ml

Indications, route, and dosage
Diagnostic test of adrenocortical function
Children and adults: Up to 80 units I.M. or S.C. in divided doses; or a single dose of repository form; or 10 to 25 units (aqueous form) in 500 ml of dextrose 5% in water I.V. over 8 hours, between blood samplings.

Individual dosages vary with adrenal glands' sensitivity to stimulation and with the specific disease. Infants and younger children require larger doses per kilogram than do older children and adults.
Severe allergic reactions, collagen disorders, dermatologic disorders, inflammation
†*Children:* 1.6 units/kg or 50 units/m² I.M., I.V., or S.C. daily, divided into three or four equal doses. Alternatively, administer repository corticotropin at a dosage of 0.8 units/kg or 25 units/m² in one or two doses.
Adults: 40 to 80 units/day I.M. or S.C. Adjust dosage based upon patient response.
†*Infantile spasms*
Infants: 40 units I.M. daily or 80 units I.M. every other day using I.M. ACTH Gel, until seizures subside or symptoms of toxicity occur. Then discontinue by tapering off gradually.

---

*Canada only   †Unlabeled clinical use   Italicized adverse reactions have been observed in children.

Action and kinetics

• *Diagnostic action:* Corticotropin is used to test adrenocortical function. Corticotropin binds with a specific receptor in the adrenal cell plasma membrane, stimulating the synthesis of the entire spectrum of adrenal steroids, one of which is cortisol. The effect of corticotropin is measured by analyzing plasma cortisol before and after drug administration. In patients with primary adrenocortical insufficiency, corticotropin does not increase plasma cortisol concentrations significantly.

• *Anti-inflammatory action:* In nonsuppurative thyroiditis and acute exacerbations of multiple sclerosis, corticotropin stimulates release of adrenal cortex hormones, which combat tissue responses to inflammatory processes.

• *Kinetics in adults:* Corticotropin is absorbed rapidly after I.M. administration; absorption occurs over 8 to 16 hours after I.M. administration of zinc or repository form. Maximum stimulation occurs after infusing 1 to 6 units of corticotropin over 8 hours. Peak cortisol levels are achieved within 1 hour of I.M. or rapid I.V. administration of corticotropin. Peak 17-hydroxycorticosteroid levels are achieved within 7 to 24 hours with zinc and 3 to 12 hours with the repository form. The exact distribution of corticotropin is unknown, but it is removed rapidly from plasma by many tissues. Corticotropin probably is excreted by the kidneys. Its duration of action is about 2 hours with zinc form and up to 3 days with the repository form. Half-life is about 15 minutes.

Contraindications and precautions

Corticotropin is contraindicated in patients with known hypersensitivity to corticotropin, primary adrenocortical insufficiency, or congenital adrenogenital syndrome (because corticotropin will be ineffective) and in any condition associated with adrenocortical hyperfunction (which may become exacerbated). Corticotropin also may exacerbate CHF or hypertension (because of sodium and fluid retention), ocular herpes simplex (because of the risk of corneal perforation), sensitivity to proteins of porcine origin (because corticotropin often is obtained from pigs), osteoporosis, and scleroderma.

Corticotropin should be used cautiously in patients with acquired immunodeficiency syndrome (AIDS) or a predisposition to AIDS because of an increased risk of uncontrollable infection or neoplasms; in patients with diabetes mellitus, which may become exacerbated; in patients with ulcerative colitis, diverticulitis, peptic ulcer, or gastritis, because symptoms of disease progression may be masked or perforation may occur without warning; and in patients with systemic fungal or tuberculosis infection, which may become exacerbated.

Use in hypothyroidism and cirrhosis may result in an enhanced corticotropin effect. Use in gouty arthritis should be limited to a few days because rebound attacks may follow withdrawal after prolonged use. Corticotropin may aggravate existing emotional instability or psychotic tendencies. Corticotropin should be used cautiously in patients with myasthenia gravis because it may cause muscle weakness.

Interactions

Concomitant use of corticotropin with diuretics ma accentuate the electrolyte loss associated with di uretic therapy; use with amphotericin B or carboni anhydrase inhibitors may cause severe hypokalemia Amphotericin B also decreases adrenal responsive ness to corticotropin. Concurrent use with insulin ma require increased dosage of the hypoglycemic agent use with hepatic enzyme-inducing agents may in crease corticotropin metabolism resulting from in duction of hepatic microsomal enzymes; use with digitalis glycosides may increase the risk of dys rhythmias or digitalis toxicity associated with hy pokalemia; and use with cortisone, hydrocortisone, or estrogens may elevate plasma cortisol levels abnormally.

Effects on diagnostic tests

Corticotropin therapy alters blood and urinary glucose levels; sodium and potassium levels; protein-bound iodine levels; radioactive iodine (^{131}I) uptake and liothyronine (T_3) uptake; total protein values; serum amylase, urine amino acid, serotonin, uric acid, calcium, and 17-ketosteroid levels; and leukocyte counts.

High plasma cortisol concentrations may be reported erroneously in patients receiving spironolactone, cortisone, or hydrocortisone when fluorometric analysis is used. This does not occur with the radioimmunoassay or competitive protein-binding method. However, therapy can be maintained with prednisone, dexamethasone, or betamethasone because they are not detectable by the fluorometric method.

Adverse reactions

Uncontrollable adverse reactions may be associated with chronic use of more than 40 units/day.

• CNS: convulsions, dizziness, papilledema, headache, euphoria, insomnia, mood swings, personality changes, depression, psychosis, vertigo.

• CV: hypertension, CHF, necrotizing angiitis.

• DERM: impaired wound healing; thin, fragile skin; petechiae; ecchymoses; facial erythema; increased sweating; acne; hyperpigmentation; allergic skin reactions; hirsutism.

• EENT: cataracts, glaucoma, exophthalmos.

• GI: peptic ulcer with perforation and hemorrhage; pancreatitis; abdominal distention; ulcerative esophagitis; nausea; vomiting.

• GU: menstrual irregularities.

• Metabolic: sodium and fluid retention, calcium and potassium loss, hypokalemic alkalosis, negative nitrogen balance.

• Other: muscle weakness, steroid myopathy, loss of muscle mass, osteoporosis, vertebral compression fractures, cushingoid state, suppression of growth in children, activation of latent diabetes mellitus, progressive increase in antibodies, loss of corticotropin stimulatory effect, hypersensitivity.

Overdose and treatment

Specific information unavailable. Treatment is supportive, as appropriate.

▶ **Special considerations**
• Use with caution in children because prolonged use of corticotropin will inhibit skeletal growth. Intermittent administration is recommended.
• Use with caution if surgery or emergency treatment is required.
• If administering gel, warm it to room temperature, draw into large needle, and give slowly, deep I.M. with a 22G needle.
• Cosyntropin is less antigenic and less likely to cause allergic reactions than corticotropin. However, allergic reactions occur rarely with corticotropin.
• In patient with suspected sensitivity to porcine proteins, skin testing should be performed. To decrease the risk of anaphylactic reaction in patient with limited adrenal reserves, 1 mg of dexamethasone may be given at midnight before the corticotropin test and 0.5 mg at start of test.
• Counteract edema by low-sodium, high-potassium intake; nitrogen loss by high-protein diet; and psychotic symptoms by reducing corticotropin dosage or administering sedatives.
• Corticotropin may mask signs of chronic disease and decrease host resistance and ability to localize infection.
• Insulin dosages may need to be increased during corticotropin therapy.
• Monitor weight, fluid exchange, and resting blood pressure levels until minimal effective dosage is achieved.
• Refrigerate reconstituted product and use within 24 hours.
• Corticotropin must not be discontinued abruptly, especially after prolonged therapy. An addisonian crisis may occur.

Information for parents and patient
• Tell parents and patient that injection is painful.
• Tell parents to report marked fluid retention, weight gain, muscle weakness, abdominal pain, seizures, headache, or GI distress.
• Tell parents that patient should not be vaccinated during corticotropin therapy.
• Show parents and patient how to monitor for edema, and explain the need for fluid and salt restriction as appropriate.
• Warn parents not to discontinue medication except as prescribed because abrupt discontinuation may provoke severe adverse reactions. Patient should not take any other drugs without medical approval.
• Advise parents or patient to inform new physician or dentist that patient is taking this drug.
• Patient should wear a Medic Alert bracelet or necklace that identifies the disease and drug dosage.
• Explain to parents of adolescents the importance of reporting suspected pregnancy immediately.

cortisone acetate
Cortelan*, Cortistab*, Cortone

• Classification: anti-inflammatory, replacement therapy (glucocorticoid, mineralocorticoid)

How supplied
Available by prescription only
Tablets: 5 mg, 10 mg, 25 mg
Injection: 25 mg/ml, 50 mg/ml suspension

Indications, route, and dosage
Adrenal insufficiency, allergy, inflammation
Adults: 25 to 300 mg P.O. or I.M. daily or on alternate days. Doses highly individualized, depending on severity of disease.
Adrenal insufficiency
Children: 700 mcg/kg or 20 to 25 mg/m²/daily in divided doses; or 700 mcg/kg to 37.5mg/m² I.M. every 3rd day; or 233.33 to 350 mg/kg or 12.5 mg/m² I.M. daily.
Allergy inflammation
Children: 2.5 to 10 mg/kg or 75 to 300 mg/m² P.O. in divided doses; or 833 mcg to 5 mg/kg or 25 to 150 mg/m² every 12 to 24 hours.

Action and kinetics
• *Adrenocorticoid replacement:* Cortisone acetate is an adrenocorticoid with both glucocorticoid and mineralocorticoid properties. A weak anti-inflammatory agent, cortisone acetate has only about 80% of the anti-inflammatory activity of an equal weight of hydrocortisone. It is a potent mineralocorticoid, however, having twice the potency of prednisone. Cortisone (or hydrocortisone) is usually the drug of choice for replacement therapy in patients with adrenal insufficiency. It is usually not used for inflammatory or immunosuppressant activity because of the extremely large doses that must be used and because of the unwanted mineralocorticoid effects. The injectable form has a slow onset but a long duration of action. It is usually used only when the oral dosage form cannot be used.
• *Kinetics in adults:* Cortisone is absorbed readily after oral administration, with peak effects in about 1 to 2 hours. The suspension for injection has a variable onset of 24 to 48 hours.
    Cortisone is distributed rapidly to muscle, liver, skin, intestines, and kidneys. Cortisone is extensively bound to plasma proteins (transcortin and albumin). Only the unbound portion is active. Cortisone is distributed into breast milk and through the placenta.
    Cortisone is metabolized in the liver to the active metabolite hydrocortisone, which in turn is metabolized to inactive glucuronide and sulfate metabolites.
    The inactive metabolites and small amounts of unmetabolized drug are excreted by the kidneys. Insignificant quantities of the drug are also excreted in feces. The biological half-life of cortisone is 8 to 12 hours.

Contraindications and precautions

Cortisone is contraindicated in patients with systemic fungal infections (except in adrenal insufficiency) or a hypersensitivity to ingredients of adrenocorticoid preparations. Patients who are receiving cortisone should not be given live virus vaccines because cortisone suppresses the immune response.

Cortisone should be used with extreme caution in patients with GI ulceration, renal disease, hypertension, osteoporosis, diabetes mellitus, thromboembolic disorders, seizures, myasthenia gravis, congestive heart failure (CHF), tuberculosis, hypoalbuminemia, hypothyroidism, cirrhosis of the liver, emotional instability, psychotic tendencies, hyperlipidemias, glaucoma, or cataracts, because the drug may exacerbate these conditions.

Because adrenocorticoids increase the susceptibility to and mask symptoms of infection, cortisone should not be used (except in life-threatening situations) in patients with viral or bacterial infections not controlled by anti-infective agents.

Interactions

When used concomitantly, cortisone may decrease the effects of oral anticoagulants by unknown mechanisms (rarely); increase the metabolism of isoniazid and salicylates; and cause hyperglycemia, requiring dosage adjustment of insulin in diabetic patients.

Use with barbiturates, phenytoin, or rifampin may cause decreased corticosteroid effects because of increased hepatic metabolism. Use with cholestyramine, colestipol, or antacids decreases cortisone's effect by adsorbing the corticosteroid, decreasing the amount absorbed.

Cortisone may enhance hypokalemia associated with diuretic or amphotericin B therapy. The hypokalemia may increase the risk of toxicity in patients concurrently receiving digitalis glycosides.

Concomitant use with estrogens may reduce the metabolism of cortisone by increasing the concentration of transcortin. The half-life of cortisone is then prolonged because of increased protein binding. Concomitant administration of ulcerogenic drugs, such as the nonsteroidal anti-inflammatory agents, may increase the risk of GI ulceration.

Effects on diagnostic tests

Cortisone therapy suppresses reactions to skin tests; causes false-negative results in the nitroblue tetrazolium test for systemic bacterial infections; and decreases ^{131}I uptake and protein-bound iodine concentrations in thyroid function tests.

It may increase glucose and cholesterol levels; decrease serum potassium, calcium, thyroxine, and triiodothyronine levels; and increase urine glucose and calcium levels.

Adverse reactions

When administered in high doses or for prolonged therapy, cortisone suppresses release of adrenocorticotropic hormone (ACTH) from the pituitary gland; in turn, the adrenal cortex stops secreting endogenous corticosteroids. The degree and duration of hypothalamic-pituitary-adrenal (HPA) axis suppression produced by the drug is highly variable among patients and depends on the dose, frequency and time of administration, and duration of cortisone therapy.

• CNS: euphoria, insomnia, headache, psychotic behavior, pseudotumor cerebri, mental changes, nervousness, restlessness, *psychoses.*
• CV: CHF, *hypertension,* edema.
• DERM: delayed healing, *acne,* skin eruptions, striae.
• EENT: *cataracts,* glaucoma, thrush.
• GI: *peptic ulcer,* irritation, increased appetite.
• Immune: immunosuppression, *increased susceptibility to infection.*
• Metabolic: *hypokalemia,* sodium retention, fluid retention, weight gain, hyperglycemia, *osteoporosis,* growth suppression in children, *glycosuria.*
• Musculoskeletal: muscle atrophy, weakness, *myopathy.*
• Local: atrophy at I.M. injection sites.
• Other: pancreatitis, *hirsutism, cushingoid symptoms,* withdrawal syndrome (nausea, fatigue, anorexia, dyspnea, hypotension, hypoglycemia, myalgia, arthralgia, fever, dizziness and fainting). Sudden withdrawal may be fatal or may exacerbate the underlying disease. Acute adrenal insufficiency may follow increased stress (infection, surgery, trauma) or abrupt withdrawal after long-term therapy.

Overdose and treatment

Acute ingestion, even in massive doses, is rarely a clinical problem. Toxic signs and symptoms rarely occur if the drug is used for less than 3 weeks, even at large dosage ranges. However, chronic use causes adverse physiologic effects, including suppression of the HPA axis, cushingoid appearance, muscle weakness, and osteoporosis.

▶ Special considerations

• Chronic use of cortisone in children and adolescents may delay growth and maturation.
• If possible, avoid long-term administration of pharmacologic dosages of glucocorticoids in children because these drugs may retard bone growth. Manifestations of adrenal suppression in children include retardation of linear growth, delayed weight gain, low plasma coritsol concentrations, and lack of response to corticotropin stimulation. In children who require prolonged therapy, closely monitor growth and development. Alternate-day therapy is recommended to minimize growth-suppression.
• Establish baseline blood pressure, fluid intake and output, weight, and electrolyte status. Watch for any sudden patient weight gain, edema, change in blood pressure, or change in electrolyte status.
• During times of physiologic stress (trauma, surgery, infection), the patient may require additional steroids and may experience signs of steroid withdrawal, patients who were previously steroid-dependent may need systemic corticosteroids to prevent adrenal insufficiency.
• After long-term therapy, the drug should be reduced gradually. Rapid reduction may cause withdrawal symptoms.
• Be aware of the patient's psychological history and watch for any behavioral changes.
• Observe for signs of infection or delayed wound healing.

• Acute withdrawal of drug may result in fever, myalgia, arthralgia, malaise, hypotension, hypoglycemia shock.

Information for parents and patient
• Be sure that the parents and patient understand the need to take the adrenocorticosteroid as prescribed. Give patients instructions on what to do if a dose is inadvertently missed.
• Warn the parents and patient not to discontinue the drug abruptly.
• Inform the parents and patient of the possible therapeutic and adverse effects of the drug, so that they may report any complication promptly.
• Advise parents that the patient should wear a Medic Alert bracelet or necklace indicating the need for supplemental adrenocorticoids during times of stress.
• Patient may take drug with food or milk to reduce GI upset.
• Patient should reduce salt (sodium) intake and increase potassium intake through dietary sources or prescribed supplements.
• Patient should not take any other drugs, not even aspirin, without medical approval.
• Parents and patient should inform new physician or dentist that patient is taking this drug.

cosyntropin
Cortrosyn

• Classification: diagnostic agent (anterior hormone)

How supplied
Available by prescription only
Injection: 0.25 mg/vial

Indications, route, and dosage
Diagnostic test of adrenocortical function
Children under age 2: 0.125 mg I.M. or I.V.
Children age 2 and over and adults: 0.25 to 1 mg I.M. or I.V. (unless label prohibits I.V. administration) between blood samplings. To administer as I.V. infusion, dilute 0.25 mg in dextrose 5% in water or normal saline solution, and infuse over 6 to 8 hours (40 mcg/hour).

Action and kinetics
• *Diagnostic action:* Cosyntropin is used to test adrenal function. The drug binds with a specific receptor in the adrenal cell plasma membrane to initiate synthesis of its entire spectrum of hormones, one of which is cortisol. In patients with primary adrenocortical insufficiency, cosyntropin does not increase plasma cortisol levels significantly.
• *Kinetics in adults:* Cosyntropin is inactivated by the proteolytic enzymes in the GI tract. After I.M. administration, cosyntropin is absorbed rapidly. After rapid I.V. administration, plasma cortisol levels begin to rise within 5 minutes and double within 15 to 30 minutes. Peak levels occur within 1 hour after I.M. or rapid I.V. administration. Distribution of cosyntropin is not fully understood, but the drug is removed

rapidly from plasma by many tissues. Metabolism is unknown. Cosyntropin probably is excreted by the kidneys.

Contraindications and precautions
Cosyntropin is contraindicated in patients with known hypersensitivity to the drug; however, it is less antigenic than corticotropin and less likely to produce allergic reactions.

Cosyntropin should be used cautiously in patients with preexisting allergic disease or a history of allergic reactions to corticotropin, because hypersensitivity reactions are possible.

Interactions
Concomitant use of cosyntropin with cortisone, hydrocortisone, or estrogens may cause abnormally elevated plasma cortisol levels. High plasma cortisol levels may be reported erroneously in patients receiving spironolactone, cortisone, or hydrocortisone when fluorometric analysis is used. This does not occur with the radioimmunoassay or competitive protein-binding method. However, therapy can be maintained with prednisone, dexamethasone, or betamethasone because these are not detectable by the fluorometric method.

Effects on diagnostic tests
Cosyntropin therapy alters blood glucose levels.

Adverse reactions
Except for hypersensitivity reactions, short-term administration of cosyntropin is unlikely to produce adverse reactions. Discontinue if hypersensitivity reaction occurs.

Overdose and treatment
Acute overdose probably requires no therapy other than symptomatic treatment and supportive care, as appropriate.

▶ Special considerations
• More cortisol is secreted if dosage is given slowly, not rapidly I.V.
• Cosyntropin is less antigenic than corticotropin and less likely to produce allergic reactions.
• Some clinicians prefer to determine plasma cortisol concentration 60 minutes after injection of cosyntropin.
• Determine if patient is taking medications containing spironolactone, cortisone, hydrocortisone, or estrogen because these drugs may alter plasma cortisol levels.
• Reconstitute powder by adding 1 ml of normal saline solution to 0.25-mg vial to yield a solution containing 0.25 mg/ml.
• Reconstituted solution remains stable at room temperature for 24 hours or for 21 days at 2° to 8° C. (36° to 46° F.).
• A normal response to cosyntropin includes morning control cortisol level exceeding 5 mcg/100 ml plasma; 30 minutes after the injection, cortisol levels rise by at least 7 mcg/100 ml above control and exceed 18 mcg/100 ml.

Information for parents and patient
Advise parents and patient of test procedure.

---

co-trimoxazole (trimethoprim-sulfamethoxazole)
Apo-Sulfatrim*, Bactrim, Bactrim DS, Bactrim I.V. Infusion, Bethaprim SS, Cotrim, Novotrimel*, Protrin*, Roubac*, Septra, Septra DS, Septra I.V. Infusion, SMZ-TMP, Sulfatrim, Sulmeprim

• Classification: antibiotic (sulfonamide and folate antagonist)

How supplied
Available by prescription only
Tablets: trimethoprim 80 mg and sulfamethoxazole 400 mg; trimethoprim 160 mg and sulfamethoxazole 800 mg
Suspension: trimethoprim 40 mg and sulfamethoxazole 200 mg/5 ml
Injectable: trimethoprim 16 mg and sulfamethoxazole 80 mg/ml (5ml/ampule)

Indications, route, and dosage
Urinary tract infections and shigellosis
Children up to 40 kg: 4 mg/kg trimethoprim per 20 mg/kg sulfamethoxazole P.O. q 12 hours (10 days for urinary tract infections; 5 days for shigellosis).
Children 40 kg and over and adults: 160 mg trimethoprim per 800 mg sulfa-methoxazole (double-strength tablet) q 12 hours for 10 to 14 days in urinary tract infections and for 5 days in shigellosis. For simple cystitis or acute urethral syndrome, may give one to three double-strength tablets as a single dose.
Otitis media
Children up to 40 kg: 4 mg/kg trimethoprim per 20 mg/kg sulfamehoxazole P.O. q 12 hours for 10 days.
Pneumocystis carinii pneumonia
Infants, children, and adults: 5 mg Trimethoprim per 25 mg sulfamethoxazole/kg P.O. q. 6 hours.
Dosage in renal failure (parenteral form)
In children with impaired renal function, doses or frequency of administration must be modified according to degree of renal impairment, severity of infection, and susceptibility of organism.

Creatinine clearance (ml/min/1.73 m²)	Dosage in children
>30	Usual pediatric dose
20 to 30	One half the usual pediatric dose
<20	Use is contraindicated

Creatinine clearance (ml/min/1.73 m²)	Dosage in adults
>30	Usual adult dose
15 to 30	One half the usual adult dose
<15	Use is not recommended

Action and kinetics
• *Antibacterial action:* Co-trimoxazole is generally bactericidal; it acts by sequential blockade of folic acid enzymes in the synthesis pathway. The sulfamethoxazole component inhibits formation of dihydrofolic acid from para-aminobenzoic acid (PABA), whereas trimethoprim inhibits dihydrofolate reductase. Both drugs block folic acid synthesis, preventing bacterial cell synthesis of essential nucleic acids.
   Co-trimoxazole is effective against *Escherichia coli, Klebsiella, Enterobacter, Proteus mirabilis, Hemophilus influenzae, Streptococcus pneumoniae, Staphylococcus aureus, Acinetobacter, Salmonella, Shigella,* and *Pneumocystis carinii.*
• *Kinetics in adults:* Co-trimoxazole is well absorbed from the GI tract after oral administration and is distributed widely into body tissues and fluids, including middle ear fluid, prostatic fluid, bile, aqueous humor, and CSF. Co-trimoxazole crosses the placenta.
   Co-trimoxazole is metabolized by the liver and is excreted primarily in urine by glomerular filtration and renal tubular secretion.

Contraindications and precautions
Do not give co-trimoxazole to children with known hypersensitivity to sulfonamides (or any other drug containing sulfur, such as thiazides, furosemide, and oral sulfonylureas); to children with known hypersensitivity to trimethoprim; or to children with severe renal or hepatic dysfunction or porphyria.
   Co-trimoxazole should be used cautiously in children with acquired immunodeficiency syndrome (AIDS), because of the increased incidence of adverse reactions; and in children with mild to moderate renal or hepatic impairment or urinary obstruction, because of the hazard of drug accumulation; and in those with severe allergies, asthma, blood dyscrasias, and folate or glucose-6-phosphate dehydrogenase deficiency. In neonates, co-trimoxazole may displace unconjugated bilirubin from plasma albumin and increase the risk of kernicterus.

Interactions
Co-trimoxazole may inhibit hepatic metabolism of oral anticoagulants, displacing them from binding sites and enhancing anticoagulant effects. Concomitant use of co-trimoxazole with PABA antagonizes sulfonamide effects. Concomitant use with oral sulfonylureas enhances their hypoglycemic effects, probably by displacement of sulfonylureas from protein-binding sites.
   Concomitant use of urinary acidifying agents (ammonium chloride or ascorbic acid) decreases urinary

---

pH and sulfonamide solubility, thereby increasing the risk of crystalluria.

Effects on diagnostic tests

Co-trimoxazole alters urine glucose test results utilizing cupric sulfate (Benedict's reagent or Clinitest).

Co-trimoxazole may elevate liver function test results; it may decrease serum concentration levels of erythrocytes, platelets, or leukocytes.

Adverse reactions

• CNS: headache, mental depression, seizures, hallucinations.
• DERM: erythema multiforme *(Stevens-Johnson syndrome)*, generalized skin eruption, epidermal necrolysis, exfoliative dermatitis, photosensitivity, urticaria, pruritus, petechiae.
• GI: nausea, vomiting, diarrhea, abdominal pain, anorexia, stomatitis.
• GU: toxic nephrosis with oliguria and anuria, crystalluria, hematuria.
• HEMA: agranulocytosis, aplastic anemia, megaloblastic anemia, thrombocytopenia, leukopenia, hemolytic anemia.
• Hepatic: jaundice.
• Other: hypersensitivity, serum sickness, drug fever, *anaphylaxis*.

Note: Patients with AIDS have a much higher incidence of all adverse reactions, especially hypersensitivity, rash, fever, hematologic toxicity, and liver function test abnormalities.

Drug should be discontinued if signs of toxicity or hypersensitivity occur; if hematologic abnormalities are accompanied by sore throat, pallor, fever, jaundice, purpura, or weakness; if crystalluria is accompanied by renal colic, hematuria, oliguria, proteinuria, urinary obstruction, urolithiasis, increased blood urea nitrogen levels, or anuria; or if severe diarrhea indicates pseudomembranous colitis. If signs of megaloblastic anemia develop, drug should be discontinued and folinic acid administered to rescue the bone marrow.

Overdose and treatment

Clinical signs of overdose include mental depression, confusion, headache, nausea, vomiting, diarrhea, facial swelling, slight elevations in liver function test results, and bone marrow depression.

Treat by emesis or gastric lavage, followed by supportive care (correction of acidosis, forced fluids, and/or urinary alkalinization to enhance solubility and excretion). Treatment of renal failure may be required; transfuse appropriate blood products in severe hematologic toxicity; use folinic acid to rescue bone marrow. Hemodialysis has limited ability to remove co-trimoxazole.

▶ Special considerations

• Assess patient's history of allergies; do not give a sulfonamide to any patient with a history of hypersensitivity reactions to sulfonamides or to any other drug containing sulfur (such as thiazides, furosemide, and oral sulfonylureas).
• Sulfonamides are also contraindicated in the child with severe renal or hepatic dysfunction, or porphyria.

Sulfonamides may cause kernicterus in infants, because they displace bilirubin at the binding site. Infants under age 2 months should receive sulfonamides only if there is no therapeutic alternative.
• Administer sulfonamides with caution to children with the following conditions: mild to moderate renal or hepatic impairment, urinary obstruction (because of the risk of drug accumulation), severe allergies, asthma, blood dyscrasias, or G6PD deficiency.
• Give sulfonamides with caution to children with fragile X chromosome associated with mental retardation, because they are vulnerable to psychomotor depression from folate depletion.
• Monitor continuously for possible hypersensitivity reactions or other untoward effects; patients with AIDS have a much higher incidence of adverse reactions.
• Obtain results of cultures and sensitivity tests before first dose, but therapy may begin before laboratory tests are complete. Check test results periodically to assess drug efficacy. Monitor urine cultures, CBC, and urinalysis before and during therapy.
• Monitor patients on long-term therapy or those who are receiving immunosuppressants or radiation therapy for possible superinfection.
• Co-trimoxale has been used to prevent recurrent urinary tract infections and other infections — for example, in children with cancer.
• Give oral dosage with adequate water. Keep patient well hydrated.
• Tablet may be swallowed with water to facilitate passage into stomach and maximum absorption.
• Always consult manufacturer's directions for reconstitution, and storage of drugs; check expiration dates.
• Give oral sulfonamide at least 1 hour before or 2 hours after meals for maximum absorption.
• For I.V. use, dilute infusion in dextrose 5% in water. Do not mix with other drugs. Do not administer by rapid infusion or bolus injection. Infuse slowly over 60 to 90 minutes. Change infusion site every 48 to 72 hours.
• Use solution within 2 hours after preparation. Do not refrigerate solution.
• Check solution carefully for precipitate before starting infusion. Do not use solution containing a precipitate.
• Assess I.V. site for signs of phlebitis or infiltration.
• Note that DS means double-strength.

Information for parents and patient

• Advise parents that patient should avoid exposure to direct sunlight because of possible photosensitivity reaction. Recommend use of sunscreen.
• Tell parents to give oral sulfonamides at least 1 hour before and 2 hours after meals for maximum absorption. Shake oral suspensions well before administering to ensure correct dosage.
• Be sure patient and parents understand how and when to administer drug; urge them to complete entire prescribed regimen, to comply with instructions for around-the-clock dosage, and to keep follow-up appointments.
• Teach signs and symptoms of hypersensitivity and other adverse reactions, and emphasize need to report these. Specifically urge parents to report bloody urine,

difficult breathing, rash, fever, chills, or severe fatigue.
• Teach signs and symptoms of bacterial and fungal superinfection to patients and parents; if low resistance from immunosuppressants or irradiation is evident, emphasize need to report them. Instruct parents regarding oral hygiene and care of diaper area to prevent yeast infection.
• Advise parents of diabetic children not to monitor urine glucose levels with Clinitest; sulfonamides alter results of tests utilizing cupric sulfate.
• Advise patient or parents to tell new physician or dentist of sulfonamide therapy.

---

cromolyn sodium
Intal Aerosol Spray, Intal Nebulizer Solution, Intal Powder for Inhalation (contained in capsules), Nasalcrom, Opticrom

• Classification: mast cell stabilizer, antiasthmatic (chromone derivative)

How supplied
Available by prescription only
Aerosol: 800 mcg/metered spray
Solution: 20 mg/2 ml for nebulization
Ophthalmic solution: 4% (with benzalkonium chloride 0.01%, EDTA 0.01%, and phenylethyl alcohol 0.4%)
Nasal solution: 5.2 mg/metered spray (40 mg/ml)

Indications, route, and dosage
Adjunct in treatment of severe perennial bronchial asthma
Children over age 5 and adults: Contents of 20-mg capsule inhaled q.i.d. at regular intervals. Or, administer two metered sprays using inhaler q.i.d. at regular intervals. Also available as an aqueous solution administered through a nebulizer.
Prevention and treatment of allergic rhinitis
Children over age 5 and adults: 1 spray (5.2 mg) of the nasal solution in each nostril t.i.d or q.i.d. May give up to 6 times daily.
Prevention of exercise-induced bronchospasm
Children over age 5 and adults: Patient should inhale contents of 20-mg capsule or inhale two metered sprays no more than 1 hour before anticipated exercise.
    Inhalation of 20 mg of the oral inhalation solution may be used in adults or children age 2 and over. Repeat inhalation as required for protection during long exercise.
Allergic ocular disorders (giant papillary conjunctivitis, vernal keratoconjunctivitis, vernal keratitis, and allergic keratoconjunctivitis)
Children over age 4 and adults: Instill 1 to 2 drops in each eye 4 to 6 times daily at regular intervals. One drop contains approximately 1.6 mg cromolyn sodium.

Action and kinetics
• *Antiasthmatic action:* Cromolyn prevents release of the mediators of Type I allergic reactions, including histamine and slow-reacting substance of anaphylaxis (SRS-A), from sensitized mast cells after the antigen-antibody union has taken place. Cromolyn does not inhibit the binding of the IgE to the mast cell nor the interaction between the cell-bound IgE and the specific antigen. It does inhibit the release of substances (such as histamine and SRS-A) in response to the IgE binding to the mast cell. The main site of action occurs locally on the lung mucosa, nasal mucosa, and eyes.
• *Bronchodilating action:* Besides the mast cell stabilization, recent evidence suggests that the drug may have a bronchodilating effect by an unknown mechanism. Comparative studies have shown cromolyn and theophylline to be equally efficacious but less effective than orally inhaled B_2-adrenergic agonist in preventing this bronchospasm.
• *Ocular antiallergy action:* Cromolyn inhibits the degranulation of sensitized mast cells that occurs after exposure to specific antigens, preventing the release of histamine and SRS-A.
    Cromolyn has no direct anti-inflammatory, vasoconstrictor, antihistamine, antiserotonin, or corticosteroid-like properties.
    Cromolyn dissolved in water and given orally has been found to be effective in managing food allergy, inflammatory bowel disease (Crohn's disease, ulcerative colitis), and systemic mastocytosis.
• *Kinetics in adults:* Only 0.5% to 2% of an oral dose is absorbed. After inhalation using capsules via an oral inhaler (Spinhaler), approximately 7.5% (range 5% to 10%) of a dose of cromolyn powder reaches the lungs and is absorbed readily into the systemic circulation. The amount reaching the lungs depends on the patient's ability to use the inhaler correctly, the amount of bronchoconstriction, and the size or presence of mucous plugs. The degree of absorption depends on the method of administration; the most absorption occurs with the powder via the Spinhaler, next the aerosol via metered-dose inhaler, and the lowest administration of the solution via power-operated nebulizer. Less than 7% of an intranasal dose of cromolyn as a solution is absorbed systemically. Only minimal absorption (0.03%) of an ophthalmic dose occurs after instillation into the eye. The absorption half-life from the lung is 1 hour. A plasma concentration of 9 mcg/ml can be achieved 15 minutes after following a 20-mg dose. Cromolyn does not cross most biological membranes because it is ionized and lipid-insoluble at the body's pH. Less than 0.1% of a cromolyn dose crosses to the placenta; it is not known if the drug is distributed into breast milk. Cromolyn is not metabolized; it is excreted unchanged in urine (50%) and bile (approximately 50%). Small amounts may be excreted in the feces or exhaled. The elimination half-life is 81 minutes.

Contraindications and precautions
Cromolyn is contraindicated in patients with a hypersensitivity to cromolyn or any ingredient (lactose) in these products. It should be not be used to treat acute asthma, especially status asthmaticus, because

---

‡May contain sulfites   ◆May contain tartrazine   ◆◆May contain benzyl alcohol

it is a prophylactic drug with no benefit in acute situations.

Cromolyn's safety in pregnancy has not been established. It should be used only when benefit clearly outweighs the risk to the fetus.

Interactions
None reported.

Effects on diagnostic tests
None reported.

Adverse reactions
• CNS: dizziness, headache, vertigo, neuritis.
• DERM: *rash*, urticaria, dermatitis.
• EENT: lacrimation, swollen parotid gland, irritation of the throat and trachea, *cough, bronchospasm* after inhalation of dry powder; esophagitis; *nasal congestion;* pharyngeal irritation; wheezing.
• GI: nausea, dry mouth, vomiting, esophagitis.
• GU: dysuria, urinary frequency, nephrosis.
• Other: joint swelling and pain, angioedema, myalgia.
  The adverse effect related to the cromolyn capsule delivery system is inhalation of gelatin particles.

Overdose and treatment
No information available.

▶ Special considerations
• Cromolyn use in children under age 5 is limited to the inhalation route of administration; the capsule form and the Spinhaler are not recommended. The safety of the nebulizer solution in children under age 2 and of the nasal solution in children under age 6 has not been established.
• Pulmonary status should be monitored before and immediately after therapy.
• Capsules are not to be swallowed. Insert capsule into Spinhaler or use Nasalmatic device provided; follow manufacturer's directions and assist patient in proper technique.
• Bronchospasm or cough occasionally occurs after inhalation and may require discontinuation of cromolyn therapy. Prior bronchodilation may help but discontinuation of cromolyn may still be necessary.
• Asthma symptoms may recur if cromolyn dosage is reduced below the recommended dosage.
• Patients with impaired renal or hepatic function should receive reduced dosage.
• Eosinophilic pneumonia or pulmonary infiltrates with eosinophilia requires stopping the drug.
• Nasal solution may cause nasal stinging or sneezing immediately after instillation of the drug but this reaction rarely requires discontinuation of the drug.
• Watch for recurrence of asthmatic symptoms when corticosteroids are also used. Use only when acute episode has been controlled, airway is cleared, and patient is able to inhale.
• Patients considered for cromolyn therapy should have pulmonary function tests to confirm significant bronchodilator-reversible component of airway obstruction.
• Protect capsules, oral solution, and ophthalmic solution from direct sunlight.

• Therapeutic effects may not be seen for 2 to 4 weeks after initiating therapy.

Information for parents and patient
• Teach correct use of Spinhaler: Insert capsule in device properly, exhale completely before placing mouthpiece between lips, then inhale deeply and rapidly with steady, even breath; remove inhaler from mouth, hold breath a few seconds, and exhale. Repeat until all powder has been inhaled.
• Instruct parents and patient to avoid excessive handling of capsule.
• Urge parents to call if drug causes wheezing or coughing.
• Instruct parents of patients with asthma or seasonal or perennial allergic rhinitis to administer the drug at regular intervals to ensure clinical effectiveness.
• Advise patient that gargling and rinsing mouth after administration can help reduce mouth dryness.
• The patient who is taking prescribed adrenocorticoids should continue taking them during cromolyn therapy, if appropriate.
• Tell parents and patient who uses a bronchodilator inhaler to administer a dose about 5 minutes before taking cromolyn (unless otherwise indicated); explain that this step helps reduce adverse reactions.
• Tell parents to store capsules at room temperature in a tightly closed container; protect from moisture and temperatures higher than 104° F. (40° C.).

crotamiton
Eurax

• Classification: scabicide and antipruritic (synthetic chloroformate salt)

How supplied
Available by prescription only
Cream: 10%
Lotion: 10% (emollient base)

Indications, route, and dosage
Scabicide
Children and adults: Wash thoroughly and scrub away loose scales, then towel dry; massage drug onto skin of the entire body from the neck to the toes (with special attention to skin folds, creases, and interdigital spaces). Repeat application in 24 hours. Take a cleansing bath 48 hours after the final application.
Antipruritic
Children and adults: Apply locally b.i.d. or t.i.d.

Action and kinetics
The mechanisms of crotamiton's scabicidal and antipruritic actions are unknown. Crotamiton is toxic to the parasitic mite *Sarcoptes scabiei.*
• *Kinetics in adults:* Unknown.

Contraindications and precautions
Do not apply crotamiton to acutely inflamed or raw skin.

  Crotamiton is contraindicated in patients with a

---

history of hypersensitivity to the drug and in those who exhibit primary irritation after application of the drug.

Interactions
None reported.

Effects on diagnostic tests
None reported.

Adverse reactions
• Local: irritation, contact dermatitis.
Note: Drug should be discontinued if sensitization develops.

Overdose and treatment
Discontinue therapy.

▶ Special considerations
• Avoid applying crotamiton to the face, eyes, mucous membranes, or urethral meatus.
• Patients may require isolation and special care of linens until treatment is complete.
• If primary irritation or hypersensitivity occurs, discontinue treatment and remove drug with soap and water.

Information for parents and patient
• All contaminated clothing and bed linen should be machine-washed in hot water and dried in hot dryer or dry-cleaned.
• Patient should reapply drug if accidentally washed off but should avoid overuse.
• Advise parents or patient that pruritus may persist after treatment.

---

cyanocobalamin (vitamin B₁₂)
Bay Bee-12, Berubigen, Betalin 12, Cabadon-M, Cobex, Crystimin-1000, Cyanoject, Cyomin, Kaybovite-1000, Pernavit, Redisol, Rubesol-1000, Rubramin PC, Sytobex, Vibal

hydroxocobalamin (vitamin B₁₂ₐ)
Alphamin, AlphaRedisol, Codroxomin, Droxomin, Hybalamin, Hydrobexan, Hydro-Cobex, Hydroxo-12, Hydroxocobalamin, LA-12, Vibal L.A.

• Classification: vitamin, nutrition supplement

How supplied
Available by prescription only
Injection: 30-ml vials (30 mcg/ml, 100 mcg/ml, 120 mcg/ml with benzyl alcohol, 1,000 mcg/ml, 1,000 mcg/ml with benzyl alcohol), 10-ml vials (100 mcg/ml, 100 mcg/ml with benzyl alcohol, 1,000 mcg/ml, 1,000 mcg/ml with benzyl alcohol, 1,000 mcg/ml with methyl and propyl parabens), 5-ml vials (1,000 mcg/ml with benzyl alcohol), 1-ml vials (1,000 mcg/ml with benzyl alcohol), 1-ml unimatic (1,000 mcg/ml with benzyl alcohol)

Tablets: 25 mcg, 50 mcg, 100 mcg, 250 mcg, 500 mcg, 1,000 mcg

Indications, route, and dosage
Vitamin B₁₂ deficiency from any cause except malabsorption related to pernicious anemia or other GI disease
Children: 1 mcg P.O. daily as dietary supplement, or 1 to 30 mcg S.C. or I.M. daily for 5 to 10 days, depending on severity of deficiency.
Maintenance dose: At least 60 mcg I.M. or S.C. monthly. For subsequent prophylaxis, advise adequate nutrition and recommended daily allowance (RDA) vitamin B₁₂ supplements.
Adults: 25 mcg P.O. daily as dietary supplement, or 30 to 100 mcg S.C. or I.M. daily for 5 to 10 days, depending on severity of deficiency.
Maintenance dose: 100 to 200 mcg I.M. monthly. For subsequent prophylaxis, advise adequate nutrition and RDA of vitamin B₁₂ supplements.
Pernicious anemia or vitamin B₁₂ malabsorption
Children: 1,000 to 5,000 mcg I.M. or S.C. given over 2 or more weeks in 100-mcg increments; then 60 mcg I.M. or S.C. monthly for life.
Adults: Initially, 100 to 1,000 mcg I.M. daily for 2 weeks, then 100 to 1,000 mcg I.M. monthly for life. If neurologic complications are present, follow initial therapy with 100 to 1,000 mcg I.M. once every 2 weeks before starting monthly regimen.
Methylmalonic aciduria
Neonates: 1,000 mcg I.M. daily for 11 days with a protein-restricted diet.
Diagnostic test for vitamin B₁₂ deficiency without concealing folate deficiency in patients with megaloblastic anemias
Children and adults: 1 mcg I.M. daily for 10 days with diet low in vitamin B₁₂ and folate. Reticulocytosis between days 3 and 10 confirms diagnosis of vitamin B₁₂ deficiency.
Schilling test flushing dose
Children and adults: 1,000 mcg I.M. in a single dose.

Action and kinetics
• *Nutritional action:* Vitamin B₁₂ can be converted to coenzyme B₁₂ in tissues and, as such, is essential for conversion of methyl-malonate to succinate and synthesis of methionine from homocysteine, a reaction that also requires folate. Without coenzyme B₁₂, folate deficiency occurs. Vitamin B₁₂ is also associated with fat and carbohydrate metabolism and protein synthesis. Cells characterized by rapid division (epithelial cells, bone marrow, and myeloid cells) appear to have the greatest requirement for vitamin B₁₂.
Vitamin B₁₂ deficiency may cause megaloblastic anemia, GI lesions, and neurologic damage; it begins with an inability to produce myelin followed by gradual degeneration of the axon and nerve. Parenteral administration of vitamin B₁₂ completely reverses the megaloblastic anemia and GI symptoms of vitamin B₁₂ deficiency.
• *Kinetics in adults:* After oral administration, vitamin B₁₂ is absorbed irregularly from the distal small intestine. Vitamin B₁₂ is protein-bound, and this bond must be split by proteolysis and gastric acid before

---

‡May contain sulfites   ♦May contain tartrazine   ♦♦May contain benzyl alcohol

absorption. Absorption depends on sufficient intrinsic factor and calcium. Vitamin B_{12} is inadequate in malabsorptive states and in pernicious anemia. Vitamin B_{12} is absorbed rapidly from I.M. and S.C. injection sites; the plasma level peaks within 1 hour. After oral administration of doses below 3 mcg, peak plasma levels are not reached for 8 to 12 hours.

Vitamin B_{12} is distributed into the liver, bone marrow, and other tissues, including the placenta. At birth, the vitamin B concentration in neonates is three to five times that in the mother. Vitamin B_{12} is distributed into breast milk in concentrations approximately equal to the maternal vitamin B_{12} concentration. Unlike cyanocobalamin, hydroxocobalamin is absorbed more slowly parenterally and may be taken up by the liver in larger quantities; it also produces a greater increase in serum cobalamin levels and less urinary excretion. Cyanocobalamin and hydroxocobalamin are metabolized in the liver.

In healthy persons receiving only dietary vitamin B_{12}, approximately 3 to 8 mcg of the vitamin is secreted into the GI tract daily, mainly from bile, and all but about 1 mcg is reabsorbed; less than 0.25 mcg is usually excreted in the urine daily. When vitamin B_{12} is administered in amounts that exceed the binding capacity of plasma, the liver, and other tissues, it is free in the blood for urinary excretion.

Contraindications and precautions

Vitamin B_{12} is contraindicated in patients with known hypersensitivity to cobalt, vitamin B_{12}, or any component of these medications. An intradermal test dose is recommended. After starting vitamin B_{12} therapy, serum potassium concentrations should be monitored to avoid fatal hypokalemia. Vitamin B_{12} should be administered cautiously to persons who are susceptible to gout (because of the potential for increased nucleic acid degeneration) and to those with heart disease (because of the potential for increased blood volume).

Vitamin B_{12} should not be used in patients with hereditary optic nerve atrophy (Leber's disease) because rapid optic nerve atrophy has been reported as an adverse effect.

Interactions

Concomitant use of the following drugs decreases vitamin B_{12} absorption from the GI tract: aminoglycosides, colchicine, extended-release potassium preparations, aminosalicylic acid and its salts, anticonvulsants, cobalt irradiation of the small bowel, and excessive alcohol intake. Concurrent administration of colchicine may increase neomycin-induced malabsorption of vitamin B_{12}. Large amounts of ascorbic acid should not be administered within 1 hour of taking vitamin B_{12} because ascorbic acid may destroy vitamin B_{12}. In patients with pernicious anemia, vitamin B_{12} absorption and intrinsic factor secretion may be increased. Chloramphenicol and other hematopoietic suppressants may block the action of vitamin B_{12} because they interfere with maturation of erythrocytes.

Effects on diagnostic tests

Vitamin B_{12} therapy may cause false-positive results for intrinsic factor antibodies, which are present in the blood of half of all patients with pernicious anemia.

Methotrexate, pyrimethamine, and most anti-infectives invalidate diagnostic blood assays for vitamin B_{12}.

Adverse reactions

• CV: pulmonary edema, CHF (early in treatment), peripheral vascular thrombosis.
• DERM: itching, transitory exanthema, urticaria.
• EENT: severe optic nerve atrophy in patients with early Leber's disease.
• GI: mild, transient diarrhea.
• HEMA: polycythemia vera.
• Local: pain at injection site.
• Other: anaphylactic shock and death, feeling that entire body is swelling, hypokalemia.

Overdose and treatment

Not applicable. Even in large doses, oral vitamin B_{12} is usually nontoxic.

▶ Special considerations

• Safety and efficacy of vitamin B_{12} for use in children have not been established. The RDA for vitamin B_{12} is 0.5 to 3 mcg in children and 3 mcg in adults, as recommended by the Food and Nutrition Board of the National Academy of Sciences — National Research Council.
• Some of these products contain benzyl alcohol, which has been associated with a fatal "gasping syndrome" in premature infants.
• Patients with a history of sensitivities and those suspected of being sensitive to vitamin B_{12} should receive an intradermal test dose before therapy begins. Sensitization to vitamin B_{12} may develop after as many as 8 years of treatment.
• Determine patient's diet and drug history, including patterns of alcohol use, to identify poor nutritional habits.
• Administer oral vitamin B_{12} with meals to increase absorption. Oral solution should be administered promptly after mixing with fruit juice. Ascorbic acid causes instability of vitamin B_{12}.
• Monitor bowel function because regularity is essential for consistent absorption of oral preparations.
• Do not mix the parenteral form with dextrose solutions, alkaline or strongly acidic solutions, or oxidizing and reducing agents, because anaphylactic reactions may occur with I.V. use. Check compatibility with pharmacist.
• Parenteral therapy is preferred for patients with pernicious anemia because oral administration may be unreliable. In patients with neurologic complications, prolonged inadequate oral therapy may lead to permanent spinal cord damage. Oral therapy is appropriate for mild conditions without neurologic signs and for those patients who refuse or are sensitive to the parenteral form.
• Expect therapeutic response to occur within 48 hours; it is measured by laboratory values and effect on fatigue, GI symptoms, anorexia, pallid or yellow complexion, glossitis, distaste for meat, dyspnea on

exertion, palpitation, neurologic degeneration (paresthesias, loss of vibratory and position sense and deep reflexes, incoordination), psychotic behavior, anosmia, and visual disturbances.

• Therapeutic response to vitamin B_{12} may be impaired by concurrent infection, uremia, folic acid or iron deficiency, or drugs having bone marrow suppressant effects. Large doses of vitamin B_{12} or B_{12a} may improve folate-deficient megaloblastic anemia.

• Expect reticulocyte concentration to rise in 3 to 4 days, peak in 5 to 8 days, and then gradually decline as erythrocyte count and hemoglobin rise to normal levels (in 4 to 6 weeks).

• Monitor potassium levels during the first 48 hours, especially in patients with pernicious anemia or megaloblastic anemia. Potassium supplements may be required. Conversion to normal erythropoiesis increases erythrocyte potassium requirement and can result in fatal hypokalemia in these patients.

• Monitor vital signs in patients with cardiac disease and those receiving parenteral vitamin B_{12}. Watch for symptoms of pulmonary edema, which tend to develop early in therapy.

• Patients with mild peripheral neurologic defects may respond to concomitant physical therapy. Usually, neurologic damage that does not improve after 12 to 18 months of therapy is considered irreversible. Severe vitamin B_{12} deficiency that persists for 3 months or longer may cause permanent spinal cord degeneration.

• Continue periodic hematologic evaluations throughout the patient's lifetime.

Information for parents and patient

• Emphasize the importance of a well-balanced diet. To prevent progression of subacute combined degeneration, patient should not use folic acid instead of vitamin B_{12} to prevent anemia.

• Tell parents that patients should not smoke; smoking appears to increase the requirement for vitamin B_{12}.

• Tell parents to report infection or disease in case patient's condition requires increased dosage of vitamin B_{12}.

• Tell parents that patient with pernicious anemia must have lifelong treatment with vitamin B_{12} to prevent recurring symptoms and the risk of incapacitating and irreversible spinal cord damage.

cyclacillin
Cyclapen-W

• Classification: antibiotic (aminopenicillin)

How supplied

Available by prescription only
Suspension: 125 mg/5 ml, and 250 mg/5 ml (after reconstitution)
Tablets: 250 mg, 500 mg

Indications, route, and dosage
Systemic and urinary tract infections, otitis media, and skin and skin structure infections caused by susceptible organisms

Children: 50 to 100 mg/kg daily in equally spaced doses q 6 to 8 hours.
Adults: 250 to 500 mg P.O. q.i.d. in equally spaced doses.

Tonsilitis, pharyngitis

Children 2 months of age and older weighing less than 20 kg: 125 mg q 8 hours.
Children 2 months of age and older weighing more than 20 kg: 250 mg P.O. q 8 hours.

Dosage in renal failure

In patients with impaired renal function, doses or frequency of administration must be modified according to degree of renal impairment, severity of infection, and susceptibility of organism.

Creatinine clearance (ml/min/1.73 m²)	Dosage in adults
>50	Up to 500 mg q 6 hours
30 to 50	Up to 500 mg q 12 hours
15 to 30	Up to 500 mg q 18 hours
10 to 15	Up to 500 mg q 24 hours
≤10	Serum determinations are recommended to determine dose and frequency.

Action and kinetics

• *Antibiotic action:* Cyclacillin is bactericidal; it adheres to bacterial penicillin-binding proteins, thus inhibiting bacterial cell wall synthesis.

Cyclacillin's spectrum of activity includes nonpenicillinase-producing gram-positive bacteria, *Neisseria gonorrhoeae, N. meningitidis, Hemophilus influenzae, Escherichia coli, Proteus mirabilis, Salmonella,* and *Shigella.*

• *Kinetics in adults:* Cyclacillin is well absorbed after oral administration; peak plasma concentrations occur 30 to 60 minutes after an oral dose. Cyclacillin distribution is not clearly defined; drug is about 18% to 25% protein-bound. Cyclacillin is only partially metabolized. Cyclacillin is excreted in urine by renal tubular secretion and glomerular filtration. Elimination half-life in adults is ½ to 1 hour, and 0.7 to 0.8 hours in children age 4 to 39 months, extended to 10 hours in patients with extensive renal impairment.

Contraindications and precautions

Cyclacillin is contraindicated in patients with known hypersensitivity to any other penicillin or to cephalosporins.

Cyclacillin should be used with caution in patients with renal impairment because it is excreted in urine; decreased dosage is required in moderate to severe renal failure.

Interactions
Probenecid inhibits renal tubular secretion of cyclacillin, raising its serum concentration levels.

Effects on diagnostic tests
None reported.

Adverse reactions
• GI: nausea, vomiting, diarrhea.
• GU: acute interstitial nephritis.
• HEMA: anemia, thrombocytopenia, thrombocytopenic purpura, leukopenia, neutropenia, eosinophilia.
• Other: hypersensitivity reactions (edema, fever, chills, rash, pruritus, urticaria, anaphylaxis), bacterial or fungal superinfection.
   Note: Drug should be discontinued if immediate hypersensitivity reaction occurs, or if bone marrow toxicity or acute interstitial nephritis develops.

Overdose and treatment
Clinical signs of overdose include neuromuscular sensitivity or seizures. After recent ingestion (4 hours or less), empty the stomach by induced emesis or gastric lavage; follow with activated charcoal to reduce absorption. Cyclacillin can be removed by hemodialysis.

▶ Special considerations
• Safety in infants under age 2 months has not been established.
• Assess patient's history of allergies; do not give cyclacillin to any patient with a history of hypersensitivity reactions to cephalosporins. Try to determine whether previous reactions were true hypersensitivity or another reaction, such as GI distress, which the patient has interpreted as allergy.
• Keep in mind that a negative history for penicillin hypersensitivity does not preclude future allergic reactions; monitor patient continuously for possible allergic reactions or other untoward effects.
• In patients with renal impairment, dosage should be reduced if creatinine clearance is below 10 ml/minute.
• Assess level of conciousness, neurologic status, and renal function when high doses are used, because excessive blood levels can cause CNS toxicity.
• Obtain results of cultures and sensitivity tests before first dose, but therapy may begin before test results are complete. Repeat tests periodically to assess drug efficacy.
• Monitor vital signs, electrolytes, and renal function studies; monitor body weight for fluid retention.
• Coagulation abnormalities, even frank bleeding, can follow high doses; monitor prothrombin times and platelet counts, and assess for signs of occult or frank bleeding.
• Monitor patients on long-term therapy for possible superinfection, especially debilitated patients and others receiving immunosuppressants or radiation therapy; monitor closely for fever.
• Give penicillins at least 1 hour before giving bacteriostatic antibiotics (tetracyclines, erythromycins, and chloramphenicol); these drugs inhibit bacterial cell growth, decreasing rate of penicillin uptake by bacterial cell walls.

• Cyclacillin is as effective as amoxicillin in otitis media and causes less diarrhea.
• Oral suspension is stable for 7 days at room temperature, and 14 days under refrigeration; check expiration date.
• Because cyclacillin is dialyzable, patients undergoing hemodialysis may need dosage adjustments.

Information for parents and patient
• Teach signs and symptoms of hypersensitivity and other adverse reactions, and emphasize need to report any unusual reactions.
• Teach signs and symptoms of bacterial and fungal superinfection to patients and parents, especially to debilitated patients and others with low resistance because of immunosuppressants or irradiation; emphasize need to report signs of infection.
• Be sure parents understand how and when to give drug; urge them to complete entire prescribed regimen, to comply with instructions for around-the-clock dosage, and to keep follow-up appointments.
• Counsel parents to check expiration date and to discard unused drug.

---

cyclopentolate hydrochloride
AK-Pentolate, Cyclogyl, I-Pentolate, Minims Cyclopentolate*, Pentolair

• Classification: cyloplegic, mydriatic (anticholinergic agent)

How supplied
Available by prescription only
Ophthalmic solution: 0.5%, 1%, 2%

Indications, route, and dosage
Diagnostic procedures requiring mydriasis and cycloplegia
Children: Instill 1 drop of 0.5%, 1%, or 2% solution in each eye, followed by 1 drop of 0.5% or 1% solution in 5 minutes, if necessary, 40 to 50 minutes before procedure.
Adults: Instill 1 drop of 1% solution in eye, followed by another drop in 5 minutes 40 to 50 minutes before procedure. Use 2% solution in heavily pigmented irises.

Action and kinetics
• *Cycloplegic and mydriatic action:* Anticholinergic action prevents the sphincter muscle of the iris and the muscle of the ciliary body from responding to cholinergic stimulation. This results in unopposed adrenergic influence, producing pupillary dilation (mydriasis) and paralysis of accommodation (cycloplegia).
• *Kinetics in adults:* Peak mydriatic effect occurs within 30 to 60 minutes and cycloplegic effect within 25 to 75 minutes. Recovery from mydriasis usually occurs in about 24 hours; recovery from cycloplegia may occur in 6 to 24 hours.

Contraindications and precautions

Cyclopentolate is contraindicated in patients with narrow-angle glaucoma and in patients with hypersensitivity to any component of the preparation. It should be used with caution in patients in whom increased intraocular pressure may occur; and in children because of increased risk of cardiovascular and CNS effects. Do not use solutions more concentrated than 0.5% in neonates.

Interactions

Cyclopentolate may increase the bioavailability of nitrofurantoin from the anticholinergic effect of delayed gastric emptying. It also may interfere with the antiglaucoma action of pilocarpine, carbachol, or cholinesterase inhibitors.

Effects on diagnostic tests

None reported.

Adverse reactions

• CNS: *ataxia,* irritability, *incoherent speech,* confusion (failure to identify people), somnolence, hallucinations, seizures, *and behavioral disturbances in children.*
• CV: flushing, *tachycardia.*
• Eye: burning sensation on instillation, increased intraocular pressure, blurred vision, exudate, photophobia, ocular congestion, contact dermatitis, conjunctivitis.
• Other: dry skin and mouth, fever, urinary retention.
   Note: Drug should be discontinued if behavioral disturbances occur.

Overdose and treatment

Clinical manifestations of overdose include flushing, warm dry skin, dry mouth, dilated pupils, delirium, hallucinations, tachycardia, bladder distention, ataxia, hypotension, respiratory depression, coma, and death. Induce emesis or give activated charcoal. Use physostigmine to antagonize cyclopentolate's anticholinergic activity, and in severe toxicity; propranolol may be used to treat symptomatic tachydysrhythmias unresponsive to physostigmine.

▶ Special considerations

• Avoid getting the preparation in a child's mouth while administering.
• Infants and young children may experience an increased sensitivity to the cardiopulmonary and CNS effects of cyclopentolate.
• Neonates should not be given any solution more concentrated than 0.5%.
• Superior to homatropine hydrobromide, cyclopentolate has a shorter duration of action.
• To avoid systemic absorption, finger pressure should be applied to lacrimal sac during and for 1 to 2 minutes after instillation.
• Recovery from mydriasis and cycloplegia usually occurs within 24 hours. Pilocarpine 1% or 2% solution will reduce recovery time to 3 to 6 hours.

Information for parents and patient

• Warn parents and patient that drug will cause burning sensation when instilled.

• Advise parents to protect patient's eyes from bright illumination; dark glasses may reduce sensitivity.

---

cyclophosphamide
Cytoxan, Neosar

• Classification: antineoplastic (alkylating agent [cell cycle-phase nonspecific])

How supplied

Available by prescription only
Tablets: 25 mg, 50 mg
Injection: 100-mg, 200-mg, 500-mg, 1-g, 2-g vials

Indications, route, and dosage

Dosage and indications may vary. Check literature for recommended protocols.
†*Breast, head, neck, lung, and ovarian carcinoma; Hodgkin's disease; chronic lymphocytic or myelocytic and acute lymphoblastic leukemia; neuroblastoma; retinoblastoma; non-Hodgkin's lymphomas; multiple myeloma; mycosis fungoides; sarcomas; severe rheumatoid disorders; glomerular and nephrotic syndrome (in children); systemic lupus erythematosus; immunosuppression after transplants*
Children: 2 to 8 mg/kg or 60 to 250 mg/m² P.O. or I.V. daily for 6 days (dosage depends on susceptibility of neoplasm); divide oral dosages; give I.V. dosages once weekly. Maintenance dosage is 2 to 5 mg/kg or 50 to 150 mg/m² P.O. twice weekly.
Adults: 40 to 50 mg/kg P.O. or I.V. in single dose or in two to five doses, then adjust for maintenance; or 2 to 4 mg/kg P.O. daily for 10 days, then adjust for maintenance. Maintenance dosage, 1 to 5 mg/kg P.O. daily; 10 to 15 mg/kg I.V. q 7 to 10 days; or 3 to 5 mg/kg I.V. twice weekly.
†*Polymyositis*
Adults: 1 to 2 mg/kg P.O. daily.
†*Rheumatoid arthritis*
Adults: 1.5 to 3 mg/kg P.O. daily.
†*Wegener's granulomatosis*
Adults: 1 to 2 mg/kg P.O. daily (usually administered with prednisone).

Action and kinetics

• *Antineoplastic action:* The cytotoxic action of cyclophosphamide is mediated by its two active metabolites. These metabolites function as alkylating agents, preventing cell division by cross-linking DNA strands and leading to cell death. Cyclophosphamide also has significant immunosuppressive activity.
• *Kinetics in adults:* Cyclophosphamide is almost completely absorbed from the GI tract at doses of 100 mg or less. Higher doses (300 mg) are approximately 75% absorbed.
   Cyclophosphamide is distributed throughout the body, although only minimal amounts have been found in saliva, sweat, and synovial fluid. The concentration in the cerebrospinal fluid is too low for treatment of meningeal leukemia. Cyclophosphamide is metabo-

---

‡May contain sulfites   ◆May contain tartrazine   ◆◆May contain benzyl alcohol

lized to its active form by hepatic microsomal enzymes. The active metabolites are approximately 50% bound to plasma proteins. The activity of these metabolites is terminated by metabolism to inactive forms.

Cyclophosphamide and its metabolites are eliminated primarily in urine, with 15% to 30% excreted as unchanged drug. The plasma half-life ranges from 4 to 6½ hours.

Contraindications and precautions
Use cyclophosphamide with caution in patients of childbearing age because it may impair fertility; in patients with myelosuppression or infections because of potentially severe immunosuppression; and in patients who have had pelvic radiation because they have an increased risk of hemorrhagic cystitis.

Interactions
Concomitant use of cyclophosphamide with barbiturates, phenytoin, or chloral hydrate increases the rate of metabolism of cyclophosphamide to toxic metabolites. These agents are known to be inducers of hepatic microsomal enzymes. These drugs should be discontinued before cyclophosphamide therapy. Concurrent use with allopurinol prolongs the half-life of cyclophosphamide.

Corticosteroids are known to initially inhibit the metabolism of cyclophosphamide, reducing its effect. Eventual reduction of dose or discontinuation of steroids may increase metabolism of cyclophosphamide to a toxic level.

Patients on cyclophosphamide therapy who receive succinylcholine as an adjunct to anesthesia may experience prolonged respiratory distress and apnea. This may occur up to several days after the discontinuation of cyclophosphamide. The mechanism of this interaction is that cyclophosphamide depresses the activity of pseudocholinesterases, the enzyme responsible for the inactivation of succinylcholine. Use succinylcholine with caution or not at all.

Concomitant use of cyclophosphamide may potentiate the cardiotoxic effects of doxorubicin.

Effects on diagnostic tests
Cyclophosphamide may suppress positive reaction to Candida, mumps, tricophyton, and tuberculin TB skin tests. A false-positive result for the Papanicolaou test may occur. Cyclophosphamide therapy may also increase serum uric acid concentrations and decrease serum pseudocholinesterase concentrations.

Adverse reactions
• CV: *cardiotoxicity* (with very high doses and in combination with doxorubicin), thrombophlebitis.
• GI: anorexia; *nausea and vomiting* beginning within 6 hours, may last for 24 hours; mucositis; diarrhea.
• GU: *gonadal suppression* (may be irreversible), *hemorrhagic cystitis* (may develop in approximately 10% of patients because of poor hydration), bladder fibrosis, nephrotoxicity.
• HEMA: *bone marrow depression* (dose-limiting); *leukopenia* (nadir between days 8 and 15, recovery in 17 to 28 days); thrombocytopenia; anemia.

• Metabolic: hyperuricemia syndrome of inappropriate ADH secretion (with high doses), *hyponatremia*.
• Other: reversible alopecia in 50% of patients, especially with high doses; secondary malignancies; pneumonitis, *pulmonary infiltrates and fibrosis* (with high doses); fever; anaphylaxis, dermatitis.
   Note: Drug should be discontinued if hemorrhagic cystitis develops.

Overdose and treatment
Clinical manifestations of overdose include myelosuppression, alopecia, nausea, vomiting, and anorexia. Treatment is generally supportive and includes transfusion of blood components and antiemetics. Cyclophosphamide is dialyzable.

▶ Special considerations
• Follow all established procedures for safe handling, administration, and disposal.
• Vital signs and patency of catheter or I.V. line throughout administration should be monitored.
• Treat extravasation promptly.
• Reconstitute vials with appropriate volume of bacteriostatic or sterile water for injection to give a concentration of 20 mg/ml.
• Reconstituted solution is stable 7 days refrigerated or 24 hours at room temperature.
• Cyclophosphamide can be given by direct I.V. push into a running I.V. line or by infusion in normal saline solution or dextrose 5% in water.
• Avoid all I.M. injections when platelet counts are low.
• Oral medication should be taken with or after a meal.
• Administration with cold foods such as ice cream may improve toleration of oral dose. Alternatively, the powder for injection may be mixed in an aromatic elixir for oral administration. Contact pharmacist for further information.
• Push fluid (3 liters daily) to prevent hemorrhagic cystitis. Drug should not be given at bedtime, because voiding afterward is too infrequent to avoid cystitis. If hemorrhagic cystitis occurs, discontinue drug. Cystitis can occur months after therapy has been discontinued.
• Reduce dosage of cyclophosphamide if patient is concomitantly receiving corticosteroid therapy and develops viral or bacterial infections.
• Monitor for cyclophosphamide toxicity if patient's corticosteroid therapy is discontinued.
• Monitor BUN, hematocrit, platelet count, ALT (SGPT), AST (SGOT), LDH, serum bilirubin, serum creatinine, uric acid total and differential leukocyte, CBC, renal and hepatic function.
• Observe for hematuria and ask patient if he has dysuria.
• Nausea and vomiting are most common with high doses of I.V. cyclophosphamide. Administer antiemetics p.r.n.
• Use cautiously in severe leukopenia, thrombocytopenia, malignant cell infiltration of bone marrow, after recent radiation therapy or chemotherapy, and in hepatic or renal disease.
• The dosage of cyclophosphamide should be adjusted for renal impairment.
• Has been used successfully to treat many nonma-

---

*Canada only   †Unlabeled clinical use   Italicized adverse reactions have been observed in children.

lignant conditions, for example, multiple sclerosis, because of its immunosuppresive activity.

Information for parents and patient

• Emphasize the importance of continuing drug despite nausea and vomiting. Advise parents to report vomiting that occurs shortly after an oral dose.

• Warn parents and patient that alopecia is likely to occur, but that it is reversible.

• Encourage adequate fluid intake to prevent hemorrhagic cystitis and to facilitate uric acid excretion. Patient should empty bladder frequently. Parents may need to wake patient during the night to empty bladder.

• Patient should avoid exposure to persons with bacterial or viral infections because chemotherapy can increase susceptibility to infection. Parents should watch for and report any signs of infection promptly. They should check temperature of neutropenic patient every 4 hours and should report fever or cough immediately

• Advise parents that patient's dental work should be completed before initiation of therapy whenever possible or should be deferred until blood counts are normal.

• Warn parents that patient may bruise easily because of drug's effect on blood count. Patient may need to limit activity when thrombocytopenic.

• Advise parents that immunizations should be avoided if possible.

• Good oral hygiene, including frequent rinsing, may minimize stomatitis.

• Advise patients of childbearing age who are sexually active to practice contraception while taking this drug and for 4 months after; drug is potentially teratogenic. Patient may experience amenorrhea but should continue contraception.

---

cyclosporine
Sandimmune

• Classification: immunosuppressant (polypeptide antibiotic)

How supplied
Available by prescription only
Oral solution: 100 mg/ml
Injection: 50 mg/ml

Indications, route, and dosage
Prophylaxis of organ rejection in kidney, liver, and heart transplants
Children and adults: 15 mg/kg P.O. daily (oral solution) 4 to 12 hours before transplantation. Continue this daily dose postoperatively for 1 to 2 weeks. Then, gradually reduce dosage by 5% per week to maintenance level of 5 to 10 mg/kg/day. Alternatively, administer 5 to 10 mg/kg/day I.V. divided q 12 to 24 hours. Postoperatively, administer this dose daily as an I.V. dilute solution infusion (50 mg per 20 to 100 ml infused over 2 to 6 hours) until patient can tolerate oral solution. Adjust dosage to maintain trough concentration for the specific assay used.

Action and kinetics
• *Immunosuppressant action:* The exact mechanism is unknown; purportedly, its action is related to the inhibition of interleukin II, which plays a role in both cellular and humoral immune responses.

• *Kinetics in adults:* Absorption after oral administration varies widely between patients and in the same individual. Only 30% of an oral dose reaches systemic circulation; peak levels occur at 3 to 4 hours. Cyclosporine is distributed widely outside the blood volume. About 33% to 47% is found in plasma; 4% to 9%, in leukocytes; 5% to 12%, in granulocytes; and 41% to 58%, in erythrocytes. In plasma, approximately 90% is bound to proteins, primarily lipoproteins. Cyclosporine crosses the placenta; cord blood levels are about 60% those of maternal blood. Cyclosporine enters breast milk. It is metabolized extensively in the liver and is eliminated primarily in feces (biliary excretion) with only 6% of the drug found in urine.

Contraindications and precautions
Cyclosporine is contraindicated in patients with known hypersensitivity to the drug or to polyoxyethylated castor oil. It should be used cautiously in patients with renal or hepatic toxicity or hypertension because drug may exacerbate the signs and symptoms of these conditions.

Interactions
Concomitant use with amphotericin B is likely to increase nephrotoxicity because both drugs are nephrotoxic, and amphotericin may increase cyclosporine blood levels.

Except for corticosteroids, cyclosporine should not be used concomitantly with immunosuppressive agents because of the increased risk of malignancy (lymphoma) and susceptibility to infection.

Erythromycin, ketoconazole, diltiazem, verapamil, and possibly corticosteroids impair hepatic enzyme metabolism and increase plasma cyclosporine levels; reduced dosage of cyclosporine may be necessary. Phenytoin, rifampin, phenobarbital, and cotrimoxazole increase hepatic metabolism and may lower plasma levels of cyclosporine.

Effects on diagnostic tests
Cyclosporine therapy may alter CBC and differential blood tests and may increase serum lipids levels; drug elevation of serum BUN and creatinine levels and liver function tests may signal nephrotoxicity or hepatotoxicity.

Adverse reactions
• CNS: tremor, seizures, headache, paresthesias, ataxia, depression.
• CV: hypertension, chest pain.
• DERM: acne, hirsutism, oily skin, brittle nails.
• EENT: gum hyperplasia, oral thrush, mouth ulcers, visual disturbances, sore throat.
• GI: nausea, vomiting, diarrhea, anorexia, difficulty swallowing, constipation.

---

‡May contain sulfites ◆May contain tartrazine ◆◆May contain benzyl alcohol

- GU: nephrotoxicity, increased BUN and serum creatinine levels, acute or chronic renal failure.
- HEMA: leukopenia, thrombocytopenia, anemia.
- Hepatic: hepatotoxicity.
- Other: anaphylaxis (with I.V. only), flushing, night sweats, gynecomastia, joint pains.
  Note: Drug should be discontinued if hypersensitivity occurs.

Overdose and treatment

Clinical manifestations of overdose include extensions of common adverse effects. Hepatotoxicity and nephrotoxicity often accompany nausea and vomiting; tremor and seizures may occur. Up to 2 hours after ingestion, empty stomach by induced emesis or lavage; thereafter, treat supportively. Monitor vital signs and fluid and electrolyte levels closely. Cyclosporine is not removed by hemodialysis or charcoal hemoperfusion.

▶ Special considerations

- Safety and efficacy in children have not been established; however, drug has been used in children as young as 6 months. Use with caution.
- Cyclosporine usually is prescribed with corticosteroids.
- Possible kidney rejection should be considered before discontinuation of drug for suspected nephrotoxicity.
- Monitor hepatic and renal function tests routinely; hepatotoxicity may occur in the first month after transplantation, but renal toxicity may be delayed for 2 to 3 months.
- Dose should be given at same time each day. Oral doses should be measured carefully in oral syringe and mixed with plain or chocolate milk or fruit juice to increase palatability; it should be served in a glass to minimize drug adherence to container walls. Drug can be taken with food to minimize nausea.
- Drug levels are assay specific.

Information for parents and patient

- Explain rationale for therapy, possible side effects, and importance of reporting them, especially fever, sore throat, mouth sores, abdominal pain, unusual bleeding or bruising, pale stools, or dark urine.
- Encourage compliance with prescribed therapy and follow-up care.
- Teach parents and patient how and when to take medication for optimal benefit and minimal discomfort; caution against discontinuing drug without medical approval.
- Advise parents that they can make oral solution more palatable by diluting with room-temperature milk, chocolate milk, or orange juice.

cyclothiazide
Anhydron, Fluidil

- Classification: diuretic, antihypertensive (thiazide)

How supplied

Available by prescription only
Tablets: 2 mg

Indications, route, and dosage
Edema

Children: 0.02 to 0.04 mg/kg or 0.6 to 1.2 mg/m² P.O. once daily in the morning. Reduce to lowest effective dose for maintenance therapy.
Adults: 1 to 2 mg P.O. daily; may be used on alternate days as maintenance dose.
Hypertension

Adults: 2 mg P.O. daily; up to 2 mg b.i.d. or t.i.d.

Action and kinetics

- *Diuretic action:* Cyclothiazide increases urinary excretion of sodium and water by inhibiting sodium reabsorption in the cortical diluting tubule of the nephron, thus relieving edema.
- *Antihypertensive action:* The exact mechanism of cyclothiazide's antihypertensive effect is unknown. This effect may partially result from direct arteriolar vasodilation and a decrease in total peripheral resistance.
- *Kinetics in adults:* Cyclothiazide is absorbed from the GI tract; diuresis begins within 2 hours. Cyclothiazide is distributed into extracellular space throughout the body; duration of diuretic effect is 18 to 24 hours. Drug is excreted in urine.

Contraindications and precautions

Cyclothiazide is contraindicated in patients with anuria and in those with known hypersensitivity to the drug or to other sulfonamide derivatives.

Cyclothiazide should be used cautiously in patients with severe renal disease, because it may decrease glomerular filtration rate and precipitate azotemia; in patients with impaired hepatic function or liver disease, because drug-induced electrolyte alterations may induce hepatic coma; and in patients taking digoxin, because electrolyte changes in such patients may predispose them to digitalis toxicity.

Interactions

Cyclothiazide potentiates the hypotensive effects of most other antihypertensive drugs; this may be used to therapeutic advantage.

Cyclothiazide may potentiate hyperglycemic, hypotensive, and hyperuricemic effects of diazoxide, and its hyperglycemic effect may increase insulin requirements in diabetic patients.

Cyclothiazide may reduce renal clearance of lithium, elevating serum lithium levels, and may necessitate a 50% reduction in lithium dosage.

Cyclothiazide turns urine slightly more alkaline and may decrease urinary excretion of some amines, such as amphetamine and quinidine; alkaline urine also may decrease therapeutic efficacy of methenamine compounds, such as methenamine mandelate.

Cholestyramine and colestipol may bind cyclothiazide, preventing its absorption; give drugs 1 hour apart.

Effects on diagnostic tests

Cyclothiazide therapy may alter serum electrolyte levels and may increase serum urate, glucose, amylase, cholesterol, and triglyceride levels; drug may decrease urine estrogen and corticosteroid levels.

Cyclothiazide may interfere with tests for parathyroid function and should be discontinued for 48 hours before such tests.

Adverse reactions

• CV: volume depletion and dehydration, orthostatic hypotension, hypercholesterolemia, hypertriglyceridemia.
• DERM: dermatitis, photosensitivity, rash.
• GI: anorexia, nausea, pancreatitis.
• HEMA: aplastic anemia, agranulocytosis, leukopenia, thrombocytopenia.
• Hepatic: hepatic encephalopathy.
• Metabolic: asymptomatic hyperuricemia; gout; hyperglycemia and impairment of glucose tolerance; fluid and electrolyte imbalances, including hypokalemia, dilutional hyponatremia and hypochloremia, and hypercalcemia; metabolic alkalosis.
• Other: hypersensitivity reactions, such as pneumonitis and vasculitis.
   Note: Drug should be discontinued if rising BUN and serum creatinine levels indicate renal impairment or if patient shows signs of hypersensitivity or impending coma.

Overdose and treatment

Clinical signs of overdose include diuresis, leading to electrolyte imbalance, and lethargy that may progress to coma; other symptoms include nausea, vomiting, diarrhea, hypermotility, seizures, and cardiac dysrhythmias.

Treatment is mainly supportive; monitor and assist respiratory, cardiovascular, and renal function as indicated. Monitor fluid and electrolyte balance. Induce vomiting with syrup of ipecac in conscious patient; otherwise, use gastric lavage to avoid aspiration. Do not give cathartics; these promote additional loss of fluids and electrolytes.

▶ Special considerations

• Inspect skin and mucous membranes of patients on prolonged therapy for petechiae, which require reduced dosage or discontinuation of drug.
• Monitor weight and serum electrolyte levels regularly.
• Monitor serum potassium levels; encourage high-potassium diet. Foods rich in potassium include citrus fruits, tomatoes, bananas, dates, and apricots. Watch for signs of hypokalemia (for example, muscle weakness or cramps). Patients also taking digitalis have an increased risk of digitalis toxicity from the potassium-depleting effect of cyclothiazide.
• Drug may be used with potassium-sparing diuretics to attenuate potassium loss.

• Check insulin requirements in patients with diabetes.
• Monitor serum creatinine and BUN levels regularly. Drug is not as effective if these levels are more than twice normal.
• Monitor blood uric acid levels.
• A.M. administration is recommended to prevent nocturia.
• Antihypertensive effects persist for approximately 1 week after discontinuation of the drug.
• Instruct parents to watch for and report any joint swelling, pain, or redness; these signs may indicate hyperuricemia.
• Cyclothiazide is distributed in breast milk; safety and effectiveness in breast-feeding women have not been established.

Information for parents and patient

• Explain rationale of therapy and diuretic effects of drug.
• Advise parents to watch for and promptly report signs of electrolyte imbalance: weakness, fatigue, muscle cramps, paresthesias, confusion, nausea, vomiting, diarrhea, headache, dizziness, and palpitations.
• Tell parents to report any increased edema or excess diuresis (more than a 2% weight loss or gain) and to record the child's weight each morning after voiding and before breakfast, on the same scale wearing the same type of clothing.
• Advise parents to give drug with food to minimize gastric irritation; to encourage child to eat potassium-rich foods, such as citrus fruits, potatoes, dates, raisins, and bananas; and to restrict child's access to salt and high-sodium foods, such as lunch meat, smoked meats, and processed cheeses. Inform them that low-sodium formulas are available for infants.
• Tell parents to seek medical approval before giving the patient nonprescription drugs; many contain sodium and potassium and can cause electrolyte imbalances.
• Explain photosensitivity reactions. In thiazide-related photosensitivity, ultraviolet radiation alters drug structure, causing allergic reactions in some persons; such reactions occur 10 days to 2 weeks after initial sun exposure.
• Caution patient to change position slowly, especially when rising to upright position, to prevent dizziness from orthostatic hypotension.
• Warn parents to supervise the child's activities closely to prevent falls and other injuries that may result from dizziness, especially at beginning of therapy.
• Advise parents to watch the patient closely for signs of chest, back, and leg pain, or shortness of breath, and to call immediately if they occur.
• Advise parents to administer the drug only as prescribed and at the same time each day, to prevent nighttime diuresis and interrupted sleep.
• Emphasize importance of regular medical follow-up to monitor effectiveness of diuretic therapy.

cyproheptadine hydrochloride
Periactin

- Classification: antihistamine, H_1-receptor antagonist, antipruritic agent (piperidine derivative)

How supplied
Available by prescription only
Tablets: 4 mg
Syrup: 2 mg/5 ml

Indications, route, and dosage
Allergy symptoms, pruritus, cold urticaria, allergic conjunctivitis, †appetite stimulant, †vascular cluster headaches
Children age 2 to 6: 2 mg P.O. b.i.d. or t.i.d. Maximum dosage is 12 mg daily.
Children age 7 to 14: 4 mg P.O. b.i.d. or t.i.d. Maximum dosage is 16 mg daily.
Adults: 4 mg P.O. t.i.d. or q.i.d. Maximum dosage is 0.5 mg/kg daily.

Drug also has been used experimentally to stimulate appetite and increase weight gain in children.

Action and kinetics
- *Antihistamine action:* Antihistamines compete with histamine for histamine H_1-receptor sites on smooth muscle of the bronchi, GI tract, uterus, and large blood vessels; they bind to cellular receptors, preventing access of histamine, thereby suppressing histamine-induced allergic symptoms. They do not directly alter histamine or its release.

Cyproheptadine also displays significant anticholinergic and antiserotonin activity.
- *Kinetics in adults:* Cyproheptadine is well absorbed from the GI tract and appears to be almost completely metabolized in the liver. Metabolites are excreted primarily in urine; small amounts of unchanged cyproheptadine and metabolites are excreted in feces.

Contraindications and precautions
Cyproheptadine is contraindicated in children with known hypersensitivity to this drug or other antihistamines with similar chemical structures, such as azatadine; in patients experiencing asthmatic attacks, because cyproheptadine thickens bronchial secretions; and in patients who have taken MAO inhibitors within the preceding 2 weeks.

Cyproheptadine should be used with caution in patients with narrow-angle glaucoma; in those with pyloroduodenal obstruction or urinary bladder obstruction from prostatic hyperthophy or narrowing of the bladder neck, because of their marked anticholinergic effects; in patients with cardiovascular disease, hypertension, or hyperthyroidism, because of the risk of palpitations and tachycardia; and in patients with renal disease, diabetes, bronchial asthma, urinary retention, or stenosing peptic ulcers.

Interactions
MAO inhibitors interfere with the detoxification of antihistamines and thus prolong and intensify their central depressant and anticholinergic effects; additive sedative effects result when cyproheptadine is used concomitantly with alcohol or other CNS depressants, such as barbiturates, tranquilizers, sleeping aids, and antianxiety agents.

Serum amylase and prolactin concentrations may be increased when these drugs are administered with thyrotropin-releasing hormone.

Effects on diagnostic tests
Cyproheptadine should be discontinued 4 days before diagnostic skin tests. Antihistamines can prevent, reduce, or mask positive skin test response.

Adverse reactions
- CNS: stimulation, sedation, drowsiness, headache, fatigue, excitability, appetite stimulation, agitation, confusion, visual hallucinations, ataxia, tremors, disturbed coordination.
- CV: hypotension, palpitations, tachycardia.
- DERM: urticaria, photosensitivity.
- EENT: dry nose and throat, blurred vision, tinnitus.
- GI: dry mouth, constipation, jaundice.
- GU: urinary frequency and retention.
- HEMA: hemolytic anemia, leukopenia, thrombocytopenia, appetite stimulation, agranulocytosis.
- Metabolic: weight gain.

Overdose and treatment
Clinical manifestations of overdose may include either CNS depression (sedation, reduced mental alertness, apnea, and cardiovascular collapse) or CNS stimulation (insomnia, hallucinations, tremors, or convulsions). Anticholinergic symptoms, such as dry mouth, flushed skin, fixed and dilated pupils, and GI symptoms, are common, especially in children.

Treat overdose by inducing emesis with ipecac syrup (in conscious patient), followed by activated charcoal to reduce further drug absorption. Use gastric lavage if patient is unconscious or ipecac fails. Treat hypotension with vasopressors, and control seizures with diazepam or phenytoin. *Do not give stimulants.*

▶ Special considerations
- Drug is contraindicated during an acute asthma attack because it may not alleviate the symptoms and because antimuscarinic effects can cause thickening of secretions.
- CNS stimulation (agitation, confusion, tremors, hallucinations) is more common in children and may require dosage reduction. Children, especially those under age 6, may experience paradoxical hyperexcitability with restlessness, insomnia, nervousness, euphoria, tremors, and seizures.
- Cyproheptadine can cause weight gain. Monitor weight.
- In some patients, sedative effect disappears within 3 or 4 days.
- Drug is not indicated in newborn or premature infants.
- Reduce GI distress by giving drug with food; give sugarless gum, lollipops, or ice chips to relieve dry mouth; increase fluid intake (if allowed) or humidify air to decrease adverse effect of thickened secretions.

★Canada only   †Unlabeled clinical use   Italicized adverse reactions have been observed in children.

Information for parents and patient
• Advise patient to take drug with meals or snack to prevent gastric upset and to use any of the following measures to relieve dry mouth; warm water rinses, artificial saliva, ice chips, or sugarless gum or candy. Patient should avoid overusing mouthwash, which may add to dryness (alcohol content) and destroy normal flora.
• Warn parents that child should avoid hazardous activities which require balance or alertness until extent of CNS effects are known.
• They should seek medical approval before administering tranquilizers, sedatives, pain relievers, or sleeping medications.
• Warn parents to discontinue drug 4 days before diagnostic skin tests, to preserve accuracy of tests.

---

cytarabine (ARA-C, cytosine arabinoside)
Cytosar-U

• Classification: antineoplastic (antimetabolite [cell cycle-phase specific, S phase])

How supplied
Available by prescription only
Injection: 100-mg, 500-mg vials, 1g, 2g vials

Indications, route, and dosage
Dosage and indications may vary. Check literature for recommended protocols.
Acute myelocytic and other acute leukemias
Children and adults: 100 to 200 mg/m² or 3 mg/kg daily by continuous I.V. infusion or rapid I.V. injection in divided doses for 5 days at 2-week intervals for remission induction; or 30 mg/m² intrathecally (range: 5 to 75 mg/m²) q 4 days until cerebrospinal fluid findings are normal. Doses up to 3 g/m² q 12 hours for 12 days have been given by intermittent infusion for refractory acute leukemias.

Action and kinetics
• *Antineoplastic action:* Cytarabine requires conversion to its active metabolite within the cell. This metabolite acts as a competitive inhibitor of the enzyme DNA polymerase, disrupting the normal synthesis of DNA.
• *Kinetics in adults:* Cytarabine is poorly absorbed (less than 20%) across the GI tract because of rapid deactivation in the gut lumen. After I.M. or subcutaneous administration, peak plasma levels are less than after I.V. administration.
Cytarabine rapidly distributes widely through the body. Approximately 13% of the drug is bound to plasma proteins. The drug penetrates the blood-brain barrier only slightly after a rapid I.V. dose; however, when the drug is administered by a continuous I.V. infusion, cerebrospinal fluid levels achieve a concentration 40% to 60% of that of plasma levels.
Cytarabine is metabolized primarily in the liver but also in the kidneys, GI mucosa, and granulocytes.

The elimination of cytarabine has been described as biphasic, with an initial half-life of 8 minutes and a terminal phase half-life of 1 to 3 hours. Cytarabine and its metabolites are excreted in urine. Less than 10% of a dose is excreted as unchanged drug in urine.

Contraindications and precautions
Cytarabine is contraindicated in patients with a history of hypersensitivity to the drug.

Interactions
When used concomitantly, cytarabine decreases the cellular uptake of methotrexate, reducing its effectiveness.

Effects on diagnostic tests
Cytarabine therapy may increase blood and urine levels of uric acid. It may also increase serum alkaline phosphatase, AST (SGOT), and bilirubin concentrations, which indicate drug-induced hepatotoxicity.

Adverse reactions
• CNS: neurotoxicity; neuritis and peripheral neuropathy (with high-doses), *encephalitis-like symptoms* (lethargy, confusion), arachnoiditis (after intrathecal use).
• DERM: rash, photosensitivity.
• EENT: keratitis, *conjunctivitis.*
• GI: *nausea; vomiting; diarrhea;* dysphagia; reddened area at juncture of lips, followed by sore mouth, *oral ulcers* in 5 to 10 days; high dose given via rapid I.V. may cause projectile vomiting.
• HEMA: leukopenia (nadir 5 to 7 days after drug stopped), anemia, thrombocytopenia, reticulocytopenia (platelet nadir occurring on day 10), *bone marrow depression* (dose-limiting) *megaloblastosis.*
• Hepatic: *hepatotoxicity* (usually mild and reversible).
• Metabolic: hyperuricemia.
• Other: *flulike syndrome (malaise, myalgia),* anaphylaxis, fever, alopecia.
Note: Drug should be discontinued if the polymorphonuclear granulocyte count falls below 1,000/mm³; if the platelet count falls below 50,000/mm³ during maintenance therapy (not during remission induction therapy).

Overdose and treatment
Clinical manifestations of overdose include myelosuppression, nausea, vomiting, and megaloblastosis.
Treatment is usually supportive and includes transfusion of blood components and antiemetics.

▶ Special considerations
• Follow all established procedures for the safe handling, administration, and disposal. Patient may develop a fever shortly after administration.
• Monitor vital signs and patency of catheter or I.V. line throughout administration.
• Extravasations should be treated promptly.
• Monitor BUN, hematocrit, platelet count, ALT (SGPT), AST (SGOT), LDH, serum bilirubin, serum creatinine, uric acid, total and different leukocyte, and others as required.
• To reconstitute the 100-mg vial for I.V. administra-

---

‡May contain sulfites   ◆May contain tartrazine   ◆ ◆ May contain benzyl alcohol

tion use 5 ml bacteriostatic water for injection (20 mg/ml) and for the 500-mg vial with 10 ml bacteriostatic water for injection (50 mg/ml).

• Drug may be further diluted with dextrose 5% in water or normal saline solution for continuous I.V. infusion.

• For intrathecal injection, dilute the drug in 5 to 15 ml of lactated Ringer's solution, Elliot's B solution, or normal saline solution with no preservative, and administer after withdrawing an equivalent volume of cerebrospinal fluid.

• Do not reconstitute the drug with bacteriostatic diluent for intrathecal administration because the preservative, benzyl alcohol, has been associated with a higher incidence of neurologic toxicity.

• Infusion solutions up to a concentration of 5 mg/ml are stable for 7 days at room temperature. Discard cloudy reconstituted solution.

• Dose modification may be required in thrombocytopenia, leukopenia, renal or hepatic disease, and after other chemotherapy or radiation therapy.

• Watch for signs of infection (cough, fever, sore throat). Monitor CBC before and after therapy.

• Excellent mouth care can help prevent oral adverse reactions.

• Nausea and vomiting are more frequent when large doses are administered rapidly by I.V. push. These reactions are less frequent with infusion. To reduce nausea, give antiemetic before administering.

• Monitor intake and output carefully. Maintain high fluid intake and give allopurinol, if ordered, to avoid urate nephropathy in leukemia induction therapy. Monitor uric acid levels.

• Monitor hepatic function.

• Monitor patients receiving high doses for cerebellar dysfunction. Assess CNS status before and during therapy. Watch for lethargy and confusion.

• Prescribe steroid eye drops (dexamethasone) to prevent drug-induced keratitis.

• Avoid I.M. injections of any drugs in patients with severely depressed platelet count (thrombocytopenia) to prevent bleeding.

Information for parents and patient

• Teach proper oral hygiene including caution when using toothbrush or dental floss. Recommend use of toothettes and frequent rinsing with a soothing solution to promote healing of stomatitis. Chemotherapy can increase incidence of microbial infection, delayed healing, and bleeding gums.

• Tell parents that patient's dental work should be completed before initiation of therapy whenever possible, or delayed until blood counts are normal.

• Warn parents that patient may bruise easily because of drug's effect on platelets and may have to limit activity to prevent injury.

• Warn parents to prevent child's exposure to persons who have taken oral poliovirus vaccine and to avoid exposure to persons with bacterial or viral infection, because chemotherapy may increase susceptibility to infection. Instruct them to report signs of infection and exposure to chicken pox in susceptible patients.

• Advise parents that patient should not receive immunizations during therapy and for several weeks after therapy. Members of the same household should not receive live-virus immunizations during the same period.

• Tell parents to watch for and to report immediately any redness, pain, or swelling at injection site. Local injury and scarring may result from tissue infiltration at the infusion site.

• Advise parents to encourage adequate fluid intake to increase urine output and facilitate excretion of uric acid.

• Instruct patient who receives intrathecal administration to report headache or tingling.

• Instruct patient to wear sunscreen when outdoors.

---

dacarbazine (DTIC)
DTIC-Dome

• Classification: antineoplastic (alkylating agent)

How supplied
Available by prescription only
Injection: 100-mg, 200-mg vials

Indications, route, and dosage
Dosage and indications may vary. Check current literature for recommended protocols.
Metastatic malignant melanoma
Adolescents and adults: 2 to 4.5 mg/kg or 70 to 160 mg/m² I.V. daily for 10 days, then repeat q 4 weeks as tolerated; or 250 mg/m² I.V. daily for 5 days, repeated at 3-week intervals.
Hodgkin's disease
Adolescents and adults: 150 mg/m² for 5 days, repeated q 4 weeks; or 375 mg/m² on day 1, repeated q 15 days (usually used in combination with other drugs).

Action and kinetics
• *Antineoplastic action:* Three mechanisms have been proposed to explain the cytotoxicity of dacarbazine: alkylation, in which DNA and RNA synthesis are inhibited; antimetabolite activity as a false precursor for purine synthesis; and binding with protein sulfhydryl groups.
• *Kinetics in adults:* Because of poor absorption from the GI tract, dacarbazine is not administered orally. Dacarbazine is thought to localize in body tissues, especially the liver. The drug crosses the blood-brain barrier to a limited extent. It is minimally bound to plasma proteins and is rapidly metabolized in the liver to several compounds, some of which may be active. The elimination of dacarbazine is biphasic, with an initial phase half-life of 19 minutes and terminal phase of 5 hours in patients with normal renal and hepatic function. Approximately 30% to 45% of a dose is excreted in urine.

Contraindications and precautions
Dacarbazine is contraindicated in patients with a history of hypersensitivity to the drug.

Interactions
When used concomitantly, barbiturates and phenytoin may increase the metabolism of dacarbazine, reducing its effect through inducement of hepatic microsomal enzymes. Barbiturates and phenytoin should be discontinued before treatment with dacarbazine.

Effects on diagnostic tests
Dacarbazine therapy causes transient increases in serum BUN, ALT (SGPT), AST (SGOT), and alkaline phosphatase levels.

Adverse reactions
• CNS: confusion, headache, *paresthesia.*
• DERM: phototoxicity, urticaria.
• EENT: blurred vision.
• GI: *severe nausea and vomiting* (beginning within 1 to 3 hours in 90% of patients and lasting 1 to 12 hours), anorexia, *diarrhea.*
• HEMA: *bone marrow depression* (dose-limiting), leukopenia and thrombocytopenia (nadir between 3 and 4 weeks), anemia.
• Local: *severe pain if I.V. solution infiltrates or if solution is too concentrated;* tissue damage.
• Other: *flulike syndrome* (fever, malaise, myalgia beginning 7 days after treatment is stopped and possibly lasting 7 to 21 days), *alopecia, anaphylaxis, facial flushing, photosensitivity, renal impairment, hepatic necrosis.*
  Note: Drug should be discontinued if hematopoietic toxicity is evident.

Overdose and treatment
Clinical manifestations of overdose include myelosuppression and diarrhea. Treatment is usually supportive and includes transfusion of blood components and monitoring of hematologic parameters.

▶ Special considerations
• Follow established procedures for safe, proper handling, administration, and disposal of chemotherapeutic agents.
• Vital signs and patency of catheter or I.V. line should be monitored throughout administration.
• Attempt to ease anxiety in parents and patient before treatment.
• To reconstitute the drug for I.V. administration, use a volume of sterile water for injection that gives a concentration of 10 mg/ml (9.9 ml for 100-mg vial, 19.7 ml for 200-mg vial).
• Drug may be diluted further with dextrose 5% in water to a volume of 100 to 200 ml for I.V. infusion over 30 minutes. Increase volume or slow the rate of infusion to decrease pain at infusion site.
• Drug may be administered I.V. push over 1 to 2 minutes.
• A change in solution color from ivory to pink indicates some drug degradation. During infusion, protect the solution from light to avoid possible drug breakdown.
• Treatment of extravasation with application of hot packs may relieve burning sensation, local pain, and irritation.
• Discard refrigerated solution after 72 hours and room temperature solution after 8 hours.
• Nausea and vomiting may be minimized by admin-

istering dacarbazine by I.V. infusion and by hydrating patient 4 to 6 hours before therapy.
• Monitor platelet count and BUN, hematocrit, ALT (SGPT), AST (SGOT), lactic dehydrogenase, serum bilirubin, serum creatinine, uric acid total, and differential leukocyte levels.
• Reduce dosage when giving repeated doses to a patient with severely impaired renal function.
• Use lower dose if renal function or bone marrow is impaired. Stop drug if WBC count falls to 3,000/mm³ or if platelet count drops to 100,000/mm³. Monitor CBC.
• Monitor daily temperature. Observe for signs of infection.
• Avoid all I.M. injections when platelet count is below 100,000/mm³.
• Anticoagulants and aspirin products should be used cautiously. Watch closely for signs of bleeding.

Information for parents and patient
• Advise parents to have child avoid sunlight and sunlamps for first 2 days after treatment.
• Reassure parents and child that hair growth should return after treatment has ended.
• Advise parents that flulike syndrome may be treated with mild antipyretics such as acetaminophen.
• Tell parents to avoid administering aspirin and aspirin-containing products because of their anti-coagulant effects. Urge them to report signs and symptoms of bleeding promptly.
• Advise parents that immunizations should be avoided if possible.
• Advise parents to have patient avoid exposure to persons with bacterial or viral infections because chemotherapy can increase susceptibility to infection. Parents should watch for and report any signs of infection promptly.
• Instruct parents and patient about oral hygiene, including need for caution when using toothbrush and dental floss.
• Advise parents that the patient's dental work should be completed before therapy whenever possible or delayed until blood counts are normal.
• Warn parents and patient that patient may bruise easily because of drug's effect on blood count.

---

dactinomycin (actinomycin D)
Cosmegen

• Classification: antineoplastic (antibiotic antineoplastic [cell cycle-phase nonspecific])

How supplied
Available by prescription only
Injectable: 500-mcg vial

Indications, route, and dosage
Dosage and indications may vary. Check current literature for recommended protocols.

Melanomas, sarcomas, †trophoblastic tumors in women, testicular cancer
Adults: 10 to 15 mcg/kg I.V. for a maximum of 5 days every 4 to 6 weeks; or 500 mcg/m² I.V. once a week (maximum 2 mg per week) for 3 weeks
Testicular or endometrial carcinoma, trophoblastic tumors, †ovarian carcinoma, sarcoma botryoides, Wilms' tumor, rhabdomyosarcoma, Ewing's sarcoma
Children: 10 to 15 mcg/kg/day or 450 mcg/m²/day I.V. (maximum dose: 500 mcg/day for 5 days or 2.4 mg/m² in divided doses over 7 days). If all signs of toxicity have disappeared, may be repeated in 4 to 6 weeks.
Note: Use body surface area calculation in obese or edematous patients and patients with cancer. Dosage reduction may be required in patients who have received radiation.
For isolation-perfusion, use 50 mcg/kg for lower extremity or pelvis; 35 mcg/kg for upper extremity.

Action and kinetics
• *Antineoplastic action:* Dactinomycin exerts its cytotoxic activity by intercalating between DNA base pairs and uncoiling the DNA helix. The result is inhibition of DNA synthesis and DNA-dependent RNA synthesis.
• *Kinetics in adults:* Due to its vesicant properties, dactinomycin must be administered intravenously.
Dactinomycin is widely distributed into body tissues, with the highest levels found in the bone marrow and nucleated cells. The drug does not cross the blood-brain barrier to any significant extent. It is minimally metabolized in the liver. Dactinomycin and its metabolites are excreted in the urine and bile. The plasma elimination half-life of the drug is 36 hours.

Contraindications and precautions
Dactinomycin is contraindicated in patients with chicken pox or herpes zoster and in infants under age 12 months. Dactinomycin treatment of such patients may lead to serious generalized disease and death.
Drug also is contraindicated in patients with renal, hepatic, or bone marrow impairment and viral infections. Use cautiously in combination with chlorambucil and methotrexate therapy because such use may cause extreme bone marrow and GI toxicity.
Use with caution in patients who have received cytotoxic drugs or radiation therapy within 6 weeks, or in patients with a history of gout, infection, or hematologic compromise because of increased potential for adverse effects.

Interactions
None reported.

Effects on diagnostic tests
Dactinomycin therapy may increase blood and urine concentrations of uric acid.

Adverse reactions
Bone marrow depression and GI reactions are the dose-limiting toxicity factors.
• DERM: *erythema; desquamation; hyperpigmentation of skin, especially in previously irradiated areas;* acnelike eruptions (reversible), folliculitis.

• GI: anorexia, *nausea, vomiting,* abdominal pain, *diarrhea, stomatitis, esophagitis, pharyngitis, oral ulcers.*
• HEMA: anemia, leukopenia, thrombocytopenia, pancytopenia, agranulocytosis.
• Local: *phlebitis,* severe damage to soft tissue.
• Other: reversible alopecia.

Note: Drug should be discontinued if diarrhea and stomatitis develop. Therapy may be resumed when these conditions subside.

Overdose and treatment
Clinical manifestations of overdose include myelosuppression, nausea, vomiting, glossitis, and oral ulceration.

Treatment is generally supportive and includes antiemetics and transfusion of blood components.

▶ Special considerations
• Restrict use of dactinomycin in infants to those age 6 months and older; adverse reactions are more frequent in infants under age 6 months.
• To reconstitute for I.V. administration, add 1.1 ml of sterile water for injection to drug to give a concentration of 0.5 mg/ml. Do not use a preserved diluent, as precipitation may occur. Protect solution from light. This mixture should be used within 24 hours.
• Use gloves when preparing and administering this drug. Follow institutional procedures for safe preparation, administration, and disposal.
• May dilute further with dextrose 5% in water or normal saline for administration by I.V. infusion. May administer by I.V. push injection into the tubing of a freely flowing I.V. infusion.
• Drug is vesicant. Avoid placement of I.V. site at or near a joint that may become immobilized if extravasation occurs. During I.V. administration, monitor continuously for extravasation. If it occurs, stop infusion, remove I.V., and treat promptly according to institutional policy. Treatment of extravasation may include topical administration of dimethylsulfoxide and cold compresses.
• To reduce nausea, give antiemetic before administering. Nausea usually occurs within 30 minutes of a dose.
• Premedicating with an antiemetic may prevent nausea and vomiting. If vomiting occurs, administer antiemetics p.r.n.
• Patients who have received drugs with strong emetic properties may experience anticipatory nausea and vomiting at subsequent treatments. They may benefit from treatment with an anxiolytic drug.
• Monitor patient's intake, output, and weight.
• Continue I.V. hydration until patient resumes sufficient oral intake.
• Monitor CBC daily and platelet counts every third day. Observe for signs of bleeding.
• Monitor renal and hepatic functions.
• Vital signs and patency of catheter or I.V. line should be monitored throughout administration.
• Monitor BUN, hematocrit; platelet count, ALT (SGPT), AST (SGOT), LDH, serum bilirubin, serum creatinine, uric acid, and total and differential leukocytes.

Information for parents and patient
• Tell parents that dental work should be completed before initiation of therapy whenever possible, or delayed until blood counts are normal.
• Advise parents that patient should not receive immunizations during therapy and for several weeks after therapy. Members of the same household should not receive immunizations during the same period.
• Advise parents and child that alopecia may occur but is usually reversible; transient acne may develop.
• Tell parents and patient to promptly report sore throat, fever, or any signs of bleeding.
• Stress importance of keeping follow-up appointments for monitoring hematologic status.
• Instruct parents to monitor neutropenic patient's temperature every 4 hours (not rectally) and to report fever, cough and other signs of infection *promptly.*
• Explain importance of promptly reporting susceptible patient's exposure to chicken pox.
• Patient should avoid contact with persons who have received live immunizations (polio, measles/mumps/rubella).
• Teach parents and patient to check for signs of bleeding and bruising. Parents may need to restrict child's participation in contact sports. Such activity is dangerous when patient's platelets are low.
• Explain "radiation recall." Previously irradiated areas may become erythematous after administration of drug.

dantrolene sodium
Dantrium

• Classification: skeletal muscle relaxant (hydantoin derivative)

How supplied
Available by prescription only
Capsules: 25 mg, 50 mg, 100 mg
Injection: 20 mg parenteral (contains 3 g mannitol)

Indications, route, and dosage
Spasticity resulting from upper motor neuron disorders
Children over age 5: 0.5 mg/kg daily P.O. b.i.d., increased gradually as needed by 0.5 mg/kg b.i.d. to q.i.d. to maximum of 100 mg q.i.d.
Adults: 25 mg P.O. daily, increased gradually in increments of 25 mg at 4- to 7-day intervals, up to 100 mg b.i.d. to q.i.d., to maximum of 400 mg daily.
Prevention of malignant hyperthermia in susceptible patients who require surgery
Children and adults: 4 to 8 mg/kg/day P.O. given in three to four divided doses for 1 to 2 days before procedure. Administer last dose 3 to 4 hours before procedure.
Management of malignant hyperthermia crisis
Children and adults: 1 mg/kg I.V. initially; may repeat dose up to cumulative dose of 10 mg/kg.

Prevention of recurrence of malignant hyperthermia after I.V. therapy

Children and adults: 4 to 8 mg/kg/day P.O. given in four divided doses for up to 3 days after crisis.

Action and kinetics

• *Skeletal muscle relaxant action:* A hydantoin derivative, dantrolene is chemically and pharmacologically unrelated to other skeletal muscle relaxants. It directly affects skeletal muscle, reducing muscle tension. It interferes with the release of calcium ion from the sarcoplasmic reticulum, resulting in decreased muscle contraction. This mechanism is of particular importance in malignant hyperthermia when increased myoplasmic calcium ion concentrations activate acute catabolism in the skeletal muscle cell. Dantrolene prevents or reduces the increase in myoplasmic calcium concentrations associated with malignant hyperthermia crises.

• *Kinetics in adults:* 35% of oral dose is absorbed through GI tract, with peak concentrations reached within 5 hours. Therapeutic effect in patients with upper motor neuron disorders may take 1 week or more.

Dantrolene is substantially plasma protein-bound, mainly to albumin.

Dantrolene is metabolized in the liver to its less active 5-hydroxy derivatives, and to its amino derivative by reductive pathways.

Dantrolene is excreted in urine as metabolites.

Contraindications and precautions

Dantrolene is contraindicated in patients with active hepatic disease (hepatitis, cirrhosis), upper motor neuron disorders, and those in whom spasticity helps maintain upright posture and balance.

Administer cautiously to patients with cardiac function impairment (may cause pleural effusion), pulmonary function impairment (especially chronic obstructive pulmonary disease), or preexisting hepatic disease. Also administer cautiously to patients receiving other drugs (especially estrogens) concomitantly, because of increased risk of hepatotoxicity.

There are no contraindications to the use of I.V. dantrolene in management of malignant hyperthermia crisis.

Interactions

Concomitant use with other CNS depressant drugs, including alcohol, narcotics, anxiolytics, antipsychotics, and tricyclic antidepressants, may increase CNS depression. Reduce dosage of one or both if used concurrently.

Effects on diagnostic tests

Dantrolene therapy alters liver function test results (increased ALT [SGPT], AST [SGOT], alkaline phosphatase, and lactic dehydroginase), blood urea nitrogen levels, and total serum bilirubin.

Adverse reactions

• CNS: muscle weakness, drowsiness, dizziness, lightheadedness, mental depression, confusion, fatigue, malaise, speech disturbance, headache, increased nervousness, hallucinations.

• CV: tachycardia, erratic blood pressure, phlebitis, pleural effusion with pericarditis.

• DERM: pruritus, urticaria, acneiform rash, eczematoid eruption, photosensitivity reactions.

• EENT: excessive tearing, visual and auditory disturbances.

• GI: nausea, severe diarrhea, anorexia, vomiting, gastric irritation, abdominal cramps, constipation, difficulty swallowing, GI bleeding, alteration of taste.

• GU: urinary frequency, incontinence, nocturia, crystalluria, hematuria, difficulty achieving erection.

• Hepatic: hepatitis.

• Other: sweating, backache, myalgia, chills, fever, drooling.

Note: Drug should be discontinued if hypersensitivity or liver function test abnormality occurs, or if improvement does not occur after 45 days of oral therapy.

Overdose and treatment

Clinical manifestations of overdose include exaggeration of adverse reactions, particularly CNS depression, and nausea and vomiting.

Treatment includes supportive measures, gastric lavage, and observation of symptoms. Maintain adequate airway, have emergency ventilation equipment on hand, monitor ECG, and administer large quantities of I.V. solutions to prevent crystalluria. Monitor vital signs closely. The benefit of dialysis is not known.

▶ Special considerations

• Not recommended for long-term use in children under age 5.

• To prepare suspension for single oral dose, dissolve contents of appropriate number of capsules in fruit juice or other suitable liquid.

• Before therapy begins, check patient's baseline neuromuscular functions—posture, gait, coordination, range of motion, muscle strength and tone, presence of abnormal muscle movements, and reflexes—for later comparisons.

• Walking should be supervised until patient's reaction to drug is known. With relief of spasticity, patient may lose ability to maintain balance.

• Improvement may require a week or more of drug therapy.

• Because of the risk of hepatic injury, drug should be discontinued if improvement is not evident within 45 days.

• Perform baseline and regularly scheduled liver function tests (alkaline phosphatase, ALT [SGPT], AST [SGOT], and total bilirubin), blood cell counts, and renal function tests.

• Risk of hepatotoxicity may be greater in patients taking other medications, and patients taking high dantrolene doses (400 mg or more daily) for prolonged periods.

• Clinical signs of malignant hyperthermia include skeletal muscle rigidity (often the first sign), sudden tachycardia, cardiac dysrhythmias, cyanosis, tachypnea, unstable blood pressure, rapidly rising temperature, acidosis, and shock.

• In malignant hyperthermia crisis, drug should be given by rapid I.V. injection as soon as reaction is recognized.

---

*Canada only   †Unlabeled clinical use   Italicized adverse reactions have been observed in children.

• To reconstitute, add 60 ml sterile water for injection to 20-mg vial. Do not use bacteriostatic water for injection.
• Treating malignant hyperthermia requires continual monitoring of body temperature, management of fever, correction of acidosis, maintenance of fluid and electrolyte balance, monitoring of intake and output, adequate oxygenation, and seizure precautions.

Information for parents and patient
• Instruct parents and patient to report promptly the onset of jaundice: yellow skin or sclerae, dark urine, clay-colored stools, itching, and abdominal discomfort. Hepatotoxicity occurs more frequently between the 3rd and 12th month of therapy.
• Advise parents of patients susceptible to malignant hyperthermia that patients should wear Medic Alert bracelet or necklace indicating diagnosis, physician's name and telephone number, drug causing reaction, and treatment used.
• Because hepatotoxicity occurs more commonly after concurrent use of other drugs with dantrolene, warn parents to avoid administering nonprescription medications, alcoholic beverages, and other CNS depressants to the patient except as prescribed.
• Photosensitivity reactions are possible. Advise patient to avoid excessive or unnecessary exposure to sunlight and to use protective clothing and a sunscreen agent.
• Drug may cause drowsiness. Warn parents that child should to avoid hazardous activities that require alertness until CNS depressant effects are determined.
• Advise parents to report any adverse reactions immediately.
• Tell parents to store drug away from heat and direct light (not in bathroom medicine cabinet). Keep out of reach of children.

---

dapsone*
Avlosulfon*

• Classification: antileprotic, antimalarial agent (synthetic sulfone)

How supplied
Available by prescription only
Tablets: 25 mg, 100 mg

Indications, route, and dosage
All forms of leprosy (Hansen's disease)
Children: 1 to 1.5 mg/kg P.O. daily.
Adults: 50 to 100 mg P.O. daily for indefinite period, plus rifampin 600 mg daily for 6 months.
Prophylaxis for leprosy patient's close contacts
Infants under age 6 months: 6 mg P.O. three times weekly.
Infants age 6 to 23 months: 12 mg P.O. three times weekly.
Children age 2 to 5: 25 mg P.O. three times weekly.
Children age 6 to 12: 25 mg P.O. daily.

Children over age 12 and adults: 50 mg P.O. daily.
Dermatitis herpetiformis
Children over age 12 and adults: Initially, 50 mg P.O. daily; may increase up to 400 mg/day.
Malaria suppression or prophylaxis
Children: 2 mg/kg P.O. weekly, with pyrimethamine 0.25 mg/kg weekly.
Adults: 100 mg P.O. weekly, with pyrimethamine 12.5 mg P.O. weekly.
Continue prophylaxis throughout exposure and 6 months postexposure.
†Pneumocystis carinii pneumonia
Adults: 100 mg P.O. daily. Usually administered with trimethoprim, 20 mg/kg daily divided q.i.d.

Action and kinetics
• *Antibiotic action:* Dapsone is bacteriostatic and bactericidal; like sulfonamides, it is thought to act principally by inhibition of folic acid. It acts against *Mycobacterium leprae* and *M. tuberculosis*, and has some activity against *Pneumocystis carinii* and *Plasmodium*.
• *Kinetics in adults:* Dapsone is absorbed completely, but rather slowly, from the GI tract after oral administration; peak serum levels occur 2 to 8 hours after ingestion. Dapsone is distributed widely into most body tissues and fluids. Dapsone is 50% to 80% protein-bound.
  Dapsone undergoes acetylation by liver enzymes; rate varies and is genetically determined. Almost 50% of blacks and whites are slow acetylators, whereas over 80% of Chinese, Japanese, and Eskimos are fast acetylators. Dosage adjustment may be required. Dapsone and metabolites are excreted primarily in urine; small amounts of drug are excreted in feces and possibly in breast milk. Dapsone undergoes enterohepatic circulation; half-life in adults ranges between 10 and 50 hours (average 28 hours). Orally administered charcoal may enhance excretion. Dapsone is dialyzable.

Contraindications and precautions
Dapsone is contraindicated in patients with known hypersensitivity to dapsone or its derivatives and in patients with severe anemia.
  Dapsone should be used cautiously in patients with glucose-6-phosphate dehydrogenase (G6PD) deficiency, methemoglobin reductase deficiency, or hemoglobin M; in patients predisposed to hemolysis induced by other drugs or conditions (certain infections or diabetic ketosis) because of potential adverse hematologic effects; and in patients taking probenecid because of decreased excretion and drug accumulation. Special care must be taken to recognize leprosy reactional states.

Interactions
Concomitant use of dapsone with nitrite, phenyhydrazine, nitrofurantoin, or primaquine increases hazard of hemolysis in patients with G6PD deficiency; with probenecid may increase dapsone serum levels by blocking renal tubular secretion; with para-aminobenzoic acid (PABA) antagonizes dapsone's antibacterial effect.

---

‡May contain sulfites ♦ May contain tartrazine ♦♦ May contain benzyl alcohol

Rifampin-induced hepatic enzymes increase metabolic rate and reduce dapsone serum levels.

Effects on diagnostic tests
None reported.

Adverse reactions
• CNS: psychosis, headache, dizziness, lethargy, severe malaise, paresthesias.
• DERM: allergic dermatitis (generalized or fixed maculopapular rash).
• EENT: tinnitus, allergic rhinitis.
• GI: anorexia, abdominal pain, nausea, vomiting.
• HEMA: aplastic anemia, agranulocytosis, hemolytic anemia, methemoglobinemia, possible leukopenia.
• Hepatic: hepatitis, cholestatic jaundice.
• Other: fever, phototoxicity.
   Note: Drug should be discontinued if patient shows signs of hypersensitivity reaction, dermatologic toxicity, muscle weakness, hepatotoxicity, or marked hematologic abnormalities (leukopenia, thrombocytopenia, anemia); reduce dosage or temporarily discontinue dapsone if hemoglobin level falls below 9 g/dl, if leukocyte level falls below 5,000/mm^3, or if erythrocyte count falls below 2.5 million/mm^3 or remains low.

Leprosy reactional states
When treating leprosy with dapsone, it is essential to recognize two types of leprosy reactional states that are related to effectiveness of dapsone therapy.
   Type I, reversal reaction, includes erythema, followed by swelling of skin and nerve lesions in tuberculoid patients; skin lesions may ulcerate and multiply, and acute neuritis may cause neural dysfunction. Severe cases require hospitalization, analgesics, corticosteroids, and nerve trunk decompression while dapsone therapy is continued.
   Type II, erythema nodosum leprosum, occurs primarily in lepromatous leprosy, with an incidence of about 50% during the first year of therapy. Signs and symptoms include tender erythematous skin nodules, fever, malaise, arthritis, neuritis, albuminuria, iritis, joint swelling, epistaxis, and depression; skin lesions may ulcerate. Treatment includes corticosteroids and analgesics.
   Additional treatment guidelines are available from National Hansen's Disease Center, (504) 642-7771.

Overdose and treatment
Signs of overdose include nausea, vomiting, and hyperexcitability, occurring within minutes or up to 24 hours after ingestion; methemoglobin-induced depression, cyanosis, and convulsions may occur. Hemolysis is a late complication (up to 14 days after ingestion).
   Treat by gastric lavage, followed by activated charcoal; treat dapsone-induced methemoglobinemia in G6PD patients with methylene blue. Hemodialysis may also be used to enhance elimination.

▶ **Special considerations**
• Use with caution in children.
• Give drug with or after meals to avoid gastric irritation.

• Obtain specimens for culture and sensitivity testing before first dose, but therapy may begin before test results are complete; repeat periodically to detect drug resistance.
• Observe patient for adverse effects and monitor hematologic and liver function studies to minimize toxicity.
• Monitor dapsone serum concentrations periodically to maintain effective levels. Levels of 0.1 to 0.7 mg per 100 ml are usually effective and safe.
• Observe skin and mucous membranes for early signs of allergic reactions or leprosy reactional states.
• Isolation of patient with inactive leprosy is not required; however, surfaces in contact with discharge from nose or skin lesions should be disinfected.
• Therapeutic effect on leprosy may not be evident until 3 to 6 months after start of therapy.
• Monitor vital signs frequently during early weeks of drug therapy. Frequent or high fever may require reduced dosage or discontinuation of drug.
• Because dapsone is dialyzable, patients undergoing hemodialysis may require dosage adjustments.

Information for parents and patient
• Explain disease process and rationale for long-term therapy; emphasize that improvement may not occur for 3 to 6 months.
• Teach signs and symptoms of hypersensitivity and other adverse reactions, and emphasize need to report these promptly; explain possibility of cumulative effects; urge parents to report *any* unusual effects or reactions and to report loss of appetite, nausea, or vomiting promptly.
• Emphasize the need to comply with prescribed regimen. Encourage parents to report no improvement or worsening of symptoms after 3 months of drug treatment. Warn against discontinuing drug without medical approval. Explain importance of follow-up visits and need to monitor close contacts at 6- to 12-month intervals for 10 years.
• Teach sanitary disposal of nasal or skin secretions.
• Assure parents and patient that inactive leprosy is no barrier to employment or school attendance.
• New mothers need not be separated from infant during therapy; teach signs of cyanosis and methemoglobinemia.

---

daunorubicin hydrochloride
Cerubidine

• Classification: antineoplastic (antibiotic antineoplastic [cell cycle-phase nonspecific])

How supplied
Available by prescription only
Injection: 20-mg vials

Indications, route, and dosage
Dosage and indications may vary. Check current literature for recommended protocols.

Remission induction in acute nonlymphocytic leukemia (myelogenous, monocytic, erythroid), acute lymphocytic leukemia

Children: 25 mg/m² once a week, usually combined with vincristine and prednisone.

Adults: As a single agent — 30 to 60 mg/m² I.V. daily on days 1, 2, and 3 q 3 to 4 weeks; or 800 mcg to 1 mg/kg for 3 to 6 days, repeated q 3 to 4 weeks. Maximum dosage is 550 mg/m² (450/m² for patients who have received chest irradiation). In combination — 45 mg/m² I.V. daily on days 1, 2, and 3 of the first course and on days 1 and 2 of subsequent courses with cytosine arabinoside infusions.

Note: Dose should be reduced if hepatic function is impaired.

Action and kinetics

• *Antineoplastic action:* Daunorubicin exerts its cytotoxic activity by intercalating between DNA base pairs and uncoiling the DNA helix. The result is inhibition of DNA synthesis and DNA-dependent RNA synthesis. The drug may also inhibit polymerase activity.

• *Kinetics in adults:* Because of its vesicant nature, daunorubicin must be given intravenously. Daunorubicin is widely distributed into body tissues, with the highest concentrations found in the spleen, kidneys, liver, lungs, and heart. The drug does not cross the blood-brain barrier. The drug is extensively metabolized in the liver by microsomal enzymes. One of the metabolites has cytotoxic activity. Daunorubicin and its metabolites are primarily excreted in bile, with a small portion excreted in urine. Plasma elimination has been described as biphasic, with an initial phase half-life of 45 minutes and a terminal phase half-life of 18½ hours.

Contraindications and precautions

Daunorubicin is contraindicated in patients with severe myelosuppression, preexisting cardiac disease, severe infections, or hepatic or renal dysfunction, because the drug may worsen these conditions. It should not be used in pregnant patients because of significant risk to the fetus.

Interactions

When used concomitantly, other hepatotoxic drugs may increase the risk of hepatotoxicity with daunorubicin.

Do not mix daunorubicin with either heparin sodium or dexamethasone phosphate. Admixture of these agents results in the formation of a precipitate.

Effects on diagnostic tests

Daunorubicin therapy may increase blood and urine concentrations of uric acid.

Daunorubicin therapy may also cause an increase in serum alkaline phosphatase, AST (SGOT), and bilirubin levels, indicating drug-induced hepatotoxicity.

Adverse reactions

• CV: irreversible cardiomyopathy (dose-related), *ECG changes, dysrhythmias,* pericarditis, myocarditis, *cardiotoxicity.*
• DERM: rash.

• GI: *nausea, vomiting,* stomatitis, esophagitis, anorexia, *diarrhea.*
• GU: nephrotoxicity, transient red urine.
• HEMA: *bone marrow depression* (dose-limiting), anemia, pancytopenia (nadir between 10 and 14 days), leukopenia, thrombocytopenia.
• Hepatic: hepatotoxicity, *red urine (not hematuric).*
• Local: *severe cellulitis or tissue slough if drug extravasates.*
• Other: generalized alopecia, fever, chills, *anaphylactoid reaction, conjunctivitis.*

Note: Drug should be discontinued if patient develops signs of congestive heart failure or cardiomyopathy.

Overdose and treatment

Clinical manifestations of overdose include myelosuppression, nausea, vomiting, and stomatitis.

Treatment is usually supportive and includes transfusion of blood components and antiemetics.

▶ Special considerations

• Vital signs and patency of catheter or I.V. line should be monitored throughout administration.

• Carefully follow all established procedures for the safe and proper handling, administration, and disposal of chemotherapy.

• Monitor BUN, hematocrit, platelet count, ALT (SGPT), AST (SGOT), LDH, serum bilirubin, serum creatinine, uric acid, and total and differential leukocytes.

• To reconstitute the drug for I.V. administration, add 4 ml of sterile water for injection to a 20-mg vial to give a concentration of 5 mg/ml.

• Drug may be diluted further into 100 ml of dextrose 5% in water or normal saline solution and infused over 30 to 45 minutes.

• For I.V. push administration, withdraw reconstituted drug into syringe containing 10 to 15 ml of normal saline solution, and inject over 2 to 3 minutes into the tubing of a freely flowing I.V. infusion. Reconstituted solution is stable for 24 hours at room temperature.

• Reddish color of drug looks similar to that of doxorubicin (Adriamycin). Do not confuse the two drugs.

• Erythematous streaking along the vein or flushing in the face indicate that the drug is being administered too rapidly.

• Drug is a vesicant. Avoid placement of I.V. site at or near a joint that may become immobilized if extravasation occurs. During I.V. administration, monitor continuously for extravasation. If it occurs, stop infusion, remove I.V., and treat promptly according to institutional policy. NIH recommendations include S.C. injection of Solucortef and topical hydrocortisone.

• Antiemetics may be used to prevent or treat nausea and vomiting. Nausea and vomiting may be very severe and last 24 to 48 hours.

• Patients who have received drugs with strong emetic properties may experience anticipatory nausea and vomiting at subsequent treatments. They may benefit from treatment with an anxiolytic drug.

• Monitor patient's intake, output, and weight. Continue I.V. hydration until patient resumes sufficient oral intake.

‡May contain sulfites   ♦May contain tartrazine   ♦ ♦May contain benzyl alcohol

• Children have an increased incidence of drug-induced cardiotoxicity, which may occur at lower doses. The total lifetime dosage for children over age 2 is 300 mg/m², for children under age 2, 10 mg/kg.
• Monitor ECG before treatment and monthly during treatment. Note if resting pulse rate is high (a sign of cardiac adverse reactions).
• Monitor CBC and hepatic function.
• Do not use a scalp tourniquet or apply ice to prevent alopecia, because this may compromise effectiveness of drug.

Information for parents and patient
• Patient should avoid exposure to persons with bacterial or viral infections as chemotherapy can make the patient more susceptible to infection. Urge parents to report signs of infection and exposure to chicken pox immediately.
• Advise parents to have child use caution when using toothbrush or dental floss. Chemotherapy can increase incidence of microbial infection, delayed healing, and bleeding gums.
• Instruct patient to perform frequent oral hygiene. Patient should avoid using commercial mouthwashes, which may contain alcohol and have an irritating effect. Solutions of sodium bicarbonate or hydrogen peroxide are more appropriate rinses.
• Instruct patient to avoid foods that are spicy and extremely hot or cold. Topical anesthetics administered before meals (swish and spit) may relieve mouth discomfort.
• Tell parents that patient's dental work should be completed before initiation of therapy whenever possible, or delayed until blood counts are normal.
• Warn parents and patient that bruising may easily occur because of drug's effects on blood count. Patient may have to limit activity to prevent injury.
• Tell parents and patient to immediately report redness, pain, or swelling at injection site. Injury and scarring may result if I.V. infiltrates.
• Advise parents that patient should not receive immunizations during therapy and for several weeks after therapy. Members of the same household should not receive live-virus immunization during the same period.
• Warn parents and patient that urine may be red for 1 to 2 days and that this is a drug effect, not bleeding.
• Advise parents and patient that alopecia may occur, but that it is usually reversible.
• Advise parents to encourage child to drink plenty of fluids to increase urine output and facilitate excretion of uric acid.
• Warn parents and patient that nausea and vomiting may be severe and may last for 24 to 48 hours.
• Tell parents to call if the child develops a sore throat, fever, or any signs of bleeding and to report shortness of breath or swollen ankles, which may indicate cardiac toxicity.
• Inform parents and patient that fever may follow drug administration; however, they should report fever that persists for 24 hours after the drug has been given.

demecarium bromide
Humorsol

• Classification: miotic (cholinesterase inhibitor)

How supplied
Available by prescription only
Ophthalmic solution: 0.125% and 0.25% in 5-ml ocumeter

Indications, route, and dosage
Glaucoma
Children: Instill 1 drop of 0.125% or 0.25% solution in eyes twice weekly up to b.i.d., depending on intraocular pressure.
Adults: Instill 1 or 2 drops of 0.125% or 0.25% solution in eyes twice weekly up to b.i.d., depending on intraocular pressure.
Accommodative esotropia (convergent strabismus)
Children: Instill 1 drop of 0.125% solution in each eye daily for 2 to 3 weeks; taper to 1 drop q 2 days for 3 to 4 weeks, then 1 drop twice weekly. Therapy should be discontinued after 4 months if control of condition still requires every-other-day therapy or if patient shows no response.

Drug is antidote for atropine in glaucoma or preglaucoma patients and is used to control postoperative rise in intraocular pressure.

Action and kinetics
• *Miotic action:* Demecarium inhibits the enzymatic destruction of acetylcholine by inactivating cholinesterase. This leaves acetylcholine free to act on the effector cells of the iridic sphincter and ciliary muscles, causing pupillary constriction and accommodation spasm.
• *Kinetics in adults:* Although demecarium is a reversible inhibitor of cholinesterase, its duration of action is similar to that of irreversible cholinesterase inhibitors. Maximal decrease in intraocular pressure occurs in 24 hours and may persist for over a week.

Contraindications and precautions
Demecarium is contraindicated in patients with active uveal inflammation, narrow-angle glaucoma, secondary glaucoma resulting from iridocyclitis, ocular hypertension, vasomotor instability, bronchial instability, bronchial asthma, spastic GI conditions, peptic ulcer, severe bradycardia, hypotension, recent myocardial infarction, epilepsy, or history of retinal detachment, because the drug may aggravate the signs or symptoms of these disorders. It should be used with caution in patients with myasthenia gravis who are also receiving systemic anticholinesterase therapy and in patients exposed to organophosphorus insecticides.

Interactions
When used concomitantly, demecarium may increase neuromuscular blocking effects of succinylcholine, antagonize antiglaucoma effect of cyclopentolate and belladonna alkaloids, interfere with pilocarpine-in-

duced miosis, increase the toxicity of carbamate or-ganophosphate insecticides, add to effects of systemic anticholinesterase agents used for myasthenia gravis, and decrease duration of echothiophate-induced miosis; echothiophate usually is tried first.

Effects on diagnostic tests
None reported.

Adverse reactions
• CNS: muscle weakness, headache
• CV: bradycardia, dysrhythmias.
• DERM: contact dermatitis.
• Eye: iris cysts (reversible with discontinuation), lens opacity, blurred vision, eye or brow pain, retinal detachment, vitreous hemorrhage, eyelid twitching, iritis, conjunctival and intraocular hyperemia, ocular pain, paradoxical increased intraocular pressure.
• GI: nausea, vomiting, abdominal pain, diarrhea, salivation.
• GU: urinary incontinence.
• Respiratory: dyspnea.
  Note: Drug should be discontinued immediately if excessive salivation, sweating, urinary incontinence, diarrhea, or muscle weakness occurs.

Overdose and treatment
Clinical manifestations of overdose include nausea, vomiting, abdominal pain, diarrhea, increased salivation, headache, syncope, tremors, urinary incontinence, dyspnea, hypotension, bradycardia, and dysrhythmias. When swallowed accidentally, vomiting is usually spontaneous; if not, induce emesis and follow with activated charcoal or a cathartic. Treat cardiovascular or blood pressure responses with epinephrine; treat accidental dermal exposure by washing the area twice with water. Atropine sulfate, given S.C. or I.V., is the antidote of choice.

▶ Special considerations
• Demecarium is a potent, long-acting drug capable of producing cumulative systemic side effects. Follow prescribed concentration and dosage schedule closely; monitor patient.
• Wash hands immediately before and after administering; if solution contacts skin, wash promptly with large amount of water.
• Check patient for lenticular opacities every 6 months.
• Store in tightly closed original container.
• Finger pressure should be applied to lacrimal sac for 1 to 2 minutes after instillation to decrease risk of absorption and systemic reactions.

Information for parents and patient
• Teach parents correct way to use and store medication and adequate safety measures; stress compliance with schedule and importance of close, constant medical supervision. Warn parents and patient never to exceed recommended dosage.
• Warn parents to stop drug at least 2 weeks before scheduled ophthalmic surgery or other surgery involving general anesthesia.
• Instruct parents to have patient use drug at bedtime because drug blurs vision.

• Reassure parents and patient that blurred vision usually diminishes with prolonged use.
• Instruct parent to apply finger pressure to patient's lacrimal sac during and for 1 to 2 minutes after instillation of solution.
• In case of emergency surgery or general anesthesia, inform the anesthesiologist that this drug is being used.

---

demeclocycline hydrochloride
Declomycin, Ledermycin

• Classification: antibiotic (tetracycline)

How supplied
Available by prescription only
Oral: 150-mg capsules; 150- and 300-mg tablets
Capsules: 150 mg
Tablets: 150 mg, 300 mg

Indications, route, and dosage
Infections caused by susceptible organisms
Children over age 8: 6 to 12 mg/kg P.O. daily, divided q 6 to 12 hours.
Adults: 150 mg P.O. q 6 hours, or 300 mg P.O. q 12 hours.
Gonorrhea
Adults: 600 mg P.O. initially, then 300 mg P.O. q 12 hours for 4 days (total 3 g).
Uncomplicated urethral, endocervical, or rectal infection
Adults: 300 mg P.O. q.i.d. for at least 7 days.
†Syndrome of inappropriate antidiuretic hormone (a hyposmolar state)
Adults: 600 to 1,200 mg P.O. daily in divided doses.

Action and kinetics
• *Antibacterial action:* Demeclocycline is bacteriostatic. Tetracyclines bind reversibly to ribosomal subunits, thereby inhibiting bacterial protein synthesis. Demeclocycline is active against many gram-negative and gram-positive organisms, *Mycoplasma, Rickettsia, Chlamydia,* and spirochetes.
• *Kinetics in adults:* Demeclocycline is 60% to 80% absorbed from the GI tract after oral administration; peak serum levels occur at 3 to 4 hours. Food or milk reduces absorption by 50%; antacids chelate with tetracyclines and further reduce absorption.
  Demeclocycline has the greatest affinity of all tetracyclines for calcium ions. It is distributed widely into body tissues and fluids, including synovial, pleural, prostatic, and seminal fluids; bronchial secretions; saliva; and aqueous humor. CSF penetration is poor. Demeclocycline crosses the placenta; it is 36% to 91% protein-bound. Demeclocycline is not metabolized and is excreted primarily unchanged in urine by glomerular filtration; some drug may be excreted in breast milk. Plasma half-life is 10 to 17 hours in adults with normal renal function. Hemodialysis and peritoneal dialysis remove only minimal amounts of demeclocycline.

Contraindications and precautions

Demeclocycline is contraindicated in patients with known hypersensitivity to any tetracycline. It also is contraindicated during the second half of pregnancy because it may cause fatty infiltration of the liver in the mother and may cause permanent discoloration or hypoplasia of tooth enamel or impaired skeletal growth in the fetus. It is contraindicated in children under age 8 because it may cause permanent discoloration of teeth, enamel defects, and retardation of bone growth.

Use demeclocycline with caution in patients with decreased renal function, because it may elevate BUN levels and exacerbate renal dysfunction, and in patients likely to be exposed to direct sunlight or ultraviolet light because of the risk of photosensitivity reactions.

Interactions

Oral absorption of tetracycline is impaired by concomitant use with antacids containing aluminum, calcium, or magnesium or laxatives containing magnesium because of chelation; absorption of tetracycline is also impaired by food, milk and other dairy products, iron products, and sodium bicarbonate.

Tetracyclines may antagonize bactericidal effects of penicillin, inhibiting cell growth because of bacteriostatic action; administer penicillin 2 to 3 hours before tetracycline.

Concomitant use of tetracycline increases the risk of nephrotoxicity from methoxyflurane. When used concomitantly with oral anticoagulants, it necessitates lowered dosages of oral anticoagulants because of enhanced effects; and when used with digoxin, lowered dosages of digoxin because of increased bioavailability.

Effects on diagnostic tests

Demeclocycline causes false-negative results in urine tests using glucose oxidase reagent (Clinistix or Tes-Tape). It also causes false elevations in fluorometric tests for urinary catecholamines.

Demeclocycline may elevate serum BUN levels in patients with decreased renal function.

Adverse reactions

• CV: pericarditis.
• DERM: maculopapular and erythematous rashes, photosensitivity, increased pigmentation, urticaria, discolored nails and teeth.
• EENT: dysphagia, glossitis.
• GI: anorexia, nausea, vomiting, diarrhea, enterocolitis, anogenital inflammation.
• GU: reversible nephrotoxicity (Fanconi's syndrome) with outdated tetracyclines, progressive renal dysfunction in patients with preexisting renal impairment.
• HEMA: neutropenia, eosinophilia.
• Metabolic: increased BUN levels, diabetes insipidus syndrome (polyuria, polydipsia and weakness).
• Other: hypersensitivity, bacterial and fungal superinfection.

Note: Drug should be discontinued if signs of toxicity, hypersensitivity, progressive renal dysfunction,

or superinfection occur; if erythema follows exposure to sunlight or ultraviolet light; or if severe diarrhea indicates pseudomembranous colitis.

Overdose and treatment

Clinical signs of overdose are usually limited to the GI tract. Treatment may include antacids or gastric lavage if ingestion occurred within the preceding 4 hours.

▶ Special considerations

• Drug should not be used in children under age 9.
• Demeclocycline is usually reserved for patients intolerant of other antibiotics.
• A reversible diabetes insipidus syndrome has been reported with long-term use; monitor for weakness, polyuria, and polydipsia.

Information for parents and patient

• Warn patient to avoid direct sunlight and ultraviolet light. A suncreen may help prevent photosensitivity reactions. Photosensitivity may persist for some time after discontinuing drug.
• Administration with milk or dairy products, food, antacids, or iron products reduces effectiveness. Be sure patient takes drug with sufficient water at least 1 hour before meals or 2 hours afterward. Give at least 1 hour before bedtime to avoid esophagitis.
• Be sure patient takes the drug exactly as prescribed, even if feeling better.
• Tell patient to discard any unused medication.
• Stress good oral hygiene to prevent overgrowth of non-susceptible organisms.

---

deslanoside
Cedilanid-D Injection

• Classification: antiarrhythmic, inotropic (digitalis glycoside)

How supplied
Available by prescription only
Injection: 0.2 mg/ml

Indications, route, and dosage
CHF, paroxysmal atrial tachycardia, atrial fibrillation and flutter
Premature and full-term neonates: 22 mcg/kg I.M. or I.V. divided into two or three doses at 3- or 4-hour intervals.
Children age 2 weeks to 3 years: 25 mcg/kg I.M. or I.V. divided into two or three doses at 3- or 4-hour intervals.
Children age 3 and older: 22.5 mcg/kg I.M. or I.V. divided into two or three doses at 3- or 4-hour intervals.
Adults: Loading dosage is 1.2 to 1.6 mg I.M. or I.V. in 2 divided doses over 24 hours; for maintenance, use another cardiac glycoside.

Action and kinetics

Deslanoside has effects similar to those of digoxin but may have a slightly faster onset of action. Its clinical usefulness is somewhat limited because its therapeutic serum level profile has not yet been defined and because an oral dosage form is unavailable.

Deslanoside's effects on the myocardium are dose-related and involve both direct and indirect mechanisms. The drug directly increases the force and velocity of myocardial contraction, AV node refractory period, and total peripheral resistance. At higher doses, increased sympathetic outflow occurs. The drug indirectly depresses the SA node and prolongs conduction to the AV node.

• *Inotropic action:* In patients with heart failure, increased contractile force boosts cardiac output, improves systolic emptying, and decreases diastolic heart size. It also increases ventricular end-diastolic pressure and consequently decreases pulmonary and systemic venous pressures. Increased myocardial contractility and cardiac output reflexively reduce sympathetic tone in patients with CHF. This compensates for the drug's direct vasoconstrictive action and thereby reduces total peripheral resistance; it also slows the heart rate and causes diuresis in edematous patients.

• *Antiarrhythmic action:* Deslanoside-induced heart rate slowing in patients without CHF is negligible and stems mainly from vagal (cholinergic) and sympatholytic effects on the SA node; however, with toxic doses, heart-rate slowing results from direct depression of SA node automaticity. Although therapeutic doses produce little effect on the action potential, toxic doses increase automaticity (increased spontaneous diastolic depolarization) in all heart regions except the SA node.

• *Kinetics in adults:* Deslanoside is inconsistently and incompletely absorbed from the GI tract. After I.V. administration, effects occur in about 10 minutes; peak effects occur in about 20 minutes. Deslanoside is widely distributed in body tissues; highest concentrations occur in the heart, kidneys, intestine, stomach, liver, and skeletal muscle; lowest concentrations are in the plasma and brain. Deslanoside crosses both the blood-brain barrier and the placenta; consequently, fetal and maternal serum drug levels are presumably similar. About 25% of drug is bound to plasma proteins. Drug's metabolism is minimal. Deslanoside is excreted unchanged in the urine; elimination half-life is about 33 hours.

Contraindications and precautions

Deslanoside is contraindicated in patients with ventricular fibrillation, because it may cause ventricular asystole; in patients with digitalis toxicity, because of potential for additive toxicity; and in patients with hypersensitivity to the drug.

Deslanoside should be used with extreme caution, if at all, in patients with idiopathic hypertrophic subaortic stenosis, because the drug may increase obstruction of left ventricular outflow; in patients with incomplete AV block who do not have an artificial pacemaker (especially those with Stokes-Adams syndrome), because the drug may induce advanced or complete AV block; in patients with hypersensitive

carotid sinus syndrome, because the drug increases vagal tone (carotid sinus massage has induced ventricular fibrillation in patients receiving cardiac glycosides); in patients with Wolff-Parkinson-White syndrome, because the drug may increase conduction through accessory pathways; in patients with sinus node disease (for example, sick sinus syndrome), because the drug may worsen sinus bradycardia or SA block; and in patients with acute glomerulonephritis and CHF, because the drug may accumulate rapidly to toxic levels.

Deslanoside should be used with caution in patients with severe pulmonary disease, hypoxia, myxedema, acute myocardial infarction, severe heart failure, acute myocarditis, or an otherwise damaged myocardium, because of the increased risk of drug-induced dysrhythmias in these patients; in patients with chronic constrictive pericarditis, because such patients may respond unfavorably to the drug; in patients with frequent premature ventricular contractions or ventricular tachycardia (especially if these dysrhythmias are not caused by heart failure), because the drug may induce additional dysrhythmias; in patients with low cardiac output states caused by valvular stenosis, chronic pericarditis, or chronic cor pulmonale, because the drug may decrease heart rate and subsequently further reduce cardiac output; in patients with conditions that increase cardiac sensitivity to cardiac glycosides, including hypokalemia, chronic pulmonary disease, and acute hypoxemia; and in patients with hypertension, because I.V. administration may transiently increase blood pressure.

Interactions

Concomitant use of deslanoside with other drugs that affect AV conduction (such as procainamide, propranolol, and verapamil) may have additive cardiac effects. Concomitant use with sympathomimetics (such as ephedrine, epinephrine, and isoproterenol), rauwolfia, or succinylcholine may increase the risk of cardiac dysrhythmias.

Concomitant use with I.V. calcium preparations may cause synergistic cardiac effects, precipitating dysrhythmias; use with electrolyte-altering agents may increase or decrease serum electrolyte levels, in turn predisposing the patient to deslanoside toxicity. For example, concomitant use with diuretics (such as ethacrynic acid, furosemide, and bumetanide) may cause hypokalemia and hypomagnesemia; thiazides may cause hypercalcemia. Fatal cardiac dysrhythmias may result. Concomitant use with amphotericin B, corticosteroids, corticotropin, edetate disodium, laxatives, or sodium polystyrene sulfonate may deplete total body potassium levels. Concomitant use with glucagon, high-dose dextrose, or dextrose-insulin infusions reduces extracellular potassium. Patients receiving these drugs may be predisposed to digitalis toxicity.

Effects on diagnostic tests

None reported.

Adverse reactions

• CNS: fatigue, generalized weakness, agitation, hallucinations, headache, malaise, dizziness, vertigo, stupor, paresthesias.

• CV: increased severity of CHF, dysrhythmias (most commonly conduction disturbances with or without AV block, premature ventricular contractions, and supraventricular dysrhythmias), hypotension. (These effects may be life-threatening and require immediate attention.)
• EENT: yellow-green halos around visual images, blurred vision, light flashes, photophobia, diplopia.
• GI: anorexia, nausea, vomiting, diarrhea.
Note: Drug should be discontinued if signs of digitalis toxicity are present (nausea, vomiting, dysrhythmias).

Overdose and treatment
Clinical effects of overdose mainly involve the gastrointestinal, CNS, and cardiovascular systems.

Hyperkalemia may occur with severe intoxication and may develop rapidly, possibly resulting in life-threatening cardiac effects. Signs of cardiac toxicity may occur with or without other toxicity signs and commonly precede other toxic manifestations. Because most toxic cardiac effects also may be manifestations of heart disease, it may be difficult to determine whether these result from underlying heart disease or from drug therapy. Patients with chronic drug toxicity commonly have ventricular dysrhythmias and/or AV conduction disturbances. In patients with digoxin-induced ventricular tachycardia, mortality is high; this condition may progress to ventricular fibrillation or asystole.

If toxicity is suspected, the drug should be discontinued immediately and the serum drug concentration measured. (Usually, the drug requires at least 6 hours to equilibrate between plasma and tissue; therefore, plasma levels drawn earlier may show higher levels than those present after the drug is distributed to the tissues.)

Any interacting drugs probably also should be discontinued. Ventricular dysrhythmias may be treated with I.V. potassium, I.V. phenytoin, I.V. lidocaine, or I.V. propranolol. Refractory ventricular tachydysrhythmias may be controlled with overdrive pacing. Procainamide may be used for ventricular dysrhythmias that do not respond to the above treatments. In severe AV block, asystole, and hemodynamically significant sinus bradycardia, atropine may restore normal heart rate.

▶ Special considerations
• Pediatric patients have poorly defined serum drug level ranges; however, toxicity apparently does not occur at same concentrations considered toxic in adults. Divided daily dosing is recommended for infants and children under age 10. Children over age 10 require adult doses proportional to body weight.
• Do not administer calcium salts to patient receiving deslanoside because this may cause serious dysrhythmias. Because deslanoside predisposes to postcardioversion dysrhythmias, it is commonly withheld 1 to 2 days before elective cardioversion in patients with atrial fibrillation. (However, consider consequences of increased ventricular response to atrial fibrillation while deslanoside is withheld.)
• Elective cardioversion should be postponed in patients with signs of drug toxicity.

• Hypothyroid patients are sensitive to drug; hyperthyroid patients may need larger doses.
• Obtain baseline heart rate and rhythm, blood pressure, and serum electrolytes levels before giving first dose.
• Find out if patient used cardiac glycosides within previous 2 to 3 weeks before administering loading dose.
• Always divide loading dose over first 24 hours unless clinical situation indicates otherwise. Use only for rapid digitalization, not maintenance therapy.
• Dosage must be adjusted to patient's clinical condition; ECG and serum levels of drug, calcium, potassium, and magnesium must be monitored. Serum potassium should be maintained at 4 to 5 mEq/liter to prevent ventricular irritability.
• Monitor clinical status. Take apical and radial pulses for full minute. Watch for significant changes (sudden rate increase or decrease, pulse deficit, irregular beats, and especially regularization of a previously irregular rhythm). Check blood pressure and obtain 12-lead ECG if these changes occur.
• Excessive slowing of pulse rate may be a sign of drug toxicity. Withhold drug and reevaluate therapy if this occurs.
• Observe patient's eating patterns. Monitor for nausea, vomiting, anorexia, visual disturbances, or other toxicity symptoms.
• I.M. injection is painful; give I.V. if possible.
• Monitor serum potassium levels. Take corrective action before hypokalemia occurs.
• Higher-than-usual doses and serum drug levels may be needed to adequately control atrial tachydysrhythmias.
• Before prescribing or administering additional drugs for patient currently receiving cardiac glycosides, review drug interactions, which are numerous and may seriously affect therapy.

Information for parents and patient
• Instruct parents to report loss of appetite, stomach pain, nausea, vomiting, diarrhea, unusual fatigue or weakness, drowsiness, headache, blurred or yellow vision, rash or hives, or depression.
• Warn parents that patient should not stop taking drug without medical approval.

desmopressin acetate
DDAVP, Stimate

• Classification: antidiuretic, hemostatic agent (posterior pituitary hormone)

How supplied
Available by prescription only
Nasal solution: 2.5-ml vials, 0.1 mg/ml
Injection: 10-ml vials, 4 mcg/ml

Indications, route, and dosage
Nonnephrogenic diabetes insipidus, temporary polyuria, and polydipsia associated with pituitary trauma

Children age 3 months to 12 years: 5 mcg (0.05 ml of a 0.01% solution,) preferably in the evening. Dosage adjustments are based on urine output. Usual dosage range is 5 to 30 mcg daily in a single dose or in divided doses.

Adults: 5 to 40 mcg (0.05 to 0.4 ml of a 0.01% solution) intranasally daily in one to three doses. Adjust morning and evening doses separately for adequate diurnal rhythm of water turnover. Alternatively, may administer injectable form in dosage of 0.5 to 1 ml I.V. or S.C. daily, usually in two divided doses.

Hemophilia A and von Willebrand's disease
Children and adults: 0.3 mcg/kg diluted in normal saline solution and infused I.V. slowly over 15 to 30 minutes. May repeat dosage, if necessary, as indicated by laboratory response and the patient's clinical condition.

Enuresis
†*Children:* 5 to 40 mcg of DDAVP administered intranasally at bedtime.

Evaluation of renal concentrating function
†*Infants to age 3 months:* 10 mcg intranasally.
Infants over age 3 months and children: 20 mcg intranasally.
Adults: 10 to 40 mcg intranasally. Collect urine 1 to 5 hours after administration of desmopressin to determine specific gravity.

Action and kinetics
• *Antidiuretic action:* Desmopressin is used to control or prevent signs and complications of neurogenic diabetes insipidus. The site of action is primarily at the renal tubular level. Desmopressin increases cyclic 3′,5′-adenosine monophosphate, which increases water permeability at the renal tubule and collecting duct, resulting in increased urine osmolality and decreased urinary flow rate.

• *Hemostatic action:* Desmopressin increases Factor VIII activity by releasing endogenous Factor VIII from plasma storage sites.

• *Kinetics in adults:* Desmopressin is destroyed in the GI tract. After intranasal administration, 10% to 20% of the dose is absorbed through nasal mucosa; antidiuretic action occurs within 1 hour and peaks in 1 to 5 hours. After I.V. infusion, plasma Factor VIII activity increases within 15 to 30 minutes and peaks between 1½ and 3 hours. Plasma levels decline in two phases: the half-life of the fast phase is about 8 minutes; the slow phase, 75½ minutes. Duration of action after intranasal administration is 8 to 20 hours; after I.V. administration, it is 12 to 24 hours for mild hemophilia and approximately 3 hours for von Willebrand's disease.

Contraindications and precautions
Desmopressin is contraindicated in patients with known hypersensitivity to the drug. It should be used cautiously in patients with allergic rhinitis, nasal congestion, or upper respiratory infection, because these states may interfere with the drug's absorption. Large doses of desmopressin may produce a slight rise in blood pressure when used in patients with coronary artery disease or hypertension.

Interactions
Concomitant use of desmopressin with carbamazepine, chlorpropamide, or clofibrate may potentiate desmopressin's antidiuretic action. Concomitant use with lithium, epinephrine, norepinephrine, demeclocycline, heparin, or alcohol may decrease the antidiuretic effect.

Effects on diagnostic tests
None reported.

Adverse reactions
• CNS: headache, seizures, confusion, drowsiness, coma.
• CV: slight rise in blood pressure at high doses, hypotension with rapid I.V. injection.
• EENT: nasal congestion, rhinitis.
• GI: nausea, abdominal cramps.
• GU: anuria, vulval pain, problems with urination.
• Local: pain, redness at injection site.
• Other: weight gain, flushing, anaphylaxis.
  Note: Drug should be discontinued if signs or symptoms of anaphylaxis, hypersensitivity, or water intoxication occur.

Overdose and treatment
Clinical manifestations of overdose include drowsiness, listlessness, headache, confusion, anuria, and weight gain (water intoxication). Treatment requires water restriction and temporary withdrawal of desmopressin until polyuria occurs. Severe water intoxication may require osmotic diuresis with mannitol, hypertonic dextrose, or urea—alone or with furosemide.

▶ Special considerations
• Use of desmopressin in infants under age 3 months is not recommended because of infants' increased tendency to develop hyponatremia and water intoxication.

• Desmopressin is usually administered intranasally through a flexible catheter called a rhinyle. A measured quantity is drawn up into the catheter, one end is inserted into the patient's nose, and the patient blows on the other end to deposit drug into nasal cavity.

• Patients may be switched from intranasal to subcutaneous desmopressin (for example, during episodes of rhinorrhea). They should receive one-tenth of their usual dosage parenterally.

• Observe for early signs and symptoms of water intoxication—drowsiness, listlessness, headache, confusion, anuria, and weight gain—to prevent seizures, coma, and death.

• Overdose may cause oxytocic or vasopressor activity. If patient develops uterine cramps, increased GI activity, fluid retention, or hypertension, withhold drug until effects subside. Furosemide may be used if fluid retention is excessive.

• Adjust patient's fluid intake to reduce risk of water intoxication and sodium depletion, especially in young patients.

• Patient should be weighed daily and observed for edema.

• Desmopressin is not indicated for hemophilia A patients with Factor VIII levels up to 5% or in patients with severe von Willebrand's disease.

• Desmopressin therapy may enable some patients to avoid the hazards of contaminated blood products.

Information for parents and patient

• Teach parents correct administration technique, then evaluate administration technique and accurate measurement on return visits. Emphasize that dosage should not be increased or decreased unless it is prescribed.

• Review with parents and patient fluid intake measurement and methods for measuring fluid output.

• Tell parents to call if signs or symptoms of water intoxication (drowsiness, listlessness, headache, confusion, weight gain, or shortness of breath) develop.

• Tell parents to store drug away from heat and direct light, not in bathroom, where heat and moisture can cause drug to deteriorate.

---

desonide
DesOwen, Tridesilon

• Classification: anti-inflammatory (topical adrenocorticoid)

How supplied
Available by prescription only
Cream, ointment: 0.05%

Indications, route, and dosage
Adjunctive therapy for inflammation in acute and chronic corticosteroid-responsive dermatoses
Children: Apply cream or lotion sparingly to affected area once a day.
Adults: Apply sparingly to affected area b.i.d. to q.i.d.

Action and kinetics
• *Anti-inflammatory action:* Desonide stimulates the synthesis of enzymes needed to decrease the inflammatory response. Desonide is a group IV nonfluorinated glucocorticoid with a potency similar to that of alclometasone dipropionate 0.05% and fluocinolone acetonide 0.01%.

• *Kinetics in adults:* Absorption depends on the amount applied and on the nature of the skin at the application site. It ranges from about 1% in areas with a thick stratum corneum (such as the palms, soles, elbows, and knees) to as much as 36% in the thinnest areas (face, eyelids, and genitals). Absorption increases in skin areas that are damaged, inflamed, or under occlusion. Some systemic absorption occurs, especially through the oral mucosa.

After topical application, desonide is distributed throughout the local skin layer. Any drug that is absorbed into circulation is removed rapidly from the blood and distributed into muscle, liver, skin, intestines, and kidneys.

After topical administration, desonide is metabolized primarily in the skin. The small amount that is absorbed is metabolized primarily in the liver to inactive compounds.

Inactive metabolites are excreted by the kidneys, primarily as glucuronides and sulfates, but also as unconjugated products. Small amounts of the metabolites are also excreted in feces.

Contraindications and precautions
Desonide is contraindicated in patients who are hypersensitive to any component of the preparation and in patients with viral, fungal, or tubercular skin lesions.

Desonide should be used with extreme caution in patients with impaired circulation, because the drug may increase the risk of skin ulceration.

Interactions
None significant.

Effects on diagnostic tests
None reported.

Adverse reactions
• Local: burning, itching, irritation, dryness, folliculitis, hypertrichosis, acneiform eruptions, hypopigmentation, perioral dermatitis, allergic contact dermatitis, maceration, secondary infection, atrophy, striae, miliaria.

Significant systemic absorption may produce the following effects.

• CNS: euphoria, insomnia, headache, psychotic behavior, pseudotumor cerebri, mental changes, nervousness, restlessness.

• CV: congestive heart failure, hypertension, edema.

• EENT: cataracts, glaucoma, thrush.

• GI: peptic ulcer, irritation, increased appetite.

• Immune: increased susceptibility to infection.

• Metabolic: hypokalemia, sodium retention, fluid retention, weight gain, hyperglycemia, osteoporosis, growth suppression in children.

• Musculoskeletal: muscle atrophy.

• Other: withdrawal syndrome (nausea, fatigue, anorexia, dyspnea, hypotension, hypoglycemia, myalgia, arthralgia, fever, dizziness, and fainting).

Note: Drug should be discontinued if local irritation, infection, systemic absorption, or hypersensitivity reaction occurs.

Overdose and treatment
No information available.

▶ Special considerations
• Children may have greater susceptibility to topical corticosteroid-induced HPA axis suppression and Cushing's syndrome than mature patients because of a higher ratio of skin surface area to body weight. Hypothalamic-pituitary-adrenal (HPA) axis suppression, Cushing's syndrome, and intracranial hypertension have been reported in children receiving topical corticosteroids. Signs of adrenal suppression in children include linear growth retardation, delayed weight gain, low plasma cortisol levels, and absence of response to ACTH stimulation. Signs of intracranial

---

★Canada only   †Unlabeled clinical use   Italicized adverse reactions have been observed in children.

hypertension includ bulging fontanelles, headaches, and bilateral papilledema.

• Administration of topical corticosteroids to children should be limited to the least effective amount. Chronic corticosteroid therapy may interfere with growth and development.

• Stop drug if the patient develops signs of systemic absorption (including Cushing's syndrome, hyperglycemia, or glucosuria), skin irritation or ulceration, hypersensitivity, or infection. (If antifungals or antibiotics are being used with corticosteroids and the infection does not respond immediately, corticosteroids should be stopped until infection is controlled.)

• Monitor patient response. Observe area of inflammation and elicit patient comments concerning pruritus. Inspect skin for infection, striae, and atrophy. Skin atrophy is common and may be clinically significant within 3 to 4 weeks of treatment with high-potency preparations; it also occurs more readily at sites where percutaneous absorption is high.

• Do not apply occlusive dressings over desonide because this may lead to secondary infection, maceration, atrophy, striae, or miliaria caused by increasing steroid penetration and potency.

Information for parents and patient
Instruct parents and patient in application of the drug. Tell them the following:

Method for applying topical preparations
• Wash your hands before and after applying the drug.
• Gently cleanse the area of application. Washing or soaking the area before application may increase drug penetration.
• Apply sparingly in a light film; rub in lightly. Avoid contact with patient's eyes, unless using an ophthalmic product.
• Avoid prolonged application in areas near the eyes, genitals, rectum, on the face, and in skin folds. High-potency topical corticosteroids are more likely to cause striae in these areas because of their higher rates of absorption.
• If an occlusive dressing is necessary, minimize adverse reactions by using it intermittently. Do not leave it in place longer than 16 hours each day.
• Warn patient not to use nonprescription topical preparations other than those specifically recommended.
• Advise parents not to use tight-fitting diapers or plastic pants on a child being treated in the diaper area, since such garments may serve as occlusive dressings.

---

desoximetasone
Topicort

• Classification: anti-inflammatory (topical adrenocorticoid)

How supplied
Available by prescription only
Cream: 0.05%, 0.25%
Gel: 0.05%
Ointment: 0.25%

Indications, route, and dosage
Inflammation of corticosteroid-responsive dermatoses
Children: Apply cream, gel, or ointment to affected areas once daily.
Adults: Apply cream sparingly in a very thin film and rub in gently to the affected area once daily to t.i.d.

Action and kinetics
• *Anti-inflammatory action:* Desoximetasone stimulates the synthesis of enzymes needed to decrease the inflammatory response. Desoximetasone is a synthetic fluorinated corticosteroid. The 0.05% gel and cream have a potency of group III; the 0.25% cream and ointment have a potency of group II.

• *Kinetics in adults:* The amount of desoximetasone absorbed depends on the strength of the preparation, the amount applied, and the nature of the skin at the application site. It ranges from about 1% in areas with a thick stratum corneum (such as the palms, soles, elbows, and knees) to as much as 36% in the thinnest areas (face, eyelids, and genitals). Absorption increases in skin areas that are damaged, inflammed, or under occlusion. Some systemic absorption of topical steroids, especially through the oral mucosa, may occur.

After topical application, desoximetasone is distributed throughout the local skin. Any drug that is absorbed is removed rapidly from the blood and distributed into muscle, liver, skin, intestines, and kidneys.

After topical administration, desoximetasone is metabolized primarily in the skin. The small amount that is absorbed is metabolized primarily in the liver to inactive compounds.

Inactive metabolites are excreted by the kidneys, primarily as glucuronides and sulfates, but also as unconjugated products. Small amounts of the metabolites are also excreted in feces.

Contraindications and precautions
Desoximetasone is contraindicated in patients who are hypersensitive to any component of the preparation and in patients with viral, fungal, or tubercular skin lesions.

Desoximetasone should be used with extreme caution in patients with impaired circulation, because the drug may increase the risk of skin ulceration.

Interactions
None significant.

Effects on diagnostic tests
None reported.

Adverse reactions
• Local: burning, itching, irritation, dryness, folliculitis, hypertrichosis, acneiform eruptions, hypopigmentation, perioral dermatitis, allergic contact dermatitis, maceration, secondary infection, atrophy, striae, miliaria.

Significant systemic absorption may produce the following reactions.
• CNS: euphoria, insomnia, headache, psychotic be-

---

‡May contain sulfites   ◆May contain tartrazine   ◆◆May contain benzyl alcohol

havior, pseudotumor cerebri, mental changes, nervousness, restlessness.
• CV: congestive heart failure, hypertension, edema.
• DERM: delayed healing, acne, skin eruptions, striae.
• EENT: cataracts, glaucoma, thrush.
• GI: peptic ulcer, GI irritation, increased appetite.
• Immune: immunosuppression, increased susceptibility to infection.
• Metabolic: hypokalemia, sodium retention, fluid retention, weight gain, hyperglycemia, osteoporosis, growth suppression in children.
• Musculoskeletal: muscle atrophy.
• Other: withdrawal syndrome (nausea, fatigue, anorexia, dyspnea, hypotension, hypoglycemia, myalgia, arthralgia, fever, dizziness, and fainting).
  Note: Drug should be discontinued if local irritation, infection, systemic absorption, or hypersensitivity reaction occurs.

Overdose and treatment
No information available.

▶ **Special considerations**
• Children may have greater susceptibility to topical corticosteroid-induced HPA axis suppression and Cushing's syndrome than mature patients because of higher ratio of skin surface area to body weight. Hypothalamic-pituitary-adrenal (HPA) axis suppression, Cushing's syndrome, and intracranial hypertension have been reported in children receiving topical corticosteroids. Signs of adrenal suppression in children include linear growth retardation, delayed weight gain, low plasma cortisol levels, and absence of response to ACTH stimulation. Signs of intracranial hypertension include bulging fontanelles, headaches, and bilateral papilledema.
• Administration of desoximetasone to children should be limited to the least effective amount. Chronic corticosteroid therapy may interfere with growth and development.
• Stop drug if the patient develops signs of systemic absorption (including Cushing's syndrome, hyperglycemia, or glucosuria), skin irriation or ulceration, hypersensitivity, or infection. (If antifungals or antibiotics are being used with desoximetasone and the infection does not respond immediately, drug should be discontinued until infection is controlled.)
• Monitor patient response. Observe area of inflammation and elicit patient comments concerning pruritus. Inspect skin for infection, striae, and atrophy. Skin atrophy is common and may be clinically significant within 3 to 4 weeks of treatment with high-potency preparations; it also occurs more readily at sites with percutaneous absoprtion is high.
• Do not apply occlusive dressings over desoximetasone because this may lead to secondary infection, maceration, atrophy, striae, or miliaria caused by increasing steroid penetration and potency.

Information for parents and patient
• Instruct parents and patient in application of the drug. Tell them the following:
Method for applying topical preparations
• Wash your hands before and after applying the drug. Gently cleanse the area of application. Washing or

soaking the are before application may increase drug penetration.
• Apply sparingly in a light film; rub in lightly. Avoid contact with patient's eyes.
• Avoid prolonged application on the face, in skin folds, and in areas near the eyes, genitals, and rectum. High-potency topical corticosteroids are more likely to cause striae in these areas because of their higher rates of absorption.
• If an occlusive dressing is necessary, minimize adverse reactions by using it intermittently. Do not leave it in place longer than 16 hours a day.
• Warn parents and patient not to use nonprescription topical preparations other than those specifically recommended.
• Advise parents not to use tight-fitting diapers or plastic pants on a child being treated in the diaper area, since such garments may serve as occlusive dressings.

dexamethasone
Systemic: Decadron, Deronil*, Dexasone*, Dexone, Hexadrol, SK-Dexamethasone

Topical: Aeroseb-Dex, Decaderm, Decaspray

Ophthalmic: Maxidex

dexamethasone acetate
Systemic: Dalalone D.P., Decadron L.A., Decaject L.A., Decameth L.A., Dexacen, Dexasone L.A., Dexon L.A., Solurex L.A.

dexamethasone sodium phosphate
Systemic: AK-Dex, Dalalone, Decadrol, Decadron, Decaject, Decameth, Dexacen, Dexasone, Dexon, Dexone, Hexadrol Phosphate, Oradexon*, Solurex

Topical: Decadron Cream

Ophthalmic: AK-Dex, Decadron, Dexair, Maxidex, 1-Methasone, Ocu-Dex

Nasal inhalant: Decadron Phosphate Turbinaire

Oral inhalant: Decadron Phosphate Respihaler

• Classification: anti-inflammatory, immunosuppressant (glucocorticoid)

How supplied
Available by prescription only

Dexamethasone
Tablets: 0.25 mg, 0.5 mg, 0.75 mg, 1 mg, 1.5 mg, 2 mg, 4 mg, 6 mg
Elixir: 0.5 mg/5 ml
Oral solution: 0.5 mg/5 ml, 0.5 mg/0.5 ml
Topical aerosol: 0.01%, 0.04%
Gel: 0.1%
Ophthalmic suspension: 0.01%
Dexamethasone acetate
Injection: 8 mg/ml, 16 mg/ml suspension
Dexamethasone sodium phosphate
Injection: 4 mg/ml, 10 mg/ml, 20 mg/ml, 24 mg/ml
Topical cream: 0.1%
Ophthalmic ointment: 0.5%
Solution: 0.1%
Nasal aerosol: 84 mcg metered spray, 170 doses per canister
Oral inhalation aerosol: 84 mcg metered spray, 170 doses per canister

Indications, route, and dosage
Cerebral edema
Dexamethasone sodium phosphate
Children: 0.5 to 1.5 mg/kg I.V. or I.M., then 0.2 to 0.5 mg/kg daily I.V. or I.M. for 5 days; then gradually taper. Alternatively, give 0.2 mg/kg P.O. daily in divided doses.
Adults: Initially, 10 mg I.V., then 4 to 6 mg I.M. q 6 hours for 2 to 4 days, then taper over 5 to 7 days.
Inflammatory conditions, allergic reactions, neoplasias
Children: 0.0833 to 0.333 mg/kg daily in three divided doses.
Adults: 0.5 to 9 mg P.O. b.i.d., t.i.d., or q.i.d.
Dexamethasone sodium phosphate
Children: 0.02776 to 0.16665 mg/kg I.M.
Adults: 0.2 to 6 mg intra-articularly, intralesional, or into soft tissue; or 0.5 to 9 mg I.M.
Adrenal insufficiency
Dexamethasone sodium phosphate
Children: 0.0233 mg/kg I.M. in three divided doses; or 0.00776 to 0.01165 mg/kg I.M. daily.
Inflammation of corticosteroid-responsive dermatoses
Dexamethasone
Children: Apply gel or topical aerosol once or twice daily. Apply cream once a day.
Adults: Apply gel or aerosol sparingly t.i.d. to q.i.d.
For aerosol use on scalp, shake can well and apply to dry scalp after shampooing. Hold can upright. Slide applicator tube under hair so that it touches scalp. Spray while moving tube to all affected areas, keeping tube under hair and in contact with scalp throughout spraying, which should take about 2 seconds. Inadequately covered areas may be spot sprayed. Slide applicator tube through hair to touch scalp, press and immediately release spray button. Do not massage medication into scalp or spray forehead or eyes.

Uveitis; iridocyclitis; inflammation of eyelids, conjunctiva, cornea, anterior segment of globe; corneal injury from burns or penetration by foreign bodies
Dexamethasone; Dexamethasone sodium phosphate
Children and adults: Instill 1 to 2 drops into conjunctival sac. For initial therapy of severe cases, instill the solution or suspension into the conjunctival sac every hour during the day and every 2 hours during the night. Instill the ointment into the conjunctival sac three or four times daily initially and once or twice daily thereafter. The ointment may also be used at night with daytime use of the suspension or solution. The duration of treatment depends on the type and severity of the disease.
Control of bronchial asthma in patients with steroid-dependent asthma
Oral inhaler
Children: 2 inhalations t.i.d. or q.i.d., to a maximum dosage of 8 inhalations daily.
Adults: 3 inhalations t.i.d. or q.i.d., to a maximum dosage of 12 inhalations daily.
Relief of symptoms of perennial or seasonal rhinitis; prevention of recurrence of nasal polyps after surgical removal
Nasal inhaler
Children age 6 to 12: 1 or 2 sprays (84 to 168 mcg) into each nostril b.i.d. Maximum dosage is 8 sprays daily (672 mcg).
Adults: 2 sprays (168 mcg) into each nostril b.i.d. or t.i.d. Maximum dosage of 12 sprays daily (1,008 mcg).

Action and kinetics
• *Anti-inflammatory action:* Dexamethasone stimulates the synthesis of enzymes needed to decrease the inflammatory response. It causes suppression of the immune system by reducing activity and volume of the lymphatic system, producing lymphocytopenia (primarily T-lymphocytes), decreasing passage of immune complexes through basement membranes, and possibly by depressing reactivity of tissue to antigen-antibody interactions.

Dexamethasone is a long-acting synthetic adrenocorticoid with strong anti-inflammatory activity and minimal mineralocorticoid properties. It is 25 to 30 times more potent than an equal weight of hydrocortisone.

The acetate salt is a suspension and should not be used I.V. It is particularly useful as an anti-inflammatory agent in intra-articular, intradermal, and intralesional injections.

The sodium phosphate salt is highly soluble and has a more rapid onset and a shorter duration of action than does the acetate salt. It is most commonly used for cerebral edema and unresponsive shock. It can also be used in intra-articular, intralesional, or soft tissue inflammation.

• *Antiasthmatic action:* Dexamethasone is used as a nasal inhalant for the symptomatic treatment of seasonal or perennial rhinitis and nasal polyposis. It is used as an oral inhalant to treat bronchial asthma in patients who require corticosteroids to control symptoms.

• *Kinetics in adults:* After oral administration, dexamethasone is absorbed readily, and peak effects occur in about 1 to 2 hours. The suspension for injection has a variable onset and duration of action (ranging from 2 days to 3 weeks), depending on whether it is injected into an intra-articular space, a muscle, or the blood supply to the muscle.

Absorption after topical application depends on the potency of the preparation, the amount applied, and site of application. Topical absorption ranges from about 1% in areas with a thick stratum corneum (such as the palms, soles, elbows, and knees) to as high as 36% in the thinnest areas (face, eyelids, and genitals). Absorption increases in skin areas that are damaged, inflamed, or under occlusion. Some systemic absorption occurs, especially through the oral mucosa.

After topical application, dexamethasone is distributed throughout the local skin layer and metabolized primarily in the skin. After ophthalmic administration, dexamethasone is absorbed through the aqueous humor and is distributed throughout the local tissue layers. Because only low doses are administered, little if any systemic absorption occurs. Approximately 30% to 50% of an orally inhaled dose is systemically absorbed. Onset of action usually occurs within a few days but may take as long as 7 days in some patients. Distribution following intranasal aerosol administration has not been described. After oral aerosol administration, most of the drug is distributed into the mouth and throat. The remainder is distributed through the trachea and bronchial tissue.

Dexamethasone is removed rapidly from the blood and distributed to muscle, liver, skin, intestines, and kidneys. It is bound weakly to plasma proteins (transcortin and albumin). Only the unbound portion is active. Adrenocorticoids are distributed into breast milk and through the placenta.

Dexamethasone is metabolized primarily in the liver to inactive glucuronide and sulfate metabolites. Some drug may be metabolized locally in the lung tissue. The inactive metabolites and small amounts of unmetabolized drug are excreted by the kidneys. Insignificant quantities of drug are excreted in feces. The biological half-life of dexamethasone is 36 to 54 hours.

Contraindications and precautions

Dexamethasone is contraindicated in patients who are hypersensitive to ingredients of adrenocorticoid preparations and in those with systemic fungal infections (except in adrenal insufficiency). Patients who are receiving dexamethasone should not be given live-virus vaccines because dexamethasone suppresses the immune response.

Dexamethasone should be used with extreme caution in patients with GI ulceration, renal disease, hypertension, osteoporosis, diabetes mellitus, thromboembolytic disorders, seizures, myasthenia gravis, CHF, tuberculosis, hypoalbuminemia, hypothyroidism, cirrhosis of the liver, emotional instability, psychotic tendencies, hyperlipidemias, glaucoma, or cataracts, because the drug may exacerbate these conditions.

Because adrenocorticoids increase susceptibility to and mask symptoms of infection, dexamethasone should not be used (except in life-threatening situa-tions) in patients with viral or bacterial infections not controlled by anti-infective agents.

The ophthalmic form is contraindicated in patients with fungal infections of the eye and in patients with acute, untreated purulent bacterial, viral, or fungal ocular infections. It should be used cautiously in patients with corneal abrasions. If a bacterial infection does not respond promptly to appropriate anti-infective therapy, dexamethasone should be discontinued and other therapy applied. The topical forms should be used with extreme caution in patients with impaired circulation, because the drug may increase the risk of skin ulceration.

Intraocular pressure should be measured every 2 to 4 weeks for the first 2 months of ophthalmic corticosteroid therapy and then, if no increase in intraocular pressure has occurred, every 1 to 2 months thereafter. Dexamethasone is more likely than other ophthalmic products to increase intraocular pressure in susceptible patients.

Prolonged use of dexamethasone may produce posterior subcapsular cataracts or glaucoma with possible damage to the optic nerves, and may enhance the establishment of secondary ocular infections from fungi or viruses.

Dexamethasone inhalant is contraindicated in patients with acute status asthmaticus, hypersensitivity to any component of the preparation, or nasal infections. It should be used with caution in patients receiving systemic corticosteroids, because of increased risk of hypothalamic-pituitary-adrenal axis suppression; when switching inhalant for oral systemic administration, because withdrawal symptoms may occur; and in patients with healing nasal septal ulcers, oral or nasal surgery, or trauma.

Interactions

When used concomitantly, dexamethasone may in rare cases decrease the effects of oral anticoagulants by unknown mechanisms.

Dexamethasone increases the metabolism of isoniazid and salicylates; causes hyperglycemia, requiring dosage adjustment of insulin in diabetic patients; and may enhance hypokalemia associated with diuretic or amphotericin B therapy. The hypokalemia may increase the risk of toxicity in patients concurrently receiving digitalis glycosides.

Concomitant use of barbiturates, phenytoin, and rifampin may cause decreased corticosteroid effects because of increased hepatic metabolism. Cholestyramine, colestipol, and antacids decrease the corticosteroid effect by adsorbing the corticosteroid, decreasing the amount absorbed.

Concomitant use with estrogens may reduce the metabolism of dexamethasone by increasing the concentration of transcortin. The half-life of the corticosteroid is then prolonged because of increased protein-binding. Concomitant administration of ulcerogenic drugs, such as the nonsteroidal anti-inflammatory agents, may increase the risk of GI ulceration.

Effects on diagnostic tests

Dexamethasone suppresses reactions to skin tests; causes false-negative results in the nitroblue tetrazolium test for systemic bacterial infections; and decreases ^{131}I uptake and protein-bound iodine concentrations in thyroid function tests.

Dexamethasone may increase glucose and cholesterol levels; may decrease levels of serum potassium, calcium, thyroxine, and triiodothyronine; and may increase urine glucose and calcium levels.

Adverse reactions

When administered in high doses or for prolonged periods, dexamethasone suppresses the release of adrenocorticotropic hormone (ACTH) from the pituitary gland, stopping secretion of endogenous corticosteroids from the adrenal cortex. The degree and duration of hypothalamic-pituitary-adrenal (HPA) axis suppression produced by glucocorticoids is highly variable among patients and depends on the dose, frequency, and time of administration, and duration of glucocorticoid therapy.

• CNS: euphoria, insomnia, headache, psychotic behavior, pseudotumor cerebri, mental changes, nervousness, restlessness, *psychoses*.
• CV: CHF, *hypertension*, edema.
• DERM: delayed healing, *acne*, skin eruptions, striae.
• ENT: (after oral inhalation) flushing, rash, dry mouth, hoarseness, irritation of the tongue or throat, and impaired sense of taste; (after nasal inhalation) itchy nose, dryness, burning, irritation and sneezing, infrequent epistaxis, bloody mucus; fungal overgrowth and infections of the nose, mouth, or throat; headache, nausea, GI upset.
• Eye: transient burning or stinging on administration; mydriasis, ptosis, epithelial punctate keratitis, and possible corneal or scleral malacia; increased intraocular pressure, thinning of the cornea, interference with corneal wound healing, increased susceptibility to viral or fungal corneal infection, and corneal ulceration; glaucoma, cataracts, defects in visual acuity and visual field long-term use.
• GI: *peptic ulcer*, irritation, increased appetite.
• Immune: immunosuppression, *increased susceptibility to infection*.
• Metabolic: *hypokalemia, sodium retention, fluid retention*, weight gain, hyperglycemia, osteoporosis, growth suppression in children, *glycosuria*.
• Musculoskeletal: muscle atrophy, weakness, *myopathy*.
• Local: atrophy at I.M. injection sites, burning, itching, dryness, folliculitis, hypertrichosis, acneiform eruptions, hypopigmentation, perioral dermatitis, and allergic contact dermatitis. Use of occlusive dressings may result in maceration, secondary infection, skin atrophy, striae, and miliaria.
• Other: pancreatitis, *hirsutism, cushingoid symptoms*, withdrawal syndrome (nausea, fatigue, anorexia, dyspnea, hypotension, hypoglycemia, myalgia, arthralgia, fever, dizziness, and fainting). Sudden discontinuation may be fatal or may exacerbate the underlying disease. Acute adrenal insufficiency may follow increased stress (infection, surgery, trauma) or abrupt withdrawal after long-term therapy.

Note: Drug should be discontinued if topical application results in local irritation, infection, significant systemic absorption, or hypersensitivity reaction; if visual acuity decreases or visual field is diminished; if burning, stinging, or watering of eyes does not quickly resolve after administration; or after inhalant use if no improvement is evident after 7 to 10 days, or if nasal or oral infections develop.

Overdose and treatment

Acute ingestion, even in massive doses, rarely poses a clinical problem. Toxic signs and symptoms rarely occur if drug is used for less than 3 weeks, even at large dosage ranges. However, chronic use causes adverse physiologic effects, including suppression of the HPA axis, cushingoid appearance, muscle weakness, and osteoporosis.

▶ Special considerations

• This drug is being used investigationally to prevent hyaline membrane disease (respiratory distress syndrome) in premature infants. The suspension (acetate salt) is administered I.M. to the mother two or three times daily for 2 days before delivery.
• If possible, avoid long-term administration of pharmacologic dosages of dexamethasone in children because these drugs may retard bone growth. Manifestations of adrenal suppression in children include retardation of linear growth, delayed weight gain, low plasma cortisol concentrations, and lack of response to corticotropin stimulation. In children who require prolonged therapy, closely monitor growth and development. Alternate-day therapy is recommended to minimize growth suppression.
• Establish baseline blood pressure, fluid intake and output, weight, and electrolyte status. Watch for any sudden patient weight gain, edema, change in blood pressure, or change in electrolyte status.
• During times of physiologic stress (trauma, surgery, infection), the patient may require additional steroids and may experience signs of steroid withdrawal, patients who were previously steroid-dependent may need systemic corticosteroids to prevent adrenal insufficiency.
• After long-term therapy, the drug should be reduced gradually. Rapid reduction may cause withdrawal symptoms.
• Be aware of the patient's psychological history and watch for any behavioral changes.
• Observe for signs of infection or delayed wound healing.
• Acute withdrawal of drug may result in fever, myalgia, arthralgia, malaise, hypotension, hypoglycemic shock.

Topical administration

• *Children may have greater susceptibility to topical corticosteroid-induced HPA axis suppression and Cushing's syndrome than mature patients because of a higher ratio of skin surface area to body weight.* Hypothalamic-pituitary-adrenal (HPA) axis suppression, Cushing's syndrome, and intracranial hypertension have been reported in children receiving topical corticosteroids. Signs of intracranial hypertension include bulging fontanelles, headaches, and bilateral papilledema.
• Administration of topical dexamethasone to children should be limited to the least effective amount. Chronic corticosteroid therapy may interfere with growth and development.
• Stop topical use if the patient develops signs of

---

systemic absorption (including Cushing's syndrome, hyperglycemia, or glucosuria), skin irritation or ulceration, hypersensitivity, or infection. (If antifungals or antibiotics are being used with corticosteroids and the infection does not respond immediately, discontinue drug until infection is controlled.)

• Monitor patient response. Observe area of inflammation and elicit patient comments concerning pruritus. Inspect skin for infection, striae, and atrophy. Skin atrophy is common and may be clinically significant within 3 to 4 weeks of treatment with high-potency preparations; it also occurs more readily at sites where percutaneous absorption is high.

• Do not apply occlusive dressing over topical drug because this may lead to secondary infection, maceration, atrophy, striae, or miliaria caused by increasing steroid penetration and potency.

• Ophthalmic products may initially cause sensitivity to bright light. This may be minimized by wearing sunglasses. Monitor the patient's response by observing the area of inflammation and eliciting patient comments concerning pruritus and vision. Inspect the eye and surrounding tissues for infection and additional irritation.

• The therapeutic effects of intranasal inhalants, unlike those of sympathomimetic decongestants, are not immediate. Full therapeutic benefit requires regular use and is usually evident within a few days, although a few patients may require up to 3 weeks of therapy for maximum benefit. Use of nasal or oral inhalation therapy may occasionally allow a patient to discontinue systemic corticosteroid therapy. Systemic corticosteroid therapy should then be discontinued by gradually tapering the dosage while carefully observing the patient for signs of adrenal insufficiency (joint pain, lassitude, depression).

Information for parents and patient

• Chronic use of dexamethasone in children and adolescents may delay growth and maturation.

• Be sure that parents and patient understand the need to take the drug as prescribed. Give the parents and patient instructions on what to do if a dose is inadvertently missed.

• Recommend restriction of sodium intake.

• Warn the parents and patient not to discontinue the drug abruptly.

• Inform the parents and patient of the possible therapeutic and adverse effects of the drug, so that they may report any complications as soon as possible.

• Advise the parents that the patient should carry a Medic Alert bracelet or necklace indicating the need for supplemental adrenocorticoids during times of stress.

• Instruct parents and patient in application of the drug. Tell them the following:

Method for applying topical preparations
• Wash hands before and after applying the drug.

• Gently cleanse the area of application. Washing or soaking in the area before application may increase drug penetration.

• Apply sparingly in a light film; rub in lightly. Avoid contact with patient's eyes, unless using an ophthalmic product.

• Avoid prolonged application in areas near the eyes,

genitals, rectum, on the face, and in skin folds. High-potency topical corticosteroids are more likely to cause striae in these areas because of their higher rates of absorption.

• If an occlusive dressing is necessary, apply cream. Minimize adverse reactions by using it intermittently. Do not leave it in place longer than 16 hours each day.

• Warn patient not to use nonprescription topical preparations other than those specifically recommended.

• Advise parents not to use tight-fitting diapers or plastic pants on a child being treated in the diaper area, since such garments may serve as occlusive dressings.

Method for administering eye drops
Advise the parents and patient to use the following steps when administering eye drops:

• Wash hands well.

• Shake solution or suspension well.

• Tilt head back or lie down.

• Lightly pull lower eyelid down by applying gentle pressure at the lid base at the bony rim of the orbit.

• Approach the eye from below with the dropper; do not touch dropper to any tissue.

• Holding dropper no more than 1″ above the eye, drop medication inside lower lid while looking up.

• Try to keep eye open for 30 seconds.

• Apply light finger pressure inward and down to the side of the bridge of the nose (the lacrimal canaliculi) for 1 to 2 minutes after instillation to prevent drainage of solution into nasal passages, where more of the drug is absorbed systemically.

• If using more than one ophthalmic kind of drug at the same time, wait at least 5 minutes before applying the other drops.

Method for administering ophthalmic ointments
Advise the parents and patient to use the following steps when administering ophthalmic ointments:

• Wash hands well. Hold the tube in your hand several minutes before use to warm it and improve flow of ointments.

• When opening the ointment tube for the first time, squeeze out the first ¼″ of ointment and discard (using sterile gauze) because it may be too dry.

• Apply a small "ribbon" or strip of ointment (¼″ to ½″) to the inside of the lower eyelid. Do not touch any part of the eye with the tip of the tube. Close the eye gently and roll the eyeball in all directions to spread the ointment.

• If using a second eye ointment, wait at least 10 minutes before applying it.

For patients taking any form of eye medication
• Instruct parents to observe for adverse effects. The parents should call if no improvement occurs after 7 to 8 days, if the condition worsens, or if pain, itching, or swelling of the eye occurs.

• Warn parents not to administer nonprescription ophthalmic preparations other than those specifically recommended. Nonprescription ophthalmic solutions should not be used for more than 7 days or in children under age 2.

• Warn the parents not to use leftover medication for a new eye inflammation and never to share eye medication with others. Tell them to store all eye medications in original container.

---

*Canada only   †Unlabeled clinical use   Italicized adverse reactions have been observed in children.

• Parents should call for specific instructions before discontinuing therapy.

For patients using a nasal inhaler

• Instruct patient to use only as directed. Inform him that full therapeutic effect is not immediate but requires regular use of inhaler.

• Encourage a patient with blocked nasal passages to use an oral decongestant ½ hour before intranasal corticosteroid administration to ensure adequate penetration. Advise patient to clear nasal passageway of secretions before using the inhaler.

• Ask parents and patient to read manufacturer's instruction and have patient demonstrate use of inhaler. Assist patient until proper use of inhaler is demonstrated.

• Instruct patient to clean inhaler according to manufacturer's instructions.

For patients using an oral inhaler

• Instruct patient to use only as directed.

• Advise patient receiving bronchodilators by inhalation to use the bronchodilator before the corticosteroid inhalant to enhance penetration of the corticosteroid into the bronchial tree. Patient should wait several minutes to allow time for the bronchodilator to relax the smooth muscle.

• Ask patient to read manufacturer's instructions and demonstrate use of inhaler. Assist patient until proper use of inhaler is demonstrated.

• Instruct patient to hold breath for a few seconds to enhance placement and action of the drug and to wait 1 minute before taking subsequent puffs of medication.

• Tell patient to rinse mouth with water after using the inhaler to decrease the chance of oral fungal infections. Tell him to check nasal and oral mucous membranes frequently for signs of fungal infection.

• Instruct patient to clean inhaler according to manufacturer's instructions.

• Warn asthma patients not to increase use of corticosteroid inhaler during a severe asthma attack but to call physician for adjustment of therapy, possibly by adding a systemic steroid.

For patients using either type of inhaler

• Tell patient to report decreased response; an adjustment in dosage or discontinuation of the drug may be necessary.

---

dexchlorpheniramine maleate
Polaramine, Polaramine Repetabs

• Classification: antihistamine H_1-receptor antagonist, antipruritic (alkylamine derivative)

How supplied
Available by prescription only
Tablets: 2 mg
Tablets (repeat-action): 4 mg, 6 mg
Syrup: 2 mg/5 ml

Indications, route, and dosage
Rhinitis, allergy symptoms, contact dermatitis, pruritus, allergic conjunctivitis, adjunct to epinephrine for anaphylaxis after control of acute manifestations
Children under age 12: 0.15 mg/kg or 4.5 mg/m² daily in four divided doses. Alternatively, adjust dosage according to age:
Children age 2 to 5: 0.5 mg every 4 to 6 hours; do not use repeat-action form.
Children age 6 to 11: 1 mg every 4 to 6 hours or 4 mg repeat-action tablet at bedtime.
Children age 12 and over and adults: 1 to 2 mg P.O. (tablets or syrup) t.i.d. or q.i.d.; or 4 to 6 mg (timed-release) b.i.d. or t.i.d.

Action and kinetics
• *Antihistamine action:* Antihistamines compete with histamine for histamine H_1-receptor sites on smooth muscle of the bronchi, GI tract, uterus, and large blood vessels; they bind to cellular receptors, preventing access of histamine, thereby suppressing histamine-induced allergic symptoms. They do not directly alter histamine or its release.

• *Kinetics in adults:* Dexchlorpheniramine is well absorbed from the GI tract. Action begins within 30 to 60 minutes. Dexchlorpheniramine is distributed extensively throughout the body and is 70% protein-bound. Plasma half-life ranges from 20 to 24 hours. Drug is metabolized by the liver. Drug and metabolites are excreted in urine.

Contraindications and precautions
Dexchlorpheniramine is contraindicated in children with known hypersensitivity to this drug or other antihistamines with similar chemical structures (brompheniramine, chlorpheniramine, and triprolidine); during an acute asthmatic attack, because dexchlorpheniramine thickens bronchial secretions; and in patients who have taken MAO inhibitors within the preceding 2 weeks, because these drugs prolong and intensify the effects of antihistamines.

Dexchlorpheniramine should be used with caution in patients with narrow-angle glaucoma; in those with pyloroduodenal obstruction or urinary bladder obstruction from narrowing of the bladder neck, because of their marked anticholinergic effects; in patients with cardiovascular disease, hypertension, or hyperthyroidism, because of the risk of palpitations and tachycardia; and in patients with renal disease, diabetes, bronchial asthma, urinary retention, or stenosing peptic ulcers. Repeat-action tablets are not recommended for use in children under age 6. Infants and children under age 6 may experience paradoxical hyperexcitability.

Interactions
MAO inhibitors interfere with detoxification of antihistamines and thus prolong and intensify their central depressant and anticholinergic effects; additive CNS depression may occur when dexchlorpheniramine is given concomitantly with other CNS depressants, such as alcohol, barbiturates, tranquilizers, sleeping aids, and antianxiety agents.

Dexchlorpheniramine may diminish the effects of

---

sulfonylureas, enhance the effects of epinephrine, and may partially counteract the anticoagulant effects of heparin.

Effects on diagnostic tests

Dexchlorpheniramine should be discontinued 4 days before diagnostic skin tests; antihistamines can prevent, reduce, or mask positive skin test response.

Adverse reactions

- CNS: drowsiness, dizziness, stimulation, weakness.
- CV: palpitations, tachycardia, hypotension.
- DERM: eruptions, urticaria, photosensitivity.
- EENT: blurred vision, tinnitus.
- GI: dry mouth, nausea, vomiting, diarrhea, constipation, anorexia.
- GU: polyuria, dysuria, urinary retention.

Overdose and treatment

Clinical manifestations of overdose may include either CNS depression (sedation, reduced mental alertness, apnea, and cardiovascular collapse) or CNS stimulation (insomnia, hallucinations, tremors, or convulsions). Anticholinergic symptoms, such as dry mouth, flushed skin, fixed and dilated pupils, and GI symptoms, are common, especially in children.

Treat overdose by inducing emesis with ipecac syrup (in conscious patient), followed by activated charcoal to reduce further drug absorption. Use gastric lavage if patient is unconscious or ipecac fails. Treat hypotension with vasopressors, and control seizures with diazepam or phenytoin. *Do not give stimulants.*

▶ Special considerations

- Drug is not indicated for use in neonates or premature infants.
- Children, especially those under age 6, may experience paradoxical hyperexcitably with restlessness, insomnia, nervousness, euphoria, tremors, and seizures.
- Drug is contraindicated during an acute asthma attack, because it may not alleviate the symptoms and because antimuscarinic effects can cause thickening of secretions.
- Monitor blood counts during long-term therapy; watch for signs of blood dyscrasias.
- Reduce GI distress by giving drug with food; give sugarless gum, sour hard candy, or ice chips to relieve dry mouth; increase fluid intake (if allowed) or humidify air to decrease adverse effects of thickened secretions.
- Repeat-action dexchlorpheniramine tablets must be swallowed whole. Do not crush or permit patient to chew tablet. Regular tablets may be crushed or mixed with food.

Information for parents and patients

- Advise patient to take drug with meals or snack to prevent gastric upset and to use any of the following measures to relieve dry mouth: warm water rinses, artificial saliva, ice chips, or sugarless gum or candy. Patient should avoid overusing mouthwash, which may add to dryness (alcohol content) and destroy normal flora.
- Warn parents that child should avoid hazardous ac-

tivities that require balance or alertness until extent of CNS effects are known. Tell them to seek medical approval before administering tranquilizers, sedatives, pain relievers, or sleeping medications.
- Warn parents to discontinue drug 4 days before diagnostic skin tests, to preserve accuracy of tests.

---

dexpanthenol
Ilopan, Intrapan, Panthoderm (topical), Tonestat

- Classification: GI stimulant, emollient (vitamin B complex analog)

How supplied

Available by prescription only
Injection: 250 mg/ml in vials, ampules, and prefilled syringes
Topical cream: 2% cream

Indications, route, and dosage

Emollient and protectant: colostomy area or other surgical sites
Children and adults: Apply p.r.n.
Itching, wounds, insect bites, poison ivy, poison oak, diaper rash, chafing, mild eczema, decubitus ulcers, dry lesions
Children and adults: Apply topically p.r.n.
Prevention of postoperative adynamic ileus
Adults: 250 to 500 mg I.M.; repeat in 2 hours. Then give q 6 hours, as needed.
Treatment of adynamic ileus
Adults: 500 mg I.M., repeat in 2 hours. Then give q 6 hours, as needed.

Action and kinetics

- *Emollient action:* By stimulating granulation and epithelialization, dexpanthenol promotes healing and relieves itching.
- *GI stimulant action:* Dexpanthenol stimulates the acetylation of choline to acetylcholine, which increases peristalsis. The exact mechanism of this action is unknown.
- *Kinetics in adults:* Dexpanthenol is absorbed from I.M. sites. After conversion to pantothenic acid, drug is distributed widely, mainly as coenzyme A. Some concentration occurs in the liver, adrenal glands, heart, and kidneys. Conversion to pantothenic acid occurs readily. Most metabolites are excreted in urine; remainder in feces.

Contraindications and precautions

Dexpanthenol is contraindicated in patients with ileus due to obstruction, because of potential for severe cramping and worsening of condition; and on wounds in patients with hemophilia, because of potential for severe bleeding.

Interactions

When used concomitantly, antibiotics, barbiturates, and narcotics have stimulated an allergic response to dexpanthenol. Succinylcholine's actions are prolonged in the presence of dexpanthenol; therefore, give these drugs at least 1 hour apart.

Effects on diagnostic tests
None reported.

Adverse reactions
• CV: slight decreases in blood pressure.
• DERM: itching, red patches, dermatitis, tingling.
• GI: intestinal colic, vomiting, diarrhea.
  Note: Drug should be discontinued if hypersensitivity reactions occur.

Overdose and treatment
No information available.

▶ Special considerations
• Safety of parenteral form has not been established for pediatric use.
• For I.V. administration, dilute in glucose or lactate Ringer's solutions and infuse slowly.
• Be sure to monitor fluid and electrolytes (especially potassium) in patients with adynamic ileus. Anemia, hypoproteinemia, and infection may contribute to the condition.
• Avoid concomitant use with drugs that decrease GI motility.

Information for parents and patient
Advise parents and patient of potential adverse reactions.

---

dextran, low molecular weight
Dextran 40, Gentran 40, 10% LMD
Rheomacrodex

dextran, high molecular weight
Dextran 70, Dextran 75, Gentran 75, Macrodex

• Classification: plasma volume expander (glucose polymer)

How supplied
Available by prescription only
Injection: 10% Dextran 40 in dextrose 5% in water (D_5W) or 0.9% sodium chloride; 6% Dextran 70 in 0.9% sodium chloride or D_5W; 6% Dextran 75 in 0.9% sodium chloride or D_5W

Indications, route, and dosage
Plasma volume expansion
Dosage depends on amount of fluid loss.
Children: The total dosage of Dextran 70 or 75 should not exceed 1.2 g/kg (20 ml/kg), with the dose based on the body weight or surface area. If therapy is continued, dosage should not exceed 0.6 g/kg (10 ml/kg) daily.
Adults: Initially, 500 ml of Dextran 40 with central venous pressure monitoring. Infuse remaining dose slowly. Total daily dose should not exceed 2 g/kg body weight. If therapy continues past 24 hours, do not

exceed 1 g/kg daily. Continue for no longer than 5 days.
  The usual dose of Dextran 70 or 75 solution is 30 g (500 ml of 6% solution) I.V. In emergency situations, may be administered at a rate of 1.2 to 2.4 g (20 to 40 ml)/minute. Total dose during the first 24 hours is not to exceed 1.2 g/kg; actual dose depends on the amount of fluid loss and resultant hemoconcentration and must be determined individually. In normovolemic patients, the rate of administration should not exceed 240 mg (4 ml/minute).
Priming pump oxygenators
Children and adults: Dextran 40 can be used as the only priming fluid or as an additive to other primers in pump oxygenators. Dextran 40 is added to the perfusion circuit as the 10% solution in a dose of 1 to 2 g/kg (10 to 20 ml/kg); total dose should not exceed 2 g/kg (20 ml/kg).
Prophylaxis of venous thrombosis and pulmonary embolism
Adults: Dextran 40 therapy should usually be given during the surgical procedure. On the day of surgery, Dextran 40 (10% solution) is given at the dose of 50 to 100 g (500 to 1,000 ml or approximately 10 ml/kg). Treatment is continued for 2 to 3 days at a dose of 50 g (500 ml) daily. Then, if needed, 50 g (500 ml) may be given q 2 or 3 days for up to 2 weeks to reduce the risk of thromboembolism (deep venous thrombosis [DVT]) or pulmonary embolism.
Reduction of blood sludging
Adults: 500 ml of 10% solution by I.V. infusion.

Action and kinetics
• *Plasma expanding action:* Dextran 40 (10%) has an average molecular weight of 40,000, the osmotic equivalent of twice the volume of plasma. Dextran 40 has a duration of action of 2 to 4 hours. Dextran 70 has an average molecular weight of 70,000; the I.V. infusion results in an expansion of the plasma volume slightly in excess of the volume infused. This effect, useful in treating shock, lasts for approximately 12 hours.
  Dextran 40, 70, and 75 enhance the blood flow, particularly in the microcirculation. Dextran 40 can be used to prime oxygenator pumps, as the only fluid or in combination with other fluids.
• *Prophylaxis of venous thrombosis and pulmonary embolism:* Dextran 40 inhibits vascular stasis and platelet adhesiveness and alters the structure and lysability of fibrin clots. Dextran 40 increases cardiac output, arterial, venous, and microcirculatory flow, and reduces mean transit time, mainly by expanding plasma volume and by reducing blood viscosity through hemodilution and reducing red cell aggregation.
• *Kinetics in adults:* Dextran 40 and 70 are given by I.V. infusion. The plasma concentration depends on the rate of infusion and the rate of disappearance of the drug from the plasma. Dextran 40 is distributed throughout the vascular system.
  Dextran molecules with molecular weights above 50,000 are enzymatically degraded by dextranase to glucose at a rate of about 70 to 90 mg/kg/day. This is a variable process. Dextran molecules with molecular weights below 50,000 are eliminated by renal excretion, with 40% of Dextran 70 appearing in the

---

urine within 24 hours. Approximately 50% of Dextran 40 is excreted in the urine within 3 hours, 60% within 6 hours, and 75% within 24 hours. The remaining 25% is hydrolyzed partially and excreted in urine, excreted partially in feces, and partially oxidized.

Contraindications and precautions
Dextran 40 and 70 are contraindicated in patients with a known hypersensitivity to dextran; in patients with marked hemostatic defects of all types (such as thrombocytopenia and hypofibrinogenemia), including those caused by drugs (such as heparin and warfarin); in patients with marked cardiac decompensation; and in patients with renal disease with severe oliguria or anuria.

Interactions
None reported.

Effects on diagnostic tests
Falsely elevated blood glucose levels may occur in patients receiving Dextran 40 or 70 if the test uses high concentrations of acid. Dextran may cause turbidity, which interferes with bilirubin assays that use alcohol, total protein levels using biuret reagent, and blood glucose levels using the ortho-toluidine method. Blood typing and cross-matching using enzyme techniques may give unreliable readings if the samples are taken after the dextran infusion.

Dextran 40 administration has been associated with abnormal renal and hepatic function test results.

Adverse reactions
• DERM: hypersensitivity reaction (rash, pruritus, nasal congestion, mild hypotension, dyspnea) occurs rarely (Dextran 40 has less antigenic potential than Dextran 70); urticaria.
• GI: nausea, vomiting.
• GU: tubular stasis and blocking, increased viscosity and specific gravity of urine in patients having diminished urine flow, which may lead to acute tubular failure that is usually associated with dehydration or shock.
• HEMA: decreased level of hemoglobin and hematocrit; increased bleeding times caused by interference with platelet function can occur, especially when the higher-molecular-weight product is used in doses exceeding 1.5 liters.
• Hepatic: increased serum transaminase levels with Dextran 40.
• Other: anaphylactic reaction, fever, infection at injection site, venous thrombosis or phlebitis extending from injection site, extravasation, hypervolemia.

Overdose and treatment
No information available.

▶ Special considerations
• Dextran in sodium chloride solution is hazardous when given to patients with heart failure, severe renal failure, and clinical states in which edema exists with sodium restriction. (Dextrose 5% in water should be used.)
• Dextran works as a plasma expander via colloidal osmotic effect, thereby drawing fluid from interstitial

to intravascular space. It provides plasma expansion slightly greater than volume infused. Observe for circulatory overload or a rise in central venous pressure readings.
• Dextran 1 (Promit) may be given to prevent Dextran-induced anaphylaxis. Usual dose is 20 ml of Dextran 1 over 60 seconds, given 1 to 2 minutes before Dextran 40.
• Avoid doses that exceed the recommendations because dose-related increases in the incidence of wound hematoma, wound seroma, wound bleeding, distant bleeding (such as hematuria and melena), and pulmonary edema have been observed.
• Monitor urine flow rate during administration. If oliguria or anuria occurs or is not reversed by the initial infusion (500 ml), administration should be discontinued.
• Monitor urine or serum osmolarity; urine specific gravity will be increased by urine dextran concentration.
• Check hemoglobin and hematocrit; do not allow to fall below 30% by volume.
• Observe patient closely during early phase of infusion; check for infiltration, phlebitis, and anaphylactic reactions.
• Dextran may interfere with analysis of blood grouping, cross-matching, bilirubin, blood glucose, and protein.
• Store at constant 77° F. (25° C.). Solution may precipitate in storage. Discard any solution that is not clear.
• Avoid concomitant use of drugs that can affect platelet function.

Information for parents and patient
• Explain therapy and need for frequent monitoring to parents and patient. Advise parents to monitor for adverse reactions.

dextranomer
Debrisan

• Classification: topical debriding agent (synthetic polysaccharide)

How supplied
Available by prescription only
Beads: 4 g, 25 g, 60 g, 120 g
Paste: 10 g

Indications, route, and dosage
To clean exudative wounds
Children and adults: Apply to affected area daily or more often if area becomes wet. Apply to ⅛″ or ¼″ thickness, and cover with sterile gauze.

Action and kinetics
• *Debriding action:* Dextranomer cleanses wound surfaces by capillary action, drawing wound exudate, bacteria, and contaminants into the beads and therefore enhancing formation of granulative tissue and promoting wound healing.

• *Kinetics in adults:* Absorption is limited with topical use.

Contraindications and precautions
Dextranomer is contraindicated in deep fistulas, sinus tracts, or any area where complete removal is not ensured; and in dry wounds, because it is ineffective in cleaning these wounds.

Interactions
Dextranomer should not be used concomitantly with topical antibiotics or debriding enzymes.

Effects on diagnostic tests
None reported.

Adverse reactions
• Local: transient pain at site, bleeding, erythema, contact dermatitis.
   Note: Drug should be discontinued if sensitization develops.

Overdose and treatment
No information available.

▶ Special considerations
• Use strict aseptic technique when applying dextranomer.
• Dextranomer is not an enzyme and cannot be used for dry wounds.
• Clean wound before applying, leaving area moist; cover wound to a thickness of at least ¼"; then bandage lightly to hold beads in place. Be sure to leave room for expansion (1 g of beads absorbs 4 ml of exudate).
• When product is saturated and grayish yellow, irrigate wound and remove beads or paste; beads must be removed thoroughly, especially before any surgical treatment, and vigorous irrigation or soaking may be necessary.
• If dressing becomes dry, do not remove it without prior wetting to loosen bandage and beads.
• Stop treatment when area is free of exudate.

Information for parents and patient
• Teach parents or patient how to perform dressing changes before discharge.
• Patient should avoid drug contact with eyes and should wash hands well after application.
• Paste may be used for hard-to-reach areas or irregular body surfaces.

dextroamphetamine sulfate
Dexampex, Dexedrine, Ferndex, Oxydess II, Robese, Spancap #1

• Classification: CNS stimulant, short-term adjunctive anorexigenic agent, sympathomimetic amine (amphetamine)
• Controlled substance schedule II

How supplied
Available by prescription only
Tablets: 5 mg, 10 mg
Elixir: 5 mg/5 ml
Capsules (sustained-release): 5 mg, 10 mg, 15 mg

Indications, route, and dosage
Narcolepsy
Children age 6 to 12: 5 mg P.O. daily, with 5-mg increments weekly, p.r.n.
Children over age 12: 10 mg P.O. daily, with 10-mg increments weekly, p.r.n.
Adults: 5 to 60 mg P.O. daily in divided doses. Long-acting dosage forms allow once-daily dosing.
Attention deficit disorders with hyperactivity
Children age 3 to 5: 2.5 mg P.O. daily, with 2.5-mg increments weekly, p.r.n.; not recommended for children under age 3.
Children age 6 and older: 5 mg once daily or b.i.d., with 5-mg increments weekly, p.r.n.

Action and kinetics
• *CNS stimulant action:* Amphetamines are sympathomimetic amines with CNS stimulant activity; in hyperactive children, they have a paradoxical calming effect.
   The cerebral cortex and reticular activating system appear to be the primary sites of activity; amphetamines release nerve terminal stores of norepinephrine, promoting nerve impulse transmission. At high dosages, effects are mediated by dopamine.
   Amphetamines are used to treat narcolepsy and as adjuncts to psychosocial measures in attention deficit disorder in children. Their precise mechanism of action in these conditions is unknown.
• *Kinetics in adults:* Dextroamphetamine sulfate is rapidly absorbed from the GI tract; peak serum concentrations occur 2 to 4 hours after oral administration; long-acting capsules are absorbed more slowly and have a longer duration of action. Dextroamphetamine sulfate is distributed widely throughout the body and is excreted in urine.

Contraindications and precautions
Dextroamphetamine is contraindicated in children with hypersensitivity or idiosyncratic reaction to amphetamines; in patients with hyperthyroidism, angina pectoris, any degree of hypertension, or other severe cardiovascular disease; and in patients with a history of substance abuse. It also is contraindicated for concomitant use with monoamine oxidase (MAO) inhibitors or within 14 days of discontinuing MAO inhibitors.
   It should be used with caution in patients with

diabetes mellitus; in debilitated, or hyperexcitable patients; and in children with Gilles de la Tourette's syndrome. Amphetamine-induced CNS stimulation superimposed on CNS depression can cause seizures. Some formulations (Dexedrine) contain tartrazine, which may induce allergic reactions in hypersensitive individuals.

Interactions

Concomitant use with MAO inhibitors (or drugs with MAO-inhibiting activity, such as furazolidone) or within 14 days of such therapy may cause hypertensive crisis; use with antihypertensives may antagonize antihypertensive effects.

Concomitant use with antacids, sodium bicarbonate, or acetazolamide enhances reabsorption of dextroamphetamine and prolongs duration of action; use with ascorbic acid enhances dextroamphetamine excretion and shortens duration of action.

Concomitant use with phenothiazines or haloperidol decreases dextroamphetamine effects; barbiturates antagonize dextroamphetamine by CNS depression; use with theophylline, caffeine, or other CNS stimulants produces additive effects.

Dextroamphetamine may alter insulin requirements.

Effects on diagnostic tests

Dextroamphetamine may elevate plasma corticosteroid levels and may interefere with urinary steroid determinations.

Adverse reactions

• CNS: restlessness, tremor, hyperactivity, talkativeness, insomnia, irritability, dizziness, headache, chills, overstimulation, dysphoria, psychosis.
• CV: tachycardia, palpitations, hypertension, hypotension.
• DERM: urticaria.
• GI: nausea, vomiting, cramps, dry mouth, diarrhea, constipation, metallic taste, anorexia, weight loss.
• Other: impotence, changes in libido.
Note: Drug should be discontinued if signs of hypersensitivity or idiosyncrasy occur.

Overdose and treatment

Individual responses to overdose vary widely. Toxic symptoms may occur at 15 mg and 30 mg and can cause severe reactions; however, doses of 400 mg or more have not always proved fatal.

Symptoms of overdose include restlessness, tremor, hyperreflexia, tachypnea, confusion, aggressiveness, hallucinations, and panic; fatigue and depression usually follow excitement stage. Other symptoms may include dysrhythmias, shock, alterations in blood pressure, nausea, vomiting, diarrhea, and abdominal cramps; death is usually preceded by seizures and coma.

Treat overdose symptomatically and supportively: If ingestion is recent (within 4 hours), use gastric lavage or emesis and sedate with a barbiturate; monitor vital signs and fluid and electrolyte balance. Urinary acidification may enhance excretion. Saline catharsis (magnesium citrate) may hasten GI evacuation of unabsorbed sustained-release drug.

▶ Special considerations

• Amphetamines should be used cautiously in children who are debilitated, hyperexcitable, or with diabetes mellitus; and in children with Gilles de la Tourette's syndrome. Avoid long-term therapy when possible because of the risk of a psychic dependence or habituation.
• Children should receive lowest effective dose with dosage adjusted individually according to response; after long-term use, dosage should be lowered gradually to prevent acute rebound depression.
• Amphetamines may impair ability to perform tasks requiring mental alertness, such as schoolwork or driving a car.
• Vital signs should be checked regularly for increased blood pressure or other signs of excessive stimulation; avoid late-day or evening dosing, especially of long-acting dosage forms, to minimize insomnia.
• Monitor blood and urine glucose levels. Drug may alter daily insulin requirement in patient with diabetes.
• For narcolepsy, patient should take first dose on awakening.
• Encourage patient to get adequate rest; unusual, compensatory fatigue may result as drug wears off.
• Amphetamine use for analeptic effect is discouraged; CNS stimulation superimposed on CNS depression may cause neuronal instability and seizures.
• Carefully follow manufacturer's directions for reconstitution, storage, and administration of all preparations. Prolonged administration of CNS stimulants to children with attention deficit disorders may be associated with temporary decreased growth.
• Amphetamines have a high potential for abuse; they are not recommended to combat the fatigue of exhaustion or the need for sleep, but are often abused for this purpose by students, athletes, and truck drivers.
• In the event of overdose, protect patient from excessive noise or stimulation.

Information for parents and patient

• Explain rationale for therapy and the potential risks and benefits.
• Patient should avoid drinks containing caffeine, to prevent added CNS stimulation, and should not increase dosage.
• Advise narcoleptic patients to take first dose on awakening.
• Tell patient not to chew or crush sustained-release dosage forms.
• Warn patient not to use drug to mask fatigue, to be sure to obtain adequate rest, and to report excessive CNS stimulation.
• Advise diabetic patients and parents to monitor blood glucose levels carefully, because drug may alter insulin needs.
• Advise patient to avoid tasks that require mental alertness until degree of cognitive impairment is determined.

dextrose (D-glucose)
$D_{2.5}W$, D_5W, $D_{10}W$, $D_{20}W$, $D_{25}W$, $D_{30}W$, $D_{38.5}W$, $D_{40}W$, $D_{50}W$, $D_{60}W$, $D_{70}W$

- Classification: total parenteral nutrition (TPN) component, caloric agent, fluid volume replacement (carbohydrate)

How supplied
Available by prescription only
Injection: 1,000 ml (2.5%, 5%, 10%, 20%, 30%, 40%, 50%, 60%, 70%); 650 ml (38.5%); 500 ml (5%, 10%, 20%, 30%, 40%, 50%, 60%, 70%); 400 ml (25%); 250 ml (5%, 10%); 100 ml (5%); 70-ml pin-top vial (70% for additive use only); 50 ml (5% and 50% available in vial, ampule, and Bristoject); 10 ml (25%); 5-ml ampule (10%); 3-ml ampule (10%)

Indications, route, and dosage
Fluid replacement and caloric supplementation in patient who cannot maintain adequate oral intake or who is restricted from doing so
Children and adults: Dosage depends on fluid and caloric requirements. Use peripheral I.V. infusion of 2.5%, 5%, or 10% solution, or central I.V. infusion of 20% solution for minimal fluid needs. Use 50% solution to treat insulin-induced hypoglycemia. Solutions from 40% to 70% are used diluted in admixtures, normally with amino acid solutions, because TPN should be given through a central vein.

Action and kinetics
- *Metabolic action:* Dextrose is a rapidly metabolized source of calories and fluids in patients with inadequate oral intake. While increasing blood glucose concentrations, dextrose may decrease body protein and nitrogen losses, promote glycogen deposition, and decrease or prevent ketosis if sufficient doses are given. Dextrose also may induce diuresis. Parenterally injected doses of dextrose undergo oxidation to carbon dioxide and water. A 5% solution is isotonic and is administered peripherally. Concentrated dextrose infusions provide increased caloric intake with less fluid volume; they may be irritating if given by peripheral infusions. Concentrated solutions (greater than 12.5%) should be administered only by central venous catheters.
- *Kinetics in adults:* After oral administration, dextrose (a monosaccharide) is absorbed rapidly by the small intestine, principally by an active mechanism. In patients with hypoglycemia, blood glucose concentrations increase within 10 to 20 minutes after oral administration. Peak blood concentrations may occur 40 minutes after oral administration. As a source of calories and water for hydration, dextrose solutions expand plasma volume. Dextrose is metabolized to carbon dioxide and water. In some patients, dextrose solutions may produce diuresis.

Contraindications and precautions
Dextrose is contraindicated in patients with diabetic coma while blood glucose levels are excessively high. Concentrated solutions should not be used in the presence of intracranial or intraspinal hemorrhage. Dextrose is contraindicated in patients with delirium tremens and in dehydrated patients with glucose-galactose malabsorption syndrome. Hypertonic solutions also are contraindicated in patients with a known corn allergy.

Dextrose solutions must be used cautiously in patients with diabetes mellitus or carbohydrate intolerance. I.V. administration may cause fluid or solute overload and resultant congestive conditions with peripheral or pulmonary edema; risk is directly proportional to the electrolyte concentration. Hypomagnesemia, hypokalemia, and hypophosphatemia may result from I.V. dextrose administration. Rapid administration of hypertonic dextrose solutions may lead to hyperglycemia and hyperosmolar syndrome.

Interactions
Dextrose should be administered cautiously, especially if it contains sodium ions, to patients receiving corticosteroids or corticotropin. Dextrose administration may cause vitamin B_6 deficiency. Additives must be introduced aseptically, mixed thoroughly, and not stored; incompatibility is possible. Dextrose must not be administered with blood through the same infusion set because of possible pseudoagglutination of red blood cells.

Effects on diagnostic tests
None reported.

Adverse reactions
- CNS: confusion, *unconsciousness, hyperosmolar syndrome* (with concentrated solutions).
- CV: (with fluid overload) pulmonary edema, exacerbated hypertension, and congestive heart failure in susceptible patients. Prolonged or concentrated infusions may cause phlebitis and sclerosis of vein, especially with peripheral route of administration.
- DERM: *sloughing and tissue necrosis if extravasation occurs* with concentrated solutions.
- GU: *glycosuria,* osmotic diuresis.
- Metabolic: (with rapid infusion of concentrated solution or prolonged infusion) *hyperglycemia,* hypervolemia, hyperosmolarity. Rapid termination of long-term infusions may cause *hypoglycemia* from rebound hyperinsulinemia.
- Other: *fever, hypervolemia, hypovolemia.*

Overdose and treatment
If fluid or solute overload occurs during I.V. therapy, reevaluate the patient's condition and institute appropriate corrective treatment.

▶ Special considerations
- Use with caution in infants of diabetic women, except as may be indicated in neonates who are hypoglycemic.
- Monitor infusion rate for maximum dextrose infusion of 0.5g/kg/hour, using the largest available peripheral vein and a well-placed needle or catheter.
- Injection site should be checked frequently during the day to prevent irritation, tissue sloughing, necrosis, and phlebitis.

---

‡May contain sulfites   ◆May contain tartrazine   ◆◆May contain benzyl alcohol

• Avoid rapid administration, which may cause hyperglycemia, hyperosmolar syndrome, or glycosuria. Infuse concentrated solutions slowly; rapid infusion can cause hyperglycemia and fluid shifts.

• Hypertonic solutions are more likely than isotonic or hypotonic solutions to cause irritation; they should be administered into larger central veins.

• Carefully monitor patient's vital signs, intake, output, and body weight, especially in patients with renal dysfunction.

• Monitor serum glucose levels during long-term treatment.

• Depletion of pancreatic insulin production and secretion can occur. To avoid an adverse effect on insulin production, patient may need to have insulin added to infusions.

• Fluid imbalance or changes in electrolyte concentrations and acid-base balance should be evaluated clinically by periodic laboratory determinations during prolonged therapy. Additional electrolyte supplementation may be required.

• Excessive administration of potassium-free solutions may result in hypokalemia. Potassium should be added to dextrose solutions and administered to fasting patients with good renal function; special precautions should be taken with patients receiving digitalis.

• To avoid rebound hypoglycemia, dextrose 5% or 10% solution is advisable upon discontinuation of concentrated dextrose infusions.

Information for parents and patient

• Explain therapy and the need for restraints to safely maintain I.V. infusion to parents and patient. Advise them to monitor for adverse reactions.

• Encourage parents to hold and comfort the child during I.V. therapy.

---

dextrothyroxine sodium
Choloxin

• Classification: antilipemic (thyroid hormone)

How supplied
Available by prescription only
Tablets: 1 mg, 2 mg, 4 mg, 6 mg

Indications, route, and dosage
Primary type II hyperlipoproteinemia
Children: Initial dose 0.05 mg/kg daily, increased slowly by 0.05 mg/kg daily at monthly intervals to a total of 4 mg daily.
Adults: Initial dose 1 to 2 mg daily, increased gradually by 1 to 2 mg daily at monthly intervals to a total of 4 to 8 mg daily.

Action and kinetics
• *Antilipemic action:* Dextrothyroxine accelerates hepatic catabolism of cholesterol and increases bile secretion to lower cholesterol and low-density lipoprotein levels.

• *Kinetics in adults:* Dextrothyroxine is 25% absorbed from the GI tract. Drug is almost completely protein-

bound. Metabolism is not completely understood; some drug is deiodinated in peripheral tissues, and a small amount is metabolized by the liver. Drug is excreted in urine and feces; half-life is 18 hours. Serum lipids return to pretreatment levels 6 weeks to 3 months after discontinuing therapy.

Contraindications and precautions
Dextrothyroxine is contraindicated in patients with heart disease or a history of hypertension or rheumatic heart disease because drug increases myocardial oxygen demand and such patients are at increased risk of angina or myocardial infarction; in patients with advanced liver or kidney disease or a history of iodism because the drug may exacerbate these conditions; and in pregnant or lactating patients because thyroid hormones cross the placenta and enter breast milk.

Dextrothyroxine tablets may contain tartrazine dye (FD&C Yellow No. 5), which may cause allergic reactions in some individuals, usually patients sensitive to aspirin.

Interactions
Dextrothyroxine may potentiate effects of oral anticoagulants (warfarin); if concomitant use is unavoidable, reduce anticoagulant dose by one third and monitor prothrombin time frequently, readjusting dose as needed. Dextrothyroxine can also increase blood glucose levels, necessitating increased insulin dosage in patients with diabetes mellitus. Dextrothyroxine may enhance effects of other thyroid preparations; it may increase myocardial stimulant effects of cardiac glycosides. Patients with coronary artery disease receiving dextrothyroxine may be more susceptible to dysrhythmias after administration of catecholamines. Cholestyramine and colestipol may decrease absorption of dextrothyroxine.

Effects on diagnostic tests
Dextrothyroxine therapy alters serum levels of thyroxine (T_4), alkaline phosphatase, aspartate aminotransferase, and bilirubin; it may also decrease radioactive iodine uptake and alter urinary and blood glucose levels.

Adverse reactions
Adverse reactions are most common in patients with hypothyroidism, with heart disease, and at dosages greater than 8 mg/day; they may not occur until 1 to 6 weeks after initiation of therapy.

• CNS: headache, tinnitus, dizziness, psychic changes, paresthesia.

• CV: palpitations, tachycardia, peripheral edmea, angina pectoris, dysrhythmias, ischemic ECG changes, myocardial infarction.

• EENT: visual disturbances, ptosis, hoarseness.

• GI: dyspepsia, nausea, vomiting, diarrhea, constipation, bitter taste, decreased appetite.

• Metabolic: insomnia, weight loss, sweating, flushing, hyperthermia, hair loss, menstrual irregularities.

• Other: malaise, tiredness, muscle pain.

Note: Drug should be discontinued if signs or symptoms of heart disease develop.

Overdose and treatment
Clinical signs of overdose include signs and symptoms of hyperthyroidism — palpitations, diarrhea, abdominal cramps, nervousness, sweating, heat intolerance, fever, increased pulse and blood pressure, dysrhythmias, and congestive heart failure.

Empty stomach by induced emesis or gastric lavage. Give oxygen and treat fever, fluid loss, and congestive heart failure. Propranolol is useful to treat increased sympathetic activity.

▶ Special considerations
• Children with familial hypercholesterolemia have been treated for 1 year or longer without adverse effects on growth. However, continue the drug in children only if it has lowered serum cholesterol level significantly.
• Observe patient for signs of hyperthyroidism.
• Some preparations contain tartrazine, which may precipitate allergic reactions, especially in persons allergic to aspirin.
• Dextrothyroxine therapy is an adjunct to adequate dietary management and patients receiving the drug should continue to reduce total saturated fat and cholesterol intake.
• Because it may cause adverse hormonal and cardiac effects, the use of dextrothyroxine is limited to euthyroid patients with no history of cardiovascular disease.

Information for parents and patient
• Explain disease process and rationale for therapy; stress importance of close monitoring and of reporting any adverse reactions.
• Encourage compliance with prescribed regimen and appropriate diet; dextrothyroxine is not curative.
• Patient should not exceed prescribed dosage.
• Recommend taking with food to minimize GI discomfort.

---

diazepam
Apo-Diazepam★, E-Pam★, Meval★, Neo-Calme★, Novodipam★, Rival★, Valium, Valrelease, Vivol★

• Classification: antianxiety agent; skeletal muscle relaxant; amnesic agent; anticonvulsant; sedative-hypnotic (benzodiazepine)
• Controlled substance schedule IV

How supplied
Available by prescription only
Tablets: 2 mg, 5 mg, 10 mg
Capsules (extended-release): 15 mg
Oral solution: 5 mg/ml; 5 mg/5 ml
Oral suspension: 5 mg/5 ml
Injection: 5 mg/ml in 2-ml ampules or 10-ml vials
Disposable syringe: 2-ml Tel-E-Ject

Indications, route, and dosage
Sedation; adjunct to skeletal muscle spasm
Children: 0.04 to 0.2 mg/kg I.M. or I.V. q 2 to 4 hours. Maximum dose: 0.6 mg/kg within an 8-hour period.

Alternatively, give 0.12 to 0.8 mg/kg P.O. daily divided q 6 to 8 hours.
Adults: 2 to 10 mg P.O. b.i.d. to q.i.d.; or 2 to 5 mg I.M. or I.V., repeated in 3 to 4 hours as needed.
Tetanus
Neonates: 0.83 to 1.67 mg/kg/hour I.V. as a continuous infusion, or 20 to 40 mg/kg/day, divided q 2 hours.
Infants age 1 month to children age 5: 1 to 2 mg I.M. or I.V., repeated q 3 to 4 hours.
Children age 5 and older: 5 to 10 mg q 3 to 4 hours, as needed; or 15 mg/kg/day, divided q 2 hours.
Adjunct to convulsive disorders
Children over age 6 months: 1 to 2.5 mg P.O. t.i.d. or q.i.d.
Adults: 2 to 10 mg b.i.d. to q.i.d.
Adjunct to anesthesia; endoscopic procedures
Adults: 5 to 10 mg I.M. before surgery; or administer slowly I.V. just before procedure, titrating dose to effect. Usually, less than 10 mg is used, but up to 20 mg may be given.
Status epilepticus
Neonates: 0.15 to 0.5 mg/kg I.V. q 2 to 5 minutes.
Infants age 1 month to children age 5: 0.1 to 0.4 mg/kg I.V. repeated q 2 to 5 minutes to maximum of 1 mg/kg.
Children age 5 and over: 1 mg I.V. q 2 to 5 minutes to a maximum of 10 mg; repeat in 2 to 4 hours, as needed.
Adults: 5 to 10 mg I.V., repeated at 10- to 15-minute intervals to a maximum dose of 30 mg. Repeat q 3 to 4 hours, if needed.

Action and kinetics
• *Anxiolytic and sedative-hypnotic actions:* Diazepam depresses the CNS at the limbic and subcortical levels of the brain. It produces an anti-anxiety effect by influencing the effect of the neurotransmitter gamma-aminobutyric acid (GABA) on its receptor in the ascending reticular activating system, which increases inhibition and blocks cortical and limbic arousal.
• *Anticonvulsant action:* Diazepam suppresses the spread of seizure activity produced by epileptogenic foci in the cortex, thalamus, and limbic structures by enhancing presynaptic inhibition.
• *Amnesic action:* The exact mechanism of action is unknown.
• *Skeletal muscle relaxant action:* The exact mechanism is unknown, but it is believed to involve inhibiting polysynaptic afferent pathways.
• *Kinetics in adults:* When administered orally, diazepam is absorbed through the GI tract. Onset of action occurs within 30 to 60 minutes, with peak action in 1 to 2 hours. I.M. administration results in erratic absorption of the drug; onset of action usually occurs in 15 to 30 minutes. After I.V. administration, rapid onset of action occurs 1 to 5 minutes after injection.

Diazepam is distributed widely throughout the body. Approximately 85% to 95% of an administered dose is bound to plasma protein.

Diazepam is metabolized in the liver to the active metabolite desmethyldiazepam.

Most metabolites of diazepam are excreted in urine, with only small amounts excreted in feces. Duration of effect is 3 hours; this may be prolonged up to 90 hours in elderly patients and in patients with hepatic or renal dysfunction.

Contraindications and precautions

Diazepam is contraindicated in patients with known hypersensitivity to the drug; in patients with acute narrow-angle glaucoma or untreated open-angle glaucoma, because of the drug's possible anticholinergic effect; in patients in shock or coma, because the drug's hypnotic or hypotensive effect may be prolonged or intensified; in patients with acute alcohol intoxication who have depressed vital signs, because the drug will worsen CNS depression; and in infants younger than age 30 days, in whom slow metabolism of the drug causes it to accumulate.

Diazepam should be used cautiously in patients with psychoses, because the drug is rarely beneficial in such patients and may induce paradoxical reactions; in patients with myasthenia gravis or Parkinson's disease, because it may exacerbate the disorder; in patients with impaired renal or hepatic function, which prolongs elimination of the drug; in elderly or debilitated patients, who are usually more sensitive to the drug's CNS effects; and in individuals prone to addiction or drug abuse. Abrupt withdrawal of diazepam may precipitate seizures in patients with seizure disorders. Use of I.V. diazepam in patients with petit mal or Lennox-Gastaut syndrome may precipitate tonic status epilepticus.

Interactions

Diazepam potentiates the CNS depressant effects of phenothiazines, narcotics, barbiturates, alcohol, antihistamines, monoamine oxidase inhibitors, general anesthetics, and antidepressants. Concomitant use with cimetidine and possibly disulfiram causes diminished hepatic metabolism of diazepam, which increases its plasma concentration. Use with antacids may decrease the rate of absorption of diazepam.

Haloperidol may change the seizure patterns of patients treated with diazepam; benzodiazepines also may reduce the serum levels of haloperidol.

Diazepam reportedly can decrease digoxin clearance; monitor patients for digoxin toxicity.

Patients receiving diazepam and nondepolarizing neuromuscular blocking agents such as pancuronium and succinylcholine have intensified and prolonged respiratory depression.

Heavy smoking accelerates diazepam's metabolism, thus lowering clinical effectiveness. Oral contraceptives may impair the metabolism of diazepam. Diazepam may inhibit the therapeutic effect of levodopa.

Effects on diagnostic tests

Diazepam therapy may elevate liver function test results. Minor changes in EEG patterns, usually low-voltage, fast activity, may occur during and after diazepam therapy.

Adverse reactions

• CNS: confusion, depression, drowsiness, lethargy, hangover effect, ataxia, dizziness, syncope, nightmares, fatigue, slurred speech, tremors, vertigo, headache, muscle cramps, paresthesias, nervousness, euphoria.
• CV: cardiovascular collapse, *hypotension*, bradycardia, dysrhythmias (with I.V.), *tachycardia*.
• DERM: rash, urticaria.
• EENT: diplopia, blurred vision, photosensitivity, nystagmus.
• GI: *constipation,* salivation changes, anorexia, metallic taste, depressed gag reflex (with I.V.), nausea, vomiting, abdominal discomfort.
• GU: urinary retention or incontinence.
• Local: pain, *phlebitis at the injection site,* desquamation of the skin at the I.V. site, *hypotonia, increased respiratory rate.*
• Other: blood dyscrasias, *respiratory depression,* dysarthria, hepatic dysfunction, changes in libido, tissue necrosis (with intra-arterial administration), lactic acidosis (high-dose I.V. use), *hyperbilirubinemia.*
Note: Drug should be discontinued if hypersensitivity and the following paradoxical reactions occur: acute hyperexcited state, anxiety, hallucinations, increased muscle spasticity, insomnia, or rage.

Overdose and treatment

Clinical manifestations of overdose include somnolence, confusion, coma, hypoactive reflexes, dyspnea, labored breathing, hypotension, bradycardia, slurred speech, and unsteady gait or impaired coordination.

Support blood pressure and respiration until drug effects subside; monitor vital signs. Mechanical ventilatory assistance via endotracheal tube may be required to maintain a patent airway and support adequate oxygenation. Use I.V. fluids and vasopressors such as dopamine and phenylephrine to treat hypotension as needed. If the patient is conscious, induce emesis; use gastric lavage if ingestion was recent, but only if an endotracheal tube is present to prevent aspiration. After emesis or lavage, administer activated charcoal with a cathartic as a single dose. Dialysis is of limited value.

▶ Special considerations

• Safe use of oral diazepam in infants less than age 6 months and of parenteral diazepam in infants younger than age 30 days has not been established.
• Because children, particularly young ones, are sensitive to the CNS depressant effects of benzodiazepines, caution must be exercised. A neonate whose mother took diazepam during pregnancy may exhibit withdrawal symptoms.
• Closely observe neonates of mothers who took diazepam for a prolonged period during pregnancy; the infants may show withdrawal symptoms. Use of diazepam during labor may cause neonatal flaccidity.
• Administer with milk or immediately after meals to prevent GI upset. Give antacid, if needed, at least 1 hour before or after dose to prevent interaction and ensure maximum drug absorption and effectiveness.
• Crush tablet or empty capsule and mix with food if patient has difficulty swallowing.
• Capsule form is not recommended for use in children.

• Assess level of consciousness and neurologic status before and frequently during therapy for changes. Monitor for paradoxical reactions, especially early in therapy.

• Assess sleep patterns and quality. Institute seizure precautions. Assess for changes in seizure character, frequency, or duration.

• Assess vital signs frequently during therapy. Significant changes in blood pressure and heart rate may indicate impending toxicity.

• Monitor renal and hepatic function periodically to ensure adequate drug removal and prevent cumulative effects. During prolonged therapy, periodically monitor blood counts and liver function studies.

• Comfort measures – such as back rubs and relaxation techniques – may enhance drug effectiveness.

• As needed, institute safety measures – raised side rails and ambulatory assistance – to prevent injury. Anticipate possible rebound excitement reactions.

• Patient should be observed to prevent drug hoarding or self-dosing, especially in depressed or suicidal patients or those who are, or who have a history of being, drug-dependent. Patient's mouth should be checked to be sure tablet or capsule was swallowed.

• After prolonged use, abrupt continuation may cause withdrawal symptoms, discontinue gradually.

• To enhance taste, oral solution can be mixed with liquids or semisolid foods, such as applesauce or puddings, immediately before administration.

• Shake oral suspension well before administering.

• When prescribing with opiates for endoscopic procedures, reduce opiate dose by at least one third. Assess gag reflex postendoscopy and before resuming oral intake to prevent aspiration.

• Parenteral forms of diazepam may be diluted in normal saline solution; a slight precipitate may form; the solution can still be used.

• Diazepam interacts with plastic. Do not store diazepam in plastic syringes or administer it in plastic administration sets, which will decrease availability of the infused drug.

• I.V. route is preferred because of rapid and more uniform absorption.

• For I.V. administration, drug should be infused slowly, directly into a large vein, at a rate not exceeding 5 mg/minute for adults or 0.25 mg/kg of body weight over 3 minutes for children. Do not inject diazepam into small veins to avoid extravasation into subcutaneous tissue. Observe the infusion site for phlebitis. If direct I.V. administration is not possible, inject diazepam directly into I.V. tubing at point closest to vein insertion site to prevent extravasation.

• Administration by continuous I.V. infusion is not recommended.

• Inject I.M. dose deep into deltoid muscle. Aspirate for backflow to prevent inadvertent intraarterial administration. Use I.M. route only if I.V. or oral routes are unavailable.

• Patients should remain in bed under observation for at least 3 hours after parenteral administration of diazepam to prevent potential hazards; keep resuscitation equipment nearby.

• Lower doses are effective in patients with renal or hepatic dysfunction.

• Anticipate possible transient increase in frequency or severity of seizures when diazepam is used as adjunctive treatment of convulsive disorders. Impose seizure precautions.

• Do not mix diazepam with any other drug in a syringe or infusion container.

• Solution contains sodium benzoate which may interfere with bilirubin binding to albumin.

Information for parents and patient

• Warn parents that patient should avoid use of alcohol or other CNS depressants, such as antihistamines, analgesics, monoamine oxidase (MAO) inhibitors, antidepressants, and barbiturates, while taking benzodiazepines to prevent additive depressant effects.

• Patient should take the drug exactly as prescribed and not give medication to others. Parents should not increase the dose or frequency and should call the physician before giving any nonprescription cold or allergy preparations.

• Warn parents that patient should avoid activities requiring alertness and good psychomotor coordination until the CNS response to the drug is determined. Instruct patient in safety measures to prevent injury.

• Patient should avoid using antacids, which may delay drug absorption, unless prescribed.

• Be sure parents and patient understand that diazepam can cause physical and psychological dependence with prolonged use.

• Warn parents that patient should not stop taking the drug abruptly to prevent withdrawal symptoms after prolonged therapy.

• Tell parents and patient that smoking decreases the drug's effectiveness. Encourage patient to stop smoking during therapy.

• Tell parents to report any adverse effects. These are often dose-related and can be relieved by dosage adjustments.

• Explain to adolescent patient and her parents the importance of reporting suspected pregnancy immediately.

• Warn parents and patient that sudden changes of position can cause dizziness. Advise parents that patient should dangle legs for a few minutes before getting out of bed to prevent falls and injury.

diazoxide
Hyperstat I.V., Proglycem

• Classification: antihypertensive, antihypoglycemic (peripheral vasodilator)

How supplied
Available by prescription only
Injection: 300 mg/20 ml
Capsule: 50 mg
Oral suspension: 50 mg/ml in 30-ml bottle

Indications, route, and dosage
Hypertensive crisis
Children: 3 to 5 mg/kg I.V. push; may repeat in 30 minutes.
Adults: 1 to 3 mg/kg I.V. (up to a maximum of 150

mg) every 5 to 15 minutes until an adequate reduction in blood pressure is achieved.

Note: The use of 300-mg I.V. bolus push is no longer recommended. Switch to therapy with oral antihypertensives as soon as possible.

Hypoglycemia from hyperinsulinism

Infants and neonates: Usual daily dosage is 8 to 15 mg/kg P.O. b.i.d. or t.i.d.

Children and adults: Usual daily dosage is 3 to 8 mg/kg P.O. b.i.d. or t.i.d.

Action and kinetics

• *Antihypertensive action:* Diazoxide is a nondiuretic congener of thiazide diuretics. It directly relaxes arteriolar smooth muscle, causing vasodilation and reducing peripheral vascular resistance, thus reducing blood pressure.

• *Antihypoglycemic action:* Diazoxide increases blood glucose levels by inhibiting pancreatic secretion of insulin, by stimulating catecholamine release, or by increasing hepatic release of glucose.

• *Kinetics in adults:* After I.V. administration, blood pressure should decrease promptly, with maximum decrease in less than 5 minutes. After oral administration, hyperglycemic effect begins in 1 hour. Diazoxide is distributed throughout the body; highest concentration is found in kidneys, liver, and adrenal glands; diazoxide crosses placenta and blood-brain barrier. Drug is approximately 90% protein-bound; it is metabolized partially in the liver. Diazoxide and its metabolites are excreted slowly by the kidneys. Duration of antihypertensive effect varies widely, ranging from 30 minutes to 72 hours (average 3 to 12 hours) after I.V. administration; after oral administration, antihypoglycemic effect persists for about 8 hours. Antihypertensive and antihypoglycemic effects may be prolonged in patients with renal dysfunction.

Contraindications and precautions

Diazoxide is contraindicated in patients with known hypersensitivity to the drug or to other thiazide derivatives. I.V. diazoxide is contraindicated in patients with coarctation of the aorta or an atrioventricular shunt; oral diazoxide is contraindicated in patients with functional hypoglycemia.

Diazoxide should be used cautiously in patients who may be harmed by sodium and water retention and in patients with impaired cerebral, cardiac, or renal function, because the drug may reduce blood pressure abruptly, resulting in decreased perfusion.

Interactions

Diazoxide may potentiate antihypertensive effects of other antihypertensive agents, especially if I.V. diazoxide is administered within 6 hours after patient has received another antihypertensive agent.

Concomitant use of diazoxide with phenytoin may increase metabolism and decrease the plasma protein binding of phenytoin.

Concomitant use of diazoxide with diuretics may potentiate antihypoglycemic, hyperuricemic, or antihypertensive effects of diazoxide.

Diazoxide may displace warfarin, bilirubin, or other highly protein-bound substances from protein-binding sites.

Concomitant use with other thiazides may enhance effects of diazoxide. Diazoxide may alter insulin requirements in previously stable diabetic patients.

Effects on diagnostic tests

Diazoxide inhibits glucose-stimulated insulin release and may cause false-negative insulin response to glucagon. Prolonged use of oral diazoxide may decrease hemoglobin and hematocrit levels.

Adverse reactions

• CNS: headache, dizziness, light-headedness, euphoria.

• CV: *sodium and water retention,* orthostatic hypotension, sweating, flushing, warmth, angina, myocardial ischemia, *dysrhythmias, ECG changes.*

• GI: *nausea, vomiting, abdominal discomfort.*

• Metabolic: *hyperglycemia, hyperuricemia,* ketoacidosis, hyponatremia.

• Other: *hypertrichosis* (ceases when treatment stops).

Overdose and treatment

Overdose is manifested primarily by hyperglycemia; ketoacidosis and hypotension may occur.

Treat acute overdose supportively and symptomatically. If hyperglycemia develops, give insulin and replace fluid and electrolyte losses; use vasopressors if hypotension fails to respond to conservative treatment. Prolonged monitoring may be necessary because of diazoxide's long half-life.

▶ Special considerations

• Diazoxide is used to treat only hypoglycemia resulting from hyperinsulinism; it is not used to treat functional hypoglycemia. It may be used temporarily to control preoperative or postoperative hypoglycemia in patients with hyperinsulinism.

• I.V. use of diazoxide is seldom necessary for more than 4 or 5 days.

• After I.V. injection, monitor blood pressure every 5 minutes for 15 to 30 minutes, then every hour when patient is stable. Discontinue if severe hypotension develops or if blood pressure continues to fall 30 minutes after drug infusion; keep patient recumbent during this time and have norepinephrine available. Monitor I.V. site for infiltration or extravasation.

• Monitor patient's intake and output carefully. If fluid or sodium retention develops, diuretics may be given 30 to 60 minutes after diazoxide. Keep patient recumbent for 8 to 10 hours after diuretic administration.

• Monitor daily blood glucose and electrolyte levels, watching diabetic patients closely for severe hyperglycemia or hyperglycemic hyperosmolar nonketotic coma; also monitor daily urine glucose and ketone levels, intake and output, and weight. Check serum uric acid levels frequently.

• Protect solutions from light, heat, or freezing; do not administer solutions that have darkened or that contain particulate matter.

• Significant hypotension does not occur after oral administration in doses used to treat hypoglycemia.

• Drug may be given by constant I.V. infusion until adequate blood pressure reduction occurs.

Information for parents and patient
• Explain that orthostatic hypotension can be minimized by rising slowly and avoiding sudden position changes.
• Tell parents to report any adverse effect immediately, including pain and redness at injection site, which may indicate infiltration.
• Have parents check patient's weight daily and report gains of over 5 lb (2.3 kg) per week, because diazoxide causes sodium and water retention.
• Reassure parents and patient that excessive hair growth is a common reaction that subsides when drug treatment is completed.

dicloxacillin sodium
Dycill, Dynapen, Pathocil

Classification: antibiotic (penicillinase-resistant penicillin)

How supplied
Available by prescription only
Capsules: 125 mg, 250 mg, 500 mg
Oral suspension: 62.5 mg/5 ml (after reconstitution)

Indications, route, and dosage
Systemic infections caused by susceptible organisms
Neonates: 4 to 8 mg/kg P.O. every 6 hours.
Children older than age 1 month weighing less than 40 kg: 25 to 50 mg/kg P.O. daily, divided into doses given q 6 hours.
Adults and children 40 kg and over: 1 to 2 g P.O. daily, divided into doses given q 6 hours.

Action and kinetics
• *Antibiotic action:* Dicloxacillin is bactericidal; it adheres to bacterial penicillin-binding proteins, thus inhibiting bacterial cell wall synthesis. Dicloxacillin resists the effects of penicillinases — enzymes that inactivate penicillin — and is thus active against many strains of penicillinase-producing bacteria; this activity is most important against penicillinase-producing staphylococci; some strains may remain resistant. Dicloxacillin is also active against a few gram-positive aerobic and anaerobic bacilli but has no significant effect on gram-negative bacilli.
• *Kinetics in adults:* Dicloxacillin is absorbed rapidly but incompletely (35% to 76%) from the GI tract; it is relatively acid stable. Peak plasma levels occur ½ to 2 hours after an oral dose. Food may decrease both rate and extent of absorption. Dicloxacillin is distributed widely into bone, bile, and pleural and synovial fluids. CSF penetration is poor but is enhanced by meningeal inflammation. Dicloxacillin crosses the placenta; it is 95% to 99% protein-bound. Dicloxacillin is metabolized only partially. Dicloxacillin and metabolites are excreted in urine by renal tubular secretion and glomerular filtration; they are also excreted in breast milk. Elimination half-life in adults is ½ to 1 hour, extended minimally to 2½ hours in patients with renal impairment.

Contraindications and precautions
Dicloxacillin is contraindicated in patients with known hypersensitivity to any other penicillin or to cephalosporins.
   Dicloxacillin should be used cautiously in patients with renal impairment because it is excreted in urine; decreased dosage is required in moderate to severe renal failure.

Interactions
Concomitant use with aminoglycosides produces synergistic bactericidal effects against *Staphylococcus aureus.* Probenecid blocks renal tubular secretion of dicloxacillin, raising its serum levels.

Effects on diagnostic tests
Dicloxacillin alters test results for urine and serum proteins; it produces false-positive or elevated results in turbidimetric urine and serum protein tests using sulfosalicylic acid or trichloroacetic acid; it also reportedly produces false results on the Bradshaw screening test for Bence Jones protein.
   Dicloxacillin may cause transient elevations in liver function study results and transient reductions in red blood cell, white blood cell, and platelet counts. Elevated liver function test results may indicate drug-induced cholestasis or hepatitis.
   Dicloxacillin may falsely decrease serum aminoglycoside concentrations.

Adverse reactions
• CNS: neuromuscular irritability, seizures.
• GI: nausea, vomiting, epigastric distress, flatulence, diarrhea, pseudomembranous colitis, intrahepatic cholestasis.
• GU: acute interstitial nephritis.
• HEMA: eosinophilia, leukopenia, granulocytopenia, thrombocytopenia, agranulocytosis.
• Other: hypersensitivity reaction (pruritus, urticaria, rash, anaphylaxis), bacterial or fungal superinfection.
   Note: Drug should be discontinued if immediate hypersensitivity reactions occur or if signs of interstitial nephritis or pseudomembranous colitis occur. Patient may require alternate therapy if any of the following occurs: drug fever, eosinophilia, hematuria, neutropenia, or unexplained elevations in serum creatinine levels, BUN levels, or liver function studies.

Overdose and treatment
Clinical signs of overdose include neuromuscular irritability or seizures. No specific recommendations. Treatment is supportive. After recent ingestion (4 hours or less), empty the stomach by induced emesis or gastric lavage; follow with activated charcoal to reduce absorption. Dicloxacillin is not appreciably dialyzable.

▶ Special considerations
• Assess patient's history of allergies; do not give dicloxacillin to any patient with a history of hyper-

sensitivity reactions to either penicillins or cephalosporins. Try to determine whether previous reactions were true hypersensitivity reactions or another reaction, such as GI distress, which the patient has interpreted as allergy.

• Keep in mind that a negative history for penicillin hypersensitivity does not preclude future allergic reactions; monitor patient continuously for possible allergic reactions or other untoward effects.

• In patients with renal impairment, dosage should be reduced if creatinine clearance is below 10 ml/minute.

• Assess level of consciousness, neurologic status, and renal function when high doses are used, because excessive blood levels can cause CNS toxicity.

• Obtain results of cultures and sensitivity tests before first dose; however, therapy may begin before test results are complete. Repeat tests periodically to assess drug efficacy.

• Monitor vital signs, electrolytes, and renal function studies; monitor body weight for fluid retention with extended-spectrum penicillins for possible hypokalemia or hypernatremia.

• Coagulation abnormalities, even frank bleeding, can follow high doses, especially of extended-spectrum penicillins; monitor prothrombin times and platelet counts, and assess patient for signs of occult or frank bleeding.

• Monitor patients on long-term therapy for possible superinfection, especially debilitated patients and others receiving immunosuppressants or radiation therapy; monitor closely for fever.

Oral and parenteral administration

• Give penicillins at least 1 hour before giving bacteriostatic antibiotics (tetracyclines, erythromycins, and chloramphenicol); these drugs inhibit bacterial cell growth, decreasing rate of penicillin uptake by bacterial cell walls.

• Give oral penicillin at least 1 hour before or 2 hours after meals to enhance gastric absorption; food may or may not decrease absorption. Give drug with water only; acid in fruit juice or carbonated beverage may inactivate drug.

• Refrigerate oral suspensions (stable for 14 days); shake well before administering to ensure correct dosage.

• Always consult manufacturer's directions for reconstitution, dilution, and storage of drugs; check expiration dates.

• Regularly assess renal, hepatic, and hematopoietic function during prolonged therapy.

Information for parents and patient

• Instruct parents to shake suspension to ensure correct dosage.

• Tell parents to report severe diarrhea, rash, or itching promptly.

• Teach signs and symptoms of hypersensitivity and other adverse reactions, and emphasize need to report any unusual reactions.

• Teach signs and symptoms of bacterial and fungal superinfection to parents and patients, especially debilitated patients and others with low resistance from immunosuppressants or irradiation; emphasize need to report signs of infection. To prevent fungal infections in infants, instruct parents to keep diaper area clean and dry and to avoid use of plastic pants.

• Be sure parents understand how and when to give drugs; urge them to complete entire prescribed regimen, to comply with instructions for around-the-clock dosage, and to keep follow-up appointments.

• Counsel parents to check expiration date of drug and to discard unused drug.

---

diflorasone diacetate
Florone, Flutone*, Maxiflor

• Classification: anti-inflammatory (topical adrenocorticoid)

How supplied
Available by prescription only
Cream, ointment: 0.05%

Indications, route, and dosage
Inflammation of corticosteroid-responsive dermatoses
Children: Apply sparingly to affected area once a day.
Adults: Apply ointment sparingly in a thin film once a day to q.i.d.; apply cream once a day to q.i.d.

Action and kinetics
• *Anti-inflammatory action:* Diflorasone stimulates the synthesis of enzymes needed to decrease the inflammatory response. Diflorasone is a high-potency (group II) anti-inflammatory agent similar in potency to triamcinolone acetonide 0.5%.

• *Kinetics in adults:* The amount of diflorasone absorbed depends on the amount applied and on the nature of the skin at the application site. It ranges from about 1% in areas with a thick stratum corneum (such as the palms, soles, elbows, and knees) to as high as 36% in areas of the thinnest stratum corneum (face, eyelids, and genitals). Absorption increases in areas of skin damage, inflammation, or occlusion. Some systemic absorption of topical steroids occurs, especially through the oral mucosa.

After topical application, diflorasone is distributed throughout the local skin and metabolized primarily in the skin. Any drug absorbed into the circulation is distributed rapidly into muscle, liver, skin, intestines, and kidneys. The small amount absorbed is metabolized primarily in the liver to inactive compounds.

Inactive metabolites are excreted by the kidneys, primarily as glucuronides and sulfates, but also as unconjugated products. Small amounts of the metabolites are also excreted in feces.

Contraindications and precautions
Diflorasone is contraindicated in patients who are hypersensitive to any component of the preparation and in patients with viral, fungal, or tubercular skin lesions.

Diflorasone should be used with extreme caution in patients with impaired circulation, because its use may increase the risk of skin ulceration.

Interactions
None significant.

Effects on diagnostic tests
None reported.

Adverse reactions
• Local: burning, itching, irritation, dryness, folliculitis, hypertrichosis, acneiform eruptions, hypopigmentation, perioral dermatitis, allergic contact dermatitis, maceration, secondary infection, atrophy, striae, miliaria.

Significant systemic absorption may produce the following reactions.
• CNS: euphoria, insomnia, headache, psychotic behavior, pseudotumor cerebri, mental changes, nervousness, restlessness.
• CV: congestive heart failure, hypertension, edema.
• EENT: cataracts, glaucoma, thrush.
• GI: peptic ulcer, irritation, increased appetite.
• Immune: immunosuppression, increased susceptibility to infection.
• Musculoskeletal: muscle atrophy.
• Other: withdrawal syndrome (nausea, fatigue, anorexia, dyspnea, hypotension, hypoglycemia, myalgia, arthralgia, fever, dizziness, and fainting).
Note: Drug should be discontinued if local irritation, infection, systemic absorption, or hypersensitivity reaction occurs.

Overdose and treatment
No information available.

▶ Special considerations
• *Children may show greater susceptibility to topical corticosteroid-induced HPA axis suppression and Cushing's syndrome than mature patients because of a higher ratio of skin surface area to body weight.* Hypothalamic-pituitary-adrenal (HPA) axis suppression, Cushing's syndrome, and intracranial hypertension have been reported in children receiving topical corticosteroids. Signs of adrenal suppression in children include linear growth retardation, delayed weight gain, low plasma cortisol levels and absence of response to ACTH stimulation. Signs of intracranial hypertension include bulging fontanelles, headaches, and bilateral papilledema.
• Administration of diflorasone to children should be limited to the least effective amount. Chronic corticosteroid therapy may interfere with growth and development.
• Stop drug if the patient develops signs of systemic absorption (including Cushing's syndrome, hyperglycemia, or glucosuria), skin irritation or ulceration, hypersensitivity, or infection. (If antifungals or antibiotics are being used with diflorasone and the infection does not respond immediately, drug should be discontinued until infection is controlled.)
• Monitor patient response. Observe area of inflammation and elicit patient comments concerning pruritus. Inspect skin for infection, striae, and atrophy. Skin atrophy is common and may be clinically significant within 3 to 4 weeks of treatment with high-potency preparations; it also occurs more readily at sites where percutaneous absorption is high.

• Do not apply occlusive dressing over diflorasone because this may lead to secondary infection, maceration, atrophy, striae, or miliaria caused by increasing steroid penetration and potency.

Information for parents and patient
• Instruct parents and patients in application of the drug.
Method for applying topical preparations
• Wash hands before and after applying the drug.
• Gently cleanse the area of application. Washing or soaking the area before application may increase drug penetration.
• Apply sparingly in a light film; rub in lightly. Avoid contact with patient's eyes, unless using an ophthalmic product.
• Avoid prolonged application in areas near the eyes, genitals, rectum, on the face, and in skin folds. High-potency topical corticosteroids are more likely to cause striae in these areas because of their higher rates of absorption.
• If an occlusive dressing is necessary, minimize adverse reactions by using it intermittently. Do not leave it in place longer than 16 hours each day.
• Warn patient not to use nonprescription topical preparations other than those specifically recommended.
• Advise parents not to use tight-fitting diapers or plastic pants on a child being treated in the diaper area, since such garments may serve as occlusive dressings.

---

digitoxin
Crystodigin, Purodigin

• Classification: antiarrhythmic agent, inotropic agent (digitalis glycoside)

How supplied
Available by prescription only
Tablets: 0.05 mg, 0.1 mg, 0.15 mg, 0.2 mg
Injection: 0.2 mg/ml

Indications, route, and dosage
CHF, paroxysmal atrial tachycardia, atrial fibrillation and flutter
Premature infants, neonates, and severely ill older infants: Loading dose is 0.022 mg/kg I.M., I.V., or P.O. in divided doses over 24 hours; maintenance dosage is 0.0022 mg/kg daily. Monitor closely for toxicity.
Children age 2 weeks to 1 year: Loading dose is 0.045 mg/kg I.M., I.V., or P.O. in divided doses over 24 hours; maintenance dosage is 0.0045 mg/kg daily. Monitor closely for toxicity.
Children age 1 to 2: Loading dose is 0.04 mg/kg over 24 hours in divided doses; maintenance dosage is 0.004 mg/kg daily. Monitor closely for toxicity.
Children age 2 to 12: Loading dose is 0.03 mg/kg or 0.75 mg/m^2 I.M., I.V., or P.O. in divided doses over 24 hours; maintenance dosage is ¹⁄₁₀ loading dose or 0.003 mg/kg or 0.075 mg/m^2 daily. Monitor closely for toxicity.

---

‡May contain sulfites   ◆May contain tartrazine   ◆ ◆May contain benzyl alcohol

Adults: Loading dose is 1.2 to 1.6 mg I.V. or P.O. in divided doses over 24 hours; maintenance dosage is 0.1 mg daily.

Action and kinetics

• *Inotropic action:* Digitoxin's effect on the myocardium is dose-related and involves both direct and indirect mechanisms. It directly increases the force and velocity of myocardial contraction, AV node refractory period, and total peripheral resistance; at higher doses, it also increases sympathetic outflow. It indirectly depresses the SA node and prolongs conduction to the AV node. In patients with heart failure, increased contractile force boosts cardiac output, improves systolic emptying, and decreases diastolic heart size. Digitoxin also reduces ventricular end diastolic pressure and, consequently, pulmonary and systemic venous pressures. Increased myocardial contractility and cardiac output reflexively reduce sympathetic tone in patients with CHF. This compensates for the drug's direct vasoconstrictive action, thereby reducing total peripheral resistance. It also slows increased heart rate and causes diuresis in edematous patients.

• *Antiarrhythmic action:* Digitoxin-induced heart-rate slowing in patients without CHF is negligible and stems mainly from vagal (cholinergic) and sympatholytic effects on the SA node; however, with toxic doses, heart-rate slowing results from direct depression of SA node automaticity. Therapeutic doses produce little effect on the action potential, but toxic doses increase the automaticity (spontaneous diastolic depolarization) of all cardiac regions except the SA node.

• *Kinetics in adults:* Digitoxin is absorbed rapidly and completely from the GI tract. After oral administration, therapeutic effects appear in 1 to 2 hours, with peak effects occurring in 8 to 12 hours. After I.V. administration, clinical effects appear in 30 minutes to 2 hours, with peak effects occurring in 4 to 12 hours. Digitoxin is distributed widely in body tissues; highest concentrations appear in the heart, kidneys, intestine, stomach, liver, and skeletal muscle; lowest concentrations appear in the plasma and brain. Little of the drug crosses the blood-brain barrier. About 97% is bound to plasma proteins. Usual therapeutic steady-state serum levels range from 40 to 45 ng/ml. Digitoxin is metabolized extensively, apparently in the liver, to active metabolites (one of which is digoxin) and inactive metabolites. Dosage reduction may be necessary in patients with hepatic impairment. After it is metabolized and enters the enterohepatic recirculation, digitoxin is eventually excreted in urine. Elimination half-life ranges from 5 to 14 days.

Contraindications and precautions

Digitoxin is contraindicated in patients with ventricular fibrillation, because the drug may induce dysrhythmias; in patients with digitoxin toxicity; and in patients with hypersensitivity to the drug.

Digitoxin should be used with extreme caution, if at all, in patients with idiopathic hypertrophic subaortic stenosis, because the drug may cause increased obstruction of left ventricular outflow; in patients with incomplete AV block who do not have an artificial pacemaker (especially those with Stokes-Adams syndrome), because the drug may induce advanced or complete AV block; in patients with hypersensitive carotid sinus syndrome, because the drug increases vagal tone (carotid sinus massage has induced ventricular fibrillation in patients receiving cardiac glycosides); in patients with Wolff-Parkinson-White syndrome, because the drug may cause fatal ventricular dysrhythmias; in patients with sinus node disease (such as sick sinus syndrome), because the drug may worsen sinus bradycardia or SA block; in patients with severe pulmonary disease, hypoxia, myxedema, acute myocardial infarction, severe heart failure, acute myocarditis, or an otherwise damaged myocardium, because the drug increases the risk of dysrhythmias in these patients; in patients with chronic constrictive pericarditis, because such patients may respond unfavorably to the drug; in patients with frequent premature ventricular contractions or ventricular tachycardia (especially if these dysrhythmias do not result from heart failure), because the drug may induce dysrhythmias; in patients with low cardiac output states caused by valvular stenosis, chronic pericarditis, or chronic cor pulmonale, because the drug may decrease heart rate, which, in turn, may reduce cardiac output; and in patients with conditions that increase cardiac sensitivity to digitalis, including hypokalemia, chronic pulmonary disease, and acute hypoxemia.

Interactions

Concomitant use of digitoxin with antacids containing aluminum and/or magnesium hydroxide, magnesium trisilicate, kaolin-pectin, aminosalicylic acid, and sulfasalazine interferes with absorption of orally administered digitoxin. Cholestyramine and colestipol may bind digitoxin in the GI tract and impair absorption.

Concomitant use with other cardiac drugs that may affect AV conduction (such as procainamide, propranolol, and verapamil) may have additive cardiac effects. Concomitant use with sympathomimetics (such as ephedrine, epinephrine, and isoproterenol), rauwolfia alkaloids, or succinylcholine may increase the risk of dysrhythmias. Concomitant use with I.V. calcium preparations may cause synergistic effects that precipitate dysrhythmias.

Concomitant use with electrolyte-altering agents may increase or decrease serum electrolyte concentrations, predisposing the patient to digitoxin toxicity. For example, such diuretics as ethacrynic acid, furosemide, and bumetanide may cause hypokalemia and hypomagnesemia; thiazides may cause hypercalcemia. Fatal cardiac dysrhythmias may result. Amphotericin B, corticosteroids, corticotropin, edetate disodium, laxatives, and sodium polystyrene sulfonate deplete total body potassium levels, possibly leading to drug toxicity. Glucagon, large dextrose doses, and dextrose-insulin infusions reduce extracellular potassium levels, possibly causing digitoxin toxicity.

Concomitant use with barbiturates, hydantoins, rifampin, and phenylbutazone may stimulate microsomal enzymes that metabolize digitoxin in the liver, possibly causing decreased serum digitoxin levels.

Effects on diagnostic tests

Digitoxin may interfere with the Zimmerman reaction, causing falsely-elevated urinary 17-ketogenic steroid levels.

Adverse reactions

• CNS: fatigue, generalized weakness, agitation, hallucinations, headache, malaise, dizziness, vertigo, stupor, paresthesias.
• CV: increased severity of CHF, dysrhythmias (most commonly, conduction disturbances with or without AV block, premature ventricular contractions, and supraventricular dysrhythmias), hypotension. (Toxic cardiac effects may be life-threatening and require immediate attention.)
• EENT: yellow-green halos around visual images, blurred vision, light flashes, photophobia, diplopia.
• GI: anorexia, nausea, vomiting, diarrhea.
   Note: Drug should be discontinued if signs of digitalis toxicity are present (nausea, vomiting, dysrhythmias).

Overdose and treatment

Clinical effects of overdose are primarily gastrointestinal, CNS, and cardiac reactions. Severe intoxication may cause hyperkalemia, which may develop rapidly and result in life-threatening cardiac manifestations. Cardiac signs of digitoxin toxicity may occur with or without other toxicity signs and commonly precede other toxic effects. Because toxic cardiac effects also may occur as manifestations of heart disease, determining whether these effects result from underlying heart disease or digitoxin toxicity may be difficult. Digitoxin has caused almost every kind of dysrhythmia; various combinations of dysrhythmias may occur in the same patient. Patients with chronic digitoxin toxicity commonly have ventricular dysrhythmias and/or AV conduction disturbances. Patients with digitoxin-induced ventricular tachycardia have a high mortality because ventricular fibrillation or asystole may result.

Treatment requires immediate discontinuation of the drug and measurement of serum drug levels. Usually, drug takes at least 6 hours to equilibrate between plasma and tissue; plasma levels drawn earlier may show higher digitoxin levels than those present after the drug distributes into the tissues.

Other treatment measures include immediate emesis induction, gastric lavage, and administration of activated charcoal to reduce absorption of drug remaining in the gut. Multiple doses of activated charcoal (such as 50 gm q 6 hours) may help reduce further absorption, especially of any drug undergoing enterohepatic recirculation. Any interacting drugs should probably be discontinued. Ventricular dysrhythmias may be treated with I.V. potassium (replacement doses; but not in patients with significant AV block), I.V. phenytoin, I.V. lidocaine, or I.V. propranolol. Refractory ventricular tachydysrhythmias may be controlled with overdrive pacing. Procainamide may be used for ventricular dysrhythmias that do not respond to the above treatments. In severe AV block, asystole, and hemodynamically significant sinus bradycardia, atropine restores a normal rate.

Administration of specific antibody fragments (digoxin immune Fab [Digibind]) is a new treatment for life-threatening digitoxin toxicity. These fragments bind digitoxin in the bloodstream and are excreted in the urine, rapidly decreasing serum levels and therefore cardiac drug concentrations. Each 40 mg of Fab fragments will bind about 0.6 mg of digoxin or digitoxin.

▶ Special considerations

• Pediatric patients have a poorly defined serum concentration level range; however, toxicity apparently does not occur at the same concentration levels considered toxic in adults. Divided daily dosing is recommended for infants and children under age 10; older children require adult doses proportional to body weight.
• Obtain baseline heart rate and rhythm, blood pressure, and serum electrolyte levels before giving first dose.
• Find out about use of cardiac glycosides within previous 2 to 3 weeks before administering loading dose. Always divide loading dose over first 24 hours unless clinical situation indicates otherwise.
• Adjust dose to patient's clinical condition; monitor ECG and serum levels of digitoxin, calcium, potassium, and magnesium. Therapeutic blood digitoxin levels range from 25 to 35 ng/ml.
• I.M. injection is painful and dose is poorly absorbed; give I.V. if parenteral route is necessary.
• Monitor clinical status. Take apical-radial pulse for a full minute. Watch for significant changes (sudden rate increase, pulse deficit, irregular beats, and especially regularization of a previously irregular rhythm). Check blood pressure and obtain 12-lead ECG if these changes occur.
• Because digitoxin predisposes patient to postcardioversion dysrhythmias, most clinicians withhold drug 1 to 2 days before elective cardioversion in patients with atrial fibrillation. (However, consider the consequences of increased ventricular response to atrial fibrillation if digitoxin is withheld.)
• Elective cardioversion should be postponed in patients with signs of digitoxin toxicity.
• Do not administer calcium salts to patient receiving digitoxin. Calcium affects cardiac contractility and excitability in much the same way that digitoxin does and may lead to serious dysrhythmias.
• Thyroid function inversely affects plasma levels of cardiac glycosides. Patients with myxedema require lower doses, while thyrotoxic patients may be relatively insensitive to cardiac glycosides.
• Monitor patient's eating patterns. Ask about nausea, vomiting, anorexia, visual disturbances, and other symptoms of toxicity. Watch closely for toxicity signs in children and elderly patients.
• Monitor serum potassium levels. Take corrective action before hypokalemia occurs.
• Digitoxin is a long-acting drug; watch for cumulative effects.
• Protect solution from light.
• Consider that different brands may not be therapeutically interchangeable.
• Ask patient if he has a history of chronic or recent cardiac glycoside use before starting therapy.
• Monitor heart rate daily because of drug's effects

on the cardiac conduction system. Slowing of heart rate may be an early sign of toxicity (except in patients with chronically slow heart rate).
• Obtain serum drug levels before administering morning dose or at least 6 to 12 hours after a dose is administered, because of drug's slow distribution.
• Higher-than-usual doses and serum drug levels may be needed to adequately control atrial tachydysrhythmias.
• Before prescribing additional drugs for patient currently receiving cardiac glycosides, review drug interactions, which are numerous and may seriously affect therapy.

Information for parents and patient
• Instruct parents and patient about drug action, medication regimen, how to take pulse, reportable signs, and follow-up plans.
• Instruct parents to have patient take drug only as directed and at same time every day.
• Teach parents and patient how to take pulse rate; advise them to call if rate drops below the patient's normal rate.
• Warn parents that patient should not take missed dose with next regularly scheduled dose. Tell them to call for instructions if patient misses more than two doses.
• Patient should avoid all nonprescription preparations, such as cough, cold, or allergy medications or diet drugs, except as directed.
• Instruct parents to watch for and report loss of appetite, stomach pain, nausea, vomiting, diarrhea, unusual fatigue or weakness, drowsiness, headache, blurred or yellow vision, rash or hives, or depression.
• Warn parents that patient should not stop taking drug without medical approval.

---

digoxin
Lanoxicaps, Lanoxin, Novodigoxin*

• Classification: antiarrhythmic, inotropic (digitalis glycoside)

How supplied
Available by prescription only
Tablets: 0.125 mg, 0.25 mg, 0.5 mg
Capsules: 0.05 mg, 0.10 mg, 0.20 mg
Elixir: 0.05 mg/ml
Injection: 0.05mg/ml*, 0.1 mg/ml (pediatric), 0.25 mg/ml

Indications, route, and dosage
CHF, atrial fibrillation and flutter, paroxysmal atrial tachycardia
Premature neonates: Loading dose is 0.015 to 0.025 mg/kg I.V. Maintenance dosage is 20% to 30% of the total loading dose daily, in two or three divided doses.
Full-term neonates: Loading dose is 0.03 to 0.05 mg/kg I.V. Maintenance dosage is 25% to 35% of the total loading dose daily, in two or three divided doses.
Infants age 1 month to 2 years: Loading dose is 0.03 to 0.05 mg/kg I.V. Maintenance dosage is 25% to 35%

of the total loading dose daily, in two or three divided doses.
Children age 2 to 5: Loading dose is 0.025 to 0.035 mg/kg I.V. Maintenance dosage is 25% to 35% of the total loading dose daily, in two or three divided doses.
Children age 5 to 10: Loading dose is 0.015 to 0.03 mg/kg I.V. Maintenance dosage is 25% to 35% of the total loading dose daily, in two or three divided doses.
Children age 10 and over: Loading dose is 0.008 to 0.012 mg/kg I.V. Maintenance dosage is 25% to 35% of the total loading dose daily, in two or three divided doses.
Adults: Loading dose is 0.4 to 0.6 mg I.V. or P.O. with additional doses of 0.1 to 0.3 mg q 4 to 8 hours as tolerated and needed up to 1 mg over 24 hours. Maintenance dosage is 0.125 to 0.5 mg I.V. or P.O. daily in a single dose or in divided doses.

Action and kinetics
Digoxin is the most widely used cardiac glycoside. Multiple oral forms and a parenteral form are available, facilitating the drug's use in both acute and chronic clinical settings.
• *Inotropic action:* Digoxin's effect on the myocardium is dose-related and involves both direct and indirect mechanisms. It directly increases the force and velocity of myocardial contraction, AV node refractory period, and total peripheral resistance; at higher doses, it also increases sympathetic outflow. It indirectly depresses the SA node and prolongs conduction to the AV node. In patients with heart failure, increased contractile force boosts cardiac output, improves systolic emptying, and decreases diastolic heart size. It also reduces ventricular end-diastolic pressure and, consequently, pulmonary and systemic venous pressures. Increased myocardial contractility and cardiac output reflexively reduce sympathetic tone in patients with CHF. This compensates for the drug's direct vasoconstrictive action, thereby reducing total peripheral resistance. It also slows increased heart rate and causes diuresis in edematous patients.
• *Antiarrhythmic action:* Digoxin-induced heart-rate slowing in patients without CHF is negligible and stems mainly from vagal (cholinergic) and sympatholytic effects on the SA node; however, with toxic doses, heart-rate slowing results from direct depression of SA node automaticity. Therapeutic doses produce little effect on the action potential, but toxic doses increase the automaticity (spontaneous diastolic depolarization) of all cardiac regions except the SA node.
• *Kinetics in adults:* With tablet or elixir administration, 60% to 85% of dose is absorbed. With capsule form, bioavailability increases. About 90% to 100% of a dose is absorbed. With I.M. administration, about 80% of dose is absorbed. With oral administration, onset of action occurs in 30 minutes to 2 hours, with peak effects occurring in 6 to 8 hours. With I.M. administration, onset of action occurs in 30 minutes, with peak effects in 4 to 6 hours. With I.V. administration, action occurs in 5 to 30 minutes, with peak effects in 1 to 5 hours. Digoxin is distributed widely in body tissues; highest concentrations occur in the heart, kidneys, intestine, stomach, liver, and skeletal muscle; lowest concentrations are in the plasma and

brain. Digoxin crosses both the blood-brain barrier and the placenta; fetal and maternal digoxin levels are equivalent at birth. About 20% to 30% of drug is bound to plasma proteins. Usual therapeutic range for steady-state serum levels is 0.5 to 2 ng/ml. In treatment of atrial tachydysrhythmias, higher serum levels (such as 2 to 4 ng/ml) may be needed. Because of drug's long half-life, achievement of steady-state levels may take 7 days or longer, depending on patient's renal function. Toxic symptoms may appear within the usual therapeutic range; however, these are more frequent and serious with levels above 2.5 ng/ml. In most patients, a small amount of digoxin apparently is metabolized in the liver and gut by bacteria. This metabolism varies and may be substantial in some patients. Drug undergoes some enterohepatic recirculation (also variable). Metabolites have minimal cardiac activity. Most of dose is excreted by the kidneys as unchanged drug. Some patients excrete a substantial amount of metabolized or reduced drug. In patients with renal failure, biliary excretion is a more important excretion route. In healthy patients, terminal half-life is 30 to 40 hours. In patients lacking functioning kidneys, half-life increases to at least 4 days.

Contraindications and precautions
Digoxin is contraindicated in patients with ventricular fibrillation, because the drug may induce dysrhythmias; in patients with digoxin toxicity; and in patients with hypersensitivity to the drug.

Digoxin should be used with extreme caution, if at all, in patients with idiopathic hypertrophic subaortic stenosis, because the drug may cause increased obstruction of left ventricular outflow; in patients with incomplete AV block who do not have an artificial pacemaker (especially those with Stokes-Adams syndrome), because the drug may induce advanced or complete AV block; in patients with hypersensitive carotid sinus syndrome, because the drug increases vagal tone (carotid sinus massage has induced ventricular fibrillation in patients receiving cardiac glycosides); in patients with Wolff-Parkinson-White syndrome, because the drug may cause fatal ventricular dysrhythmias; in patients with sinus node disease (such as sick sinus syndrome), because the drug may worsen sinus bradycardia or SA block; in patients with severe pulmonary disease, hypoxia, myxedema, acute myocardial infarction, severe heart failure, acute myocarditis, or an otherwise damaged myocardium, because the drug increases the risk of dysrhythmias in these patients; in patients with chronic constrictive pericarditis, because such patients may respond unfavorably to the drug; in patients with frequent premature ventricular contractions or ventricular tachycardia (especially if these dysrhythmias do not result from heart failure), because the drug may induce dysrhythmias; in patients with low cardiac output states caused by valvular stenosis, chronic pericarditis, or chronic cor pulmonale, because the drug may decrease heart rate, which, in turn, may reduce cardiac output; and in patients with conditions that increase cardiac sensitivity to digitalis, including hypokalemia, chronic pulmonary disease, and acute hypoxemia.

I.V. digoxin should be used with caution in patients with hypertension, because I.V. administration may increase blood pressure transiently.

Interactions
Concomitant use of digoxin with antacids containing aluminum and/or magnesium hydroxide, magnesium trisilicate, kaolin-pectin, aminosalicylic acid, and sulfasalazine decreases absorption of orally administered digoxin. Cholestyramine and colestipol may bind digoxin in the GI tract and impair absorption.

Concomitant use with cytotoxic agents or radiation therapy may decrease digoxin absorption if the intestinal mucosa is damaged. (Use of digoxin elixir or capsules is recommended in this situation.) Concomitant use with amiodarone, diltiazem, flecainide, nifedipine, verapamil, or quinidine may cause increased serum digoxin levels, predisposing the patient to toxicity. Concomitant use with cardiac drugs affecting AV conduction (such as procainamide, propranolol, and verapamil) may cause additive cardiac effects. Concomitant use with sympathomimetics (such as ephedrine, epinephrine, and isoproterenol) or rauwolfia alkaloids may increase the risk of dysrhythmia.

When used concomitantly, erythromycin and tetracycline may interfere with bacterial flora that allow formation of inactive reduction products in the GI tract, possibly causing a significant increase in digoxin bioavailability and, consequently, increased serum digoxin levels.

Concomitant use with I.V. calcium preparations may cause synergistic effects that precipitate dysrhythmias. Concomitant use with electrolyte-altering agents may increase or decrease serum electrolyte concentrations, predisposing the patient to digoxin toxicity. For example, such diuretics as ethacrynic acid, furosemide, and bumetanide may cause hypokalemia and hypomagnesemia; thiazides may cause hypercalcemia. Fatal cardiac dysrhythmias may result. Amphotericin B, corticosteroids, corticotropin, edetate disodium, laxatives, and sodium polystyrene sulfonate deplete total body potassium, possibly causing digoxin toxicity. Glucagon, large dextrose doses, and dextrose-insulin infusions reduce extracellular potassium, possibly leading to digitalis toxicity. Concomitant use with succinylcholine may precipitate cardiac dysrhythmias by potentiating digoxin's effects.

Effects on diagnostic tests
None reported.

Adverse reactions
• CNS: fatigue, generalized weakness, agitation, hallucinations, headache, malaise, dizziness, vertigo, stupor, paresthesias.
• CV: *increased severity of CHF, dysrhythmias* (most commonly, conduction disturbances with or without AV block, premature ventricular contractions, and supraventricular dysrhythmias), hypotension, *bradycardia.* (Toxic cardiac effects may be life-threatening and require immediate attention.)
• EENT: yellow-green halos around visual images, blurred vision, light flashes, photophobia, diplopia.

• GI: *anorexia, nausea, vomiting, diarrhea, feeding intolerance, weight loss.*

Note: Drug should be discontinued if signs of digitalis toxicity are present (nausea, vomiting, dysrhythmias).

Overdose and treatment

Clinical effects of overdose are primarily gastrointestinal, CNS, and cardiac reactions.

Severe intoxication may cause hyperkalemia, which may develop rapidly and result in life-threatening cardiac manifestations. Cardiac signs of digoxin toxicity may occur with or without other toxicity signs and commonly precede other toxic effects. Because toxic cardiac effects also can occur as manifestations of heart disease, determining whether these effects result from underlying heart disease or digoxin toxicity may be difficult. Digoxin has caused almost every kind of dysrhythmia; various combinations of dysrhythmias may occur in the same patient. Patients with chronic digoxin toxicity commonly have ventricular dysrhythmias and/or AV conduction disturbances. Patients with digoxin-induced ventricular tachycardia have a high mortality, because ventricular fibrillation or asystole may result.

If toxicity is suspected, the drug should be discontinued and serum drug level measurements obtained. Usually, the drug takes at least 6 hours to equilibrate between plasma and tissue; plasma levels drawn earlier may show higher digoxin levels than those present after the drug distributes into the tissues.

Other treatment measures include immediate emesis induction, gastric lavage, and administration of activated charcoal to reduce absorption of drug remaining in the gut. Multiple doses of activated charcoal (such as 50 g q 6 hours) may help reduce further absorption, especially of any drug undergoing enterohepatic recirculation. Any interacting drugs probably should be discontinued. Ventricular dysrhythmias may be treated with I.V. potassium (replacement doses; but not in patients with significant AV block), I.V. phenytoin, I.V. lidocaine, or I.V. propranolol. Refractory ventricular tachydysrhythmias may be controlled with overdrive pacing. Procainamide may be used for ventricular dysrhythmias that do not respond to the above treatments. In severe AV block, asystole, and hemodynamically significant sinus bradycardia, atropine restores a normal rate.

Administration of digoxin-specific antibody fragments (digoxin immune Fab [Digibind]) is a promising new treatment for life-threatening digoxin toxicity. Each 40 mg of digoxin immune Fab binds about 0.6 mg of digoxin in the bloodstream. The complex is then excreted in the urine, rapidly decreasing serum levels and therefore cardiac drug concentrations.

▶ Special considerations

• Pediatric patients have a poorly defined toxic serum concentration range; however, toxicity apparently does not occur at same concentrations considered toxic in adults. Divided daily dosing is recommended for infants and children under age 10; older children require adult doses proportional to body weight.
• Obtain baseline heart rate and rhythm, blood pressure, and serum electrolyte levels before giving first dose.
• Question patient about use of cardiac glycosides within the previous 2 to 3 weeks before administering a loading dose. Always divide loading dose over first 24 hours unless clinical situation indicates otherwise.
• Adjust dose to patient's clinical condition; monitor ECG and serum levels of digoxin, calcium, potassium, and magnesium. Therapeutic serum digoxin levels range from 0.5 to 2 ng/ml. Serum concentration exceeding 3.5 ng/ml are considered toxic. Take corrective action before hypokalemia occurs.
• Monitor clinical status. Take apical-radial pulse for a full minute. Watch for significant changes (sudden rate increase or decrease, pulse deficit, irregular beats, and especially regularization of a previously irregular rhythm). Check blood pressure and obtain 12-lead ECG if these changes occur.
• GI absorption may be reduced in patients with CHF, especially right heart failure.
• Digoxin dosage generally should be reduced and serum level monitoring performed if patient is receiving digoxin concomitantly with amiodarone, diltiazem, flecainide, nifedipine, verapamil, or quinidine. Also monitor patient closely for signs and symptoms of digoxin toxicity. Obtain serum digoxin levels if you suspect toxicity.
• Because digoxin may predispose patients to postcardioversion asystole, most clinicians withhold digoxin 1 or 2 days before elective cardioversion in patients with atrial fibrillation. (However, consider consequences of increased ventricular response to atrial fibrillation if drug is withheld.)
• Elective cardioversion should be postponed in patients with signs of digoxin toxicity.
• Do not administer calcium salts to patient receiving digoxin. Calcium affects cardiac contractility and excitability in much the same way that digoxin does and may lead to serious dysrhythmias.
• Hypothyroid patients are highly sensitive to glycosides; hyperthyroid patients may need larger doses.
• Monitor patient's eating patterns. Ask him about nausea, vomiting, anorexia, visual disturbances, and other evidence of toxicity.
• Consider that different brands may not be therapeutically interchangeable.
• Digoxin solution is enclosed in newly available soft capsule (Lanoxicaps). Because these capsules are better absorbed than tablets, dose is usually slightly smaller.
• Avoid adult preparations of digoxin; only use vials marked "for pediatric use."
• I.V. digoxin can be diluted with dextrose 5% in water, normal saline solution, or sterile water using a fourfold or greater volume and administered over a period of 5 minutes or longer.
• Calculation of dosage and dose in syringe should be performed by at least two separate persons.
• Ask patient if he has a history of chronic or recent cardiac glycoside use before starting therapy.
• Monitor heart rate daily because of drug's effects on the cardiac conduction system. Slowing of the heart rate (60 to 70 beats/minute or less in older children; less than 90 to 110 beats/minute in neonates and

infants) may be an early sign of toxicity (except in patients with chronically slow heart rate).

• Obtain serum drug levels before administering morning dose or at least 6 to 12 hours after a dose is administered, because of drug's slow distribution.

• Higher-than-usual doses and serum drug levels may be needed to adequately control atrial tachydysrhythmia.

• Before prescribing additional drugs for patient currently receiving cardiac glycosides, review drug interactions, which are numerous and may seriously affect therapy.

• Hypokalemia associated with diuretic therapy may increase effects and toxicity.

Information for parents and patient
• Instruct parents and patient about drug action, medication regimen, how to take pulse, reportable signs, and follow-up plans.

• Instruct parents to have patient take drug only as directed and at same time every day.

• Teach parents and patient how to take pulse rate; advise them to call if rate drops below the patient's normal rate.

• Warn parents that patient should not take missed dose with next regularly scheduled dose. Tell them to call for instructions if patient misses more than two doses.

• Patient should avoid all nonprescription preparations, such as cough, cold, or allergy medications or diet drugs, except as directed.

• Instruct parents to report loss of appetite, stomach pain, nausea, vomiting, diarrhea, unusual fatigue or weakness, drowsiness, headache, blurred vision or yellow haloes, rash or hives, or depression.

• Warn parents that patient should not stop taking the drug without medical approval.

---

dihydrotachysterol
DHT, Hytakerol

• Classification: antihypocalcemic (vitamin D analog)

How supplied
Available by prescription only
Tablets: 0.125 mg, 0.2 mg, 0.4 mg
Capsules: 0.125 mg
Solution: 0.2 mg/ml (Intensol), 0.2 mg/5 ml (in 4% alcohol), 0.25 mg/ml (in sesame oil)

Indications, route, and dosage
Familial hypophosphatemia
Children and adults: 0.5 to 2 mg P.O. daily. Maintenance dose is 0.3 to 1.5 mg daily.
Hypocalcemia associated with hypoparathyroidism and pseudohypoparathyroidism
Children: Initially, 1 to 5 mg P.O. for several days. Maintenance dose is 0.2 to 1 mg daily, as required for normal serum calcium levels.
Adults: Initially, 0.8 to 2.4 mg P.O. daily for several days. Maintenance dose is 0.2 to 2 mg daily, as re-

quired for normal serum calcium levels. Average dose is 0.6 mg daily.
Renal osteodystrophy in chronic uremia
Adults: 0.1 to 0.6 mg P.O. daily.

Action and kinetics
• *Antihypocalcemic action:* Once activated to its 25-hydroxy form, dihydrotachysterol works with parathyroid hormone to regulate levels of calcium. It appears to have little activity as the parent compound.
• *Kinetics in adults:* Drug is absorbed readily from the small intestine and is distributed widely; it is largely protein-bound. Drug is metabolized in the liver and has a duration of action up to 9 weeks. It is excreted in urine and bile.

Contraindications and precautions
Dihydrotachysterol is contraindicated in patients with hypercalcemia or sensitivity to vitamin D.

Interactions
Antacids may alter absorption of dihydrotachysterol. Barbiturates, phenytoin, and primidone may increase metabolism and therefore reduce activity of dihydrotachysterol. The resulting increases in calcium may potentiate the effects of digitalis glycosides.

Effects on diagnostic tests
Drug alters serum alkaline phosphatase concentrations and cholesterol levels and may alter electrolytes, such as magnesium, phosphate, and calcium, in serum and urine.

Adverse reactions
Signs and symptoms of hypercalcemia:
• CNS: headache, lethargy, depression, amnesia, disorientation, hallucinations, syncope and coma.
• EENT: vertigo, tinnitus.
• GI: nausea, vomiting, abdominal cramps, constipation, anorexia.
• Other: weakness, polyuria and polydipsia (with impairment of renal function).
  Note: Drug should be discontinued if patient develops signs or symptoms of hypercalcemia.

Overdose and treatment
Hypercalcemia is the only clinical manifestation of overdose. Treatment involves discontinuing therapy, instituting a low-calcium diet, increasing fluid intake, and providing supportive measures. In severe cases, death from cardiac and renal failure has occurred. Calcitonin administration may help reverse hypercalcemia.

▶ Special considerations
• Some infants may be hyperreactive to drug.
• Monitor serum and urine calcium levels. Observe patient for signs and symptoms of hypercalcemia.
• Adequate dietary calcium intake is necessary; it is usually supplemented with 10 to 15 g oral calcium lactate or gluconate daily.
• One milligram of dihydrotachysterol is equal to 120,000 units ergocalciferol (vitamin D_2).
• Store in tightly closed, light-resistant containers. Do not refrigerate.

Information for parents and patient
Explain the importance of a calcium-rich diet.

dimenhydrinate
Apo-Dimenhydrinate*, Calm X, Dimentabs, Dinate, Dommanate, Dramamine, Dramilin, Dramocen, Dramoject, Dymenate, Gravol*, Hydrate, Marmine, Motion-Aid, Nauseatol*, Novodimenate*, PMS-Dimenhydrinate*, Reidamine, Travamine*, Wehamine

- Classification: antihistamine, H_1-receptor antagonist, antiemetic, antivertigo agent (ethanolamine derivative)

How supplied
Available with or without prescription
Tablets: 50 mg
Liquid: 12.5 mg/4 ml
Injection: 50 mg/ml
Rectal: 50 mg, 100 mg

Indications, route, and dosage
Nausea, vomiting, dizziness of motion sickness (prophylaxis and treatment)
Children: 5 mg/kg/day P.O. I.M. or rectally in four divided doses; or 150 mg/m²/day P.O. in four divided doses, not to exceed 300 mg/day, or according to the following schedule:
Children under age 2: 1.25 mg/kg I.M. or I.V.; or 37.5 mg/m² I.M. or I.V. Do not use in neonates and premature infants.
Children age 2 to 6: 12.5 to 25 mg P.O. q 6 to 8 hours; maximum dosage is 75 mg/day.
Children age 6 to 12: 25 to 50 mg P.O. q 6 to 8 hours; maximum dosage is 150 mg/day.
Children age 12 and over and adults: 50 to 100 mg q 4 hours P.O., I.V., or I.M. (and rectally where available). For I.V. administration, dilute each 50-mg dose in 10 ml of normal saline solution and inject slowly over 2 minutes.
Drug has been used to treat Meniere's disease. Dosage is 50 mg I.M. for acute attack, 25 to 50 mg t.i.d. for maintenance.

Action and kinetics
- *Antiemetic and antivertigo action:* Dimenhydrinate probably inhibits nausea and vomiting by centrally depressing sensitivity of the labyrinth apparatus that relays stimuli to the chemoreceptor trigger zone and stimulates the vomiting center in the brain.
- *Kinetics in adults:* Dimenhydrinate is well absorbed. The drug is well distributed throughout the body and crosses the placenta. It is metabolized in the liver and excreted in urine.

Contraindications and precautions
Dimenhydrinate is contraindicated in children with known hypersensitivity to this drug or to other antiemetic antihistamines with a similar chemical structure, such as diphenhydramine; and in those sensitive to theophylline, because dimenhydrinate is the 8-chlorotheophylline salt of diphenhydramine.

Dimenhydrinate should be used with caution in patients with narrow-angle glaucoma, asthma, or GU or GI obstruction, because of the drug's anticholinergic effects; and in patients with seizure disorders. Drug may mask signs of brain tumor or intestinal obstruction.

Safety in neonates has not been established. Infants and children under age 6 may experience paradoxical hyperexcitability. I.V. dosage for children has not been established.

Interactions
Additive CNS sedation and depression may occur when drug is used concomitantly with other CNS depressants, such as alcohol, barbiturates, tranquilizers, sleeping agents, and antianxiety agents.

Dimenhydrinate may mask the signs of ototoxicity caused by known ototoxic agents, including the aminoglycosides, salicylates, vancomycin, loop diuretics, and cisplatin.

Effects on diagnostic tests
Dimenhydrinate may alter or confuse test results for xanthines (caffeine, aminophylline) because of its 8-chlorotheophylline content; discontinue dimenhydrinate 4 days before diagnostic skin tests, to avoid preventing, reducing, or masking test response.

Adverse reactions
- CNS: drowsiness, dizziness, headache, *incoordination, convulsions.*
- CV: palpitations, hypotension.
- EENT: blurred vision, tinnitus, dry mouth and respiratory passages.
- GI: constipation, diarrhea, anorexia.
- GU: urinary frequency, dysuria.

Overdose and treatment
Clinical manifestations of overdose may include either CNS depression (sedation, reduced mental alertness, apnea, and cardiovascular collapse) or CNS stimulation (insomnia, hallucinations, tremors, or convulsions). Anticholinergic symptoms, such as dry mouth, flushed skin, fixed and dilated pupils, and GI symptoms, are likely to occur, especially in children.

Use gastric lavage to empty stomach contents; emetics may be ineffective. Diazepam or phenytoin may be used to control seizures. Treat supportively.

▶ Special considerations
- Children, especially those under age 6, may experience paradoxical hyperexcitability with restlessness, insomnia, nervousness, euphoria, tremors, and seizures.
- Antihistamines are contraindicated during an acute asthma attack, because they may not alleviate the symptoms and because antimuscarinic effects can cause thickening of secretions.
- Reduce GI distress by giving antihistamines with food; give sugarless gum, sour hard candy, or ice chips to relieve dry mouth; increase fluid intake (if allowed)

---

*Canada only †Unlabeled clinical use Italicized adverse reactions have been observed in children.

or humidify air to decrease adverse effect of thickened secretions.
- If tolerance develops, another antihistamine may be substituted.
- Dimenhydrinate may mask ototoxicity from high doses of aspirin and other salicylates.
- Incorrectly administered or undiluted I.V. solution is irritating to veins and may cause sclerosis.
- Parenteral solution is incompatible with many drugs; do not mix other drugs in the same syringe.
- Advise safety measures for all patients; dimenhydrinate has a high incidence of drowsiness. Tolerance to CNS depressant effects usually develops within a few days.
- To prevent motion sickness, patient should take medication ½ hour before traveling and again before meals and at bedtime.
- Antiemetic effect may diminish with prolonged use.

Information for parents and patient
- Advise patient to take drug with meals or snack to prevent gastric upset and to use any of the following measures to relieve dry mouth: warm water rinses, artificial saliva, ice chips, or sugarless gum or candy. Patient should avoid overusing mouthwash, which may add to dryness (alcohol content) and destroy normal flora.
- Warn parents that child should avoid hazardous activities until extent of CNS effects are known. Tell them to seek medical approval before administering tranquilizers, sedatives, pain relievers, or sleeping medications.
- Warn parents to discontinue drug 4 days before diagnostic skin tests, to preserve accuracy of tests.

diphenhydramine hydrochloride
Beldin, Benadryl, Benadryl Children's Allergy, Benadryl Complete Allergy, Bendylate, Benylin, Compoz, Diahist, Diphen, Diphenadril, Fenylhist, Fynex, Hydramine, Hydril, Insomnal∗, Nervine Nighttime Sleep-Aid, Noradryl, Nordryl, Nytol with DPH, Robalyn, Sleep-Eze 3, Sominex Formula 2, Tusstat, Twilite, Valdrene

- Classification: antihistamine, H_1-receptor antagonist, antiemetic, antivertigo agent, antitussive, sedative-hypnotic, topical anesthetic, anticholinergic antidyskinetic agent (ethanolamine derivative)

How supplied
Available with or without prescription
Tablets: 25 mg, 50 mg
Capsules: 25 mg, 50 mg
Elixir: 12.5 mg/5 ml (14% alcohol)
Syrup: 12.5 mg/5 ml, 13.3 mg/5 ml (5% alcohol)
Injection: 10 mg/ml, 50 mg/ml
Cream: 1%, 2%
Lotion: 2%

Indications, route, and dosage
Allergic rhinitis, urticaria, allergic reactions to blood or plasma (antihistamine)
Children: 1.25 mg/kg P.O. every 4 to 6 hours; or 37.5 mg/m² P.O. every 4 to 6 hours, not to exceed 300 mg/day. (For children weighing less than 9.1 kg, 6.25 to 12.5 mg P.O. every 4 to 6 hours. For children weighing 9.1 kg and over, 12.5 to 25 mg P.O. every 4 to 6 hours.) Or 1.25 mg/kg or 37.5 mg/m² I.M. q.i.d., not to exceed 300 mg/day.
Adults: 25 to 50 mg P.O. every 4 to 6 hours p.r.n.; or 10 to 50 mg I.V. or deep I.M.
Motion sickness or vertigo
Children: 1 to 1.5 mg/kg P.O. every 4 to 6 hours p.r.n.; or 1 to 1.5 mg/kg I.M. every 6 hours, not to exceed 300 mg/day.
Adults: 25 to 50 mg P.O. every 4 to 6 hours p.r.n.; or 10 mg I.M. or I.V. initially, then 20 to 50 mg I.M. or I.V. every 2 to 3 hours p.r.n.
Cough
Children age 2 to 5: 6.25 mg P.O. q 4 to 6 hours; maximum dosage is 25 mg/day.
Children age 6 to 12: 12.5 mg P.O. q 4 to 6 hours; maximum dosage is 50 mg/day.
Adults: 25 mg P.O. q 4 to 6 hours.
Control of dyskinetic movement
Children: 5 mg/kg/day divided t.i.d. or q.i.d.
Adults: Initially, 25 mg t.i.d., increased to 50 mg q.i.d.; or 10 to 50 mg I.M. or I.V.

Action and kinetics
- *Antihistamine action:* Antihistamines compete for histamine H_1-receptor sites on the smooth muscle of the bronchi, GI tract, uterus, and large blood vessels; by binding to cellular receptors, they prevent access of histamine and suppress histamine-induced allergic symptoms, even though they do not prevent its release.
- *Antivertigo, antiemetic, and antidyskinetic action:* Central antimuscarinic actions of antihistamines probably are responsible for these effects of diphenhydramine.
- *Antitussive action:* Diphenhydramine suppresses the cough reflex by a direct effect on the cough center.
- *Sedative action:* Mechanism of the CNS depressant effects of diphenhydramine is unknown.
- *Anesthetic action:* Diphenhydramine is structurally related to local anesthetics, which prevent initiation and transmission of nerve impulses; this is the probable source of its topical and local anesthetic effects.
- *Kinetics in adults:* Diphenhydramine is well absorbed from the GI tract. Action begins within 15 to 30 minutes and peaks in 1 to 4 hours. Diphenhydramine is distributed widely throughout the body, including the CNS; drug crosses the placenta and is excreted in breast milk. Diphenhydramine is approximately 82% protein-bound. About 50% to 60% of an oral dose of diphenhydramine is metabolized by the liver before reaching the systemic circulation (first-pass effect); virtually all available drug is metabolized by the liver within 24 to 48 hours. Plasma elimination half-life of diphenhydramine is about 3½ hours; drug and metabolites are excreted primarily in urine.

Contraindications and precautions

Diphenhydramine is contraindicated in patients with known hypersensitivity to this drug or antihistamines with similar chemical structures (carbinoxamine and clemastine); during an acute asthma attack, because diphenhydramine thickens bronchial secretions; and in patients who have taken MAO inhibitors within the past 2 weeks. (See Interactions.)

Diphenhydramine should be used with caution in patients with narrow-angle glaucoma; in those with pyloroduodenal obstruction or urinary bladder obstruction from narrowing of the bladder neck, because of their marked anticholinergic effects; in patients with cardiovascular disease, hypertension, or hyperthyroidism, because of the risk of palpitations and tachycardia; and in patients with renal disease, diabetes, bronchial asthma, urinary retention, or stenosing peptic ulcers.

Benadryl 25 contains bisulfites, which can cause severe reactions in individuals allergic to these chemicals.

Diphenhydramine should not be used in premature infants or neonates. Infants and children, especially those under age 6, may experience paradoxical hyperexcitability.

Interactions

MAO inhibitors interfere with the detoxification of diphenhydramine and thus prolong their central depressant and anticholinergic effects; additive CNS depression may occur when carbinoxamine is given concomitantly with other CNS depressants, such as alcohol, barbiturates, tranquilizers, sleeping aids, and antianxiety agents.

Diphenhydramine may diminish the effects of sulfonylureas, enhance the effects of epinephrine, and partially counteract the anticoagulant effects of heparin.

Effects on diagnostic tests

Discontinue diphenhydramine 4 days before diagnostic skin tests; antihistamines can prevent, reduce, or mask positive skin test response.

Adverse reactions

• CNS: drowsiness, sedation, dizziness, disturbed coordination, confusion, headache, *insomnia, restlessness, vertigo;* (in children) fever, ataxia, *excitement, seizures,* hallucinations.
• CV: hypotension, palpitations, tachycardia, extrasystoles.
• DERM: photosensitivity, urticaria.
• EENT: blurred vision, diplopia, dry nose and throat.
• GI: dry mouth, nausea, vomiting, diarrhea, constipation, epigastric distress, anorexia.
• GU: urinary frequency, dysuria, urinary retention.
• HEMA: leukopenia, agranulocytosis, hemolytic anemia.
• Respiratory: chest tightness, wheezing, thickened bronchial secretions, anaphylaxis.

Overdose and treatment

Drowsiness is the usual clinical manifestation of overdose. Seizures, coma, and respiratory depression may occur with profound overdose. Anticholinergic symptoms, such as dry mouth, flushed skin, fixed and dilated pupils, and GI symptoms, are common, especially in children.

Treat overdose by inducing emesis with ipecac syrup (in conscious patient), followed by activated charcoal to reduce further drug absorption. Use gastric lavage if patient is unconscious or ipecac fails. Treat hypotension with vasopressors, and control seizures with diazepam or phenytoin. *Do not give stimulants.*

▶ Special considerations

• Children, especially those under age 6, may experience paradoxical hyperexcitability with restlessness, insomnia, nervousness, euphoria, tremors, and seizures.
• Drug is contraindicated during an acute asthma attack, because it may not alleviate the symptoms and because antimuscarinic effects can cause thickening of secretions.
• Diphenhydramine injection is compatible with most I.V. solutions but is *incompatible* with some drugs; check compatibility before mixing in the same I.V. line.
• Alternate injection sites to prevent irritation. Administer deep I.M. into large muscle.
• Drowsiness is the most common side effect during initial therapy but usually disappears with continued use of the drug.
• Injectable and elixir solutions are light-sensitive; protect from light.

Information for parents and patients

• Advise patient to take drug with meals or snack to prevent gastric upset and to use any of the following measures to relieve dry mouth: warm water rinses, artificial saliva, ice chips, or sugarless gum or candy. Patient should avoid overusing mouthwash, which may add to dryness (alcohol content) and destroy normal flora.
• Warn parents that child should avoid hazardous activities until extent of CNS effect are known. Tell them to seek medical approval before administering tranquilizers, sedatives, pain relievers, or sleeping medications.
• Warn parents to discontinue drug 4 days before diagnostic skin tests, to preserve accuracy of tests.

---

diphenoxylate hydrochloride (with atropine sulfate)
Diphenatol, Latropine, Lofene, Lomanate, Lomotil, Lonox, Lo-Quel, Lo-Trol, Nor-Mil

• Classification: antidiarrheal (opiate)
• Controlled substance schedule V

How supplied

Available by prescription only
Tablets: 2.5 mg diphenoxylate hydrochloride and 0.025 mg atropine sulfate per tablet
Liquid: 2.5 mg diphenoxylate hydrochloride and 0.025 mg atropine sulfate/5 ml

---

Indications, route, and dosage
Acute, nonspecific diarrhea
Children age 2 and over: 0.3 to 0.4 mg/kg/day diphenoxylate component in divided doses; or administer according to diphenoxylate component, as follows:
Children age 2 to 3 (11 to 14 kg): 0.75 to 1.5 mg q.i.d.
Children age 3 to 4 (12 to 16 kg): 1 to 1.5 mg q.i.d.
Children age 4 to 5 (14 to 20 kg): 1 to 2 mg q.i.d.
Children age 5 to 6 (16 to 23 kg): 1.25 to 2.25 mg q.i.d.
Children age 6 to 9 (17 to 32 kg): 1.25 to 2.5 mg q.i.d.
Children age 9 to 12 (23 to 55 kg): 1.75 to 2.5 mg q.i.d.
Children over age 12: Give usual adult dose.
Adults: 1 to 2 tablets or tsp t.i.d. or q.i.d. initially; decrease dose to 1 tablet or tsp b.i.d. or t.i.d.

Action and kinetics
• *Antidiarrheal action:* Diphenoxylate is a meperidine analogue that inhibits GI motility locally and centrally. In high doses, it may produce an opiate effect. Atropine is added in subtherapeutic doses to prevent abuse by deliberate overdose.
• *Kinetics in adults:* About 90% of an oral dose is absorbed. Action begins in 45 to 60 minutes. Drug is distributed in breast milk and metabolized extensively by the liver. Metabolites are excreted mainly in feces via the biliary tract, with lesser amounts excreted in urine. Duration of effect is 3 to 4 hours.

Contraindications and precautions
Diphenoxylate is contraindicated in patients with known hypersensitivity to this drug, atropine, or meperidine; in patients with obstructive jaundice, because of potential for hepatic coma; and in patients with diarrhea caused by pseudomembranous colitis, because of potential for toxic megacolon. Use cautiously in patients with diarrhea caused by poisoning or by infection by *Shigella, Salmonella,* and some strains of *Escherichia coli,* because expulsion of intestinal contents may be a protective mechanism.

Diphenoxylate should be used with extreme caution in patients with impaired hepatic function, cirrhosis, advanced hepatorenal disease, or abnormal liver function test results, because the drug may precipitate hepatic coma.

Interactions
Diphenoxylate may precipitate hypertensive crisis in patients receiving MAO inhibitors. Concomitant use with such CNS depressants as barbiturates, tranquilizers, and alcohol may result in an increased depressant effect.

Effects on diagnostic tests
Diphenoxylate may decrease urinary excretion of phenolsulfonphthalein (PSP) during the PSP excretion test; drug may increase serum amylase levels.

Adverse reactions
• CNS: sedation, dizziness, headache, drowsiness, lethargy, restlessness, depression, euphoria.
• CV: tachycardia.
• DERM: pruritus, giant urticaria, rash, dryness.
• EENT: mydriasis.
• GI: dry mouth, nausea, vomiting, abdominal discomfort or distention, paralytic ileus, anorexia, fluid retention in bowel (may mask depletion of extracellular fluid and electrolytes, especially in young children treated for acute gastroenteritis), abdominal cramps, toxic megacolon, constipation.
• GU: urinary retention.
• Other: possible physical dependence in long-term use, angioedema, *respiratory depression,* flushing, fever, dry mucous membranes.
Note: Drug should be discontinued if signs of CNS depression develop or if response does not occur within 48 hours.

Overdose and treatment
Overdose in children is particularly hazardous. Clinical effects of overdose include drowsiness, low blood pressure, marked seizures, apnea, blurred vision, miosis, flushing, dry mouth and mucous membranes, and psychotic episodes.

Treatment is supportive; maintain airway and support vital functions. A narcotic antagonist, such as naloxone, may be given. Gastric lavage may be performed. Monitor patient for 48 to 72 hours.

▶ Special considerations
• Drug is contraindicated in children under age 2; some children may experience respiratory depression. Children, especially those with Down's syndrome, appear to be particularly sensitive to atropine content of this medication.
• Children age 2 to 12 should be given the oral solution rather than the tablet.
• Monitor vital signs and intake and output; observe patient for adverse reactions, especially CNS reactions.
• Monitor bowel function. Observe for signs of paralytic ileus.
• Drug is usually ineffective in treating antibiotic-induced diarrhea.
• Reduce dosage as soon as symptoms are controlled. Withdrawal symptoms may occur after prolonged use.
• Uncomplicated diarrhea in children is often better left untreated. Especially in young children, inhibition of peristalsis can cause retention of fluid in the bowel, worsening dehydration and electrolyte imbalance; it may also change response to the drug.

Information for parents and patient
• Warn parents to give drug exactly as ordered and not to exceed recommended dose.
• Explain that patient should maintain adequate fluid intake during course of diarrhea. Teach parents about diet and fluid replacement.
• Caution parents that patient should avoid hazardous activities that require alertness because drug may cause drowsiness and dizziness; warn parents that patient should avoid alcohol while taking this drug because additive depressant effect may occur.
• Advise parents to call physician if drug is not effective within 48 hours.
• Warn parents that prolonged use may result in tol-

erance and that use of larger-than-recommended doses may result in drug dependence.

diphtheria and tetanus toxoids, adsorbed, combined

• Classification: diphtheria and tetanus prophylaxis agent (toxoid)

How supplied
Available by prescription only
Available in pediatric (DT) and adult (Td) strengths
Injection: pediatric — 6.6 to 15 Lf units of inactivated diphtheria and 5 to 10 Lf units of inactivated tetanus per 0.5 ml, in 5-ml vials; adult — 1.4 to 2 Lf units of inactivated diphtheria and 5 to 10 Lf units of inactivated tetanus per 0.5 ml, in 5-ml vials

Indications, route, and dosage
Primary immunization
Infants age 6 weeks to 1 year: Use pediatric strength. Give three 0.5-ml doses I.M. at least 8 weeks apart. Give booster dose 6 to 12 months after third injection.
Children age 1 to 6: Use pediatric strength. Give two 0.5-ml doses I.M. at least 8 weeks apart. Give booster dose 6 to 12 months after the second injection. If the final immunizing dose is given after the 7th birthday, use the adult strength.
Children over age 7 and adults: Use adult strength. Give 0.5 ml I.M. 4 to 8 weeks apart for two doses and a third dose 1 year later. Booster dosage is 0.5 ml I.M. q 10 years.

Action and kinetics
• *Diphtheria and tetanus prophylaxis:* Diphtheria and tetanus toxoids promote active immunization to diphtheria and tetanus by inducing production of antitoxins.
• *Kinetics in adults:* No information available.

Contraindications and precautions
Diphtheria and tetanus toxoids are contraindicated in patients with an acute respiratory infection or any other active infection. Defer elective immunization during these situations and during outbreaks of poliomyelitis. Defer immunization until the 2nd year of life in an infant with a history of seizures or CNS damage. (Use single antigen when immunizing such patients.) This preparation also is contraindicated in patients with a known hypersensitivity to thimerosal, a component of the toxoid, and in immunosuppressed patients (those with congenital immunodeficiencies, cancer, or acquired immunodeficiency syndrome and those being treated with corticosteroids, antineoplastic agents, or radiation).

Interactions
Concomitant use with corticosteroids or immunosuppressants may impair the immune response to diphtheria and tetanus toxoids. Avoid elective immunization under these circumstances.

Effects on diagnostic tests
None reported.

Adverse reactions
• Local: stinging, edema, erythema, pain, induration; a nodule may develop and last several weeks.
• Systemic: fretfulness, drowsiness, anorexia, vomiting, chills, fever, flushing, malaise, arthralgia, myalgia, anaphylaxis.

Overdose and treatment
No information available.

▶ Special considerations
• Obtain a thorough history of allergies and reactions to immunizations.
• Epinephrine solution 1:1,000 should be available to treat allergic reactions.
• Diphtheria and tetanus toxoids are used primarily when pertussis vaccine is contraindicated or used separately.
• These toxoids are not used to treat active tetanus or diphtheria infections.
• Although teratogenicity has not been reported, immunization during pregnancy is generally not recommended.
• Administer in site not previously used for vaccines or toxoids.
• To prevent sciatic nerve damage, avoid administration in gluteal muscle.
• Store toxoids between 36° and 46° F. (2° and 8° C.). Do not freeze.

Information for parents and patient
• Inform parents that child may experience discomfort at the injection site and that a nodule may develop there and persist for several weeks after immunization. He also may develop fever, headache, upset stomach, general malaise, or body aches and pains. Tell parents to relieve such effects with acetaminophen and to report any distressing adverse reactions.
• Stress the importance of keeping all scheduled appointments for subsequent doses because full immunization requires a series of injections.

diphtheria antitoxin, equine

• Classification: diphtheria antitoxin

How supplied
Available by prescription only
Injection: not less than 500 units/ml in 10,000-unit and 20,000-unit vials

Indications, route, and dosage
Diphtheria prevention
Children and adults: 1,000 to 10,000 units I.M. (dose dependent on length of time since exposure, extent of exposure, and individual's medical condition).
Diphtheria treatment
Children and adults: 20,000 to 120,000 units slow I.V. infusion in normal saline solution (dose based on

---

extent of disease). A 1:20 dilution of the antitoxin is infused at 1 ml/minute. Additional doses may be given in 24 hours. I.M. route may be used in mild cases. Begin antibiotic therapy.

Action and kinetics
• *Antitoxin action:* Diphtheria antitoxin neutralizes and binds toxin.
• *Kinetics in adults:* Absorption, distribution, metabolism, and excretion have not been described.

Contraindications and precautions
Because this product is derived from horses immunized with diphtheria toxin, an intradermal or scratch skin test and a conjunctival test for sensitivity to equine serum (against a control of normal saline solution) should be performed before administering diphtheria antitoxin. If sensitivity test is positive, check desensitization schedule.

Interactions
None reported.

Effects on diagnostic tests
None reported.

Adverse reactions
• Local: erythema, tenderness, and induration at injection site.
• Systemic: hypersensitivity, anaphylaxis; serum sickness (urticaria, pruritus, fever, malaise, and arthralgia) may occur within 7 to 12 days. Discontinue if severe systemic reactions occur.

Overdose and treatment
No information available.

▶ Special considerations
• Obtain a thorough patient history of allergies, especially to horses and horse immune serum; of asthma; and of previous reactions to immunizations.
• Epinephrine solution 1:1,000 should be available to treat allergic reactions.
• All asymptomatic nonimmunized contacts of patients with diphtheria should receive prompt prophylaxis with antibiotic therapy and have cultures taken before and after treatment. The patient should receive diphtheria toxoid and be monitored for 7 days thereafter.
• Therapy should begin immediately, without waiting for culture and sensitivity test results, if patient has clinical symptoms of diphtheria (sore throat, fever, and tonsillar membrane involvement).
• Refrigerate the antitoxin at 36° to 46° F. (2° to 8° C.). It also may be warmed to 90° to 93° F. (32° to 34° C.); higher temperatures will diminish potency.

Information for parents and patient
• Tell parents that patient may experience allergic reactions (such as rash, joint swelling or pain, or difficulty breathing) but that he will be monitored closely and will receive medication, as needed, to relieve such effects.
• Delayed effects associated with this antitoxin may

occur in 7 to 12 days after treatment. Encourage parents to report all unusual symptoms.

---

diphtheria toxoid, adsorbed

• Classification: diphtheria prophylaxis agent (toxoid)

How supplied
Available by prescription only
Injection: Suspension of 15 Lf units inactivated diphtheria per 0.5 ml, in 5-ml vials

Indications, route, and dosage
Diphtheria immunization
Children under age 6: 0.5 ml I.M. 6 to 8 weeks apart for two doses and a third dose 1 year later. Booster dosage is 0.5 ml I.M. at 5- to 10-year intervals. Not advised for adults or for children over age 6; instead, use adult strength of diphtheria toxoid (usually available as diphtheria and tetanus toxoids, adsorbed combined).

Action and kinetics
• *Diphtheria prophylaxis:* Diphtheria toxoid promotes active immunity to diphtheria by inducing production of antitoxin.
• *Kinetics in adults:* No information available.

Contraindications and precautions
Diphtheria toxoid is contraindicated in patients with an acute respiratory infection or any other active infection. Defer elective immunization during these situations and during outbreaks of poliomyelitis.

Defer immunization until the 2nd year of life in infants with a history of seizures or CNS damage. (Alternatively, one-tenth the recommended initial dosage may be used, followed by standard doses if no untoward effect occurs.)

Diphtheria toxoid is not recommended for adults or for children over age 6. This preparation also is contraindicated in patients with known hypersensitivity to thimerosal, a component of the toxoid, and in immunosuppressed patients (those with congenital immunodeficiencies, cancer, or acquired immune deficiency syndrome and those undergoing treatment with corticosteroids, antineoplastic agents, or radiation).

Interactions
Concomitant use of diphtheria toxoid with corticosteroids or immunosuppressants may impair the immune response to the toxoid. Avoid elective immunization under these circumstances.

Effects on diagnostic tests
None reported.

Adverse reactions
• Local: erythema, pain, and induration at injection site; a nodule may develop and persist for several weeks.
• Systemic: fever, malaise, urticaria, tachycardia,

---

flushing, pruritus, hypotension, myalgia, arthralgia, anaphylaxis.

Overdose and treatment
No information available.

▶ **Special considerations**
• Obtain a thorough history of allergies and reactions to immunizations.
• Epinephrine solution 1:1,000 should be available to treat allergic reactions.
• This preparation is used primarily when products containing tetanus toxoid or pertussis vaccine would not be advisable.
• Shake well before using.
• Do not use diphtheria toxoid to treat active diphtheria infections.
• Store between 36° and 46° F. (2° and 8° C.). Do not freeze.

Information for parents and patient
• Explain to parents that child may experience discomfort at the injection site after immunization and may develop a nodule there that can persist for several weeks. The child also may develop fever, general malaise, or body aches and pains. Recommend acetaminophen to relieve minor discomfort.
• Tell parents to report any worrisome or intolerable adverse reactions promptly.
• Emphasize the importance of keeping scheduled appointments for subsequent doses. Full immunization requires a series of injections.

---

disopyramide phosphate
Napamide, Norpace, Norpace CR, Rythmodon∗, Rythmodon-LA∗

• *Classification:* ventricular antiarrhythmic, supraventricular antiarrhythmic, atrial antitachyarrhythmic (pyridine derivative)

How supplied
Available by prescription only
Capsules: 100 mg, 150 mg
Capsules (extended-release): 100 mg, 150 mg

Indications, route, and dosage
Premature ventricular contractions (unifocal, multifocal, or coupled); ventricular tachycardia not severe enough to require electrocardioversion
Children age 1 and under: 10 to 30 mg/kg/day.
Children age 1 to 4: 10 to 20 mg/kg/day.
Children age 4 to 12: 10 to 15 mg/kg/day.
Children age 12 to 18: 6 to 15 mg/kg/day.
    All children's doses should be divided into equal amounts and given every 6 hours. Extended-release capsules not recommended for use in children.
Adults: Usual maintenance dosage is 150 to 200 mg P.O. q 6 hours; for patients who weigh less than 50 kg or those with renal, hepatic, or cardiac impairment, dosage is 100 mg P.O. q 6 hours. May give sustained-release capsule q 12 hours. Recommended dosages in advanced renal insufficiency: creatinine clearance 15 to 40 ml/minute—100 mg q 10 hours; creatinine clearance 5 to 15 ml/minute—100 mg q 20 hours; creatinine clearance 1 to 5 ml/minute—100 mg q 30 hours.

Action and kinetics
• *Antiarrhythmic action:* A Class IA antiarrhythmic agent, disopyramide depresses phase 0 of the action potential. It is considered a myocardial depressant because it decreases myocardial excitability and conduction velocity and may depress myocardial contractility. It also possesses anticholinergic activity that may modify the drug's direct myocardial effects. In therapeutic doses, disopyramide reduces conduction velocity in the atria, ventricles, and His-Purkinje system. By prolonging the effective refractory period (ERP), it helps control atrial tachyarrhythmias (however, this indication is unapproved in the United States). Its anticholinergic action, which is much greater than quinidine's, may increase AV node conductivity.
    Disopyramide also has a greater myocardial depressant (negative inotropic) effect than quinidine. It helps manage premature ventricular beats by suppressing automaticity in the His-Purkinje system and ectopic pacemakers. At therapeutic doses, it usually does not prolong the QRS segment duration and PR interval but may prolong the QT interval.
• *Kinetics in adults:* Disopyramide is rapidly and well absorbed from the GI tract; about 60% to 80% of the drug reaches systemic circulation. Onset of action usually occurs in 30 minutes; peak blood levels occur approximately 2 hours after administration of conventional capsules and 5 hours after administration of extended-release capsules. Disopyramide is well distributed throughout extracellular fluid but is not extensively bound to tissues. Plasma protein binding varies, depending on drug concentration levels, but generally ranges from about 50% to 65%. Usual therapeutic serum level ranges from 2 to 4 mcg/ml, although some patients may require up to 7 mcg/ml. Levels above 9 mcg/ml generally are considered toxic. Disopyramide is metabolized in the liver to one major metabolite that possesses little antiarrhythmic activity but greater anticholinergic activity than the parent compound. About 90% of an orally administered dose is excreted in the urine as unchanged drug and metabolites; 40% to 60% is excreted as unchanged drug. Usual elimination half-life is about 7 hours but lengthens in patients with renal and/or hepatic insufficiency. Duration of effect is usually 6 to 7 hours.

Contraindications and precautions
Disopyramide is contraindicated in patients with second- or third-degree heart block (unless a pacemaker is in place), because of the drug's effects on AV conduction; in patients with myasthenia gravis, because the drug's anticholinergic effect may precipitate a myasthenic crisis; in patients with untreated glaucoma or urinary retention because of the drug's anticholinergic effect (however, disopyramide may be used with caution in such patients if they are treated

appropriately and monitored carefully); in patients with uncompensated CHF and cardiogenic shock, because of the drug's negative inotropic effect; and in patients with known hypersensitivity to the drug.

Disopyramide should be used with caution in patients with sick sinus syndrome, Wolff-Parkinson-White syndrome, or bundle branch block, because of the drug's unpredictable effects on AV conduction; and in patients with renal or hepatic insufficiency, because decreased drug elimination may cause toxicity.

Interactions
When used concomitantly, other antiarrhythmic agents may cause additive or antagonistic cardiac effects and additive toxicity. Concomitant use with enzyme inducers, such as rifampin, may impair disopyramide's antiarrhythmic activity. Concomitant use with anticholinergic agents may cause additive anticholinergic effects. Concomitant use with warfarin may potentiate anticoagulant effects. Insulin may cause additive hypoglycemia.

Effects on diagnostic tests
The physiologic effects of disopyramide may cause a decrease in blood glucose concentrations.

Adverse reactions
• CNS: dizziness, agitation, depression, fatigue, muscle weakness, syncope.
• CV: hypotension, CHF, heart block, edema, chest pain.
• DERM: rash (1% to 3%).
• EENT: blurred vision, dry eyes and nose.
• GI: nausea, vomiting, anorexia, bloating, abdominal pain, constipation, dry mouth.
• GU: urinary retention and hesitancy (particularly in males).
• Hepatic: cholestatic jaundice.
• Metabolic: hypoglycemia.
   Note: Drug should be discontinued if hypotension, progressive heart failure, or heart block occurs; if the QRS complex widens by 25% to 50% over baseline; or if the QT interval lengthens.

Overdose and treatment
Clinical manifestations of overdose include anticholinergic effects, severe hypotension, widening of QRS complex and QT interval, ventricular dysrhythmias, cardiac conduction disturbances, bradycardia, CHF, asystole, loss of consciousness, seizures, apnea episodes, and respiratory arrest.

Treatment involves general supportive measures (including respiratory and cardiovascular support) and hemodynamic and ECG monitoring. If ingestion was recent, gastric lavage, emesis induction, and administration of activated charcoal may decrease absorption. Isoproterenol or dopamine may be administered to correct hypotension, after adequate hydration has been ensured. Digoxin and diuretics may be administered to treat heart failure. Hemodialysis and charcoal hemoperfusion may effectively remove disopyramide. Some patients may require intraaortic balloon counterpulsation, mechanically assisted respiration, and/or endocardial pacing.

▶ Special considerations
• Although drug's safety and effectiveness in children has not been established, current recommendations call for total daily dosage given in equally divided doses every 6 hours or at intervals based on individual requirements.
• Monitor pediatric patients during initial titration period; dose titration should begin at lower end of recommended ranges. Monitor serum drug levels and therapeutic response carefully.
• Correct any underlying electrolyte abnormalities, especially hypokalemia, before administering drug, because disopyramide may be ineffective in patients with these problems.
• Do not give sustained-release capsules for rapid control of ventricular dysrhythmias if therapeutic blood drug levels must be attained rapidly or if patient has cardiomyopathy, possible cardiac decompensation, or severe renal impairment.
• Watch for signs of developing heart block, such as QRS complex widening by more than 25% or QT interval lengthening by more than 25% above baseline.
• Disopyramide may cause hypoglycemia in some patients; monitor serum glucose levels in patients with altered serum glucose regulatory mechanisms.
• If drug causes constipation, administer laxatives and encourage proper diet.
• Disopyramide is commonly prescribed for patients with heart failure who cannot tolerate quinidine or procainamide.
• Pharmacist may prepare disopyramide suspension; 100-mg capsules are used with cherry syrup to prepare suspension (this may be best form for young children).
• Disopyramide is removed by hemodialysis. Dosage adustments may be necessary in patients undergoing dialysis.

Information for parents and patient
• When changing from immediate-release to sustained-release capsules, advise parents that patient should begin taking sustained-release capsule 6 hours after last immediate-release capsule.
• Emphasize the importance of taking drug on time, exactly as prescribed. To do this, parents or patient may have to use an alarm clock for night doses.
• Advise patient to use sugarless gum or candy to relieve dry mouth.

---

dobutamine hydrochloride
Dobutrex

• Classification: inotropic agent (adrenergic beta$_1$ agonist)

How supplied
Available by prescription only
Injection: 12.5 mg/ml in 20-ml vials (parenteral)

---

‡May contain sulfites   ◆May contain tartrazine   ◆◆May contain benzyl alcohol

Indications, route, and dosage
To increase cardiac output in short-term treatment of cardiac decompensation caused by depressed contractility
†*Children:* 2.5 to 15 mcg/kg/minute as an I.V. infusion. Maximum recommended dose 40 mcg/kg/minute.
Adults: 2.5 to 10 mcg/kg/minute as an I.V. infusion. Rarely, infusion rates up to 40 mcg/kg/minute may be needed. Titrate dosage carefully to patient response.

Action and kinetics
• *Inotropic action:* Dobutamine selectively stimulates beta$_1$-adrenergic receptors to increase myocardial contractility and stroke volume, resulting in increased cardiac output (a positive inotropic effect in patients with normal hearts or in CHF). At therapeutic doses, dobutamine decreases peripheral resistance (afterload), reduces ventricular filling pressure (preload), and may facilitate AV node conduction. Systolic blood pressure and pulse pressure may remain unchanged or increased from increased cardiac output. Increased myocardial contractility results in increased coronary blood flow and myocardial oxygen consumption. Heart rate usually remains unchanged; however, excessive doses do have chronotropic effects. Dobutamine does not appear to affect dopaminergic receptors, nor does it cause renal or mesenteric vasodilation; however, urine flow may increase because of increased cardiac output.
• *Kinetics in adults:* After I.V. administration, onset of action occurs within 2 minutes, with peak concentrations achieved within 10 minutes. Effects persist a few minutes after I.V. is discontinued. Dobutamine is widely distributed throughout the body; it is metabolized by the liver and by conjugation to inactive metabolites. Dobutamine is excreted mainly in urine, with minor amounts in feces, as its metabolites and conjugates.

Contraindications and precautions
Dobutamine is contraindicated in patients with idiopathic hypertrophic subaortic stenosis or known hypersensitivity to the drug or its ingredients. Use with extreme caution after myocardial infarction (may intensify or extend myocardial ischemia). Dobutamine increases AV conduction; therefore, patients with atrial fibrillation should have therapeutic levels of a cardiac glycoside before administration of dobutamine.
   Drug contains sodium bisulfite and may trigger allergic reaction in patients with sulfite sensitivity.

Interactions
Concomitant use with inhalation hydrocarbon anesthetics, especially halothane and cyclopropane, may trigger ventricular dysrhythmias. Beta-adrenergic blockers may antagonize the cardiac effects of dobutamine, resulting in increased peripheral resistance and predominance of alpha-adrenergic effects.
   Dobutamine may decrease the hypotensive effects of guanadrel and guanethidine; however, these agents may potentiate the pressor effects of dobutamine, possibly resulting in hypertension and cardiac dysrhythmias. Concomitant use with nitroprusside may cause higher cardiac output and lower pulmonary wedge pressure. Theoretically, rauwolfia alkaloids may prolong the actions of dobutamine (a denervation supersensitivity response).

Effects on diagnostic tests
None reported.

Adverse reactions
• CV: *ectopic heart beats,* increased heart rate, angina, chest pain, palpitation, *hypertension,* dysrhythmias.
• GI: nausea, vomiting.
• Other: tingling sensation, paresthesias, dyspnea, headache, mild leg cramps.
   Note: Drug should be discontinued if hypersensitivity reaction to drug or sulfites or if cardiac dysrhythmia occurs.

Overdose and treatment
Clinical manifestations of overdose include nervousness and fatigue. No treatment is necessary beyond dosage reduction or withdrawal of drug.

▶ Special considerations
• Before administration of dobutamine, correct hypovolemia with appropriate plasma volume expanders.
• Monitor ECG, blood pressure, cardiac output, and pulmonary wedge pressure via central venous pressure line or Swan-Ganz catheter. Assess vital signs, including level of consciousness and urine output carefully during therapy.
• Before giving dobutamine, administer digitalis if patient has atrial fibrillation (dobutamine increases AV conduction).
• Most patients experience an increase of 10 to 20 mm Hg in systolic blood pressure; some show an increase of 50 mm Hg or more. Most also experience an increase in heart rate of 5 to 15 beats/minute; some show increases of 30 or more beats/minute. Premature ventricular dysrhythmias may also occur in about 5% of patients. Dosage reduction may be necessary when these occur.
• Dose should be adjusted to meet individual needs and achieve desired clinical response. Drug must be administered by I.V. infusion using an infusion pump or other device to control flow rate.
• Concentration of infusion solution should not exceed 5 mg/ml; the solution should be used within 24 hours. Rate and duration of infusion depend on patient response.
• Pink discoloration of solution indicates slight oxidation but no significant loss of potency.
• Dobutamine is incompatible with alkaline solution (sodium bicarbonate). Also, do not mix with or give through same I.V. line as heparin, hydrocortisone sodium succinate, cefazolin, cefamandole, neutral cephalothin, penicillin, or ethacrynate sodium.

Information for parents and patient
• Advise parents and patient to report any adverse reactions.
• Inform parents that patient will need frequent monitoring of vital signs.

Dopamine hydrochloride
Dopastat, Intropin

Classification: inotropic, vasopressor (adrenergic)

How supplied
Available by prescription only

Injection: 40 mg/ml, 80 mg/ml, and 160 mg/ml parenteral concentrate for injection for I.V. infusion; 0.8 mg/ml (200 or 400 mg) in dextrose 5%; 1.6 mg/ml (400 or 800 mg) in dextrose 5%, and 3.2 mg/ml (800 mg) in dextrose 5% parenteral injection for I.V. infusion.

Indications, route, and dosage

Adjunct in shock to increase cardiac output, blood pressure, and urine flow

Children and adults: 1 to 5 mcg/kg/minute I.V. infusion, up to 50 mcg/kg/minute. Infusion rate may be increased by 1 to 4 mcg/kg/minute at 10- to 30-minute intervals until optimum response is achieved. In severely ill patient, infusion may begin at 5 mcg/kg/minute and gradually increase by increments of 5 to 10 mcg/kg/minute until optimum response is achieved.

Short-term treatment of severe, refractory, chronic CHF

Children and adults: Initially, 0.5 to 2 mcg/kg/minute I.V. infusion. Dosage may be increased until desired renal response occurs. Average dosage, 1 to 3 mcg/kg/minute.

Action and kinetics
Vasopressor action: An immediate precursor of norepinephrine, dopamine stimulates dopaminergic, beta-adrenergic, and alpha-adrenergic receptors of the sympathetic nervous system. The main effects produced are dose-dependent. It has a direct stimulating effect on beta_1 receptors (in I.V. doses of 2 to 10 mg/g/minute) and little or no effect on beta_2 receptors. In I.V. doses of 0.5 to 2 mcg/kg/minute it acts on dopaminergic receptors, causing vasodilation in the renal, mesenteric, coronary, and intracerebral vascular beds; in I.V. doses above 10 mcg/kg/minute, it stimulates alpha receptors.

Low to moderate doses result in cardiac stimulation (positive inotropic effects) and renal and mesenteric vasodilation (dopaminergic response). High doses result in increased peripheral resistance and renal vasoconstriction.

Kinetics in adults: Onset of action after I.V. administration occurs within 5 minutes and persists for less than 10 minutes. The drug is widely distributed throughout the body; however, it does not cross the blood-brain barrier. The drug is metabolized in the liver, kidneys, and plasma by monoamine oxidase to inactive compounds. About 25% is metabolized to norepinephrine within adrenergic nerve terminals. Dopamine is excreted in urine, mainly as its metabolites.

Contraindications and precautions
Dopamine is contraindicated in patients with pheochromocytoma and in those with uncorrected tachydysrhythmias or ventricular fibrillation because of potential for severe cardiovascular effects.

Commercially available dopamine solutions containing sulfites should be administered cautiously to patients with asthma and other patients with known hypersensitivity to them. Administer cautiously to patients with ischemic heart disease. Monitor patients with a history of occlusive vascular disease for decreased circulation to extremities.

Interactions
Concomitant use with MAO inhibitors may prolong and intensify the effects of dopamine. Use with beta-adrenergic blockers antagonizes the cardiac effects of dopamine; use with alpha-adrenergic blockers may antagonize the peripheral vasoconstriction caused by high doses of dopamine.

Combined use with general anesthetics, especially halothane and cyclopropane, may cause ventricular dysrhythmias and hypertension. Use with I.V. phenytoin may cause hypotension and bradycardia; use with diuretics increases diuretic effects of both agents. Use with oxytocics may cause advanced vasoconstriction. Dosage adjustments may be needed.

Dopamine decreases hypotensive effects of guanadrel, guanethidine, methyldopa, and trimethaphan through potentiated pressor effects of dopamine. Use with digitalis glycosides, levodopa, and sympathomimetics increases risk of cardiac dysrhythmias.

Effects on diagnostic tests
Dopamine may cause an elevation in serum glucose levels, although level usually doesn't rise above normal limits.

Adverse reactions
• CV: *ectopic heartbeats, tachycardia,* angina, palpitation, *vasoconstriction,* hypotension, cardiac conduction abnormalities, widened QRS complex, *bradycardia, hypertension,* ventricular dysrhythmias (high doses).
• GI: nausea, *vomiting.*
• Other: dyspnea, headache, *azotemia,* anxiety, and piloerection. *Extravasation can cause local necrosis and sloughing of tissue.*

Note: Drug should be discontinued if patient develops signs of hypersensitivity to drug or sulfite preservative, cardiac dysrhythmias, or tachyphylaxis.

Overdose and treatment
Clinical manifestations of overdose include excessive, severe hypertension. No treatment is necessary beyond dosage reduction or withdrawal of drug. If that fails to lower blood pressure, a short-acting alpha-adrenergic blocking agent may be helpful.

▶ Special considerations
• Hypovolemia should be corrected with appropriate plasma volume expanders before administration of dopamine.
• Dopamine is administered by I.V. infusion using an infusion device to control rate of flow.
• Administer dopamine into a large vein to prevent the possibility of extravasation. If necessary to administer in hand or ankle veins, change injection site

to larger vein as soon as possible. Monitor continuously for free flow. Central venous access is recommended.

• Adjust dose to meet individual needs of patient and to achieve desired clinical response. If dose required to obtain desired systolic blood pressure exceeds optimum rate of renal response, reduce dose as soon as hemodynamic condition is stabilized.

• Significant hypokalemia may result with excessive administration of potassium-free solutions. Monitor electrolyte levels.

• Severe hypotension may result with abrupt withdrawal of infusion; therefore, reduce dose gradually.

• If extravasation occurs, stop infusion and infiltrate site promptly with 10 to 15 ml of normal saline solution injection containing 5 to 10 mg of phentolamine. Use syringe with a fine needle, and infiltrate area liberally with phentolamine solution.

• Do not mix other drugs in dopamine solutions. Discard solutions after 24 hours. Drug may be diluted in dextrose 5% in water, dextrose 10% in water, or normal saline solution. Do not mix with alkaline solutions, such as sodium bicarbonate. Solution is stable for 24 hours. Discoloration of solution indicates decomposition and should be discarded.

• Monitor blood pressure, cardiac output, ECG, and intake and output during infusion, especially if dose exceeds 50 mcg/kg/minute. Watch for cold extremities.

• Tachyphylaxis (tolerance) may develop after prolonged or excessive use.

Information for the patient
• Advise parents to report any adverse reactions.
• Inform parents of need for frequent monitoring of the patient's vital signs and condition.

---

doxapram hydrochloride
Dopram

• Classification: CNS and respiratory stimulant (analeptic)

How supplied
Available by prescription only
Injection: 20 mg/ml (benzyl alcohol 0.9%)

Indications, route, and dosage
Postanesthesia respiratory stimulation, drug-induced CNS depression, acute hypercapnia associated with chronic obstructive pulmonary disease
Adults: 0.5 to 1 mg/kg of body weight (up to 2 mg/kg in CNS depression) I.V. injection or infusion. Maximum dosage is 4 mg/kg, up to 3 g in 1 day. Infusion rate is 1 to 3 mg/minute (initial dose is 5 mg/minute for postanesthesia).

Action and kinetics
• *Respiratory stimulant action:* Doxapram increases respiratory rate by direct stimulation of the medullary respiratory center and possibly by indirect action on

chemoreceptors in the carotid artery and aortic arch. Doxapram causes increased release of catecholamines.

• *Kinetics in adults:* After I.V. administration, action begins within 20 to 40 seconds; peak effect occurs in 1 to 2 minutes. Plasma half-life ranges from about 2½ to 4 hours; pharmacologic action persists for 5 to 12 minutes. Doxapram is distributed throughout the body. Drug is 99% metabolized by the liver. Metabolites are excreted in urine.

Contraindications and precautions
Doxapram is contraindicated in patients with head trauma and epilepsy or other seizure disorders because of the risk of drug-induced convulsions; in patients with acute bronchial asthma, pulmonary embolism, pneumothorax, pulmonary fibrosis, airway obstruction, severe dyspnea and respiratory failure from muscle paresis, because of risk of hypoxia and subsequent dysrhythmias; and in patients with coronary artery disease, severe hypertension, frank uncompensated heart failure, or cerebrovascular accident, because of drug's vasopressor effects.

Doxapram should be used with caution in patients with a history of severe tachycardia or cardiac dysrhythmia, because of the risk of hypoxia and subsequent dysrhythmia; and in patients with increased cerebrospinal fluid pressure or cerebral edema, pheochromocytoma, or hyperthyroidism, because of drug's vasopressor effects.

Interactions
Concomitant use with MAO inhibitors or sympathomimetic drugs may produce added pressor effects.

Discontinue anesthetics, such as halothane, cyclopropane, and enflurane, at least 10 minutes before giving doxapram; these agents sensitize the myocardium to catecholamines. Doxapram temporarily may mask residual effects of neuromuscular blockers used after anesthesia.

Effects on diagnostic tests
Doxapram may cause T-wave depression on ECG, decreased erythrocyte and leukocyte counts, reduced hemoglobin and hematocrit levels, increased BUN levels, and albuminuria.

Adverse reactions
• CNS: seizures, headache, dizziness, apprehension disorientation, pupillary dilatation, bilateral Babinski's signs, flushing, sweating, paresthesias.
• CV: chest pain and tightness, dysrhythmias, hypertension, phlebitis.
• DERM: pruritus.
• GI: nausea, vomiting, diarrhea, urge to defecate.
• GU: urinary retention, stimulation of bladder with incontinence.
• Respiratory: cough, sneezing, hiccups, bronchospasm, rebound hypoventilation.
Note: Drug should be discontinued if hypotension or dyspnea occurs.

Overdose and treatment

Signs of overdose include hypertension, tachycardia, dysrhythmias, skeletal muscle hyperactivity, and dyspnea.

Treatment is supportive. Keep oxygen and resuscitative equipment available, but use oxygen with caution, because rapid increase in partial pressure of oxygen (Po_2) levels can suppress carotid chemoreceptor activity. Keep I.V. anticonvulsants available to treat seizures.

▶ Special considerations

• Safety in children under age 12 has not been established. Drug is contraindicated in infants because it contains benzyl alcohol. However, clinicians report rare, last-resort use in infants with central apnea.
• Doxapram's use as an analeptic is strongly discouraged; drug should be used only in surgery or emergency room.
• Establish adequate airway before administering drug; prevent aspiration of vomitus by placing patient on his side.
• Monitor blood pressure, heart rate, deep tendon reflexes, and arterial blood gas (ABG) levels before giving drug and every 30 minutes afterward. Discontinue drug if ABG levels deteriorate or mechanical ventilation is started.
• Do not infuse doxapram faster than recommended rate because hemolysis may occur. Drug should be used only on an intermittent basis; maximum infusion period is 2 hours.
• Avoid repeated injections in the site for long periods, because of risk of thrombophlebitis or local skin irritation.
• Do not combine doxapram, which is acidic, with alkaline solutions, such as thiopental sodium; solution is compatible with dextrose 5% or 10% and 0.9% sodium chloride.
• Give concomitant oxygen cautiously to patients who have just undergone surgery; doxapram-stimulated respiration increases oxygen demand.
• Monitor patient (especially hypertensive patient) for signs of toxicity—tachycardia, muscle tremor, spasticity, and hyperactive reflexes—and blood pressure changes.

Information for parents and patient

Inform parents about purpose of therapy and potential benefits and adverse reactions.

---

doxorubicin hydrochloride
Adriamycin RDF

• Classification: antineoplastic (antineoplastic antibiotic [cell cycle-phase nonspecific])

How supplied

Available by prescription only
Injection: 10-mg, 20-mg, 50-mg vials

Indications, route, and dosage

Dosage and indications may vary. Check current literature for recommended protocol.

Cancer of bladder, kidney, breast, cervix, head, neck, liver, lungs, ovary, prostate, stomach, testes, brain, or blood and lymph system; sarcomas; neuroblastoma
Children under age 2 may have a higher risk of cardiotoxicity.
Children: 30 mg/m² I.V. daily on 3 successive days of 3 weeks.
Adults: 60 to 75 mg/m² I.V. as a single dose q 3 weeks; or 25 to 30 mg/m² I.V. as a single daily dose on days 1 to 3 of 4-week cycle. Alternatively, 20 mg/m² I.V. once weekly. Maximum cumulative dosage is 550 mg/m² (450 mg/m² in patients who have received chest irradiation).

Action and kinetics

• *Antineoplastic action:* Doxorubicin exerts its cytotoxic activity by intercalating between DNA base pairs and uncoiling the DNA helix. The result is inhibition of DNA synthesis and DNA-dependent RNA synthesis. Doxorubicin also inhibits protein synthesis.
• *Kinetics in adults:* Because of its vesicant effects, doxorubicin must be administered intravenously. Doxorubicin distributes widely into body tissues, with the highest concentrations found in the liver, heart, and kidneys. The drug does not cross the blood-brain barrier. Doxorubicin is extensively metabolized by hepatic microsomal enzymes to several metabolites, one of which possesses cytotoxic activity. Doxorubicin and its metabolites are excreted primarily in bile. A minute amount is eliminated in urine. The plasma elimination of doxorubicin is described as triphasic with a half-life of about ½ hour in the initial phase and 16½ hours in the terminal phase.

Contraindications and precautions

Doxorubicin is contraindicated in patients with hepatic dysfunction, depressed bone marrow function or impaired cardiac function and in patients who have previously received lifetime cumulative doses of doxorubicin or daunorubicin because of increased potential for cardiac or hematopoietic toxicity.

Interactions

Concomitant use with streptozocin may increase the plasma half-life of doxorubicin by an unknown mechanism, increasing the activity of doxorubicin. Concomitant use of daunorubicin or cyclophosphamide may potentiate the cardiotoxicity of doxorubicin through additive effects on the heart. Doxorubicin should not be mixed with heparin sodium, dexamethasone phosphate, or hydrocortisone sodium phosphate. Mixing these agents with doxorubicin will result in a precipitate.

Effects on diagnostic tests

Doxorubicin therapy may increase blood and urine concentrations of uric acid.

Adverse reactions
• CV: *cardiotoxicity, transient* ECG changes, *dysrhythmias;* irreversible cardiomyopathy, sometimes with pulmonary edema.
• DERM: hyperpigmentation, especially in previously irradiated areas.
• GI: *nausea, vomiting, diarrhea, stomatitis, anorexia, esophagitis.*
• GU: transient red urine.
• HEMA: leukopenia, especially agranulocytosis, during days 10 to 15, with recovery by day 21; thrombocytopenia; bone marrow depression (dose-limiting).
• Local: *severe cellulitis.*
• Other: hyperpigmentation of nails and dermal creases, complete alopecia, *anaphylactoid reaction, fever and chills, photosensitivity.*
  Note: Drug should be discontinued if hematopoietic toxicity becomes severe.

Overdose and treatment
Clinical manifestations of overdose include myelosuppression, nausea, vomiting, mucositis, and irreversible myocardial toxicity.
  Treatment is usually supportive and includes transfusion of blood components, antiemetics, antibiotics for infections which may develop, symptomatic treatment of mucositis, and digitalis preparations.

▶ Special considerations
• Vital signs and patency of catheter or I.V. line should be monitored throughout administration.
• Carefully follow all established procedures for safe handling, administration, and disposal.
• Monitor BUN, hematocrit, platelet count, ALT (SGPT), AST (SGOT), LDH, serum bilirubin, serum creatinine, uric acid, and total and differential leukocytes.
• To reconstitute, add 5 ml of normal saline solution to the 10-mg vial, 10 ml to the 20-mg vial, and 25 ml to the 50-mg vial, to yield a concentration of 2 mg/ml. Drug is also available ready to use.
• Drug may be further diluted with normal saline solution or dextrose 5% in water and administered by I.V. infusion.
• Drug may be administered by I.V. push injection over 5 to 10 minutes into the tubing of a freely flowing I.V. infusion.
• The alternative dosage schedule (once-weekly dosing) causes a lower incidence of cardiomyopathy.
• For continuous infusion, administer only through a central venous catheter.
• Continuous infusions of doxorubicin or treatment for 5 to 7 days decreases the total daily dose and the subsequent incidence of cardiotoxicity associated with its administration. Patients with no history of congestive heart failure have tolerated cumulative doses up to 800 mg/m² without complication.
• If cumulative dose exceeds 550 mg/m² body surface area, 30% of patients develop cardiac adverse reactions, which begin 2 weeks to 6 months after stopping drug. Monitor chest X-ray and ECG before and after therapy.
• Premedicating with an antiemetic may prevent nausea and vomiting. If vomiting occurs, administer antiemetics p.r.n.

• Patients who have received drugs with strong emetic properties may experience anticipatory nausea and vomiting at subsequent treatments. They may benefi from treatment with an anxiolytic drug.
• Monitor patient's intake, output, and weight.
• Continue I.V. hydration until patient resumes suf ficient oral intake.
• The occurrence of streaking along a vein or facia flushing indicates that the drug is being administere too rapidly.
• Applying a scalp tourniquet or ice may decrease alopecia. However, *do not* use these if treating leu kemias or other neoplasms where tumor stem cell may be present in scalp.
• Drug should be discontinued or rate of infusion slowed if tachycardia develops. Treat extravasation with topical application of dimethyl sulfoxide and ic packs.
• Monitor CBC and hepatic function.
• Decrease dosage as follows if serum bilirubin leve increases: 50% of dose when bilirubin level is 1.2 t 3 mg/100 ml; 25% of dose when bilirubin level exceed 3 mg/100 ml.
• Esophagitis is common in patients who have als received radiation therapy.

Information for parents and patient
• Instruct patient to clean teeth with toothettes gauze,or soft toothbrush when platelets are low. Che motherapy can increase incidence of microbial infec tion, delayed healing, and bleeding gums.
• Tell parents that patient's dental work should be completed before therapy if possible, or delayed unti blood counts are normal.
• Warn parents and patient that bruising may easily occur because of drug's effects on blood count.
• Teach parents and patient to check for signs of bleed ing and bruising. Parents may need to restrict child's activity to prevent injury when platelets are low.
• Stress importance of keeping follow-up appoint ments for monitoring hematologic status.
• Instruct parents to monitor neutropenic patient's temperature every 4 hours (not rectally) and to repor fever, cough, and other signs of infection *promptly.*
• Explain importance of promptly reporting suscep tible patient's exposure to chicken pox. Patient shoulc avoid contact with persons who have received live immunizations (polio, measles/mumps/rubella).
• Tell parents and patient to immediately report red ness, pain, or swelling at injection site. Local injur y and scarring may result if I.V. infiltrates.
• Advise parents to encourage patient's fluid intake to increase urine output and facilitate excretion o uric acid.
• Warn parents and patient that alopecia will occur but hair growth should resume 2 to 5 months afte drug is stopped.
• Advise parents and patient that urine will become reddish for 1 to 2 days after the dose and does no indicate bleeding. The urine may stain clothes.
• Tell parents to have patient avoid exposure to per sons with bacterial or viral infections as chemother apy can make the patient more susceptible to infection Urge parents to report infection immediately.
• Patient should not receive any immunizations during

therapy and for several weeks after. Other members of the patient's household should also not receive live-virus immunizations during the same period.
• Explain radiation recall. Previously irradiated areas may become erythematous after administration of drug.

doxycycline hyclate
Doxy-100, Doxy-200, Doxy-Caps, Doxychel, Doxy-Lemmon, Doxy-Tabs, Vibramycin, Vibra-Tabs, Vivox

• Classification: antibiotic (tetracycline)

How supplied
Available by prescription only
Capsules: 50 mg, 100 mg
Tablets: 50 mg, 100 mg
Injection: 100 mg, 200 mg

Indications, route, and dosage
Infections caused by sensitive organisms
Children over age 8 weighing less than 45 kg: 4.4 mg/kg P.O. I.V. daily, divided q 12 hours 1st day, then 2.2 to 4.4 mg/kg daily. For children weighing more than 45 kg, dosage is same as adults.
Adults: 100 mg P.O. q 12 hours on 1st day, then 100 mg P.O. daily; or 200 mg I.V. on 1st day in one or two infusions, then 100 to 200 mg I.V. daily.

Action and kinetics
• *Antibacterial action:* Doxycycline is bacteriostatic; it binds reversibly to ribosomal units, thereby inhibiting bacterial protein synthesis.
    Doxycycline's spectrum of activity includes many gram-negative and gram-positive organisms, *Mycoplasma, Rickettsia, Chlamydia,* and spirochetes.
• *Kinetics in adults:* Doxyciline is 90% to 100% absorbed after oral administration; Doxycycline has the least affinity for calcium of all tetracyclines; its absorption is insignificantly altered by milk or other dairy products.
    Doxycycline is distributed widely into body tissues and fluids, including synovial, pleural, prostatic, and seminal fluids; bronchial secretions; saliva; and aqueous humor. CSF penetration is poor. Doxycycline readily crosses the placenta.
    Doxycycline is insignificantly metabolized; and is excreted primarily unchanged in urine by glomerular filtration; some drug may be excreted in breast milk. Plasma half-life is 22 to 24 hours after multiple dosing in adults with normal renal function; 20 to 30 hours in patients with severe renal impairment.
• *Kinetics in children:* Tetracyclines form a stable complex in bone-forming tissue, and may cause permanent enamel hypoplasia or yellow-gray discoloration of teeth in children under age 8.

Contraindications and precautions
Doxycycline is contraindicated in children with known hypersensitivity to any tetracycline; and those under age 8 because of the risk of permanent discoloration of teeth, enamel defects, and retardation of bone growth.
    Use doxycycline with caution in children with impaired renal function, as serum half-life is prolonged; and in children likely to be exposed to direct sunlight or ultraviolet light because of the risk of photosensitivity reactions.

Interactions
Concomitant use of doxycycline with antacids containing aluminum, calcium, or magnesium or laxatives containing magnesium decreases oral absorption of doxycycline because of chelation; oral iron products and sodium bicarbonate also impair absorption of tetracyclines.
    Doxycycline may antagonize bactericidal effects of penicillin, inhibiting cell growth because of bacteriostatic action; administer penicillin 2 to 3 hours before tetracycline.
    Concomitant use of doxycycline with oral anticoagulants necessitates lowered dosage of oral anticoagulants because of enhanced effects; when used with digoxin, lowered dosages of digoxin because of increased bioavailability.

Effects on diagnostic tests
Doxycycline causes false-negative results in urine tests using glucose oxidase reagent (Clinistix or TesTape); parenteral dosage form may cause false-negative Clinitest results.
    Doxycycline also causes false elevations in fluorometric tests for urinary catecholamines.

Adverse reactions
• CNS: intracranial hypertension.
• CV: pericarditis.
• DERM: maculopapular and erythematous rashes, photosensitivity, increased pigmentation, urticaria, discolored nails.
• EENT: sore throat, glossitis, dysphagia.
• GI: anorexia, epigastric distress, nausea, vomiting, diarrhea, enterocolitis, anogenital inflammation.
• GU: reversible nephrotoxicity (Fanconi's syndrome) with outdated tetracyclines.
• HEMA: neutropenia, eosinophilia.
• Local: thrombophlebitis.
• Other: hypersensitivity, bacterial and fungal superinfection, discolored teeth.
    Note: Drug should be discontinued if signs of toxicity or hypersensitivity or superinfection occur; if erythema follows exposure to sunlight or ultraviolet light; or if severe diarrhea indicates pseudomembranous colitis.

Overdose and treatment
Clinical signs of overdose are usually limited to the GI tract; give antacids or empty stomach by gastric lavage if ingestion occurred within the preceding 4 hours.

▶ Special considerations
• Assess child's allergic history; do not give doxycycline to a patient with a history of hypersensitivity reactions to any other tetracycline. Monitor continuously for this and other adverse reactions.

‡May contain sulfites   ◆May contain tartrazine   ◆◆May contain benzyl alcohol

• Obtain results of cultures and sensitivity tests before first dose, but do not delay therapy; check cultures periodically to assess drug efficacy.
• Monitor vital signs, electrolytes and renal function studies before and during therapy.
• Monitor for bacterial and fungal superinfection, especially in debilitated children and those who are receiving immunosuppressants or radiation therapy; watch especially for oral candidiasis. If symptoms occur, discontinue drug.
• Children age 8 and under should not receive tetracyclines unless there is no alternative. Tetracyclines can cause permanent discoloration of teeth, enamel hypoplasia, and a reversible decrease in bone calcification.
• Reversible decreases in bone calcification have been reported in infants.

Administration
• Give I.V. infusion slowly (minimum 1 hour). Infusion must be completed within 12 hours (within 6 hours in lactated Ringer's solution or dextrose 5% in lactated Ringer's solution).
• Give oral drug 1 hour before or 2 hours after meals for maximum absorption; do not give with food, milk, or other dairy products, sodium bicarbonate, iron compounds, or antacids, which may impair absorption. Give water with and after oral drug to facilitate passage to stomach, because incomplete swallowing can cause severe esophageal irritation; do not administer within 1 hour of bedtime, to prevent esophageal reflux.
• Reconstitute powder for injection with sterile water for injection. Use 10 ml in a 100-mg vial and 20 ml in a 200-mg vial. Dilute solution to 100 to 1,000 ml for I.V. infusion. Do not infuse solutions more concentrated than 1mg/ml.
• Reconstituted solution is stable for 72 hours if refrigerated and protected from light.
• Do not inject S.C. or I.M.
• Doxycycline may be used in patients with impaired renal function; it does not accumulate or cause a significant rise in BUN levels.
• Monitor I.V. injection sites and rotate routinely to minimize local irritation. I.V. administration may cause severe phlebitis.

Information for parents and patient
• Teach signs and symptoms of adverse reactions, and emphasize need to report these promptly; urge parents to report any unusual effects.
• Teach parents of children with low resistance from immunosuppressants or irradiation how to recognize signs and symptoms of bacterial and fungal superinfection. To prevent fungal infection, parents of infants should keep diaper area clean and dry and avoid use of plastic pants.
• Advise parents to prevent child's direct exposure to sunlight and to apply a sunscreen to help prevent photosensitivity reactions.
• Patient should take doxycycline with enough water to facilitate passage to the stomach, 1 hour before or 2 hours after meals for maximum absorption, and not less than 1 hour before bedtime (to prevent irritation from esophageal reflux).
• Emphasize that taking the drug with food, milk or other dairy products, sodium bicarbonate, or iron compounds may interfere with absorption. Patients who need antacids should take them 3 hours after tetracycline.
• Emphasize importance of completing prescribed regimen exactly as ordered and keeping follow-up appointments.
• Tell parents to check expiration dates and discard any expired drug.
• Tell parents of diabetic child that drug may interfere with urine test for glucose.

---

dronabinol (delta 9 tetrahydrocannabinol; THC)
Marinol

• Classification: antiemetic (cannabinoid)
• Controlled substance schedule II

How supplied
Available by prescription only
Capsules: 2.5 mg, 5 mg, 10 mg

Indications, route, and dosage
Nausea and vomiting associated with cancer chemotherapy
Children and adults: 5 mg/m^2 P.O. 1 to 3 hours before administration of chemotherapy; then same dose q 2 to 4 hours after chemotherapy for a total of 4 to 6 doses daily. Dose may be increased in increments of 2.5 mg/m^2 to a maximum of 15 mg/m^2 per dose.

Action and kinetics
• *Antiemetic action:* Dronabinol is a synthetic cannabinoid that inhibits vomiting centers in the brain and possibly in the chemoreceptor trigger zone and other sites.
• *Kinetics in adults:* About 10% to 20% of dose is absorbed; action begins in 30 to 60 minutes, with peak action in 1 to 3 hours. Dronabinol is distributed rapidly into many tissue sites. Drug is 97% to 99% protein-bound. Dronabinol undergoes extensive metabolism in the liver. Metabolite activity is unknown. Dronabinol is excreted primarily in feces, via the biliary tract. Drug effect may persist for several days after treatment ends; duration varies considerably among patients.

Contraindications and precautions
Dronabinol is contraindicated in patients with nausea and vomiting not secondary to cancer chemotherapy or not refractory to conventional antiemetics; and in patients with hypersensitivity to sesame oil or dronabinol.
Dronabinol should be used cautiously in children and in patients with hypertension, cardiac disease, or psychiatric illness, because of possible CNS and cardiovascular adverse effects. Drug may exacerbate underlying psychiatric illness.

Interactions
When used concomitantly with alcohol or other sedatives or psychotomimetic drugs, dronabinol may have

additive sedative effect. Dronabinol may alter
anol elimination, increasing it in some patients and
creasing it in others. Concomitant use with anti-
olinergics may cause tachycardia.

fects on diagnostic tests
ne reported.

dverse reactions
NS: drowsiness, dizziness, euphoria, altered think-
g, mood changes, psychosis, hallucinations, im-
ired coordination, irritability, anxiety, ataxia, visual
tortions, confusion, depression, weakness, pares-
esias.
V: orthostatic hypotension, tachycardia.
I: dry mouth, diarrhea.
ther: muscle pain.
Note: Drug should be discontinued if blood pressure
ops.

verdose and treatment
information available.

Special considerations
Dronabinol is used only in patients with nausea and
miting resulting from cancer chemotherapy who do
t respond to other treatment; drug should be given
fore chemotherapy infusion.
• Monitor frequency and degree of vomiting.
• Monitor pulse, blood pressure, and fluid intake and
tput to help prevent dehydration; observe for signs
confusion.
• Dronabinol is the major active ingredient of *Cannabis*
tiva (marijuana) and therefore has a potential for
use.

formation for parents and patient
• Warn parents that patient should avoid hazardous
tivities requiring alertness until extent of CNS de-
essant effects are known.
• Urge parents to ensure that patient is supervised
a responsible person during and immediately after
eatment.
• Caution parents and patient and family to anticipate
ug's mood-altering effects.

---

roperidol
apsine

Classification: tranquilizer (butyrophenone deriva-
ive)

ow supplied
vailable by prescription only
jection: 2.5 mg/ml

dications, route, and dosage
nesthetic premedication
hildren age 2 to 12: 0.088 to 0.165 mg/kg I.V. or
M.
dults: 2.5 to 10 mg I.M. or I.V. 30 to 60 minutes
efore induction of general anesthesia.

Adjunct for induction of general anesthesia
Children: 0.088 to 0.165 mg/kg I.V. or I.M.
Adults: 0.22 to 0.275 mg/kg I.V. (preferably) or I.M.
concomitantly with an analgesic, a general anesthetic, or both.

Action and kinetics
• *Tranquilizer action:* Droperidol produces marked sedation by directly blocking subcortical receptors. Droperidol also blocks CNS receptors at the chemoreceptor
trigger zone, producing an antiemetic effect.
• *Kinetics in adults:* Droperidol is well absorbed after
I.M. injection. Sedation begins in 3 to 10 minutes,
peaks at 30 minutes, and lasts for 2 to 4 hours; some
alteration of consciousness may persist for 12 hours.
Drug crosses the blood-brain barrier and is distributed in the CSF. It also crosses the placenta. Droperidol is metabolized by the liver to p-fluoro-
phenylacetic acid and p-hydroxypiperidine. Droperidol
and its metabolites are excreted in urine and feces.

Contraindications and precautions
Droperidol is contraindicated in patients with known
hypersensitivity or intolerance to the drug. It should
be used cautiously in patients with hypotension and
other cardiovascular disease, because of its vasodilatory effects; in patients with hepatic or renal disease, in whom drug clearance may be impaired; and
in patients taking other CNS depressants, including
alcohol, opiates, and sedatives, because droperidol
may potentiate the effects of these drugs.

Interactions
Droperidol potentiates the CNS depressant effects of
opiate or other analgesics and has an additive or potentiating effect when used concomitantly with other
CNS depressants, such as alcohol, barbiturates, tranquilizers, and sedative-hypnotics.

Effects on diagnostic tests
Droperidol temporarily alters the EEG pattern, which
returns slowly to normal after administration of the
drug. Droperidol may decrease pulmonary artery
pressure.

Adverse reactions
• CNS: sedation, altered consciousness, respiratory
depression, postoperative hallucinations, extrapyramidal reactions (dystonia [extended tongue, stiff rotated neck, upward rotation of eyes], akathesia
[restlessness], fine tremors of limbs).
• CV: hypotension with rebound tachycardia, bradycardia (occasional), hypertension when combined with
fentanyl or other parenteral analgesics (rare).
Note: Drug should be discontinued if patient shows
signs of hypersensitivity, severe persistent hypotension, respiratory depression, paradoxical hypertension, or dystonia.

Overdose and treatment
Clinical signs of overdose include extension of the
drug's pharmacologic actions. Treat overdose symptomatically and supportively.

▶ **Special considerations**
• Safety and efficacy in children under age 2 have not been established.
• Monitor vital signs and watch carefully for extrapyramidal reactions. Droperidol is related to haloperidol and is more likely than other antipsychotics to cause extrapyramidal symptoms.
• If opiates are required during recovery from anesthesia, they should be used initially in reduced doses (as low as one-quarter to one-third of the usual recommended dosage).
• Droperidol has been used for its antiemetic effects in preventing or treating cancer chemotherapy-induced nausea and vomiting, especially that produced by cisplatin.
• Observe for postoperative hallucinations or emergence delirium and drowsiness.
• Be prepared to treat severe hypotension.

Information for parents and patient
Advise parents and patient of possible postoperative effects.

---

dyclonine hydrochloride
Dyclone, Sucrets

• Classification: local anesthetic

How supplied
Available by prescription only
Solution: 0.5%, 1%

Available without a prescription
Lozenges: 1.2 mg, 3 mg

Indications, route, and dosage
Relief of pain and itching from minor burns, insect bites, or irritations, or anogenital lesions; to anesthetize mucous membranes before endoscopic procedures
Children and adults: Dosage varies with area to be anesthetized and technique used. Generally, apply to affected area as needed. If used before urologic endoscopy, instill 6 to 30 ml of the solution into the urethra before the procedure. Have patient retain the solution for 5 to 10 minutes.
Local anesthesia before laryngoscopy, bronchoscopy, esophagoscopy, or endotracheal procedures
Children and adults: Dosage should be individualized. Dyclonine should be used sparingly because it is absorbed through the oral mucosa. Before bronchoscopy, 2 ml of the 1% dyclonine hydrochloride solution (20 mg) may be sprayed into the larynx and trachea every 5 minutes until the laryngeal reflex is abolished; 2 or 3 applications usually are required. Five minutes should elapse before bronchoscopy is performed. For esophagoscopy after pharyngeal anesthesia, 10 to 15 ml of the 0.5% solution (50 to 75 mg) is swallowed. To produce local analgesia in the throat and oral cavity, 5 to 10 ml of the 0.5% or 1% solution (25 to 100 mg) may be swabbed, gargled, or sprayed and then expectorated. For relief of esophageal pain, 5 15 ml of the 0.5% solution (25 to 75 mg) may swallowed.
For temporary relief of minor sore throat pa or mouth irritation
Children over age 12 and adults: Dissolve one lozen slowly in the mouth; may be repeated q 2 hours needed.

Action and kinetics
• *Anesthetic action:* Dyclonine blocks conduction nerve impulses at the sensory nerve endings by tering cell membrane permeability to ionic transfe
• *Kinetics in adults:* Absorption is limited with sho term topical use. Topical application produces loc anesthesia within 2 to 10 minutes, lasting for abo 30 minutes.

Contraindications and precautions
Dyclonine hydrochloride is contraindicated in patier with hypersensitivity to the drug or in patients u dergoing cystoscopic procedures after excretion ur raphy, because visualization may be impaired. It shou be used with caution on ulcerated or inflamed are or for prolonged periods, as increased absorption n selectively increases drug effectiveness, untoward fects, and systemic toxicity.

Interactions
None reported.

Effects on diagnostic tests
None reported.

Adverse reactions
• CNS: stimulation or depression.
• Local: irritation or stinging.
   Note: Drug should be discontinued if sensitizati occurs.

Overdose and treatment
No information available.

▶ **Special considerations**
• If used as an oral topical anesthetic, dyclonine ma impair patient's swallowing ability. Watch for asp ration.
• Lozenges are not recommended for children und age 12.

Information for parents and patient
• Explain correct use of drug, and stress avoidan of contact with eyes; emphasize need to wash han thoroughly after use.
• Caution parents to apply drug sparingly, to minimi systemic effects.
• Advise keeping drug out of reach of children.

econazole nitrate
Spectazole

Classification: antifungal (synthetic imidazole derivative)

How supplied
Available by prescription only
Cream: 1% (water-soluble base)

Indications, route, and dosage
Tinea pedis, tinea cruris, and tinea corporis; cutaneous candidiasis
Children and adults: Gently rub sufficient quantity into affected areas b.i.d. in the morning and evening.
Tinea versicolor
Children and adults: Gently rub into affected area once daily.

Action and kinetics
Antifungal action: Although exact mechanism of action is unknown, econazole is thought to exert its effects by altering cellular membranes and interfering with intracellular enzymes. Econazole is active against many fungi, including dermatophytes and yeasts, as well as some gram-positive bacteria.
Kinetics in adults: Percutaneous absorption is minimal but rapid. Distribution is minimal.

Contraindications and precautions
Econazole nitrate is contraindicated in patients with known hypersensitivity and during the first trimester of pregnancy. It should be used in second and third trimesters only if deemed essential to patient's welfare.

Interactions
None reported.

Effects on diagnostic tests
None reported.

Adverse reactions
Local: chemical irritation, burning, itching, stinging, erythema.
Note: Drug should be discontinued if sensitization develops, condition persists or worsens, or irritation occurs.

Overdose and treatment
Discontinue therapy.

Special considerations
Wash affected area with soap and water, and dry thoroughly before applying drug.

• Do not apply econazole to the eye or administer intravaginally.

Information for parents and patient
• Instruct parents or patient to wash hands well after application.
• Patient should use medication for entire treatment period (usually 2 to 4 weeks) even if symptoms lessen. Relief of symptoms usually occurs within the first week or two of therapy.
• Patient with tinea pedis (athlete's foot) should wear well-fitting, well-ventilated shoes and should change shoes and all-cotton socks daily.

edetate disodium (EDTA)
Chealamide, Disotate, Endrate

• Classification: heavy metal antagonist (chelating agent)

How supplied
Available by prescription only
Injection: 150 mg/ml

Indications, route, and dosage
Hypercalcemia
Children: 40 to 70 mg/kg daily added to a sufficient amount of dextrose 5% in water or normal saline solution so that drug concentration is no greater than 30 mg/ml. This solution is administered by slow I.V. infusion over 3 to 4 hours.
Adults: 50 mg/kg daily by slow I.V. infusion. Dilute in 500 ml of dextrose 5% in water or normal saline solution. Give over 3 or more hours.
Digitalis-induced cardiac dysrhythmias
Children and adults: I.V. infusion of 15 mg/kg/hour; maximum dosage is 60 mg/kg daily. Dilute in dextrose 5% in water.

Action and kinetics
• *Chelating agent:* Edetate disodium binds many divalent and trivalent ions but has the strongest affinity for calcium, with which it forms a stable complex readily excreted by the kidney. Edetate disodium also chelates magnesium, zinc, and other trace metals, increasing their urinary excretion; it does not decrease CSF calcium concentrations.
• *Kinetics in adults:* Edetate disodium is absorbed poorly from the GI tract. Drug does not enter the CSF in significant amounts but distributes widely throughout the rest of the body. After I.V. administration, edetate disodium is excreted rapidly in urine.

Contraindications and precautions
Edetate disodium is contraindicated in patients with severe renal failure or anuria; in patients with sus-

pected or known hypocalcemia, active or healed tuberculosis, or severe heart, renal, or coronary artery disease; and in patients with a history of seizures, because drug may exacerbate the signs and symptoms of these conditions.

Edetate disodium should be used cautiously in patients with renal impairment; in patients with incipient CHF, because its effect on calcium concentration depresses cardiac function and because large sodium and fluid loads are delivered during therapy; and in patients with hypokalemia or hypomagnesemia, because drug may lower total body stores via increased renal excretion.

Drug should not be used to treat lead poisoning; edetate calcium disodium should be used instead.

Interactions
Edetate disodium interferes with the cardiac effects of digitalis glycosides indirectly by decreasing intracellular calcium by both chelation and urinary excretion of extracellular calcium.

Drug may decrease insulin requirements in diabetic patients by chelation of zinc in exogenous insulin.

Effects on diagnostic tests
Edetate disodium lowers serum calcium concentrations when measured by oxalate or other precipitation methods and by colorimetry. The drug also lowers blood glucose concentration in diabetic patients. Edetate disodium-induced hypomagnesemia decreases serum alkaline phosphatase levels.

Adverse reactions
- CNS: seizures, headache, circumoral paresthesia, numbness.
- CV: *severe cardiac dysrhythmias*, hypotension.
- DERM: erythema, exfoliative dermatitis.
- GI: nausea, diarrhea, vomiting, abdominal cramps, anorexia.
- GU: urinary urgency, nocturia, polyuria, proteinuria, *acute tubular necrosis*.
- Metabolic: *severe hypocalcemia*, hypomagnesemia.
- Local: pain at infusion site, erythema, dermatitis.
- Other: fever, chills, back pain, muscle pain and weakness.
  Note: Drug should be discontinued if hypocalcemia, cardiac dysrhythmias, tetany, or seizures occur.

Overdose and treatment
Clinical signs of overdose may include hypotension, cardiac dysrhythmias, and cardiac arrest. Treat hypotension with fluids, if necessary. Treat dysrhythmias with lidocaine, and seizures and tetany with calcium replacement; use I.V. diazepam for refractory seizures. Replace magnesium and potassium, as needed.

▶ Special considerations
- Safety and efficacy in children have not been established; give recommended dose slowly, over at least 3 hours.
- Monitor infusion site closely. Extravasation severely irritates tissue; rotate infusion sites with multiple doses or chronic therapy.
- Do not exceed recommended rate of infusion or dos-

age; rapid infusion and/or high concentrations of edetate disodium may precipitously decrease serum calcium levels, causing seizures and death. Therefore have I.V. calcium replacement readily available whenever drug is administered.
- Monitor calcium levels, and observe patient for seizures or altered vital signs and ECG during infusion. Administer infusion over at least 3 hours; have patient remain supine for 20 to 30 minutes after infusion because of possible postural hypotension. Drug also exerts a negative inotropic effect on the heart.
- Assess renal function before drug is administered. Perform urinalysis daily during therapy.
- Edetate disodium also has been used topically or by iontophoresis to treat corneal calcium deposits.
- Although once considered useful in treating digitalis-induced dysrhythmias, edetate disodium has been replaced by digoxin immune FAB as the drug of choice for digoxin toxicity.

Information for parents and patient
- Explain possible adverse reactions; stress importance of reporting signs and symptoms of adverse reactions promptly.
- Diabetic patients may need adjustment of insulin dosage.

---

edrophonium chloride
Enlon, Tensilon

- Classification: cholinergic agonist, diagnostic agent (cholinesterase inhibitor)

How supplied
Available by prescription only
Injection: 10 mg/ml in 1-ml ampule or 10-ml vial

Indications, route, and dosage
Diagnostic aid in myasthenia gravis
Children: 0.2 mg/kg or 6 mg/m² I.V. Give 20% of the calculated dose in the first minute; if no response within 45 seconds, give remaining drug. Alternatively, some clinicians administer according to the following schedule:
Infants weighing < 34 kg: no more than 0.5 mg I.V. or 2 mg I.M.
Infants weighing > 34 kg: no more than 0.5 mg I.V. or 5 mg I.M. After I.M. use, reaction is delayed for 2 to 10 minutes.
Children up to 75 pounds (34 kg): 1 mg I.V. If no response within 45 seconds, give 1 mg q 45 seconds to maximum of 5 mg.
Children over 75 pounds (34 kg): 2 mg I.V. If no response within 45 seconds, give 1 mg q 45 seconds to maximum of 10 mg.
Adults: 1 to 2 mg I.V. within 15 to 30 seconds, then 8 mg if no response (increase in muscular strength).
To differentiate myasthenic crisis from cholinergic crisis
Adults: 1 mg I.V. If no response in 1 minute, repeat dose once. Increased muscular strength confirms

myasthenic crisis; no increase or exaggerated weakness confirms cholinergic crisis.

†Paroxysmal supraventricular tachycardia
Children: 0.1 to 0.2 mg/kg (up to 2 mg) I.V. slowly.
Adults: 10 mg I.V. given over 1 minute or less.

Action and kinetics
• *Cholinergic action:* Edrophonium blocks acetylcholine's hydrolysis by cholinesterase, resulting in acetylcholine accumulation at cholinergic synapses. That leads to increased cholinergic receptor stimulation at the neuromuscular junction and vagal sites. Edrophonium is a short-acting agent which makes it particularly useful for the diagnosis of myasthenia gravis.
• *Kinetics in adults:* Action begins 30 to 60 seconds after I.V. administration and 2 to 10 minutes after I.M. administration.

Edrophonium may cross the placenta; little else is known about distribution.

Exact metabolic fate is unknown; drug is not hydrolyzed by cholinesterases. Duration of effect ranges from 5 to 10 minutes after I.V. administration and 5 to 30 minutes after I.M. administration. Exact excretion mode is unknown.

Contraindications and precautions
Edrophonium is contraindicated in patients with mechanical obstruction of the GI or urinary tract because of its stimulatory effect on smooth muscle and in patients with bradycardia, hyperthyroidism, or hypotension, because it may exacerbate these conditions.

Administer edrophonium cautiously to patients with cardiac disease because of stimulating effects on cardiovascular system; to patients with peptic ulcer disease, because it may increase gastric acid secretion; and to patients with bronchial asthma, because it may precipitate asthma attacks.

Interactions
Concomitant use with procainamide or quinidine may reverse edrophonium's cholinergic effect on muscle. Use with corticosteroids may decrease edrophonium's cholinergic effects; when corticosteroids are stopped, however, cholinergic effects may increase, possibly affecting muscle strength.

Concomitant use with succinylcholine may cause prolonged respiratory depression from plasma esterase inhibition, leading to delayed succinylcholine hydrolysis. Concomitant use with ganglionic blockers, such as mecamylamine, may lead to a critical blood pressure decrease, usually preceded by abdominal symptoms. Magnesium administration has a direct depressant effect on skeletal muscle and concomitant administration may antagonize edrophonium's anticholinesterase effect. Concomitant use with other cholinergic drugs may lead to additive toxicity.

Effects on diagnostic tests
None reported.

Adverse reactions
• CNS: weakness, *respiratory paralysis*, sweating.
• CV: *hypotension, bradycardia*, palpitations.
• EENT: miosis, blurred vision.

• GI: *nausea, vomiting, diarrhea, abdominal cramps, excessive salivation.*
• Other: *increased bronchial secretions, bronchospasm,* muscle cramps, muscle fasciculation.
Note: Drug should be discontinued if hypersensitivity, difficulty breathing, or paralysis develops.

Overdose and treatment
Clinical signs of overdose include muscle weakness, nausea, vomiting, diarrhea, blurred vision, miosis, excessive tearing, bronchospasm, increased bronchial secretions, hypotension, incoordination, excessive sweating, cramps, fasciculations, paralysis, bradycardia or tachycardia, excessive salivation, and restlessness or agitation. Muscles first weakened by overdose include neck, jaw, and pharyngeal muscles, followed by muscle weakening of the shoulder, upper extremities, pelvis, outer eye, and legs.

Discontinue drug immediately. Support respiration; bronchial suctioning may be performed. Atropine may be given to block edrophonium's muscarinic effects but will not counter the drug's paralytic effects on skeletal muscle. Avoid atropine overdose, because it may lead to bronchial plug formation.

▶ Special considerations
• Children may require I.M. administration; with this route, drug effects may be delayed for 2 to 10 minutes.
• Have atropine available to reduce or reverse hypersensitivity reactions.
• Administer atropine prior to or concurrently with large doses of parenteral anticholinesterases to counteract muscarinic side effects.
• Dosage must be individualized according to severity of disease and patient response.
• Of all cholinergics, edrophonium has the most rapid onset of action but the shortest duration of effect; consequently, it is not used to treat myasthenia gravis.
• When giving edrophonium to differentiate myasthenic crisis from cholinergic crisis, evaluate patient's muscle strength closely.
• For easier administration, use a tuberculin syringe with an I.V. needle.

Information for parents and patient
• Tell parents and patient drug's adverse affects will be transient because of its short duration of effect.

---

emetine hydrochloride

• Classification: amebicide (ipecac alkaloid)

How supplied
Available by prescription only
Injection: 65 mg/ml

Indications, route, and dosage
Acute fulminating amebic dysentery
Children: 1 mg/kg daily in two doses I.M. or S.C. for up to 5 days; maximum dosage 10 mg/day in children younger than age 8, and 20 mg/day in children over age 8.

Adults: 1 mg/kg daily, up to 60 mg daily (one or two doses), deep S.C. or I.M. for 3 to 5 days to control symptoms. Give another antiamebic drug simultaneously.

Amebic hepatitis and abscess
Adults: 60 mg daily (one or two doses) deep S.C. or I.M. for 10 days.

Dosage should be decreased by 50% in debilitated patients.

Action and kinetics
• *Amebicidal action:* Emetine is amebicidal against protozoa, especially *Entamoeba histolytica;* it causes degeneration of the nucleus and reticulum of amebic cytoplasm.

• *Kinetics in adults:* Emetine causes nausea and vomiting and is absorbed erratically after oral administration; therefore, it is administered I.M. or S.C. It is distributed into the liver, lungs, kidneys, and spleen, and it crosses the placenta. Metabolism is largely unknown. Emetine is excreted slowly by the kidneys over 2 months or more. It is unknown if emetine is excreted in breast milk.

Contraindications and precautions
Emetine also is contraindicated in children, except those with severe dysentery uncontrolled by other amebicides.

Emetine is contraindicated in patients with organic heart disease because it may cause cardiac abnormalities; in patients with kidney disease because of its slow renal elimination; in patients with recent polyneuropathy or muscle disease because it can exacerbate these conditions; and during pregnancy because of possible hazard to the fetus. I.V. administration of emetine is dangerous and contraindicated. Drug should be used with caution in patients about to undergo surgery.

Because it accumulates over time, emetine should not be used in patients who have received it during the preceding 6 weeks. Such vulnerable patients should receive emetine only if safer agents have failed.

Interactions
None reported. However, emetine's GI effects may decrease absorption of orally administered drugs.

Effects on diagnostic tests
Emetine may alter ECG tracings for 6 weeks: It may widen the QRS complex, prolong the PR or QT interval, or cause inversion or flattening of the T wave, increased amplitude of the P wave, ST deformation, premature beats, AV junctional rhythm, or transient atrial fibrillation. Decreased serum potassium levels, increased serum transaminase levels, and thrombocytopenia have also been reported.

Adverse reactions
• CNS: dizziness, headache, mild sensory disturbances, central or peripheral nerve function changes, neuromuscular symptoms (weakness, aching, stiffness, tenderness, pain, tremors).
• CV: acute toxicity (hypotension, tachycardia, precordial pain, dyspnea, ECG abnormalities, gallop rhythm, cardiac dilatation, severe acute degenerative myocarditis, pericarditis, congestive heart failure), palpitations.
• DERM: eczematous, urticarial purpuric lesions.
• GI: nausea, vomiting, diarrhea, abdominal cramps, loss of sense of taste, epigastric burning or pain, constipation.
• Metabolic: decreased serum potassium levels.
• Local: skeletal muscle stiffness, aching, tenderness, muscle weakness at injection site, cellulitis, tissue necrosis.
• Other: edema.
  Note: Acute toxicity can occur at any dosage. Drug should be discontinued if signs of hypersensitivity or toxicity occur.

Overdose and treatment
Overdose is characterized by tremors, weakness, and muscle pain. Nausea, vomiting, and diarrhea are common. Purpura, dermatitis, hemoptysis, or dysrhythmias and heart failure may occur.

Treatment of emetine overdose is supportive: Fluid management and blood pressure stabilization are important.

▶ Special considerations
• ECG should be taken before therapy, after the fifth dose, at completion of therapy, and 1 week after discontinuation.
• Emetine should not be administered I.V. The I.M. route is acceptable, but deep S.C. is preferred. Rotate injection sites and apply warm soaks to relieve local discomfort.
• Patients should be confined to bed during treatment and for several days thereafter.
• Monitor vital signs and record pulse rate and blood pressure two or three times daily.
• Assess cardiac and pulmonary status closely; be alert for shortness of breath, dyspnea on exertion, chest pain, or signs of congestive heart failure.
• Also monitor neuromuscular function, especially neck and extremities; fatigue, listlessness, and muscle stiffness usually precede more serious signs of toxicity.
• Monitor intake and output, odor and consistency of stools, and presence of mucus, blood, or other foreign matter in stools.
• Send fecal specimens to laboratory promptly; infection is detectable only in warm specimens. Repeat fecal examinations at 3-month intervals to ensure elimination of amebae.
• Also check family members and suspected contacts for infestation. Patients with acute amebic dysentery often become asymptomatic carriers.
• Isolation of patient is not required.
• This drug is irritating; avoid contact with eyes or mucous membranes.
• Suspect an emetine-induced reaction if diarrhea recurs after initial relief.
• Do not exceed recommended dose or extend therapy beyond 10 days.

Information for parents and patient
• Explain importance of medical follow-up after discharge.
• Advise parents to report any adverse reactions.

• Instruct parents and patient about limiting activities during treatment.
• Advise use of liquid soap or reserved bar of soap to prevent cross contamination.
• Encourage other household members and suspected contacts to be tested and, if necessary, treated.
• Isolation is not required, but patient must refrain from preparing, processing, or serving food until treatment is complete.
• To help prevent reinfection, instruct parents and patient in proper hygiene, including disposal of feces and hand washing after defecation and before handling, preparing, or eating food, and about the risks of eating raw food and the control of contamination by flies.

---

ephedrine
Bofedrol

ephedrine hydrochloride
Efedron

ephedrine sulfate
Ectasule Minus, Ephed II, Slo-Fedrin, Vicks Va-tro-nol

• Classification: bronchodilator, vasopressor, nasal decongestant (adrenergic)

How supplied
Available without prescription as appropriate
Capsules: 25 mg, 50 mg
Capsules (extended-release): 15 mg, 30 mg, 60 mg
Solution: 11 mg/5 ml, 20 mg/5 ml
Nasal solution: 0.6% jelly; 0.5% and 1%
Injection: 5 mg/ml, 20 mg/ml, 25 mg/ml, 50 mg/ml (parenteral)

Indications, route, and dosage
To correct hypotensive states
Children: 3 mg/kg S.C. or 100 mg/m² I.V. daily, divided into four to six doses.
Adults: 25 to 50 mg I.M. or S.C., or 10 to 25 mg slow I.V. bolus. If necessary, a second I.M. dose of 50 mg or I.V. dose of 25 mg may be administered. Additional I.V. doses may be given in 5 to 10 minutes. Maximum dosage, 150 mg daily.
Orthostatic hypotension
Children: 3 mg/kg P.O. daily, divided into four to six doses.
Adults: 25 mg P.O. once daily to q.i.d.
Bronchodilator or nasal decongestant
Children: 2 to 3 mg/kg or 100 mg/m² P.O. daily in four to six divided doses.
Adults: 25 mg to 50 mg q 3 to 4 hours as needed; or 15 to 60 mg extended-release capsules q 8 to 12 hours. As nasal decongestant, 0.5% to 1% solution topically to nasal mucosa as drops, or on a nasal pack. Instill no more often than q 4 hours.
Severe, acute bronchospasm
Children: 3 mg/kg or 100 mg/m² I.V. or S.C. daily in four to six divided doses.

Adults: 12.5 to 25 mg I.M., S.C., or I.V.

Action and kinetics
Ephedrine is both a direct- and indirect-acting sympathomimetic that stimulates alpha- and beta-adrenergic receptors. Release of norepinephrine from its storage sites is one of its indirect effects. In therapeutic doses, ephedrine relaxes bronchial smooth muscle and produces cardiac stimulation with increased systolic and diastolic blood pressure when norepinephrine stores are not depleted.
• *Bronchodilator action:* Ephedrine relaxes bronchial smooth muscle by stimulating beta₂-adrenergic receptors, resulting in increased vital capacity, relief of mild bronchospasm, improved air exchange, and decreased residual volume.
• *Vasopressor action:* Ephedrine produces positive inotropic effects with low doses by action on beta₁-adrenergic receptors in the heart. Vasodilation results from its effect on beta₂-adrenergic receptors; vasoconstriction from its alpha-adrenergic effects. Pressor effects may result from vasoconstriction or cardiac stimulation; however, when peripheral vascular resistance is decreased, blood pressure elevation results from increased cardiac output.
• *Nasal decongestant action:* Ephedrine stimulates alpha-adrenergic receptors in blood vessels of nasal mucosa, producing vasoconstriction and nasal decongestion.
• *Kinetics in adults:* Ephedrine is rapidly and completely absorbed after oral, S.C., or I.M. administration. After oral administration, onset of action occurs within 15 to 60 minutes and persists 2 to 4 hours. Pressor and cardiac effects last 1 hour after I.V. dose of 10 to 25 mg or I.M. or S.C. dose of 25 to 50 mg; they last up to 4 hours after oral dose of 15 to 50 mg. Ephedrine is widely distributed throughout the body.
  Ephedrine is slowly metabolized in the liver by oxidative deamination, demethylation, aromatic hydroxylation, and conjugation. Most of a dose is excreted unchanged in urine. Rate of excretion depends on urine pH.

Contraindications and precautions
Ephedrine is contraindicated in patients with narrow-angle glaucoma or psychoneurosis, because the drug may exacerbate these conditions. The injectable form is contraindicated during general anesthesia with cyclopropane or halothane, because the patient may experience cardiac dysrhythmias.
  Administer with extreme caution to hypertensive or hyperthyroid patients (increased incidence of adverse reactions), diabetic patients, and those with cardiovascular disease or a history of sensitivity to ephedrine or other sympathomimetics.

Interactions
Concomitant use of other sympathomimetic agents may add to their effects and toxicity. Use with alpha-adrenergic blocking agents may decrease vasopressor effects of ephedrine. Concomitant beta-adrenergic blocking agents may block cardiovascular and bronchodilating effects of ephedrine. Use with general anesthetics (especially cyclopropane or halothane) and

---

:May contain sulfites   ◆May contain tartrazine   ◆◆May contain benzyl alcohol

digitalis glycosides may sensitize myocardium to effects of ephedrine, causing cardiac dysrhythmias.

MAO inhibitors may potentiate the pressor effects of ephedrine, possibly resulting in hypertensive crisis. Allow 14 days to lapse after withdrawal of MAO inhibitor before using ephedrine. Reserpine, guanethidine, methyldopa, and diuretics may decrease ephedrine's pressor effects.

Concomitant use with atropine blocks reflex bradycardia and enhances pressor effects. Administration with a theophylline derivative such as aminophylline reportedly produces a greater incidence of adverse reactions than either drug when used alone.

Effects on diagnostic tests
None reported.

Adverse reactions
• CNS: nervousness, anxiety, apprehension, fear, tension, agitation, excitation, restlessness, insomnia, weakness, irritability, talkativeness, dizziness, lightheadedness, vertigo, tremor, hyperactive reflexes, confusion, delirium, hallucinations, euphoria.
• CV: hypertension, palpitations, tachycardia, dysrhythmias, precordial pain.
• GI: nausea, vomiting, mild epigastric distress, anorexia.
• GU: urinary retention, difficult urination, priapism.
• Other: fever; pallor; dryness of mouth, throat, and nose; respiratory difficulty; sweating; rebound congestion; and tachyphylaxis.

Overdose and treatment
Clinical manifestations of overdose include exaggeration of common adverse reactions, especially cardiac dysrhythmias, extreme tremors or convulsions, nausea and vomiting, fever, and CNS and respiratory depression.

Treatment requires supportive and symptomatic measures. If patient is conscious, induce emesis with ipecac followed by activated charcoal. If patient is depressed or hyperactive, perform gastric lavage. Maintain airway and blood pressure. Do not administer vasopressors. Monitor vital signs closely.

A beta blocker (such as propranolol) may be used to treat cardiac dysrhythmias. A cardioselective beta blocker is recommended in asthmatic patients. Phentolamine may be used for hypertension; paraldehyde or diazepam for convulsions; dexamethasone for pyrexia.

▶ **Special considerations**
• As a pressor agent, ephedrine is not a substitute for blood, plasma, fluids, or electrolytes. Correct fluid volume depletion before administration.
• Tolerance may develop after prolonged or excessive use. Increased dose may be needed. Also, if drug is discontinued for a few days and readministered, effectiveness may be restored.
• To prevent insomnia, last dose should be taken at least 2 hours before bedtime.
• With parenteral dosing, monitor blood pressure, pulse, respirations, and urine output closely during infusion. Tachycardia is common. Tachyphylaxis or tolerance may develop after prolonged or excessive use.

Information for parents and patient
• Tell parents administering nonprescription product to follow directions on label. Patient should take last dose a few hours before bedtime to reduce possibility of insomnia, take only as directed, and not increase dose or frequency.
• Warn parents and patient not to crush, break, or chew extended-release capsules. If capsule is too large to swallow, patient may open it and mix contents with applesauce, jelly, honey, or syrup and swallow without chewing.
• Instruct parents and patient on proper method of instillation.
— Drops: Tell patient to tilt head back while sitting or standing up; or to lie on bed with head over side. Stay in position a few minutes to permit medication to spread through nose.
— Spray: With head upright, squeeze bottle quickly and firmly to produce one or two sprays into each nostril; wait 3 to 5 minutes, blow nose, and repeat dose.
— Jelly: Place in each nostril and sniff it well back into nose.
• Instruct patient to blow nose gently (with both nostrils open) to clear nasal passages before administration of medication.
• Instruct parents that patient who misses a dose should take it as soon as remembered if within 1 hour. If beyond 1 hour, patient should skip dose and return to regular schedule.
• Teach patient to be aware of palpitations and significant pulse rate changes.

---

epinephrine
Bronkaid Mist, Bronkaid Mistometer*, Dysne-Inhal*, EpiPen, EpiPen Jr., Primatene Mist Solution, Sus-Phrine

epinephrine bitartrate
AsthmaHaler, Bronitin Mist, Bronkaid Mist Suspension, Epitrate, Medihaler-Epi, Primatene Mist Suspension

epinephrine hydrochloride
Adrenalin Chloride, Epifrin, Glaucon

racemic epinephrine (racepinephrine)
AsthmaNefrin, microNEFRIN, S-2 Inhalant, Vaponefin

• Classification: bronchodilator, vasopressor, cardiac stimulant, local anesthetic, topical antihemorrhagic, antiglaucoma agent (adrenergic)

How supplied
Available without prescription
Nebulizer inhaler: 1% (1:100), 1.25%, 2.25%

Aerosol inhaler: 160 mcg, 200 mcg, 250 mcg/metered spray

Available by prescription only
Injection: 0.01 mg/ml (1:100,000), 0.1 mg/ml (1:10,000), 0.5 mg/ml (1:2,000), 1 mg/ml (1:1,000) parenteral; 5 mg/ml (1:200) parenteral suspension

Indications, route, and dosage
Severe anaphylaxis or asthma
Children: 0.01 mg/kg (0.01 ml/kg of a 1:1000 solution) or 0.3 mg/m² (0.3 ml/m² of a 1:1000 solution) S.C. Dosage not to exceed 0.5 mg. May be repeated at 20-minute to 4-hour intervals as needed. Alternatively, 0.02 to 0.025 mg/kg (0.004 to 0.005 ml/kg) or 0.625 mg/m² (0.125 ml/m²) of a 1:200 solution. May be repeated but not more often than every 6 hours. Alternatively, 0.1 mg (10 ml of a 1:100,000 dilution) I.V. slowly over 5 to 10 minutes followed by a 0.1 to 1.5 mcg/kg/minute I.V. infusion.
Adults: Initially, 0.1 to 0.5 mg (0.1 to 0.5 mg of a 1:1000 solution) S.C. or I.M.; may be repeated if needed. Alternatively, 0.1 to 0.25 mg (1 to 2.5 ml of a 1:10,000 solution) I.V. slowly over 5 to 10 minutes. May be repeated every 5 to 15 minutes if needed or followed by a 1 to 4 mcg/minute I.V. infusion.
Bronchodilator
Epinephrine
Children and adults: One inhalation via metered aerosol, repeated once if needed after 1 minute; subsequent doses should not be repeated for at least 4 hours. Alternatively, one or two deep inhalations via hand-bulb nebulizer of a 1% (1:100) solution; may be repeated at 1-to 2-minute intervals. Alternatively, 0.03 ml (0.3 mg) of a 1% solution via IPPB.
Racemic epinephrine
Children over age 4 and adults: Two or three inhalations of a 2.25% solution followed in 5 minutes by an additional two or three inhalations. Repeat four to six times daily.
To restore cardiac rhythm in cardiac arrest
Infants: Initially, 0.01 to 0.03 mg/kg (0.1 to 0.3 ml/kg of a 1:10,000 solution) I.V. bolus or intratracheal. May be repeated q 5 minutes if needed.
Children: Initially, 0.01 mg/kg (0.1 ml/kg of a 1:10,000 solution) I.V. bolus or intratracheally; may be repeated q 5 minutes if needed.
Alternatively, initially, 0.1 mcg/kg/minute; may increase in increments of 0.1 mcg/kg/minute to a maximum of 1 mcg/kg/minute. Alternatively, 0.005 to 0.01 mg/kg (0.05 to 0.1 ml of a 1:10,000 solution) intracardiac.
Adults: Initially, 0.5 to 1 mg (range: 0.1 to 1 mg [1 to 10 ml of a 1:10,000 solution]) I.V. bolus; may be repeated q 5 minutes if needed. Alternatively, initial dose followed by 0.3 mg S.C. or 1 to 4 mcg/minute I.V. infusion. Alternatively, 1 mg (10 ml of a 1:10,000 solution) intratracheally, or 0.1 to 1 mg (1 to 10 ml of a 1:10,000 solution) intracardiac.
Hemostatic use
Children and adults: 1:50,000 to 1:1,000, applied topically.
To prolong local anesthetic effect
Children and adults: 1:500,000 to 1:50,000 mixed with local anesthetic.

Action and kinetics
Epinephrine acts directly by stimulating alpha- and beta-adrenergic receptors in the sympathetic nervous system. Its main therapeutic effects include relaxation of bronchial smooth muscle, cardiac stimulation, and dilation of skeletal muscle vasculature.
• *Bronchodilator action:* Epinephrine relaxes bronchial smooth muscle by stimulating beta₂-adrenergic receptors. Epinephrine constricts bronchial arterioles by stimulating alpha-adrenergic receptors, resulting in relief of bronchospasm, reduced congestion and edema, and increased tidal volume and vital capacity. By inhibiting histamine release, it may reverse bronchiolar constriction, vasodilation, and edema.
• *Cardiovascular and vasopressor actions:* As a cardiac stimulant, epinephrine produces positive chronotropic and inotropic effects by action on beta₁ receptors in the heart, increasing cardiac output, myocardial oxygen consumption, and force of contraction, and decreasing cardiac efficiency. Vasodilation results from its effect on beta₂ receptors; vasoconstriction results from alpha-adrenergic effects.
• *Local anesthetic (adjunct) action:* Epinephrine acts on alpha receptors in skin, mucous membranes, and viscera; it produces vasoconstriction, which reduces absorption of local anesthetic, thus prolonging its duration of action, localizing anesthesia, and decreasing risk of anesthetic's toxicity.
• *Local vasoconstricting action:* Epinephrine's effect results from action on alpha receptors in skin, mucous membranes, and viscera, which produces vasoconstriction and hemostasis in small vessels.
• *Kinetics in adults:* Well absorbed after S.C. or I.M. injection, epinephrine has a rapid onset of action and short duration of action. Bronchodilation occurs within 5 to 10 minutes and peaks in 20 minutes after S.C. injection; onset after oral inhalation is within 1 minute.
Topical administration or intraocular injection usually produces local vasoconstriction within 5 minutes and lasts less than 1 hour. After topical application to the conjunctiva, reduction of intraocular pressure occurs within 1 hour, peaks in 4 to 8 hours, and persists up to 24 hours. Epinephrine is distributed widely throughout the body.
Drug is metabolized at sympathetic nerve endings, liver, and other tissues to inactive metabolites. Epinephrine is excreted in urine, mainly as its metabolites and conjugates.

Contraindications and precautions
Epinephrine is contraindicated in patients with shock (except anaphylactic shock), cardiac heart disease, cardiac dilatation, and dysrhythmias, because it increases myocardial oxygen demand; in patients with organic brain damage or cerebral arteriosclerosis, because of potential adverse CNS effects; in patients with narrow-angle glaucoma, because the drug may worsen the condition; and in patients with known sensitivity to the drug. Epinephrine is contraindicated in conjunction with local anesthetics in fingers, toes, ears, nose, or genitalia, because vasoconstriction in these extremities may induce tissue necrosis.
Administer with extreme caution to patients with hypertension or hyperthyroidism; and to diabetic pa-

‡May contain sulfites   ♦ May contain tartrazine   ♦ ♦ May contain benzyl alcohol

tients, and those with cardiovascular diseases, history of sensitivity to sympathomimetics, bronchial asthma, or psychoneurotic disorders. Use with extreme caution in patients receiving inhalational anesthetics because of the potential for cardiac dysrhythmias. Use cautiously in patients with sulfite hypersensitivity; some epinephrine preparations contain sulfites.

Interactions
Concomitant use with other sympathomimetics may produce additive effects and toxicity. Beta-adrenergic blockers antagonize cardiac and bronchodilating effects of epinephrine; alpha-adrenergic blockers antagonize vasoconstriction and hypertension. Use with general anesthetics (especially cyclopropane and halothane) and digitalis glycosides may sensitize the myocardium to epinephrine's effects, causing dysrhythmias. Use with tricyclic antidepressants, antihistamines, and thyroid hormones may potentiate adverse cardiac effects of epinephrine. Concomitant use with oxytocics or ergot alkaloids may cause severe hypertension.

Because phenothiazines may cause reversal of its pressor effects, epinephrine should not be used to treat circulatory collapse or hypotension caused by phenothiazines; such use may cause further lowering of blood pressure.

Use with guanethidine may decrease its hypotensive effects while potentiating epinephrine's effects, resulting in hypertension and cardiac dysrhythmias.

Concomitant use of ophthalmic epinephrine with topical miotics, topical beta-adrenergic blocking agents, osmotic agents, and carbonic anhydrase inhibitors may cause additive lowering of intraocular pressure. Concomitant use with miotics offers the advantage of reducing the ciliary spasm, mydriasis, blurred vision, and increased intraocular pressure that may occur with miotics or epinephrine alone.

Effects on diagnostic tests
Epinephrine therapy alters blood glucose and serum lactic acid levels (both may be increased), increases BUN levels, and interferes with tests for urinary catecholamines.

Adverse reactions
• CNS: fear, anxiety, tenseness, restlessness, *headache*, tremor, dizziness, light-headedness, *nervousness*, sleeplessness, excitability, irritability, weakness, psychomotor agitation, disorientation, impaired memory, panic, hallucinations, suicidal tendencies, *cerebral hemorrhage*.
• CV: ECG changes (decreased T-wave amplitude), *disturbances in cardiac rhythm and rate* (palpitations, tachycardia), angina, *dysrhythmias*, syncope, *hypertension, vasoconstriction, pulmonary edema*.
• EENT: ocular discomfort, conjunctival irritation, lacrimation, blurred vision, mydriasis, localized melanin-like pigmentary deposits in the conjunctiva or eyelids (prolonged ophthalmic use).
• GI: *nausea, vomiting*.
• Other: sweating, pallor, respiratory difficulty, rebound nasal congestion, respiratory weakness, apnea, *hyperglycemia, hypokalemia*, contact dermatitis. Ex-

travasation can cause local necrosis and bleeding at injection site.
Note: Drug should be discontinued if hypersensitivity occurs.

Overdose and treatment
Clinical manifestations of overdose may include a sharp increase in systolic and diastolic blood pressure, rise in venous pressure, severe anxiety, irregular heartbeat, severe nausea or vomiting, severe respiratory distress, unusually large pupils, unusual paleness and coldness of skin, pulmonary edema, renal failure, and metabolic acidosis.

Treatment includes symptomatic and supportive measures, because epinephrine is rapidly inactivated in the body. Monitor vital signs closely. Trimethaphan or phentolamine may be needed for hypotension; beta blockers (such as propranolol), for dysrhythmias.

▶ Special considerations
• Ensure correct dilution dosage.
• After S.C. or I.M. injection, massaging the site may hasten absorption.
• Epinephrine is destroyed by oxidizing agents, alkalies (including sodium bicarbonate), halogens, permanganates, chromates, nitrates, and salts of easily reducible metals, such as iron, copper, and zinc.
• A tuberculin syringe may assure greater accuracy in measurement of parenteral doses.
• To avoid hazardous medication errors, check carefully type of solution prescribed, concentration, dosage, and route before administration. Do not mix with alkali.
• Before withdrawing epinephrine suspension into syringe, shake vial or ampule thoroughly to disperse particles; then inject promptly. Do not use solution that is discolored or contains a precipitate.
• Repeated injections may cause tissue necrosis from vascular constriction. Rotate injection sites, and observe for signs of blanching.
• Avoid I.M. injection into buttocks. Epinephrine-induced vasoconstriction favors growth of the anaerobe *Clostridium perfringens*.
• Monitor blood pressure, pulse, respirations, and urine output, and observe patient closely. Epinephrine may widen pulse pressure. If dysrhythmias occur, discontinue epinephrine immediately. Watch for changes in intake/output ratio.
• Patients receiving I.V. epinephrine should be on cardiac monitor. Keep resuscitation equipment available.
• When drug is administered I.V., check patient's blood pressure repeatedly during first 5 minutes, then every 3 to 5 minutes until patient is stable.
• Intracardiac administration requires external cardiac massage to move drug into coronary circulation.
• Drying effect on bronchial secretions may make mucus plugs more difficult to dislodge. Bronchial hygiene program, including postural drainage, breathing exercises, and adequate hydration, may be necessary.
• Epinephrine may increase blood glucose levels. Closely observe patients with diabetes for loss of diabetes control.
• Monitor amount, consistency, and color of sputum.

---

arenteral preparations

f used as a pressor agent, correct fluid volume de-
etion before administration. Adrenergics are not a
bstitute for blood, plasma, fluid, or electrolytes.
achyphylaxis (tolerance) may develop after pro-
nged or excessive use.

halation

Treatment should start with first symptoms of bron-
ospasm. Patient should use the least number of
halations that provides relief. To prevent excessive
sage, at least 1 or 2 minutes should elapse before
king additional inhalations of epinephrine. Dosage
quirements vary. Warn patient that overuse or too-
equent use can cause severe adverse reactions.

The preservative sodium bisulfite is present in many
lrenergic formulations. Patients with a history of
lergy to sulfites should avoid preparations that con-
in this preservative.

Therapy should be administered when patient arises
morning and before meals to reduce fatigue by
iproving lung ventilation.

Adrenergic inhalation may be alternated with other
lrenergics if necessary, but should not be admin-
tered simultaneously because of danger of excessive
chycardia.

Do not use discolored or precipitated solutions.

Protect solutions from light, freezing, and heat. Store
controlled room temperature.

Systemic absorption can follow applications to nasal
nd conjunctival membranes, though infrequently. If
mptoms of systemic absorption occur, patient should
op taking the drug.

Prolonged or too-frequent use may cause tolerance
bronchodilating and cardiac stimulant effect. Re-
ound bronchospasm may follow end of drug effect.

asal

Instill nose drops with patient's head in lateral,
ead-low position to prevent entry of drug into throat.

formation for parents and patient

Urge patient to report diminishing effect. Repeated
prolonged use of epinephrine can cause tolerance
the drug's effects. Continuing to take epinephrine
espite tolerance can be hazardous. Interrupting drug
erapy for 12 hours to several days may restore re-
onsiveness to drug.

halation

Instruct patient to rinse mouth and throat with water
mediately after inhalation to avoid swallowing re-
dual drug (the propellant in the aerosol preparation
ay cause epigastric pain and systemic effects) and
prevent dryness of oropharyngeal membranes.

Treatment should start with first symptoms of bron-
ospasm.

Dosage and recommended method of inhaling may
ary with type of nebulizer and formulation used.
Information and instructions are furnished with the
erosol forms of these drugs. Urge parents or patient
read them carefully and ask questions if necessary.

Carefully instruct parents and patient in correct use
nebulizer. Patient should take no more than two
halations at a time with 1- to 2-minute intervals
etween.

Teach parents and patient that a single aerosol treat-
ent is usually enough to control an asthma attack.

Tell them to call promptly if the patient requires more
than three aerosol treatments in 24 hours, and to
call immediately if patient receives no relief within
20 minutes or if condition worsens.

• Explain that overuse of adrenergic bronchodilators
may cause tachycardia, palpitations, headache, nausea and dizziness, loss of effectiveness, possible paradoxical reaction, and cardiac arrest.

• Tell parents to call if bronchodilator causes dizziness, chest pain, or lack of therapeutic response to
usual dose.

• Patient should avoid other adrenergic medications
unless they are prescribed.

• Tell parents and patient that increased fluid intake
facilitates clearing of secretions. Inform them that
saliva and sputum may appear pink after inhalation
treatment.

• Teach parents and patient how to accomplish postural drainage, to cough productively, and to clap and
vibrate to promote good respiratory hygiene.

• Tell patient not to discard drug applicator. Refill
units are available.

• Inform parents and patient taking repeated doses
about adverse reactions, and advise them to report
such reactions promptly.

Nasal

• Tell parents to call if patient's symptoms are not
relieved in 20 minutes or if they become worse, and
to report bronchial irritation, nervousness, or sleeplessness, which require reduced dosage.

• Warn parents or patient that intranasal applications
may sting slightly and cause rebound congestion or
drug-induced rhinitis after prolonged use. Nose drops
should be used for 3 or 4 days only. Encourage patient
to use drug exactly as prescribed.

• Advise rinsing nose dropper or spray tip with hot
water after each use to avoid contaminating the solution.

• To avoid excessive systemic absorption, parent or
patient should gently press finger against patient's
nasolacrimal duct for at least 1 or 2 minutes immediately after drug instillation.

ergocalciferol
Calciferol, Deltalin Gelseals, Drisdol,
Vitamin D Capsules

• Classification: antihypocalcemic (vitamin)

How supplied

Available without prescription
Liquid: 8,000 units/ml in 60 ml dropper bottle

Available by prescription only
Capsules: 0.625 mg (25,000 units), 1.25 mg (50,000
units)
Tablets: 1.25 mg (50,000 units)
Injection: 12.5 mg (500,000 units)/ml

Indications, route, and dosage
Nutritional rickets or osteomalacia
Children: 25 to 125 mcg P.O. daily if patient has normal GI absorption. With malabsorption, 250 to 625 mcg.

Adults: 25 to 125 mcg P.O. daily if patient has normal GI absorption. With severe malabsorption, 250 mcg to 7.5 mg P.O. or 250 mcg I.M. daily.

Familial hypophosphatemia
Children: 1 to 2 mg P.O. daily with phosphate supplements. Increase daily dosage in 250- to 500-mg increments at 3- to 4-month intervals until adequate response is obtained.

Adults: 250 mcg to 1.5 mg P.O. daily with phosphate supplements.

Vitamin D-dependent rickets
Children: 75 to 125 mcg P.O. daily.

Adults: 250 mcg to 1.5 mg P.O. daily.

Anticonvulsant-induced rickets and osteomalacia
Adults: 50 mcg to 1.25 mg P.O. daily.

Hypoparathyroidism and pseudohypoparathyroidism
Children: 1.25 to 5 mg P.O. daily with calcium supplements.

Adults: 625 mcg to 5 mg P.O. daily with calcium supplements.

Action and kinetics
• *Antihypocalcemic action:* Once activated, ergocalciferol acts to regulate the serum concentrations of calcium by regulating absorption from the GI tract and resorption from bone.
• *Kinetics in adults:* Drug is absorbed readily in the small intestine. Onset of action is 10 to 24 hours. Drug is distributed widely and bound to proteins. It is metabolized in the liver and kidneys. It has an average half-life of 24 hours and a duration of up to 6 months. Bile (feces) is the primary excretion route. A small percentage is excreted in urine.

Contraindications and precautions
Ergocalciferol is contraindicated in patients with hypercalcemia or vitamin D toxicity, malabsorption syndrome, or abnormal sensitivity to vitamin D effects.

Use with extreme caution in patients with impaired renal function, heart disease, renal stones, arteriosclerosis; and in patients receiving cardiac glycosides.

Interactions
Concomitant use of ergocalciferol and cardiac glycosides may result in cardiac dysrhythmias. Concomitant use with thiazide diuretics may cause hypercalcemia in patients with hypoparathyroidism; with magnesium-containing antacids may lead to hypermagnesemia; with verapamil may induce recurrence of atrial fibrillation when supplemental calcium and calciferol have induced hypercalcemia. Corticosteroids counteract the drug's effects. Administration of phenobarbital or phenytoin may increase the drug's metabolism to inactive metabolites. Cholestyramine, colestipol, and excessive use of mineral oil may interfere with the absorption of ergocalciferol.

Effects on diagnostic tests
Ergocalciferol may falsely increase serum cholesterol levels and may elevate AST (SGOT) and ALT (SGPT) levels.

Adverse reactions
Adverse reactions listed are usually seen in vitamin D toxicity only.
• CNS: headache, dizziness, ataxia, irritability, weakness, somnolence, decreased libido, overt psychosis, seizures.
• CV: calcifications of soft tissues, including the heart, hypertension, dysrhythmias.
• DERM: pruritus.
• EENT: dry mouth, metallic taste, rhinorrhea, conjunctivitis (calcific), photophobia, tinnitus.
• GI: anorexia, nausea, vomiting, constipation, diarrhea.
• GU: polyuria, albuminuria, hypercalciuria, nocturia, impaired renal function, renal calculi.
• Metabolic: hypercalcemia, hyperphosphatemia.
• Other: bone and muscle pain, bone demineralization, weight loss, weakness, fever, overt psychosis, polydipsia.

Note: Drug should be discontinued if adverse reactions become severe.

Overdose and treatment
Clinical manifestations of overdose include hypercalcemia, hypercalciuria, and hyperphophotemia, which may be treated by stopping therapy, starting a low calcium diet, and increasing fluid intake. A loop diuretic, such as furosemide, may be given with saline I.V. infusion to increase calcium excretion. Supportive measures should be provided. In severe cases, death from cardiac or renal failure may occur. Calcitonin may decrease hypercalcemia.

▶ Special considerations
• Some infants may be hyperreactive to this drug.
• I.M. injection of ergocalciferol dispersed in oil is preferable in patients who cannot absorb the oral form.
• If I.V. route is necessary, use only water-miscible solutions intended for dilution in large-volume parenteral solutions. Use cautiously in cardiac patients, especially if they are receiving cardiotonic glycosides. In such patients, hypercalcemia may precipitate dysrhythmias.
• Monitor eating and bowel habits; dry mouth, nausea, vomiting, metallic taste, and constipation can be early signs of toxicity.
• Patients with hyperphosphatemia require dietary phosphate restrictions and binding agents to avoid metastatic calcifications and renal calculi.
• When high therapeutic doses are used, frequent serum and urine calcium, potassium, and urea determinations should be made.
• Malabsorption caused by inadequate bile or hepatic dysfunction may require addition of exogenous bile salts.
• Doses of 60,000 IU daily can cause hypercalcemia.
• Patients taking ergocalciferol should restrict their intake of magnesium-containing antacids.

Information for parents and patient
• Explain the importance of a diet rich in calcium.
• Caution parents that patient should not increase daily dose on his own initiative. Vitamin D is a fat-soluble vitamin; vitamin D toxicity is thus more likely to occur.
• Patient should avoid magnesium-containing antacids and mineral oil.
• Patient should swallow tablets whole without crushing or chewing.

---

ergotamine tartrate
Ergomar, Ergostat, Medihaler-Ergotamine, Wigrettes

• Classification: vasoconstrictor (ergot alkaloid)

How supplied
Available without prescription, as appropriate
Tablets (sublingual): 2 mg
Aerosal inhaler: 360 mcg/metered spray

Indications, route, and dosage
To prevent or abort vascular headache, including migraine and cluster headaches
†*Older children and adolescents:* 1 mg S.L. as needed. May repeat once in 30 minutes.
Adults: Initially, 2 mg S.L., then 1 to 2 mg S.L. q ½ hour, to maximum 6 mg daily and 10 mg weekly. Alternatively, initially, inhalation; if not relieved in 5 minutes, repeat inhalation. May repeat inhalations at least 5 minutes apart up to maximum of six inhalations per 24 hours or fifteen inhalations weekly.

Action and kinetics
• *Vasoconstricting action:* By stimulating alpha-adrenergic receptors, ergotamine in therapeutic doses causes peripheral vasoconstriction (if vascular tone is low); however, if vascular tone is high, it produces vasodilation. In high doses, it is a competitive alpha-adrenergic blocker. In therapeutic doses, it inhibits the reuptake of norepinephrine, which increases the vasoconstricting activity of ergotamine. A weaker serotonin antagonist, it reduces the increased rate of platelet aggregation caused by serotonin.

In the treatment of vascular headaches, ergotamine probably causes direct vasoconstriction of dilated carotid artery beds while decreasing the amplitude of pulsations. Its serotoninergic and catecholamine effects also seem to be involved.
• *Kinetics in adults:* Ergotamine is rapidly absorbed after inhalation and variably absorbed after oral administration. Peak concentrations are reached within ½ to 3 hours. Caffeine may increase rate and extent of absorption. Drug undergoes first-pass metabolism after oral administration. Ergotamine is widely distributed throughout the body and is extensively metabolized in the liver. 4% of a dose is excreted in urine within 96 hours; remainder of a dose presumed to be excreted in feces. Ergotamine is dialyzable. Onset of action depends on how promptly drug is given after onset of headache.

Contraindications and precautions
Ergotamine is contraindicated in patients with sepsis or peripheral vascular disease, because of adverse vascular effects; in patients with impaired renal or hepatic function, because of the potential for accumulation and toxicity; and in patients with malnutrition, severe pruritus, severe hypertension, or known hypersensitivity to drug or ergot alkaloids. Ergotamine is also contraindicated in patients who are or who may become pregnant.

Interactions
Concomitant use with propranolol or other beta blockers may intensify ergotamine's vasoconstrictor effects. Use with troleandomycin appears to interfere with the detoxification of ergotamine in the liver; use concurrently with caution.

Effects on diagnostic tests
None reported.

Adverse reactions
• CV: numbness or tingling in fingers and toes, transient sinus tachycardia or bradycardia, arterial spasm, symptoms of impaired peripheral circulation (cold, numb, painful extremities with or without paresthesia; diminished or absent pulse in affected extremity; claudication of legs), coronary insufficiency, precipitation or aggravation of angina pectoris.
• GI: nausea, vomiting, abdominal pain, diarrhea, epigastric pain, ischemic colitis.
• Other: weakness in legs, localized edema, muscle pain or stiffness, fatigue, polydipsia, itching.
   Note: Drug should be discontinued if patient develops hypersensitivity, signs and symptoms of impaired circulation, severe headaches, or worsening of migraine.

Overdose and treatment
Clinical manifestations of overdose include adverse vasospastic effects, nausea, vomiting, lassitude, impaired mental function, delirium, severe dyspnea, hypotension, hypertension, rapid and weak pulse, unconsciousness, spasms of the limbs, seizures, and shock.

Treatment requires supportive and symptomatic measures, with prolonged and careful monitoring. If patient is conscious and ingestion is recent, empty stomach by emesis or gastric lavage; if comatose, perform gastric lavage after placement of endotracheal tube with cuff inflated. Activated charcoal and a saline (magnesium sulfate) cathartic may be used. Provide respiratory support. Apply warmth (not direct heat) to ischemic extremities if vasospasm occurs. As needed, administer vasodilators (nitroprusside, prazosin, or tolazoline) and if necessary, I.V. diazepam to treat convulsions. Dialysis may be helpful.

▶ Special considerations
• Safety and efficacy of ergotamine in young children have not been established.
• Monitor vital signs, especially blood pressure.
• Administer dose at bedtime to reduce potential of dizziness or light-headedness.
• Ergotamine is most effective when used in prodromal

---

stage of headache or as soon as possible after onset. Provide quiet, low-light environment to relax patient after dose is administered.
• Store drug in light-resistant container.
• Sublingual tablet is preferred during early stage of attack because of its rapid absorption.
• Obtain an accurate dietary history to determine possible relationship between certain foods and onset of headache.
• Rebound headache or an increase in duration or frequency of headache may occur when drug is withdrawn.
• If patient experiences severe vasoconstriction with tissue necrosis, administer I.V. sodium nitroprusside or intraarterial tolazoline. I.V. heparin and 10% dextran 40 in 5% dextrose injection also may be administered to prevent vascular stasis and thrombosis.

Information for parents and patient
• Warn parents and patient about postural hypotension. Patient should avoid sudden changes to upright position.
• Tell parents to call promptly if patient develops dizziness or irregular heartbeat.
• Advise parents to have patient take dose at bedtime to reduce potential for dizziness or light-headedness.
• Warn parents that patient should avoid hazardous tasks that require mental alertness until effects of medication are established.
• Reassure parents and patient that adverse effects should lessen after several doses.
• Tell parents and patient that the use of alcohol, excessive exercise, prolonged standing, and exposure to heat will intensify adverse effects.
• Advise parents against giving patient any other medication, including any that can be purchased without a prescription.
• Instruct parents and patient in correct use of inhaler.
• Urge parents to report immediately any feelings of numbness or tingling in fingers or toes, or red or violet blisters on hands or feet.
• Warn parents that patient should avoid prolonged exposure to very cold temperatures, which may increase adverse effects of drug.
• Tell parent to promptly report illness or infection, which may increase sensitivity to drug effects.
• Tell the parents and patient that the body may need time to adjust, depending on the amount used and length of time involved, after discontinuing the medication.
• Advise parents of patients who use inhaler to call promptly if mouth, throat, or lung infection occurs, or if condition worsens. Cough, hoarseness, or throat irritation may occur. Patient should gargle and rinse mouth after each dose to help prevent hoarseness and irritation.
• Advise parents to call promptly if persistent numbness or tingling and chest, muscle, or abdominal pain occur.
• Advise parents and patient not to exceed recommended dosage.

erythromycin base
E-Mycin, Eryc, Eryc Sprinkle*, Erythrocin, Erythromycin Base Filmtabs, Robimycin, Ethril 500

erythromycin estolate
Ilosone

erythromycin ethylsuccinate
E.E.S., E-Mycin E, Pediamycin, Pediazole, Wyamycin E

erythromycin gluceptate
Ilotycin Gluceptate

erythromycin lactobionate
Erythrocin Lactobionate

erythromycin stearate
Apo-Erythro-S*, Erypar Filmseal, Erythrocin Stearate, Ethril, Novorythro*, Wyamycin S

erythromycin (topical)
Akne-Mycin, A/T/S, Eryvette, EryDerm, Erymax, Sansac*, Staticin, T-Stat

• Classification: antibiotic (macrolide)

How supplied
Available by prescription only
Oral suspension: 200 mg/5 ml, 125 mg/5 ml, 400 mg/5 ml
Erythromycin base
Tablets (enteric-coated): 250 mg, 330 mg, 500 mg
Pellets (enteric-coated): 250 mg
Erythromycin estolate
Tablets: 250 mg, 500 mg
Tablets (chewable): 125 mg, 250 mg
Capsules: 125 mg, 250 mg
Drops: 100 mg/ml
Suspension: 125 mg/5 ml, 250 mg/5 ml
Erythromycin ethylsuccinate
Tablets (chewable): 200 mg, 400 mg
Topical solution: 1.5%, 2%
Ophthalmic ointment: 5 mg/g
Erythromycin gluceptate
Injection: 250-mg, 500-mg, and 1-g vials
Erythromycin lactobionate
Injection: 500-mg and 1-g vials
Erythromycin stearate
Tablets (film-coated): 250 mg, 500 mg

Indications, route, and dosage
Acute pelvic inflammatory disease caused by Neisseria gonorrhoeae
Adults: 500 mg I.V. (erythromycin gluceptate, lactobionate) q 6 hours for 3 days, then 250 mg (erythromycin base, estolate, stearate) or 400 mg (erythromycin ethylsuccinate) P.O. q 6 hours for 7 days.

Endocarditis prophylaxis for dental procedures in patients allergic to penicillin
Erythromycin base, estolate, stearate
Adults: 1 g P.O. 1 hour before procedure, then 500 mg P.O. 6 hours later.

Intestinal amebiasis
Erythromycin base, estolate, stearate
Children: 30 to 50 mg/kg P.O. daily, divided q 6 hours for 10 to 14 days.
Adults: 250 mg P.O. q 6 hours for 10 to 14 days.

Mild to moderately severe respiratory tract, skin, and soft-tissue infections caused by susceptible organisms
Erythromycin base, estolate, stearate
Adults: 250 to 500 mg P.O. q 6 hours.
Erythromycin ethylsuccinate
Adults: 400 to 800 mg P.O. q 6 hours; or 15 to 20 mg/kg I.V. daily, as continuous infusion or divided q 6 hours.
Oral erythromycin salts
Children: 30 to 50 mg/kg P.O. daily, divided q 6 hours; or 15 to 20 mg/kg I.V. daily, divided q 4 to 6 hours.

Syphilis
Erythromycin base, estolate, stearate
Adults: 500 mg P.O. q.i.d. for 15 days.

Legionnaire's disease
Adults: 500 mg to 1 g I.V. or P.O. q 6 hours for 21 days.

Uncomplicated urethral, endocervical, or rectal infections when tetracyclines are contraindicated
Adults: 500 mg P.O. q.i.d. for at least 7 days.

Conjunctivitis caused by C. trachomatis in neonates
Neonates: 50 mg/kg/day in four divided doses for at least 2 weeks.

Pneumonia of infancy caused by C. trachomatis
Infants: 50 mg/kg/day in four divided doses for 14 to 21 days.

Topical treatment of acne vulgaris
Children and adults: Apply to the affected area b.i.d.

Prophylaxis of ophthalmia neonatorium
Neonates: Apply ointment no later than 1 hour after birth. Use new tube for each infant and do not flush after instillation. Infants born to women with gonorrhea should also be given ceftriaxone, 125 mg I.M. or I.V.

Action and kinetics
• *Antibacterial action:* Erythromycin inhibits bacterial protein synthesis by binding to ribosome's 50S subunit. It is used in the treatment of *Haemophilus influenzae, Entamoeba histolytica, Mycoplasma pneumoniae, Corynebacterium diptheriae,* and *C. minutissimum, Legionella pneumophilia,* and *Bordetella pertussis.* It may be used as an alternate to penicillins or tetracycline in the treatment of *streptococcus pneumoniae, S. veridans, Listeria monocytogenes, Staphylococcus aureus, Chlamydia trachomatis, Neisseria gonorrheae,* and *Treponema pallidium.*
• *Kinetics in adults:* Because base salt is acid-sensitive, it must be buffered or have enteric coating to prevent destruction by gastric acids. Acid salts and esters (estolate, ethylsuccinate, and stearate) are not affected by gastric acidity and therefore are well absorbed. Base and stearate preparations should be given on empty stomach. Absorption of estolate and ethylsuccinate preparations is unaffected or possibly even enhanced by presence of food. When administered topically, drug is absorbed minimally.

Erythromycin is distributed widely to most body tissues and fluids except CSF, where it appears only in low concentrations. Drug crosses the placenta. About 80% of erythromycin base and 96% of erythromycin estolate are protein-bound.

Erythromycin is metabolized partially in the liver to inactive metabolites and is excreted mainly unchanged in bile. Only small drug amounts (less than 5%) are excreted in urine; some drug is excreted in breast milk. In patients with normal renal function, plasma half-life is about 1½ hours. Peritoneal hemodialysis does not remove drug.

Contraindications and precautions
Erythromycin is contraindicated in patients with known hypersensitivity to drug. Erythromycin estolate is contraindicated in patients with hepatic disease because drug may be hepatotoxic.

Other erythromycin forms should be administered cautiously to patients with preexisting hepatic disease because drug may exacerbate hepatic dysfunction.

Interactions
Concomitant use of erythromycin may inhibit metabolism of theophylline (possibly leading to elevated serum theophylline levels), warfarin (causing excessive anticoagulant effect), carbamazepine (possibly causing toxicity), and cyclosporine (resulting in elevation of serum cyclosporine levels to nearly nephrotoxic ranges).

When used concomitantly with topical desquamating or abrasive acne preparations, topical erythromycin has a cumulative irritant effect.

Effects on diagnostic tests
Erythromycin may interfere with fluorometric determination of urinary catecholamines. Liver function test results may become abnormal during erythromycin therapy (rare).

Adverse reactions
• DERM: urticaria; rashes; erythema, burning, dryness, pruritus (with topical application).
• EENT: eye irritation (with topical application), hearing loss (with high I.V. doses, especially in patients with renal failure).
• GI: *abdominal pain and cramps, nausea, vomiting, diarrhea.*
• Hepatic: cholestatic jaundice (with estolate).
• Local: *venous irritation,* thrombophlebitis (both after I.V. injection).
• Other: *overgrowth of nonsusceptible bacteria or fungi,* anaphylaxis, fever, *sensitivity reaction* (with topical application).
Note: Drug should be discontinued if patient develops hypersensitivity reaction.

Overdose and treatment
No information available.

▶ **Special considerations**
• Erythromycin ethylsuccinate is not recommended for use in infants less than 2 months old.
• Culture and sensitivity tests should be performed before treatment starts and then as needed.
• Base and stearate preparations should be given on empty stomach. Estolate and ethylsuccinate preparations are unaffected or possibly enhanced by presence of food. When administered topically, drug is minimally absorbed.
• If patient is receiving erythromycin concomitantly with theophylline, monitor serum theophylline levels; with warfarin, monitor for prolonged prothrombin time and abnormal bleeding.
• Reconstitute injectable form (lactobionate) according to manufacturer's instructions and dilute every 250 mg in at least 100 ml of normal saline solution. Continuous infusions are preferred, but drug may be given by intermittent infusion at a maximum concentration of 5 mg/ml infused over 20 to 60 minutes.
• Replace I.M. or I.V. use with oral route as soon as possible to minimize discomfort.
• Do not administer erythromycin lactobionate with other drugs because of chemical instability. Reconstituted solutions are acidic and should be completely administered within 8 hours of preparation.
• Drug may cause overgrowth of nonsusceptible bacteria or fungi.
• Drug is bacteriostatic, but high concentrations may be bactericidal against highly susceptible organisms.

Information for parents and patient
• For best absorption, patient should take oral form with full glass of water 1 hour before or 2 hours after meals and should not take drug with fruit juice. (However, patient receiving enteric-coated tablets may take them with meals). Patient who is taking chewable tablets should not swallow them whole; patient who is taking enteric-coated tablets should not chew them.
• Advise parents that if patient is using topical solution, instruct them to wash, rinse, and dry affected areas before applying it. Warn them not to apply solution near eyes, nose, mouth, or other mucous membranes. Caution them to avoid sharing washcloths and towels with family members.
• Advise parents applying ophthalmic ointment to wash hands before and after applying ointment. Instruct them to cleanse eye area of excess exudate before applying ointment and not to allow tube to touch the eye or surrounding tissue. Instruct them to promptly report signs of sensitivity, such as itching eyelids and constant burning.
• Patient should take drug exactly as directed and continue taking it for prescribed period, even after he feels better.
• Instruct parents to report adverse reactions promptly. They should report nausea and vomiting that may interfere with drug administration.

ethacrynate sodium
ethacrynic acid
Edecrin

Classification: loop diuretic

How supplied
Available by prescription only
Tablets: 25 mg, 50 mg
Injectable: 50 mg (with 62.5 mg of mannitol and 0.1 mg of thimerosal)

Indications, route, and dosage
Acute pulmonary edema
†*Neonates and children:* 1 to 2 mg/kg I.V. slowly over 5 to 10 minutes. Do not exceed 3 mgk/kg in a 30-minute period. Repeat q 8 hours if needed.
Adults: 50 to 100 mg of ethacrynate sodium I.V. slowly over several minutes.
Edema
Neonates: 0.5 to 1 mg/kg P.O. q 8 to 12 hours. Use with caution. Dosage for infants is not well established.
Children: Initially, 25 mg P.O., given cautiously and increased in 25-mg increments daily until desired effect is achieved.
Adults: 50 to 200 mg P.O. daily. Refractory cases may require up to 200 mg b.i.d.

Action and kinetics
• *Diuretic action:* Ethacrynic acid inhibits sodium and chloride reabsorption in the proximal part of the ascending loop of Henle, promoting the excretion of sodium, water, chloride, and potassium.
• *Kinetics in adults:* Ethacrynic acid is absorbed rapidly from the GI tract; diuresis occurs in 30 minutes and peaks in 2 hours. After I.V. administration of ethacrynate sodium, diuresis occurs in 5 minutes and peaks in 15 to 30 minutes. In animal studies, ethacrynic acid was found to accumulate in the liver. Drug does not enter the cerebrospinal fluid, and its distribution into breast milk or the placenta is unknown. In animals, ethacrynic acid is metabolized by the liver to a potentially active metabolite. Animal studies show that 30% to 65% of ethacrynate sodium is excreted in urine and 35% to 40% is excreted in bile, as the metabolite. Duration of action is 6 to 8 hours after oral administration and about 2 hours after I.V. administration.

Contraindications and precautions
Ethacrynic acid is contraindicated in patients with known hypersensitivity, anuria, hypotension, dehydration with low serum sodium levels, or metabolic alkalosis with hypokalemia, because the drug may exacerbate these conditions.

Ethacrynic acid should be used with caution in patients with hearing impairment or cirrhosis, especially those with a history of electrolyte imbalance or hepatic encephalopathy; in patients with diabetes, because it may alter carbohydrate metabolism; in patients with increasing azotemia or oliguria; and in patients receiving cardiac glycosides (digoxin, digitoxin), because ethacrynic acid-induced hypokalemia may predispose such patients to digitalis toxicity.

Interactions

Concomitant use of ethacrynic acid with other diuretics may enhance the diuretic effect of the other drugs; reduce dosage when adding ethacrynic acid to a diuretic regimen. Concomitant use of potassium-sparing diuretics (spironolactone, triamterene, amiloride) may decrease the potassium loss induced by ethacrynic acid and may be a therapeutic advantage; severe potassium loss may occur if ethacrynic acid is administered with other potassium-depleting drugs, such as steroids and amphotericin B. Ethacrynic acid may reduce renal clearance of lithium, elevating serum lithium levels; monitor lithium levels and adjust dosage.

Diabetic patients may need increased dosages of insulin when taking ethacrynic acid. Ethacrynic acid may potentiate the hypotensive effect of antihypertensive agents; patients may require dosage reduction.

Concomitant administration of ethacrynic acid and aminoglycosides or other ototoxic drugs may increase the incidence of deafness; avoid use of such combinations.

Effects on diagnostic tests

Ethacrynic acid therapy alters electrolyte balance and liver and renal function tests.

Adverse reactions

- CV: volume depletion and dehydration, orthostatic hypotension.
- CNS: *vertigo.*
- DERM: dermatitis.
- EENT: transient deafness with too-rapid I.V. injection, *ototoxicity.*
- GI: abdominal discomfort and pain, diarrhea, upper GI bleeding.
- HEMA: agranulocytosis, neutropenia, thrombocytopenia.
- Metabolic: *hypochloremic alkalosis;* asymptomatic hyperuricemia; *fluid and electrolyte imbalances,* including *hypokalemia,* hypocalcemia, hypomagnesemia, and *dilutional hyponatremia; hyperglycemia* and impairment of glucose tolerance.

Note: Drug should be discontinued if excessive diuresis, electrolyte abnormalities, increasing azotemia, oliguria, hematuria, bloody stools, or severe or watery diarrhea occurs.

Overdose and treatment

Clinical manifestations of overdose include profound electrolyte and volume depletion, which may precipitate circulatory collapse.

Treatment of ethacrynic acid overdose is primarily supportive; replace fluid and electrolytes as needed.

▶ Special considerations

- Use ethacrynate sodium or ethacrynic acid with caution in neonates. The usual pediatric dosage can be used, but dosage intervals should be extended.
- Safety for use in children has not been established.
- Monitor blood pressure and pulse rate (especially

during rapid diuresis), establish baseline values before therapy, and watch for significant changes.
- Do not give ethacrynate sodium either I.M. or S.C. because it may cause severe local pain and irritation. When giving I.V., check infusion site frequently for infiltration (edema or skin blanching).
- Infuse ethacrynate sodium slowly over 20 to 30 minutes, by I.V. infusion or by direct I.V. injection over a period of several minutes; rapid injection may cause hypotension. Use a solution of 1 to 2 mg/ml diluted with normal saline solution or 5% dextrose in water.
- Do not administer ethacrynate sodium simultaneously with whole blood or blood products; hemolysis may occur.
- Advise safety measures for all ambulatory patients until response to the diuretic is known.
- Establish baseline and periodically review CBC, including WBC count; serum electrolytes, CO_2, BUN, and creatinine levels; and results of liver function tests.
- Administer diuretics in the morning so major diuresis occurs before bedtime. To prevent nocturia, do not prescribe diuretics for use after 6 p.m.
- Consider possible dosage adjustment in the following circumstances; reduced dosage for patients with hepatic dysfunction; increased dosage in patients with renal impairment, oliguria, or decreased diuresis (inadequate urine output may result in circulatory overload, causing water intoxication, pulmonary edema, and CHF); increased doses of insulin in diabetic patients; and reduced dosages of other antihypertensive agents.
- Monitor patient for edema and ascites. Observe lower extremities of ambulatory children and the sacral area of infants and those on bed rest.
- Patient should be weighed each morning immediately after voiding and before breakfast in same type of clothing and on the same scale. Weight helps evaluate clinical response to diuretic therapy.
- Consult dietitian on possible need for dietary potassium supplementation.
- Patients taking digitalis are at increased risk of digitalis toxicity from potassium depletion.
- Ototoxicity may follow prolonged use or administration of large doses.
- Patients with liver disease are especially susceptible to diuretic-induced electrolyte imbalance; in extreme cases, stupor, coma, and death can result.
- Patient should have urinal or commode readily available.
- I.V. ethacrynate sodium has been used to treat hypercalcemia and to manage ethylene glycol poisoning and bromide intoxication.
- Periodically assess hearing function in patients receiving high-dose therapy.

Information for parents and patient

- Explain to the parents and patient the rationale for therapy and the diuretic effect of drug.
- Teach parents signs of adverse effects, especially hypokalemia (weakness, fatigue, muscle cramps, paresthesias, confusion, nausea, vomiting, diarrhea, headache, dizziness, or palpitations), and importance of reporting such symptoms promptly.
- Advise parents to have patient eat potassium-rich

foods, such as citrus fruits, potatoes, dates, raisins, and bananas; to avoid high-sodium foods, such as lunch meat, smoked meats, and processed cheeses; and not to add salt to other foods. Recommend salt substitutes. Inform parents that low-sodium formulas are available for infants.
• Emphasize importance of keeping follow-up appointments to monitor effectiveness of diuretic therapy.
• Tell parents to report if patient experiences increased edema or excess diuresis (more than 2% weight loss or gain).
• With initial doses, caution patient to change position slowly, especially when rising to upright position, to prevent dizziness from orthostatic hypotension.
• Instruct parents to call at once if patient develops chest, back, or leg pain, or shortness of breath.

---

ethambutol hydrochloride
Myambutol

• Classification: antitubercular agent (semisynthetic antitubercular)

How supplied
Available by prescription only
Tablets: 100 mg, 400 mg

Indications, route, and dosage
Adjunctive treatment in pulmonary tuberculosis
Children age 13 and older and adults: Initial treatment for patients who have not received previous antitubercular therapy, 15 mg/kg P.O. daily single dose. Retreatment, 25 mg/kg P.O. daily single dose for 60 days with at least one other antitubercular drug; then decrease to 15 mg/kg P.O. daily single dose.

Action and kinetics
• *Antitubercular action:* Ethambutol is bacteriostatic; it interferes with ribonucleic acid synthesis, inhibiting protein metabolism and cell replication. Ethambutol is active against *Mycobacterium tuberculosis, M. bovis,* and *M. marinum,* and some strains of *M. kansasii, M. avium, M. fortuitum,* and *M. intracellulare.* Ethambutol is considered adjunctive therapy in tuberculosis and is combined with other antituberculosis agents to prevent or delay development of drug resistance.
• *Kinetics in adults:* Ethambutol is absorbed rapidly from the GI tract; peak serum levels occur 2 to 4 hours after ingestion. It is distributed widely into body tissues and fluids, especially into lungs, erythrocytes, saliva, and kidneys; lesser amounts distribute into brain, ascitic, pleural, and cerebrospinal fluids. Ethambutol is 8% to 22% protein-bound.
Ethambutol undergoes partial hepatic metabolism. After 24 hours, about 50% of an oral dose of ethambutol and 8% to 15% of its metabolites are excreted in urine; 20% to 25% is excreted in feces. Small amounts of drug may be excreted in breast milk. Elimination half-life in adults is about 3½ hours; half-life is prolonged in decreased renal or hepatic function.

Ethambutol can be removed by peritoneal dialysis and to a lesser extent by hemodialysis.

Contraindications and precautions
Ethambutol is contraindicated in patients with known hypersensitivity to ethambutol.
Ethambutol should be used cautiously in patients with preexisting visual disturbances, in whom ethambutol-induced visual changes are difficult to identify; monthly vision tests are mandatory at high dosage levels. Use drug with caution in patients with gout and in patients with decreased renal or hepatic function.

Interactions
Ethambutol may potentiate adverse effects of agents that produce neurotoxicity.

Effects on diagnostic tests
Ethambutol may elevate serum urate levels and liver function test results.

Adverse reactions
• CNS: headache, dizziness, mental confusion, possible hallucinations, peripheral neuritis (numbness and tingling of extremities).
• EENT: *optic neuritis (vision loss and loss of color discrimination,* especially red and green).
• GI: anorexia, *nausea, vomiting,* abdominal pain, impaired liver function.
• Metabolic: *elevated uric acid levels.*
• Other: anaphylactoid reactions, fever, malaise, bloody sputum, joint pain.
  Note: Drug should be discontinued if patient shows signs of hypersensitivity reaction or substantive visual changes.

Overdose and treatment
No specific recommendation is available. Treatment is supportive. After recent ingestion (4 hours or less), empty stomach by induced emesis or gastric lavage. Follow with activated charcoal to decrease absorption.

▶ Special considerations
• Not recommended for use in children under age 13. Drug is not used in children who are too young for vision testing.
• Give drug with food if necessary to prevent gastric irritation; food does not interfere with absorption.
• Obtain specimens for culture and sensitivity testing before first dose, but therapy can begin before test results are complete; repeat periodically to detect drug resistance.
• Assess visual status before therapy; test visual acuity and color discrimination monthly in patients taking more than 15 mg/kg/day. Visual disturbances are dose-related and reversible if detected in time.
• Monitor blood (including serum uric acid), renal, and liver function studies before and periodically during therapy to minimize toxicity.
• Monitor for change in renal function. Dosage reduction may be necessary.

Information for parents and patient
• Explain disease process and rationale for long-term therapy.
• Teach signs and symptoms of hypersensitivity and other adverse reactions, and emphasize need to notify physician if these occur; urge parents to report *any* unusual reactions, especially blurred vision, red-green color blindness, or changes in urinary elimination.
• Assure parents and patient that visual alterations will disappear within several weeks or months after drug is discontinued.
• Urge parents to have patient to complete entire prescribed regimen, to comply with instructions for around-the-clock dosage, to avoid missing doses, and not to discontinue drug without medical approval. Explain importance of keeping follow-up appointments.
• Teach preventive measures for avoiding intercurrent infections and tuberculosis re-infection.

ethionamide
Trecator-SC

• Classification: antitubercular agent (isonicotinic acid derivative)

How supplied
Available by prescription only
Tablets: 250 mg

Indications, route, and dosage
Adjunctive treatment in pulmonary or extrapulmonary tuberculosis (streptomycin and isoniazid cannot be used or have failed)
Children: Optimum dosage has not been established. Some clinicians use 15 to 20 mg/kg P.O. daily (up to a maximum dose of 1 g).
Adults: 500 mg to 1 g P.O. daily in divided doses. Concomitant administration of other effective antitubercular drugs and pyridoxine is recommended.
Leprosy
Children: 4 to 5 mg/kg P.O. daily.
Adults: 250 to 500 mg P.O. daily.

Action and kinetics
• *Antitubercular action:* Ethionamide appears to disrupt bacterial peptide synthesis; its exact mechanism of antibacterial action is unknown. It is either bacteriostatic or bactericidal, depending on organism susceptibility and drug concentration at infection site. Ethionamide is active against *Mycobacterium tuberculosis, M. bovis, M. kansasii,* and some strains of *M. avium* and *M. intracellulare.* Ethionamide is considered adjunctive therapy in tuberculosis and is given with another antitubercular agent to prevent or delay development of drug resistance by *M. tuberculosis.*
• *Kinetics in adults:* About 80% of an oral dose of ethionamide is absorbed from the GI tract; peak serum levels occur 3 hours after ingestion. Ethionamide is distributed widely into body tissues and fluids, and has good CSF penetration. Ethionamide crosses the placenta; it is 10% protein-bound. Ethionamide is me-

tabolized extensively, probably in the liver, and is excreted primarily in urine; 1% to 5% is excreted unchanged in 24 hours; the rest is excreted as metabolites. Plasma half-life is about 3 hours.

Contraindications and precautions
Ethionamide is contraindicated in patients with severe hepatic impairment and in patients with known hypersensitivity to drug. It should be used cautiously in patients with known hypersensitivity to chemically related drugs, such as isoniazid or pyrazinamide, to avoid cross-hypersensitivity; and in patients with diabetes, because drug may hinder stabilization of serum glucose. Incidence of ethionamide-induced hepatic dysfunction is higher in diabetic patients.

Interactions
Ethionamide may intensify adverse reactions of concomitantly used antitubercular drugs.
Concomitant use with cycloserine or alcohol increases hazard of neurotoxicity.

Effects on diagnostic tests
Ethionamide may cause transient elevations of liver function test results; it may decrease serum protein-bound iodine and thyroxine (T_4) values.

Adverse reactions
• CNS: peripheral neuritis, psychic disturbances (especially mental depression), tremors, paresthesias, seizures, dizziness, olfactory disturbances, blurred vision.
• CV: postural hypotension, ganglionic blockade.
• DERM: rash, photosensitivity, acne.
• GI: anorexia, metallic taste in mouth, nausea, vomiting, sialorrhea, epigastric distress, diarrhea, stomatitis, weight loss.
• HEMA: thrombocytopenia.
• Hepatic: jaundice, hepatitis, elevated AST (SGOT) and ALT (SGPT) levels.
• Other: hypoglycemia, gynecomastia, impotence, acute rheumatic symptoms.
Note: Drug should be discontinued if patient shows signs of hypersensitivity reaction, hepatic dysfunction, or acute bleeding disorder.

Overdose and treatment
No specific recommendation is available. Treatment is supportive. After recent ingestion (within 4 hours), empty stomach by induced emesis or gastric lavage. Follow with activated charcoal to decrease absorption. For further information, contact your poison information center.

▶ Special considerations
• When necessary, drug may be used in children even though optimal dose has not been established.
• Give drug with or after meals to avoid gastric irritation. Severe irritation requires adjustment.
• Obtain specimens for culture and sensitivity testing before first dose, but therapy may begin before test results are complete; repeat periodically to detect drug resistance.
• Monitor renal and liver function studies before and

---

every 2 to 4 weeks during therapy to detect and minimize toxicity.

• Observe patient for adverse reactions, especially hepatic dysfunction and CNS toxicity; vitamin B_6 may be prescribed to prevent or relieve peripheral neuritis or neurotoxicity.

• Closely monitor the diabetic patient for hyperglycemia.

• Establish safety measures in case postural hypotension occurs.

Information for parents and patient

• Explain disease process and rationale for long-term therapy.

• Teach signs and symptoms of hypersensitivity and other adverse reactions, and emphasize need to report *any* unusual effects.

• Encourage parents to call if GI distress persists or becomes severe, if rash develops, or if patient develops signs or symptoms of hepatic dysfunction: loss of appetite, fatigue, malaise, jaundice, or dark urine.

• Patient should take drug with food to minimize gastric irritation.

• Advise parents that patient should avoid alcohol.

• Be sure parents and patient understand how and when to take drug; urge them to complete entire prescribed regimen, to comply with instructions for around-the-clock dosage, and to keep follow-up appointments.

ethosuximide
Zarontin

• Classification: anticonvulsant (succinimide derivative)

How supplied
Available by prescription only
Capsules: 250 mg
Syrup: 250 mg/5 ml

Indications, route, and dosage
Absence (petit mal) seizures
Children: 20 to 40 mg/kg daily in divided doses. Alternatively, administer the following dosage according to age:
Children age 3 to 6: 250 mg P.O. daily in a single dose or divided b.i.d. May increase by 250 mg q 4 to 7 days. Alternatively, may build up to 20 to 30 mg/kg/day. Total maximum dose is 1 g/day.
Children over age 6 and adults: Initially, 250 mg P.O. b.i.d. May increase by 250 mg q 4 to 7 days up to 1.5 g daily.

Action and kinetics
• *Anticonvulsant action:* Ethosuximide raises the seizure threshold; it suppresses characteristic spike-and-wave pattern by depressing neuronal transmission in the motor cortex and basal ganglia. It is indicated for absence (petit mal) seizures refractory to other drugs.

• *Kinetics in adults:* Ethosuximide is absorbed from the GI tract; steady-state plasma levels occur in 4 to

7 days. Drug is distributed widely throughout the body; protein binding is minimal. Ethosuximide is metabolized extensively in the liver to several inactive metabolites. Ethosuximide is excreted in urine, with small amounts excreted in bile and feces.

Contraindications and precautions
Ethosuximide is contraindicated in patients with known hypersensitivity to succinimides. It should be used with extreme caution in patients with hepatic or renal disease and in those taking other CNS depressants or anticonvulsants. Ethosuximide may increase the incidence of generalized tonic-clonic seizures if used alone to treat patient with mixed seizures; abrupt withdrawal may precipitate petit mal seizures. Anticonvulsants have been associated with an increased incidence of birth defects.

Interactions
Concomitant use of ethosuximide and other CNS depressants (alcohol, narcotics, anxiolytics, antidepressants, antipsychotics, and other anticonvulsants) causes additive CNS depression and sedation.

Effects on diagnostic tests
Ethosuximide may elevate liver enzyme levels and may cause false-positive Coombs' test results. It may also cause abnormal results of renal function tests.

Adverse reactions
• CNS: drowsiness, headache, fatigue, dizziness, *ataxia*, irritability, hiccups, euphoria, lethargy, psychotic behavior.

• DERM: urticaria, *pruritic and erythematous rashes*, hirsutism, Stevens-Johnson syndrome, lupus-like syndromes.

• EENT: myopia.

• GI: *nausea, vomiting,* diarrhea, gum hypertrophy, weight loss, cramps, tongue swelling, *anorexia*, epigastric and abdominal pain.

• GU: vaginal bleeding.

• HEMA: *leukopenia, eosinophilia, agranulocytosis, pancytopenia, aplastic anemia.*

   Note: Drug should be discontinued if signs of hypersensitivity, rash, or unusual skin lesions or any of the following signs of blood dyscrasia occur: joint pain, fever, sore throat, or unusual bleeding or bruising.

Overdose and treatment
Symptoms of ethosuximide overdose, when used alone or with other anticonvulsants, include CNS depression, ataxia, stupor, and coma. Treatment is symptomatic and supportive. Carefully monitor vital signs and fluid and electrolyte balance. Contact local or regional poison control center for more information.

▶ Special considerations
• Ethosuximide is not recommended for children under age 3.

• Monitor baseline liver and renal function studies and blood studies; repeat CBCs every 3 months and urinalysis and liver function tests every 6 months.

• Observe patient closely for dermatologic reactions at initiation of therapy.

• Monitor closely for signs and symptoms of hyper-

---

sensitivity, hematologic reactions, or other adverse reactions: skin rash, sore throat, joint pain, unexplained fever, or unusual bleeding or bruising.
• Drug adds to CNS depressant effects of alcohol, narcotics, anxiolytics, antidepressants, and tranquilizers.
• Administer ethosuximide with food to minimize GI distress.
• Avoid abrupt discontinuation of drug. This may precipitate petit mal seizures.
• Therapeutic levels: 40 to 100 mg/liter.

Information for parents and patient
• Tell patient to take drug with food or milk to prevent GI distress, to avoid use with alcoholic beverages, and to avoid hazardous tasks that require alertness if drug causes drowsiness, dizziness, or blurred vision.
• Tell parents to protect pediatric syrup from freezing.
• Teach parents and patient signs and symptoms of hypersensitivity, liver dysfunction, and blood dyscrasias and advise patient to report them promptly.
• Warn parents and patient never to discontinue drug or change dosage without medical approval.
• Encourage parents to have patient wear a Medic Alert bracelet or necklace, listing drug and seizure disorder.
• Explain to parents of adolescents the importance of reporting suspected pregnancy immediatley.

---

ethotoin
Peganone

• Classification: anticonvulsant (hydantoin derivative)

How supplied
Available by prescription only
Tablets: 250 mg, 500 mg

Indications, route, and dosage
Generalized tonic-clonic (grand mal) or complex-partial (psychomotor) seizures
Children: Initially, 250 mg P.O. b.i.d.; may increase up to 250 mg P.O. q.i.d.
Adults: Initially, 250 mg P.O. q.i.d. after meals; may increase slowly over several days to 3 g daily divided q.i.d.

Action and kinetics
• *Anticonvulsant action:* Like other hydantoin derivatives, ethotoin stabilizes neuronal membranes and limits seizure activity by increasing efflux of sodium ions across cell membranes in the motor cortex during generation of nerve impulses. However, ethotoin lacks the antiarrhythmic effects of phenytoin.
Ethotoin is indicated for tonic-clonic (grand mal) and partial seizures.
• *Kinetics in adults:* Ethotoin is absorbed rapidly from the GI tract.
Ethotoin is distributed widely throughout the body; its therapeutic range is believed to be 15 to 50 mcg/ml.

Ethotoin is metabolized by the liver, probably by a saturable mechanism (at high doses, a small increase in dosage may produce a large increase in plasma levels).
Ethotoin is excreted in urine and feces; small amounts appear in saliva and breast milk.

Contraindications and precautions
Ethotoin is contraindicated in patients with hepatic dysfunction or hematologic disorders. It should be used with caution in patients taking other hydantoin derivatives; concomitant use with phenacemide has caused extreme paranoid symptoms.

Interactions
Concomitant use of ethotoin with phenacemide may cause extreme paranoia. Use of ethotoin with oral contraceptives may decrease the efficacy of oral contraceptives.
The use of anticonvulsants during pregnancy has been associated with an increased incidence of birth defects.

Effects on diagnostic tests
Ethotoin may raise liver enzyme levels.

Adverse reactions
• CNS: fatigue, insomnia, dizziness, headache, numbness.
• CV: chest pain.
• DERM: rash.
• EENT: diplopia, nystagmus.
• GI: nausea, vomiting, diarrhea, gingival hyperplasia (rare).
• HEMA: thrombocytopenia, leukopenia, agranulocytosis, pancytopenia, megaloblastic anemia.
• Other: fever, lymphadenopathy.
Note: Drug should be discontinued if signs of hypersensitivity occur, if a lymphoma-like syndrome develops, or if laboratory tests show hepatic or hematologic changes.

Overdose and treatment
Symptoms of overdose may include drowsiness, nausea, nystagmus, ataxia, and dysarthria; hypotension, respiratory depression, and coma may follow.
Treat overdose with gastric lavage or emesis and follow with supportive treatment. Carefully monitor vital signs and fluid and electrolyte balance. Hemodialysis or total exchange transfusion has been used for managing severe overdose, especially in children.

▶ Special considerations
• Drug should not be discontinued abruptly but slowly over 6 weeks; abrupt discontinuation may cause status epilepticus.
• Drug interactions are frequently a problem, primarily with hepatically cleared drugs, such as chloramphenicol, digitoxin, isoniazid, and griseofulvin; be especially alert for toxic symptoms or breakthrough seizures in patients taking any of these drugs.
• Carefully follow manufacturer's directions for reconstitution, storage, and administration of all preparations.

---

‡May contain sulfites   ◆May contain tartrazine   ◆◆May contain benzyl alcohol

• Obtain complete blood count and urinalysis at start of therapy and monthly thereafter. Monitor baseline liver function and hematologic laboratory studies and repeat at monthly intervals.

• Administer ethotoin after meals. Schedule doses as evenly as possible over 24 hours.

• Ethotoin generally produces milder adverse effects than phenytoin; however, larger doses needed to maintain therapeutic effect frequently cause GI distress.

• Ethotoin does not usually cause gingival hyperplasia. It is commonly used in patients who cannot tolerate adverse reactions to phenytoin.

• Use cautiously in patients receiving phenacemide.

• Ethotoin may be removed by hemodialysis. Dosage adjustments may be necessary in patients undergoing dialysis.

Information for parents and patient

• Tell parents that patient should avoid alcohol-containing beverages or elixirs while taking drug, as it may decrease drug's effectiveness and may increase CNS adverse reactions.

• Advise parents that patient should avoid hazardous tasks that require mental alertness until degree of CNS sedative effect is determined.

• Patient should take oral drug with food if GI distress occurs.

• Teach parents signs and symptoms of hypersensitivity, liver dysfunction, and blood dyscrasias and to call the physician at once if any of the following occurs: sore throat, fever, bleeding, easy bruising, swollen glands, yellow skin or eyes, infection, or rash.

• Explain to adolescent patient and her parents the need to report pregnancy immediately.

• Warn parents that patient should never discontinue drug suddenly or without medical supervision.

• Encourage parents to have patient wear a Medic Alert bracelet or necklace, indicating drug taken and seizure disorders.

• Explain that drug may increase gum growth and sensitivity (gingival hyperplasia); teach proper oral hygiene and urge parents and patient to establish good mouth care.

• Assure parents and patient that pink or reddish brown discoloration of urine is normal and harmless.

---

ethylestrenol
Maxibolin

• Classification: antianemic, antiosteoporotic, antiarthritic (anabolic steroid)

How supplied
Available by prescription only
Tablets: 2 mg
Elixir: 2 mg/5 ml

Indications, route, and dosage
Promote weight gain; combat tissue depletion, refractory anemias, and catabolic effects of corticosteroids, osteoporosis, immobilization, and debilitation
Children: 1 to 3 mg P.O. daily for 6 weeks, followed by a 4-week drug-free period.
Adults: 4 mg P.O. daily for 6 weeks, followed by a 4-week drug-free period.

Action and kinetics
• *Erythropoietic action:* Ethylestrenol stimulates the kidneys' production of erythropoietin, leading to increases in red blood cell mass and volume. It increases serum calcium and phosphate levels, and decreases the bone pain of osteoporosis by an unknown mechanism. Ethylestrenol is of questionable value in treating advanced arthritis. Reversal of catabolism, improved nitrogen and calcium balance, and a sense of well-being are possible beneficial effects.

• *Kinetics in adults:* The pharmacokinetics of ethylestrenol are not well described.

Contraindications and precautions
Ethylestrenol is not recommended for use in neonates. It should be used with extreme caution in pediatric patients to avoid premature induction of puberty and closure of the epiphyses.

Ethylestrenol is contraindicated in patients with severe renal, cardiac, or hepatic disease (this drug may cause fluid and electrolyte retention); elimination of this drug may be impaired in the presence of severe hepatic disease. Drug is also contraindicated in male patients with prostatic or breast cancer (drug can stimulate the growth of cancerous breast or prostate tissue in males); in patients with undiagnosed abnormal genital bleeding; and in pregnant or breast-feeding patients (animal studies have shown that administration of anabolic steroids during pregnancy causes masculinization of the fetus). Administer ethylestrenol cautiously in patients with a history of coronary artery disease because the drug has hypercholesterolemic effects.

Interactions
In patients with diabetes, decreased blood glucose levels may require adjustment of insulin dosage.

Concomitant use with anticoagulants may potentiate the effects of warfarin-type anticoagulants, causing increases in prothrombin time. Use with adrenocorticosteroids or adrenocorticotropic hormone increases the potential for fluid and electrolyte retention.

Effects on diagnostic tests
Ethylestrenol may cause abnormal results of the fasting plasma glucose test, glucose tolerance test, and metyrapone test. It may increase sulfobromophthalein retention. Thyroid function test results (protein-bound iodine, radioactive iodine uptake, thyroid-binding capacity) and 17-ketosteroid levels may decrease. Liver function test results, prothrombin time (especially in patients receiving anticoagulant therapy), and serum creatinine levels may be elevated. Because of this agent's anabolic activity, serum sodium, potassium,

---

calcium, phosphate, and cholesterol levels may all rise.

Adverse reactions
• Androgenic: *in females:* deepening of voice, clitoral enlargement, changes in libido; *in males:* prepubertal—premature epiphyseal closure, priapism, phallic enlargement; postpubertal—testicular atrophy, oligospermia, decreased ejaculatory volume, impotence, gynecomastia, epididymitis.
• CNS: headache, mental depression.
• CV: edema.
• DERM: acne, oily skin, hirsutism, flushing, sweating.
• GI: gastroenteritis, nausea, vomiting, diarrhea, constipation, change in appetite, weight gain.
• GU: bladder irritability, vaginitis, menstrual irregularities.
• Hepatic: reversible jaundice, hepatotoxicity.
• Other: hypercalcemia.
   Note: Drug should be discontinued if hypercalcemia, edema, hypersensitivity reaction, priapism, or excessive sexual stimulation occurs; or if virilization occurs in females.

Overdose and treatment
No information available.

▶ Special considerations
• Anabolic steroids should be used with caution in prepubertal children. Boys should be closely observed for precocious development of male sexual characteristics.
• In children, X-rays of wrist bones should establish level of bone maturation before therapy begins. During treatment, bone maturation may proceed more rapidly than linear growth. Intermittent dosage and periodic X-rays are recommended to monitor skeletal effects.
• Watch female patients for signs of virilization. If possible, discontinue therapy when virilization first becomes apparent because some adverse effects (deepening of voice, clitoral enlargement) are irreversible.
• If patient develops menstrual irregularity, therapy should be discontinued pending etiologic determination.
• Anabolic steroids do not improve athletic performance. Risks associated with their use for this purpose far outweigh any possible benefits. Proof of anabolic steroid use is grounds for disqualification in many athletic events.
• Hypercalcemia symptoms may be difficult to distinguish from symptoms of condition being treated unless anticipated and thought of as a cluster.
• Edema usually is controllable with salt restriction, diuretics, or both. Monitor weight routinely.
• Watch for jaundice. Dosage adjustment may reverse condition. Periodic liver function tests are recommended.
• Observe patient on concomitant anticoagulant therapy for ecchymotic areas, petechiae, or abnormal bleeding. Monitor prothrombin time.
• Watch for symptoms of hypoglycemia in patients with diabetes. Adjustment of antihypoglycemic drug dosage may be required.
• Anabolic steroids may alter many laboratory studies

during therapy and for 2 to 3 weeks after therapy is stopped.
• Use with therapeutic diet high in calories high in protein unless contraindicated. Give small, frequent meals.
• Anabolic steroids are contraindicated in patients with hepatic, or renal decompensation, nephrosis, and in premature infants. Use cautiously in prepubertal males; in patients with diabetes or coronary diseases; and in patients taking adrenocorticotropic hormones, corticosteroids, or anticoagulants.
• A single course of therapy in both adults and children should not exceed 6 weeks; may be reinstituted after 4-week interval.

Information for parents and patient
• Advise parents to administer drug with foods or meals if GI upset occurs.
• Tell female patient to report menstrual irregularities.
• Discuss adverse reactions that affect body image (hirsutism, acne, weight gain) with adolescent patient.
• Tell patient to avoid excess sodium intake and to watch for hidden sources of sodium (soft drinks, processed foods).

---

etomidate
Amidate

• Classification: I.V. anesthetic, sedative (nonbarbiturate hypnotic)

How supplied
Available by prescription only
Injection: 2 mg/ml

Indications, route, and dosage
Induction of general anesthesia
Children over age 10 and adults: 0.2 to 0.06 mg/kg I.V. over a period of 30 to 60 seconds.

Action and kinetics
• *Anesthetic and sedative actions:* Etomidate, like naturally occurring gamma-aminobutyric acid, decreases the firing rate of neurons within the ascending reticular activating system.
• *Kinetics in adults:* Etomidate is only given I.V. Onset of action is rapid, usually beginning in 60 seconds; duration of action is usually 3 to 5 minutes. Etomidate distributes widely into body tissue and is highly protein-bound (76%). Etomidate is metabolized rapidly in the liver. About 75% of a given dose is excreted in urine as an active metabolite; 10% of drug is excreted in bile and 13% in feces.

Contraindications and precautions
Etomidate is contraindicated in patients allergic to the drug. It should be used cautiously in debilitated patients with underlying pulmonary disease, because of increased respiratory depression. Monitor patients on prolonged use for signs of adrenal insufficiency,

because etomidate may block adrenal steroid production.

Interactions
None significant.

Effects on diagnostic tests
Reduced cortisol plasma levels have been reported, lasting for 6 to 8 hours after induction.

Adverse reactions
• CNS: transient skeletal muscle movements (chiefly myoclonic, some tonic), averting movements.
• CV: hypertension, hypotension, tachycardia, bradycardia, dysrhythmias.
• GI: postoperative nausea or vomiting after induction of anesthesia.
• Local: transient venous pain on injection.
• Other: hiccups, snoring, transient apnea.
  Note: Drug should be discontinued if patient shows signs of hypersensitivity or adrenal insufficiency or if prolonged apnea occurs.

Overdose and treatment
Clinical signs include CNS depression and respiratory arrest. Treat patient supportively, using mechanical ventilation if necessary, until drug effects subside.

▶ **Special considerations**
• Use is not recommended in patients younger than age 10.
• Etomidate is compatible with commonly used preanesthetic agents.
• Transient muscle movements may be reduced by injection of 0.1 mg of fentanyl before giving etomidate, probably by reducing total dose of etomidate.
• Muscle movements are more common in patients with transient venous irritation and pain.
• Etomidate has a much lower incidence of cardiovascular and respiratory effects and is therefore used to advantage in high-risk surgical patients.

Factor IX complex
Konyne-HT, Profilnine Heat-Treated,
Proplex SX-T, Proplex T

• Classification: systemic hemostatic (blood derivative)

How supplied
Available by prescription only
Injection: Vials, with diluents. Units specified on label.

Indications, route, and dosage
Factor IX deficiency (hemophilia B or Christmas disease), anticoagulant overdose
Children and adults: Determine units required by multiplying 0.8 to 1 by body weight (in kg), then by percentage of desired Factor IX level increase; administer by slow I.V. infusion or I.V. push. Dosage is highly individualized, depending on degree of deficiency, desired level of Factor IX, body weight, and severity of bleeding.

Factor IX complex can also be used to reverse coumarin anticoagulation when emergency situations such as surgery preclude less hazardous therapy.

One unit of Factor IX complex (Factor IX units) equals the average of Factor II, VII, IX, and X activity in 1 ml of normal fresh pooled plasma less than 1 hour old.

Action and kinetics
• *Hemostatic action:* Factor IX complex directly replaces deficient clotting factor.
• *Kinetics in adults:* Factor IX complex must be given parenterally for systemic effect. Equilibration within extravascular space takes 4 to 6 hours. Factor IX complex is rapidly cleared by plasma. Half-life is approximately 24 hours.

Contraindications and precautions
Factor IX complex is contraindicated in hepatic disease, intravascular coagulation, or fibrinolysis.

Administer Factor IX complex cautiously to neonates and infants susceptible to hepatitis, which Factor IX complex may transmit; presently available heat-treated products lessen this risk.

Interactions
None significant.

Effects on diagnostic tests
None reported.

Adverse reactions
• CNS: headache, tingling sensation.
• CV: thromboembolic reactions, hypotension, tachycardia, possible intravascular hemolysis in patients with blood types A, B, and AB.
• Other: transient fever, chills, flushing, hypersensitivity, viral hepatitis, disseminated intravascular coagulation (DIC).
Note: Drug should be discontinued if signs of allergic reaction appear.

Overdose and treatment
Clinical manifestations of overdose include a risk of DIC on repeated use because of increased levels of Factors II, IX, and X.

▶ Special considerations
• Administer cautiously to neonates and other infants because of increased risk of hepatitis; only heat-treated products are now available, thus decreasing the risk.
• Refrigerate vials until needed; before reconstituting, warm to room temperature. Use 20 ml sterile water for injection of each vial of lyophilized drug. To mix, gently roll vial between hands; do not shake or mix with other I.V. solutions. Keep product away from heat (but do not refrigerate, because this may cause precipitation of active ingredient), and use within 3 hours.
• Adverse reactions are usually related to too-rapid infusion. Take baseline pulse rate before I.V. administration; if pulse rate increases significantly during infusion, reduce flow rate or stop drug. If patient complains of tingling sensation, fever, chills, or headache, decrease flow rate. A rate of 100 units/minute is usually well-tolerated; do not give drug faster than 3 ml/minute.
• Monitor coagulation studies before and during therapy; monitor vital signs regularly, and be alert for allergic reactions.
• Patient should be immunized with hepatitis B vaccine to decrease the risk of transmission of hepatitis.

Information for parents and patient
Teach or review proper storage, preparation, and injection technique for the specific product the patient uses.

ferrous fumarate

Femiron, Feostat, Fumasorb, Fumerin, Hemocyte, Ircon-FA, Neo-Fer★, Novofumar★, Palafer★, Palmiron, Span-FF

ferrous gluconate

Apo-Ferrous Gluconate★, Fergon, Ferralet, Fertinic★, Novoferrogluc★, Simron

ferrous sulfate

Apo-Ferrous Sulfate★, Feosol, Fer-In-Sol, Fer-Iron, Fero-Grad★, Fero-Gradumet, Ferralyn, Fesofor★, Mol-Iron, Novoferrosulfa★, PMS Ferrous Sulfate★, Slow Fe

• Classification: hematinic (iron supplement)

How supplied
Ferrous fumarate
Ferrous fumarate is 33% elemental iron. All products are available without prescription.
Tablets: 63 mg, 195 mg, 200 mg, 325 mg
Tablets (chewable): 100 mg
Tablets (extended-release): 325 mg
Suspension: 100 mg/5 ml, 45 mg/0.6 ml
Ferrous gluconate
Ferrous gluconate is 11.6% elemental iron. All products are available without prescription.
Tablets: 300 mg, 320 mg, 325 mg (320-mg tablet contains 37 mg Fe +)
Capsules: 86 mg, 325 mg, 435 mg
Elixir: 300 mg/5 ml (contains 35 mg Fe +)
Ferrous sulfate
Ferrous sulfate is 20% elemental iron; dried and powdered (exsiccated), it is about 32% elemental iron. All products are available without a prescription.
Tablets: 195 mg, 300 mg, 325 mg; 200 mg (exsiccated); 160 mg (exsiccated, extended-release)
Capsules: 150 mg, 225 mg, 250 mg, 390 mg, 525 mg (extended-release); 190 mg (exsiccated); 150 mg, 167 mg (exsiccated, extended-release)
Syrup: 90 mg/5 ml
Elixir: 220 mg/5 ml
Liquid: 75 mg/0.6 ml

Indications, route, and dosage
Iron deficiency
Ferrous fumarate
Children: 3 mg/kg P.O. daily in one or more doses.
*Adults:*200 mg P.O.t.i.d. or q.i.d. Dosage is adjusted gradually, as needed and as tolerated. For extended-release tablet, 300 mg P.O. b.i.d.
Ferrous gluconate
Children under age 2: Dosage must be individualized; 5 ml of elixir contains 300 mg ferrous gluconate (35 mg elemental iron).
Children age 2 and older: 16 mg/kg P.O. t.i.d.
Adults: 325 mg P.O. q.i.d.; dosage increased as needed and tolerated, up to 650 mg q.i.d.

Ferrous sulfate
Children: 10 mg/kg P.O. t.i.d.
Adults: 300 mg P.O. b.i.d.; dosage gradually increased to 300 mg q.i.d. as needed and tolerated. For extended-release capsule, 150 to 250 mg P.O. one or two times daily; for extended-release tablets, 160 to 525 mg one or two times daily.
Prophylaxis for iron-deficiency anemia
Children: 5 mg/kg P.O. daily in divided doses.
Adults: 300 mg P.O. daily.

Action and kinetics
• *Hematinic action:* Ferrous sulfate replaces iron, an essential component in the formation of hemoglobin.
• *Kinetics in adults:* Iron is absorbed from the entire length of the GI tract, but primary absorption sites are the duodenum and proximal jejunum. Up to 10% of iron is absorbed by healthy individuals; patients with iron-deficiency anemia may absorb up to 60%. Enteric-coated and some extended-release formulas have decreased absorption, because they are designed to release iron past the points of highest absorption; food may decrease absorption by 33% to 50%.

Iron is transported through GI mucosal cells directly into the blood, where it is immediately bound to a carrier protein, transferrin, and transported to the bone marrow for incorporation into hemoglobin. Iron is highly protein-bound. Iron is liberated by the destruction of hemoglobin but is conserved and reused by the body. Healthy individuals lose very little iron each day. Men and postmenopausal women lose about 1 mg/day, and premenopausal women about 1.5 mg/day. The loss usually occurs in nails, hair, feces, and urine; trace amounts are lost in bile and sweat.

Contraindications and precautions
Ferrous salts are contraindicated in patients with hemochromatosis, hemosiderosis, hemolytic anemia, or known hypersensitivity to any components of the product. Ferrous salts should be administered with extreme caution to patients with peptic ulcer, regional enteritis, ulcerative colitis, or hepatitis because of iron's irritant effects on the GI mucosa.

Interactions
Ascorbic acid (vitamin C) increases absorption of ferrous salts. Antacids, cholestyramine, pancreatic extracts, and vitamin E decrease ferrous sulfate absorption (separate doses by 1- to 2-hour intervals); doxycycline may interfere with ferrous sulfate absorption even when doses are separated; chloramphenicol delays response to iron therapy. Concomitant use of ferrous sulfate and tetracycline inhibits absorption of both drugs; give tetracycline 3 hours after or 2 hours before iron supplement.

Ferrous salts decrease penicillamine absorption; separate doses by at least 2 hours.

Effects on diagnostic tests
Ferrous salts blacken feces and may interfere with tests for occult blood in the stool; the guaiac test and orthotoluidine test may yield false-positive results, but benzidine test is usually not affected.

Iron overload may decrease uptake of technetium 99m and thus interfere with skeletal imaging.

verse reactions

I: *nausea, vomiting,* anorexia, *constipation, dark
ols* (green or black), *diarrhea, epigastric pain.*
EMA: hemosiderosis (with long-term use).
ther: *liquid preparations may stain teeth, rickets
th* prolonged use of high doses).
Note: GI symptoms are exacerbated with long-term
.

erdose and treatment

e lethal dose of iron is between 200 to 250 mg/kg;
alities have occurred with lower doses. Symptoms
y follow ingestion of 20 to 60 mg/kg. Clinical signs
acute overdose may occur as follows.
Between ½ hour to 8 hours after ingestion, patient
y experience lethargy, nausea and vomiting, green
en tarry stools, weak and rapid pulse, hypotension,
ydration, acidosis, and coma. If death does not
mediately ensue, symptoms may clear for about 24
urs. At 12 to 48 hours, symptoms may return, ac-
npanied by diffuse vascular congestion, pulmonary
ema, shock, convulsions, anuria, and hyperther-
a. Death may follow.
Treatment requires immediate support of airway,
spiration, and circulation. In conscious patient with
act gag reflex, induce emesis with ipecac; if not,
pty stomach by gastric lavage. Follow emesis with
age, using a 1% sodium bicarbonate solution, to
vert iron to less irritating, poorly absorbed form.
hosphate solutions have been used, but carry haz-
d of other adverse effects.) Take abdominal X-ray
determine continued presence of excess iron; if
rum iron levels exceed 350 mg/dl, deferoxamine
y be used for systemic chelation. Survivors are
ely to sustain organ damage, including pyloric or
tral stenosis, hepatic cirrhosis, CNS damage, and
estinal obstruction.

Special considerations

n premature infants, drug may cause increased red
ll hemolysis and hemolytic anemia because of low
rum values of vitamin E. When given with vitamin
response to iron therapy is decreased.
sually not indicated during first 2 to 3 months of
e or in patients weighing less than 1,800 g.
ron extended-release capsules or tablets are usually
t recommended for children. *Overdose may be fatal.*
Dilute liquid preparations in juice (preferably orange
ce, which promotes absorption of iron) or water, but
t in milk or antacids. Administer antacids 1 hour
fore or 2 hours after iron, if possible, to prevent
terference with absorption. To avoid staining teeth,
ve liquid preparations through a straw.
Tablets or capsules should not be crushed; if patient
s trouble swallowing, liquid form can be used.
GI upset is dose-related, based on amount of ele-
ental iron; between-meal dosage is preferred but
ay increase GI intolerance.
Food decreases absorption by 33% to 50%. Enteric-
ated formulas and some sustained-release formulas
ay also decrease absorption significantly, because
ey transport iron past primary site of absorption.
Monitor effect on bowel function.
Oral iron may turn stools black. This is unabsorbed
on and is harmless but may mask GI bleeding.

• Monitor hemoglobin and reticulocyte counts during
therapy.

Information for parents and patient

• Explain toxicity of iron, and emphasize importance
of keeping iron preparations away from children because of hazard of fatal iron poisoning.
• Explain rationale for therapy; teach possible adverse
effects, and emphasize importance of reporting diarrhea or constipation for adjustment in dose, diet, or
further work-up. Patient may need iron for 2 to 4
months after anemia resolves; encourage compliance.
• Advise diluting liquid dosage in juice (preferably
orange juice) or water, not milk or antacids, and drinking through a straw to avoid staining teeth.
• Teach parents dietary measures to help prevent constipation.
• Tell parents and patient that oral iron may turn
stools black; this is unabsorbed iron and is harmless.

fibrinolysin and
deoxyribonuclease, combined
(bovine)
Elase

• Classification: topical debriding agent (proteolytic
enzyme)

How supplied

Available by prescription only
Dry powder: 25 units fibrinolysin and 15,000 units
deoxyribonuclease in a 30-ml vial
Ointment: 30 units fibrinolysin and 20,000 units deoxyribonuclease in 30-g tube

Indications, route, and dosage
Topical debridement of inflamed and infected
skin lesions and wounds

Children and adults: Apply ointment or solution as a
spray at intervals for as long as enzyme action is
desired, usually at least once daily, but two or three
times daily may be preferred; apply solution as a wet
dressing three or four times daily.
Irrigating agent for the treatment of ab-
scesses, empyema cavities, fistulae, sinus
tracts, or subcutaneous hematomas

Children and adults: Irrigate and replace solution every 6 to 10 hours.

Action and kinetics

• *Debriding action:* Digests necrotic tissues by proteolytic action; fibrinolysis is directed toward denatured proteins in devitalized tissues. Produces clear
surfaces and facilitates wound healing.
• *Kinetics in adults:* Absorption is limited with topical
use.

Contraindications and precautions

Fibrinolysin is contraindicated in patients with hypersensitivity to bovine products or mercury compounds.

Interactions
None reported.

Effects on diagnostic tests
None reported.

Adverse reactions
• Local: hyperemia, irritation.
Note: Drug should be discontinued if hypersensitivity reaction occurs.

Overdose and treatment
No specific recommendations available.

▶ Special considerations
• To prepare solution, reconstitute contents of each vial with 10 ml of isotonic sodium chloride solution. Higher or lower concentrations can be prepared by varying the amount of diluent.
• Use solution promptly after preparation; do not use after 24 hours.
• Enzyme must be in constant contact with substrate surface for optimal activity. Therefore, remove dense, dry skin before applying drug.
• To apply ointment, clean wound and skin area carefully with normal saline solution, hydrogen peroxide, or water; moisten thoroughly, then gently dry area. Apply a thin layer of ointment to the affected area, and cover with loose-fitting, nonadhering or petrolatum gauze dressing.
• Change dressing at least once daily; flush away enzyme and debris before reapplication.
• Solution may be applied topically as a spray or as a wet dressing. As a spray, apply using an atomizer; as a wet dressing, saturate gauze dressing with solution and pack affected area.
• Avoid using spray near eyes or mucous membranes.

Information for parents and patient
Be sure parents or patient understands how to use product; teach correct application.

---

flavoxate hydrochloride
Urispas

• Classification: urinary tract spasmolytic (flavone derivative)

How supplied
Available by prescription only
Tablets: 100 mg

Indications, route, and dosage
Symptomatic relief of dysuria, frequency, urgency, nocturia, incontinence, and suprapubic pain associated with urologic disorders
Children over age 12 and adults: 100 to 200 mg P.O. t.i.d. or q.i.d.

Action and kinetics
• *Spasmolytic action:* Flavoxate exerts a direct spasmolytic effect on smooth muscle, primarily in the urinary tract. Acting on the detrusor muscle, th agent increases bladder capacity in patients with bla der spasticity; drug also has antihistaminic, an muscarinic, local anesthetic, and analgesic effects
• *Kinetics in adults:* Flavoxate is absorbed well fro the GI tract; peak levels occur in approximately hours. Flavoxate is excreted in urine; 10% to 30 appears in urine within 6 hours.

Contraindications and precautions
Flavoxate is contraindicated in patients with pylor or duodenal obstruction, GI hemorrhage, obstructi uropathies of the lower urinary tract, and obstructi lesions of the intestine or ileus, because it may e acerbate of these symptoms of illnesses. Exercise ca tion when using drug in patients with glaucoma a in those performing hazardous tasks.

Interactions
Flavoxate enhances the antimuscarinic effects of atr pine and related compounds. It may also potentia the effects of CNS depressants.

Effects on diagnostic tests
None reported.

Adverse reactions
• CNS: nervousness, vertigo, confusion, headache, d ziness, drowsines, mental confusion (especially in derly patients).
• CV: tachycardia, palpitations.
• DERM: urticaria, dermatoses.
• GI: nausea, vomiting, abdominal pain, constipati (at high doses).
• Ocular: blurred vision, increased intraocular tensi disturbed accommodation.
• Other: dysuria, hyperpyrexia, eosinophilia, d mouth and throat.

Overdose and treatment
Clinical manifestations of overdose include clums ness, dizziness, drowsiness, fever, flushing, halluc nations, shortness of breath, nervousnes restlessness, or irritability. Treatment begins wi gastric lavage or emesis and may include slow I. physostigmine 0.4 to 2 mg up to 5 mg total dose. appropriate, excitement may be controlled with 2 thiopental I.V. drip or a rectal infusion of 2% chlor hydrate 100 to 200 ml. Treat fever symptomaticall Respiratory depression may require artificial resp ration.

▶ Special considerations
• Safety has not been established in children und age 12.
• Dosage may be reduced as symptoms improve.

Information for parents and patient
• Tell parents and patient that flavoxate may be tak on an empty stomach or with food or milk if gastr irritation occurs.
• Warn of possible increased sensitivity to light.

---

ucytosine (5FC)
ncobon

Classification: antifungal (fluorinated pyrimidine)

ow supplied
vailable by prescription only
apsules: 250 mg and 500 mg

dications, route, and dosage
evere fungal infections caused by suscepti-
le strains of Candida *and* Cryptococcus
hildren weighing less than 50 kg: 1.5 to 4.5 g/m²/
ay in four divided doses q 6 hours P.O.
hildren weighing more than 50 kg and adults: 50 to
50 mg/kg daily divided q 6 hours P.O.
Severe infections, such as meningitis, may require
ses up to 250 mg/kg.
osage in renal failure
patients with a creatinine clearance of 10 to 50
l/minute/1.73 m², reduce dose by 50% to 70%, or
crease dosage interval to every 12 to 24 hours. In
atients with a creatinine clearance of < 10 ml/min-
e/1.73m², reduce dose by 20% to 80% or increase
osage interval to 24 to 48 hours. If possible, serum
vels should be monitored. Flucytosine is removed by
emodialysis and peritoneal dialysis. Patients under-
oing hemodialysis every 48 to 72 hours should re-
eive a supplemental dose of 20 to 50 mg/kg
mmediately after dialysis.

ction and kinetics
Antifungal action: Flucytosine penetrates fungal
ells, where it is converted to fluorouracil, which in-
rferes with pyrimidine metabolism; it also may be
onverted to fluorodeoxyuredylic acid, which inter-
res with DNA synthesis. Because human cells lack
e enzymes needed to convert the drug to these toxic
etabolites, flucytosine is selectively toxic to fungal,
ot host cells. It is active against some strains of
ryptococcus and *Candida.*
Kinetics in adults: About 75% to 90% of an oral dose
flucytosine is absorbed. Peak serum concentrations
ccur at 2 to 6 hours after a dose. Food decreases
e rate of absorption. Flucytosine is distributed widely
to the liver, spleen, heart, bronchial secretions,
ints, peritoneal fluid, and aqueous humor. CSF levels
ary from 60% to 100% of serum levels. Drug is 2%
4% bound to plasma proteins. Only small amounts
flucytosine are metabolized. About 75% to 95% of
dose is excreted unchanged in urine; less than 10%
excreted unchanged in feces. Serum half-life is 2½
6 hours with normal renal function; as long as
160 hours with creatinine clearance below 2 ml/
inute.

ontraindications and precautions
ucytosine is contraindicated in patients with known
persensitivity to the drug. It should be used with
aution in patients with bone marrow depression (re-
ardless of origin), as it may exacerbate this condi-
on; and in patients with impaired renal function, to

prevent toxic drug accumulation. In patients with impaired renal function, serum concentrations should
be determined to maintain therapeutic range (25 to
120 mcg/ml).

Interactions
Flucytosine potentiates the efficacy and toxicity of
amphotericin B.

Effects on diagnostic tests
Flucytosine causes falsely elevated creatinine values
on iminohydrolase enzymatic assay.
  Flucytosine may increase alkaline phosphatase,
AST (SGOT), ALT (SGPT), BUN, and serum creatinine
levels and may decrease WBC, RBC, and platelet
counts.

Adverse reactions
• CNS: dizziness, *drowsiness,* confusion, headache,
vertigo, hallucinations.
• DERM: *occasional rash.*
• GI: *nausea, vomiting, diarrhea,* abdominal bloating.
• HEMA: *anemia, leukopenia, bone marrow depres-
sion, thrombocytopenia.*
• Hepatic: *elevated AST (SGOT) and ALT (SGPT) lev-
els.*
• Metabolic: *elevated serum alkaline phosphatase,
BUN, and serum creatinine levels.*

Overdose and treatment
Flucytosine overdose may affect cardiovascular and
pulmonary function. Treatment is largely supportive.
Induced emesis or lavage may be useful within 4 hours
after ingestion. Activated charcoal and osmotic cathartics also may be helpful. Flucytosine is readily
removed by either hemodialysis or peritoneal dialysis.

▶ Special considerations
• Susceptibility tests to determine sensitivity of organism should precede therapy.
• Hematologic studies and renal and hepatic function
studies should also precede therapy and should be
repeated frequently thereafter to evaluate dosage and
monitor for adverse reactions. Prolonged elevated blood
levels (> 100 mcg/ml) are associated with an increased risk of bone marrow suppression.
• Give capsules over a 15-minute period to reduce
nausea, vomiting, and GI distress.
• Monitor intake and output to ensure adequate renal
function.
• Flucytosine is usually given concomitantly with amphotericin B because they are synergistic.
• Protect drug from light.
• Because flucytosine is removed by hemodialysis,
dosage adjustments should be made in patients undergoing hemodialysis.

Information for parents and patient
• Teach parents the signs and symptoms of adverse
reactions and the need to report them. Parents should
call promptly if patient's urine output decreases or if
signs of bleeding or bruising occur.
• Explain that adequate response may require several
weeks or months of therapy. Advise compliance with
medical regimen and scheduled follow-up visits.

fludrocortisone acetate
Florinef

- Classification: mineralocorticoid replacement therapy (mineralocorticoid, glucocorticoid)

How supplied
Available by prescription only
Tablets: 0.1 mg

Indications, route, and dosage
Adrenal insufficiency (partial replacement), salt-losing adrenogenital syndrome
Children: 0.05 to 0.1 mg P.O. daily.
Adults: 0.1 to 0.2 mg P.O. daily.

Action and kinetics
- *Adrenal hormone replacement:* Fludrocortisone, a synthetic glucocorticoid with potent mineralocorticoid activity, is used for partial replacement of steroid hormones in adrenocortical insufficiency and in salt-losing forms of congenital adrenogenital syndrome. In treating adrenocortical insufficiency, an exogenous glucocorticoid must also be administered for adequate control. (Cortisone or hydrocortisone are usually the drugs of choice for replacement because they produce both mineralocorticoid and glucocorticoid activity.) Fludrocortisone is administered on a variable schedule ranging from three times weekly to twice daily, depending on individual requirements.
- *Kinetics in adults:* Fludrocortisone is absorbed readily from the GI tract, reaching peak concentrations in about 1½ hours.

Fludrocortisone is removed rapidly from the blood and distributed to muscle, liver, skin, intestines, and kidneys. It has a plasma half-life of about 30 minutes. It is extensively bound to plasma proteins (transcortin and albumin). Only the unbound portion is active. Adrenocorticoids are distributed into breast milk and through the placenta.

Fludrocortisone is metabolized in the liver to inactive glucuronide and sulfate metabolites.

The inactive metabolites and small amounts of unmetabolized drug are excreted by the kidneys. Insignificant quantities of drug are also excreted in feces. The biological half-life is 18 to 36 hours.

Contraindications and precautions
Fludrocortisone is contraindicated in patients with hypersensitivity to fludrocortisone acetate. It should be used with extreme caution in patients with hypertension, congestive heart failure (CHF), or cardiac disease and should be discontinued if a significant increase in weight or blood pressure, edema, or cardiac enlargement occurs.

The use of fludrocortisone should be accompanied by adequate glucocorticoid therapy in adrenal insufficiency or the salt-losing form of adrenogenital syndrome.

Patients with Addison's disease are more sensitive to the action of fludrocortisone and may develop adverse reactions to an exaggerated degree. Stop treatment in the event of a significant increase in weight or blood pressure, or the development of edema or cardiac enlargement.

Sodium retention and potassium loss are accelerated by a high sodium intake. If edema develops, restriction of dietary sodium and administration of potassium supplements may be necessary.

Interactions
Concomitant use with barbiturates, phenytoin, or rifampin may cause decreased corticosteroid effects because of increased hepatic metabolism. Fludrocortisone may enhance hypokalemia associated with diuretic or amphotericin B therapy. The hypokalemia may increase the risk of toxicity in patients concurrently receiving digitalis glycosides. Fludrocortisone may increase the metabolism of isoniazid and salicylates.

Effects on diagnostic tests
Fludrocortisone therapy increases serum sodium levels and decreases serum potassium levels. Glucose tolerance tests should be performed only if necessary because addisonian patients tend to develop severe hypoglycemia within 3 hours of the test.

Adverse reactions
- CNS: frontal and occipital headaches, dizziness.
- CV: sodium and water retention, leading to increased blood volume, edema, hypertension, CHF, cardiac dysrhythmias, and cardiomegaly.
- Metabolic: hypokalemia, unusual weight gain.
- Musculoskeletal: arthralgias and tendon contractures, extreme weakness of extremities with ascending paralysis secondary to low potassium.

Note: Drug should not be discontinued without direct medical supervision; rapid discontinuation may cause an addisonian crisis.

Overdose and treatment
Acute toxicity is manifested as an extension of the therapeutic effect, such as disturbances in fluid and electrolyte balance, hypokalemia, edema, hypertension, and cardiac insufficiency. In acute toxicity, administer symptomatic treatment and correct fluid and electrolyte imbalance.

▶ Special considerations
- Dosage must be carefully adjusted for individual replacement need.
- Chronic use of fludrocortisone in children and adolescents may delay growth and maturation.
- If possible, avoid long-term administration of pharmacologic dosages of glucocorticoids in children because these drugs may retard bone growth. Manifestations of adrenal suppression in children include retardation of linear growth, delayed weight gain, low plasma cortisol concentrations, and lack of response to corticotropin stimulation. In children who require prolonged therapy, closely monitor growth and development. Alternate-day therapy is recommended to minimize growth suppression.
- Establish baseline blood pressure, fluid intake and output, weight, and electrolyte status. Watch for and

---

sudden weight gain, edema, change in blood pressure, or change in electrolyte status.
• During times of physiologic stress (trauma, surgery, infection), the patient may require additional steroids and may experience signs of steroid withdrawal; patients who were previously steroid-dependent may need systemic corticosteroids to prevent adrenal insufficiency.
• After long-term therapy, the drug should not be reduced gradually. Rapid reduction may cause withdrawal symptoms.
• Be aware of the patient's psychological history and watch for any behavioral changes.
• Observe for signs of infection or delayed wound healing.
• Acute withdrawal of drug may result in fever, myalgia, arthralgia, malaise, hypotension, hypoglycemic shock.
• Plasma renin activity is usually the most sensitive laboratory test used to evaluate the adequacy of drug therapy. It is profoundly abnormal before clinical signs and symptoms become apparent.
• Use only with other supplemental measures, such as glucocorticoids, control of electrolytes, and control of infection.
• Supplemental dosages may be required in times of physiologic stress from serious illness, trauma, or surgery.

Information for parents and patient
• Teach parents and patient to recognize signs of electrolyte imbalance: muscle weakness, paresthesias, numbness, fatigue, anorexia, nausea, altered mental status, increased urination, altered heart rhythm, severe or continuing headaches, unusual weight gain, or swelling of the feet.
• Tell parents that patient should take missed dose as soon as possible, unless it is almost time for the next dose, and not to double the dose.
• Be sure that the parents and patient understand the need to take the adrenocorticosteroid as prescribed. Give instructions on what to do if a dose is inadvertently missed.
• Explain the importance of reporting patient's suspected pregnancy promptly.
• Warn the parents and patient not to discontinue the drug abruptly or without medical approval.
• Inform the parents and patient of the possible therapeutic and adverse effects of the drug so that they may report any complications promptly.
• Advise the parents that the patient should wear a Medic Alert bracelet or necklace indicating the need for supplemental adrenocorticoids during times of stress.
• Parents and patient should inform new physician or dentist that patient is taking this drug.

flunisolide

Nasal inhalant
Nasalide

Oral inhalant
AeroBid

• Classification: anti-inflammatory, antiasthmatic agent (glucocorticoid)

How supplied
Available by prescription only
Nasal inhalant: 25 mcg/metered spray; 200 doses/bottle
Oral inhalant: 250 mcg/metered spray; 50 doses/inhaler

Indications, route, and dosage
Steroid-dependent asthma
Children age 6 and older: One inhalation t.i.d. Do not exceed four inhalations a day.
Adults: Two inhalations b.i.d. Do not exceed eight inhalations a day.

Action and kinetics
• *Anti-inflammatory action:* Flunisolide stimulates the synthesis of enzymes needed to decrease the inflammatory response. The anti-inflammatory and vasoconstrictor potency of topically applied flunisolide is several hundred times greater than that of hydrocortisone and about equal to that of an equal weight of triamcinolone; the metabolite, 6-beta-hydroxyflunisdolide, has about three times the activity of hydrocortisone.
• *Antiasthmatic action:* The nasal inhalant form of flunisolide is used in the symptomatic treatment of seasonal or perennial rhinitis. In patients who require corticosteroids to control symptoms, the oral inhalant form is used to treat bronchial asthma.
• *Kinetics in adults:* Approximately 50% of a nasally inhaled dose is absorbed systemically. Peak plasma concentrations occur within 10 to 30 minutes. After oral inhalation, about 70% of the dose is absorbed from the lungs and GI tract. Only about 20% of an orally inhaled dose of flunisolide reaches systemic circulation unmetabolized because of extensive metabolism in the liver. Onset of action usually occurs in a few days but may take as long as 4 weeks in some patients.
   Distribution following intranasal administration has not been described. After oral inhalation, 10% to 25% of the drug is distributed to the lungs; the remainder is deposited in the mouth and swallowed. No evidence exists of tissue storage of flunisolide or its metabolites. When absorbed, it is 50% bound to plasma proteins.
   Flunisolide that is swallowed undergoes rapid metabolism in the liver or GI tract to a variety of metabolites, one of which has glucocorticoid activity. Flunisolide and its 6-beta-hydroxy metabolite are

---

‡May contain sulfites   ◆May contain tartrazine   ◆◆May contain benzyl alcohol

eventually conjugated in the liver, by glucuronic acid or surface sulfate, to inactive metabolites.

Excretion of inhaled flunisolide has not been described. When the drug is administered systemically, the metabolites are excreted in approximately equal portions in feces and urine. The biological half-life of flunisolide averages about 2 hours.

Contraindications and precautions
Flunisolide is contraindicated in patients with acute status asthmaticus; in patients with tuberculosis or viral, fungal, or bacterial respiratory infections; and in patients who are hypersensitive to any component of the preparation.

It should be used cautiously in patients receiving systemic corticosteroids because of increased risk of hypothalamic-pituitary-adrenal axis suppression; when substituting inhalant for oral systemic administration (because withdrawal symptoms may occur); and in patients with healing nasal septal ulcers, oral or nasal surgery, or trauma.

Interactions
None reported.

Effects on diagnostic tests
None reported.

Adverse reactions
• EENT: (after oral inhalation) flushing, rash, dry mouth, hoarseness, irritation of the tongue or throat, and impaired sense of taste; (after nasal inhalation) itchy nose, dryness, burning, irritation and sneezing, infrequent epistaxis, bloody mucus.
• Immune: suppression of immune response; fungal overgrowth and infections of the nose, mouth, or throat.
• Other: restlessness, anxiety, altered taste.
Note: Drug should be discontinued if no improvement is evident after 4 weeks, or if nasal or oral infections develop.

Overdose and treatment
No information available.

▶ Special considerations
• In children, systemic corticosteroid therapy may be successfully substituted with nasal or oral inhalant corticosteroid therapy, thus reducing the risk of adverse systemic effects. However, the risk of HPA axis suppression and Cushing's syndrome still exists, particularly if excessive dosages are used. Manifestations of adrenal suppression in children include retardation of linear growth, delayed weight gain, low plasma cortisol concentrations, and lack of response to corticotropin stimulation.
• The therapeutic effects of intranasal inhalants, unlike those of sympathomimetic decongestants, are not immediate. Full therapeutic benefit requires regular use and is usually evident within a few days, although a few patients may require up to 3 weeks of therapy for maximum benefit.
• Use of nasal or oral inhalation therapy may occasionally allow a patient to discontinue systemic corticosteroid therapy. Systemic corticosteroid therapy should be discontinued by gradually tapering the dosage while carefully observing the patient for signs of adrenal insufficiency (joint pain, lassitude, depression).
• After the desired clinical effect is obtained, maintenance dose should be reduced to the smallest amount necessary to control symptoms.
• The drug should be discontinued if the patient develops signs of systemic absorption (including Cushing's syndrome, hyperglycemia, or glycosuria), mucosal irritation or ulceration, hypersensitivity, or infection. (If antifungals or antibiotics are being used with corticosteroids and the infection does not respond immediately, discontinue corticosteroids unil the infection is controlled.)

Information for the parents and patient
• Instruct patient to use nasal inhaler only as directed. Inform patient that full therapeutic effect is not immediate but requires regular use of inhaler. Patient with blocked nasal passages should use an oral decongestant ½ hour before intranasal corticosteroid administration to ensure adequate penetration. Advise patient to clear nasal passages of secretions before using the inhaler.
• Ask parents and patient to read manufacturer's instructions and demonstrate correct use of inhaler. Assist patient until proper use of inhaler is demonstrated.
• Advise patient receiving bronchodilators by inhalation to use the bronchodilator before using the corticosteroid inhalant to enhance penetration of the corticosteroid into the bronchial tree. Patient should wait several minutes to allow time for the bronchodilator to relax the smooth muscle.
• Instruct patient to hold breath for a few seconds to enhance placement and action of the drug and to wait 1 minute before taking subsequent puffs of drug.
• Patient should rinse mouth with water after using the inhaler to decrease the chance of oral fungal infections, and should check nasal and oral mucuous membranes frequently for signs of fungal infection.
• Warn asthma patients not to increase use of corticosteroid inhaler during a severe asthma attack, but to call for adjustment in dosage or discontinuation of the drug if necessary.
• Instruct parents to observe for adverse effects, and if fever or local irritation develops, to discontinue use and report the effect promptly.

fluocinolone acetonide
Fluoderm★, Fluolar★, Fluonid, Fluonide★, Flurosyn, Synalar, Synamol★, Synandone★, Synemol

• Classification: anti-inflammatory (adrenocorticoid)

How supplied
Available by prescription only
Cream: 0.01%, 0.025%, 0.2%
Ointment: 0.025%
Solution: 0.01%

Indications, route, and dosage

Inflammation of corticosteroid-responsive dermatoses

Children: Apply 0.01% cream or topical solution one to two times a day; apply 0.025% or 0.25 cream or ointment once a day.

Adults: Apply cream, ointment, or solution sparingly b.i.d. to q.i.d. Treat multiple or extensive lesions sequentially, applying to only small areas at any one time. Occlusive dressings may be used for severe or resistant dermatoses.

Action and kinetics

Anti-inflammatory action: Fluocinolone stimulates the synthesis of enzymes needed to decrease the inflammatory response. It is a high-potency fluorinated glucocorticoid. Preparations of 0.01% potency are in group V; 0.025% potency in group III; and 0.2% potency in group II.

Kinetics in adults: The amount absorbed depends on the strength of the preparation, the amount applied, and the nature of the skin at the application site. It ranges from about 1% in areas with a thick stratum corneum (such as the palms, soles, elbows, and heels) to as high as 36% in areas of the thinnest stratum corneum (face, eyelids, and genitals). Absorption increases in areas that are damaged, inflamed, or under occlusion. Some systemic absorption of topical steroids occurs, especially through the oral mucosa.

After topical application, fluocinolone is distributed throughout the skin and metabolized primarily locally. Any drug absorbed into the circulation is distributed rapidly into muscle, liver, skin, intestines, and kidneys and is metabolized primarily in the liver to inactive compounds.

Inactive metabolites are excreted by the kidneys, primarily as glucuronides and sulfates, but also as unconjugated products. Small amounts of the metabolites are also excreted in feces.

Contraindications and precautions

Fluocinolone is contraindicated in patients who are hypersensitive to any component of the preparation and in patients with viral, fungal, or tubercular skin lesions.

Fluocinolone should be used with extreme caution in patients with impaired circulation because the drug may increase the risk of skin ulceration.

Interactions

None significant.

Effects on diagnostic tests

None significant.

Adverse reactions

Local: burning, itching, irritation, dryness, folliculitis, hypertrichosis, acneiform eruptions, hypopigmentation, perioral dermatitis, allergic contact dermatitis, maceration, secondary infection, atrophy, striae, miliaria.

Significant systemic absorption can produce the following reactions.

CNS: euphoria, insomnia, headache, psychotic behavior, pseudotumor cerebri, mental changes, nervousness, restlessness.
• CV: congestive heart failure, hypertension, edema.
• EENT: cataracts, glaucoma, thrush.
• GI: peptic ulcer, irritation, increased appetite.
• Immune: immunosuppression, increased susceptibility to infection.
• Metabolic: hypokalemia, sodium retention, fluid retention, weight gain, hyperglycemia, osteoporosis, growth suppression in children.
• Musculoskeletal: muscle atrophy.
• Other: withdrawal syndrome (nausea, fatigue, anorexia, dyspnea, hypotension, hypoglycemia, myalgia, arthralgia, fever, dizziness, and fainting).

Note: Drug should be discontinued if local irritation, infection, systemic absorption, or hypersensitivity reaction occurs.

Overdose and treatment

No information available.

▶ Special considerations

• Children may show greater susceptibility to topical corticosteroid-induced HPA axis suppression and Cushing's syndrome than mature patients because of a higher ratio of skin surface area to body weight. Hypothalamic-pituitary-adrenal (HPA) axis suppression, Cushing's syndrome, and intracranial hypertension have been reported in children receiving topical corticosteroids. Signs of adrenal suppression in children include linear growth retardation, delayed weight gain, low plasma cortisol levels, and absence of response to ACTH stimulation. Signs of intracranial hypertension include bulging fontanells, headaches, and bilateral papilledema.
• Administration of topical corticosteroids to children should be limited to the least effective amount. Chronic corticosteroid therapy may interfere with growth and development.
• Stop drug if the patient develops signs of systemic absorption (including Cushing's syndrome, hyperglycemia, or glucosuria), skin irritation or ulceration, hypersensitivity, or infection. (If antifungals or antibiotics are being used with corticosteroids and the infection does not respond immediately, corticosteroids should be stopped until infection is controlled.)
• Monitor patient response. Observe area of inflammation and elicit patient comments concerning pruritus. Inspect skin for infection, striae, and atrophy. Skin atrophy is common and may be clinically significant within 3 to 4 weeks of treatment with high-potency preparations; it also occurs more readily at sites where percutaneous absorption is high.
• Do not apply occlusive dressings over topical steroids because this may lead to secondary infection, maceration, atrophy, striae, or miliaria caused by increasing steroid penetration and potency.

Information for parents and patient

• Instruct parents and patient in application of the drug. Tell them the following:
Method for applying topical preparations
• Wash your hands before and after applying the drug.
• Gently cleanse the area of application. Washing or

■May contain sulfites   ◆May contain tartrazine   ◆◆May contain benzyl alcohol

soaking the area before application may increase drug penetration.
• Apply sparingly in a light film; rub in lightly. Avoid contact with patient's eyes, unless using an ophthalmic product.
• Avoid prolonged application in areas near the eyes, genitals, rectum, on the face, and in skin folds. High-potency topical corticosteroids are more likely to cause striae in these areas because of their higher rates of absorption.
• If an occlusive dressing is necessary, minimize adverse reactions by using it intermittently. Do not leave it in place longer than 16 hours each day.
• Warn patient not to use nonprescription topical preparations other than those specifically recommended.
• Advise parents not to use tight-fitting diapers or plastic pants on a child being treated in the diaper area, since such garments may serve as occlusive dressings.

fluocinonide
FAPG, Lidemol*, Lidex, Lidex-E, , Lyderm*, Metosyn*

• Classification: anti-inflammatory (topical adrenocorticoid)

How supplied
Available by prescription only
Cream, gel, ointment, solution: 0.05%

Indications, route, and dosage
Inflammation of corticosteroid-responsive dermatoses
Children: Apply sparingly to affected areas once a day.
Adults: Apply sparingly b.i.d. to q.i.d. Occlusive dressings may be used for severe or resistant dermatoses.

Action and kinetics
• *Anti-inflammatory action:* Fluocinonide stimulates the synthesis of enzymes needed to decrease the inflammatory response. Fluocinonide is a high-potency fluorinated glucocorticoid categorized as a group II topical steroid.
• *Kinetics in adults:* The amount absorbed depends on the amount applied and on the nature of the skin at the application site. It ranges from about 1% in areas of thick stratum corneum (such as the palms, soles, elbows, and knees) to as high as 36% in areas of thin stratum corneum (face, eyelids, and genitals). Absorption increases in areas that are damaged, inflamed, or under occlusion. Some systemic absorption of steroids occurs, especially through the oral mucosa.
After topical application, fluocinonide is distributed and metabolized primarily in the skin. Any absorbed drug is removed rapidly from the blood and distributed into muscle, liver, skin, intestines, and kidneys, and the small amount absorbed into systemic circulation is metabolized primarily in the liver to inactive compounds.
Inactive metabolites are excreted by the kidneys,

primarily as glucuronides and sulfates, but also unconjugated products. Small amounts of the metabolites are excreted in feces.

Contraindications and precautions
Fluocinonide is contraindicated in patients who are hypersensitive to any component of the preparation and in patients with viral, fungal, or tubercular skin lesions.
Fluocinonide should be used with extreme caution in patients with impaired circulation because the drug may increase the risk of skin ulceration.

Interactions
None significant.

Effects on diagnostic tests
None reported.

Adverse reactions
• Local: burning, itching, irritation, dryness, folliculitis, hypertrichosis, acneiform eruptions, hypopigmentation, perioral dermatitis, allergic contact dermatitis, maceration, secondary infection, atrophy, striae, miliaria.
Significant systemic absorption may cause the following reactions.
• CNS: euphoria, insomnia, headache, psychotic behavior, pseudotumor cerebri, mental changes, nervousness, restlessness.
• CV: congestive heart failure, hypertension, edema.
• DERM: delayed healing, acne, skin eruptions, striae.
• EENT: cataracts, glaucoma, thrush.
• GI: peptic ulcer, irritation, increased appetite.
• Immune: immunosuppression, increased susceptibility to infection.
• Metabolic: hypokalemia, sodium retention, fluid retention, weight gain, hyperglycemia, osteoporosis, growth suppression in children.
• Musculoskeletal: muscle atrophy.
• Other: withdrawal syndrome (nausea, fatigue, anorexia, dyspnea, hypotension, hypoglycemia, myalgia, arthralgia, fever, dizziness, and fainting).
Note: Drug should be discontinued if local irritation, infection, systemic absorption, or hypersensitivity reaction occurs.

Overdose and treatment
No information available.

▶ Special considerations
• Children may show greater susceptibility to topical corticosteroid-induced HPA axis suppression and Cushing's syndrome than mature patients because a higher ratio of skin surface area to body weight. Hypothalamic-pituitary-adrenal (HPA) axis suppression, Cushing's syndrome, and intracranial hypertension have been reported in children receiving topical corticosteroids. Signs of adrenal suppression in children include linear growth retardation, delayed weight gain, low plasma cortisol levels, and absence of response to ACTH stimulation. Signs of intracranial hypertension include bulging fontanelles, headache, and bilateral papilledema.
• Administration of topical corticosteroids to children

should be limited to the least effect amount. Chronic corticosteroid therapy may interfere with growth and development.

• Stop drug if the patient develops signs of systemic absorption (including Cushing's syndrome, hyperglycemia, or glucosuria), skin irritation or ulceration, hypersensitivity, or infection. (If antifungals or antibiotics are being used with corticosteroids and the infection does not respond immediately, corticosteroids should be stopped until infection is controlled.)

• Monitor patient response. Assess for inflammation and pruritus. Inspect skin for infection, striae, and atrophy. Skin atrophy is common and may be clinically significant within 3 to 4 weeks of treatment with high-potency preparations; it also occurs more readily at sites where percutaneous absorption is high.

• Do not apply occlusive dressings over topical steroids becuase this may lead to secondary infection, maceration, atrophy, striae, or miliaria caused by increasing steroid penetration and potency.

Information for parents and patient

• Instruct parents and patient in application of the drug. Tell them the following:

Method for applying topical medication

Wash your hands before and after applying the drug. Gently cleanse the area of application. Washing or soaking the area before application may increase drug penetration. Then apply sparingly in a light film; rub in lightly. Avoid contact with patient's eyes.

• Avoid prolonged application on the face, in skin folds, and in areas near the eyes, genitals, and rectum. High-potency topical corticosteroids are more likely to cause striae in these areas because of their higher rates of absorption.

• If an occlusive dressing is necessary, minimize adverse reactions by using it intermittently. Do not leave it in place longer than 16 hours each day.

• Warn patient not to use nonprescription topical preparations other than those specifically recommended.

• Advise parents not to use tight-fitting diapers or plastic pants on a child being treated in the diaper area, since such garments may serve as occlusive dressings.

---

fluorometholone
Fluor-Op Ophthalmic, FML Liquifilm Ophthalmic, FML Ointment

• Classification: ophthalmic anti-inflammatory (corticosteroid)

How supplied
Available by prescription only
Ointment: 0.1%
Suspension: 0.1%, 0.25%

Indications, route, and dosage
Inflammatory and allergic conditions of cornea, conjunctiva, sclera, anterior uvea
Children and adults: Instill 1 to 2 drops in conjunctival sac b.i.d. to q.i.d. May use q hour during first 1 to 2

days if needed. In severe cases, apply ½″ of the ointment in the conjunctival sac q 4 hours during the first 24 to 48 hours of therapy.

Action and kinetics
• *Anti-inflammatory action:* Fluorometholone stimulates the synthesis of enzymes needed to decrease the inflammatory response. Fluorometholone is a synthetic fluorinated corticosteroid that is less likely than hydrocortisone, prednisolone, or dexamethasone to cause intraocular hypertension.

• *Kinetics in adults:* After ophthalmic administration, fluorometholone is absorbed mainly into the aqueous humor. Slight systemic absorption typically occurs. Fluorometholone is distributed throughout the local tissue layers. Any absorbed drug is removed rapidly from the blood, distributed into muscle, liver, skin, intestines, and kidneys and primarily metabolized locally. The small amount absorbed is metabolized primarily in liver to inactive compounds. Inactive metabolites are excreted by the kidneys, primarily as glucuronides and sulfates, but also as unconjugated products. Small amounts of the metabolites are also excreted in the feces.

Contraindications and precautions
Fluorometholone is contraindicated in patients who are hypersensitive to any component of the preparation; in patients with fungal infections of the eye; and in patients with acute, untreated purulent bacterial, viral, or fungal ocular infections. If a bacterial infection does not respond promptly to appropriate anti-infective therapy, fluorometholone should be discontinued and another therapy applied.

Intraocular pressure should be measured every 2 to 4 weeks for the first 2 months of ophthalmic corticosteroid therapy; then, if no increase in intraocular pressure has occurred, every 1 to 2 months thereafter.

Interactions
None reported.

Effects on diagnostic tests
None reported.

Adverse reactions
• Eye: transient burning or stinging on administration; mydriasis, ptosis, epithelial punctate keratitis, and corneal or scleral malacia (rare); increased intraocular pressure, thinning of the cornea, interference with corneal wound healing, increased susceptibility to viral or fungal corneal infection, corneal ulceration; glaucoma, cataracts, and defects in visual acuity and visual field (with long-term use).

• Systemic: rare, but may occur with excessive doses or long-term use.

Note: Drug should be discontinued if topical application results in local irritation, infection, significant systemic absorption, or hypersensitivity reaction; if visual acuity decreases or visual field diminishes; or if burning, stinging, or watering of eyes does not quickly resolve after administration.

Overdose and treatment
No information available.

---

‡May contain sulfites   ◆ May contain tartrazine   ◆◆ May contain benzyl alcohol

▶ Special considerations

• Because of their greater ratio of skin surface area to body weight, children may be more susceptible than adults to topical corticosteroid-induced hypothalamic-pituitary-adrenal axis suppression and Cushing's syndrome. Although such reactions occur extremely rarely with ophthalmic use, it is still advisable to limit corticosteroid therapy in children to the minimum effective dosage.

• Ophthalmic products may initially cause sensitivity to bright light. This may be minimized by wearing sunglasses.

• Monitor the patient's response by observing the area of inflammation and eliciting patient comments concerning pruritus and vision. Inspect the eye and surrounding tissues for infection and additional irritation.

• Discontinue the drug if the patient develops signs of systemic absorption (including Cushing's syndrome, hyperglycemia, or glucosuria), skin irritation or ulceration, hypersensitivity, or infection. (If antivirals or antibiotics are being used with corticosteroids and the infection is doese not respond immediately, corticosteroids should be stopped until the infection is controlled.)

Information for parents and patient

Advise the parents and patient to use the following steps when administering eye drops:

Method for applying eye drops

Wash hands well. Shake solution or suspension well. Tilt head back or lie down. Then, lightly pull lower eyelid down by applying gentle pressure at the lid base at the bony rim of orbit. Approach the eye from below with the dropper, do not touch dropper to any tissue. Holding dropper no more than 1″ above the eye, drop medication inside lower lid while looking up. Then, try to keep eye open for 30 seconds. After instillation, apply light finger pressure inward and down to the side of the bridge of the nose (the lacrimal canaliculi) for 1 to 2 minutes to prevent drainage of solution into nasal passages, where most of the drug is absorbed systemically.

• Wait at least 5 minutes before applying another ophthalmic medication.

• When administering opthalmic ointments: Wash hands well. Hold the tube several minutes before use to warm it and improve flow of ointment. If opening the ointment tube for the first time, squeeze out the first ¼″ of ointment and discard (using sterile gauze) because it may be too dry.

• Apply a small "ribbon" or strip of ointment (¼″ to ½″) to the inside of the lower eyelid without touching any part of the eye with the tip of the tube. Close the eye gently and roll the eyeball in all directions to spread the ointment.

• Wait at least 10 minutes before applying a second eye ointment.

• Instruct parents to observe for adverse effects. They should call if no improvement occurs after 7 to 8 days, if the condition worsens, or if pain, itching, or swelling of the eye occurs.

• Warn parents not to administer nonprescription ophthalmic preparations other than those specifically recommended. Nonprescription ophthalmic solutions should not be used for more than 7 days or in children under age 2.

• Warn parents not to use leftover medication for a new eye inflammation and never to share eye medication with others. Tell them to store all eye medications in original container.

• Parents should call for specific instructions before discontinuing therapy.

---

fluorouracil (5-FU)
Adrucil, Efudex, Fluroplex

• Classification: antineoplastic (antimetabolite [cell cycle-phase specific, S phase])

How supplied

Available by prescription only
Injection: 50 mg/ml in 10-ml and 20-ml vials and 1,000 mg/20 ml vials
Cream: 1%, 5%
Topical solution: 1%, 2%, 5%

Indications, route, and dosage

Dosage and indications may vary. Check current literature for recommended protocol.

Colon, rectal, breast, ovarian, cervical, gastric, esophageal, bladder, liver, pancreatic, and unknown primary cancers

†*Children and adults:* 7 to 12 mg/kg I.V. for 4 days, then (after 3 days) 7 to 10 mg/kg q 3 to 4 days for 2 weeks. Alternatively, 12 mg/kg I.V. for 5 days, followed (after 1 day) by 6 mg/kg I.V. every other day for 4 or 5 doses, for a total course of 2 weeks. Maintenance infusion is 7 to 12 mg/kg I.V. q 7 to 10 days or 300 to 500 mg/m² every 4 to 5 days, repeated monthly. Do not exceed 800 mg/day (400 mg/day in severely ill patients).

Action and kinetics

• *Antineoplastic action:* Fluorouracil exerts its cytotoxic activity by acting as an antimetabolite, competing for the enzyme that is important in the synthesis of thymidine, an essential substrate for DNA synthesis. Therefore, DNA synthesis is inhibited. The drug also inhibits RNA synthesis to a lesser extent.

• *Kinetics in adults:* Fluorouracil is absorbed poorly after oral administration. Fluorouracil distributes widely into all areas of body water and tissues, including tumors, bone marrow, liver, and intestinal mucosa. Fluorouracil crosses the blood-brain barrier to a significant extent. A small amount of drug is converted in the tissues to the active metabolite, with a majority of the drug degraded in the liver. Metabolites of fluorouracil are primarily excreted through the lungs as carbon dioxide. A small portion of a dose is excreted in urine as unchanged drug.

Contraindications and precautions

Fluorouracil is contraindicated in patients with poor nutritional status, depressed bone marrow function, recent major surgery, or serious infections because of

---

the increased potential for toxicity; and in pregnant patients because the drug may be fetotoxic.

Interactions
When used concomitantly, leucovorin calcium given as a continuous infusion causes increased binding of fluorouracil to substrate, increased fluorouracil cell uptake and increased inhibition of thymidine synthetase.

Effects on diagnostic tests
Fluorouracil may decrease plasma albumin concentration because of drug-induced protein malabsorption.

Adverse reactions
• CNS: *acute cerebellar syndrome,* drowsiness, euphoria, aphagia.
• CV: mild angina, ECG changes.
• DERM: maculopapular rash, dryness, erythema, hyperpigmentation (especially in blacks), nail changes, pigmented palmar creases, pruritus, suppuration, burning, swelling, scarring.
• GI: anorexia, proctitis, paralytic ileus, *oral and GI ulcers,* stomatitis, *diarrhea* (GI ulcer may precede leukopenia), *nausea, vomiting,* GI toxicity (dose-limiting).
• HEMA: *bone marrow depression* (dose-limiting), leukopenia (nadir in 7 to 14 days), anemia.
• Other: photosensitivity, lacrimation, reversible alopecia, weakness, malaise, *hypersensitivity reaction.*
   Note: Drug should be discontinued if intractable vomiting, stomatitis, diarrhea, GI ulceration, or GI bleeding occurs; if the leukocyte count falls below 3,000/mm³; or if the platelet count falls below 100,000/mm³.

Overdose and treatment
Clinical manifestations of overdose include myelosuppression, diarrhea, alopecia, dermatitis, hyperpigmentation, nausea, and vomiting.
   Treatment is usually supportive and includes transfusion of blood components, antiemetics, and antidiarrheals.

▶ Special considerations
• Follow established procedures for the safe handling, administration, and disposal of chemotherapy.
• Monitor vital signs and patency of catheter or I.V. line throught administration.
• Attempt to alleviate or reduce anxiety in patient and family before treatment.
• Monitor BUN, hematocrit, platelet count, ALT (SGPT), AST (SGOT), LDH, serum bilirubin, serum creatinine, uric acid, total and differential leukocyte, and others as required.
• To reconstitute, withdraw solution through a 5-micron filter and add to vial.
• Drug may be administered I.V. push over 1 to 2 minutes.
• Drug may be further diluted in dextrose 5% in water or normal saline solution for infusions up to 24 hours in duration.
• Use plastic I.V. containers for administering continuous infusions. Solution is more stable in plastic I.V. bags than in glass bottles.
• Do not use cloudy solution. If crystals form, redissolve by warming at a temperature of 140° F. (60° C.).
• Give antiemetic before administering to decrease nausea.
• Premedicating with an antiemetic may prevent nausea and vomiting. If vomiting occurs, administer antiemetics p.r.n.
• Monitor patient's intake, output, and weight.
• If extravasation occurs, treat as a chemical phlebitis with warm compresses.
• Do not refrigerate fluorouracil.
• Drug can be diluted in 120 ml of a 0.2 M sodium bicarbonate solution and administered orally.
• General photosensitivity occurs for 2 to 3 months after a dose.
• Ingestion and systemic absorption may cause leukopenia, thrombocytopenia, stomatitis, diarrhea or GI ulceration, bleeding, and hemorrhage. A topical local anesthetic may be used to soothe mouth lesions. Encourage good and frequent mouth care.
• Monitor intake and output, CBC, and renal and hepatic function.
• Avoid I.M. injections in patients with low platelet counts.
• Apply topical drug while using plastic gloves. Wash hands immediately after handling medication. Avoid topical use with occlusive dressings.
• Apply topical solution with caution near eyes, nose, and mouth.
• Topical application to larger ulcerated areas may cause systemic toxicity.
• For superficial basal cell carcinoma confirmed by biopsy, use 5% strength. Apply 1% concentration on the face. Reserve higher concentrations for thicker-skinned areas or resistant lesions. Occlusion may be required.
• Do not continue to treat lesions resistant to fluorouracil; they should be biopsied.

Information for parents and patient
• Tell parents that child's dental work should be completed before therapy whenever possible, or delayed until blood counts are normal.
• Stress importance of keeping follow-up appointments for monitoring hematologic status.
• Instruct parents to monitor neutropenic patient's temperature every 4 hours (not rectally) and to report fever, cough, and other signs of infection *promptly.*
• Warn parents that child may bruise easily because of drug's effect on platelets. Teach them to check for signs of bleeding and bruising. Parents may need to restrict child's participation in contact sports. Such activity is dangerous when patient's platelets are low.
• Patient should avoid contact with persons who have bacterial or viral infections or who have received live-virus immunizations (polio, measles/mumps/rubella). Explain importance of promptly reporting susceptible patient's exposure to chicken pox.
• Advise parents that patient should not receive immunizations during therapy and for several weeks after therapy. Members of the same household should not receive live-virus immunizations during the same period.

• Instruct patient to clean teeth with toothettes, gauze, or soft toothbrush when platelets are low. Patient should perform frequent oral hygiene and should avoid using commercial mouthwashes, which may contain alcohol and have an irritating effect. Solutions of sodium bicarbonate or hydrogen peroxide are more appropriate rinses.

• Patient should watch for and immediately report any redness, pain, or swelling that occurs at injection site. Tissue injury and scarring may result from infiltration at the infusion site.

• Instruct patient to avoid foods that are spicy and extremely hot or cold. Topical anesthetics administered before meals (swish and spit) may relieve mouth discomfort.

• Patient should avoid exposure to strong sunlight or ultraviolet light because it will intensify the skin reaction. Encourage use of sunscreens.

• Reassure parents and patient that hair should grow back after treatment is discontinued.

• Tell parents and patient to apply topical fluorouracil with gloves and to wash hands thoroughly after application. Warn them that treated area may be unsightly during therapy and for several weeks after therapy is stopped. Complete healing may not occur until 1 or 2 months after treatment is stopped.

---

fluoxymesterone
Android-F, Halotestin, Hysterone, Oratestryl

• Classification: androgen replacement, antineoplastic

How supplied
Available by prescription only
Tablets: 2 mg, 5 mg, 10 mg

Indications, route, and dosage
Treatment of delayed puberty in males
Adolescents: 2.5 to 10 mg P.O. daily for up to 6 months
Male hypogonadism
Adults: 5 to 20 mg P.O. daily, in a single dose or in three or four divided doses.
†Stimulation of erythropoiesis
Adults: 10 mg P.O. b.i.d. Doses up to 40 mg daily have been used.

Action and kinetics
• *Androgenic action:* Fluoxymesterone mimics the action of the endogenous androgen testosterone by stimulating receptors in androgen-responsive organs and tissues. It exerts inhibitory, anti-estrogenic effects on hormone-responsive breast tumors and metastases.
• *Antianemic action:* Fluoxymesterone enhances the production of erythropoietic stimulating factors, thereby increasing the production of red blood cells.
• *Kinetics in adults:* Fluoxymesterone is eliminated primarily by hepatic metabolism.

Contraindications and precautions
Fluoxymesterone is contraindicated in patients with severe renal or cardiac disease (fluid and sodium retention caused by fluoxymesterone may aggravate renal and cardiac disease); in patients with hepatic disease, because impaired elimination of the drug may cause its accumulation; in male patients with prostate or breast cancer or benign prostatic hypertrophy with obstruction; in patients with undiagnosed abnormal genital bleeding, because drug can stimulate the growth of cancerous breast or prostate tissue; in pregnant and breast-feeding women, because administration of androgens during pregnancy causes masculinization of the fetus; and in patients with known hypersensitivity to the drug.

The brands Halotestin and Ora-Testryl contain the dye tartrazine. Rare individuals, particularly those who are known to be sensitive to aspirin and who have nasal polyps, may suffer severe hypersensitivity reactions (for example, anaphylaxis) after ingesting tartrazine.

Interactions
In patients with diabetes, decreased blood glucose levels may require adjustment of insulin dosage.

Fluoxymesterone may potentiate the action of anticoagulants, resulting in increased prothrombin time. Concurrent administration with oxyphenbutazone may increase serum oxyphenbutazone concentrations.

Effects on diagnostic tests
Fluoxymesterone may cause abnormal results of the glucose tolerance test. Thyroid function test results (protein-bound iodine, radioactive iodine uptake, thyroid-binding capacity) may decrease. Prothrombin time (especially in patients on anticoagulant therapy) may be prolonged. Abnormal liver function test may occur. Because of this agent's anabolic activity, serum sodium, potassium, calcium, phosphate, and cholesterol levels may all rise.

Adverse reactions
• Androgenic: *in females:* deepening of voice, clitoral enlargement, changes in libido; *in males:* prepubertal—premature epiphyseal closure, priapism, phallic enlargement; postpubertal—testicular atrophy, oligospermia, decreased ejaculatory volume, impotence, gynecomastia, epididymitis.
• CNS: headache, anxiety, mental depression, generalized paresthesia.
• CV: edema.
• DERM: acne, oily skin, hirsutism, flushing, sweating, male pattern baldness.
• GI: gastroenteritis, nausea, vomiting, diarrhea, constipation, change in appetite, weight gain.
• GU: bladder irritability, priapism, virilization in females, vaginitis, menstrual irregularities.
• HEMA: polycythemia; suppression of clotting factors II, V, VII, and X.
• Hepatic: cholestatic hepatitis, jaundice.
• Other: hypercalcemia, hepatocellular cancer (with long-term use).

Note: Drug should be discontinued if hypercalcemia, edema, hypersensitivity reaction, priapism, or excessive sexual stimulation develops; or if virilization occurs in females.

Overdose and treatment
No information available.

▶ Special considerations
• Children receiving androgens must be observed carefully for excessive virilization and precocious puberty. Androgen therapy may cause premature epiphyseal closure and short stature. Regular X-ray examinations of hard bones may be used to monitor skeletal maturation during therapy.
• Do not administer androgens to males with breast or prostatic cancer, or symptomatic prostatic hypertrophy; to patients with severe cardiac, renal, or hepatic disease; or to patients with undiagnosed abnormal genital bleeding.
• Administration of androgens during pregnancy may cause masculinization of the female fetus and is therefore contraindicated.
• Hypercalcemia symptoms may be difficult to distinguish from symptoms of the condition being treated unless anticipated and thought of as a cluster.
• Priapism in males indicates that dosage is excessive. Serious acute toxicities have not been reported from large overdoses.
• Yellowing of the sclera of the eyes, or of the skin, may indicate hepatic dysfunction resulting from administration of androgens.
• Androgens do not improve athletic performance, but they are abused for this purpose by some athletes. Risks associated with their use for this purpose far outweigh any possible benefits.
• Observe female patients carefully for signs of excessive virilization. If possible, therapy should be discontinued at the first sign of virilization because some adverse effects (deepening of the voice, clitoral enlargement) are not reversible.
• When drug is used in breast cancer, subjective effects may not appear for about 1 month; objective improvement not for 3 months.
• Watch for symptoms of hypoglycemia in patients with diabetes. Insulin dosage may need adjustment.
• If patient is receiving anticoagulants concurrently with fluoxymesterone, monitor for ecchymoses, petechiae, and other signs of bleeding.
• Halotestin and Ora-Testryl contain tartrazine. Observe for signs of allergic reactions in patients sensitive to aspirin or tartrazine.

Information for parents and patient
• Administer drug with food to minimize GI upset.
• Reassure parents and female patients that growth of facial hair and development of acne are reversible once the drug is withdrawn.
• Explain to parents and female patients that medication may cause menstrual cycle irregularities. Advise them to report such effects and to discontinue therapy until their causes have been determined.
• Advise parents and male patient to report frequent or persistent penile erections.
• Advise parents and patient to report persistent GI distress, diarrhea, or the onset of jaundice.

• Discuss changes in body image that may result from drug's effects in adolescent patients.

---

fluphenazine decanoate
Modecate Decanoate*, Prolixin Decanoate

fluphenazine enanthate
Moditen Enanthate*, Prolixin Enathate

fluphenazine hydrochloride
Permitil Hydrochloride, Prolixin Hydrochloride

• Classification: antipsychotic (phenothiazine [piperazine derivative])

How supplied
Available by prescription only
Fluphenazine hydrochloride
Tablets: 1 mg, 2.5 mg, 5 mg, 10 mg
Oral concentrate: 5 mg/ml (contains 14% alcohol)
Elixir: 2.5 mg/5 ml (with 14% alcohol)
I.M. injection: 2.5 mg/ml
Fluphenazine enanthate
Depot injection: 25 mg/ml
Fluphenazine decanoate
Depot injection: 25 mg/ml

Indications, route, and dosage
Psychotic disorders
Children age 5 to 12: 3.125 to 12.5 mg fluphenazine decanoate I.M. or S.C. q 1 to 3 weeks, as needed and tolerated.
Children over age 12: 6.25 to 18.75 mg fluphenazine decanoate I.M. or S.C. weekly. Increase to 12.5 to 25 mg I.M. or S.C. q 1 to 3 weeks, as needed and tolerated. Alternatively, give fluphenazine enanthate 25 mg I.M. or S.C. q 1 to 3 weeks as needed and tolerated.
Children age 12 and under: 0.25 to 0.75 mg fluphenazine hydrochloride P.O. one to four times a day; or one third to one half of oral dose I.M.; maximum dosage is 10 mg daily.
Children over age 12 and adults: 12.5 to 25 mg of long-acting esters (fluphenazine decanoate and enanthate) I.M. or S.C. q 1 to 6 weeks. Maintenance dosage is 25 to 100 mg, p.r.n.
Adults: Initially, 0.5 to 10 mg fluphenazine hydrochloride P.O. daily in divided doses q 6 to 8 hours; may increase cautiously to 20 mg. Maintenance dosage is 1 to 5 mg P.O. daily. I.M. doses are one third to one half that of oral doses.

Actions and kinetics
• *Antipsychotic action:* Fluphenazine is thought to exert its antipsychotic effects by postsynaptic blockade of CNS dopamine receptors, thereby inhibiting dopamine-mediated effects.

Fluphenazine has many other central and peripheral effects; it produces both alpha and ganglionic blockade and counteracts histamine- and serotonin-

---

‡May contain sulfites   ◆May contain tartrazine   ◆◆May contain benzyl alcohol

mediated activity. Its most prominent adverse reactions are extrapyramidal.

• *Kinetics in adults:* Rate and extent of absorption vary with route of administration; oral tablet absorption is erratic and variable. Oral and I.M. dosages have an onset of action within ½ to 1 hour. Long-acting decanoate and enanthate salts act within 24 to 72 hours.

Fluphenazine is distributed widely into the body, including breast milk. CNS concentrations are usually higher than those in plasma. Drug is 91% to 99% protein-bound. Peak effects of oral dose usually occur at 2 hours; steady-state serum levels are achieved within 4 to 7 days.

Fluphenazine is metabolized extensively by the liver, but no active metabolites are formed; duration of action is about 6 to 8 hours after oral administration; 1 to 6 weeks (average, 2 weeks) after I.M. depot administration.

Most of drug is excreted in urine via the kidneys; some is excreted in feces via the biliary tract.

Contraindications and precautions

Fluphenazine is contraindicated in patients with known hypersensitivity to phenothiazines and related compounds, including allergic reactions involving hepatic function; in patients with blood dyscrasias and bone marrow depression because of possible agranulocytosis; in patients with disorders accompanied by coma, brain damage, or CNS depression because of additive CNS depression; in patients with circulatory collapse or cerebrovascular disease because of its hypotensive effect; and for use with adrenergic blocking agents or spinal or epidural anesthetics because of potential hypotension and alpha blockade.

Fluphenazine should be used cautiously in patients with cardiac disease (dysrhythmias, congestive heart failure, angina pectoris, valvular disease, or heart block), encephalitis, Reye's syndrome, head injury, respiratory disease, epilepsy and other seizure disorders, glaucoma, prostatic hypertrophy, urinary retention, hepatic or renal dysfunction, Parkinson's disease, pheochromocytoma, or hypocalcemia. Some oral preparations of fluphenazine contain tartrazine; use of such products may cause allergic reaction in patients with aspirin allergy.

Interactions

Concomitant use of fluphenazine with sympathomimetics, including epinephrine, phenylephrine, phenylpropanolamine, and ephedrine (often found in nasal sprays), and appetite suppressants may decrease their stimulatory and pressor effects.

Fluphenazine may inhibit blood pressure response to centrally acting antihypertensive drugs such as guanethidine, guanabenz, guanadrel, clonidine, methyldopa, and reserpine. Additive effects are likely after concomitant use of fluphenazine with CNS depressants, including alcohol, analgesics, barbiturates, narcotics, tranquilizers, and general, spinal, or epidural anesthetics, or parenteral magnesium sulfate (oversedation, respiratory depression, and hypotension); antiarrhythmic agents, quinidine, disopyramide, and procainamide (increased incidence of cardiac dysrhythmias and conduction defects); atropine or other anticholinergic drugs, including antidepressants, monoamine oxidase (MAO) inhibitors, phenothiazines, antihistamines, meperidine, and antiparkinsonian agents (oversedation, paralytic ileus, visual changes, and severe constipation); nitrates (hypotension); and metrizamide (increased risk of convulsions).

Beta-blocking agents may inhibit fluphenazine metabolism, increasing plasma levels and toxicity.

Concomitant use with propylthiouracil increases risk of agranulocytosis; concomitant use with lithium may result in severe neurologic toxicity with an encephalitis-like syndrome, and a decreased therapeutic response to fluphenazine.

Pharmacokinetic alterations and subsequent decreased therapeutic response to fluphenazine may follow concomitant use with phenobarbital (enhanced renal excretion), aluminum- and magnesium-containing antacids and antidiarrheals (decreased absorption), or caffeine, and with heavy smoking (increased metabolism).

Fluphenazine may antagonize therapeutic effect of bromocriptine on prolactin secretion; it also may decrease the vasoconstricting effects of high-dose dopamine, and may decrease effectiveness and increase toxicity of levodopa (by dopamine blockade). Fluphenazine may inhibit metabolism and increase toxicity of phenytoin and tricyclic antidepressants.

Effects on diagnostic tests

Fluphenazine causes false-positive test results for urinary porphyrins, urobilinogen, amylase, and 5-hydroxyindoleacetic acid (5-HIAA), because of darkening of urine by metabolites; it also causes false-positive urine pregnancy test results using human chorionic gonadotropin.

Fluphenazine elevates test results for liver enzymes and protein-bound iodine, and causes quinidine-like ECG effects.

Adverse reactions

• CNS: extrapyramidal symptoms—dystonia, akathisia, torticollis, tardive dyskinesia, sedation (low incidence), pseudoparkinsonism, drowsiness (frequent), neuroleptic malignant syndrome (dose-related; fatal respiratory failure in over 10% of patients if untreated), dizziness, headache, insomnia, *exacerbation of psychotic symptoms.*

• CV: asystole, orthostatic hypotension, tachycardia, dizziness and fainting, dysrhythmias, ECG changes, increased anginal pain after I.M. injection.

• EENT: blurred vision, tinnitus, mydriasis, increased intraocular pressure, ocular changes (retinal pigmentary change with long-term use).

• GI: dry mouth, constipation, nausea, vomiting, anorexia, diarrhea.

• GU: urinary retention, gynecomastia, hypermenorrhea, inhibited ejaculation.

• HEMA: transient leukopenia, agranulocytosis, thrombocytopenia, anemia (within 30 to 90 days).

• Local: contact dermatitis from concentrate or injectable form, muscle necrosis from I.M. injection

• Other: hyperprolactinemia, photosensitivity, increased appetite or weight gain, hypersensitivity (rash, urticaria, drug fever, edema, cholestatic jaundice [in 2% to 4% of patients within first 30 days]).

After abrupt withdrawal of long-term therapy, patient may develop gastritis, nausea, vomiting, dizziness, tremors, feeling of heat or cold, sweating, tachycardia, headache or insomnia.

Note: Drug should be discontinued immediately if any of the following occurs: hypersensitivity, jaundice, agranulocytosis, neuroleptic malignant syndrome (marked hyperthermia, extrapyramidal effects, autonomic dysfunction), or if severe extrapyramidal symptoms occur even after dosage is lowered. Drug should be discontinued 48 hours before and 24 hours after myelography utilizing metrizamide because of the risk of convulsions. When feasible, drug should be withdrawn slowly and gradually; many drug effects persist after withdrawal.

Overdose and treatment

CNS depression is characterized by deep, unarousable sleep and possible coma, hypotension or hypertension, extrapyramidal symptoms, dystonia, abnormal involuntary muscle movements, agitation, seizures, dysrhythmias, ECG changes, hypothermia or hyperthermia, and autonomic nervous system dysfunction.

Treatment is symptomatic and supportive, including maintaining vital signs, airway, stable body temperature, and fluid and electrolyte balance.

Do not induce vomiting: drug inhibits cough reflex, and aspiration may occur. Use gastric lavage, then activated charcoal and saline cathartics; dialysis does not help. Regulate body temperature as needed. Treat hypotension with I.V. fluids: *do not give epinephrine.* Treat seizures with parenteral diazepam or barbiturates; dysrhythmias with parenteral phenytoin (1 mg/kg with rate titrated to blood pressure); extrapyramidal reactions with barbiturates, benztropine, or parenteral diphenhydramine at 2 mg/kg/minute.

▶ Special considerations

• Fluphenazine may be used in children over age 6.
• Note that two parenteral forms are available: depot injection (25 mg/ml) and I.M. injection (2.5 mg/ml).
• The depot injection form is not recommended for patients who are not stabilized on a phenothiazine. This form has a prolonged elimination; its action could not be terminated in case of adverse reactions.
• Check vital signs regularly for decreased blood pressure (especially before and after parenteral therapy) or tachycardia; observe patient carefully for other adverse reactions.
• Check intake and output for urinary retention or constipation, which may require dosage reduction.
• Monitor bilirubin levels weekly for first 4 weeks; monitor complete blood count, ECG (for quinidine-like effects), liver and renal function studies, electrolyte levels (especially potassium) and eye examinations at baseline and periodically thereafter, especially in patients on long-term therapy.
• Observe patient for mood changes to monitor progress; benefits may not be apparent for several weeks.
• Monitor for involuntary movements. Check patient receiving prolonged treatment at least once every 6 months.

• Do not withdraw drug abruptly; although physical dependence does not occur with antipsychotic drugs, rebound exacerbation of psychotic symptoms may occur, and many drug effects persist.
• Carefully follow manufacturer's instructions for reconstitution, dilution, administration, and storage of drugs; slightly discolored liquids may or may not be all right to use. Check with pharmacist.

Information for parents and patient

• Explain rationale and anticipated risks and benefits of therapy, and that full therapeutic effect may not occur for several weeks.
• Teach signs and symptoms of adverse reactions and importance of reporting *any* unusual effects, especially involuntary movements.
• Tell parents that patient should avoid beverages and drugs containing alcohol, and should not take any other drug (especially CNS depressants) including nonprescription products without medical approval.
• Instruct parents of diabetic children to monitor blood glucose levels, because drug may alter insulin needs.
• Teach parents or patient how and when to administer drug, not to increase dose without medical approval, and never to discontinue drug abruptly; suggest taking full dose at bedtime if daytime sedation is troublesome.
• Patient should lie down for 30 minutes after first dose (1 hour if I.M.) and to rise slowly from sitting or supine position to prevent orthostatic hypotension.
• Patient should avoid hazardous activities requiring mental alertness and psychomotor coordination, until full effects of drug are established.
• Drugs are locally irritating; advise taking with milk or food to minimize GI distress. Warn that oral concentrates and solutions will irritate skin, and patient should not crush or open sustained-release products, but swallow them whole.
• Warn parents that patient's excessive exposure to sunlight, heat lamps, or tanning beds may cause photosensitivity reactions (burn, hyperpigmentation).
• Patient should avoid exposure to extremes of heat or cold, because of risk of hypothermia or hyperthermia induced by alteration in thermoregulatory function.
• Recommend sugarless gum, hard candy, or ice chips to relieve dry mouth.
• Explain that phenothiazines may cause pink to brown discoloration of urine.

---

flurandrenolide
Cordran, Cordran SP, Drenison★

• Classification: anti-inflammatory (adrenocorticoid)

How supplied

Available by prescription only
Cream: 0.025%, 0.05%
Lotion: 0.05%
Ointment: 0.025%, 0.05%
Tape: 4 mcg/cm^2

Indications, route, and dosage
Inflammation of corticosteroid-responsive dermatoses
Children: Apply 0.025% cream or ointment once or twice daily; apply 0.05% cream, lotion, or ointment, and tape once a day.

Adults: Apply cream, lotion, or ointment sparingly b.i.d. or t.i.d. Apply tape q 12 to 24 hours.

Occlusive dressings may be used for severe or resistant dermatoses. The tape is usually applied as an occlusive dressing to clean, dry affected areas.

Action and kinetics
• *Anti-inflammatory action:* Flurandrenolide stimulates the synthesis of enzymes needed to decrease the inflammatory response. Depending on strength, flurandrenolide is either a group III (0.05%) or group IV (0.025%) fluorinated glucocorticoid.

• *Kinetics in adults:* The amount absorbed depends on concentration, the amount applied, and the nature of the skin at the application site. It ranges from about 1% in areas with a thick stratum corneum (such as the palms, soles, elbows, and knees) to as high as 36% in areas of the thinnest stratum corneum (face, eyelids, and genitals). Absorption increases in skin areas that are damaged, inflamed or under occlusion. Some systemic absorption may occur, especially through the oral mucosa.

After topical application, drug is distributed throughout the local skin and metabolized primarily in the skin. Any drug that is absorbed is removed rapidly from the blood; distributed into muscle, liver, skin, intestines, and kidneys; and metabolized primarily in the liver to inactive compounds. Inactive metabolites are excreted by the kidneys, primarily as glucuronides and sulfates, but also as unconjugated products. Small amounts of the metabolites are also excreted in feces.

Contraindications and precautions
Flurandrenolide is contraindicated in patients who are hypersensitive to any component of the preparation and in patients with viral, fungal, or tubercular skin lesions.

Flurandrenolide should be used with extreme caution in patients with impaired circulation because it may increase the risk of skin ulceration.

Interactions
None significant.

Effects on diagnostic tests
None significant.

Adverse reactions
• Local: burning, itching, irritation, dryness, folliculitis, hypertrichosis, acneiform eruptions, hypopigmentation, perioral dermatitis, allergic contact dermatitis, maceration, secondary infection, atrophy, striae, miliaria.

Significant systemic absorption can produce the following reactions.
• CNS: euphoria, insomnia, headache, psychotic behavior, pseudotumor cerebri, mental changes, nervousness, restlessness.

• CV: congestive heart failure, hypertension, edema.
• EENT: cataracts, glaucoma, thrush.
• GI: peptic ulcer, irritation, increased appetite.
• Immune: immunosuppression, increased susceptibility to infection.
• Metabolic: hypokalemia, sodium retention, fluid retention, weight gain, hyperglycemia, osteoporosis, growth suppression in children.
• Musculoskeletal: muscle atrophy.
• Other: withdrawal syndrome (nausea, fatigue, anorexia, dyspnea, hypotension, hypoglycemia, myalgia, arthralgia, fever, dizziness, and fainting).

Note: Drug should be discontinued if local irritation, infection, systemic absorption, or hypersensitivity reaction occurs.

Overdose and treatment
No information available.

▶ Special considerations
• Children may show greater susceptibility to topical corticosteroid-induced HPA axis suppression and Cushing's syndrome than mature patients because of a higher ratio of skin surface area to body weight. Hypothalamic-pituitary-adrenal (HPA) axis suppression, Cushing's syndrome, and intracranial hypertension have been reported in children receiving topical corticosteroids. Signs of adrenal suppression in children include linear growth retardation, delayed weight gain, low plasma cortisol levels, and absence of response to ACTH stimulation. Signs of intracranial hypertension include bulging fontanelles, headaches, and bilateral papilledema.
• Administration of topical corticosteroids to children should be limited to the least effective amount. Chronic corticosteroid therapy may interfere with growth and development.
• Stop drug if the patient develops signs of systemic absorption (including Cushing's syndrome, hyperglycemia, or glucosuria), skin irritation or ulceration, hypersensitivity, or infection. (If antifungals or antibiotics are being used with corticosteroids and the infection does not respond immediately, corticosteroids should be stopped until infection is controlled.)
• Monitor patient response. Observe area of inflammation and elicit patient comments concerning pruritus. Inspect skin for infection, striae, and atrophy. Skin atrophy is common and may be clinically significant within 3 to 4 weeks of treatment with high-potency preparations; it also occurs more readily at sites where percutaneous absorption is high.
• Do not apply occlusive dressings over topical steroids because this may lead to secondary infection, maceration, atrophy, striae, or miliaria caused by increasing steroid penetration and potency.

Information for parents and patient
Instruct parents and patient in application of the drug. Tell them the following:
Method for applying topical preparations
• Wash hands before and after applying the drug.
• Gently cleanse the area of application. Washing or soaking the area before application may increase drug penetration.
• Apply sparingly in a light film; rub in lightly. Avoid

---

ntact with patient's eyes, unless using an ophthalic product.

Avoid prolonged application on the face, in skin folds, nd in areas near the eyes, genitals and rectum. High-tency topical corticosteroids are more likely to cause riae in these areas because of their higher rates of sorption.

f an occlusive dressing is necessary, minimize ad-rse reactions by using it intermittently. Do not leave in place longer than 16 hours each day.

Warn patient not to use nonprescription topical prep-ations other than those specifically recommended.

Advise parents not to use tight-fitting diapers or astic pants on a child being treated in the diaper ea, since such garments may serve as occlusive essings.

olic acid (vitamin B₉)
olvite

Classification: vitamin supplement (folic acid de-rivative)

ow supplied
vailable by prescription only
jection: 10-ml vials (5 mg/ml with 1.5% benzyl al-hol or 10 mg/ml with 1.5% benzyl alcohol and 0.2% DTA)
ablets: 0.1 mg, 0.4 mg, 0.8 mg, 1 mg

dications, route, and dosage
**egaloblastic or macrocytic anemia second-
ry to folic acid deficiency, hepatic disease,
lcoholism, intestinal obstruction, excessive
emolysis**
hildren under age 4: Up to 0.3 mg P.O., S.C., or I.M. aily.
hildren age 4 and older and adults: 1 mg P.O., S.C., r I.M. daily for 4 to 5 days. After anemia secondary folic acid deficiency is corrected, proper diet and ecommended daily allowance (RDA) of supplements re necessary to prevent recurrence.
**revention of megaloblastic anemia of preg-
ancy and fetal damage**
dults: 1 mg P.O., S.C., or I.M. daily throughout preg-ancy.
utritional supplement
hildren: 0.05 mg P.O. daily.
dults: 0.1 mg P.O., S.C., or I.M. daily.
ropical sprue
dults: 3 to 15 mg P.O. daily.
**est of megaloblastic anemia patients to de-
ect folic acid deficiency without masking
ernicious anemia**
hildren and adults: 0.1 to 0.2 mg P.O. or I.M. for 10 ays while maintaining a diet low in folate and vi-amin B₁₂. (Reticulosis, reversion to normoblastic he-atopoiesis, and return to normal hemoglobin levels dicate folic acid deficiency.)

Action and kinetics
• *Nutritional action:* Exogenous folate is required to maintain normal erythropoiesis and to perform nu-cleoprotein synthesis. Folic acid stimulates produc-tion of red and white blood cells and platelets in certain megaloblastic anemias.

Dietary folic acid is present in foods, primarily as reduced folate polyglutamate. This vitamin may be absorbed only after hydrolysis, reduction, and meth-ylation occur in the GI tract. Conversion to active tetrahydrofolate may require vitamin B₁₂.

The oral synthetic form of folic acid is a mono-glutamate and is absorbed completely after admin-istration, even in malabsorption syndromes.
• *Kinetics in adults:* Folic acid is absorbed rapidly from the GI tract, mainly from the proximal part of the small intestine. Peak folate activity in blood occurs within 30 to 60 minutes after oral administration. Normal serum folate concentrations range from 0.005 to 0.015 mcg/ml. Usually, serum levels below 0.005 mcg/ml indicate folate deficiency; those below 0.002 mcg/ml usually result in megaloblastic anemia. The active tetrahydrofolic acid and its derivatives are dis-tributed into all body tissues; the liver contains about half of the total body folate stores. Folate is actively concentrated in the CSF; normal CSF concentrations range from 0.175 to 0.316 mcg/ml. Folic acid is dis-tributed into breast milk.

Folic acid is metabolized in the liver to N^5-meth-yltetrahydrofolic acid—the main form of folate storage and transport. A single 0.1-mg to 0.2-mg dose of folic acid usually results in only a trace amount of the drug in the urine. After administering large doses, exces-sive folate is excreted unchanged in urine. Small amounts of folic acid have been recovered in feces. About 0.05 mg/day of normal body folate stores is lost by a combination of urinary and fecal excretion and oxidative cleavage of the molecule.

Contraindications and precautions
Folic acid is contraindicated in patients with perni-cious, aplastic, or normocytic anemias. Folic acid may obscure the diagnosis of pernicious anemia, which can cause disabling neurologic complications.

Interactions
Concomitant use of folic acid (15 to 20 mg/day) de-creases serum phenytoin levels to subtherapeutic con-centrations, possibly with increased frequency of seizures. Folic acid appears to increase the metabolic clearance of phenytoin and cause redistribution of phenytoin in the CSF and brain.

Conversely, phenytoin and primidone may decrease serum folate levels and produce symptoms of folic acid deficiency in long-term therapy. Para-aminosal-icylic acid and sulfasalazine may cause a similar de-ficiency. Although oral contraceptives may also impair folate metabolism and produce folate depletion, they are unlikely to induce anemia or megaloblastic changes.

Folic acid may interfere with the antimicrobial ac-tions of pyrimethamine against toxoplasmosis.

Folic acid antagonists, pyrimethamine, trimetho-prim, or triamterene may cause dihydrofolate reductase deficiency, which may interfere with folic acid utilization.

Effects on diagnostic tests

Folic acid therapy alters serum and erythrocyte folate concentrations; falsely low serum and erythrocyte folate levels may occur with the *Lactobacillus casei* assay method in those patients receiving anti-infectives, such as tetracycline, which suppress the growth of this organism.

Adverse reactions
• DERM: rash, pruritus, erythema.
• Other: allergic bronchospasm, general malaise, anaphylaxis.

Overdose and treatment

Folic acid is relatively nontoxic. Adverse GI and CNS effects have been reported rarely in patients receiving 15 mg of folic acid daily for 1 month.

▶ Special considerations
• The RDA for folic acid is 30 to 400 mcg in children and 400 to 800 mcg in adults; 100 mcg/day is considered an adequate oral supplement.
• Take a careful dietary history because many drugs, such as oral contraceptives and alcohol, can cause folate deficiencies.
• Ensure that patients do not also have vitamin B_{12} deficiency; folic acid can improve hematologic measurements while allowing progression of neurologic damage. Do not use as sole treatment of pernicious anemia.
• Patients undergoing renal dialysis are at risk for folate deficiency.
• Monitor complete blood counts to measure effectiveness of drug treatment.
• Protect folic acid injections from light.

Information for parents and patient
• Teach parents and patient about dietary sources of folic acid, such as yeast, whole grains, leafy vegetables, beans, nuts, and fruit.
• Explain that folate is destroyed by overcooking and canning.
• Stress the importance of administering folic acid only under medical supervision.

---

furazolidone
Furoxone

• Classification: antibacterial, antiprotozoal agent (nitrofuran derivative)

How supplied
Available by prescription only
Tablets: 100 mg
Liquid: 50 mg/15 ml

Indications, route, and dosage
Giardiasis
Children age 1 month to 1 year: 8 to 17 mg P.O. q.i.d.
Children over age 1 to 4 years: 17 to 25 mg P.O. q.i.d.
Children age 5 years and older: 28 to 50 mg P.O .q.i.d.
Adults: 100 mg or 1.25 mg/kg P.O. q.i.d.

Dosage should not exceed 8.8 mg/kg daily. Although another drug should be considered if no response is seen in 7 days, therapy should continue for 10 days.

Action and kinetics
• *Antibacterial and antiprotozoal action:* Furazolidone presumably works by inhibiting several vital enzymatic reactions; its activity includes monoamine oxidase (MAO) inhibition. Spectrum of activity includes many gram-positive and gram-negative enteric organisms, including *Vibrio cholerae*. It is also effective against protozoa, including *Giardia lamblia* and *Trichomonas.*
• *Kinetics in adults:* Furazolidone is absorbed poorly after oral administration and is inactivated in the intestine. Distribution is unknown.

Furazolidone is metabolized via intestinal degradation and is excreted mainly in feces, with approximately 5% excreted in urine.

Contraindications and precautions
Furazolidone is contraindicated in infants under age 1 month because of the possibility of inducing hemolytic anemia, and in patients with known hypersensitivity to the drug.

Furazolidone should be administered cautiously to patients with glucose-6-phosphate dehydrogenase (G6PD) deficiency because it may cause hemolytic anemia.

Interactions
When used concomitantly with alcohol, furazolidone may lead to a disulfiram-type reaction, possibly causing flushing, nausea, vomiting, hypotension, sweating, and tachycardia. Concomitant use with sympathomimetic drugs and tyramine-containing foods or beverages may lead to hypertensive crisis (from furazolidone's MAO-inhibiting properties). Concomitant use with tricyclic antidepressants may cause toxic psychosis.

Effects on diagnostic tests
Furazolidone therapy may cause false-positive results on some urine glucose tests using Benedict's reagent (for example, Clinitest).

Adverse reactions
• CNS: headache, malaise.
• GI: nausea and vomiting, colitis, pruritus ani.
• HEMA: hemolysis (with G6PD deficiency).
• Other: disulfiram-type reaction (with alcohol).
   Note: Drug should be discontinued if signs or symptoms of hemolytic anemia occur or if adverse effects become intolerable. Dosage reduction may alleviate nausea and vomiting.

Overdose and treatment
No information available.

▶ **Special considerations**

• Furazolidone is contraindicated in infants under age 1 month because it increases the risk of drug-induced hemolytic anemia.

• Culture and sensitivity tests should be done before initiating therapy.

• Diarrhea usually resolves within 2 to 5 days after therapy begins.

• Monitor hydration status, weight, intake, and output.

• Monitor blood and urine tests in patients with G6PD deficiency.

• Store drug in dark place at 35.6° to 59° F. (2° to 15°C.).

• Drug may turn urine brown.

Information for parents and patient

• Instruct parents to have patient continue taking drug exactly as directed, even if he feels better.

• Tell parents that patient should avoid beverages and medications containing alcohol during therapy and for 4 days afterward to avoid disulfiram-type reactions (nausea, sweating, flushing, tachycardia). Warn them to check for alcohol content before administering any medication.

• If patient is taking high doses (more than 400 mg/day) or is on long-term therapy, patient should avoid all drugs containing stimulants or decongestants and tyramine-rich foods and beverages.

• Advise parents and patient that drug may turn urine brown.

---

furosemide
Lasix, Novosemide*, Apo-Furosemide*, Myrosemide, Uritol*

• Classification: loop diuretic, antihypertensive

How supplied
Available by prescription only
Tablets: 20 mg, 40 mg, 80 mg
Oral solution: 10 mg/ml, 40 mg/5 ml
Injection: 10 mg/ml

Indications, route, and dosage
Acute pulmonary edema
Infants and children: 1 mg/kg I.M. or I.V. Increase dosage by 1 mg/kg q 2 hours until response is achieved; maximum dosage is 6 mg/kg/day.
Adults: 40 mg I.V. injected slowly; then 80 mg I.V. within 1 hour if needed.
Edema
Infants and children: 2 mg/kg P.O. increased by 1 to 2 mg/kg in 6 to 8 hours if needed, carefully titrated not to exceed 6 mg/kg/day.
Adults: 20 to 80 mg P.O. daily in morning, with second dose given in 6 to 8 hours, carefully titrated up to 600 mg daily if needed; or 20 to 40 mg I.M. or I.V. Increase by 20 mg q 2 hours until desired response is achieved. I.V. dosage should be given slowly over 1 to 2 minutes.

Action and kinetics
• *Diuretic action:* Loop diuretics inhibit sodium and chloride reabsorption in the proximal part of the ascending loop of Henle, promoting the excretion of sodium, water, chloride, and potassium.

• *Antihypertensive action:* This drug effect may be the result of renal and peripheral vasodilatation and a temporary increase in glomerular filtration rate and a decrease in peripheral vascular resistance.

• *Kinetics in adults:* About 60% of a given furosemide dose is absorbed from the GI tract after oral administration. Food delays oral absorption but does not alter diuretic response. Diuresis begins in 30 to 60 minutes; peak diuresis occurs 1 to 2 hours after oral administration. Diuresis follows I.V. administration within 5 minutes and peaks in 20 to 60 minutes. Furosemide is about 95% plasma protein-bound. It crosses the placenta and distributes into breast milk. Furosemide is metabolized minimally by the liver. About 50% to 80% of a furosemide dose is excreted in urine; plasma half-life is about 30 minutes. Duration of action is 6 to 8 hours after oral administration and about 2 hours after I.V. administration.

Contraindications and precautions
Furosemide is contraindicated in patients with known hypersensitivity, anuria, hepatic coma, or electrolyte depletion and in the presence of rising BUN and serum creatinine levels or oliguria, even though it is used to produce diuresis in patients with renal impairment, because rapid fluid and electrolyte changes can exacerbate these conditions.

Furosemide should be used with caution in patients hypersensitive to sulfonamides; in patients with hepatic cirrhosis and ascites, because changes in electrolyte balance may precipitate hepatic encephalopathy; and in patients receiving cardiac glycosides (digoxin, digitoxin), because furosemide-induced hypokalemia may predispose them to digitalis toxicity. Rapid I.V. administration of furosemide increases risk of ototoxicity.

Interactions
Furosemide potentiates the hypotensive effect of most other antihypertensive agents and of other diuretics; both actions are used to therapeutic advantage.

Concomitant use with potassium-sparing diuretics (spironolactone, triamterene, amiloride) may decrease furosemide-induced potassium loss; use with other potassium-depleting drugs, such as steroids and amphotericin B, may cause severe potassium loss.

Furosemide may reduce renal clearance of lithium and increase lithium levels; lithium dosage may require adjustment.

Indomethacin and probenecid may reduce furosemide's diuretic effect; their combined use is not recommended. However, if there is no therapeutic alternative, an increased furosemide dosage may be required.

Concomitant administration of furosemide with ototoxic or nephrotoxic drugs may result in enhanced toxicity.

Furosemide could prolong neuromuscular blockade by muscle relaxants.

Patients receiving I.V. furosemide within 24 hours

---

of a dose of chloral hydrate have experienced sweating, flushing, and blood pressure fluctuations; if possible, use an alternative sedative in patients receiving I.V. furosemide.

Effects on diagnostic tests
Furosemide therapy alters electrolyte balance and liver and renal function tests.

Adverse reactions
• CV: volume depletion and dehydration, *orthostatic hypotension,* cardiac arrest.
• DERM: dermatitis, photosensitivity, *rash.*
• EENT: transient deafness with too-rapid I.V. injection, *ototoxicity* (rare).
• GI: abdominal discomfort and pain, diarrhea (with oral solution), *nephrotoxicity.*
• HEMA: agranulocytosis, transient leukopenia, thrombocytopenia.
• Metabolic: hypochloremic alkalosis; asymptomatic hyperuricemia; *fluid and electrolyte imbalances,* including hypocalcemia, hypokalemia, hypomagnesemia, and dilutional hyponatremia; hyperglycemia and impairment of glucose tolerance; *metabolic acidosis.*
• Other: *thrombophlebitis.*
    Note: Drug should be discontinued if dehydration or hypotension occurs or if BUN and creatinine levels rise.

Overdose and treatment
Clinical manifestations of overdose include profound electrolyte and volume depletion, which may precipitate circulatory collapse.

    Treatment is chiefly supportive; replace fluids and electrolytes.

▶ Special considerations
• Use furosemide with caution in neonates. The usual pediatric dosage can be used, but dosing intervals should be extended.
• Sorbitol content of oral preparations may cause diarrhea, especially at high dosages. It can cause necrotizing enterocolitis in neonates.
• Monitor blood pressure and pulse rate (especially during rapid diuresis), establish baseline values before therapy, and watch for significant changes.
• Advise safety measures for all ambulatory patients until response to the diuretic is known.
• Establish baseline and periodically review CBC, including WBC count; serum electrolytes, CO_2, BUN, and creatinine levels; and results of liver function tests.
• Administer diuretics in the morning so major diuresis occurs before bedtime. To prevent nocturia, do not prescribe diuretics for use after 6 p.m.
• Consider possible dosage adjustment in the following circumstances: reduced dosage for patients with hepatic dysfunction; increased dosage in patients with renal impairment, oliguria, or decreased diuresis (inadequate urine output may result in circulatory overload, causing water intoxication, pulmonary edema, and CHF); increased doses of insulin in diabetic patients; and reduced dosages of other antihypertensive agents.
• Monitor patient for edema and ascites. Observe lower extremities of ambulatory children and the sacral area of those on bed rest.
• Patient should be weighed each morning immediately after voiding and before breakfast, in same type of clothing and on the same scale. Weight helps evaluate clinical response to diuretic therapy.
• Consult dietitian on possible need for dietary potassium supplementation.
• Patients taking digitalis are at increased risk of digitalis toxicity from potassium depletion.
• Ototoxicity may follow prolonged use or administration of large doses.
• Patients with liver disease are especially susceptible to diuretic-induced electrolyte imbalance; in extreme cases, stupor, coma, and death can result.
• Patient should have urinal or commode readily available.
• Give I.V. furosemide slowly, over 1 to 2 minutes, at a rate not to exceed 4 mg/minute; for I.V. infusion, dilute furosemide in dextrose 5% in water, normal saline solution, or lactated Ringer's solution, and use within 24 hours.
• Furosemide has been used to treat hypercalcemia at dosages of 80 to 100 mg I.V., given every 1 to 2 hours.

Information for parents and patient
• Explain to the parents and patient the rationale for therapy and the diuretic effect of drug.
• Teach parents signs of adverse effects, especially hypokalemia (weakness, fatigue, muscle cramps, paresthesias, confusion, nausea, vomiting, diarrhea, headache, dizziness, or palpitations), and importance of reporting such symptoms promptly.
• Advise parents to have patient eat potassium-rich foods, such as citrus fruits, potatoes, dates, raisins, and bananas; to avoid high-sodium foods, such as lunch meat, smoked meats, and processed cheeses; and not to add salt to other foods. Recommend salt substitutes. Inform parents that low-sodium formulas are available for infants.
• Tell parents to report if patient experiences increased edema or excess diuresis (more than 2% weight loss or gain).
• With initial doses, caution patient to change position slowly, especially when rising to upright position, to prevent dizziness from orthostatic hypotension.
• Instruct parents to watch for and promptly report chest, back, or leg pain, or shortness of breath.
• Warn parents and patient about photosensitivity reaction. Explain that this reaction is a photoallergy in which ultraviolet radiation alters drug structure causing allergic reactions in some persons. Tell them that photosensitivity reactions occur 10 days to 2 weeks after initial sun exposure.
• Emphasize importance of regular medical follow-up to monitor effectiveness of diuretic therapy.

gentamicin sulfate‡
Cidomycin*, Garamycin Pediatric‡, Jenamicin

• Classification: antibiotic (aminoglycoside)

How supplied
Available by prescription only
Injection: 40 mg/ml (adult), 10 mg/ml (pediatric), 2 mg/ml (intrathecal)
Topical: 0.1% ointment, 0.1% cream

Indications, route, and dosage
Serious infections caused by susceptible organisms
Premature infants age 1 to 7 days and < 28 weeks' gestation: 2.5 mg/kg q 24 hours.
Premature infants age 1 to 7 days and 28 to 34 weeks' gestation: 2.5 mg/kg q 18 hours.
Premature infants over age 7 days and < 28 weeks' gestation: 2.5 mg/kg q 18 hours.
Premature infants over age 7 days and 28 to 34 weeks' gestation: 2.5 mg/kg q 12 hours.
Neonates age 1 to 7 days: 2.5 mg/kg I.V. q 12 hours.
For I.V. infusion, dilute in normal saline solution or dextrose 5% in water and infuse over 30 minutes to 2 hours.
Infants and neonates over age 1 week with normal renal function: 2.5 mg/kg I.M. or I.V. infusion q 8 hours.
Children with normal renal function: 2 to 2.5 mg/kg I.M. or I.V. infusion q 8 hours.
Adults with normal renal function: 3 mg/kg I.M. or I.V. infusion (in 50 to 200 ml of normal saline solution or dextrose 5% in water infused over 30 minutes to 2 hours) daily in divided doses q 8 hours. May be given by direct I.V. push if necessary. For life-threatening infections, patient may receive up to 5 mg/kg/day in three to four divided doses.
Meningitis
Neonates age 8 days or older: 2.5 mg/kg I.V. or I.M. q 8 hr.
Children over age 3 months: systemic therapy as above; may also use 1 to 2 mg intrathecally daily.
Adults: systemic therapy as above; may also use 4 to 8 mg intrathecally daily.
Endocarditis prophylaxis for GI or GU procedure or surgery
Children: 2.5 mg/kg I.M. or I.V. 30 to 60 minutes before procedure or surgery and q 8 hours after, for two doses. Given separately with aqueous penicillin G or ampicillin.
Adults: 1.5 mg/kg I.M. or I.V. 30 to 60 minutes before procedure or surgery and q 8 hours after, for two doses. Given separately with aqueous penicillin G or ampicillin.

External ocular infections caused by susceptible organisms
Children and adults: Instill 1 to 2 drops in eye q 4 hours. In severe infections, may use up to 2 drops q 1 hour. Apply ointment to lower conjunctival sac b.i.d. or t.i.d.
Primary and secondary bacterial infections; superficial burns; skin ulcers; and infected lacerations, abrasions, insect bites, or minor surgical wounds
Children over age 1 and adults: Rub in small amount gently t.i.d. or q.i.d., with or without gauze dressing.
Dosage in renal failure
Initial dose is same as for those with normal renal function. Subsequent doses and frequency determined by renal function studies and blood concentrations; keep peak serum concentrations between 4 and 10 mcg/ml, and trough serum concentrations between 1 and 2 mcg/ml.
Posthemodialysis to maintain therapeutic blood levels
Children: 2 to 2.5 mg/kg I.M. or I.V. infusion after each dialysis.
Adults: 1 to 1.7 mg/kg I.M. or I.V. infusion after each dialysis.

Action and kinetics
• *Antibiotic action:* Gentamicin is bactericidal; it binds directly to the 30S ribosomal subunit, thus inhibiting bacterial protein synthesis. Its spectrum of activity includes many aerobic gram-negative organisms (including most strains of *Pseudomonas aeruginosa*) and some aerobic gram-positive organisms. Gentamicin may act against some bacterial strains resistant to other aminoglycosides; bacterial strains resistant to gentamicin may be susceptible to tobramycin, netilmicin, or amikacin.
• *Kinetics in adults:* Gentamicin is absorbed poorly after oral administration and is given parenterally; after I.M. administration, peak serum concentrations occur at 30 to 90 minutes.
Gentamicin is distributed widely after parenteral administration; intraocular penetration is poor. CSF penetration is low even in patients with inflamed meninges. Intraventricular administration produces high concentrations throughout the CNS. Protein-binding is minimal. Gentamicin crosses the placenta.
Gentamicin is excreted primarily in urine by glomerular filtration; small amounts may be excreted in bile and breast milk. Elimination half-life in adults is 2 to 3 hours. In patients with severe renal damage, half-life may extend to 24 to 60 hours.
• *Kinetics in children:* Plasma elimination half-life is estimated to be 5.5 hours in neonates less than 1 week old and in large premature infants. In children age 1 week to 6 months, gentamicin plasma half-life is similar to adults (3 to 3.5 hours).

---

‡May contain sulfites   ◆May contain tartrazine   ◆◆May contain benzyl alcohol

Contraindications and precautions

Gentamicin is contraindicated in patients with known hypersensitivity to gentamicin or any other aminoglycoside.

Gentamicin should be used cautiously in neonates and other infants, because of decreased renal clearance; in patients with decreased renal function because of potential for decreased drug clearance; in patients with tinnitus, vertigo, or high-frequency hearing loss, who are susceptible to ototoxicity; with dehydration because of increased risk of ototoxicity and nephrotoxicity; and with myasthenia gravis, parkinsonism, or hypocalcemia because it may aggravate muscle weakness.

Interactions

Concomitant use with the following drugs may increase the hazard of nephrotoxicity, ototoxicity, or neurotoxicity: methoxyflurane, polymyxin B, vancomycin, capreomycin, cisplatin, cephalosporins, amphotericin B, and other aminoglycosides; hazard of ototoxicity is also increased during use with ethacrynic acid, furosemide, bumetanide, urea, or mannitol. Dimenhydrinate and other antiemetic and antivertigo drugs may mask gentamicin-induced ototoxicity.

Concomitant use with a penicillin results in synergistic bactericidal effect against *Pseudomonas aeruginosa, Escherichia coli, Klebsiella, Citrobacter, Enterbacter, Serratia,* and *Proteus mirabilis*; however, the drugs are physically and chemically incompatible and are inactivated when mixed or given together.

Gentamicin may potentiate neuromuscular blockade produced by general anesthetics, neuromuscular blocking agents such as succinylcholine and tubocurarine, or botulism toxin.

Effects on diagnostic tests

Gentamicin-induced nephrotoxicity may elevate levels of blood urea nitrogen (BUN), nonprotein nitrogen, or serum creatinine, and increase urinary excretion of casts.

Adverse reactions

• CNS: headache, *lethargy, neuromuscular blockade with respiratory depression, muscle twitching, arachnoiditis (rare).*
• DERM: small percentage of minor skin irritation; possible photosensitivity; allergic contact dermatitis.
• EENT: *ototoxicity (tinnitus, vertigo, hearing loss),* burning, stinging, transient irritation from ophthalmic ointment or solution.
• GI: diarrhea.
• GU: *nephrotoxicity (cells or casts in the urine); oliguria; proteinuria; decreased creatinine clearance; increased BUN, nonprotein nitrogen, and serum creatinine levels).*
• HEMA: *blood dyscrasias (rare).*
• Hepatic: *elevated SGOT*
• Local: *pain and irritation at I.M. injection site.*
• Other: hypersensitivity reactions (eosinophilia, fever, rash, urticaria, pruritus), *bacterial and fungal superinfections, phlebitis (rare).*
Note: Drug should be discontinued if signs of ototoxicity, nephrotoxicity, or hypersensitivity occur.

Overdose and treatment

Clinical signs of overdose include ototoxicity, nephrotoxicity, and neuromuscular toxicity. Drug can be removed by hemodialysis or peritoneal dialysis. Treatment with calcium salts or anticholinesterases reverses neuromuscular blockade.

▶ Special considerations

• Assess patient's allergic history; do not give gentamicin to a patient with a history of hypersensitivity reactions to any aminoglycoside; monitor patient continuously for this and other adverse reactions.
• Obtain results of culture and sensitivity test before first dose; however, therapy must begin before tests are completed. Repeat test periodically to assess drug efficacy.
• Increased risk of toxicity is associated with prolonged peak serum concentration greater than 10 mcg/ml and/or trough serum concentration greater than 2 mcg/ml.
• Keep peak serum levels and trough serum levels at recommended concentrations, especially in patients with decreased renal function. Draw blood for peak level 1 hour after I.M. injection (30 minutes to 1 hour after I.V. infusion); for trough level, draw sample just before the next dose. Time and date all blood samples. Do not use heparinized tube to collect blood samples; it interferes with results.
• For local application to skin infections, remove crusts by gently soaking with warm water and soap or wet compresses before applying ointment or cream; cover with protective gauze.
• Because gentamicin is dialyzable, patients undergoing hemodialysis may need dosage adjustments.
• Gentamicin (without preservatives) has been administered intrathecally or intraventricularly. Many clinicians prefer intraventricular administration to ensure adequate CSF levels in the treatment of ventriculitis.
• Monitor vital signs, electrolyte levels, and renal function studies before and during therapy; be sure patient is well hydrated to minimize chemical irritation of renal tubules; watch for signs of declining renal function.
• Monitor patient's CNS status when administering into CSF for meningitis.
• Evaluate patient's hearing before and during therapy; monitor for complaints of tinnitus, vertigo, or hearing loss. Avoid concomitant use with other ototoxic or nephrotoxic drugs.
• Usual duration of therapy is 7 to 10 days; if no response occurs in 3 to 5 days drug should be discontinued and cultures repeated for reevaluation of therapy.
• Closely monitor patients on long-term therapy — especially debilitated patients and others receiving immunosuppressant or radiation therpay — for possible bacterial or fungal superinfection; monitor especially for fever.

Parenteral administration

• Consult manufacturer's directions for reconstitution, dilution, and storage of drugs; check expiration dates.
• Administer I.M. dose deep into large muscle mass (gluteal or midlateral thigh); rotate injection sites to minimize tissue injury; do not inject more than 2 g

---

of drug per injection site. Apply ice to injection site for pain.

• Do not add or mix other drugs with I.V. infusions—particularly penicillins, which will inactivate aminoglycosides; the two groups are chemically and physically incompatible. If other drugs must be given I.V., temporarily stop infusion of primary drug.

• Too-rapid I.V. administration may cause neuromuscular blockade. Infuse I.V. drug continuously or intermittently over 30 to 60 minutes for adults, 1 to 2 hours for infants; dilution volume for children is determined individually.

• Solutions should always be clear, colorless to pale yellow (in most cases, darkening indicates deterioration), and free of particles; do not give solutions containing precipitates or other particles.

Information for parents and patient

• Teach parents how to recognize signs and symptoms of hypersensitivity, bacterial or fungal superinfections (especially if the child has low resistance from immunosuppressants or irradiation); and other adverse reactions of aminioglycosides. Instruct parents and patient regarding oral hygiene. Urge them to report any unusual effects promptly.

• Teach correct procedure for ophthalmic or topical administration.

• Be sure parents and patient understand how and when to administer drug; urge them to complete entire prescribed regimen, to comply with dosage schedule, and to keep follow-up appointments.

---

gentian violet
Genapax

• Classification: topical antibacterial, antifungal (triphenylmethane [rosaniline] dye)

How supplied
Available by prescription only
Tampons: 5 mg
Available without a prescription
Solution: 1%, 2%

Indications, route, and dosage
Cutaneous or mucocutaneous infections caused by Candida albicans and other superficial skin infections
Children and adults: Apply solution to lesion with cotton b.i.d. or t.i.d. for 3 days. To treat vulvovaginal candidiasis, insert one tampon high into vagina once or twice daily for 12 consecutive days.

Action and kinetics
• *Antifungal action:* The mechanism of antifungal action is unknown; however, its antibacterial action is thought to be related to the bacterial cell characteristics that underlie the Gram stain. Gentian violet inhibits the growth of many fungi, including yeasts and dermatophytes, and is effective against some gram-positive bacteria.
• *Kinetics in adults:* Unknown.

Contraindications and precautions
Gentian violet is contraindicated in patients with known hypersensitivity to the drug and for use on ulcerated areas. Drug turns skin and clothing purple; if applied to granulation tissue, tattooing (permanent discoloration) may result.

Interactions
None reported.

Effects on diagnostic tests
None reported.

Adverse reactions
• Local: vulvovaginal burning, irritation, vesicle formation.
   Note: Drug should be discontinued if sensitization develops.

Overdose and treatment
Laryngeal obstruction may develop after prolonged or frequent use of drug. Specific treatment information is not available.

▶ Special considerations
• Store gentian violet solution in a tight container at temperature less than 104° F. (40° C.); tampons, 59° to 86° F. (15° to 30° C.).
• Tattooing of the skin may occur if drug is applied to granulation tissue.

Information for parents and patient
• Teach parents or patient how to administer drug correctly. Be sure patient understands how to use drug and to report adverse reactions.
• Patient who uses the vaginal tampon form of the drug should remove the tampon after 3 to 4 hours and continue therapy for its full course, even through menstruation.
• Tell parent or patient that drug may stain skin and clothing.

---

glucagon

• Classification: antihypoglycemic, diagnostic agent

How supplied
Available by prescription only
Powder for injection: 1 mg (1 unit)/vial, 10 mg (10 units)/vial

Indications, route, and dosage
Coma of insulin-shock therapy
Children: 0.025 mg/kg up to a maximum of 1 mg; repeated in 20 minutes if necessary.
Adults: 0.5 to 1 mg S.C., I.M., or I.V.; may repeat within 25 minutes, if necessary. In deep coma, also give glucose 10% to 50% I.V. for faster response. When patient responds, give additional carbohydrate immediately.

---

‡May contain sulfites   ◆May contain tartrazine   ◆◆May contain benzyl alcohol

Severe insulin-induced hypoglycemia during diabetic therapy
Children and adults: 0.5 to 1 mg S.C., I.M., or I.V.; may repeat q 20 minutes for 2 doses, if necessary. If coma persists, give glucose 10% to 50% I.V.

Diagnostic aid for radiologic examination
Adults: 0.25 to 2 mg I.V. or I.M. before initiation of radiologic procedure.

Action and kinetics
• *Antihypoglycemic action:* Glucagon increases plasma glucose levels and causes smooth muscle relaxation and an inotropic myocardial effect because of the stimulation of adenylate cyclase to produce cyclic 3′,5′-adenosine monophosphate (AMP). Cyclic AMP initiates a series of reactions that leads to the degradation of glycogen to glucose. Hepatic stores of glycogen are necessary for glucagon to exert an antihypoglycemic effect.
• *Diagnostic action:* The mechanism by which glucagon relaxes the smooth muscles of the stomach, esophagus, duodenum, small bowel, and colon has not been fully defined.
• *Kinetics in adults:* Glucagon is destroyed in the GI tract; therefore, it must be given parenterally. After I.V. administration, hyperglycemic activity peaks within 30 minutes; relaxation of the GI smooth muscle occurs within 1 minute. After I.M. administration, relaxation of the GI smooth muscle occurs within 10 minutes. Administration to comatose hypoglycemic patients (with normal liver glycogen stores) usually produces a return to consciousness within 20 minutes. Distribution is not fully understood.

Glucagon is degraded extensively by the liver, in the kidneys and plasma, and at its tissue receptor sites in plasma membranes. Metabolic products are excreted by the kidneys. Half-life is about 3 to 10 minutes. Duration after I.M. administration is up to 32 minutes; after I.V. administration, up to 25 minutes.

Contraindications and precautions
Glucagon is contraindicated in patients with hypersensitivity to the drug, often a result of its protein nature.

Glucagon should be used cautiously in patients with a history of insulinoma because, although it initially raises blood glucose levels in patients with insulinoma, its insulin-releasing effect subsequently may cause hypoglycemia. The drug also should be used with caution in patients with pheochromocytoma because the drug stimulates release of catecholamines.

Interactions
Concomitant use of glucagon with epinephrine increases and prolongs the hyperglycemic effect. Phenytoin appears to inhibit glucagon-induced insulin release. Use with caution as a diagnostic agent in patients with diabetes mellitus.

Effects on diagnostic tests
Glucagon lowers serum potassium levels.

Adverse reactions
• CNS: dizziness, light-headedness.
• DERM: Stevens-Johnson syndrome (one case reported).
• GI: nausea, *vomiting.*
• Other: *hypersensitivity, rebound hypoglycemia,* hypotension (rare), anaphylaxis (rare).
   Note: Drug should be discontinued if signs or symptoms of hypersensitivity, including dizziness, rash, or difficulty breathing, occur.

Overdose and treatment
Clinical manifestations of overdose include nausea, vomiting, and hypokalemia. Treat symptomatically.

▶ Special considerations
• Glucagon should not be used to treat newborn asphyxia or hypoglycemia in premature infants or in infants who have had intrauterine growth retardation.
• To prevent excessive release of insulin and rebound hypoglycemia, patient should receive a source of carbohydrates and protein immediately after administration of glucagon.
• If patient experiences nausea and vomiting from glucagon administration and cannot retain some form of sugar for 1 hour, consider administration of I.V. dextrose.
• For I.V. drip infusion, glucagon is compatible with dextrose solution but forms a precipitate in chloride solutions.
• Glucagon has a positive inotropic and chronotropic action on the heart and may be used to treat overdose of beta-adrenergic blockers.
• Glucagon may be used as a diagnostic aid in radiologic examination of the stomach, duodenum, small intestine, and colon when a hypotonic state is desirable.

Information for parents and patient
• Teach parents and patient how to mix and inject the medication properly, using an appropriate-sized syringe and injecting at a 90-degree angle.
• Explain that medication should be used within 3 months after mixing and that the mixed solution should be stored in refrigerator. Parents should store unmixed medication at room temperature, not in the bathroom, where heat and humidity can cause it to deteriorate.
• Teach parents and patient how to administer glucagon and how to recognize hypoglycemia. Urge them to call physician immediately in emergencies.
• Tell parents and patient to expect response usually within 20 minutes after injection and that injection may be repeated if no response occurs. Parents should seek medical assistance if second injection is needed.

glycopyrrolate
Robinul, Robinul Forte

• Classification: antimuscarinic, gastrointestinal antispasmodic (anticholinergic)

How supplied
Available by prescription only
Tablets: 1 mg, 2 mg
Injection: 0.2 mg/ml in 1-ml, 2-ml, 5-ml, and 20-ml vials

Indications, route, and dosage
Blockade of cholinergic effects of anticholinesterase drugs used to reverse neuromuscular blockade
Children and adults: 0.2 mg I.V. for each 1 mg neostigmine or equivalent dose of pyridostigmine. May be given I.V. without dilution or may be added to dextrose injection and given by infusion.
Preoperatively to diminish secretions and block cardiac vagal reflexes
Children under age 2: 8.8 mcg/kg I.M., 30 to 60 minutes before anesthesia.
Children age 2 and older: 4.4 to 8.8 mcg/kg I.M. 30 to 60 minutes before anesthesia.
Adults: 4.4 mcg/kg I.M. 30 to 60 minutes before anesthesia.
Dysrhythmias (intraoperative)
Children age 2 and over: 4.4 mcg/kg (up to a maximum of 100 mcg) I.V.; repeat at 2- to 3-minute intervals as needed.
Adults: 100 mcg I.V.; repeat at 2- to 3-minute intervals as needed.

Action and kinetics
• *Anticholinergic action:* Glycopyrrolate inhibits acetylcholine's muscarinic actions on autonomic effectors innervated by postganglionic cholinergic nerves. That action blocks adverse muscarinic effects associated with anticholinesterase agents used to reverse curariform-induced neuromuscular blockade. Glycopyrrolate decreases secretions and GI motility by the same mechanism. Glycopyrrolate blocks cardiac vagal reflexes by blocking vagal inhibition of the sinoatrial node.
• *Kinetics in adults:* Glycopyrrolate is poorly absorbed from the GI tract. Glycopyrrolate is rapidly absorbed when given I.M. Glycopyrrolate is rapidly distributed. It does not cross the blood-brain barrier or enter the CNS. Glycopyrrolate's exact metabolic fate is unknown. Small drug amounts are eliminated in the urine as unchanged drug and metabolites. Most of the drug is excreted unchanged in feces or bile.

Contraindications and precautions
Glycopyrrolate is contraindicated in patients with narrow-angle glaucoma, because drug-induced cycloplegia and mydriasis may increase intraocular pressure; in children with obstructive uropathy, because the drug may exacerbate urinary retention; and in patients with myasthenia gravis, paralytic ileus, intestinal atony, or toxic megacolon, because the drug may worsen these conditions.

Administer glycopyrrolate cautiously to children with hyperthyroidism, ulcerative colitis, coronary artery disease, congestive heart failure, cardiac dysrhythmias, or hypertension, because it may exacerbate these conditions; to patients with hiatal hernia associated with reflux esophagitis, because the drug may decrease lower esophageal sphincter tone, thus worsening the condition; and in hot or humid environments, because it may predispose the patient to heatstroke.

Interactions
Concurrent administration of antacids decreases oral absorption of anticholinergics. Administer glycopyrrolate at least 1 hour before antacids.

Concomitant administration of drugs with anticholinergic effects may cause additive toxicity.

Decreased GI absorption of many drugs has been reported after the use of anticholinergics (for example, levodopa and ketoconazole). Conversely, slowly dissolving digoxin tablets may yield higher serum digoxin levels when administered with anticholinergics.

Use cautiously with oral potassium supplements (especially wax-matrix formulations) because the incidence of potassium-induced GI ulcerations may be increased.

Effects on diagnostic tests
None reported.

Adverse reactions
• CNS: weakness, nervousness, drowsiness, dizziness, headache.
• CV: palpitations, tachycardia, paradoxical bradycardia, orthostatic hypotension.
• DERM: urticaria, decreased sweating or anhidrosis, other dermal manifestations.
• EENT: dilated pupils, blurred vision, photophobia, cycloplegia, increased intraocular pressure.
• GI: constipation, dry mouth, nausea, vomiting, epigastric distress, dysphagia, loss of taste, abdominal distention.
• GU: urinary hesitancy or retention.
• Other: burning at injection site, bronchial plug formation, fever.

Note: Drug should be discontinued if hypersensitivity; urinary retention; confusion; hallucinations; dilated, nonreactive pupils; or hot, dry, flushed skin occurs.

Overdose and treatment
Clinical effects of overdose include such peripheral effects as dilated, nonreactive pupils; blurred vision; flushed, hot, dry skin; dryness of mucous membranes; dysphagia; decreased or absent bowel sounds; urinary retention; hyperthermia; tachycardia; hypertension; and increased respiration.

Treatment is primarily symptomatic and supportive, as needed. If patient is alert, induce emesis (or use gastric lavage) and follow with a saline cathartic and activated charcoal to prevent further drug absorption. In severe cases, physostigmine may be administered to block glycopyrrolate's antimuscarinic effects. Give fluids, as needed, to treat shock. If urinary retention occurs, catheterization may be necessary.

▶ **Special considerations**
• Check all dosages carefully. Even slight overdose could lead to toxic effects.
• For immediate treatment of bradycardia, some clinicians prefer atropine over glycopyrrolate.
• Do not mix glycopyrrolate with I.V. solutions containing sodium chloride or bicarbonate.
• May be administered with neostigmine or physostigmine in same syringe.
• Drug is incompatible with thiopental, methohexital, secobarbital, pentobarbital, chloramphenicol, dimenhydrinate, and diazepam.
• Monitor patient's vital signs, urine output, visual changes, and for signs of impending toxicity.
• Give ice chips, cold drinks, or sugarless hard candy to relieve dry mouth.
• Constipation may be relieved by stool softeners or bulk laxatives.

___

gold sodium thiomalate
Myochrysine

• Classification: antiarthritic agent (gold salt)

___

How supplied
Available by prescription only
Injection: 10 mg/ml, 50 mg/ml with benzyl alcohol

Indications, route, and dosage
Rheumatoid arthritis
†*Children over age 2:* 0.7 to 1 mg/kg/week or one-quarter the adult dose I.M. for 20 weeks. If response is good, may be given q 3 to 4 weeks indefinitely. Maximum single dose for children younger than 12 is 50 mg.
Adults: Initially, 10 mg I.M., followed by 25 mg in 1 week and continued for second and third doses at weekly intervals. Then, 50 mg weekly until 14 to 20 doses have been given. If improvement occurs without toxicity, continue 50 mg q 2 weeks for four doses; then, 50 mg q 3 weeks for four doses; then, 50 mg/month indefinitely as maintenance therapy to cumulative dose of 800 mg to 1 g. If relapse occurs during maintenance therapy, resume injections at weekly intervals.

Action and kinetics
• *Antiarthritic action:* Gold sodium thiomalate is thought to be effective against rheumatoid arthritis by altering the immune system to reduce inflammation. Although the exact mechanism of action remains unknown, these compounds have reduced serum concentrations of immunoglobulins and rheumatoid factors in patients with arthritis.
• *Kinetics in adults:* Absorption of gold sodium thiomalate is rapid, with peak levels occurring within 3 to 6 hours. Parenteral gold salts produce higher tissue concentrations with a mean steady-state plasma level of 1 to 5 mcg/ml. Drug is distributed widely throughout the body in lymph nodes, bone marrow, kidneys, liver, spleen, and tissues. About 85% to 90% is protein-bound. Drug is not broken down into its elemental form. The half-life with cumulative dosing is 14 to 40 days. About 70% of drug is excreted in the urine, 30% in the feces.

Contraindications and precautions
Gold compounds are contraindicated in patients with uncontrolled diabetes mellitus, systemic lupus erythromatosus, Sjögren's syndrome, agranulocytosis, or blood dyscrasias; in patients who recently received radiation therapy; in breast-feeding patients, because the drug distributes into breast milk; and in patients with a history of sensitivity to gold compounds. They should be administered cautiously to patients with marked hypertension, compromised cerebral or cardiovascular function, or renal or hepatic dysfunction, because gold may exacerbate these conditions; and to patients of childbearing age, because gold compounds are teratogenic in high doses in animals.

Interactions
Concomitant use with other drugs known to cause blood dyscrasias causes an additive risk of hematologic toxicity.

Effects on diagnostic tests
Serum protein-bound iodine test, especially when done by the chloric acid digestion method, gives false readings during and for several weeks after gold therapy.

Adverse reactions
Adverse reactions to gold are considered severe and potentially life-threatening.
• CNS: dizziness, syncope, sweating.
• CV: bradycardia.
• DERM: rash, pruritus, dermatitis, exfoliative dermatitis.
• EENT: corneal gold deposition, corneal ulcers.
• GI: diarrhea, abdominal pain, nausea, vomiting, stomatitis, enterocolitis, anorexia, metallic taste, dyspepsia, flatulence.
• GU: albuminuria, proteinuria, nephrotic syndrome, nephritis, acute tubular necrosis.
• HEMA: thrombocytopenia (with or without purpura), aplastic anemia, agranulocytosis, leukopenia, eosinophilia.
• Hepatic: jaundice, elevated liver enzymes.
• Other: gold bronchitis and interstitial pneumonitis, partial or complete loss of hair, fever, anaphylaxis, angioneurotic edema.

Overdose and treatment
When severe reactions to gold occur, corticosteroids, dimercaprol (a chelating agent), or penicillamine may be given to aid in the recovery. Prednisone 40 to 100 mg/day in divided doses is recommended to manage severe renal, hematologic, pulmonary, or enterocolitic reactions to gold. Dimercaprol may be used concurrently with steroids to facilitate the removal of the gold when the steroid treatment alone is ineffective.

___

▶ Special considerations
• Use in children under age 6 is not recommended. Children age 6 to 12 may receive one-fourth the usual adult dose. Larger children (40 to 50 kg) may receive doses that approach adult dose.
• Gold salts should be administered only under close medical supervision.
• Most adverse reactions are readily reversible if drug is discontinued immediately.
• Administer all gold salts I.M., preferably intragluteally. Normal color of drug is pale yellow; do not use if it darkens.
• Remember that the gluteal muscle should not be used for I.M. injections until after the child has been walking for at least 1 year.
• Observe patient for 30 minutes after administration because of possible anaphylactic reaction.
• Patient who receives gold sodium thiomalate should remain recumbent for 10 to 20 minutes after injection.
• Patient's urine should be analyzed for protein and sediment changes before each injection.
• CBC and platelet count should be monitored monthly.
• If adverse reactions are mild, some rheumatologists resume gold therapy after 2 to 3 weeks' rest.
• Dimercaprol should be kept on hand to treat acute toxicity.
• Carefully monitor for toxic reactions (pruritus, rash, metallic taste, sore mouth, or GI reactions).
• Moderately severe skin reactions and mucous membrane reactions often benefit from a topical steroid cream, an oral antihistamine, and soothing lotions.
• Do not restart gold therapy afer a severe reaction.
• Gold therapy may alter liver function tests.

Information for parents and patient
• Explain to parents and patient the importance of taking gold sodium thiomalate according to the prescribed dosage and of having monthly follow-up blood tests.
• Tell parents and patient that joint pain may increase after a gold injection and last for 1 to 2 days but that this usually subsides afer the first few injections.
• Patient should continue taking concomitant drug therapy, such as nonsteroidal anti-inflammatory drugs, as prescribed.
• Patient should minimize exposure to sunlight or artificial ultraviolet light, because skin rash may develop or be aggravated by such exposure.
• Tell parents and patient that good oral hygiene is important.
• Urge parents and patient to have scheduled monthly platelet counts. Drug should be stopped if the platelet count falls below 100,000/mm³.
• Explain that beneficial drug effect may be delayed for 3 months. However, if response is inadequate after 6 months, gold sodium thiomalate will probably be discontinued.
• Explain that adverse reactions – faintness, weakness, dizziness, flushing, nausea, vomiting, diaphoresis – may occur immediately after injection. Advise patient to lie down until symptoms subside.
• Tell parents that patient should continue taking the drug if he experiences mild diarrhea unless it persists or becomes bloody; if so, parents should call physician immediately.
• Tell parents and patient that stomatitis is often preceded by a metallic taste. Advise parents to report this symptom immediately.
• Advise parents to report any rashes or other skin problems immediately.

---

gonadorelin hydrochloride
Factrel

• Classification: diagnostic agent (luteinizing hormone releasing hormone)

How supplied
Available by prescription only
Injection: 100 mcg, 500 mcg

Indications, route, and dosage
Diagnosis of hypogonadism
Children age 12 and older and adults: 100 mcg S.C. or I.V. In patients for whom the phase of the menstrual cycle can be established, perform the test between day 1 and day 7.

Action and kinetics
• *Gonadotropic action:* Gonadorelin stimulates the release of luteinizing hormone and follicle-stimulating hormone from the anterior pituitary. Serial measurement of luteinizing hormone levels in blood after gonadorelin injection allows assessment of pituitary gonadotropic function.
• *Kinetics in adults:* Limited information is available. Gonadorelin has a duration of action of 3 to 5 hours and a half-life of a few minutes. Distribution and metabolism are unknown. Drug is excreted primarily by the kidneys as metabolites.

Contraindications and precautions
Gonadorelin is contraindicated in patients who have demonstrated hypersensitivity to it.

Interactions
Perform diagnostic testing with gonadorelin in the absence of drugs that affect the pituitary secretion of gonadotropins, such as androgens, estrogens, progestins, adrenocorticoids, or glucocorticosteroids. Levodopa and spironolactone may elevate gonadotropin levels. Digoxin and oral contraceptives may decrease gonadotropin levels. Metoclopramide or phenothiazines also may affect test results.

Effects on diagnostic tests
Therapy with gonadorelin elevates luteinizing hormone levels.

Adverse reactions
• CNS: headache, flushing, nausea, light-headedness.
• Local: occasional pain and pruritus when administered S.C.

Overdose and treatment
Specific information unavailable. Treatment is supportive.

---

‡May contain sulfites   ◆May contain tartrazine   ◆◆May contain benzyl alcohol

▶ **Special considerations**

• As a single injection, gonadorelin can aid in evaluating the functional capacity and response of the gonadotropins of the anterior pituitary. Prolonged or repeated administration may be necessary to measure pituitary gonadotropic reserve.

• Although no hypersensitivity reactions have been reported to date, use cautiously in patients who are allergic to other drugs.

• The gonadorelin test can be performed concomitantly with other post-treatment evaluation.

• For specific test methodology and interpretation of test results, refer to the manufacturer's full product information available from pharmacist.

• Reconstitute vial with 1 ml of accompanying sterile diluent. Prepare solution immediately before use. After reconstitution, store at room temperature and use within 1 day. Discard unused reconstituted solution and diluent.

Information for parents and patient
Advise parents and patient of test procedure.

griseofulvin microsize
Fulvicin-U/F, Grifulvin V, Grisactin

• Classification: antifungal (*Penicillium* antibiotic)

How supplied
Available by prescription only
Microsize
Capsules: 125 mg, 250 mg
Tablets: 250 mg, 500 mg
Oral suspension: 125 mg/5ml
Ultramicrosize
Tablets: 125 mg, 165 mg, 250 mg, 330 mg

Indications, route, and dosage
Ringworm infections of skin, hair, and nails
Children: 11 mg/kg/day (microsize) or 7.3 mg/kg/day (ultramicrosize).
Adults: 500 mg (microsize) P.O. daily in single or divided doses. Severe infections may require up to 1 g daily. Alternatively, may give 330 to 375 mg ultramicrosize in single or divided doses. Alternatively, may give 660 to 750 mg ultramicrosize P.O. daily.

Action and kinetics
• *Antifungal action:* Griseofulvin disrupts the fungal cell's mitotic spindle, interfering with cell division; it also may inhibit DNA replication. Drug is also deposited in keratin precursor cells, inhibiting fungal invasion. It is active against *Trichophyton, Microsporum,* and *Epidermophyton.*
• *Kinetics in adults:* Griseofulvin is absorbed primarily in the duodenum and varies among individuals. Ultramicrosize preparations are absorbed almost completely; microsize absorption ranges from 25% to 70% and may be increased by giving with a high-fat meal. Peak concentrations occur at 4 to 8 hours. Griseofulvin concentrates in skin, hair, nails, fat, liver, and skeletal muscle; it is tightly bound to new keratin.

Griseofulvin is oxidatively demethylated and conjugated with glucuronic acid to inactive metabolites in the liver. About 50% of griseofulvin and its metabolites is excreted in urine and 33% in feces within 5 days. Less than 1% of a dose appears unchanged in urine. Griseofulvin is also excreted in perspiration. Elimination half-life is 9 to 24 hours.

Contraindications and precautions
Griseofulvin is contraindicated in patients with known hypersensitivity to the drug; it is also contraindicated in patients with hepatocellular failure and in patients with porphyria because it interferes with porphyrin metabolism. Griseofulvin should be used with caution in patients with penicillin hypersensitivity because both drugs are produced by *Penicillium.* It should be reserved for mycotic disease unresponsive to other topical treatment.

Interactions
Griseofulvin may potentiate the effects of alcohol, producing tachycardia and flushing; it may decrease prothrombin time in patients taking warfarin, by enzyme induction; and it may decrease the efficacy of oral contraceptives.

Concomitant use of barbiturates may impair absorption of griseofulvin and increase dosage requirements.

Effects on diagnostic tests
Griseofulvin can cause proteinuria; it also may decrease granulocyte counts.

Adverse reactions
• CNS: headaches (in early stages of treatment), transient decrease in hearing, fatigue with large doses, occasional mental confusion, impaired performance of routine activities, psychotic symptoms, dizziness, insomnia.
• DERM: rash, urticaria, *photosensitivity reactions* (may aggravate lupus erythematosus).
• GI: nausea, vomiting, excessive thirst, flatulence, diarrhea.
• HEMA: leukopenia, granulocytopenia.
• Metabolic: porphyria.
• Other: estrogen-like effects in children, oral thrush.
Note: Drug should be discontinued if granulocytopenia occurs.

Overdose and treatment
Symptoms of overdose include headache, lethargy, confusion, vertigo, blurred vision, nausea, vomiting, and diarrhea. Treatment is supportive. After recent ingestion (within 4 hours), empty stomach by induced emesis or gastric lavage. Follow with activated charcoal to decrease absorption. A cathartic may also be helpful.

▶ **Special considerations**
• Safety in children under age 2 has not been established.
• Identification of organism should be confirmed before therapy begins.
• Give drug with or after meals consisting of a high-fat content (if allowed), to minimize GI distress.

• Assess nutrition and monitor food intake; drug may alter taste sensation, suppressing appetite.
• Check CBCs regularly for possible adverse reactions; monitor renal and liver function studies periodically.
• Treatment of tinea pedis may require combined oral and topical therapy.
• Ultramicrosize griseofulvin is absorbed more rapidly and completely than microsize and is effective at one-half to two-thirds the usual dose.

Information for parents and patient
• Encourage parents to have patient maintain adequate nutritional intake; offer suggestions to improve taste of food.
• Stress importance of completing prescribed regimen to prevent relapse even though symptoms may abate quickly.
• Teach signs and symptoms of adverse reactions and hypersensitivity, and tell parents to report them immediately.
• Patient should avoid exposure to intense indoor light and sunlight to reduce the risk of photosensitivity reactions.
• Advise parents that patient should avoid alcohol during therapy because griseofulvin may potentiate alcohol effects.
• Teach correct personal hygiene and skin care.

guanabenz acetate
Wytensin

• Classification: antihypertensive (centrally acting antiadrenergic agent)

How supplied
Available by prescription only
Tablets: 4 mg, 8 mg, 16 mg

Indications, route, and dosage
Hypertension
Children age 12 and older: Initially, 0.5 to 4 mg daily; maintenance dosage ranges from 4 to 24 mg daily, administered in two divided doses.
Adults: Initially, 4 mg P.O. b.i.d. Dosage may be increased in increments of 4 to 8 mg/day every 1 to 2 weeks. The usual maintenance dosage ranges from 8 to 16 mg daily. Maximum dosage is 32 mg b.i.d.

Action and kinetics
• *Antihypertensive action:* Guanabenz lowers blood pressure by stimulating central alpha$_2$-adrenergic receptors, decreasing cerebral sympathetic outflow and thus decreasing peripheral vascular resistance. Guanabenz may also antagonize antidiuretic hormone (ADH) secretion and ADH activity in the kidney.
• *Kinetics in adults:* After oral administration, 70% to 80% of guanabenz is absorbed from the GI tract; antihypertensive effect occurs within 60 minutes, peaking at 2 to 4 hours. Guanabenz appears to be distributed widely into the body; drug is about 90% protein-bound. Guanabenz is metabolized extensively in the liver; several metabolites are formed. Guana-

benz and its metabolites are excreted primarily in urine; remaining drug is excreted in feces. Duration of antihypertensive effect varies from 6 to 12 hours.

Contraindications and precautions
Guanabenz is contraindicated in patients with known hypersensitivity to the drug. It should be used cautiously in patients with vascular insufficiency, severe coronary insufficiency, recent myocardial infarction, cerebrovascular disease, or severe hepatic or renal failure.

Interactions
Guanabenz may increase CNS depressant effects of alcohol, phenothiazines, benzodiazepines, barbiturates, and other sedatives; tricyclic antidepressants may inhibit antihypertensive effects of guanabenz.

Effects on diagnostic tests
Guanabenz may reduce serum cholesterol and total triglyceride levels slightly, but it does not alter high-density lipoprotein fraction; drug may cause nonprogressive elevations in liver enzyme levels.

Chronic use of guanabenz decreases plasma norepinephrine, dopamine, beta-hydroxylase, and plasma renin activity.

Adverse reactions
• CNS: drowsiness, sedation, dizziness, weakness, headache, ataxia, depression.
• CV: severe rebound hypertension.
• EENT: dry mouth.
Note: Drug should be discontinued if intolerable adverse reactions, such as sedation and dry mouth, do not subside.

Overdose and treatment
Clinical signs of overdose include bradycardia, CNS depression, respiratory depression, hypothermia, apnea, seizures, lethargy, agitation, irritability, diarrhea, and hypotension.

Do not induce emesis; CNS depression occurs rapidly. After adequate respiration is assured, empty stomach by gastric lavage; then give activated charcoal and a saline cathartic to decrease absorption. Follow with supportive and symptomatic care.

▶ Special considerations
• Guanabenz has been used to treat hypertension in a limited number of children over age 12; its safety and efficacy in younger children have not been established.
• To ensure overnight blood pressure control and minimize daytime drowsiness, give last dose at bedtime.
• Investigational uses include managing opiate withdrawal and adjunctive therapy in patients with chronic pain.
• Abrupt discontinuation of guanabenz will cause severe rebound hypertension; reduce dosage gradually over 2 to 4 days.
• Reduced dosages may be required in patients with hepatic impairment.

Information for parents and patient
• Explain signs and symptoms of adverse effects and importance of reporting them.
• Warn parents to have patient avoid hazardous activities that require mental alertness and to avoid alcohol and other CNS depressants.
• Suggest taking drug at bedtime until tolerance develops to sedation, drowsiness, and other CNS effects.
• Advise parents that patient should avoid sudden position changes to minimize orthostatic hypotension, and to relieve dry mouth with ice chips or sugarless gum.
• Warn parents to seek medical approval before administering nonprescription cold preparations.
• Advise parents or patient not to discontinue this drug suddenly; severe rebound hypertension may occur.

guanethidine sulfate
Ismelin

• Classification: antihypertensive (adrenergic neuron blocking agent)

How supplied
Available by prescription only
Tablets: 10 mg, 25 mg

Indications, route, and dosage
Moderate to severe hypertension
Children: Initially, 200 mcg/kg or 6 mg/m^2 P.O. daily; increase gradually every 1 to 3 weeks to maximum of five to eight times initial dose.
Adults: Initially, 10 mg P.O. once daily; increase by 10 mg at weekly to monthly intervals, as necessary. Usual dosage is 25 to 50 mg once daily; some patients may require up to 300 mg.

Action and kinetics
• *Antihypertensive action:* Guanethidine acts peripherally; it decreases arteriolar vasoconstriction and reduces blood pressure by inhibiting norepinephrine release and depleting norepinephrine stores in adrenergic nerve endings.
• *Kinetics in adults:* Guanethidine is absorbed incompletely from the GI tract. Maximal antihypertensive effects usually are not evident for 1 to 3 weeks. Guanethidine is distributed throughout the body; it is not protein-bound but demonstrates extensive tissue binding. Drug undergoes partial hepatic metabolism to pharmacologically less-active metabolites. Guanethidine and metabolites are excreted primarily in urine; small amounts are excreted in feces. Elimination half-life after chronic administration is biphasic: initial half-life is 1½ days; a second half-life is 4 to 8 days.

Contraindications and precautions
Guanethidine is contraindicated in patients with known hypersensitivity to the drug; in patients with overt CHF not caused by hypertension, because the drug may interfere with normal sympathetic compensation; and in patients with known or suspected pheo-

chromocytoma, because the drug may increase sensitivity to circulating catecholamines.
Guanethidine should be used cautiously in patients with recent myocardial infarction, severe cardiac disease, cerebrovascular disease, peptic ulcer disease, impaired renal function, or bronchial asthma, because the drug may precipitate or worsen these conditions.

Interactions
Concomitant use of guanethidine with diuretics, other antihypertensive agents, levodopa, or alcohol may potentiate guanethidine's antihypertensive effect; guanethidine potentiates pressor effects of such agents as norepinephrine, metaraminol, and oral sympathomimetic nasal decongestants.
Concomitant use with cardiac glycosides may result in additive bradycardia; use with rauwolfia alkaloids may cause excessive postural hypotension, bradycardia, and mental depression.
Concomitant administration with MAO inhibitors, tricyclic antidepressants, or oral contraceptives may antagonize the antihypertensive effect of guanethidine.

Effects on diagnostic tests
None reported.

Adverse reactions
• CNS: dizziness, weakness, syncope.
• CV: orthostatic hypotension, bradycardia, CHF, dysrhythmias, edema.
• EENT: nasal stuffiness, dry mouth.
• GI: diarrhea, weight gain.
• HEMA: anemia, thrombocytopenia, leukopenia.
   Note: Drug should be discontinued if severe diarrhea develops.

Overdose and treatment
Signs of overdose include hypotension, blurred vision, syncope, bradycardia, and severe diarrhea.
After acute ingestion, empty stomach by induced emesis or gastric lavage and give activated charcoal to reduce absorption. Further treatment is usually symptomatic and supportive.

▶ Special considerations
• Dosage requirements may be reduced in the presence of fever.
• If diarrhea develops, atropine or Paregoric may be prescribed.
• Discontinue drug 2 to 3 weeks before elective surgery, to reduce risk of cardiovascular collapse during anesthesia.
• When drug is replacing MAO inhibitors, wait at least 1 week before initiating guanethidine; if replacing ganglionic blocking agents, withdraw them slowly to prevent a spiking blood pressure response during the transfer period.
• Guanethidine has been used topically as a 5% ophthalmic solution to treat chronic open-angle glaucoma or endocrine ophthalmopathy.

Information for parents and patient
• Teach parents and patient signs and symptoms of adverse reactions and importance of reporting them;

---

*Canada only   †Unlabeled clinical use   Italicized adverse reactions have been observed in children.

parents should also report persistent diarrhea and excessive weight gain (5 lb [2.3 kg] per week or more). Advise parents not to discontinue the drug but to call for further instructions if adverse reactions occur.
• Warn parents that patient should avoid hazardous activities that require mental alertness and to take drug at bedtime until tolerance develops to sedation, drowsiness, and other CNS effects.
• Advise parents that patient should avoid sudden position changes, strenuous exercise, heat, and hot showers, to minimize orthostatic hypotension; and to relieve dry mouth with ice chips, hard candy, or gum.
• Advise parents not to double next scheduled dose if the patient misses one; he should take only the next scheduled dose.
• Advise parents to seek medical approval before administering nonprescription cold preparations.

halcinonide
Halciderm*, Halog, Halog-E

- Classification: anti-inflammatory agent (adreno-corticoid)

How supplied
Available by prescription only
Cream: 0.025%, 0.1%
Ointment: 0.1%
Topical solution: 0.1%

Indications, route, and dosage
Inflammation of acute and chronic cortico-steroid-responsive dermatoses
Children: Apply sparingly to affected areas once a day.
Adults: Apply cream, ointment, or solution sparingly b.i.d. to t.i.d. Occlusive dressing may be used for severe or resistant dermatoses.

Action and kinetics
- *Anti-inflammatory action:* Halcinonide stimulates the synthesis of enzymes needed to decrease the inflammatory response. Depending on its strength, halcinonide is a group II (0.1%) or group III (0.025%) fluorinated corticosteroid.
- *Kinetics in adults:* The amount absorbed depends on concentration, the amount applied, and the nature of the skin at the application site. It ranges from about 1% in skin with a thick stratum corneum (such as the palms, soles, elbows, and knees) to as high as 36% in areas of the thinnest stratum corneum (face, eyelids, and genitals). Absorption increases in skin areas that are damaged, inflamed, or under occlusion. Some systemic absorption of topical steroids may occur, especially through the oral mucosa.

After topical application, halcinonide is distributed throughout the local skin and metabolized primarily in the skin. Any absorbed drug is distributed into muscle, liver, skin, intestines, and kidneys; it is metabolized primarily in the liver to inactive compounds.

Inactive metabolites are excreted by the kidneys, primarily as glucuronides and sulfates, but also as unconjugated products. Small amounts of the metabolites are also excreted in feces.

Contraindications and precautions
Halcinonide is contraindicated in patients who are hypersensitive to any component of the preparation and in patients with viral, fungal, or tubercular skin lesions.

Halcinonide should be used with extreme caution in patients with impaired circulation because the drug may increase the risk of skin ulceration.

Interactions
None significant.

Effects on diagnostic tests
None reported.

Adverse reactions
- Local: burning, itching, irritation, dryness, folliculitis, hypertrichosis, acneiform eruptions, hypopigmentation, perioral dermatitis, allergic contact dermatitis, maceration, secondary infection, atrophy, striae, miliaria.

Significant systemic absorption may produce the following reactions:
- CNS: euphoria, insomnia, headache, psychotic behavior, pseudotumor cerebri, mental changes, nervousness, restlessness.
- CV: congestive heart failure, hypertension, edema.
- EENT: cataracts, glaucoma, thrush.
- GI: peptic ulcer, irritation, increased appetite.
- Immune: immunosuppression, increased susceptibility to infection.
- Metabolic: hypokalemia, sodium retention, fluid retention, weight gain, hyperglycemia, osteoporosis, growth suppression in children.
- Musculoskeletal: muscle atrophy.
- Other: withdrawal syndrome (nausea, fatigue, anorexia, dyspnea, hypotension, hypoglycemia, myalgia, arthralgia, fever, dizziness, and fainting).

Note: Drug should be discontinued if local irritation, infection, systemic absorption, or hypersensitivity reaction occurs.

Overdose and treatment
No information available.

▶ Special considerations
- Children may show greater susceptibility to topical corticosteroid-induced HPA axis suppression and Cushing's syndrome than mature patients because of a higher ratio of skin surface area to body weight. Hypothalamic-pituitary-adrenal (HPA) axis suppression, Cushing's syndrome, and intracranial hypertension have been reported in children receiving topical corticosteroids. Signs of adrenal suppression in children include linear growth retardation, delayed weight gain, low plasma cortisol levels, and absence of response to ACTH stimulation. Signs of intracranial hypertension include bulging fontanelles, headaches, and bilateral papilledema.
- Administration of topical corticosteroids to children should be limited to the least effective amount. Chronic corticosteroid therapy may interfere with growth and development.
- Stop drug if the patient develops signs of systemic absorption (including Cushing's syndrome, hyperglycemia, or glucosuria), skin irritation or ulceration, hypesensitivity, or infection. (If antifungals or antibiotics are being used with corticosteroids and the

ection does not respond immediately, corticoste-
ds should be stopped until infection is controlled.)
Monitor patient response. Observe area of inflam-
ation and elicit patient comments concerning pru-
us. Inspect skin for infection, striae, and atrophy.
in atrophy is common and may be clinically sig-
icant within 3 to 4 weeks of treatment with high-
tency preparations; it also occurs more readily at
es where percutaneous absorption is high.
o not apply occlusive dressings over topical steroids
cause this may lead to secondary infection, mac-
ation, atrophy, striae, or miliaria caused by increas-
g steroid penetration and potency.

formation for parents and patient
struct parents and patient in application of the drug.
ll them the following:

ethod for applying topical preparations
Wash hands before and after applying the drug.
Gently cleanse the area of application. Washing or
aking the area before application may increase drug
netration.
Apply sparingly in a light film; rub in lightly. Avoid
ntact with patient's eyes.
Avoid prolonged application on the face, in skin folds,
d in areas near the eyes, genitals, or rectum. High-
tency topical corticosteroids are more likely to cause
riae in these areas because of their higher rates of
sorption.
f an occlusive dressing is necessary, minimize ad-
rse reactions by using it intermittently. Do not leave
in place longer than 16 hours each day.
Warn patient not to use nonprescription topical prep-
ations other than those specifically recommended.
Advise parents not to use tight-fitting diapers or
astic pants on a child being treated in the diaper
ea, since such garments may serve as occlusive
essings.

---

aloperidol
po-Haloperidol*, Haldol,
ovoperidol*, Peridol*

aloperidol decanoate
Haldol Decanoate, Haldol LA*

aloperidol lactate
Haldol, Haldol Concentrate

Classification: antipsychotic (butyrophenone)

---

ow supplied
vailable by prescription only
aloperidol
ablets: 0.5 mg, 1 mg, 2.5 mg, 10 mg, 20 mg
jection: 5 mg/ml
aloperidol decanoate
jection: 50 mg/ml
aloperidol lactate
ral concentrate: 2 mg/ml

Indications, route, and dosage
Psychotic disorders
Children age 3 to 12 years: 0.05 to 0.15 mg/kg P.O.
daily in two or three divided doses.
Adults: Dosage varies for each patient. Initial dosage
range is 0.5 to 5 mg P.O. b.i.d. or t.i.d.; or 2 to 5 mg
I.M. q 4 to 8 hours, increased rapidly if necessary for
prompt control. Maximum dosage is 100 mg P.O. daily.
Doses over 100 mg have been used for patients with
severely resistant conditions.
Control of tics, vocal utterances in Gilles de la Tourette's syndrome
Children age 3 to 12: 0.05 to 0.075 mg/kg/day given
b.i.d. or t.i.d.
Adults: 0.5 to 5 mg P.O. b.i.d. or t.i.d., increased p.r.n.

Action and kinetics
• *Antipsychotic action:* Haloperidol is thought to exert
its antipsychotic effects by strong postsynaptic blockade of CNS dopamine receptors, thereby inhibiting
dopamine-mediated effects; its pharmacologic effects
are most similar to those of piperazine antipsychotics.
Its mechanism of action in Gilles de la Tourette's
syndrome is unknown.

Haloperidol has many other central and peripheral
effects; it has weak peripheral anticholinergic effects
and antiemetic effects, produces both alpha and ganglionic blockade, and counteracts histamine- and serotonin-mediated activity. Its most prominent adverse
reactions are extrapyramidal.
• *Kinetics in adults:* Rate and extent of absorption
vary with route of administration: oral tablet absorption yields 60% to 70% bioavailability. I.M. dose is
70% absorbed within 30 minutes. Peak plasma levels
after oral administration occur at 2 to 6 hours; after
I.M. administration, 30 to 45 minutes; and after long-
acting I.M. (decanoate) administration, 4 to 11 days.

Haloperidol is distributed widely into the body, with
high concentrations in adipose tissue. Drug is 91%
to 99% protein-bound.

Haloperidol is metabolized extensively by the liver;
there may be only one active metabolite that is less
active than the parent drug.

About 40% of a given dose is excreted in urine
within 5 days; about 15% is excreted in feces via the
biliary tract.

Contraindications and precautions
Haloperidol is contraindicated in patients with known
hypersensitivity to haloperidol, phenothiazines, and
related compounds, including that expressed by jaundice because haloperidol may impair liver function;
in patients with blood dyscrasias and bone marrow
depression because agranulocytosis can occur; in patients with disorders accompanied by coma, brain
damage, or CNS depression because of additive CNS
depression; and in circulatory collapse or cerebrovascular disease because of the drug's hypotensive
and arrhythmogenic effects.

Use haloperidol cautiously in patients with cardiac
disease (dysrhythmias, congestive heart failure, angina pectoris, valvular disease, or heart block), encephalitis, Reye's syndrome, head injury, respiratory
disease, epilepsy and other seizure disorders, glaucoma, prostatic hypertrophy, urinary retention, he-

patic or renal dysfunction, Parkinson's disease, pheochromocytoma, or hypocalcemia.

Interactions

Concomitant use of haloperidol with sympathomimetics, including epinephrine, phenylephrine, phenylpropanolamine, and ephedrine (often found in nasal sprays), and appetite suppressants may decrease their stimulatory and pressor effects.

Haloperidol may inhibit blood pressure response to centrally acting antihypertensive drugs, such as guanethidine, guanabenz, guanadrel, clonidine, methyldopa, and reserpine. Additive effects are likely after concomitant use of haloperidol with CNS depressants, including alcohol, analgesics, barbiturates, narcotics, tranquilizers, and general, spinal, or epidural anesthetics, or with parenteral magnesium sulfate (oversedation, respiratory depression, and hypotension); antiarrhythmic agents, quinidine, disopyramide, or procainamide (increased incidence of cardiac dysrhythmias and conduction defects); atropine or other anticholinergic drugs, including antidepressants, monoamine oxidase inhibitors, phenothiazines, antihistamines, meperidine, and antiparkinsonian agents (oversedation, paralytic ileus, visual changes, and severe constipation); nitrates (hypotension); and metrizamide (increased risk of convulsions).

Beta-blocking agents may inhibit haloperidol metabolism, increasing plasma levels and toxicity.

Concomitant use with propylthiouracil increases risk of agranulocytosis; concomitant use with lithium may result in severe neurologic toxicity with an encephalitis-like syndrome, and a decreased therapeutic response to haloperidol.

Pharmacokinetic alterations and subsequent decreased therapeutic response to haloperidol may follow concomitant use with phenobarbital (enhanced renal excretion); aluminum- and magnesium-containing antacids and antidiarrheals (decreased absorption); and heavy smoking (increased metabolism).

Haloperidol may antagonize therapeutic effect of bromocriptine on prolactin secretion; it also may decrease the vasoconstricting effects of high-dose dopamine, and may decrease effectiveness and increase toxicity of levodopa (by dopamine blockade). Haloperidol may inhibit metabolism and increase toxicity of phenytoin.

Effects on diagnostic tests

Haloperidol causes quinidine-like effects on the ECG.

Adverse reactions

• CNS: *extrapyramidal symptoms*—dystonia, akathisia, torticollis, tardive dyskinesia (dose-related with long-term therapy), sedation, pseudoparkinsonism, drowsiness, neuroleptic malignant syndrome (dose-related; fatal respiratory failure in over 10% of patients if untreated), dizziness, headache, insomnia, exacerbation of psychotic symptoms.
• CV: asystole, orthostatic hypotension, tachycardia, dizziness and fainting, dysrhythmias, ECG changes, increased anginal pain (after I.M. injection).
• EENT: blurred vision, tinnitus, mydriasis, increased intraocular pressure, ocular changes (retinal pigmentary change with long-term use).

• GI: dry mouth, constipation, nausea, vomiting, a[n]orexia, diarrhea.
• GU: urinary retention, gynecomastia, hypermen[o]rhea, inhibited ejaculation.
• HEMA: transient leukopenia, agranulocytos[is], thrombocytopenia, anemia (within 30 to 90 days).
• Local: contact dermatitis from concentrate or i[n]jectable form, muscle necrosis from I.M. injection mo[re] common with this drug.
• Other: hyperprolactinemia, photosensitivity, i[n]creased appetite or weight gain, hypersensitivit[y] (rash, urticaria, drug fever, edema, cholestatic jau[n]dice [in 2% to 4% of patients within first 30 days])

Note: Drug should be discontinued immediately [if] any of the following occurs: hypersensitivity, jau[n]dice, agranulocytosis; neuroleptic malignant sy[n]drome (marked hyperthermia, extrapyramidal effect[s] autonomic dysfunction); or if severe extrapyramid[al] symptoms occur even after dosage is lowered; and 4[8] hours before and 24 hours after myelography usi[ng] metrizamide because of the risk of convulsions. Whe[n] feasible, withdraw drug slowly and gradually; mar[y] drug effects persist after withdrawal.

Overdose and treatment

CNS depression is characterized by deep, unarousab[le] sleep and possible coma, hypotension or hypertensio[n,] extrapyramidal symptoms, dystonia, abnormal invo[l]untary muscle movements, agitation, seizures, dy[s]rhythmias, ECG changes (may show Q-T prolongati[on] and Torsades de Pointes), hypothermia or hype[r]thermia, and autonomic nervous system dysfunctio[n.] Overdose with long-acting decanoate requires pr[o]longed recovery time.

Treatment is symptomatic and supportive, inclu[d]ing maintaining vital signs, airway, stable body tem[]perature, and fluid and electrolyte balance. Ipec[a] may be used to induce vomiting, with due regard f[or] haloperidol's antiemetic properties and hazard of a[s]piration. Gastric lavage also may be used, followe[d] by activated charcoal and saline cathartics; dialys[is] does not help.

Regulate body temperature as needed. Treat h[y]potension with I.V. fluids: *do not give epinephrin[e.]* Treat seizures with parenteral diazepam or barbit[u]rates; dysrhythmias, with parenteral phenytoin [] mg/kg with rate titrated to blood pressure; extr[a]pyramidal reactions with barbiturates, benztropin[e,] or parenteral diphenhydramine 2 mg/kg/minute.

▶ Special considerations

• Haloperidol is not recommended for children und[er] age 3. Children are especially prone to extrapyramid[al] adverse reactions.
• Tardive dyskinesia may occur after prolonged us[e.] It may not appear until months or years later a[nd] may disappear spontaneously or persist for life.
• Protect medication from light. Slight yellowing [of] injection or concentrate is common; does not affe[ct] potency. Discard markedly discolored solutions.
• Do not withdraw drug abruptly unless required [by] severe adverse reactions.
• Higher doses in children (usually > 4 mg) may [be] associated with dysphoria, school phobia, and pe[r]sonality changes.

Dose of 2 mg is therapeutic equivalent of 100 mg chlorpromazine.

When changing from tablets to decanoate injection, patient should receive 10 to 15 times the oral dose once a month (maximum 100 mg).

Don't administer the decanoate form I.V.

Information for parents and patient

Warn parents that patients should avoid hazardous activities that require alertness and good psychomotor coordination until CNS response to drug is determined. Drowsiness and dizziness usually subside after a few weeks.

Avoid combining with alcohol or other depressants.

Explain that orthostatic hypotension may occur and should be reported if it persists longer than a few days.

Warn parents not to change dosage or discontinue drug without medical approval.

eparin calcium
Calciparine

eparin sodium
Heparin Lock Flush, Hep-Lock, Hep-lock U/P, Liquaemin Sodium

Classification: anticoagulant

ow supplied
Available products are derived from beef lung or porcine intestinal mucosa. All are injectable and available by prescription only.
Heparin calcium
Syringe: 5,000 units/0.2 ml
Ampule: 12,500 units/0.5 ml; 20,000 units/0.8 ml
Heparin sodium
Vials: 1,000 units/ml, 5,000 units/ml, 10,000 units/ml, 20,000 units/ml, 40,000 units/ml
Unit-dose ampules: 1,000 units/ml, 5,000 units/ml, 10,000 units/ml
Disposable syringes: 1,000 units/ml, 2,500 units/ml, 5,000 units/ml, 7,500 units/ml, 10,000 units/ml, 20,000 units/ml, 40,000 units/ml
Carpuject: 5,000 units/ml
Premixed I.V. solutions: 1,000 units in 500 ml normal saline solution; 2,000 units in 1,000 ml normal saline solution; 12,500 units in 250 ml 0.45% saline solution; 25,000 units in 250 ml 0.45% saline solution; 25,000 units in 500 ml 0.45% saline solution; 10,000 units in 100 ml dextrose 5% in water (D_5W); 12,500 units in 250 ml D_5W; 25,000 units in 250 ml D_5W; 25,000 units in 500 ml D_5W.
Heparin sodium flush
Vials: 10 units/ml, 100 units/ml
Disposable syringes: 10 units/ml, 25 units/2.5 ml, ,500 units/2.5 ml

ndications, route, and dosage
Deep vein thrombosis
Children: Initially, 50 units/kg I.V. drip. Maintenance dose is 50 to 100 units/kg I.V. drip every 4 hours.

Constant infusion: 20,000 units/m² daily. Dosages adjusted according to partial thromboplastin time (PTT).
Adults: Initially, 5,000 to 7,500 units I.V. push, then adjust dose according to PTT results and give dose I.V. every 4 hours (usually 4,000 to 5,000 units); or 5,000 to 7,500 units I.V. bolus, then 1,000 units hourly by I.V. infusion pump. Wait 8 hours after bolus dose, and adjust hourly rate according to PTT.
Pulmonary embolism
Children: Initially, 50 units/kg I.V. drip. Maintenance dose 50 to 100 units/kg I.V. drip every 4 hours. Constant infusion: 20,000 units/m² daily. Dosages adjusted according to PTT.
Adults: Initially, 7,500 to 10,000 units I.V. push, then adjust dose according to PTT results and give dose I.V. every 4 hours (usually 4,000 to 5,000 units); or 7,500 to 10,000 units I.V. bolus, then 1,000 units hourly by I.V. infusion pump. Wait 8 hours after bolus dose, and adjust hourly rate according to PTT.
Embolism prophylaxis
Adults: 5,000 units S.C. every 12 hours.
Open-heart surgery
Adults: (total body perfusion) 150 to 300 units/kg continuous I.V infusion.
Disseminated intravascular coagulation
Children: 25 to 50 units/kg I.V. every 4 hours, as a single injection or constant infusion. Discontinue if no improvement in 4 to 8 hours.
Adults: 50 to 100 units/kg I.V. every 4 hours as a single injection or constant infusion. Discontinue if no improvement in 4 to 8 hours.
To maintain patency of I.V. indwelling catheters
10 to 100 units as an I.V. flush (not intended for therapeutic use).

Note: Heparin dosing is highly individualized, depending upon disease state, age, and renal and hepatic status.

Action and kinetics
• *Anticoagulant action:* Heparin accelerates formation of antithrombin III-thrombin complex; it inactivates thrombin and prevents conversion of fibrinogen to fibrin.

• *Kinetics in adults:* Heparin is not absorbed from the GI tract and must be given parenterally. After I.V. use, onset of action is almost immediate; after S.C. injection, onset of action occurs in 20 to 60 minutes. Heparin is extensively bound to lipoprotein, globulins, and fibrinogen; it does not cross the placenta. Though metabolism is not completely described, heparin is thought to be removed by the reticuloendothelial system, with some metabolism occurring in the liver. Little is known; a small fraction is excreted in urine as unchanged drug. Drug is not excreted into breast milk. Plasma half-life is between 1 and 2 hours.

Contraindications and precautions
Although clearly hazardous in the following conditions, use of heparin depends on the comparative risk of failure to treat the coexisting thromboembolic disorder. Heparin is thus conditionally contraindicated in active bleeding and in patients with blood dyscrasias or bleeding tendencies, such as hemophilia, thrombocytopenia, or hepatic disease with hypopro-

thrombinemia; suspected intracranial hemorrhage; suppurative thrombophlebitis; inaccessible ulcerative lesions (especially GI); open ulcerative wounds; extensive denudation of skin; ascorbic acid deficiency and other conditions causing capillary permeability; during or after brain, eye, or spinal cord surgery; during continuous GI tube drainage; and in patients with subacute bacterial endocarditis, shock, advanced renal disease, threatened abortion, or severe hypertension.

Administer heparin cautiously during menstruation and immediately postpartum; to patients with mild hepatic or renal disease, GI ulcers, alcoholism, or occupations that risk physical injury; to patients with a history of allergy or asthma, because the drug is derived from potentially allergenic porcine or bovine sources; and to lactating patients, because osteoporosis can occur in these patients after 2 to 4 weeks of therapy.

Interactions
Concomitant use with salicylates and oral anticoagulants increases anticoagulant effect; if it is not possible to avoid using these together, monitor prothrombin time (PT) and PTT.

Large doses of vitamin C can antagonize the action of heparin.

Effects on diagnostic tests
Heparin therapy prolongs PT, may falsely elevate AST (SGOT) and serum ALT (SGPT) levels, and may cause false elevations in some tests for serum thyroxine levels.

Adverse reactions
• HEMA: *hemorrhage with excessive dosage,* overly prolonged clotting time, thrombocytopenia.
• Local: tissue irritation, mild pain, pruritus, ecchymosis, *hematomas.*
• Other: "white clot" syndrome (a type of arterial thrombosis); *hypersensitivity reactions,* including chills, fever, pruritus, rhinitis, burning of feet, conjunctivitis, lacrimation, arthralgia, and urticaria. After long-term use with large doses: *suppressed renal function,* hyperkalemia, rebound hyperlipidemia upon discontinuation of drug, osteoporosis (decrease in height, rib or back pain, spontaneous fractures), *hyperaldosteronism.*
Note: Drug should be discontinued if signs of hemorrhage or new thrombosis occur.

Overdose and treatment
The major sign of overdose is hemorrhage. Immediate withdrawal of the drug usually allows the hemorrhage to resolve; however, severe hemorrhage may require treatment with protamine sulfate. Usually, 1 mg protamine sulfate will neutralize 90 units of bovine heparin or 115 units of porcine heparin.

Heparin administered by the I.V. route disappears rapidly from the blood, so the protamine dose is dependent upon when heparin was administered. Protamine should be given slowly by I.V. injection (over 3 minutes), and not more than 50 mg should be given in any 10-minute period. Protamine should be given as a 25- to 50-mg loading dose, followed by constant infusion of the remainder of the calculated dose over 8 to 16 hours.

Heparin administered by the S.C. route will be slowly absorbed.

For severe bleeding, transfusions may be required.

▶ Special considerations
• Obtain pretherapy baseline thrombin time and PTT; measure PTT regularly. Anticoagulation is present when PTT values are 1.5 to 2 times control value; draw blood for PTT 4 to 6 hours after an I.V. bolus dose and 12 to 24 hours after an S.C. dose. Blood may be drawn at any time after 8 hours of constant I.V. infusion; if I.V. therapy is intermittent, draw blood ½ hour before next scheduled dose to avoid falsely prolonged PTT. Never draw blood for PTT from the I.V. tubing of the heparin infusion, or from vein of infusion; falsely prolonged PTT will result. Always draw blood from other arm.
• I.V. administration is preferred because of long-term effect and because S.C. and I.M. injections are irregularly absorbed. When possible, administer I.V. heparin by infusion pump for maximum safety.
• When using heparin flush solution, keep intermittent I.V. line patent by flushing it with saline solution before and after the heparin; many medications are incompatible with heparin, and may form precipitate if they come in contact with heparin.
• For S.C. injection, use one needle to withdraw solution from vial and another to inject drug. Give low-dose S.C. injections sequentially between iliac crests in lower abdomen; give slowly and deep into subcutaneous fat. Gently wipe skin with alcohol; avoid vigorous rubbing. Insert ½" to ⅝" needle (25 G) at 90° angle. After inserting needle into skin, do not withdraw plunger to check for blood, to reduce risk of tissue injury and hematoma. Alternate site every 12 hours: right for morning, left for evening. Do not massage after S.C. injection; watch for local bleeding, hematoma, or inflammation. Rotate site.
• Check patient regularly for bleeding gums, bruises on arms or legs, petechiae, nosebleeds, melena, tarry stools, hematuria, or hematemesis. Monitor platelet counts regularly.
• Check I.V. infusions regularly, even when pumps are in good working order, to prevent overdose or underdose; do not piggyback other drugs into line while heparin infusion is running, because many antibiotics and other drugs inactivate heparin. Never mix any drug with heparin in syringe when bolus therapy is used.
• Avoid excessive I.M. injection of other drugs to prevent or minimize hematomas. If possible, do not give any I.M. injections.
• Abrupt withdrawal may increase coagulability; heparin is usually followed by prophylactic oral anticoagulant therapy.

Information for parents and patient
• Teach injection technique and methods of record-keeping if parents or patient will be administering the drug.
• Encourage compliance with medication schedule, follow-up appointments, and need for routine monitoring of blood studies; teach parents and patient signs of

bleeding, and emphasize importance of calling immediately at first sign of excess bleeding.
• Caution parents that patient should not take double dose if he misses one; tell patient to call for further instructions instead.
• Warn against use of aspirin and other OTC medications; stress need to seek medical approval before taking any new medication and need to tell all physicians and dentists about use of heparin.

hepatitis B immune globulin, human (HBIG)
H-BIG, Hep-B-Gammagee, HyperHep

• Classification: hepatitis B prophylaxis product (immune serum)

How supplied
Available by prescription only
Injection: 1-ml, 4-ml, and 5-ml vials

Indications, route, and dosage
Hepatitis B exposure
Neonates born to HB_sAg-positive women: 0.5 ml into the anterolateral thigh within 24 hours of birth. Repeat dose at age 3 months and 6 months.
Children and adults: 0.06 ml/kg I.M. within 7 days after exposure. Repeat 28 days after exposure.

The American College of Obstetricians and Gynecologists recommends use of HBIG in pregnancy for postexposure prophylaxis.

Action and kinetics
• *Postexposure prophylaxis of hepatitis B:* HBIG provides passive immunity to hepatitis B.
• *Kinetics in adults:* HBIG is absorbed slowly after I.M. injection. Antibodies to hepatitis B surface antigen (HB_sAg) appear in serum within 1 to 6 days, peak within 3 to 11 days, and persist for about 2 to 6 months. Evidence suggests that HBIG probably does not cross the placenta or distribute into breast milk. No information is available about drug's metabolism. The serum half-life for antibodies to HB_sAg is reportedly 21 days.

Contraindications and precautions
HBIG is contraindicated in patients with known hypersensitivity to thimerosal, a component of this immune serum.

Interactions
Concomitant use of HBIG may interfere with immune response to vaccination with live-virus vaccines, such as measles, mumps, and rubella. Live-virus vaccines should be administered 2 weeks before or 3 months after HBIG whenever possible.

Effects on diagnostic tests
None reported.

Adverse reactions
• DERM: *rash, pruritus.*
• Local: *pain and tenderness at injection site.*
• Systemic: urticaria, angioedema, anaphylactic reactions (rare; severe, potentially fatal reactions possible with I.V. administration).
• Other: *nausea, faintness, fever, body and joint pain.*

Overdose and treatment
No information available.

▶ Special considerations
• Administer as soon as possible within 24 hours or no later than 7 days.
• Obtain a thorough history of allergies and reactions to immunizations.
• Epinephrine solution 1:1,000 should be available to treat allergic reactions.
• Administer this preparation I.M. only. Severe, even fatal, reactions may occur if it is administered I.V.
• Gluteal or deltoid areas are the preferred injection sites in larger children and adults; the anterolateral thigh is preferred in neonates and small children.
• Infants treated with HBIG should be reevaluated at age 12 to 15 months to determine success of treatment.
• HBIG may be given simultaneously, but at different sites, with hepatitis B vaccine.
• Store between 36° and 46° F. (2° and 8° C.). Do not freeze.
• Hospital staff should receive immunization if exposed to hepatitis B (for example, from a needle stick or direct contact).
• HBIG has not been associated with a higher incidence of acquired immunodeficiency syndrome (AIDS). The immune globulin is devoid of human immunodeficiency virus (HIV). Immune globulin recipients do not develop antibodies to HIV.

Information for parents and patient
• Explain to parents that the patient's chances of getting AIDS after receiving HBIG are very small.
• Inform parents that HBIG provides temporary protection against hepatitis B only.
• Tell parents and patient what to expect after vaccination: local pain, swelling, and tenderness at the injection site. Recommend acetaminophen to relieve minor discomfort.
• Encourage parents to promptly report headache, skin changes, or difficulty breathing.

hetastarch (HES, hydroxyethyl starch)
Hespan

• Classification: plasma volume expander (amylopectin derivative)

How supplied
Available by prescription only
Injection: 500 ml (6 g/100 ml in 0.9% sodium chloride solution)

Indications, route, and dosage
Plasma expander in shock and cardiopulmonary bypass surgery
†*Children and adults:* 500 to 1,000 ml I.V. dependent on amount of blood lost and resultant hemoconcentration. Total dosage usually should not exceed 1,500 ml/day. Up to 20 ml/kg (1.2 g/kg)/hour may be used in hemorrhagic shock; in burns or septic shock, the rate should be reduced.
Leukapheresis adjunct
Hetastarch is an adjunct in leukapheresis to improve harvesting and increase the yield of granulocytes.

Hetastarch 250 to 700 ml is infused at a constant fixed ratio, usually 1:8 to venous whole blood during continous flow centrifugation (CFC) procedures. Up to 2 CFC procedures/week, with a total number of 7 to 10 procedures using hetastarch, have been found safe and effective. The safety of larger numbers of procedures is unknown.

Action and kinetics
• *Plasma volume expander:* Hetastarch has an average molecular weight of 450,000 and exhibits colloidal properties similar to human albumin. After an I.V. infusion of hetastarch 6%, the plasma volume expands slightly in excess of the volume infused because of the colloidal osmotic effect. Maximum plasma volume expansion occurs in a few minutes and decreases over 24 to 36 hours. Hemodynamic status may improve for 24 hours or longer.
• *Leukapheresis adjunct:* Hetastarch enhances the yield of granulocytes by centrifugal means.
• *Kinetics in adults:* After I.V. administration, the plasma volume expands within a few minutes. Hetastarch is distributed in the blood plasma. Hetastarch molecules with a molecular weight over 50,000 are slowly degraded enzymatically to molecules that can be excreted. Forty percent of hetastarch molecules with a molecular weight under 50,000 are excreted in urine within 24 hours. Hetastarch molecules that are not hydroxyethylated are slowly degraded to glucose. Approximately 90% of the dose is eliminated from the body with an average half-life of 17 days; the remainder has a half-life of 48 days.

Contraindications and precautions
Hetastarch is contraindicated in patients with severe bleeding disorders, because it contains no clotting factors; in patients with severe congestive heart failure (CHF) or renal failure with oliguria or anuria, because it may worsen these conditions; or for treating shock in the absence of hypovolemia, because the potential for volume overload.

Hetastarch should be used cautiously in patients with impaired renal or hepatic function, pulmonary edema, or CHF, to prevent circulatory overload; and in patients with thrombocytopenia, because the compound may interfere with platelet function. Large volumes of hetastarch may prolong prothrombin time (PT), partial thromboplastin time (PTT), bleeding time, and clotting time and may decrease hematocrit and protein concentrations.

Interactions
None reported.

Effects on diagnostic tests
When added to whole blood, hetastarch increases the erythrocyte sedimentation rate.

Adverse reactions
• CNS: headache.
• CV: peripheral edema of lower extremities; circulatory overload; heart failure; elevated PT, PTT, and clotting and bleeding times.
• DERM: urticaria, pruritus.
• EENT: periorbital edema, parotid gland enlargement.
• GI: nausea, vomiting.
• Other: muscle pain; anaphylactoid reaction, including wheezing, mild fever.
  Note: Drug should be discontinued if allergic or sensitivity reaction occurs.

Overdose and treatment
Clinical manifestations of overdose include the adverse reactions. Stop the infusion if an overdose occurs and treat supportively.

▶ Special considerations
• To avoid circulatory overload, carefully monitor patients with impaired renal function and those at high risk of pulmonary edema or CHF. Hetastarch 6% in 0.9% sodium chloride contains 77 mEq sodium and chloride per 500 ml.
• Do not administer as a substitute for blood or plasma.
• Discard partially used bottle because it does not contain a preservative.
• Monitor CBC, total leukocyte and platelet counts, leukocyte differential count, hemoglobin, hematocrit, PT and PTT, and electrolyte, BUN, and creatinine levels.
• Assess vital signs and cardiopulmonary status to obtain baseline at start of infusion to prevent fluid overload.
• Monitor I.V. site for signs of infiltration and phlebitis.
• Observe patient for edema.

Information for parents and patient
• Explain therapy to parents and patient. Advise parents to monitor for adverse reactions.
• Explain that therapy carries no risk of infection because drug is not derived from blood.

---

homatropine hydrobromide
AK-Homatropine, I-Homatrine, Isopto Homatropine, Minims-Homatropine*

• Classification: cycloplegic, mydriatic (anticholinergic agent)

How supplied
Available by prescription only
Ophthalmic solution: 2%, 5%

dications, route, and dosage
ycloplegic refraction
uildren and adults: Instill 1 to 2 drops of 2% solution
 1 drop of 5% solution in eye immediately before
ocedure, and repeat in 5- to 10-minute intervals.
veitis
uildren and adults: Instill 1 to 2 drops of 2% or 5%
lution in eye b.i.d. or t.i.d. In adults, dosage fre-
.ency may be increased to q 3 to 4 hours.

ction and kinetics
• *Cycloplegic and mydriatic action:* Anticholinergic ac-
on prevents the sphincter muscle of the iris and the
uscle of the ciliary body from responding to cholin-
gic stimulation, resulting in unopposed adrenergic
fluence and producing pupillary dilation (mydriasis
d paralysis of accommodation [cycloplegia]).
• *Kinetics in adults:* Peak effect is reached in 40 to
 minutes. Recovery from cycloplegic and mydriatic
fects usually occurs within 1 to 3 days.

ontraindications and precautions
omatropine is contraindicated in patients with nar-
w-angle glaucoma or hypersensitivity to belladonna
kaloids (such as atropine) or any other component.
 should be used cautiously in patients with hyper-
nsion, cardiac disease, or increased intraocular
essure.

teractions
omatropine may interfere with the antiglaucoma ef-
cts of pilocarpine, carbachol, or cholinesterase in-
bitors.

ffects on diagnostic tests
one significant.

dverse reactions
CNS: dysarthria, hallucinations, amnesia, ataxia,
eadache, somnolence.
CV: tachycardia, hypotension, dysrhythmias, vaso-
lation.
DERM: allergic reaction, flushing, dryness, rash
hildren).
Eye: irritation, blurred vision, stinging, allergic lid
eactions, hyperemia, edema, exudate.
GI: decreased GI motility, abdominal distention (in-
.nts).
GU: bladder distention, urinary retention.
Other: fever, respiratory depression, coma, death.
  Note: Drug should be discontinued if signs of sys-
emic toxicity occur.

verdose and treatment
linical manifestations of overdose include flushed
ry skin, dry mouth, blurred vision, ataxia, dysar-
aria, hallucinations, tachycardia, and decreased
owel sounds.
  Treat accidental ingestion by emesis or activated
narcoal. Use physostigmine to antagonize homatro-
ine's anticholinergic activity in severe toxicity; pro-
ranolol may be used to treat symptomatic
achydysrhythmias unresponsive to physostigmine.

▶ Special considerations
• Drug should be used with caution in small children
and in infants. Increased chance of sensitivity exists
in children with Down's syndrome, spastic paralysis,
or brain damage.
• Homatropine may produce symptoms of atropine sulfate poisoning, such as severe mouth dryness and
tachycardia.
• Drug should not be used internally.
• Patient may be photophobic and may benefit by wearing dark glasses to minimize discomfort.
• Finger pressure should be applied to lacrimal sac
for 1 to 2 minutes after instillation to decrease risk
of absorption or systemic reaction.

Information for parents and patient
• Tell parents and patient that vision will be temporarily blurred after instillation.
• Inform parents and patient that drug may produce
drowsiness.

hyaluronidase
Wydase

• Classification: adjunctive agent to increase absorption and dispersion of injected drugs (protein enzyme)

How supplied
Available by prescription only
Injection: 150 USP units/vial, 1500 USP units/vial;
150 USP units/ml in 1-ml and 10-ml vials

Indications, route, and dosage
Adjunct to increase absorption and disper-
sion of other injected drugs
Children and adults: Add 150 USP units to solution
containing other medication.
Adjunct to increase the absorption rate of
fluids given by hypodermoclysis
Children and adults: Add 150 USP units to each liter
of clysis solution administered.
Adjunct in excretion urography
Children and adults: Administer 75 USP units S.C.
over each scapula, before administration of the contrast medium.

Action and kinetics
• *Diffusing action:* Hyaluronidase is a spreading or
diffusing substance that modifies the permeability of
connective tissue through the hydrolysis of hyaluronic
acid. The drug enhances the diffusion of substances
injected subcutaneously provided local interstitial
pressure is adequate.
• *Kinetics in adults:* Absorption, distribution, metabolism, and excretion have not been described.

Contraindications and precautions
Hyaluronidase is contraindicated in patients with
known hypersensitivity to the drug; and for injection
into infected, acutely inflamed, or cancerous areas.

May contain sulfites   ♦ May contain tartrazine   ♦ ♦ May contain benzyl alcohol

Interactions

Concomitant use with local anesthetics may increase analgesia, hasten onset, and reduce local swelling; but may also increase systemic absorption, increase toxicity, and shorten duration of action.

Effects on diagnostic tests

None reported.

Adverse reactions

• Local: irritation, hypersensitivity reaction (erythema, wheal with pseudopods and urticaria).

Note: Drug should be discontinued if hypersensitivity occurs.

Overdose and treatment

Up to 75,000 units have been administered without ill effect; local adverse effects would be anticipated. Treat symptomatically.

▶ Special considerations

• If administering hyaluronidase for hypodermoclysis, take care to avoid overhydration. In children under age 3, clysis should not exceed 200 ml; in premature neonates, clysis should not exceed 25 ml/kg and the rate should not exceed 2 ml/minute.

• Give skin test for sensitivity before use; a wheal with pseudopods appearing within 5 minutes after injection and lasting for 20 to 30 minutes along with urticaria indicates a positive reaction.

• Avoid contact with eyes; if it occurs, flood with water immediately.

• Hyaluronidase also may be used to diffuse local anesthetics at the site of injection, especially in nerve block anesthesia. It also has been used to enhance the diffusion of drugs in the management of I.V. extravasation.

Information for parents and patient

Instruct parents to report any unusual and significant reactions after injection.

---

hydralazine hydrochloride

Alazine Tabs, Apresoline

• Classification: antihypertensive (peripheral vasodilator)

How supplied

Available by prescription only
Tablets: 10 mg, 25 mg, 50 mg, 100 mg
Injection: 20 mg/ml

Indications, route, and dosage
Moderate to severe hypertension

Children: Initially, 0.75 mg/kg P.O. daily in four divided doses (25 mg/m² daily); may increase gradually to 9 mg/kg daily.

I.M. or I.V. drug dosage is 0.1 to 0.8 mg/kg q I.V. 3 to 6 hours.

Adults: Initially, 10 mg P.O. q.i.d. for 2 to 4 days, then increased to 25 mg q.i.d. for the remainder of the week. If necessary, dosage is increased to 50 mg q.i. Maximum recommended dosage is 200 mg daily, b some patients may require 300 to 400 mg daily.

For severe hypertension, 10 to 50 mg I.M. or 10 20 mg I.V. repeated as necessary. Switch to oral a tihypertensives as soon as possible.

For hypertensive crisis associated with pregnanc initially 5 mg I.V., followed by 5 to 10 mg I.V. ever 20 to 30 minutes until adequate reduction in bloc pressure is achieved (usual range is 5 to 20 mg).

†Short-term management of severe CHF

Children or adults: Initially, 50 to 75 mg P.O.; the adjusted according to patient response. Most patien respond to 200 to 600 mg daily, divided q 6 to **1** hours, but dosages as high as 3 g daily have bee used.

Action and kinetics

• *Antihypertensive action:* Hydralazine has a dire vasodilating effect on vascular smooth muscle, th lowering blood pressure. Hydralazine's effect on r sistance vessels (arterioles and arteries) is great than that on capacitance vessels (venules and veins

• *Kinetics in adults:* Hydralazine is absorbed rapid from the GI tract after oral administration; pea plasma levels occur in 1 hour. Antihypertensive effe occurs 20 to 30 minutes after oral dose, 5 to 2 minutes after I.V. administration, and 10 to 30 mi utes after I.M. administration. Food enhances a sorption. Hydralazine is distributed widely througho the body; drug is approximately 88% to 90% protei bound. Hydralazine is metabolized extensively in t GI mucosa and the liver. Most of a given dose hydralazine is excreted in urine, primarily as met: olites; about 10% of an oral dose is excreted in fece Antihypertensive effect persists 2 to 4 hours after oral dose and 2 to 6 hours after I.V. or I.M. admi istration.

Contraindications and precautions

Hydralazine is contraindicated in patients with know hypersensitivity to the drug and in patients with n tral valve rheumatic heart disease or coronary arte disease. Drug should be used cautiously in patier with a history of stroke or severe renal damage, t cause these conditions may be exacerbated by h potension.

Interactions

Hydralazine may potentiate the effects of diureti and other antihypertensive medications; profound h potension may occur if drug is given with diazoxic

Concomitant administration with MAO inhibitc may synergistically decrease blood pressure; hydr: azine may decrease the pressor response to epinep rine.

Effects on diagnostic tests

Hydralazine may cause positive antinuclear antibo (ANA) titer; positive lupus erythematosus (LE) c preparation; blood dyscrasias, including leukopen agranulocytosis, and purpura; and hematologic a normalities, including decreased hemoglobin and RI count.

Adverse reactions
• CNS: peripheral neuritis, headache, dizziness *muscle tremors, cramps.*
• CV: orthostatic hypotension, *tachycardia,* dysrhythmias, angina, palpitations, *edema.*
• DERM: rash.
• GI: nausea, *vomiting, diarrhea, anorexia,* weight gain, *GI hemorrhage.*
• HEMA: neutropenia, *leukopenia.*
• Other: *systemic lupus erythematosus (SLE) syndrome, nasal congestion, lacrimation, conjunctivitis.*
  Note: Drug should be discontinued if patient develops signs or symptoms of SLE or blood dyscrasias, a positive ANA titer, or positive LE cell preparation.

Overdose and treatment
Clinical signs of overdose include hypotension, tachycardia, headache, and skin flushing; cardiac dysrhythmias and shock may occur.
  After acute ingestion, empty stomach by emesis or gastric lavage and give activated charcoal to reduce absorption. Follow with symptomatic and supportive care.

▶ Special considerations
• Hydralazine has had limited use in children, and its safety and efficacy in children have not been established; use only if potential benefit outweighs risk.
• CBC, LE cell preparation, and ANA titer determinations should be performed before therapy and at regular intervals during long-term therapy.
• The incidence of hydralazine-induced SLE syndrome is greatest in patients receiving more than 200 mg/day for prolonged periods.
• Headache and palpitations may occur 2 to 4 hours after first oral dose but should subside spontaneously.
• Advise precautions for postural hypotension.
• Food enhances oral absorption and helps minimize gastric irritation; adhere to consistent schedule.
• Some preparations contain tartrazine, which may precipitate allergic reactions, especially in aspirin-sensitive patients.
• For I.V. administration: Monitor blood pressure every 5 minutes until stable, then every 15 minutes; put patient in Trendelenburg's position if he is faint or dizzy. Too-rapid reduction in blood pressure can cause mental changes from cerebral ischemia.
• Inject drug as soon as possible after draining through needle into syringe; drug changes color after contact with metal.
• Remember that patients with renal impairment may respond to lower maintenance doses of hydralazine.
• Sodium retention can occur with long-term use; observe for signs of weight gain and edema.

Information for parents and patient
• Teach parents and patient about the disease and therapy, and explain why the patient must take drug exactly as prescribed, even when feeling well; warn them that discontinuing the drug suddenly may cause severe rebound hypertension.
• Explain adverse effects and advise parents to report any unusual effects, especially symptoms of SLE (sore throat, fever, muscle and joint pain, and skin rash).
• Explain how to minimize impact of adverse effects:

to avoid hazardous activities until tolerance develops to sedation, drowsiness, and other CNS effects; to avoid sudden position change to minimize orthostatic hypotension; to avoid alcohol; and to take drug with meals to enhance absorption and minimize gastric irritation.
• Reassure parents and patient that headaches and palpitations occurring 2 to 4 hours after initial dose usually subside spontaneously; if not, they should report such effects.
• Instruct parents to weigh patient at least weekly. Advise them to report excessive weight gain (5 lb [2.3 kg] per week or more).
• Warn parents to seek medical approval before giving nonprescription cold preparations to the patient.

▬▬▬▬▬▬▬▬▬▬▬▬▬▬▬▬▬▬▬▬

hydrochlorothiazide
Apo-Hydro*, Aprozide, Chlorzide, Diaqua, Diuchlor-H*, Esidrix, HydroDIURIL, Hydromal, Hydro-Z-50, Hyperetic, Natrimax*, NeoCodema*, Novohydrazide*, Oretic, Ro-Hydrazide, SK-Hydrochlorothiazide, Urozide*

• Classification: diuretic, antihypertensive (thiazide)

How supplied
Available by prescription only
Tablets: 25 mg, 50 mg, 100 mg

Indications, route, and dosage
Edema
Children under age 6 months: up to 3.3 mg/kg P.O. daily divided b.i.d.
Children over age 6 months: 2.2 mg/kg or 60 mg/m² P.O. daily divided b.i.d.
  Daily dosage range in children age 2 to 12 is 3.75 to 100 mg; in children age 2 years or younger, 12.5 to 37.5 mg.

Action and kinetics
• *Diuretic action:* Hydrochlorothiazide increases urinary excretion of sodium and water by inhibiting sodium reabsorption in the cortical diluting tubule of the nephron, thus relieving edema.
• *Antihypertensive action:* The exact mechanism of hydrochlorothiazide's antihypertensive effect is unknown. It may result partially from direct arteriolar vasodilation and a decrease in total peripheral resistance.
• *Kinetics in adults:* Hydrochlorothiazide is absorbed from the GI tract. The rate and extent of absorption vary with different formulations of this drug. Hydrochlorothiazide is excreted unchanged in urine, usually within 24 hours.

Contraindications and precautions
Hydrochlorothiazide is contraindicated in patients with known hypersensitivity to the drug or to sulfonamide derivatives. Hydrochlorothiazide should be used cautiously in patients with severe renal disease, because reduced glomerular filtration rate may cause

azotemia; and in patients with impaired hepatic function or liver disease, because electrolyte alterations may precipitate hepatic coma. Hydrochlorothiazide-induced hypokalemia may predispose patients taking digoxin to digitalis toxicity.

Interactions

Hydrochlorothiazide potentiates the hypotensive effects of most other antihypertensive drugs; this may be used to therapeutic advantage.

Hydrochlorothiazide may potentiate hyperglycemic, hypotensive, and hyperuricemic effects of diazoxide, and its hyperglycemic effect may increase insulin requirements in diabetic patients.

Hydrochlorothiazide may reduce renal clearance of lithium, elevating serum lithium levels, and may necessitate reduction in lithium dosage by 50%.

Hydrochlorothiazide turns urine slightly more alkaline and may decrease urinary excretion of some amines, such as amphetamine and quinidine; alkaline urine also may decrease therapeutic efficacy of methenamine compounds such as methenamine mandelate.

Cholestyramine and colestipol may bind hydrochlorothiazide, preventing its absorption; give drugs 1 hour apart.

Effects on diagnostic tests

Hydrochlorothiazide therapy may alter serum electrolyte levels and may increase serum urate, glucose, cholesterol, and triglyceride levels. It also may interfere with tests for parathyroid function and should be discontinued before such tests.

Adverse reactions

• CV: volume depletion and dehydration, orthostatic hypotension, hypercholesterolemia, hypertriglyceridemia.
• DERM: dermatitis, photosensitivity, rash.
• GI: anorexia, nausea, pancreatitis.
• HEMA: aplastic anemia, agranulocytosis, leukopenia, thrombocytopenia.
• Hepatic: *hepatic encephalopathy, hyperbilirubinemia.*
• Metabolic: asymptomatic *hyperuricemia;* gout; *hyperglycemia* and impairment of glucose tolerance; fluid and electrolyte imbalances, including dilutional hyponatremia and hypochloremia, hypercalcemia, and *hypokalemia; metabolic alkalosis.*
• Other: hypersensitivity reactions, such as pneumonitis and vasculitis.
  Note: Drug should be discontinued if rising BUN and serum creatinine levels indicate renal impairment or if patient shows signs of impending coma.

Overdose and treatment

Clinical signs of overdose include GI irritation and hypermotility, diuresis, and lethargy, which may progress to coma.

Treatment is mainly supportive; monitor and assist respiratory, cardiovascular, and renal function as indicated. Monitor fluid and electrolyte balance. Induce vomiting with ipecac in conscious patient; otherwise, use gastric lavage to avoid aspiration. Do not give cathartics; these promote additional loss of fluids and electrolytes.

▶ Special considerations

• Monitor weight and serum electrolyte levels regularly.
• Monitor serum potassium levels; encourage high-potassium diet. Foods rich in potassium include citrus fruits, tomatoes, bananas, dates, and apricots. Watch for signs of hypokalemia (for example, muscle weakness or cramps). Patients also taking digitalis have an increased risk of digitalis toxicity from the potassium-depleting effect of these diuretics.
• Drug may be used with potassium-sparing diuretics to attenuate potassium loss.
• Check insulin requirements in patients with diabetes.
• Monitor serum creatinine and BUN levels regularly. Drug is not as effective if these levels are more than twice normal.
• Monitor blood uric acid levels.
• A.M. administration is recommended to prevent nocturia.
• Antihypertensive effects persist for approximately 1 week after discontinuation of the drug.
• Instruct parents to observe for and to report any joint swelling, pain, or redness; these signs may indicate hyperuricemia.

Information for parents and patient

• Explain rationale of therapy and diuretic effects of drug.
• Advise parents to watch for and promptly report signs of electrolyte imbalance: weakness, fatigue, muscle cramps, paresthesias, confusion, nausea, vomiting, diarrhea, headache, dizziness, and palpitations.
• Tell parents to report any increased edema or weight or excess diuresis (more than 2% gain or loss) and to record child's weight each morning after voiding and before breakfast on the same scale and wearing the same type of clothing.
• Advise parents to give drug with food to minimize gastric irritation; to encourage child to eat potassium-rich foods, such as citrus fruits, potatoes, dates, raisins, and bananas; and to restrict child's access to salt and high-sodium foods, such as lunch meat, smoked meats, and processed cheeses. Inform parents that low-sodium formulas are available for infants.
• Tell parents to seek medical approval before giving the patient nonprescription drugs; many contain sodium and potassium and can cause electrolyte imbalances.
• Explain photosensitivity reactions. In thiazide-related photosensitivity, ultraviolet radiation alters drug structure, causing allergic reactions in some persons; such reactions occurs 10 days to 2 weeks after initial sun exposure.
• Warn parents to supervise the child's activities closely to prevent falls and other injuries that may result from dizziness, especially at beginning of therapy.
• Caution patient to change position slowly, especially when rising to upright position, to prevent dizziness from orthostatic hypotension.
• Advise parents to watch patient closely for signs of

---

chest, back, or leg pain; or shortness of breath and to call immediately if they occur.
• Advise parents to administer drug only as prescribed and at the same time each day, to prevent nighttime diuresis and interrupted sleep.
• Emphasize importance of regular medical follow-up to monitor effectiveness of diuretic therapy.

hydrocortisone
Systemic: Cortef, Cortenema, Hycort*, Hydrocortone

Topical: Acticort, Barriere-HC*, Calde CORT, Cetacort, Cortate*, Cort-Dome, Cortizone, Dermacort, Dermi Cort, Dermolate, Dermtex HC, Dioderm*, Efcortelan*, Emo-Cort*, HC-Jel, Hi-Cor, H₂Cort, Hydro-Tex, Hytone, Nutracort, Penecort, Racet-SE, Rectocort*, Synacort, Unicort*

hydrocortisone acetate
Systemic: Biosone, Colifoam*, Cortifoam, Hydrocortistab*

Topical: Cortaid, Cort-Dome, Corticaine, Corticreme*, Cortiment*, Cortoderm*, Hyderm*, Lanacort, Novohydrocort*, Orabase-HCA, Pharma-Cort, Rhulicort

hydrocortisone butyrate
Topical: Locoid

hydrocortisone cypionate
Systemic: Cortef

hydrocortisone sodium phosphate
Systemic: Efcortesol*, Hydrocortone Phosphate

hydrocortisone sodium succinate
Systemic: A-hydroCort, Efcortelan Soluble*, Lifocort, Solu-Cortef

hydrocortisone valerate
Topical: Westcort

• Classification: adrenocorticoid replacement (glucocorticoid, mineralocorticoid)

How supplied
Available by prescription only
Hydrocortisone
Tablets: 5 mg, 10 mg, 20 mg
Injection: 25 mg/ml, 50 mg/ml suspension
Enema: 100 mg/60 ml
Cream: .125%, 0.25%, 0.5%, 1%, 2.5%
Ointment: 0.5%, 1%, 2.5%
Lotion: 0.125%, 0.25%, 0.5%, 1%, 2%, 2.5%

Gel: 1%
Solution: 1%
Aerosol: 0.5%
Hydrocortisone acetate
Injection: 25 mg/ml, 50 mg/ml suspension
Enema: 10% aerosol foam (provides 90 mg/application)
Aerosol foam: 0.5%
Cream: 0.5%
Ointment: 0.5%, 1%, 2.5%
Lotion: 0.5%
Suppositories: 10 mg, 15 mg, 25 mg
Hydrocortisone butyrate
Cream, ointment: 0.1%
Hydrocortisone cypionate
Oral suspension: 10 mg/5 ml
Hydrocortisone sodium phosphate
Injection: 50 mg/ml solution
Hydrocortisone sodium succinate
Injection: 100 mg, 250 mg, 500 mg, 1,000 mg/vial
Hydrocortisone valerate
Cream, ointment: 0.2%
Available without prescription
Hydrocortisone
Cream, ointment, lotion: 0.5%
Hydrocortisone acetate
Cream, ointment, lotion: 0.5%

Indications, route, and dosage
Adrenocortical insufficiency
Hydrocortisone suspension
560 mcg/kg or 30 to 37.5 mg/m² I.M. every third day; alternatively give 186 to 280 mcg/kg or 10 to 12.5 mg/m² I.M. daily.
Hydrocortisone sodium phosphate
Children: 186 to 280 mcg/kg or 10 to 12 mg/m² I.M. or I.V. daily in three divided doses.
Hydrocortisone sodium succinate
Children: 186 to 280 mcg/kg or 10 to 12 mg/m² I.M. or I.V. daily in three divided doses.
Severe inflammation
Hydrocortisone suspension
Children: 666 mcg to 4 mg/kg or 20 to 120 mg/m² I.M. q 12 to 24 hours.
Hydrocortisone sodium phosphate
Children: 666 mcg to 4 mg/kg or 20 to 120 mg/m² I.M. or I.V. q 12 to 24 hours.
Hydrocortisone sodium succinate
Children: 666 mcg to 4 mg/kg or 20 to 120 mg/m² I.M. or I.V. q 12 to 24 hours
Inflammation of corticosteroid-responsive dermatoses, including those on face, groin, armpits, and under breasts; seborrheic dermatitis of scalp
Children: Apply 0.125% to 1% cream, lotion, ointment, foam, gel, or solution once or twice a day. Or apply 2% to 2.5% ointment, lotion, or cream once a day.
Adults: Apply cream, lotion, ointment, foam, or aerosol sparingly once daily to q.i.d.

Action and kinetics
• *Adrenocorticoid replacement action:* Hydrocortisone is an adrenocorticoid with both glucocorticoid and mineralocorticoid properties. It is a weak anti-inflammatory agent but a potent mineralocorticoid, hav-

‡May contain sulfites   ◆May contain tartrazine   ◆◆May contain benzyl alcohol

ing potency similar to that of cortisone and twice that of prednisone. Hydrocortisone (or cortisone) is usually the drug of choice for replacement therapy in patients with adrenal insufficiency. It is usually not used for immunosuppressant activity because of the extremely large doses necessary and the unwanted mineralocorticoid effects.

Hydrocortisone and hydrocortisone cypionate may be administered orally. Hydrocortisone sodium phosphate may be administered by I.M., subcutaneous, or I.V. injection or by I.V. infusion, usually at 12-hour intervals. Hydrocortisone sodium succinate may be administered by I.M. or I.V. injection or I.V. infusion every 2 to 10 hours, depending on the clinical situation. Hydrocortisone acetate is a suspension that may be administered by intra-articular, intrasynovial, intrabursal, intralesional, or soft tissue injection. It has a slow onset but a long duration of action. The injectable forms are usually used only when the oral dosage forms cannot be used.

• *Anti-inflammatory action:* Hydrocortisone stimulates the synthesis of enzymes needed to decrease the inflammatory response. Hydrocortisone, a corticosteroid secreted by the adrenal cortex, is about 1.25 times more potent an anti-inflammatory agent than equivalent doses of cortisone, but both have twice the mineralocorticoid activity of the other glucocorticoids. As topical agents, hydrocortisone and hydrocortisone acetate are low-potency group VI glucocorticoids. Hydrocortisone valerate has group IV potency.

Hydrocortisone 0.5% and hydrocortisone acetate 0.5% are available without a prescription for the temporary relief of minor skin irritation, itching, and rashes caused by eczema, insect bites, soaps, and detergents.

Hydrocortisone is also administered rectally as a retention enema for the temporary treatment of acute ulcerative colitis. Hydrocortisone acetate suspension is also available as a rectal suppository or aerosol foam suspension for the temporary treatment of inflammatory conditions of the rectum such as hemorrhoids, cryptitis, proctitis, and pruritus ani.

• *Kinetics in adults:* Hydrocortisone is absorbed readily after oral administration. After oral and I.V. administration, peak effects occur in about 1 to 2 hours. The acetate suspension for injection has a variable absorption over 24 to 48 hours, depending on whether it is injected into an intra-articular space or a muscle, and the blood supply to that muscle.

Hydrocortisone is removed rapidly from the blood and distributed to muscle, liver, skin, intestines, and kidneys. Hydrocortisone is bound extensively to plasma proteins (transcortin and albumin). Only the unbound portion is active. Adrenocorticoids are distributed into breast milk and through the placenta.

After topical application, absorption of hydrocortisone depends on concentration, the amount applied, and the application site. It ranges from about 1% in areas with a thick stratum corneum (such as the palms, soles, elbows, and knees), to as high as 36% in areas where the stratum corneum is thinnest (face, eyelids, and genitals). Absorption increases in skin that is damaged, inflamed, or under occlusion. Some systemic absorption occurs, especially through the oral mucosa.

After topical application, hydrocortisone is distributed throughout the local skin layers and metabolized primarily in the skin. Any drug absorbed is removed rapidly from the blood and distributed into muscle, liver, skin, intestines, and kidneys, and metabolized primarily in the liver to inactive glucuronide and sulfate metabolites.

Inactive metabolites are excreted by the kidneys, primarily as glucuronides and sulfates, but also as unconjugated products. Small amounts of the metabolites are also excreted in feces. The biological half-life of hydrocortisone is 8 to 12 hours.

Contraindications and precautions

Hydrocortisone is contraindicated in patients with systemic fungal infections (except in adrenal insufficiency) and in those with a hypersensitivity to ingredients of adrenocorticoid preparations. Patients who are receiving hydrocortisone should not be given live virus vaccines because hydrocortisone suppresses the immune response.

Hydrocortisone should be used with extreme caution in patients with GI ulceration, renal disease, hypertension, osteoporosis, diabetes mellitus, thromboembolic disorders, seizures, myasthenia gravis, congestive heart failure (CHF), tuberculosis, hypoalbuminemia, hypothyroidism, cirrhosis of the liver, emotional instability, psychotic tendencies, hyperlipidemias, glaucoma, or cataracts, because the drug may exacerbate these conditions.

Because adrenocorticoids increase the susceptibility to and mask symptoms of infection, hydrocortisone should not be used (except in life-threatening situations) in patients with viral or bacterial infections not controlled by anti-infective agents.

Topical use of hydrocortisone is contraindicated in patients who are hypersensitive to any component of the preparation and in patients with viral, fungal, or tubercular skin lesions. Drug should be used with extreme caution in patients with impaired circulation because it may increase the risk of skin ulceration.

Interactions

When used concomitantly, systemic hydrocortisone may in rare cases decrease the effects of oral anticoagulants by unknown mechanisms. Concomitant use of barbiturates, phenytoin, or rifampin may decrease corticosteroid effects because of increased hepatic metabolism. Cholestyramine, colestipol, and antacids decrease corticosteroid effect by adsorbing the corticosteroid, thereby decreasing the amount absorbed.

Hydrocortisone increases the metabolism of isoniazid and salicylates; this causes hyperglycemia, requiring dosage adjustment of insulin in diabetic patients. It may enhance hypokalemia associated with diuretic or amphotericin B therapy. The hypokalemia may increase the risk of toxicity in patients receiving digitalis.

Concomitant use of estrogens may reduce the metabolism of corticosteroids by increasing the concentration of transcortin. The half-life of the corticosteroid is then prolonged from increased protein binding. Concomitant administration of ulcerogenic drugs, such as nonsteroidal anti-inflammatory agents, may increase the risk of GI ulceration.

Effects on diagnostic tests

Hydrocortisone suppresses reactions to skin tests; causes false-negative results in the nitroblue tetrazolium tests for systemic bacterial infections; and decreases ^{131}I uptake and protein-bound iodine concentrations in thyroid function tests.

Hydrocortisone may increase glucose and cholesterol levels; may decrease serum potassium, calcium, thyroxine, and triiodothyronine levels; and may increase urine glucose and calcium levels.

Adverse reactions

When administered in high doses or for prolonged therapy, hydrocortisone suppresses release of adrenocorticotropic hormone (ACTH) from the pituitary gland, and the adrenal cortex stops secreting endogenous corticosteroids. The degree and duration of hypothalamic-pituitary-adrenal (HPA) axis suppression produced by the drug is highly variable among patients and depends on the dose, frequency and time of administration, and duration of glucocorticoid therapy.
• CNS: euphoria, insomnia, headache, psychotic behavior, pseudotumor cerebri, mental changes, nervousness, restlessness, *psychoses*.
• CV: CHF, *hypertension*, edema.
• DERM: delayed healing, *acne*, skin eruptions, striae.
• EENT: *cataracts*, glaucoma, thrush.
• GI: *peptic ulcer*, irritation, increased appetite.
• Immune: immunosuppression, *increased susceptibility to infection*.
• Metabolic: *hypokalemia*, sodium retention, fluid retention, weight gain, hyperglycemia, osteoporosis, growth suppression in children, *glycosuria*.
• Musculoskeletal: muscle weakness, muscle atrophy, *myopathy*.
• Local: burning, itching, irritation, dryness, folliculitis, hypertrichosis, acneiform eruptions, hypopigmentation, perioral dermatitis, allergic contact dermatitis, maceration, secondary infection, atrophy, striae, miliaria.
• Other: pancreatitis, *hirsutism, cushingoid symptoms*, withdrawal syndrome (nausea, fatigue, anorexia, dyspnea, hypotension, hypoglycemia, myalgia, arthralgia, fever, dizziness, and fainting), *ecchymoses*. Sudden discontinuation of systemic use may be fatal or may exacerbate the underlying disease. Acute adrenal insufficiency may occur with increased stress (infection, surgery, trauma) or abrupt withdrawal after long-term therapy.
   Note: Topical use should be discontinued if local irritation, infection, systemic absorption, or hypersensitivity reaction occurs.

Overdose and treatment

Acute ingestion, even in massive doses, is rarely a clinical problem. Toxic signs and symptoms rarely occur if drug is used for less than 3 weeks, even at large doses. However, chronic systemic use causes adverse physiologic effects, including suppression of the HPA axis, cushingoid appearance, muscle weakness, and osteoporosis.

▶ Special considerations

• Chronic use of hydrocortisone dosage that exceeds physiologic replacement may delay growth and maturation in children and adolescents.
• If possible, avoid long-term administration of pharmacologic dosages of glucocorticoids in children because these drugs may retard bone growth. Manifestations of adrenal suppression in children include retardation of linear growth, delayed weight gain, low plasma corticol concentrations, and lack of response to corticotropin stimulation. In children who require prolonged therapy, closely monitor growth and development. Alternate-day therapy is recommended to minimize growth suppression.
• Establish baseline blood pressure, fluid intake and output, weight, and electrolyte status.
• During times of physiologic stress (trauma, surgery, infection), the patient may require additional steroids and may experience signs of steroid withdrawal, patients who were previously steroid-dependent may need systemic corticosteroids to prevent adrenal insufficiency.
• After long-term therapy, the drug should be reduced gradually. Rapid reduction may cause withdrawal symptoms.
• Be aware of the patient's psychological history and watch for any behavioral changes.
• Observe for signs of infection or delayed wound healing.
• Acute withdrawal of drug may result in fever, myalgia, arthralgia, malaise, hypotension, hypoglycemic shock.

Topical administration

• Children may show greater susceptibility to topical corticosteroid-induced HPA axis suppression and Cushing's syndrome than mature patients because of a higher ratio of skin surface area to body weight. Hypothalamic-pituitary-adrenal (HPA) axis suppression, Cushing's syndrome, and intracranial hypertension have been reported in children receiving topical corticosteroids. Signs of intracranial hypertension include bulging fontanelles, headaches, and bilateral papilledema.
• Administration of topical corticosteroids to children should be limited to the least effective amount. Chronic corticosteroid therapy may interfere with growth and development.
• Stop drug if the patient develops signs of systemic absorption (including Cushing's syndrome, hyperglycemia, or glucosuria), skin irritation or ulceration, hypersensitivity, or infection. (If antifungals or antibiotics are being used with corticosteroids and the infection does not respond immediately, corticosteroids should be stopped until infection is controlled.)
• Monitor patient response. Observe area of inflammation and elicit patient comments concerning pruritus. Inspect skin for infection, striae, and atrophy. Skin atrophy is common and may be clinically significant within 3 to 4 weeks of treatment with high-potency preparations; it also occurs more readily at sites where percutaneous absorption is high.
• Do not apply occlusive dressings over topical steroids because this may lead to secondary infection, maceration, atrophy, striae, or miliaria caused by increasing steroid penetration and potency.

Information for parents and patient
• Be sure that the parents and patient understand the need to take the adrenocorticosteroid as prescribed. Give the patient instructions on what to do if a dose is inadvertently missed.
• Warn the parents and patient not to discontinue the drug abruptly.
• Inform the parents and patient of the possible therapeutic and adverse effects of the drug, so they may report any complications as soon as possible.
• Patient may take drug with food or milk to prevent GI upset.
• Patient should reduce salt (sodium) intake and increase potassium intake.
• Parents should tell new physician or dentist that patient is taking this drug.
• Advise the parents that the patient should wear a Medic Alert bracelet or necklace indicating the need for supplemental adrenocorticoids during times of stress.
• Instruct parents and patient in application of the drug. Tell them the following:

Method for applying topical preparations
• Wash hands before and after applying the drug. Gently cleanse the area of application. Washing or soaking the area before application may increase drug penetration.
• Apply sparingly in a light film; rub in lightly. Avoid contact with patient's eyes, unless using an ophthalmic product.
• To apply the aerosol form: Shake can well. Direct spray onto affected area from a distance of 6″ (15 cm). Apply for only 3 seconds (to avoid freezing tissues). Apply to dry scalp after shampooing; no need to massage or rub medication into scalp after spraying. Apply daily until acute phase is controlled, then reduce dosage to one to three times a week as needed to maintain control.
• Avoid prolonged application on the face, in skin folds, and near the eyes, genitals and rectum. High-potency topical corticosteroids are more likely to cause striae in these areas because of their higher rates of absorption.
• If an occlusive dressing is necessary, minimize adverse reactions by using it intermittently. Do not leave it in place longer than 16 hours each day.
• Warn parents and patient to avoid exposing treated areas to extremes in temperature.
• Warn patient not to use nonprescription topical preparations other than those specifically recommended.
• Advise parents not to use tight-fitting diapers or plastic pants on a child being treated in the diaper area, because such garments may serve as occlusive dressings.

hydroflumethiazide
Diucardin, Saluron

• Classification: diuretic, antihypertensive (thiazide)

How supplied
Available by prescription only
Tablets: 50 mg

Indications, route, and dosage
Edema
Children: 1 mg/kg P.O. daily.
Adults: 25 to 200 mg P.O. daily in divided doses; maintenance doses may be on intermittent or alternate-day schedule.
Hypertension
Adults: 50 to 100 mg P.O. daily or b.i.d.

Action and kinetics
• *Diuretic action:* Hydroflumethiazide increases urinary excretion of sodium and water by inhibiting sodium reabsorption in the cortical diluting tubule of the nephron, thus relieving edema.
• *Antihypertensive action:* The exact mechanism of hydroflumethiazide's antihypertensive effect is unknown. It may be partially from direct arteriolar vasodilation and a decrease in total peripheral resistance.
• *Kinetics in adults:* Hydroflumethiazide is absorbed from the GI tract after oral administration. Limited data are available on other pharmacokinetic parameters.

Contraindications and precautions
Hydroflumethiazide is contraindicated in patients with anuria and in those with known sensitivity to the drug or to other sulfonamide derivatives.

Hydroflumethiazide should be used cautiously in patients with severe renal disease, because it may decrease glomerular filtration rate and precipitate azotemia; in patients with impaired hepatic function or liver disease, because electrolyte changes may precipitate coma; and in patients taking digoxin, because hypokalemia may predispose them to digitalis toxicity.

Interactions
Hydroflumethiazide potentiates the hypotensive effects of most other antihypertensive drugs; this may be used to therapeutic advantage.

Hydroflumethiazide may potentiate hyperglycemic, hypotensive, and hyperuricemic effects of diazoxide, and its hyperglycemic effect may increase insulin requirements in diabetic patients.

Hydroflumethiazide may reduce renal clearance of lithium, elevating serum lithium levels, and may necessitate reduction in lithium dosage by 50%.

Hydroflumethiazide turns urine slightly more alkaline and may decrease urinary excretion of some amines, such as amphetamine and quinidine; alkaline urine may also decrease therapeutic efficacy of me-

---

thenamine compounds such as methenamine mandelate.

Cholestyramine and colestipol may bind hydroflumethiazide, preventing its absorption; give drugs 1 hour apart.

Effects on diagnostic tests

Hydroflumethiazide therapy may alter serum electrolyte levels and may increase serum urate, glucose, cholesterol, and triglyceride levels. It also may interfere with tests for parathyroid function and should be discontinued before such tests.

Adverse reactions

• CV: volume depletion and dehydration, orthostatic hypotension.
• DERM: dermatitis, photosensitivity, rash.
• GI: anorexia, nausea, pancreatitis.
• HEMA: aplastic anemia, agranulocytosis, leukopenia, thrombocytopenia.
• Hepatic: hepatic encephalopathy.
• Metabolic: asymptomatic hyperuricemia; hyperglycemia and impairment of glucose tolerance; fluid and electrolyte imbalances including hypokalemia, dilutional hyponatremia and hypochloremia; metabolic alkalosis; hypercalcemia.
• Other: hypersensitivity reactions, such as pneumonitis and vasculitis.

Note: Drug should be discontinued if rising BUN and serum creatinine levels indicate renal impairment or if patient shows signs of impending coma.

Overdose and treatment

Clinical signs of overdose include GI irritation and hypermotility, diuresis, and lethargy, which may progress to coma.

Treatment is mainly supportive; monitor and assist respiratory, cardiovascular, and renal function as indicated. Monitor fluid and electrolyte balance. Induce vomiting with ipecac in conscious patient; otherwise, use gastric lavage to avoid aspiration. Do not give cathartics; these promote additional loss of fluids and electrolytes.

▶ Special considerations

• Monitor weight and serum electrolyte levels regularly.
• Monitor serum potassium levels; encourage high-potassium diet. Foods rich in potassium include citrus fruits, tomatoes, bananas, dates, and apricots. Watch for signs of hypokalemia (for example, muscle weakness or cramps). Patients also taking digitalis have an increased risk of digitalis toxicity from the potassium-depleting effect of these diuretics.
• Drug may be used with potassium-sparing diuretics to attenuate potassium loss.
• Check insulin requirements in patients with diabetes.
• Monitor serum creatinine and BUN levels regularly. Drug is not as effective if these levels are more than twice normal.
• Monitor blood uric acid levels.
• A.M. administration is recommended to prevent nocturia.

• Antihypertensive effects persist for approximately 1 week after discontinuation of the drug.
• Instruct parents to observe for and to report any joint swelling, pain, or redness; these signs may indicate hyperuricemia.

Information for parents and patients

• Explain rationale of therapy and diuretic effects of drug.
• Advise parents to watch for and promptly report signs of electrolyte imbalance: weakness, fatigue, muscle cramps, paresthesias, confusion, nausea, vomiting, diarrhea, headache, dizziness, and palpitations.
• Tell parents to report any increased edema or excess diuresis (more than a 2% weight loss or gain) and to record child's weight each morning after voiding and before breakfast on the same scale and wearing the same type of clothing.
• Advise parents to give drug with food to minimize gastric irritation; to encourage child to eat potassium-rich foods, such as citrus fruits, potatoes, dates, raisins, and bananas; and to restrict child's access to salt and high-sodium foods, such as lunch meat, smoked meats, and processed cheeses.
• Tell parents to seek medical approval before giving the patient nonprescription drugs; many contain sodium and potassium and can cause electrolyte imbalances.
• Explain photosensitivity reactions. In thiazide-related photosensitivity, ultraviolet radiation alters drug structure, causing allergic reactions in some persons; such reactions occurs 10 days to 2 weeks after initial sun exposure.
• Warn parents to supervise the child's activities closely to prevent falls and other injuries that may result from dizziness, especially at beginning of therapy.
• Caution patient to change position slowly, especially when rising to upright position, to prevent dizziness from orthostatic hypotension.
• Advise parents to watch patient closely for chest, back, or leg pain, or shortness of breath, and to call immediately if they occur.
• Advise parents to administer drug only as prescribed and at the same time each day, to prevent nighttime diuresis and interrupted sleep.
• Emphasize importance of regular medical follow-up to monitor effectiveness of diuretic therapy.

hydroxychloroquine sulfate
Plaquenil Sulfate

• Classification: antimalarial, anti-inflammatory agent (4-aminoquinoline)

How supplied

Available by prescription only
Tablets: 200 mg (150-mg base)

Indications, route, and dosage
Suppressive prophylaxis of malarial attacks
Infants and children: 10 mg/kg (calculated as the base) initially, followed by 5 mg (calculated as the base) per kg of body weight, not to exceed the adult dose (400 mg/week of the sulfate; 310 mg base). The schedule of prophylaxis is the same as for adults.
Adults: 400 mg of sulfate (310 mg base) P.O. weekly on exactly the same day each week. (Begin 2 weeks before entering and continue for 8 weeks after leaving the endemic area.) If therapy begins after exposure, *double* the initial dose to 800 mg of sulfate (620 mg base) in two divided doses, 6 hours apart.

Acute malarial attacks
Children under age 1: 100 mg (sulfate) P.O. stat, then three doses of 100 mg 6 to 9 hours apart (total of 400 mg sulfate salt).
Children age 2 to 5: 400 mg (sulfate) P.O. stat, then 200 mg 8 hours later (total of 600 mg sulfate salt).
Children age 6 to 10: 400 mg (sulfate) P.O. stat, then two doses of 200 mg at 8-hour intervals (total of 800 mg sulfate salt).
Children 11 to 15: 600 mg (sulfate) P.O. stat, then 200 mg 8 hours later, then 200 mg 24 hours later (total of 1 g sulfate salt).
Children over age 15 and adults: Initially, 800 mg (sulfate) P.O., then 400 mg after 6 to 8 hours, then 400 mg daily for 2 days (total of 2 g sulfate salt). Alternatively, a single 800-mg dose may prove effective.

†*Rheumatoid arthritis*
Adults: 400 to 600 mg P.O daily. When good response occurs (usually in 4 to 12 weeks), cut dosage in half.
Note: Safe use in juvenile arthritis has not been established.

Action and kinetics
• *Antimalarial action:* Hydroxychloroquine binds to DNA, interfering with protein synthesis. It also inhibits DNA and RNA polymerases. It is active against asexual erythrocytic forms of *Plasmodium malariae, P. ovali, P. vivax,* and many strains of *P. falciparum.*
• *Amebicidal action:* Mechanism of action is unknown.
• *Anti-inflammatory action:* Mechanism of action is unknown. Hydroxychloroquine may antagonize histamine and serotonin and inhibit prostaglandin effects by inhibiting conversion of arachidonic acid to prostaglandin F_2; it may also inhibit chemotaxis of polymorphonuclear leukocytes, macrophages, and eosinophils.
• *Kinetics in adults:* Hydroxychloroquine is absorbed readily and almost completely, with peak plasma concentrations occurring at 1 to 2 hours. Hydroxychloroquine is bound to plasma proteins. It concentrates in the liver, spleen, kidneys, heart, and brain and is strongly bound in melanin-containing cells. Hydroxychloroquine is metabolized by the liver to desethylchloroquine and desethyl hydroxychloroquine. Most of an administered dose is excreted unchanged in urine. The drug and its metabolites are excreted slowly in urine; unabsorbed drug is excreted in feces. Small amounts of the drug may be present in urine for months after the drug is discontinued. The drug is excreted in breast milk.

Contraindications and precautions
Hydroxychloroquine is contraindicated in patients who have experienced retinal or visual field changes or hypersensitivity reactions to 4-aminoquinoline compounds, unless these compounds are the only agents to which the malarial strain is sensitive.
Hydroxychloroquine should be used with caution in patients with psoriasis, porphyria, or glucose-6-phosphate dehydrogenase (G6PD) deficiency because the drug may exacerbate these conditions. Because hydroxychloroquine concentrates in the liver and may cause adverse hepatic effects, it should be used with caution in patients with hepatic disease or alcoholism and in patients receiving other hepatotoxic drugs.

Interactions
Concomitant administration of kaolin or magnesium trisilicate may decrease absorption of hydroxychloroquine. Use with digoxin may increase serum digoxin levels.

Effects on diagnostic tests
Hydroxychloroquine may cause inversion or depression of the T wave or widening of the QRS complex on ECG. Rarely, it may cause decreased WBC, RBC, or platelet counts.

Adverse reactions
• CNS: irritability, nightmares, ataxia, seizures, psychic stimulation, toxic psychosis, vertigo, tinnitus, nystagmus, lassitude, fatigue, dizziness, hypoactive deep-tendon reflexes, skeletal muscle weakness, emotional changes, headache.
• DERM: pruritus, lichen planus-like eruptions, skin and mucosal pigmentary changes, pleomorphic skin eruptions, non-light-sensitive psoriasis.
• EENT: visual disturbances (blurred vision; difficulty in focusing; reversible corneal changes; generally irreversible, sometimes progressive or delayed, retinal changes, such as narrowing of arterioles; macular lesions; pallor of optic disk; optic atrophy; visual field defects; patchy retinal pigmentation, often leading to blindness), ototoxicity (irreversible nerve deafness, tinnitus, labyrinthitis).
• GI: anorexia, abdominal cramps, diarrhea, nausea, vomiting.
• HEMA: agranulocytosis, leukopenia, thrombocytopenia, *aplastic anemia,* hemolysis in G6PD deficiency.
• Other: weight loss, bleaching of hair, alopecia, exacerbations of porphyria, immunoblastic lymphadenopathy.

Overdose and treatment
Symptoms of hydroxychloroquine overdose may appear within 30 minutes after ingestion and may include headache, drowsiness, visual changes, cardiovascular collapse, and seizures followed by respiratory and cardiac arrest.
Treatment is symptomatic. The stomach should be emptied by emesis or lavage. After lavage, activated charcoal in an amount at least five times the estimated amount of drug ingested may be helpful if given within 30 minutes of ingestion.
Ultra-short-acting barbiturates may help control seizures. Intubation may become necessary. Perito-

---

neal dialysis and exchange transfusions may also be useful. Forced fluids and acidification of the urine are helpful after the acute phase.

▶ Special considerations

• Children are extremely susceptible to toxicity; monitor closely for adverse effects.

• Give immediately before or after meals on the same day each week to minimize gastric distress.

• Be aware that chloroquine-resistant malaria is endemic in certain parts of the world. It may be necessary to also prescribe sulfadoxine/pyrimethamine (Fansidar).

• Obtain a baseline ECG, blood counts, and an ophthalmologic examination, and check periodically for changes.

• Monitor patient for signs and symptoms of cumulative effects, such as blurred vision, increased sensitivity to light, muscle weakness, impaired hearing, tinnitus, fever, sore throat, unusual bleeding or bruising, unusual pigmentation of the oral mucous membranes, and jaundice. Maximal effects may not occur for 6 months.

• Muscle weakness and alterations of deep tendon reflexes may require discontinuing the drug.

Information for parents and patient

• Counsel parents to have patient complete the entire prescribed course of therapy and to comply with follow-up blood tests and examinations.

• Tell parents to report any vision or hearing changes, muscle weakness, or darkening of urine immediately.

• Patient should take these drugs after meals to help prevent GI distress. Tell parents to report any pronounced GI distress and to separate use of magnesium or kaolin compounds from drug by at least 4 hours.

• Patient should wear sunglasses in bright light or sunlight to reduce risk of ocular damage and should avoid prolonged exposure to sunlight to avoid exacerbating drug-induced dermatoses.

• Warn parents to keep drug out of the reach of children.

---

hydroxyzine hydrochloride
Anxanil, Atarax, Atozine, Durrax, E-Vista, Hydroxacen, Hyzine, Multipax*, Orgatrax, Quiess, Vistacon, Vistaject, Vistaquel, Vistazine

hydroxyzine pamoate
Hy-Pam, Vamate, Vistaril

• Classification: antianxiety agent; sedative; antipruritic; antiemetic; antispasmodic (antihistamine [piperazine derivative])

How supplied
Available by prescription only
Hydroxyzine hydrochloride
Capsules: 10 mg, 25 mg, 50 mg
Syrup: 10 mg/5 ml
Tablets: 10 mg, 25 mg, 50 mg, 100 mg

Injection: 25 mg/ml, 50 mg/ml
Hydroxyzine pamoate
Capsules: 25 mg, 50 mg, 100 mg
Oral suspension: 25 mg/5 ml

Indications, route, and dosage
Anxiety and tension
Children: 2 mg/kg P.O. daily in divided doses q 6 hours. Alternatively, give according to age.
Children under age 6: 50 mg P.O. daily in divided doses.
Children age 6 and over: 50 to 100 mg P.O. daily in divided doses.
Adults: 25 to 100 mg P.O. t.i.d. or q.i.d.
Preoperative and postoperative adjunctive sedation
Children: 0.5 to 1 mg/kg I.M. q 4 to 6 hours.
Adults: 25 to 100 mg I.M. q 4 to 6 hours.

Action and kinetics
• *Anxiolytic and sedative actions:* Hydroxyzine produces its sedative and antianxiety effects through suppression of activity at subcortical levels; analgesia occurs at high doses.

• *Antipruritic action:* Hydroxyzine is a direct competitor of histamine for binding at cellular receptor sites.

• *Other actions:* Hydroxyzine is used as a preoperative and postoperative adjunct for its sedative, antihistaminic, and anticholinergic activity.

• *Kinetics in adults:* Hydroxyzine is absorbed rapidly and completely after oral administration. Peak serum levels occur within 2 to 4 hours. Sedation and other clinical effects are usually noticed in 15 to 30 minutes.

The distribution of hydroxyzine in humans is not well understood.

Hydroxyzine is metabolized almost completely in the liver.

Metabolites of hydroxyzine are excreted primarily in urine; small amounts of drug and metabolites are found in feces. Half-life of the drug is 3 hours. Sedative effects can last for 4 to 6 hours, and antihistaminic effects can persist for up to 4 days.

Contraindications and precautions
Hydroxyzine is contraindicated in patients with known hypersensitivity to the drug. Hydroxyzine should be used cautiously in patients with open-angle glaucoma, urinary retention, or any other condition where anticholinergic effects would be detrimental.

Interactions
Hydroxyzine may add to or potentiate the effects of opioids, barbiturates, alcohol, tranquilizers, and other CNS depressants; the dose of CNS depressants should be reduced by 50%.

Concomitant use with other anticholinergic drugs causes additive anticholinergic effects.

Hydroxyzine may block the vasopressor action of epinephrine. If a vasoconstrictor is needed, use norepinephrine or phenylephrine.

Effects on diagnostic tests
Hydroxyzine therapy causes falsely elevated urinary 17-hydroxycorticosteroid levels. It also may cause

---

‡May contain sulfites   ◆May contain tartrazine   ◆◆May contain benzyl alcohol

false-negative skin allergen tests by attenuating or inhibiting the cutaneous response to histamine.

Adverse reactions
• CNS: sedation, dizziness, *drowsiness,* ataxia, weakness, slurred speech, headache, anxiety, *tremor and seizures* at high doses (rare).
• DERM: rash, urticaria.
• EENT: *dry mouth,* blurred vision, dental problems (with prolonged use).
• GI: constipation, nausea, bitter taste.
• GU: urinary retention.
• Local: marked irritation, sterile abscess, and tissue induration (after S.C. administration).
• Other: hypersensitivity (tightness of chest, wheezing).
   Note: Drug should be discontinued if hypersensitivity with tightness of chest, wheezing, tremor, or seizures occurs.

Overdose and treatment
Clinical manifestations of overdose include excessive sedation and hypotension; seizures may occur.
   Treatment is supportive only. For recent oral ingestion, empty gastric contents through emesis or lavage. Correct hypotension with fluids and vasopressors (phenylephrine or metaraminol). Do not give epinephrine, because hydroxyzine may counteract its effect.

▶ Special considerations
• Observe patients for excessive sedation, especially those receiving other CNS depressants.
• Inject deep I.M. only; not for I.V., intraarterial, or S.C. use. Aspirate injection carefully to prevent inadvertent intravascular administration.

Information for parents and patient
• Tell parents that patient should avoid hazardous activities that require mental alertness or physical coordination until the CNS effects of the drug are known; advise against use of other CNS depressants with hydroxyzine unless prescribed. Patient should avoid alcohol ingestion, including that in liquid cough and cold preparations.
• Instruct parents to seek medical approval before administering to the patient any nonprescription cold or allergy preparations that contain antihistamine, which may potentiate the effects of hydroxyzine.
• Recommend use of sugarless gum or candy to help relieve dry mouth; advise drinking plenty of water to help with dry mouth or constipation.

ibuprofen
Advil, Amersol★, Medipren, Motrin, Nuprin, Rufen, Trendar

• Classification: nonsteroidal anti-inflammatory agent (nonnarcotic analgesic, antipyretic)

How supplied
Available without a prescription
Tablets: 200 mg

Available by prescription only
Suspension: 100 mg/5 ml
Tablets: 300 mg, 400 mg, 600 mg, 800 mg

Indications, route, and dosage
Juvenile arthritis
Children: 30 to 40 mg/kg/day P.O. divided into three or four doses. Patients with less severe disease may be controlled with 20 mg/kg/day.

Fever reduction
Children age 12 months to 12 years: If baseline temperature is > 102.5° F., the recommended dose is 10 mg/kg P.O. If the base line temperature is less than 102.5° F., give 5 mg/kg. Recommended maximum daily dosage is 40 mg/kg.
Children over age 12 and adults: 400 mg P.O. q 4 to 6 hours p.r.n.

Action and kinetics
• *Analgesic, antipyretic, and anti-inflammatory actions:* Mechanisms of action are unknown; ibuprofen is thought to inhibit prostaglandin synthesis.
• *Kinetics in adults:* Ibuprofen is absorbed rapidly and completely from the GI tract. Ibuprofen is highly protein-bound. Ibuprofen undergoes biotransformation in the liver. Ibuprofen is excreted mainly in urine, with some biliary excretion. Plasma half-life ranges from 2 to 4 hours.

Contraindications and precautions
Ibuprofen is contraindicated in patients with known hypersensitivity to the drug and in patients in whom aspirin or other nonsteroidal anti-inflammatory drugs (NSAIDs) induce symptoms of asthma, urticaria, or rhinitis.

Ibuprofen should be administered cautiously to patients with a history of GI disease, hepatic or renal disease, cardiac decompensation, systemic lupus erythematosus, or bleeding abnormalities, because the drug may worsen these conditions.

Patients with known "triad" symptoms (aspirin hypersensitivity, rhinitis/nasal polyps, and asthma) are at high risk of bronchospasm. NSAIDs may mask the signs and symptoms of acute infection (fever, myalgia, erythema); carefully evaluate patients with high risk (for example, those with diabetes).

Interactions
Concomitant use of ibuprofen with anticoagulants and thrombolytic drugs (coumarin derivatives, heparin, streptokinase, or urokinase) may potentiate anticoagulant effects. Bleeding problems may occur if ibuprofen is used with other drugs that inhibit platelet aggregation, such as azlocillin, parenteral carbenicillin, dextran, dipyridamole, mezlocillin, piperacillin, sulfinpyrazone, ticarcillin, valproic acid, cefamandole, cefoperazone, moxalactam, plicamycin, aspirin, salicylates, or other anti-inflammatory agents. Concomitant use with salicylates, anti-inflammatory agents, alcohol, corticotropin, or steroids may cause increased GI side effects, including ulceration and hemorrhage. Aspirin may decrease the bioavailability of ibuprofen. Because of the influence of prostaglandins on glucose metabolism, concomitant use with insulin or oral hypoglycemic agents may potentiate hypoglycemic effects. Ibuprofen may displace highly protein-bound drugs from binding sites. Toxicity may occur with coumarin derivatives, phenytoin, verapamil, or nifedipine. Increased nephrotoxicity may occur with gold compounds, other anti-inflammatory agents, or acetaminophen. Ibuprofen may decrease the renal clearance of methotrexate and lithium. Antacids may decrease the absorption of ibuprofen. Ibuprofen may decrease effectiveness of diuretics and antihypertensives. Concomitant use with diuretics may increase nephrotoxicity.

Effects on diagnostic tests
The physiologic effects of ibuprofen may prolong bleeding time; decrease blood glucose concentrations; increase blood urea nitrogen, serum creatinine, and serum potassium levels; decrease serum uric acid, hemoglobin, and hematocrit levels; increase prothrombin time; and increase serum alkaline phosphatase, serum lactic dehydrogenase, and serum transaminase levels.

Adverse reactions
• CNS: headache, drowsiness, dizziness, aseptic meningitis, vertigo, weakness.
• CV: peripheral edema, CHF, hypotension, palpitations, tachycardia.
• DERM: pruritus, rash, urticaria.
• EENT: visual disturbances, tinnitus.
• GI: epigastric distress, nausea, vomiting, GI bleeding, constipation, anorexia, diarrhea, occult blood loss.
• GU: reversible renal failure, hematuria, urinary tract infection, nocturia, elevated BUN, reduced creatinine clearance.
• HEMA: prolonged bleeding time.
• Other: bronchospasm, edema, elevated liver enzymes, thirst.

Note: Drug should be discontinued if hypersensitivity or renal or hepatic toxicity occurs.

Overdose and treatment
Clinical manifestations of overdose include dizziness, drowsiness, paresthesias, vomiting, nausea, abdominal pain, headache, sweating, nystagmus, apnea, and cyanosis.

To treat overdose of ibuprofen, empty stomach immediately by enducing emesis with ipecac syrup or by gastric lavage. Administer activated charcoal via nasogastric tube. Provide symptomatic and supportive measures (respiratory support and correction of fluid and electrolyte imbalances). Monitor laboratory parameters and vital signs closely. Alkaline diuresis may enhance renal excretion. Dialysis is of minimal value because ibuprofen is strongly protein-bound.

▶ Special considerations
• Do not use long-term ibuprofen therapy in children under age 14; safety of this use has not been established.
• Maximum results in arthritis may require 1 to 2 weeks of continuous therapy with ibuprofen. Improvement may be seen, however, within 7 days.
• Administer on an empty stomach, 1 hour before or 2 hours after meals for maximum absorption. However, it may be administered with meals to lessen GI upset.
• Monitor cardiopulmonary status closely; monitor vital signs, especially heart rate and blood pressure. Observe for possible fluid retention.
• Establish safety measures, including raised side rails and supervised walking, to prevent possible injury from CNS effects.
• Monitor auditory and ophthalmic functions periodically during ibuprofen therapy.

Information for parents and patient
• Instruct parents to seek medical approval before giving patient any nonprescription medications.
• Advise parents not to administer ibuprofen for longer than 10 days for analgesic use or to continue ibuprofen if fever lasts longer than 3 days unless prescribed.
• Advise parents and patient to report any adverse reactions. They are usually dose-related.
• Instruct parents in safety measures to prevent injury. Warn them that patient should avoid hazardous activities that require mental alertness until CNS effects are known.
• Encourage parents and patient to follow prescribed drug regimen. Instruct them in need for medical follow-up.

---

idoxuridine (IDU)
Herplex Liquifilm, Stoxil Ophthalmic

• Classification: antiviral agent (halogenated pyrimidine)

How supplied
Available by prescription only
Ophthalmic solution: 0.1%
Ophthalmic suspension: 0.5%

Indications, route, and dosage
Herpes simplex keratitis
Children and adults: Instill 1 drop of solution into conjunctival sac q 1 hour during day and q 2 hours at night; or if Herplex solution is used, 1 drop of solution may be instilled q minute for 5 minutes q 4 hours. Apply ointment to conjunctival sac q 4 hours or 5 times daily, with last dose at bedtime. Response should be seen within 7 days; if not, discontinue and begin alternate therapy. Therapy should not be continued longer than 21 days.

Action and kinetics
• *Antiviral action:* Idoxuridine interferes with DNA synthesis, blocking viral reproduction.
• *Kinetics in adults:* Unknown.

Contraindications and precautions
Idoxuridine is contraindicated in patients with hypersensitivity to idoxuridine or to any component of the preparation.

In superficial dendritic keratitis, concurrent application of idoxuridine and corticosteroids is contraindicated.

Interactions
When used concomitantly with boric acid preparations, precipitation of inactive ingredients or preservatives in idoxuridine may occur.

Effects on diagnostic tests
None reported.

Adverse reactions
• Eye: temporary visual haze, irritation, pain, burning, or inflammation of eye; mild edema of eyelid or cornea; photophobia; small punctate defects in corneal epithelium; slowed corneal wound healing (with ointment).
• Other: hypersensitivity.
Note: Drug should be discontinued if hypersensitivity reactions occur.

Overdose and treatment
The toxicity of ingested idoxuridine is unknown. If accidentally ingested, general measures, such as emesis, catharsis, or lavage may be used to remove drug from GI tract. Dermal exposure may be treated by washing the area with soap and water. Observe patient closely for possible signs and symptoms.

▶ Special considerations

• Drug is not intended for long-term use since it may damage corneal epithelium or inhibit ulcer healing. Do not use for more than 7 days after healing is complete, or 21 days total.

• Stoxil must be refrigerated.

• Do not mix idoxuridine with other medications; do not use old solution, which may cause ocular burning and has no antiviral activity.

• Cleanse eye area of excessive exudate before application.

Information for parents and patient

• Tell parents to watch for signs and symptoms of sensitivity, such as itching lids or constant burning and to stop drug and report such symptoms immediately.

• Inform parents that patient should avoid sharing washcloths and towels with family members.

• Advise parents and patient to wash hands before and after applying ointment or solution.

• Tell parents and patient to apply finger pressure to inside corner of the eyes for 1 minute after solution instillation, to minimize systemic absorption; patient should not close eyes tightly or blink more than usual.

imipenem-cilastatin sodium
Primaxin

• Classification: antibiotic (carbapenem [thienamycin class]; beta-lactam antibiotic)

How supplied

Available by prescription only
Injection: 250-ml and 500-ml vials

Indications, route, and dosage
Serious respiratory and urinary tract infections; intra-abdominal, gynecologic, bone, joint, or skin infections; bacterial septicemia; endocarditis

Children age 3 months to age 12 years: 15 to 25 mg/kg I.V. q 6 hours.

Some clinicians recommend 50 mg/kg/day divided q 6 to 8 hours (12.5 to 16.66 mg/kg q 6 to 8 hours)
Adults: 250 mg to 1 g by I.V. infusion q 6 to 8 hours. Maximum daily dosage is 50 mg/kg/day or 4 g/day, whichever is less.

Dosage in renal failure

• If creatinine clearance is 30 to 70 ml/minute, dosage in life-threatening infections is 500 mg q 6 hours; in moderate infections, 500 mg q 8 hours.

• If creatinine clearance is 20 to 30 ml/minute, dosage in life-threatening infections is 500 mg q 8 hours; in moderate infections, 500 mg q 12 hours.

• If creatinine clearance is 5 to 20 ml/minute, dosage in life-threatening infections is 500 mg q 12 hours; in moderate infections, 250 mg q 12 hours.

• If creatinine clearance is less than 5 ml/minute, dosage in life-threatening infections is 500 mg q 12 hours; in moderate infections, 250 mg q 12 hours.

Action and kinetics

• *Antibacterial action:* A bactericidal drug, imipenem inhibits bacterial cell-wall synthesis. Its spectrum of antimicrobial activity includes many gram-positive, gram-negative, and anaerobic bacteria, including *Staphylococcus* and *Streptococcus* species, *Escherichia coli, Klebsiella, Proteus, Enterobacter* species, *Pseudomonas aeruginosa,* and *Bacteroides* species including *B. fragilis.* Resistant bacteria include methicillin-resistant staphylococci, *Clostridium difficile,* and other *Pseudomonas* species.

Cilastatin inhibits imipenem's enzymatic breakdown in the kidneys, making it effective in treating urinary tract infections.

• *Kinetics in adults:* Imipenem-cilastatin is administered I.V. and is distributed rapidly and widely after I.V. infusion. Approximately 20% of imipenem and 40% of cilastatin is protein-bound. Peak plasma drug levels occur in about 20 minutes. Plasma half-life is about 1 hour.

Imipenem is metabolized by kidney dehydropeptidase I, resulting in low urine concentrations. Cilastatin inhibits this enzyme, thereby reducing imipenem's metabolism. About 70% of imipenem-cilastatin dose is excreted unchanged by the kidneys (when imipenem is combined with cilastatin). Imipenem is cleared by hemodialysis; therefore, a supplemental dose is required after this procedure.

Contraindications and precautions

Imipenem is contraindicated in patients with known hypersensitivity to the drug.

Imipenem should be administered cautiously to patients with a history of seizures, especially if they also have compromised renal function, because drug may induce seizures; and to patients who are allergic to penicillin or cephalosporins, because this drug is chemically similar to them. Chloramphenicol may impede the bactericidal effects of imipenem; give chloramphenicol a few hours after imipenem-cilastatin.

Interactions

Imipenem may be physically incompatible with aminoglycosides; avoid mixing together.

Effects on diagnostic tests

Serum levels of AST (SGOT), ALT (SGPT), alkaline phosphatase, lactic dehydrogenase, and bilirubin may be elevated, and erythrocyte, platelet, and leukocyte counts reduced during imipenem therapy.

Adverse reactions

• CNS: seizures, dizziness, encephalopathy, confusion.

• CV: hypotension.

• GI: *nausea,* vomiting, diarrhea, pseudomembranous colitis.

• Local: thrombophlebitis, pain at injection site.

• Other: hypersensitivity, superinfection.

Note: Drug should be discontinued if patient develops hypersensitivity reaction or if seizures or pseudomembranous colitis occurs.

Overdose and treatment

No information available.

▶ **Special considerations**
• Safety and effectiveness in children under age 12 have not been established; however, drug has been used in children age 3 months to 13 years. Dosage range is 15 to 25 mg/kg q 6 hours.
• Culture and sensitivity tests should be done before starting therapy.
• When reconstituting powder, shake until solution is clear. Solution may range from colorless to yellow; color variations within this range do not affect drug potency. After reconstitution, solution remains stable for 10 hours at room temperature and for 48 hours when refrigerated.
• Do not administer by direct I.V. bolus injection. Infuse 250- or 500-mg dose over 20 to 30 minutes; infuse 1-g dose over 40 to 60 minutes. If nausea occurs, slow infusion.
• Monitor patient for hypersensitivity reaction.
• Anticonvulsants should be continued in patients with known seizure disorders. Patients who exhibit CNS toxicity should receive phenytoin or benzodiazepines. Reduce dosage or discontinue drug if CNS toxicity continues.
• Drug has broadest antibacterial spectrum of any available beta-lactam antibiotic. It is most valuable for empiric treatment of unidentified infections and for mixed infections that would otherwise require combination of antibiotics, possibly including an aminoglycoside.
• Prolonged use may result in overgrowth of nonsusceptible organisms. In addition, use of imipenum-cilastatin as a sole antibiotic has resulted in resistance during therapy.

Information for parents and patient
• Encourage parents and patient to report any adverse effects immediately.
• Teach parents and patient how to recognize signs of superinfection and how to prevent it by practicing meticulous oral and anogenital hygiene. Parents of infants and toddlers should keep diaper area clean and dry and avoid using plastic pants.

---

imipramine hydrochloride
Apo-Imipramine*, Impril*, Janimine, Novopramine*, SK-Pramine, Tofranil, Typramine

imipramine pamoate
Tofranil-PM

• Classification: antidepressant (dibenzazepine tricyclic antidepressant)

How supplied
Available by prescription only
Tablets: 10 mg, 25 mg, 50 mg
Capsules: 75 mg, 100 mg, 125 mg, 150 mg
Injection: 12.5 mg/ml

Indications, route, and dosage
Depression, †anxiety, †neurogenic pain
Children: 0.5 mg/kg P.O. t.i.d. increasing at 3 to 4 day intervals to a maximum of 5 mg/kg daily.
Childhood enuresis
Children age 6 or over: Initially, 10 to 25 mg P.O. h.s., increasing at 1 to 2 week intervals to recommended maximum dosage based upon age:
age 6 to 8—50 mg daily; over age 8 to 10—60 mg daily; over age 10 to 12—70 mg daily; over age 12 to 14—75 mg daily.
Adults: Initially, 75 to 100 mg P.O. or I.M. daily in divided doses, with 25- to 50-mg increments, up to 200 mg. Alternatively, some patients can start with lower doses (25 mg P.O.) and titrate slowly in 25 mg increments every other day. Maximum dosage is 300 mg daily. Alternatively, the entire dosage may be given at bedtime. (I.M. route rarely used.) Maximum dosage: 200 mg/day for outpatients, 300 mg/day for inpatients.

Action and kinetics
• *Antidepressant action:* Imipramine is thought to exert its antidepressant effects by inhibiting reuptake of norepinephrine and serotonin in CNS nerve terminals (presynaptic neurons), which results in increased concentrations and enhanced activity of these neurotransmitters in the synaptic cleft. Imipramine also has anticholinergic activity and is used to treat nocturnal enuresis in children over age 6.
• *Kinetics in adults:* Imipramine is absorbed rapidly from the GI tract and muscle tissue after oral and I.M. administration.
Imipramine is distributed widely into the body, including the CNS and breast milk. Drug is 90% protein-bound. Peak effect occurs in ½ to 2 hours; steady state is achieved within 2 to 5 days. Therapeutic plasma levels (parent drug and metabolite) are thought to range from 150 to 300 ng/ml.
Imipramine is metabolized by the liver to the active metabolite desipramine. A significant first-pass effect may explain variability of serum concentrations in different patients taking the same dosage.
Most of drug is excreted in urine.

Contraindications and precautions
Imipramine is contraindicated in patients with known hypersensitivity to tricyclic antidepressants, trazodone, and related compounds; in the acute recovery phase of myocardial infarction (MI) because of its arrhythmogenic potential; in patients in coma or severe respiratory depression because of additive CNS depression; and during or within 14 days of therapy with monoamine oxidase inhibitors.
Imipramine should be used cautiously in patients with other cardiac disease (dysrhythmias, congestive heart failure [CHF], angina pectoris, valvular disease, increased QRS intervals, or heart block); respiratory disorders; epilepsy and other seizure disorders; scheduled electroconvulsive therapy; bipolar disease; glaucoma; hyperthyroidism, or in those taking thyroid replacement; Type I and Type II diabetes; prostatic hypertrophy, paralytic ileus, or urinary retention; hepatic or renal dysfunction; Parkinson's disease; and in those undergoing surgery with general anesthesia.

---

*Canada only   †Unlabeled clinical use   Italicized adverse reactions have been observed in children.

Some formulations contain tartrazine and may provoke asthma in patients with aspirin allergy.

Interactions

Concomitant use of imipramine with sympathomimetics, including epinephrine, phenylephrine, phenylpropanolamine, and ephedrine (often found in nasal sprays) may increase blood pressure; use with warfarin may increase prothrombin time and cause bleeding. Concomitant use with thyroid medication, pimozide, and antiarrhythmic agents (quinidine, disopyramide, procainamide) may increase incidence of cardiac dysrhythmias and conduction defects.

Imipramine may decrease hypotensive effects of centrally acting antihypertensive drugs, such as guanethidine, guanabenz, guanadrel, clonidine, methyldopa, and reserpine. Concomitant use with disulfiram or ethchlorvynol may cause delirium and tachycardia.

Additive effects are likely after concomitant use of imipramine with CNS depressants, including alcohol, analgesics, barbiturates, narcotics, tranquilizers, and anesthetics (oversedation); atropine or other anticholinergic drugs, including phenothiazines, antihistamines, meperidine, and antiparkinsonian agents (oversedation, paralytic ileus, visual changes, and severe constipation); or metrizamide (increased risk of convulsions).

Barbiturates and heavy smoking induce imipramine metabolism and decrease therapeutic efficacy; phenothiazines and haloperidol decrease its metabolism, decreasing therapeutic efficacy. Methylphenidate, cimetidine, oral contraceptives, propoxyphene, and beta blockers may inhibit imipramine metabolism, increasing plasma levels and toxicity.

Effects on diagnostic tests

Imipramine may prolong conduction time (elongation of QT and PR intervals, flattened T waves on ECG); it also may elevate liver function test results, decrease white blood cell counts, and decrease or increase serum glucose levels.

Adverse reactions

• CNS: *drowsiness, dizziness,* sedation, excitation, tremors, weakness, headache, nervousness, *seizures,* peripheral neuropathy, extrapyramidal symptoms, anxiety, vivid dreams, confusion (more marked in elderly patients), decreased libido, sexual dysfunction.
• CV: orthostatic hypotension, tachycardia, dysrhythmias, MI, stroke, heart block, CHF, palpitations, hypertension, ECG changes.
• EENT: blurred vision, tinnitus, mydriasis, increased intraocular pressure.
• GI: *dry mouth, constipation,* nausea, vomiting, anorexia, diarrhea, paralytic ileus, jaundice.
• GU: urinary retention.
• Other: sweating, photosensitivity, hypersensitivity (rash, urticaria, drug fever, edema).

After abrupt withdrawal of long-term therapy, nausea, headache, or malaise (does not indicate addiction) may occur.

Note: Drug should be discontinued (not abruptly) if signs of hypersensitivity occur such as urinary retention, extreme dry mouth, rash, excessive sedation, seizures, tachycardia, sore throat, fever, or jaundice.

Overdose and treatment

Imipramine overdose is frequently life-threatening, particularly when combined with alcohol. The first 12 hours after acute ingestion are a stimulatory phase characterized by excessive anticholinergic activity (agitation, irritation, confusion, hallucinations, hyperthermia, parkinsonian symptoms, seizure, urinary retention, dry mucous membranes, pupillary dilatation, constipation, and ileus). This is followed by CNS depressant effects, including hypothermia, decreased or absent reflexes, sedation, hypotension, cyanosis, and cardiac irregularities, including tachycardia, conduction disturbances, and quinidine-like effects on the ECG.

Severity of overdose is best indicated by widening of the QRS complex, which usually represents a serum level in excess of 1,000 ng/ml; serum concentrations are usually not helpful. Metabolic acidosis may follow hypotension, hypoventilation, and convulsions.

Treatment is symptomatic and supportive, including maintaining airway, stable body temperature, and fluid or electrolyte balance. Induce emesis if patient is conscious; follow with gastric lavage and repeated doses of activated charcoal/sorbitol mixture to prevent further absorption. Dialysis is of little use. Treat seizures with parenteral diazepam or phenytoin; dysrhythmias, with parenteral phenytoin or lidocaine; and acidosis, with sodium bicarbonate. Do not give barbiturates; these may enhance CNS and respiratory depressant effects.

▶ Special considerations

• Not recommended for treating depression in patients younger than age 12. Do not use pamoate salt for enuresis in children.
• Imipramine may be used to treat nocturnal enuresis in children.
• Imipramine impairs ability to perform tasks requiring mental alertness.
• Check for anticholinergic adverse reactions (urinary retention or constipation), which may require dosage reduction.
• Carefully follow manufacturer's instructions for reconstitution, dilution, and storage of drugs.
• Investigational uses include treating peptic ulcer, migraine prophylaxis, and allergy. Potential toxicity has, to date, outweighed most advantages.
• Imipramine is associated with a high incidence of orthostatic hypotension. Check sitting and standing blood pressures after initial dose.
• Do not give the full daily dosage at one time.
• I.M. administration may result in a more rapid onset of action than that with oral administration. However, oral therapy should be substituted for parenteral therapy as soon as possible.
• Drug should not be withdrawn abruptly, but tapered gradually over time.
• Do not give drug I.V.
• Tolerance to the sedative effects of this drug usually develops over several weeks.
• Drug should be discontinued at least 48 hours before surgical procedures.

---

‡May contain sulfites   ◆May contain tartrazine   ◆◆May contain benzyl alcohol

Information for parents and patient

• Explain rationale for therapy and that full thera-peutic effect may not occur for several weeks.
• Tell parents that patient should avoid beverages and drugs containing alcohol and should not take any other drug (including non-prescription products) without medical approval.
• Advise parents to have patient lie down for 30 minutes after first dose and to rise slowly to prevent orthostatic hypotension.
• Urge parents of diabetic children to monitor blood glucose levels, because drug may alter insulin needs.
• Patient should avoid hazardous activities that require mental alertness until full effect of drug is determined.
• Warn parents and patient that excessive exposure to sunlight, heat lamps, or tanning beds may cause burn and abnormal hyperpigmentation.
• Advise parents and patient that unpleasant side effects (except dry mouth) generally diminish over time.
• Patient should take the medication exactly as prescribed, not take the full daily dosage at one time, not double the dose for missed doses, and not discontinue drug abruptly.
• Suggest taking drug with food or milk if it causes stomach upset.
• Suggest relieving dry mouth with sugarless chewing gum or hard candy. Encourage good dental prophy-laxis because persistent dry mouth may lead to increased incidence of dental caries.
• Encourage parents to observe patient and report any unusual or troublesome effects immediately, including confusion, movement disorders, rapid heartbeat, dizziness, fainting, or difficulty urinating.

---

immune globulin (gamma globulin; IG; immune serum globulin; ISG)

immune globulin for I.M. use (IGIM)
Gamastan, Gammar, Immunoglobin

immune globulin for I.V. use (IGIV)
Gamimune N, Gammagard, Sandoglobulin

• Classification: immune serum

How supplied
Available by prescription only
IGIM
Injection: 2-ml and 10-ml vials
IGIV
I.V.: Gamimune N – 5% solution in 10-ml, 50-ml, and 100-ml single-use vials; Gammagard – 2.5-g and 5-g single-use vials for reconstitution; Sandoglobulin – 1-g, 3-g, and 6-g single-use vials for reconstitution

Indications, route, and dosage
Agammaglobulinemia or hypogammaglobuli-nemia
IGIV
Children and adults: For Gamimune N only, 100 to 200 mg/kg or 2 to 4 ml/kg I.V. infusion monthly. In-fusion rate is 0.01 to 0.02 ml/kg/minute for 30 min-utes. Rate can then be increased to a maximum of 0.08 ml/kg/minute for remainder of infusion. For San-doglobulin only, 200 mg/kg by I.V. infusion monthly. Start with 0.5 to 1 ml/minute of a 30 mg/ml solution, increase up to 2.5 ml/minute gradually after 15 to 30 minutes.
IGIM
Children: Initial dose 1.2 ml/kg, maximum one-time dose 20 to 30 ml.
Adults: Initial dose 1.2 ml/kg, maximum one-time dose 30 to 50 ml.
Maintenance dose (adults and children) is 0.6 ml/kg q 2 weeks.
Hepatitis A exposure
Children and adults: 0.02 to 0.04 ml/kg I.M. as soon as possible after exposure. Up to 0.1 ml/kg may be given after prolonged or intense exposure.
Serum hepatitis posttransfusion
Children and adults: 10 ml I.M. within 1 week after transfusion and 10 ml I.M. 1 month later.
Measles exposure
Children and adults: 0.02 ml/kg within 6 days after exposure.
Modification of measles
Children and adults: 0.04 ml/kg I.M. within 6 days after exposure.
Measles vaccine complications
Children and adults: 0.02 to 0.04 ml/kg I.M.
Poliomyelitis exposure
Children and adults: 0.3 to 0.4 ml/kg I.M. within 7 days after exposure.
Chicken pox exposure
Children and adults: 0.2 to 1.3 ml/kg I.M. as soon as exposed.
Rubella exposure in first trimester of preg-nancy
Women: 0.2 to 0.4 ml/kg I.M. as soon as exposed.
Idiopathic thrombocytopenic purpura
Adults: 0.4 g/kg Sandoglobulin I.V. for 5 consecutive days.

Action and kinetics
• *Immune action:* Immune globulin provides passive immunity by increasing antibody titer.
• *Kinetics in adults:* After slow I.M. absorption, serum concentrations of gamma globulin peak within 2 days. Gamma globulin distributes evenly between intra-vascular and extravascular spaces. Metabolism is un-known. The serum half-life of gamma globulin is reportedly 21 to 24 days in immunocompetent pa-tients.

Contraindications and precautions
Immune globulin is contraindicated in patients known to have had an anaphylactic or severe systemic re-sponse to immune globulin and in patients with known hypersensitivity to thimerosal, maltose, or any com-ponent of the formulation.

Interactions
Concomitant use of immune globulin may interfere with the immune response to live virus vaccines (for example, measles, mumps, and rubella). Do not administer live virus vaccines within 3 months after administration of immune globulin.

Effects on diagnostic tests
None reported.

Adverse reactions
• Local: pain, *tenderness, muscle stiffness,* erythema, and phlebitis at injection site.
• Systemic: headache, *malaise,* fever, chills, faintness, urticaria, *hypersensitivity reactions,* hypotension, dyspnea, *angioedema, fever, nephrotic syndrome, anaphylaxis.* With IGIV, *flushing, chills, anaphylaxis.*
   Note: Drug should be discontinued or the infusion rate of gamma globulin reduced if adverse reactions occur during infusion. When symptoms subside, resume at a rate the patient can tolerate.

Overdose and treatment
Excessively rapid I.V. infusion rate can precipitate an anaphylactoid reaction.

▶ Special considerations
• Obtain a thorough history of allergies and reactions to immunizations.
• Epinephrine solution 1:1,000 should be available to treat allergic reactions.
• Inject I.M. formulation into different sites, preferably into buttocks. Do not inject more than 0.5 ml per injection site.
• Do not give for hepatitis A exposure if 2 weeks or more have elapsed since exposure or after onset of clinical illness.
• Closely monitor blood pressure in patient receiving IGIV, especially if this is the patient's first infusion of immune globulin.
• Immune globulin has not been associated with an increased frequency of acquired immunodeficiency syndrome (AIDS). It is devoid of human immunodeficiency virus (HIV). Immune globulin recipients do not develop antibodies to HIV.
• Although pregnancy is not a contraindication to use, it is not known whether immune globulin can cause fetal harm.
• Store IGIM or IGIV between 36° and 46° F. (2° and 8° C.). Do not freeze. Sandoglobulin should be stored below 20° C. (68° F.).
• Immune globulin has been studied in the treatment of various conditions, including Kawasaki disease, asthma, allergic disorders, autoimmune neutropenia, myasthenia gravis, and platelet transfusion rejection. It also has been used in the prophylaxis of infections in immunocompromised patients.
• Never use I.M. preparation for I.V. use.
• Gamimune N can be diluted with dextrose 5% in water.
• Gammagard should be reconstituted with the diluent (sterile water for injection) and transfer device provided by the manufacturer. The administration set (provided) contains a 15-micron inline filter that must be used during administration.

• Sandoglobulin should be reconstituted with the diluent supplied (0.9% sodium chloride).

Information for parents and patient
• Explain to parents that the patient's chances of getting AIDS or hepatitis after receiving immune globulin are minute.
• Tell parents and patient what to expect after vaccination: some local pain, swelling, and tenderness at the injection site. Recommend acetaminophen to ease minor discomfort.
• Tell parents and patient to promptly report headache, skin changes, or difficulty breathing.

indomethacin, indomethacin sodium trihydrate
Indocid, Indocin, Indocin SR, Indo-Lemmon, Indomed, Indameth

• Classification: nonnarcotic analgesic, antipyretic, anti-inflammatory (nonsteroidal anti-inflammatory drug [NSAID])

How supplied
Available by prescription only
Injection: 1-mg vials

Indications, route, and dosage
Moderate to severe arthritis, ankylosing spondylitis
Adults: 25 mg P.O. b.i.d. or t.i.d. with food or antacids; may increase dose by 25 mg daily q 7 days up to 200 mg daily; or 50 mg rectally q.i.d. Alternatively, sustained-release capsules (75 mg) may be given: 75 mg to start, in the morning or h.s., followed, if necessary, by 75 mg b.i.d.
To close a hemodynamically significant patent ductus arteriosus in premature infants (I.V. form only)
Age less than 48 hours: 0.2 mg/kg I.V. followed by 2 doses of 0.1 mg/kg at 12- to 24-hour intervals.
Age 2 to 7 days: 0.2 mg/kg I.V. followed by 2 doses of 0.2 mg/kg at 12- to 24-hour intervals.
Over age 7 days: 0.2 mg/kg I.V. followed by 2 doses of 0.25 mg/kg at 12- to 24-hour intervals.
†Juvenile rheumatoid arthritis
Children age 2 to 14: initially 2mg/kg P.O. daily in divided doses. May increase to 4 mg/kg daily if needed and tolerated; do not exceed 200 mg daily. Reduce dosage to lowest effecive level as soon as possible.

Action and kinetics
• *Analgesic, antipyretic, and anti-inflammatory actions:* Exact mechanisms of action are unknown; indomethacin is thought to produce its analgesic, antipyretic, and anti-inflammatory effects by inhibiting prostaglandin synthesis and possibly by inhibiting phosphodiesterase.
• *Closure of patent ductus arteriosus:* The exact mechanism of action is unknown, but may be through inhibition of prostaglandin synthesis.
• *Kinetics in adults:* Indomethacin is absorbed rapidly

and completely from the GI tract. Indomethacin is highly protein-bound and is metabolized in the liver. Indomethacin is excreted mainly in urine, with some biliary excretion.

Contraindications and precautions

Indomethacin is contraindicated in patients with known hypersensitivity to the drug; in patients in whom aspirin or other nonsteroidal anti-inflammatory drugs (NSAIDs) induce symptoms of asthma, urticaria, or rhinitis; in patients with active GI disorders because it may cause GI upset; in infants with untreated infection; in patients with active bleeding; in patients with coagulation defects or thrombocytopenia; in patients with necrotizing entercolitis; and in patients with impaired renal function. Rectal form of indomethacin is contraindicated in patients with a history of recent rectal bleeding or proctitis.

The safety and effectiveness of indomethacin in children under age 14 has not been established, (except for closure of patent ductus), but some clinicians employ indomethacin if the benefits outweigh the risks. Hepatotoxicity (sometimes fatal) has appeared in children treated with the drug. Monitor liver function periodically.

Administer cautiously to patients with epilepsy, parkinsonism, hepatic or renal disease, cardiovascular disease, known intrinsic coagulation defects, infection, or a history of mental illness, because it may exacerbate the symptoms of these disorders.

Patients with known "triad" symptoms (aspirin hypersensitivity, rhinitis/nasal polyps, and asthma) are at high risk of bronchospasm. NSAIDs may mask the signs and symptoms of acute infection (fever, myalgia, erythema); carefully evaluate patients with high risk (such as those with diabetes).

Interactions

Concomitant use of indomethacin with anticoagulants and thrombolytic drugs (coumarin derivatives, heparin, streptokinase, or urokinase) may potentiate anticoagulant effects. Bleeding problems may occur if indomethacin is used with other drugs that inhibit platelet aggregation, such as azlocillin, parenteral carbenicillin, dextran, dipyridamole, mezlocillin, piperacillin, sulfinpyrazone, ticarcillin, valproic acid, cefamandole, cefoperazone, moxalactam, plicamycin, aspirin, salicylates, or other anti-inflammatory agents. Concomitant use with salicylates, anti-inflammatory agents, alcohol, corticotropin, or steroids may cause increased GI adverse effects, including ulceration and hemorrhage. Aspirin may decrease the bioavailability of indomethacin.

Because of the influence of prostaglandins on glucose metabolism, concomitant use with insulin or oral hypoglycemic agents may potentiate hypoglycemic effects. Indomethacin may displace highly protein-bound drugs from binding sites. Toxicity may occur with coumarin derivatives, phenytoin, verapamil, or nifedipine. Increased nephrotoxicity may occur with gold compounds, other anti-inflammatory agents, or acetaminophen. Indomethacin may decrease the renal clearance of methotrexate and lithium.

Concurrent use with antihypertensives and diuretics may decrease their effectiveness. Concurrent use with triamterene not recommended due to potential nephrotoxicity. Other diuretics may also predispose patients to nephrotoxicity.

Effects on diagnostic tests

Indomethacin may interfere with results of the dexamethasone suppression test. It may also interfere with urinary 5-hydroxyindoleacetic acid determinations.

Adverse reactions

- CNS: *headache*, drowsiness, dizziness, depression, confusion, peripheral neuropathy, convulsions, psychic disturbances, syncope, vertigo.
- CV: hypertension, edema.
- DERM: pruritus, rash, urticaria, *Stevens-Johnson syndrome.*
- EENT: blurred vision, corneal and retinal damage, hearing loss, tinnitus.
- GI: *nausea, vomiting,* anorexia, diarrhea, constipation, severe GI bleeding (with I.V. dose).
- GU: hematuria, hyperkalemia, *acute renal failure,* renal dysfunction (with I.V. dose).
- HEMA: hemolytic anemia, aplastic anemia, agranulocytosis, leukopenia, thrombocytopenic purpura, iron deficiency anemia, *decreased platelet aggregation* (with I.V. dose).
- Hepatic: *elevated liver enzymes, hepatotoxicity.*
- Other: hypersensitivity (shocklike symptoms, rash, respiratory distress, angioedema); hyponatremia, hyperkalemia, hypoglycemia (with I.V. dose).

Note: Drug should be discontinued if hypersensitivity, significant GI symptoms, or signs of hepatotoxicity occur.

Overdose and treatment

Clinical manifestations of overdose include dizziness, nausea, vomiting, intense headache, mental confusion, drowsiness, tinnitus, sweating, blurred vision, paresthesias, and convulsions.

To treat indomethacin overdose, empty stomach immediately by inducing emesis with ipecac syrup or by gastric lavage. Administer activated charcoal via nasogastric tube. Provide symptomatic and supportive measures (respiratory support and correction of fluid and electrolyte imbalances). Monitor laboratory parameters and vital signs closely. Dialysis may be of little value because indomethacin is strongly protein-bound.

▶ Special considerations

- Use of I.V. indomethacin in premature infants for patent ductus arteriosus is considered an alternative to surgery.
- Indocin is approved by the FDA for spondyloarthropathy in older children.
- I.V. administration should be used only for premature neonates with patent ductus arteriosus. Do not administer a second or third I.V. dose if anuria or marked oliguria is present.
- If ductus arteriosus reopens, a second course of one to three doses may be given. If ineffective, surgery may be necessary.
- Use indomethacin cautiously in patients with a history of GI disease, increased risk of GI bleeding, or

---

*Canada only   †Unlabeled clinical use   Italicized adverse reactions have been observed in children.

decreased risk of GI bleeding, or decreased renal function.

• Patients with known "triad" symptoms (aspirin hypersensitivity, rhinitis/nasal polyps, and asthma) are at high risk of bronchospasm.

• Indomethacin may mask the signs and symptoms of acute infection (fever, myalgia, erythema); carefully evaluate patients at high risk for infection (for example, those with diabetes).

• Administer indomethacin with enough water to ensure passage into stomach. Have patient sit up for 15 to 30 minutes after taking the drug to prevent lodging of the drug in the esophagus.

• Tablets may be crushed and mixed with food or fluids to aid swallowing, and with antacids to minimize gastric upset.

• Assess level of pain and inflammation before start of therapy. Evaluate patient for relief or reduction of these symptoms.

• Monitor for signs and symptoms of bleeding.

• Monitor ophthalmic and auditory function before and periodically during therapy to prevent toxicity.

• Monitor CBC, platelets, prothrombin times, and hepatic and renal function studies periodically to detect abnormalities.

• Use of indomethacin with an opioid analgesic has an additive effect. Use of lower doses of the opioid analgesic may be possible.

• The safety of long-term indomethacin use in children under age 14 has not been established.

• Do not mix oral suspension with liquids or antacids before administering.

• Patient (adults only) should retain suppository in the rectum for at least 1 hour after insertion to ensure maximum absorption.

• Reconstitute 1 mg vial of I.V. dose with 1 to 2 ml of sterile water for injection or 0.9% sodium chloride injection. Prepare solution immediately before use to prevent deterioration. Do not use solution if it is discolored or contains a precipitate.

• Administer by direct I.V. injection over 5 to 10 seconds. Use a large vein to prevent extravasation.

• Monitor I.V. site for complications.

• Monitor cardiopulmonary status for significant changes. Watch for signs and symptoms of fluid overload. Check weight and intake and output daily.

• Monitor renal and hepatic function studies before start of therapy and frequently during therapy to prevent adverse effects.

• Severe headache may occur. If headache persists, dose should be decreased.

• Monitor carefully for bleeding and for reduced urine output.

Information for parents and patient

• Tell parents to have patient take medication with 8 oz of water 30 minutes before or 2 hours after meals, or with food or milk if gastric irritation occurs.

• Explain that taking the drug as directed is necessary to achieve the desired effect; 2 to 4 weeks of treatment may be needed before benefit is seen.

• Inform parents of patients on long-term therapy that follow-up visits for laboratory studies may be necessary.

• Warn parents and patient that use of alcoholic beverages durig treatment with indomethacin may cause increased GI irritation and, possibly, GI bleeding.

---

insulin (regular)
Beef Regular Iletin II (acid neutral CZI), Humulin R, Iletin Regular★, Novolin R, Pork Regular Iletin II, Regular Iletin I, Regular (concentrated) Iletin II, Regular Pork Insulin, Velosulin, Velosulin Human

prompt insulin zinc suspension (semilente)
Iletin Semilente★, Semilente Iletin I, Insulin, Semilente Purified Pork

isophane insulin suspension (NPH)
Beef NPH Iletin II, Humulin N, Iletin NPH★, Insulatard NPH, NPH★, NPH Iletin I, Pork NPH Iletin II, Protaphane NPH, Novolin N

insulin zinc suspension (lente)
Beef Lente Iletin II, Lente Iletin I, Pork Lente Iletin II, Lentard, Monotard, Novolin L, Humulin L

protamine zinc insulin suspension (PZI)
Beef Protamine Zinc Iletin II, Iletin PZI★, Pork Protamine Zinc Iletin II, Protamine Zinc Iletin I

extended insulin zinc suspension (ultralente)
Iletin Ultralente★, Ultralente★, Ultralente Iletin I, Ultralente Insulin, Ultralente Purified Beef

• Classification: antidiabetic agent (pancreatic hormone)

How supplied
Available without prescription
Insulin (regular)
Injection (beef): 100 units/ml
Injection (pork): 100 units/ml, 500 units/ml
Injection (beef and pork): 40 units/ml, 100 units/ml
Injection (human): 100 units/ml
Prompt insulin zinc suspension (semilente)
Injection (beef): 100 units/ml
Injection (pork): 100 units/ml
Injection (beef and pork): 40 units/ml, 100 units/ml
Isophane insulin suspension (NPH)
Injection (beef): 100 units/ml
Injection (pork): 100 units/ml
Injection (beef and pork): 40 units/ml, 100 units/ml
Injection (human): 100 units/ml
Insulin zinc suspension (lente)
Injection (beef): 100 units/ml
Injection (pork): 100 units/ml

---

‡May contain sulfites   ◆May contain tartrazine   ◆◆May contain benzyl alcohol

Injection (beef and pork): 40 units/ml, 100 units/ml
Injection (human): 100 units/ml
Protamine zinc insulin (PZI)
Injection (beef): 100 units/ml
Injection (pork): 100 units/ml
Injection (beef and pork): 40 units/ml, 100 units/ml
Extended zinc insulin suspension (ultralente)
Injection (beef): 100 units/ml
Injection (pork): 100 units/ml
Injection (beef and pork): 40 units/ml, 100 units/ml

Indications, route, and dosage
Diabetic ketoacidosis (regular insulin)
Children: 0.1 unit/kg I.V. bolus, then 0.1 unit/kg/hour continuous I.V. infusion until blood glucose level drops to 250 mg/dl, then start S.C. insulin; or 0.5 to 1 unit/kg in two divided doses, one given I.V. and the other S.C., followed by 0.5 to 1 unit/kg I.V. q 1 to 2 hours. Preparation of infusion: add 100 units regular insulin to 100 ml 0.9% sodium chloride. Insulin concentration will be 1 unit/ml.
Adults: 25 to 150 units I.V. immediately, then additional doses may be given q 1 hour based on blood glucose levels until patient is out of acidosis; then give S.C. q 6 hours thereafter. Alternative dosage schedule is 50 to 100 units I.V. and 50 to 100 units S.C. immediately; additional doses may be given q 2 to 6 hours based on blood glucose levels; or 0.33 units/kg I.V. bolus, followed by 7 to 10 units/hour I.V. by continuous infusion. Continue infusion until blood glucose level drops to 250 mg/dl, then start S.C. insulin q 6 hours.
Ketosis-prone and juvenile-onset diabetes mellitus, diabetes mellitus inadequately controlled by diet and oral hypoglycemics
Children and adults: Individualized dosage adjusted according to patient's blood and urine glucose concentrations.
Hyperkalemia
Children and adults: 5 to 10 units of regular insulin with 50 ml of dextrose 50% in water over 5 minutes. Alternatively, 25 units of regular insulin given S.C. and an infusion of 1,000 ml of dextrose 10% in water with 90 mEq sodium bicarbonate; infuse 330 ml over 30 minutes and the balance over 3 hours.

Action and kinetics
• *Antidiabetic action:* Insulin is used to replace the physiologic production of endogenous insulin in patients with insulin dependent diabetes mellitus (IDDM) and diabetes mellitus inadequately controlled by diet and oral hypoglycemic agents. Insulin increases glucose transport across muscle and fat-cell membranes to reduce blood glucose levels. It also promotes conversion of glucose to its storage form, glycogen; triggers amino acid uptake and conversion to protein in muscle cells and inhibits protein degradation; stimulates triglyceride formation and inhibits release of free fatty acids from adipose tissue; and stimulates lipoprotein lipase activity, which converts circulating lipoproteins to fatty acids. Insulin is available in various forms and these differ mainly in onset, peak, and duration of action.
• *Kinetics in adults:* Insulin must be given parenterally because it is destroyed in the GI tract. Commer-

cially available preparations are formulated to differ in onset, peak, and duration after subcutaneous administration. They are classified as rapid-acting (½ to 1 hour onset), intermediate-acting (1 to 2 hour onset), and long-acting (4 to 8 hour onset). Insulin is distributed widely throughout the body. Some insulin is bound and inactivated by peripheral tissues, but the majority appears to be degraded in the liver and kidneys. Insulin is filtered by the renal glomeruli and undergoes some tubular reabsorption. The plasma half-life is about 9 minutes after I.V. administration.

Contraindications and precautions
Use only regular insulin in patients with circulatory collapse, diabetic ketoacidosis, or hyperkalemia. Do not administer regular insulin concentrated by I.V. Do not use intermediate- or long-acting insulins for coma or other emergency requiring rapid drug action.

Interactions
Alcohol, beta blockers, clofibrate, fenfluramine, MAO inhibitors, salicylates, and tetracyline can cause a prolonged hypoglycemic effect. Monitor blood glucose carefully.

Corticosteroids and thiazide diuretics can diminish insulin response. Monitor for hyperglycemia.

Effects on diagnostic tests
The physiologic effects of insulin may decrease serum magnesium, potassium, or inorganic phosphate concentrations.

Adverse reactions
• DERM: urticaria.
• Metabolic: *hypoglycemia, hyperglycemia (rebound, or Somogyi, effect).*
• Local: lipoatrophy, lipohypertrophy, itching, swelling, redness, stinging, warmth at injection site.
• Other: anaphylaxis.

Overdose and treatment
Insulin overdose may produce signs and symptoms of hypoglycemia (tachycardia, palpitations, anxiety, hunger, nausea, diaphoresis, tremors, pallor, restlessness, headache, and speech and motor dysfunction). Treatment is directed towards treating hypoglycemia. Treatment depends on the patient's symptoms. If the patient is responsive, give 10 to 15 g of a fast-acting oral carbohydrate. If the patient's signs and symptoms persist after 15 minutes, give an additional 10 g carbohydrate. If the patient is unresponsive, an I.V. bolus of dextrose 50% solution should immediately increase blood glucose. You also may give glucagon parenterally or epinephrine subcutaneously; both drugs raise blood glucose levels in a few minutes by stimulating glycogenolysis. Fluid and electrolyte imbalance may require I.V. fluids and electrolyte (such as potassium) replacement.

▶ Special considerations
• Accuracy of measurement is very important, especially with regular insulin concentrated. Aids, such as magnifying sleeve, dose magnifier, or cornwall syringe, may help improve accuracy.
• With regular insulin concentrated, a deep secondary

hypoglycemic reaction may occur 18 to 24 hours after injection.
• Dosage is always expressed in USP units.
• Do not interchange single-source beef or pork insulins without considering the need for dosage adjustment.
• Lente, semilente, and ultralente insulins may be mixed in any proportion. Regular insulin may be mixed with NPH or lente insulins in any proportion. However, in vitro binding will occur over time until an equilibrium is reached. These mixtures should be administered either immediately after preparation or after stability occurs (15 minutes for NPH regular, 24 hours for lente regular) in order to minimize variability in patient response. Note that switching from separate injections to a prepared mixture also may alter the patient's response. Advise patient not to alter the order of mixing insulins or change the model or brand of syringe or needle.
• Store insulin in cool area. Refrigeration desirable but not essential, except with regular insulin concentrated.
• Do not use insulin that has changed color or becomes clumped or granular in appearance.
• Check expiration date on vial before using contents.
• Administration route is S.C. because it allows slower absorption and causes less pain than I.M. injections. Ketosis-prone, juvenile-onset, severely ill, and newly diagnosed diabetics with very high blood sugar levels may require hospitalization and I.V. treatment with regular fast-acting insulin. Ketosis-resistant diabetics may be treated as outpatients with intermediate-acting insulin after they have received instructions on how to alter dosage according to self-performed urine or blood glucose determinations. Some patients, primarily pregnant or brittle diabetics, may use a dextrometer to perform fingerstick blood glucose tests at home.
• Press but do not rub site after injection. Rotate injection sites. Record sites to avoid overuse of one area. However, unstable diabetics may achieve better control if injection site is rotated within same anatomic region.
• To mix insulin suspension, swirl vial gently or rotate between palms or between palm and thigh. Do not shake vigorously; this causes bubbling and air in syringe.
• In pregnant diabetic patients, insulin requirements increase, sometimes drastically, then decline immediately postpartum.
• Some patients may develop insulin resistance and require large insulin doses to control symptoms of diabetes. U-500 insulin is available as Purified Pork Iletin Regular Insulin, U500 for such patients. Although every pharmacy may not normally stock it, it is readily available. Patient should notify pharmacist several days before prescription refill is needed. Give hospital pharmacy sufficient notice before refill of in-house prescription. Never store U-500 insulin in same area with other insulin preparations because of danger of severe overdose if given accidentally to other patients. U-500 insulin must be administered with a U-100 syringe because no syringes are made for this drug.
• Human insulin may be advantageous in patients who are allergic to pork or beef forms. Otherwise, these insulins offer no advantage. Humulin is synthesized by a genetically altered strain of *Escherichia coli*. Novolin brands are derived by enzymatic alteration of pork insulin.

Information for parents and patient
• Human insulin may be advantageous for patients who are allergic to pork or beef forms, for noninsulin-dependent patients requiring intermittent or short-term therapy (such as pregnancy, surgery, infection, or total parenteral nutrition), for patients with insulin resistance, or for those who develop lipoatrophy.
• Be sure parents and patient know that insulin therapy relieves symptoms but does not cure the disease.
• Explain nature of disease, importance of following therapeutic regimen, specific diet, weight reduction, exercise, personal hygiene, avoiding infection, and timing of injection and eating.
• Emphasize the importance of regular meal times and not omitting meals.
• Explain that blood glucose tests are essential guides to correct dosage and to therapeutic success.
• Emphasize the importance of recognizing hypoglycemic symptoms because insulin-induced hypoglycemia is hazardous and may cause brain damage if prolonged.
• Advise parents that patient should always wear a medical identification bracelet or pendant, carry ample insulin supply and syringes on trips, have carbohydrates (sugar or candy) on hand for emergency, and note any time-zone changes for dose schedule when traveling.
• Patient should not change the order of mixing insulins or change the model or brand of syringe or needle.
• Tell parents and patient that use of marijuana may increase insulin requirements.
• Cigarette smoking decreases the absorption of insulin administered subcutaneously. Advise patient not to smoke within 30 minutes after insulin injection.

iodoquinol (diiodohydroxyquin)
Amebaquin, Moebiquin, Yodoxin

• Classification: amebicide (iodinated 8-hydroxyquinoline)

How supplied
Available by prescription only
Tablets: 210 mg, 650 mg

Indications, route, and dosage
Intestinal amebiasis
Children: Usual dosage is 30 to 40 mg/kg of body weight daily in two or three divided doses for 20 days.
Adults: 630 to 650 mg P.O. t.i.d. for 20 days. Total daily dosage should not exceed 2 g.

Iodoquinol is usually reserved for treating resistant amebiasis. In many cases, it is combined with metronidazole (750 mg P.O. q.i.d. for 5 to 10 days) for mild to moderate intestinal disease and with several other agents for invasive disease. It is useful only against the encysted form of the parasite; hence, its use as a sole agent is limited to mild cases of asymptomatic carriers.

Additional courses of iodoquinol therapy should not be repeated before a resting interval of 2 to 3 weeks.

Action and kinetics
• *Amebicidal action:* Iodoquinol is amebicidal against protozoa, especially *Entamoeba histolytica.* It acts primarily in the intestinal lumen by an unknown mechanism.
• *Kinetics in adults:* About 8% of an oral dose is absorbed. Distribution is unknown. Most of the absorbed dose appears to be glucuronidated or sulfated in the liver. Drug is excreted primarily unchanged in feces. It is unknown if iodoquinol is excreted in breast milk.

Contraindications and precautions
Iodoquinol is contraindicated in patients with known hypersensitivity to 8-hydroxyquinolines or iodine-containing preparations because it contains iodine. It also is contraindicated in patients with hepatic or renal disease or optic neuropathy because it may exacerbate these conditions. Because of its iodine content, iodoquinol should be used with caution in patients with thyroid disease.

Long-term therapy is not recommended because of the potential hazard of visual and nerve damage.

Interactions
None reported.

Effects on diagnostic tests
Iodoquinol may increase protein-bound iodine levels and therefore interfere with thyroid function tests for up to 6 months after discontinuation of therapy.

Adverse reactions
• CNS: neurotoxicity, dysesthesia, weakness, vertigo, malaise, headache, agitation, retrograde amnesia, ataxia, peripheral neuropathy.
• DERM: pruritus, hives, papular and pustular eruptions, urticaria, discoloration of hair and nails.
• EENT: optic neuritis, optic atrophy, loss of vision.
• GI: anorexia, nausea, vomiting, abdominal cramps, diarrhea, increased motility, constipation, epigastric burning and pain, gastritis, anal irritation and itching.
• HEMA: agranulocytosis.
• Other: thyroid enlargement, fever, chills, generalized furunculosis, hair loss, muscle pain.
Note: Drug should be discontinued if signs of hypersensitivity or toxicity occur.

Overdose and treatment
Overdose with iodoquinol may affect cardiovascular and respiratory function. Treatment is largely supportive. After recent ingestion (within 4 hours), empty stomach by induced emesis or gastric lavage. Follow with activated charcoal to decrease absorption. Saline or osmotic cathartics may also be helpful.

▶ **Special considerations**
• Patients should have periodic ophthalmologic examinations during therapy to detect optic neuropathy.
• Schedule dose after meals; tablets should be crushed and mixed with applesauce or chocolate syrup to facilitate swallowing.
• Monitor intake and output and renal function.
• Send fecal specimens to laboratory promptly; infection is detectable only in warm specimens.
• Monitor for diarrhea during first 3 days of therapy; if diarrhea continues beyond 3 days, consider alternate therapy.
• Monitor serum electrolyte levels and blood counts; replace fluids and electrolytes as necessary.
• Patient may be discharged when three consecutive daily stool specimens are normal.

Information for parents and patient
• Emphasize that drug should not be discontinued prematurely.
• Tell parents to report skin rash.
• Emphasize the importance of follow-up appointments.
• Tell parents and patient that stool specimens will be checked at 1, 3, and 6 months to ensure elimination of amebae.
• To help prevent reinfection, instruct parents and patient in proper hygiene, including disposal of feces and hand washing after defecation and before eating, and about the risks of eating raw foods and the control of contamination by flies.
• Advise use of liquid soap or reserved bar of soap to prevent cross contamination.
• Advise parents that patient should not prepare, process, or handle food during treatment. Isolation of patient is unnecessary.
• Encourage other household members and suspected contacts to be tested and, if necessary, treated.

----

iron dextran
Feronim, Hematran, Hydextran, Imfergen, Imferon, Irodex, K-Feron, Nor-Feron, Proferdex

• Classification: hematinic (parenteral iron supplement)

How supplied
Available by prescription only
Injection: 50 mg elemental iron/ml

Indications, route, and dosage
Iron-deficiency anemia
Dosage is highly individualized and is based on the patient's weight and hemoglobin level.
Note: Test dose of 0.5 ml should be given before calculated therapeutic dose.

Children 5 to 15 kg, age 5 months and over:

Dose weight (12 — iron
(in ml) = 0.0476 × in kg × hemoglobin + stores.
level)

Iron stores = 1 ml/5 kg to a maximum of 14 ml.

Children over 15 kg and adults:

Dose weight (14.8 — iron
(in ml) = 0.0476 × in kg × hemoglobin + stores.
level)

Iron stores = 1 ml/5 kg to a maximum of 14 ml.

Action and kinetics

• *Hematinic action:* Iron dextran is a complex of ferric hydroxide and dextran in a colloidal solution. After I.M. injection, 10% to 50% remains in the muscle for several months; remainder enters bloodstream, increasing plasma iron concentration for up to 2 weeks. Iron is an essential component of hemoglobin.

• *Kinetics in adults:* I.M. doses are absorbed in two stages: 60% after 3 days and up to 90% by 3 weeks. Remainder is absorbed over several months or longer. During first 3 days, local inflammation facilitates passage of drug into the lymphatic system; drug is then ingested by macrophages, which enter lymph and blood. After I.M. or I.V. administration, iron dextran is cleared from plasma by reticuloendothelial cells of the liver, spleen, and bone marrow. In doses of 500 mg or less, half-life is 6 hours. Traces are excreted in breast milk, urine, bile, and feces. Drug cannot be removed by hemodialysis.

Contraindications and precautions

Iron dextran is contraindicated in patients with known hypersensitivity to any of the components and in patients with any anemia other than iron-deficiency anemia. A test dose should always be given before the therapeutic dose. Monitor patient closely and be prepared to treat a severe allergic reaction. Have epinephrine, oxygen, and emergency equipment readily available.

Administer iron dextran cautiously to patients with rheumatoid arthritis, because I.V. injections may exacerbate joint pain and swelling; and to patients with a significant history of allergies or asthma. Administer with extreme caution to patients with serious hepatic impairment because of potential for additional liver damage. *Do not administer simultaneously with oral iron.*

Interactions

None significant.

Effects on diagnostic tests

Large doses (over 100 mg iron) may color the serum brown.

Iron dextran may cause false elevations of serum bilirubin level and false reductions in serum calcium level.

Iron dextran prevents meaningful measurement of serum iron concentration and total iron binding capacity for up to 3 weeks; I.M. injection may cause dense areas of activity on bone scans using technetium 99m diphosphonate, for 1 to 6 days.

Adverse reactions

• CNS: headache, shivering, transitory paresthesias, arthralgia, myalgia, dizziness, malaise, syncope.
• CV: hypotensive reaction, peripheral vascular flushing (with overly rapid I.V. administration), tachycardia, precordial pain, fatal dysrhythmia.
• DERM: rash, urticaria.
• GI: nausea, vomiting, metallic taste, transient loss of taste.
• Local: skin discoloration, soreness, inflammation, and sterile abscess at I.M. injection site; phlebitis at I.V. injection site.
• Other: anaphylaxis; hemosiderosis; regional lymphadenopathy; I.V. administration may reactivate or exacerbate rheumatoid arthritis or ankylosing spondylitis.

Overdose and treatment

Injected iron has much greater bioavailability than oral iron, but data on acute overdose is limited.

► Special considerations

• Administer test dose of 0.5 ml iron dextrose I.M. or I.V. Be alert for anaphylaxis on test dose; monitor vital signs for drug reaction. Keep epinephrine (0.5 ml of a 1:1,000 solution) readily available for such an emergency.
• Discontinue oral iron before giving iron dextran.
• Use 10-ml multi-dose vial only for I.M. injections, because it contains phenol as a preservative; use only 2- or 5-ml ampule without preservative for I.V. administration.
• Inject I.M. preparation deeply into upper outer quadrant of buttocks (never an arm or other exposed area), using a 2″ to 3″ (5- to 8-cm), 19G or 20G needle. Use Z-track technique to avoid leakage into subcutaneous tissue and skin stains, and minimize staining by using a separate needle to withdraw drug from its container.
• I.V. use is controversial, and some hospitals do not allow it.
• Give drug I.V. if patient has insufficient muscle mass for deep injection, impaired absorption from muscle because of stasis or edema, a risk of uncontrolled I.M. bleeding from trauma (as in hemophilia), or need for massive and prolonged parenteral therapy (as in chronic substantial blood loss). Do not administer more than 50 mg of iron/minute (1 ml/minute) if using drug undiluted.
• After I.V. iron dextran administration, flush vein with 10 ml normal saline injection to minimize local irritation. Have patient rest for 15 to 30 minutes, since orthostatic hypotension may occur.
• Monitor hemoglobin, hematocrit, and reticulocyte count during therapy. An increase of about 1 g/dl/week in hemoglobin is usual.

Information for parents and patient

Warn parents or patient of potential allergic reactions and of possible skin staining with I.M. injections.
• Instruct parents about necessary adjustments of diet, especially limiting the child's excessive consumption of milk.

isoetharine hydrochloride
Arm-a-Med, Beta-2, Bisorine, Bronkosol, Dey-Dose, Dey-Lute, Dispos-a-Med

isoetharine mesylate
Bronkometer

• Classification: bronchodilator (adrenergic)

How supplied
Available by prescription only
Nebulizer inhaler: 0.062%, 0.08%, 0.1%, 0.125%, 0.14%, 0.167%, 0.17%, 0.2%, 0.25%, 0.5%, 1% solution
Aerosol inhaler: 340 mcg/metered spray

Indications, route, and dosage
Bronchial asthma and reversible bronchospasm that may occur with bronchitis and emphysema
Isoetharine hydrochloride
Children and adults: Administered by oxygen aerosolization, 0.5 to 1 ml of a 0.5% or 0.5 ml (range 0.25 to 0.5 ml) of a 1% solution diluted 1:3; or undiluted, 4 ml (range 2 to 4 ml) of a 0.125% solution, 2.5 ml of a 0.2% solution, or 2 ml of a 0.25% solution. Administered by IPPB solution, 0.5 to 1 ml of a 0.5% solution, or 0.5 ml (range 0.25 to 1 ml) of a 1% solution diluted 1:3; or undiluted 4 ml (range 2 to 4 ml) of a 0.125% solution, 2.5 ml of 0.2% solution, or 2 ml of a 0.25% solution. Administered by hand-nebulizer, four inhalations (range three to seven inhalations) of undiluted 0.5% or 1% solution.
Isoetharine mesylate
Children and adults: Administered by metered aerosol, one to two inhalations. Occasionally, more may be required.

Action and kinetics
• *Bronchodilating action:* Isoetharine relaxes bronchial smooth muscle by direct action on beta₂-adrenergic receptors, resulting in relief of bronchospasm, increased vital capacity, and decreased airway resistance. It may also inhibit release of histamine. Isoetharine also relaxes the smooth muscles of the peripheral vasculature.
• *Kinetics in adults:* Isoetharine is absorbed rapidly from the respiratory tract after oral inhalation. Bronchodilation occurs immediately, peaks in 5 to 15 minutes, and persists 1 to 4 hours. Isoetharine is distributed widely throughout the body. It is metabolized in lungs, liver, GI tract, and other tissues. Isoetharine is excreted in urine as unchanged drug and metabolites.

Contraindications and precautions
Isoetharine is contraindicated in patients with known hypersensitivity to the drug or to any ingredients in the formulation.

Administer cautiously to patients with hyperthyroidism, hypertension, acute coronary disease, an-

gina, cardiac asthma, limited cardiac reserve, and cerebral arteriosclerosis, because the drug may worsen these conditions; and to patients with sulfite sensitivity, because some formulations contain sulfite preservatives.

Interactions
Concomitant use with epinephrine or other sympathomimetics may produce additive adverse cardiovascular effects. Beta-adrenergic blocking agents (such as propranolol) antagonize isoetharine's bronchodilating, cardiac, and vasodilating effects.

Effects on diagnostic tests
None reported.

Adverse reactions
• CNS: *tremors,* weakness, *headache, anxiety,* tension, *restlessness,* insomnia, dizziness, *excitement, irritability.*
• CV: *increased heart rate,* palpitations, hypotension or *hypertension,* angina.
• GI: *nausea,* vomiting.
• Other: cough, bronchial irritation, edema, *paradoxical bronchoconstriction.*
Note: Drug should be discontinued if patient develops hypersensitivity to drug or sulfite preservatives, bronchoconstriction, or tachyphylaxis.

Overdose and treatment
Clinical manifestations of overdose include exaggeration of common adverse reactions, particularly nausea and vomiting, cardiac dysrhythmias, hypertension, and extreme tremors.

Treatment includes symptomatic and supportive measures. Monitor vital signs closely. Sedatives may be used to treat restlessness. Cardioselective beta blockers (like metoprolol) may be used to treat dysrhythmias, but with caution (may induce asthmatic attack).

▶ Special considerations
• The preservative sodium bisulfite is present in many adrenergic formulations. Patients with a history of allergy to sulfites should avoid preparations that contain this preservative. Ask parents about sensitivity to sulfites.
• Systemic absorption can follow applications to nasal and conjunctival membranes, though infrequently. If symptoms of systemic absorption occur, patient should stop the drug.
• Do not use discolored or precipitated solutions.
• Prolonged or too-frequent use may cause tolerance to bronchodilating and cardiac stimulant effect. Rebound bronchospasm may follow end of drug effect.
• Pediatric dosage recommendations not established by the manufacturer; however, some clinicians believe pediatric dosage is the same as the adult dosage.
• Therapy should be administered on arising in morning and before meals to reduce fatigue from activity by improving lung ventilation.
• Tolerance may develop after prolonged or excessive use.
• Paradoxical airway resistance (sudden worsening of dyspnea) may follow repeated excessive use. If this

---

occurs, patient or family should discontinue isoetharine and call for alternative therapy (such as epinephrine).
• Alternating therapy with isoetharine inhalation and
epinephrine may be helpful. However, these drugs
should not be administered simultaneously because
of danger of excessive cardiac stimulation.
• Protect solutions from light, freezing, and heat. Store
at controlled room temperature.

Information for parents and patient
• Treatment should start with first symptoms of bronchospasm.
• Dosage and recommended method of inhaling may
vary with type of nebulizer and formulation used.
Carefully instruct parents and patient in correct use
of nebulizer.
• Tell parents to have patient use only as directed,
and to take no more than two inhalations at one time
with 1- to 2-minute intervals between.
• Instruct patient to wait 1 full minute after initial
one to two inhalations (Bronkometer) before inhaling
another dose. Action should begin immediately and
peak within 5 to 15 minutes.
• Warn patient to keep spray away from eyes.
• Teach parents and patient that a single aerosol treatment is usually enough to control an asthma attack
and to call promptly if the patient requires more than
three aerosol treatments in 24 hours.
• If symptoms persist or worsen, patient should call
for further instructions. Excessive use may decrease
desired effect and cause distressing tachycardia, palpitations, headache, nausea, and dizziness.
• Tell parents to call if bronchodilator causes dizziness, chest pain, or lack of therapeutic response to
usual dose.
• Tell parents and patient that increased fluid intake
facilitates clearing of secretions. Inform them that
saliva and sputum may appear pink after inhalation
treatment.
• Teach parents and patient how to accomplish postural drainage, to cough productively, and to clap and
vibrate to promote good respiratory hygiene.
• Tell parents that patient should avoid other adrenergic medications unless they are prescribed.
• Information and instructions are furnished with the
aerosol forms of these drugs. Urge parents and patient
to read them carefully and ask questions if necessary.
• Tell parents and patient not to discard drug applicator. Refill units are available.
• Tell parents to store drug away from heat and light
(not in bathroom medicine cabinet where heat and
humidity can cause drug to deteriorate) and out of
small children's reach.

isoniazid (INH)
Hyzyd, Isotamine*, Laniazid, Nydrazid,
PMS-Isoniazid*, Rimifon*, Rolazid,
Teebaconin

• Classification: antitubercular agent (isonicotinic
acid hydrazine)

How supplied
Available by prescription only
Oral solution: 50 mg/5 ml
Tablets: 50 mg, 100 mg, 300 mg
Injection: 100 mg/ml

Indications, route, and dosage
*Primary treatment against actively growing
tubercle bacilli*
Infants and children: 10 to 20 mg/kg P.O. or I.M.
daily as single dose, up to 300 to 500 mg/day, continued for at least 1 year. Concomitant administration
of at least one other effective antitubercular drug is
recommended.
Adults: 5 to 10 mg/kg P.O. or I.M. daily as single
dose, up to 300 mg/day, continued for 9 months to 2
years.
*Prophylaxis against tubercle bacilli of those
closely exposed or with positive skin test
whose chest X-rays and bacteriologic studies
indicate nonprogressive tuberculosis*
Infants and children: 10 to 15 mg/kg P.O. daily as
single dose, up to 300 mg/day, continued for 9 months
to 1 year.
Adults: 300 mg P.O. daily as single dose, continued
for 1 year.

Action and kinetics
• *Antitubercular action:* Isoniazid (INH) interferes
with lipid and DNA synthesis, thus inhibiting bacterial cell wall synthesis. Its action is bacteriostatic
or bactericidal, depending on organism susceptibility
and drug concentration at infection site. INH is active
against *Mycobacterium tuberculosis, M. bovis,* and
some strains of *M. kansasii.*
   Resistance by *Mycobacterium tuberculosis* develops rapidly when INH is used to *treat* tuberculosis,
and it is usually combined with another antituberculosis agent to prevent or delay resistance. During
prophylaxis, however, resistance is not a problem and
isoniazid can be used alone.
• *Kinetics in adults:* INH is absorbed completely and
rapidly from the GI tract after oral administration;
peak serum concentrations occur 1 to 2 hours after
ingestion. Drug also is absorbed readily after I.M.
injection. INH is distributed widely into body tissues
and fluids, including ascitic, synovial, pleural, and
cerebrospinal fluids; lungs and other organs; and sputum and saliva. INH crosses the placenta.
   INH is inactivated primarily in the liver by genetically controlled acetylation. Rate of metabolism varies individually; fast acetylators metabolize drug five
times as rapidly as others. About 50% of blacks and
whites are slow acetylators of INH, whereas over 80%

---

‡May contain sulfites   ◆May contain tartrazine   ◆◆May contain benzyl alcohol

of Chinese, Japanese, and Eskimos are fast acetylators. About 75% of a dose of INH is excreted in urine as unchanged drug and metabolites in 24 hours; some drug is excreted in saliva, sputum, feces, and breast milk. Elimination half-life in adults is 1 to 4 hours, depending on metabolic rate. INH is removed by peritoneal dialysis or hemodialysis.

Contraindications and precautions
INH is contraindicated in patients with known hypersensitivity to the drug; in patients with history of INH-induced hepatic disease or other severe reactions, including arthralgias, fever, chills, or acute hepatic disease.

INH should be used cautiously in patients who ingest alcohol daily and in patients with chronic hepatic or renal disease, or a history of seizures.

Interactions
Concomitant daily use of alcohol may increase incidence of INH-induced hepatitis and seizures.

Concomitant use with cycloserine increases hazard of CNS toxicity, drowsiness, and dizziness from cycloserine.

INH-induced inhibition of metabolism and elevation of serum concentrations increases toxicity of phenytoin and carbamazepine.

Concomitant use of INH and disulfiram may cause coordination difficulties and psychotic episodes.

Concomitant use with antacids decreases oral absorption of INH; use with corticosteroids may decrease INH efficacy; use with rifampin may accelerate INH metabolism to hepatotoxic metabolites, because of rifampin-induced enzyme production.

Effects on diagnostic tests
INH alters results of urine glucose tests that use cupric sulfate method (Benedict's reagent or Clinitest).

Elevated liver function study results occur in about 15% of patients taking the drug; most abnormalities are mild and transient, but some persist throughout treatment.

Adverse reactions
• CNS: peripheral neuropathy (especially in malnourished, alcoholic, and diabetic patients, and in slow acetylators), usually preceded by paresthesias of hands and feet; psychosis; seizures.
• CV: postural hypotension.
• EENT: optic neuritis with atrophy.
• GI: nausea, vomiting, epigastric distress, constipation, dryness of the mouth.
• HEMA: agranulocytosis, hemolytic anemia, aplastic anemia, eosinophilia, leukopenia, neutropenia, thrombocytopenia, methemoglobinemia, pyridoxine-responsive hypochromic anemia.
• Hepatic: hepatitis, jaundice (rare in children).
• Metabolic: hyperglycemia, metabolic acidosis, pyridoxine deficiency, gynecomastia.
• Local: irritation at injection site.
• Other: rheumatic syndrome and systemic lupus erythematosus-like syndrome, hypersensitivity reactions (fever, rash, lymphadenopathy, vasculitis).

Note: Drug should be discontinued if patient shows signs of hypersensitivity reaction or hepatic damage.

Overdose and treatment
Early signs of overdose include nausea, vomiting, slurred speech, dizziness, blurred vision and visual hallucinations, occurring 30 minutes to 3 hours after ingestion; gross overdose causes CNS depression progressing from stupor to coma, with respiratory distress, intractable seizures, and death.

To treat, establish ventilation; control seizures with diazepam. Pyridoxine is administered to equal dose of INH. Initial dose is 1 to 4 g pyridoxine I.V., followed by 1 g every 30 minutes thereafter, until the entire dose is given. Clear drug with gastric lavage *after* seizure control, and correct acidosis with parenteral sodium bicarbonate; force diuresis with I.V. fluids and osmotic diuretics, and, if necessary, enhance clearance of the drug with hemodialysis or peritoneal dialysis.

▶ Special considerations
• Infants and children tolerate larger doses of the drug.
• Prescribe oral doses to be taken on empty stomach for maximum absorption or with food if gastric irritation occurs.
• Aluminum-containing antacids or laxatives should be taken 1 hour after oral dose of INH.
• Obtain specimens for culture and sensitivity testing before first dose, but therapy may begin before test results are complete; repeat periodically to detect drug resistance.
• Monitor blood, renal, and hepatic function studies before and periodically during therapy to minimize toxicity; assess visual function periodically.
• Observe patient for adverse effects, especially hepatic dysfunction, CNS toxicity, and optic neuritis. Establish safety measures, in case postural hypotension occurs.
• INH may hinder stabilization of serum glucose level in patients with diabetes mellitus.
• Improvement usually evident after 2 to 3 weeks of therapy.
• Some clinicians recommend pyridoxine 50 mg P.O. daily to prevent peripheral neuropathy from large doses of INH. It may also be useful in patients at risk of developing peripheral neuropathy from other causes (such as malnutrition and diabetes). Pyridoxine (50 to 200 mg daily) has been used to treat INH-induced neuropathy.
• Because INH is dialyzable, patients undergoing hemodialysis or peritoneal dialysis may need dosage adjustments.
• Hepatotoxicity is rare in children.

Information for parents and patient
• Explain disease process and rationale for long-term therapy.
• Teach signs and symptoms of hypersensitivity and other adverse reactions, particularly visual disturbances, and emphasize need to report these; urge patient to report *any* unusual effects.
• Warn parents that patient should not use alcohol; explain hazard of serious CNS toxicity and increased

---

hazard of hepatitis. Emphasize that liquid medications may contain alcohol.

• Teach parents and patient how and when to take drug; instruct patient to take INH on an empty stomach, at least 1 hour before or 2 hours after meals. If GI irritation occurs, drug may be taken with food.

• Urge compliance with complete prescribed regimen. Advise parents not to discontinue drug without medical approval; explain importance of follow-up appointments.

• INH therapy is usually continued for 18 months to 2 years for treatment of active tuberculosis; 12 months for prophylaxis; 9 months if INH and rifampin therapy are combined.

• Emphasize the importance of uninterrupted therapy to prevent relapse and spread of infection.

isopropamide iodide
Darbid

• Classification: muscarinic, gastrointestinal antispasmodic (anticholinergic)

How supplied
Available by prescription only
Tablets: 5 mg

Indications, route, and dosage
Adjunctive therapy for peptic ulcer, irritable bowel syndrome
Children over age 12 and adults: 5 mg P.O. q 12 hours. Some patients may require 10 mg or more b.i.d. Dosage should be individualized to patient's need.

Action and kinetics
• *Anticholinergic action:* Isopropamide competitively blocks acetylcholine at cholinergic neuroeffector sites, decreasing GI motility and inhibiting gastric acid secretion.

• *Kinetics in adults:* Isopropamide is poorly absorbed from the GI tract. Isopropamide does not cross the blood-brain barrier; little else is known of its distribution. Exact metabolic fate is unknown. Isopropamide is excreted in the urine as metabolites and in the feces as unchanged drug.

Contraindications and precautions
Isopropamide is contraindicated in patients with narrow-angle glaucoma, because drug-induced cycloplegia and mydriasis may increase intraocular pressure; in patients with obstructive uropathy, obstructive GI tract disease, severe ulcerative colitis, myasthenia gravis, paralytic ileus, intestinal atony, or toxic megacolon, because the drug may exacerbate these conditions; and in patients with known hypersensitivity to anticholinergics.

Administer isopropamide cautiously to children with autonomic neuropathy, hyperthyroidism, coronary artery disease, cardiac dysrhythmias, congestive heart failure, or ulcerative colitis, because the drug may exacerbate the symptoms of these disorders; to children with hepatic or renal disease, because

toxic accumulation may occur; to patients with hiatal hernia associated with reflux esophagitis, because the drug may decrease lower esophageal sphincter tone; and in hot or humid environments, because the drug may predispose the patient to heatstroke.

Interactions
Concurrent administration of antacids decreases oral absorption of anticholinergics. Administer isopropamide at least 1 hour before antacids.

Concomitant administration of drugs with anticholinergic effects may cause additive toxicity.

Decreased GI absorption of many drugs has been reported after the use of anticholinergics (for example, levodopa and ketoconazole). Conversely, slowly dissolving digoxin tablets may yield higher serum digoxin levels when administered with anticholinergics.

Use cautiously with slow-release solid oral potassium supplements (especially wax-matrix formulations) because the incidence of potassium-induced GI ulcerations may be increased.

Effects on diagnostic tests
Isopropamide may alter thyroid function test results and will suppress ^{131}I uptake; drug should be discontinued at least 1 week before such tests.

Adverse reactions
• CNS: headache, insomnia, drowsiness, dizziness, nervousness, weakness, confusion or excitement (in elderly).

• CV: palpitations, tachycardia, orthostatic hypotension.

• DERM: urticaria, decreased sweating or anhidrosis, iodine skin rash, other dermal manifestations.

• EENT: blurred vision, mydriasis, cycloplegia, increased ocular tension, photophobia.

• GI: dry mouth, dysphagia, heartburn, loss of taste, nausea, constipation, vomiting, paralytic ileus, abdominal distention.

• GU: urinary hesitancy and retention, impotence.

• Other: fever, allergic reaction.

Note: Drug should be discontinued if hypersensitivity, urinary retention, confusion or excitement, curare-like symptoms, or skin rash occurs.

Overdose and treatment
Clinical effects of overdose include curare-like symptoms and such peripheral effects as headache; dilated, nonreactive pupils; blurred vision; flushed, hot, dry skin; dryness of mucous membranes; dysphagia; decreased or absent bowel sounds; urinary retention; hyperthermia; tachycardia; hypertension; and increased respiration.

Treatment is primarily symptomatic and supportive, as needed. If patient is alert, induce emesis (or use gastric lavage) and follow with a saline cathartic and repeated doses of activated charcoal and sorbitol mixture to prevent further drug absorption. In severe cases, physostigmine may be administered to block isopropamide's antimuscarinic effects. Give fluids, as needed, to treat shock. If urinary retention develops, catheterization may be necessary.

▶ Special considerations
- Give medication 30 minutes to 1 hour before meals and at bedtime to minimize therapeutic effects.
- Monitor patient's vital signs, urine output, visual changes, and for signs of impending toxicity.
- Give ice chips, cool drinks, or sugarless hard candy to relieve dry mouth.
- Constipation may be relieved by stool softeners or bulk laxatives.
- Discontinue isopropamide at least 1 week before thyroid function tests.
- Administer cautiously to patients with iodine hypersensitivity.

Information for parents and patient
- Teach parents or patient how and when to take drug; caution patient to take drug only as prescribed and not to add other medications except as prescribed.
- Warn patient that drug may cause dizziness, drowsiness, or blurred vision.
- Patient should avoid alcoholic beverages, because they may cause additive CNS effects. Emphasize that some liquid medications contain alcohol.
- Patient should consume plenty of fluids and dietary fiber to help avoid constipation.
- Tell parents or patient to promptly report dry mouth, blurred vision, skin rash, eye pain, or any significant change in urine volume, or pain or difficulty on urination.
- Warn parents or patient that drug may cause increased sensitivity or intolerance to high temperatures; resulting in dizziness.
- Instruct parents to watch for signs of confusion and to check for rapid or pounding heartbeat and to report these effects promptly.

---

isoproterenol
Aerolone, Isuprel, Vapo-Iso

isoproterenol hydrochloride
Isuprel, Isuprel Mistometer, Norisodrine

isoproterenol sulfate
Medihaler-Iso

- Classification: bronchodilator, cardiac stimulant (adrenergic)

How supplied
Available by prescription only
Isoproterenol
Nebulizer inhaler: 0.25%, 0.5%, and 1%
Isoproterenol hydrochloride
Aerosol inhaler: 120 mcg or 131 mcg/metered spray
Tablets (sublingual): 10 mg, 15 mg
Injection: 200 mcg/ml
Isoproterenol sulfate
Aerosol inhaler: 80 mcg/metered spray

Indications, route, and dosage
Complete heart block after closure of ventricular septal defect
Children: I.V. bolus, 0.01 to 0.03 mg (0.5 to 1.5 ml of a 1:50,000 dilution).
Adults: I.V. bolus, 0.04 to 0.06 mg (2 to 3 ml of a 1:50,000 dilution).
To prevent heart block
Adults: 10 to 30 mg sublingually four to six times daily.
Bronchospasm during mild acute asthma attacks
Isoproterenol hydrochloride
Children and adults: Via aerosol inhalation, 1 inhalation initially, repeated as needed after 1 to 5 minutes, to a maximum 6 inhalations daily. Maintenance dosage is 1 to 2 inhalations four to six times daily at 3- to 4-hour intervals. Via hand-bulb nebulizer, 5 to 15 deep inhalations of a 0.5% solution; if needed, may be repeated in 5 to 10 minutes. May be repeated up to five times daily. Alternatively, 3 to 7 deep inhalations of a 1% solution, repeated once in 5 to 10 minutes if needed. May be repeated up to five times daily.
Isoproterenol sulfate
Children and adults: For acute dyspneic episodes, one inhalation initially; repeated if needed after 2 to 5 minutes. Maximum six inhalations daily. Maintenance dosage: one to two inhalations up to six times daily.
Bronchospasm in chronic obstructive pulmonary disease
Isoproterenol hydrochloride
Children and adults: Via hand-bulb nebulizer: 5 to 15 deep inhalations of a 0.5% solution, or 3 to 7 deep inhalations of a 1% solution given no more frequently than every 3 to 4 hours.
Children: Via IPPB: 2 ml of a 0.0625% solution or 2.5 ml of a 0.05% solution administered over 10 to 15 minutes up to five times daily.
Adults: Via IPPB: 2 ml of a 0.125% solution or 2.5 ml of a 0.1% solution administered over 10 to 20 minutes, up to five times daily.
Bronchospasm during mild acute asthma attacks or in chronic obstructive pulmonary disease
Isoproterenol hydrochloride
Children and adults: 6 to 12 inhalations of a 0.025% nebulized solution, repeated at 15-minute intervals to a maximum of three treatments, not to exceed eight treatments in 24 hours.
Acute asthma attacks unresponsive to inhalation therapy or control of bronchospasm during anesthesia
Isoproterenol hydrochloride
Children: 0.08 to 1.7 mcg/kg/minute as an infusion.
Adults: 0.01 to 0.02 mg (0.5 to 1 ml of a 1:50,000 dilution) I.V. Repeat if needed.
For bronchodilation
Isoproterenol hydrochloride
Children: 5 to 10 mg sublingually, not to exceed 30 mg daily.
Adults: 10 to 20 mg sublingually, not to exceed 60 mg daily.

Emergency treatment of cardiac dysrhythmias
Isoproterenol hydrochloride
Children: May give half of initial adult dose.
Adults: Initially, 0.02 to 0.06 mg I.V. bolus. Subsequent doses 0.01 to 0.2 mg I.V. Alternatively, 5 mcg/minute titrated to patient's response. Range 2 to 20 mcg/minute. Alternatively, 0.2 mg I.M. or S.C.; subsequent doses 0.02 to 1 mg I.M. or 0.15 to 0.2 mg S.C. In *extreme* cases, 0.02 mg (0.1 of 1:5,000) intracardiac injection.

Immediate temporary control of atropine-resistant hemodynamically significant bradycardia
Isoproterenol hydrochloride
Children: 0.1 mcg/kg/minute, titrated to patient's response. Maximum rate is 1 mcg/kg/minute.
Adults: 2 to 10 mcg/minute I.V. infusion, titrated to patient's response.

Adjunct in treatment of shock
Isoproterenol hydrochloride
Adults and children: 0.5 to 5 mcg/minute by continuous I.V. infusion titrated to patient's response.

Action and kinetics
• *Bronchodilator action:* Isoproterenol relaxes bronchial smooth muscle by direct action on beta$_2$-adrenergic receptors, relieving bronchospasm, increasing vital capacity, decreasing residual volume in lungs, and facilitating passage of pulmonary secretions. It also produces relaxation of GI and uterine smooth muscle via stimulation of beta$_2$ receptors. Peripheral vasodilation, cardiac stimulation, and relaxation of bronchial smooth muscle are the main therapeutic effects.
• *Cardiac stimulant action:* Isoproterenol acts on beta$_1$-adrenergic receptors in the heart, producing a positive chronotropic and inotropic effect; it usually increases cardiac output. In patients with AV block, isoproterenol AV node refractory and shortens conduction time and increases the rate and strength of ventricular contraction.
• *Kinetics in adults:* After injection or oral inhalation, isoproterenol is absorbed rapidly; after sublingual or rectal administration, absorption is variable and often unreliable. Onset of action is prompt after oral inhalation and persists up to 1 hour. Effects persist for a few minutes after I.V. injection, up to 2 hours after S.C. or sublingual administration, and up to 4 hours after rectal administration of sublingual tablet. Isoproterenol is distributed widely throughout the body. It is metabolized by conjugation in the GI tract and by enzymatic reduction in liver, lungs, and other tissues. Isoproterenol is excreted primarily in urine as unchanged drug and its metabolites.

Contraindications and precautions
Isoproterenol is contraindicated in patients with preexisting cardiac dysrhythmias, especially tachycardia (including tachycardia caused by digitalis toxicity), because of the drug's cardiac stimulant effects; and in those with known hypersensitivity to this drug or other sympathomimetics.

Administer cautiously to diabetic patients, those with renal or cardiovascular disease (hypertension, coronary insufficiency, angina, degenerative heart disease), or hyperthyroidism, because drug may worsen these conditions; and to sulfite-sensitive patients, because some formulations contain sulfite preservatives.

Interactions
Concomitant use of isoproterenol with epinephrine and other sympathomimetics may cause additive cardiovascular reactions. However, these drugs may be used together if at least 4 hours elapse between administration of the two drugs. Use with beta-adrenergic blockers antagonizes isoproterenol's cardiac-stimulating, bronchodilating, and vasodilating effects. Use with ergot alkaloids may increase blood pressure.

Dysrhythmias may occur more readily when drug is administered to patients receiving digitalis, potassium-depleting drugs, or other drugs that affect cardiac rhythm. Isoproterenol should be used with caution in patients receiving cyclopropane or halogenated hydrocarbon general anesthetics.

Effects on diagnostic tests
None reported.

Adverse reactions
• CNS: nervousness, restlessness, insomnia, anxiety, tension, fear, excitement, weakness, dizziness, *mild tremors*, light-headedness, headache, *irritability.*
• CV: palpitation, tachycardia, angina, *alterations in blood pressure, dysrhythmias, myocardial ischemia (with I.V. use).*
• GI: *nausea, vomiting, diarrhea.*
• Metabolic: hyperglycemia.
• Other: bronchial irritation and edema, sweating, flushing of face or skin, tinnitus.
Note: Drug should be discontinued if precordial distress, angina, ventricular dysrhythmias, or swelling of parotids occurs or airway resistance develops.

Overdose and treatment
Clinical manifestations of overdose include exaggeration of common adverse reactions, particularly cardiac dysrhythmias, extreme tremors, nausea and vomiting, and profound hypotension.

Treatment includes symptomatic and supportive measures. Monitor vital signs closely. Sedatives (barbiturates) may be used to treat CNS stimulation. Use cardioselective beta blocker to treat tachycardia and dysrhythmias. These agents should be used with caution; they may induce asthmatic attack.

▶ Special considerations
• Isoproterenol does not replace administration of blood, plasma, fluids, or electrolytes in patients with blood volume depletion.
• Severe paradoxical airway resistance may follow oral inhalations.
• Hypotension must be corrected before isoproterenol is administered.
• If three to five treatments within 6 to 12 hours provide minimal or no relief, re-evaluate therapy.
• Continuously monitor ECG during I.V. administration.
• Carefully monitor response to therapy by frequent

determinations of heart rate, ECG pattern, blood pressure, and central venous pressure, as well as (for patients in shock) urine volume, blood pH, and P_{CO_2} levels.

• Prescribed I.V. infusion rate should include specific guidelines for regulating flow or terminating infusion in relation to heart rate, premature beats, ECG changes, precordial distress, blood pressure, and urine flow. Because of the danger of precipitating dysrhythmias, rate of infusion is usually decreased or infusion may be temporarily discontinued if heart rate is excessively high.

• When administering drug, keep in mind the following: dilute in dextrose 5% in water; store in light-resistant containers; discard any discolored solutions; don't mix with alkaline solutions; simultaneous administration with epinephrine may lead to serious dysrhythmias; titrate when discontinuing.

• Constant-infusion pump prevents sudden infusion of excessive amounts of drug.

• Tachyphylaxis (tolerance) may develop after prolonged or excessive use.

• Sublingual doses should not be given more frequently than every 3 to 4 hours nor more than t.i.d.

• Sublingual tablet may be administered rectally, if indicated.

• Monitor for rebound bronchospasm when isoproterenol effects end.

• Isoproterenol has also been used to aid diagnosis of coronary artery disease and of mitral regurgitation.

• Do not inject solutions intended for oral inhalation.

• The preservative sodium bisulfite is present in many adrenergic formulations. Patients with a history of allergy to sulfites should avoid preparations that contain this preservative.

• Therapy should be administered when patient arises in morning and before meals to reduce fatigue by improving lung ventilation.

• Adrenergic inhalation may be alternated with other drug administration (steroids, other adrenergics) if necessary, but should not be administered simultaneously because of danger of excessive tachycardia.

• Do not use discolored or precipitated solutions.

• Protect solutions from light, freezing, and heat. Store at controlled room temperature.

• Systemic absorption can follow applications to nasal and conjunctival membranes, though infrequently. If symptoms of systemic absorption occur, patient should stop the drug.

• Prolonged or too-frequent use may cause tolerance to bronchodilating and cardiac stimulant effect. Rebound bronchospasm may follow end of drug effect.

Information for parents and patient

• Urge parents to call if symptoms persist or worsen.

• Advise parents to store oral forms away from heat and light (not in bathroom medicine cabinet where heat and moisture will cause deterioration of the drug). Keep drug out of the reach of small children.

Inhalation

• Treatment should start with first symptoms of bronchospasm.

• Dosage and recommended method of inhaling may vary with type of nebulizer and formulation used. Carefully instruct parents and patient in correct use

of nebulizer. Information and instructions are furnished with the aerosol forms of these drugs. Urge parents and patient to read them carefully and ask questions if necessary.

• Teach parents and patient that a single aerosol treatment is usually enough to control an asthma attack and to call promptly if the patient requires more than three aerosol treatments in 24 hours.

• Tell parents to call if bronchodilator causes dizziness, chest pain, or lack of therapeutic response to usual dose.

• Advise patient to rinse mouth with water after drug is absorbed completely and between doses.

• Tell parents and patient that saliva and sputum may appear red or pink after oral inhalation, because isoproterenol turns red on exposure to air.

• Tell parents that patient should avoid other adrenergic medications unless they are prescribed.

• Tell parents and patient that increased fluid intake facilitates clearing of secretions.

• Teach parents and patient how to accomplish postural drainage, to cough productively, and to clap and vibrate to promote good respiratory hygiene.

• Tell parents and patient not to discard drug applicator. Refill units are available.

• Inform parents and patient taking repeated doses about adverse reactions, and advise them to report such reactions promptly.

Sublingual use

• Tell patient to allow sublingual tablet to dissolve under tongue, without sucking, and not to swallow saliva (may cause epigastric pain) until drug has been absorbed completely.

• Warn parents and patient that frequent use of acidic sublingual tablets may damage teeth.

isotretinoin
Accutane

• Classification: antiacne agent, keratinization stabilizer (retinoic acid derivative)

How supplied

Available by prescription only
Capsules: 10 mg, 20 mg, 40 mg

Indications, route, and dosage
Severe cystic acne unresponsive to conventional therapy

Adolescents and adults: 0.5 to 1 mg/kg P.O. daily given in two divided doses and continued for 15 to 20 weeks. Maximum dose up to 2 mg/kg P.O. daily in two divided doses for severe cases or if disease is located primarily on chest and back.

Actions and kinetics

• *Antiacne action:* The exact mechanism of action is unknown; isotretinoin decreases the size and activity of sebaceous glands, which decreases secretion and probably explains the rapid clinical improvement. A reduction in *Propionibacterium acnes* in the hair fol-cles occurs as a secondary result of decreased nutrients.

Keratinizing action: Isotretinoin has anti-inflammatory and keratinizing effects. The mechanism is unknown.

Kinetics in adults: When administered orally, isotretinoin is absorbed rapidly from the GI tract. Peak concentrations occur in 3 hours, with peak concentrations of the metabolite 4-oxo-isotretinoin occurring 16 to 20 hours. The therapeutic range for isotretinoin has not been established. Isotretinoin, which has not been fully studied, is distributed widely. In animals, is found in most organs and is known to cross the placenta. In humans, the degree of placental transfer and the degree of secretion in breast milk are unknown. Isotretinoin is 99.9% protein-bound, primarily to albumin.

Isotretinoin is metabolized in the liver and possibly the gut wall. The major metabolite is 4-oxo-isotretinoin, with tretinoin and 4-oxo-tretinoin also found in the blood and urine. The elimination process is not fully known, although renal and biliary pathways are known to be used.

Contraindications and precautions

Drug is contraindicated in patients with sensitivity to isotretinoin, vitamin A, or other retinoids. Do not use in pregnant patients because of possible teratogenic effects, including hydrocephalus and microcephaly. Start therapy only after confirmation that patient is not pregnant and appropriate birth-control measures have been instituted. Any person taking isotretinoin should refrain from donating blood for at least 30 days after therapy has been discontinued.

Interactions

Isotretinoin will have a cumulative drying effect when used with medicated soaps and cleansers, medicated "cover-ups," topical peeling agents (benzoyl peroxide, resorcinol), and alcohol-containing preparations. Concurrent use of vitamin A products may have an additive toxic effect. Tetracyclines may increase the potential for the development of pseudotumor cerebri. Oral alcohol intake may increase plasma triglyceride levels.

Effects on diagnostic tests

The physiologic effects of the drug may alter liver function tests, blood counts, and blood glucose, uric acid, cholesterol, and triglyceride levels.

Adverse reactions

CNS: headache, fatigue, mood changes.
DERM: dry skin, peeling of palms and toes, skin infection, photosensitivity, skin rash, burning, redness, irritation, *pruritus, xerosis.*
EENT: conjunctivitis, corneal deposits, dry eyes.
Endocrine: hyperglycemia.
GI: nausea, vomiting, diarrhea, rectal bleeding, abdominal or stomach pain, *cheilitis* (most frequent), dry mouth, nonspecific GI symptoms, gum bleeding and inflammation.
HEMA: anemia, elevated platelet count.
Hepatic: elevated AST (SGOT), ALT (SPGT), and alkaline phosphatase.

• Other: *epistaxis, hypertriglyceridemia,* musculoskeletal pain (skeletal hyperostosis), thinning of hair.

Note: Drug should be discontinued if symptoms of inflammatory bowel disease, visual disturbances, or pseudotumor cerebri are present.

Overdose and treatment

Clinical manifestations of overdose are rare and would be extensions of adverse reactions.

▶ Special considerations

• Therapy usually lasts 15 to 20 weeks, followed by at least 8 weeks off drug before beginning a second course.
• Contact lenses may be uncomfortable during treatment; recommend use of artificial tears.
• Patient should take dose with or shortly after meals.
Special instructions for female patients
• Isotretinoin is a potent teratogen and should not be given to female patients who are pregnant or may become pregnant during therapy. Patient selection is important — informed consent must be obtained from the patient or her legal guardian before initiating therapy. The patient or responsible adult must fully understand the consequences of fetal exposure to isotretinoin.
• Reliable methods of contraception are essential for sexually active females who are taking isotretinoin.
• Negative blood tests for pregnancy must be obtained before therapy.
• Schedule follow-up visits monthly during therapy. Do not prescribe more than a 6-week supply at a time. Pregnancy tests must be repeated monthly.

Information for the parents and patient

• Recommend taking drug with or shortly after meals to ease GI discomfort; chewing gum may relieve dryness of mouth.
• Warn parents and patient that acne may worsen during the initial course of therapy and to call if the irritation becomes severe.
• Warn patient not to donate blood or become pregnant while taking this medication and for 30 days after discontinuing the drug.
• Caution against alcohol ingestion, to reduce the risk of hypertriglyceridemia.

JKL

kanamycin sulfate
Anamid*, Kantrex‡, Klebcil‡

- Classification: antibiotic (aminoglycoside)

How supplied
Available by prescription only
Capsules: 500 mg
Injection: 37.5 mg/ml (pediatric), 250 mg/ml, 333 mg/ml

Indications, route, and dosage
Serious infections caused by sensitive **Escherichia coli, Proteus, Enterobacter aerogenes, Klebsiella pneumoniae, Serratia marcescens, mycobacterium,** *and* **Acinetobacter**
Neonates age 1 to 7 days, weighing ≤ 2 kg: 7.5 mg/kg I.V. or I.M. q 12 hr
Neonates age 1 to 7 days, weighing > 2 kg: 10 mg/kg I.V. or I.M. q 12 hr
Neonates age 8 days or older, weighing ≤ 2 kg: 7.5 to 10 mg/kg I.V. or I.M. q 8 hr
Neonates age 8 days or older, weighing > 2 kg: 10 mg/kg I.V. or I.M. q 8 hr.
Children and adults with normal renal function: 15 mg/kg deep I.M. injection into upper outer quadrant of buttocks or I.V. infusion (diluted 500 mg/200 ml of normal saline solution or dextrose 5% in water infused over 30 to 60 minutes) daily divided q 8 to 12 hours. Maximum daily dose is 1.5 g.
Dosage in renal failure
Doses and/or frequency of administration should be altered. In all patients, keep peak serum concentrations between 15 and 30 mcg/ml, and trough serum concentrations between 5 and 10 mcg/ml.

Action and kinetics
- *Antibiotic action:* Kanamycin is bactericidal; it binds directly to the 30S ribosomal subunit, thus inhibiting bacterial protein synthesis. Its spectrum of activity includes many aerobic gram-negative organisms and some aerobic gram-positive organisms. Generally, kanamycin is far less active against many gram-negative organisms than are tobramycin, gentamicin, amikacin, and netilmicin. After oral administration, kanamycin inhibits ammonia-forming bacteria in the GI tract, decreasing ammonia and thus improving neurologic status of patients with hepatic encephalopathy.
- *Kinetics in adults:* Kanamycin is absorbed poorly after oral administration, although oral administration is enhanced in patients with impaired GI motility or mucosal ulcerations. Drug is usually given parenterally; peak serum concentrations occur 60 minutes after I.M. administration.

Kanamycin is distributed widely after parenteral administration; intraocular penetration is poor. CSF penetration is low, even in patients with inflamed meninges. Intraventricular administration produces high concentrations throughout the CNS. Protein binding is minimal. Kanamycin crosses the placenta.

Kanamycin is excreted unmetabolized, primarily in urine by glomerular filtration. Small amounts may be excreted in bile and breast milk. Elimination half-life in adults is 2 to 4 hours. In severe renal damage half-life may extend to 80 hours.
- *Kinetics in children:* In neonates, peak plasma levels occur with 1 hour after I.M. administration. The elimination half-life is approximately 9 hours in premature infants.

Contraindications and precautions
Kanamycin is contraindicated in patients with known hypersensitivity to kanamycin or any other aminoglycoside, and when given orally, in patients with intestinal obstruction.

Kanamycin should be used cautiously in neonates and other infants, in patients with intestinal mucosal ulcerations because of increased potential for pseudomembranous colitis; in patients with decreased renal function, tinnitus, vertigo, and high-frequency hearing loss who are susceptible to ototoxicity; in patients with dehydration, myasthenia gravis, parkinsonism, and hypocalcemia because the drug can exacerbate these symptoms or illnesses; in neonates and other infants; and in elderly patients.

Interactions
Concomitant use with the following drugs may increase the hazard of nephrotoxicity, ototoxicity, and or neurotoxicity: methoxyflurane, polymyxin B, vancomycin, amphotericin B, cisplatin, cephalosporins and other aminoglycosides; hazard of ototoxicity is also increased during use with ethacrynic acid, furosemide, bumetanide, urea, or mannitol. Dimenhydrinate and other antiemetics and antivertigo drugs may mask kanamycin-induced ototoxicity.

Concomitant use with penicillins results in a synergistic bactericidal effect against *Pseudomonas aeruginosa, E. coli, Klebsiella, Citrobacter, Enterobacter, Serratia,* and *Proteus mirabilis.* However, the drug are physically and chemically incompatible and are inactivated when mixed or given together. In vivo inactivation has been reported when aminoglycoside and penicillins are used concomitantly.

Kanamycin may potentiate neuromuscular blockade of general anesthetics or neuromuscular blocking agents such as succinylcholine and tubocurarine. Oral kanamycin inhibits vitamin K-producing bacteria in GI tract and may potentiate action of oral anticoagulants; dosage adjustment of anticoagulants may be necessary.

Effects on diagnostic tests
Kanamycin-induced nephrotoxicity may elevate levels of blood urea nitrogen (BUN), nonproton nitrogen, or

serum creatinine and increase urinary excretion of casts.

Adverse reactions
- CNS: headache, lethargy, *neuromuscular blockade with respiratory depression.*
- EENT: *ototoxicity (tinnitus, vertigo, hearing loss).*
- GI: *nausea, vomiting, diarrhea.*
- GU: *nephrotoxicity (cells or casts in the urine, oliguria, proteinuria, decreased creatinine clearance, increased BUN, serum creatinine and nonprotein nitrogen levels).*
- Other: *hypersensitivity reactions* (eosinophilia, fever, rash, urticaria, pruritus), bacterial and fungal superinfections.
  Note: Drug should be discontinued if signs of ototoxicity, nephrotoxicity, or hypersensitivity occur; if severe diarrhea indicates pseudomembranous colitis; or if intestinal obstruction develops. Drug should be discontinued or serum levels monitored if intestinal ulcerations develop, especially in renal impairment.

Overdose and treatment
Clinical signs of overdose include ototoxicity, nephrotoxicity, and neuromuscular toxicity. Remove drug by hemodialysis or peritoneal dialysis. Treatment with calcium salts or anticholinesterases may reverse neuromuscular blockade. After recent ingestion (4 hours or less), empty the stomach by induced emesis or gastric lavage; follow with activated charcoal to reduce absorption.

▶ Special considerations
- Oral kanamycin may potentiate effects of oral anticoagulants; monitor prothrombin times and adjust dosage if necessary.
- Kanamycin should not be administered to infants for more than 14 days.
- Darkening of vials does not indicate loss of potency.
- Because kanamycin is dialyzable, patients undergoing hemodialysis may need dosage adjustments.
- Kanamycin has been administered intrathecally or intraventricularly. Many clinicians prefer intraventricular administration to ensure adequate CSF levels in the treatment of ventriculitis.
- Assess patient's allergic history; do not give kanamycin to a patient with a history of hypersensitivity reactions to any aminoglycoside; monitor patient continuously for this and other adverse reactions.
- Obtain results of culture and sensitivity tests before first dose; however, therapy may begin before tests are completed. Repeat tests periodically to assess drug efficacy.
- Monitor vital signs, electrolyte levels, and renal function studies before and during therapy; be sure patient is well hydrated to minimize chemical irritation of renal tubules; watch for signs of declining renal function. Monitor intake and output. Check urine for protein.
- Keep peak serum levels and trough serum levels at recommended concentrations, especially in patients with decreased renal function. Draw blood for peak level 1 hour after I.M. injection (30 minutes to 1 hour after I.V. infusion); for trough level, draw sample just before the next dose. Time and date all blood samples.

Do not use heparized tube to collect to collect blood samples; it inteferes with results.
- Evaluate patient's hearing before and during therapy; monitor for complaints of tinnitus, vertigo, or hearing loss.
- Avoid concomitant use of aminoglycosides with other ototoxic or nephrotoxic drugs.
- Usual duration of therapy is 7 to 10 days; if no response occurs in 3 to 5 days, drug should be discontinued and cultures repeated for reevaluation of therapy.
- Closely monitor patients on long-term therapy—especially debilitated patients and others receiving immunosuppresant or radiation therapy—for possible bacterial or fungal superinfection; monitor especially for fever.

Parenteral administration
- Consult manufacturer's directions for reconstitution, dilution, and storage of drugs; check expiration dates.
- Administer I.M. dose deep into large muscle mass (gluteal or midlateral thigh); rotate injection sites in minimize tissue injury; do not inject more than 2 g of drug per injection site. Apply ice to injection site for pain.
- Too-rapid I.V. administration may cause neuromuscular blockade. Infuse I.V. drug continuously or intermittently over 30 to 60 minutes for adults, 1 to 2 hours for infants; dilution volume for children is determined individually.
- Do not add or mix other drugs with I.V. infusions—particularly penicillins, which will inactivate aminoglycosides; the two groups are chemically and physically incompatible. If other drugs must be given I.V., temporarily stop infusion of primary drug.
- Solutions should always be clear, colorless to pale yellow (in most cases, darkening indicates deterioration), and free of particles; do not give solutions containing precipitates or other foreign matter.

Information for parents and patient
- Teach parents and patients how to recognize signs and symptoms of hypersensitivity; bacterial or fungal superinfections (especially if the child has low resistance from immunosuppressants or irradiation) and other adverse reactions to aminoglycosides, urge them to report any unusual effects promptly.

---

ketoconazole
Nizoral

- Classification: antifungal (imidazole derivative)

How supplied
Available by prescription only
Tablets: 200 mg
Oral suspension: 100 mg/5 ml
Cream: 2%

Indications, route, and dosage

Severe fungal infections caused by suscepti-ble organisms

Children age 2 and over: 3.3 to 6.6 mg/kg P.O.daily as a single dose.

Adults: Initially, 200 mg P.O. daily as a single dose. Dosage may be increased to 400 mg once daily in patients who do not respond to lower dosage.

Topical treatment of tinea corporis, tinea cruris, and tinea versicolor

Children and adults: Apply once or twice daily for about 2 weeks.

Action and kinetics

• *Antifungal action:* Ketoconazole is fungicidal and fungistatic, depending on drug concentrations. It inhibits demethylation of lanosterol, thereby altering membrane permeability and inhibiting purine transport. The in vitro spectrum of activity includes most pathogenic fungi. However, CSF concentrations following oral administration are not predictable. It should not be used to treat fungal meningitis, and specimens should be obtained for susceptibility testing before therapy. Currently available tests may not accurately reflect in vivo activity, so interpret results with caution.

It is used orally to treat disseminated or pulmonary coccidiomycosis, paracoccidiomycosis, or histoplamosis; oral candidiasis and candiduria (but low renal clearance may limit its usefulness).

It is also useful in some dermatophytoses, including all forms of tinea caused by *Epidermophyton, Microsporum,* or *Trichophyton.*

• *Kinetics in adults:* Ketoconazole is converted to the hydrochloride salt before absorption. Absorption is erratic; it is decreased by raised gastric pH and may be increased in extent and consistency by food. Peak plasma concentrations occur at 1 to 4 hours. Drug is distributed into bile, saliva, cerumen, synovial fluid, and sebum; CSF penetration is erratic and considered minimal. It is 84% to 99% bound to plasma proteins. Ketoconazole is converted into several inactive metabolites in the liver. Over 50% of a ketoconazole dose is excreted in feces within 4 days; drug and metabolites are secreted in bile. About 13% is excreted unchanged in urine. It is probably excreted in breast milk.

Contraindications and precautions

Ketoconazole is contraindicated in patients with known hypersensitivity to the drug. It should be used with caution in patients with hepatic disease and in those taking other hepatotoxic drugs, because of possible added toxicity.

Because of the potential for serious hepatic toxicity, ketoconazole should be reserved for severe systemic fungal infections and should not be used for less serious fungal infections of the skin and nails.

Interactions

Concomitant use of ketoconazole with drugs that raise gastric pH (antacids, cimetidine, ranitidine, famotidine, and antimuscarinic agents) decreases absorption of ketoconazole; rifampin may decrease ketoconazole's serum concentration to ineffective levels.

Ketoconazole may enhance the toxicity of other hepatotoxic drugs and the anticoagulant effects of warfarin.

Ketoconazole may interfere with the metabolism of cyclosporine and thus raise serum levels of cyclosporine; concomitant use with phenytoin may alter serum levels of both drugs.

Effects on diagnostic tests

Ketoconazole has been reported to cause transient elevations of AST (SGOT), ALT (SGPT), and alkaline phosphatase levels; it has also been reported to cause transient alterations of serum cholesterol and triglyceride levels.

Adverse reactions

• CNS: headache, nervousness, dizziness.
• DERM: itching.
• GI: nausea, vomiting, abdominal pain, diarrhea, constipation, flatulence.
• Hepatic: elevated liver enzymes, fatal hepatotoxicity, hepatitis (in children).
• Other: gynecomastia with breast tenderness in males.

Note: Drug should be discontinued if liver function tests show marked elevation or if clinical signs of hepatocellular dysfunction occur.

Overdose and treatment

Overdose may cause dizziness, tinnitus, headache, nausea, vomiting, or diarrhea; patients with adrenal hypofunction or patients on long-term corticosteroid therapy may show signs of adrenal crisis.

Treatment includes induced emesis and sodium bicarbonate lavage, followed by activated charcoal and a cathartic, and supportive measures as needed.

▶ Special considerations

• Safe use in children under age 2 has not been established.
• Ketoconazole requires acidity for absorption and is ineffective in patients with achlorhydria.
• Identify organism, but do not delay therapy for results of laboratory tests.
• Monitor for signs of hepatotoxicity: persistent nausea, unusual fatigue, jaundice, dark urine, and pale stools.

Information for parents and patient

• Teach achlorhydric patients and their parents how to take ketoconazole: dissolve each tablet in 4 ml of aqueous solution of 0.2N hydrochloric acid, and administer through a glass or plastic straw to avoid damaging enamel on patient's teeth. Patient should drink a glass of water after each dose.
• Patient should avoid hazardous activities if drug causes dizziness or drowsiness; these symptoms often occur early in treatment but abate as treatment continues.
• Warn against changing dose or dosage interval or discontinuing drug without medical approval. Explain that therapy must continue until active fungal infection is completely eradicated, to prevent recurrence

• Reassure parents and patient that nausea will subside; to minimize reaction, patient may take drug with food or may divide dosage into two doses.
• Warn parents that self-prescribed preparations for GI distress may alter gastric pH levels and interfere with drug action. Parents should get specific medical approval before giving patient any other drugs with ketoconazole.

---

lactulose
Cephulac, Chronulac

• Classification: laxative (disaccharide)

How supplied
Available by prescription only
Oral solution: 10 g/15 ml

Indications, route, and dosage
Constipation
Adults: 15 to 30 ml P.O. daily.
To prevent and treat portal-systemic encephalopathy, including hepatic precoma and coma in patients with severe hepatic disease
Infants: 2.5 to 10 ml/day P.O. divided t.i.d. or q.i.d. P.O.
Older children and adolescents: 40 to 90 ml/day P.O. divided t.i.d. or q.i.d.
Adults: Initially, 20 to 30 g P.O. (30 to 45 ml) t.i.d. or q.i.d., until two or three soft stools are produced daily. Usual dosage is 60 to 100 g/day in divided doses; can also be given t.i.d. by retention enema in at least 100 ml of fluid.

Action and kinetics
• *Laxative action:* Because lactulose is indigestible, it passes through the GI tract to the colon unchanged; there, it is digested by normally occurring bacteria. The weak acids produced in this manner increase the stool's fluid content and cause distention, thus promoting peristalsis and bowel evacuation.
   Lactulose also is used to reduce serum ammonia levels in patients with hepatic disease. Lactulose breakdown acidifies the colon; this, in turn, converts ammonia (NH_3) to ammonium (NH_4^+), which is not absorbed and is excreted in the stool. Furthermore, this "ion trapping" effect causes ammonia to diffuse from the blood into the colon where it is excreted as well.
• *Kinetics in adults:* Lactulose is absorbed minimally. It is distributed locally, primarily in the colon, and is metabolized by colonic bacteria (absorbed portion is not metabolized). Most lactulose is excreted in feces; absorbed portion is excreted in urine.

Contraindications and precautions
Lactulose is contraindicated in patients who must restrict galactose intake and in patients with appendicitis, acute surgical abdomen, fecal impaction, or intestinal obstruction, because drug may aggravate symptoms of these disorders.
   Lactulose should be used with caution in diabetic patients because of sugar content (lactose and galactose). Because of a theoretical potential for accumulation of hydrogen gas in the GI tract, patients receiving lactulose who undergo electrocautery procedures during proctoscopy and colonoscopy should receive a thorough bowel cleansing before the procedure to minimize the risk of explosion.

Interactions
When used concomitantly, neomycin and other antibiotics may theoretically decrease lactulose effectiveness by eliminating bacteria needed to digest it into the active form. This has not been shown clinically.

Effects on diagnostic tests
None reported.

Adverse reactions
• GI: *abdominal cramps,* belching, flatulence, gaseous distention, *diarrhea.*
   Note: Drug should be discontinued if severe abdominal pain occurs.

Overdose and treatment
No cases of overdose have been reported. Clinical effects include diarrhea and abdominal cramps.

▶ Special considerations
• Drug is administered to children orally, or by nasogastric tube.
• After the drug is administered via nasogastric tube, the tube should be flushed with water to clear it and ensure drug's passage to stomach.
• Dilute drug with water or fruit juice to minimize its sweet taste.
• For administration by retention enema, 300 ml of drug should be diluted with 700 ml of water or normal saline solution and administered via rectal balloon catheter (may repeat every 4 to 6 hours). Patient should retain drug for 30 to 60 minutes. If retained less than 30 minutes, dose should be repeated immediately. Begin oral therapy before discontinuing retention enemas.
• Monitor frequency and consistency of stools. If initial dose causes diarrhea, reduce next dose. Discontinue drug if diarrhea persists.
• Monitor serum potassium levels.

Information for parents and patient
Advise taking drug with juice to improve taste.

---

leucovorin calcium (citrovorum factor or folinic acid)
Wellcovorin

• Classification: vitamin (folic acid derivative)

How supplied
Available by prescription only
Tablets: 5 mg, 25 mg
Injection: 1-ml ampule (3 mg/ml with 0.9% benzyl

---

alcohol or 5 mg/ml, with methyl and propyl parabens); 50-mg vial (10 mg/ml after reconstitution, contains no preservatives); 5-ml ampule (5 mg/ml, with methyl and propyl parabens)

Indications, route, and dosage
Overdose of folic acid antagonist
Children and adults: P.O., I.M., or I.V. dose equivalent to the weight of the antagonist given within 1 hour of the overdose.
Leucovorin rescue after large methotrexate dose in treatment of cancer
Children and adults: If patient cannot tolerate oral leucovorin, parenteral administration must be used.
   Note: Administer within 6 to 36 hours of last dose of methotrexate.
Dosage may vary with regimen. Usually, 10 mg/m² is given P.O., I.M. or I.V., followed by 10 mg/m² P.O., I.M., or I.V. q 6 hours for 72 hours. If serum creatinine level is 50% or more than the pre-methotrexate level, dosage should be increased to 100 mg/m² q 3 hours until serum methotrexate level is less than 5×10^{-8} M.
Toxic effects of methotrexate used to treat severe psoriasis
Children and adults: 4 to 8 mg I.M. 2 hours after methotrexate dose.
Hematologic toxicity from pyrimethamine therapy
Children and adults: 5 mg P.O. or I.M. daily.
Hematologic toxicity from trimethoprim therapy
Children and adults: 400 mcg to 5 mg P.O. or I.M. daily.
Megaloblastic anemia from congenital enzyme deficiency
Children and adults: 3 to 6 mg I.M. daily, then 1 mg P.O. daily for life.
Folate-deficient megaloblastic anemias
Children and adults: Up to 1 mg of leucovorin P.O. or I.M. daily. Duration of treatment depends on hematologic response.

Action and kinetics
• *Reversal of folic acid antagonist:* Leucovorin is a derivative of tetrahydrofolic acid, the reduced form of folic acid. Leucovorin performs as a cofactor in 1-carbon transfer reactions in the biosynthesis of purines and pyrimidines of nucleic acids. Impairment of thymidylate synthesis in patients with folic acid deficiency may account for defective DNA synthesis, megaloblast formation, and megaloblastic and macrocytic anemias. Leucovorin is a potent antidote for the hematopoietic and reticuloendothelial toxic effects of folic acid antagonists (trimethoprim, pyrimethamine, and methotrexate). "Leucovorin rescue" is used to prevent or decrease toxicity of massive methotrexate doses. Folinic acid "rescues" normal cells without reversing the oncolytic effect of methotrexate.
• *Kinetics in adults:* After oral administration, leucovorin is absorbed rapidly; peak serum folate concentrations occur less than 2 hours following a 15-mg dose. The increase in plasma and serum folate activity after oral administration is mainly from 5-methyltetrahydrofolate (the major transport and storage form of folate in the body). Tetrahydrofolic acid and its derivatives are distributed throughout the body; the liver contains approximately half of the total body folate stores. Leucovorin is metabolized in the liver. It is excreted by the kidneys as 10-formyl tetrahydrofolate and 5,10-methenyl tetrahydrofolate.

Contraindications and precautions
Leucovorin calcium is contraindicated in patients with allergic reactions after oral and parenteral administration of folic acid. In patients with undiagnosed anemia, leucovorin may mask pernicious anemia by alleviating its hematologic effects while allowing neurologic complications to progress. When leucovorin rescue is used with high-dose methotrexate therapy, leucovorin must be administered until the blood concentration of methotrexate declines to nontoxic levels.

Interactions
Concomitant use of leucovorin calcium with phenytoin will decrease the serum phenytoin concentrations and increase the frequency of seizures. Although this interaction has occurred solely in patients receiving folic acid, it should be considered when leucovorin is administered. The mechanism by which this occurs appears to be an increased metabolic clearance of phenytoin or a redistribution of phenytoin in the CSF and brain. Phenytoin and primidone may decrease serum folate levels, producing symptoms of folate deficiency. After chemotherapy with folic acid antagonists, parenteral administration is preferable to oral dosing because vomiting may cause loss of the leucovorin. To treat an overdose of folic acid antagonists, leucovorin should be administered within 1 hour if possible; it is usually ineffective after a 4-hour delay. Leucovorin has no effect on other methotrexate toxicities.

Effects on diagnostic tests
Leucovorin may mask the diagnosis of pernicious anemia.

Adverse reactions
• DERM: rash, pruritus, erythema.
• Other: wheezing.

Overdose and treatment
Leucovorin is relatively nontoxic; no specific recommendations for overdose are reported.

▶ Special considerations
• Drug may increase frequency of seizures in susceptible children.
• Do not use diluents containing benzyl alcohol when reconstituting drug for neonates.
• Realize that leucovorin administration continues until plasma methotrexate levels are below 5×10^{-8} M.
• To prepare leucovorin for parenteral use, add 5 ml of bacteriostatic water for injection to vial containing 50 mg of base drug.
• Do not use as sole treatment of pernicious anemia or vitamin B_{12} deficiency.
• To treat overdose of folic acid antagonists, use the

---

drug within 1 hour; it is not effective after a 4-hour delay.
• Monitor patient for rash, wheezing, pruritus, and urticaria, which can be signs of drug allergy.
• Monitor serum creatinine levels daily to detect possible renal function impairment.
• Store at room temperature in a light-resistant container, not in high-moisture areas.

Information for parents and patient
• Emphasize importance of taking leucovorin only under medical supervision.
• Emphasize the importance of leucovorin during rescue therapy. If vomiting is severe, patient may need parenteral therapy.

---

levocarnitine (L-Carnitine)
Carnitor, VitaCarn

• Classification: nutritional supplement (amino acid derivative)

How supplied
Available by prescription only
Enteral liquid: 100 mg/ml
Tablets: 330 mg
Capsules: 250 mg

Indications, route, and dosage
Primary systemic carnitine deficiency; †modification of abnormal plasma lipoprotein profile produced by loss of plasma L-carnitine; † improvement of athletic performance

Infants and children: 50 to 100 mg/kg/day P.O., divided q 3 or 4 hours, with food or dissolved in drinks or liquid food. Start dosage at 50 mg/kg/day, and increase slowly to maximum 3 g/day according to clinical response.

Adults: 1 to 3 g/day of liquid P.O. or enterally, divided one to three times a day, with meals. Start dosage at 1 g/day, increasing slowly according to clinical response. Alternatively, 990 mg P.O. (tablets) b.i.d. or t.i.d. with meals.

Action and kinetics
• *Lipid-modifying action:* Levocarnitine facilitates entry of long-chain fatty acids into cellular mitochondria, where they are used during oxidation and energy production.
• *Kinetics in adults:* Most carnitine is excreted in urine and feces. In renal failure, carnitine levels may rise.

Contraindications and precautions
D,L-carnitine, sold in health food stores as vitamin B_T, competitively inhibits L-carnitine and can cause a deficiency.

Interactions
Concurrent use with valproic acid may increase requirements for carnitine.

Effects on diagnostic tests
None reported.

Adverse reactions
• GI: nausea, vomiting, abdominal cramps, diarrhea.
• Other: body odor (drug-related)

Overdose and treatment
There are no reports of toxicity from overdosage. Treatment includes usual supportive measures.

▶ Special considerations
• Only the L isomer of carnitine (sometimes called vitamin B_T) affects lipid metabolism.
• Patient monitoring should include periodic blood chemistries, vital signs, plasma carnitine, free fatty acid and triglyceride concentrations, and overall clinical condition.
• To avoid transient GI complaints (incidence 41%), including nausea, vomiting, abdominal cramps, and diarrhea, recommend slow consumption of the dose or greater dilution of liquid. Decreasing dosage often diminishes or eliminates GI symptoms or drug-related body odor (incidence 11%).
• Monitor tolerance closely during the 1st week and after any dosage increases.
• Spacing doses evenly throughout the day (every 3 or 4 hours) will help increase tolerance of levocarnitine.
• Levocarnitine oral solution may be given alone. To reduce side effects caused by overly rapid ingestion, the solution should be dissolved in drinks or liquid foods and no more than 10 ml (1 g) should be taken at each dose.
• The dietary source of levocarnitine is foods of animal origin, such as meat and milk. Levocarnitine is also synthesized in the body, mainly in the liver and kidneys, from essential amino acids (lysine, methionine) by a process involving essential micronutrients (ascorbate, niacin, pyridoxine, iron).
• Primary systemic carnitine deficiency that impairs fatty acid metabolism produces elevated triglyceride and free fatty acid levels, diminished ketogenesis, and lipid infiltration of liver and muscle. Severe chronic deficiency may be associated with hypoglycemia, progressive myasthenia, hypotonia, lethargy, hepatomegaly, encephalopathy, hepatic coma, cardiomegaly, congestive heart failure, cardiac arrest, neurologic disturbances and, in infants, impaired growth and development.

Information for parents and patients
• Advise parents not to confuse drug with D,L-carnitine sold in health food stores.
• Advise parents to have patient take drug with meals to reduce GI adverse reactions.
• Tell parents that patient should take drug at evenly spaced times throughout the day (every 3 or 4 hours). Advise them that patient who misses a dose should wait until next scheduled time.
• Advise parents about proper storage of drug: keeping out of reach of children; storing away from heat, direct light, and moisture; protecting oral solution from freezing; not refrigerating; and discarding outdated or surplus drug.

---

‡May contain sulfites   ◆May contain tartrazine   ◆◆May contain benzyl alcohol

levothyroxine sodium (T₄ or L-thyroxine sodium)

Elthroxin*, Levothroid, Levoxine, Synthroid, Synthrox, Syroxine

• Classification: thyroid hormone replacement agent

How supplied
Available by prescription only
Tablets: 25 mcg, 50 mcg, 75 mcg, 100 mcg, 125 mcg, 150 mcg, 175 mcg, 200 mcg, 300 mcg
Injection: 200 mcg/vial, 500 mcg/vial

Indications, route, and dosage
Cretinism
Children under age 4 weeks: 25 to 50 mcg P.O. daily or 20 to 40 mcg I.V. or I.M. daily.
Thyroid hormone replacement for atrophy of gland, surgical removal, excessive radiation or anti-thyroid drugs, or congenital defect
Infants up to 6 months: 25 to 50 mcg or 8 to 10 mcg/kg/day.
Infants age 6 to 12 months: 50 to 75 mcg or 6 to 8 mcg/kg/day.
Children age 1 to 5: 75 to 100 mcg or 5 to 6 mcg/kg/day.
Children age 6 to 12: 100 to 150 mcg or 4 to 5 mcg/kg/day.
Children over age 12: Over 150 mcg or 2 to 3 mcg/kg/day.
Note: Therapy may be initiated at the full therapeutic dose. Incremental doses are not usually needed.
Adults: For mild hypothyroidism — initially, 50 mcg P.O. daily, increased by 25 to 50 mcg P.O. daily q 2 to 4 weeks until desired response is achieved; may be administered I.V. or I.M. when P.O. ingestion is precluded for long periods.

Action and kinetics
• *Thyroid hormone replacement:* Levothyroxine affects protein and carbohydrate metabolism, promotes gluconeogenesis, increases the utilization and mobilization of glycogen stores, stimulates protein synthesis, and regulates cell growth and differentiation. The major effect of levothyroxine is to increase the metabolic rate of tissue.
• *Kinetics in adults:* About 50% to 80% of levothyroxine is absorbed from the GI tract. Full effects do not occur for 1 to 3 weeks after oral therapy begins. After I.M. administration, absorption is variable and poor. After an I.V. dose in patients with myxedema coma, increased responsiveness may occur within 6 to 8 hours, but maximum therapeutic effect may not occur for up to 24 hours.

Levothyroxine distribution has not been fully described; however, the drug is distributed into most body tissues and fluids. The highest levels are found in the liver and kidneys. Levothyroxine is 99% protein-bound.

Levothyroxine is metabolized in peripheral tissues, primarily in the liver, kidneys, and intestines. About 85% of levothyroxine metabolized is deiodinated. Fecal excretion eliminates 20% to 40% of levothyroxine. Half-life is 6 to 7 days.

Contraindications and precautions
Levothyroxine is contraindicated in patients with thyrotoxicosis, acute myocardial infarction, and uncorrected adrenal insufficiency because drug increases tissue metabolic demands. Levothyroxine also is contraindicated for treating obesity because it is ineffective and can cause life-threatening adverse reactions.

Levothyroxine should be used cautiously in patients with angina or other cardiovascular disease because of the risk of increased metabolic demands; in patients with diabetes mellitus because of reduced glucose tolerance; in patients with malabsorption states because of decreased absorption; and in patients with long-standing hypothyroidism or myxedema because these patients may be more sensitive to the drug's effects.

Interactions
Concomitant use of levothyroxine with corticotropin causes changes in thyroid status. Changes in levothyroxine dosages may require dosage changes in corticotropin as well. Concomitant use with an anticoagulant may alter anticoagulant effect; an increase in levothyroxine dosage may necessitate a decrease in anticoagulant dosage. Concomitant use of levothyroxine with tricyclic antidepressants or sympathomimetics may increase the effects of any or all of these drugs and may lead to coronary insufficiency or cardiac dysrhythmias.

Concomitant use of levothyroxine with insulin may affect the dosage requirements of insulin. Beta blockers may decrease the conversion of levothyroxine to liothyronine. Cholestyramine may delay absorption of levothyroxine. Estrogens, which increase serum thyroxine-binding globulin levels, increase levothyroxine requirements. Hepatic enzyme inducers (such as phenytoin) may increase hepatic degradation of levothyroxine and raise dosage requirements of levothyroxine. Concomitant use with somatrem may accelerate epiphyseal maturation.

Effects on diagnostic tests
Levothyroxine therapy alters radioactive iodine (^{131}I) thyroid uptake, protein-bound iodine levels, and liothyronine uptake.

Adverse reactions
• CNS: nervousness, insomnia, tremor.
• CV: tachycardia, palpitations, *dysrhythmias*, angina pectoris, hypertension, widened pulse pressure, cardiac arrest.
• GI: change in appetite, nausea, diarrhea.
• Other: headache, leg cramps, weight loss, sweating, heat intolerance, allergic skin reactions, fever, menstrual irregularities, *increased metabolic rate, congestive heart failure.*
Note: Drug should be discontinued if allergic reactions or signs of hyperthyroidism occur.

Overdose and treatment
Clinical manifestations of overdose include signs and symptoms of hyperthyroidism, including weight loss,

---

increased appetite, palpitations, nervousness, diarrhea, abdominal cramps, sweating, tachycardia, increased blood pressure, widened pulse pressure, angina, cardiac dysrhythmias, tremor, headache, insomnia, heat intolerance, fever, and menstrual irregularities.

Treatment of overdose requires reduction of GI absorption and efforts to counteract central and peripheral effects, primarily sympathetic activity. Use gastric lavage or induce emesis (followed by activated charcoal up to 4 hours after ingestion). If the patient is comatose or is having seizures, inflate cuff on endotracheal tube to prevent aspiration. Treatment may include oxygen and artificial ventilation as needed to support respiration. It also should include appropriate measures to treat congestive heart failure and to control fever, hypoglycemia, and fluid loss. Propranolol (or another beta blocker) may be used to combat many of the effects of increased sympathetic activity. Levothyroxine should be gradually withdrawn over 2 to 6 days, then resumed at a lower dose.

▶ Special considerations
• During first few months of therapy, children may suffer partial hair loss. Reassure child and parents that this is temporary.
• Drug dosage varies widely among patients. Treatment should start at the lowest level, titrating to higher doses according to patient's symptoms and laboratory data until euthyroid state is reached.
• Monitor pulse rate and blood pressure.
• Monitor prothrombin time; patients taking anticoagulants usually require lower doses.
• Monitor for signs of overdose or hypothyroidism, including changes in menstrual periods, coldness, constipation, dry puffy skin, headache, listlessness, muscle aches, nausea, vomiting, weakness, fatigue, and unusual weight gain.
• Signs and symptoms of thyrotoxicosis or inadequate dosage include diarrhea, fever, irritability, listlessness, rapid heartbeat, vomiting, or weakness.
• Administer as a single dose before breakfast.
• Carefully observe patient for adverse effects during initial titration phase.
• Monitor for aggravation of concurrent diseases, such as Addison's disease or diabetes mellitus.
• Patient with a history of lactose intolerance may be sensitive to Levothroid, which contains lactose.
• Synthroid 100- and 300-mcg tablets contain tartrazine, a dye that causes allergic reactions in susceptible individuals.
• When switching from levothyroxine to liothyronine, levothyroxine dosage should stop when liothyronine treatment begins. After residual effects of levothyroxine have disappeared, liothyronine dosage can be increased in small increments. When switching from liothyronine to levothyroxine, levothyroxine therapy should begin several days before withdrawing liothyronine to avoid relapse.
• Patient taking levothyroxine who requires ^{131}I uptake studies must discontinue drug 4 weeks before test.
• Protect drug from moisture and light. Prepare I.V. dose immediately before injection. Do not mix with other I.V. solutions.

• Smaller I.V. doses may be necessary in patients with concomitant heart disease.
• Levothyroxine has predictable effects because of standard hormonal content; therefore, it is the usual drug of choice for thyroid hormone replacement.

Information for parents and patient
• Explain that drug usually must be taken for life. Warn against changing dosage or discontinuing the drug.
• Instruct parents to have patient take the medication at the same time each day; encourage morning dosing to avoid insomnia.
• Teach parents of children who can't swallow tablets the proper way to crush tablets.
• Tell parents to watch for and promptly report symptoms of excessive dosage (headache, diarrhea, nervousness, excessive sweating, heat intolerance, voracious appetite, menstrual changes, chest pain, increased pulse rate, or palpitations).
• Advise parents not to store the drug in warm, humid areas, such as the bathroom, to prevent drug deterioration.
• Parents or patient should inform new physician or dentist that patient is taking this drug.

---

lidocaine (lignocaine)
Xylocaine

lidocaine hydrochloride
Alphacaine, Anestacon, Dalcaine, Dilocaine, L-caine, Lidoject, LidoPen Auto-Injector, Nervocaine, Nulicaine, Xylocaine, Xylocaine Viscous

• Classification: ventricular antiarrhythmic, local anesthetic (amide derivative)

How supplied
Available without prescription
Ointment: 2.5%

Available by prescription only
Injection: 5 mg/ml, 10 mg/ml, 15 mg/ml, 20 mg/ml, 40 mg/ml, 100 mg/ml, and 200 mg/ml
Premixed solutions: dextrose 5% in water as 2 mg/ml, 4 mg/ml, and 8 mg/ml
Ointment: 5%
Topical solution: 2%, 4%, 10%
Jelly: 2%

Indications, route, and dosage
Ventricular dysrhythmias from myocardial infarction, cardiac manipulation, or cardiac glycosides; ventricular tachycardia
Children: 1 mg/kg by I.V. bolus, repeated q 5 to 10 minutes as needed to a maximum of 3 to 4.5 mg/kg. Follow with infusion of 20 to 40 mcg/kg/minute.
Adults: 50 to 100 mg (1 to 1.5 mg/kg) I.V. bolus at 25 to 50 mg/minute. Give half this amount to elderly or lightweight patients and to those with CHF or hepatic disease. Repeat bolus q 3 to 5 minutes until

dysrhythmias subside or side effects develop. Do not exceed 300-mg total bolus during a 1-hour period. Simultaneously, begin constant infusion: 1 to 4 mg/minute. Use lower dosage in patients with CHF or hepatic disease or those patients who weigh less than 50 kg. If single bolus has been given, repeat smaller bolus (usually one-half of the initial bolus) 15 to 20 minutes after start of infusion to maintain therapeutic serum level. After 24 hours of continuous infusion, decrease rate by half.

For I.M. administration: 200 to 300 mg in deltoid muscle has been used in early stages of acute myocardial infarction.

Local anesthesia of skin or mucous membranes, pain from dental extractions, stomatitis
Children and adults: Infiltrate area locally p.m. Maximum total dose 5 mg/kg. Alternatively, apply 2% to 5% solution or ointment or 15 ml of Xylocaine Viscous q 3 to 4 hours to oral or nasal mucosa.

Pain, burning, or itching caused by burns, sunburn, or skin irritation
Children and adults: Apply to affected areas.

Action and kinetics
• *Ventricular antiarrhythmic action:* One of the oldest antiarrhythmics, lidocaine remains among the most widely used drugs for treating acute ventricular dysrhythmias. According to the recently revised Advanced Cardiac Life Support guidelines (American Heart Association, 1986), lidocaine is the drug of choice to treat ventricular tachycardia and fibrillation. As a Class IB antiarrhythmic, it suppresses automaticity and shortens the effective refractory period and action potential duration of His-Purkinje fibers and suppresses spontaneous ventricular depolarization during diastole. Therapeutic concentrations do not significantly affect conductive atrial tissue and AV conduction. Unlike quinidine and procainamide, lidocaine does not significantly alter hemodynamics when given in usual doses. The drug seems to act preferentially on diseased or ischemic myocardial tissue; exerting its effects on the conduction system, it inhibits reentry mechanisms and halts ventricular dysrhythmias.
• *Local anesthetic action:* As a local anesthetic, lidocaine acts to block initiation and conduction of nerve impulses by decreasing the premeability of the nerve cell membrane to sodium ions.
• *Kinetics in adults:* Lidocaine is absorbed after oral administration; however, a significant first-pass effect occurs in the liver and only about 35% of the drug reaches the systemic circulation. Oral doses high enough to achieve therapeutic blood levels result in an unacceptable toxicity, probably from high concentrations of lidocaine.

Lidocaine is distributed widely throughout the body; it has a high affinity for adipose tissue. After I.V. bolus administration, an early, rapid decline in plasma levels occurs; this is associated mainly with distribution into highly perfused tissues, such as the kidneys, lungs, liver, and heart, followed by a slower elimination phase in which metabolism and redistribution into skeletal muscle and adipose tissue occur. The first (early) distribution phase occurs rapidly, calling for initiation of a constant infusion after an initial bolus dose. Distribution volume declines in patients with liver or hepatic disease, resulting in toxic concentrations with usual doses. About 60% to 80% of circulating drug is bound to plasma proteins. Usual therapeutic drug level is 1.5 to 5 mcg/ml. Although toxicity may occur within this range, levels greater than 5 mcg/ml are considered toxic and warrant dosage reduction.

Lidocaine is metabolized in the liver to two active metabolites. Less than 10% of a parenteral dose escapes metabolism and reaches the kidneys unchanged. Metabolism is affected by hepatic blood flow, which may decrease after myocardial infarction and with CHF. Liver disease also may limit metabolism. Drug's half-life undergoes a biphasic process, with an initial phase of 7 to 30 minutes followed by a terminal half-life of 1.5 to 2 hours. Elimination half-life may be prolonged in patients with CHF or liver disease. Continuous infusions longer than 24 hours also may cause an apparent half-life increase.

Contraindications and precautions
Lidocaine is contraindicated in patients with Stokes-Adams syndrome or severe degrees of sinoatrial, atrioventricular, or intraventricular heart block who do not have an artificial pacemaker, because the drug may worsen these conditions; and in patients with known hypersensitivity to this drug or other amide-type anesthetic agents.

Lidocaine is contraindicated in patients with inflammation or infection in puncture region, septicemia, severe hypertension, spinal deformities, and neurologic disorders. Use cautiously in debilitated, acutely ill, or obstetric patients; and in those with severe shock, heart block, general drug allergies, and paracervical block.

Lidocaine should be used with caution in patients with Wolff-Parkinson-White syndrome, bradycardia, or incomplete heart block, because the drug may exacerbate these conditions and precipitate other serious dysrhythmias; and in patients with atrial fibrillation, because the drug may increase the ventricular rate.

Interactions
Concomitant use of lidocaine with cimetidine or beta blockers may cause lidocaine toxicity from reduced hepatic clearance. Concomitant use of high-dose lidocaine with succinylcholine may increase succinylcholine's neuromuscular effects. Concomitant use with other antiarrhythmic agents, including phenytoin, procainamide, propranolol, and quinidine, may cause additive or antagonist effects as well as additive toxicity.

Effects on diagnostic tests
Because I.M. lidocaine therapy may increase creatine phosphokinase levels, isoenzyme tests should be performed for differential diagnosis of acute myocardial infarction.

Adverse reactions
• CNS: anxiety, apprehension, nervousness, *agitation, sedation,* unconsciousness, *respiratory arrest,* con-

---

*Canada only   †Unlabeled clinical use   Italicized adverse reactions have been observed in children.

fusion, tremors, lethargy, somnolence, stupor, restlessness, slurred speech, euphoria, depression, lightheadedness, paresthesias, *muscle twitching, seizures.*
• CV: myocardial depression, *dysrhythmias,* cardiac arrest, *hypotension, bradycardia.*
• DERM: dermatologic reactions.
• EENT: tinnitus, blurred or double vision, *ototoxicity.*
• GI: nausea, vomiting.
• Local: sensitization, rash.
• Other: edema, status asthmaticus, anaphylactoid reactions, anaphylaxis, soreness at injection site, cold sensation, diaphoresis, *diminished gag reflex.*

Overdose and treatment

Clinical effects of overdose include signs and symptoms of CNS toxicity, such as seizures or respiratory depression and cardiovascular toxicity (as indicated by hypotension).

Treatment includes general supportive measures and drug discontinuation. A patent airway should be maintained and other respiratory support measures carried out immediately. Diazepam or thiopental may be given to treat any seizures. To treat significant hypotension, vasopressors (including dopamine and norepinephrine) may be administered.

▶ Special considerations

• Use of an I.M. autoinjector device is not recommended.
• Patient who is receiving I.V. lidocaine infusion should be attended and on cardiac monitor at all times. Use infusion pump or microdrip system and timer to monitor infusion precisely. Never exceed infusion rate of 4 mg/minute, if possible. A faster rate greatly increases risk of toxicity.
• Use drug with caution in patients weighing less than 50 kg, and in patients with CHF or renal or hepatic disease. Such patients will need dosage reduction.
• Administration of lidocaine with epinephrine (for local anesthesia) to treat dysrhythmias is contraindicated. Use solutions with epinephrine cautiously in cardiovascular disorders and in body areas with limited blood supply (ears, nose, fingers, toes).
• Monitor vital signs and serum electrolyte, BUN, and creatinine levels for abnormalities.
• Monitor ECG constantly if administering drug I.V., especially in patients with liver disease, congestive heart failure, hypoxia, respiratory depression, hypovolemia, or shock, because these conditions may affect drug metabolism, excretion, or distribution volume, predisposing patient to drug toxicity.
• Monitor for signs of excessive depression of cardiac conductivity (such as sinus node dysfunction, PR-interval prolongation, QRS-interval widening, and appearance or exacerbation of dysrhythmias). If they occur, reduce dosage or discontinue drug.
• In many severely ill patients, seizures may be the first sign of toxicity. However, severe reactions are usually preceded by somnolence, confusion, and paresthesias. Regard all signs and symptoms of toxicity as serious, and promptly reduce dosage and/or discontinue therapy. Continued infusion could lead to seizures and coma. Give oxygen via nasal cannula, if

not contraindicated. Keep oxygen and CPR equipment handy.
• Doses of up to 400 mg I.M. have been advocated in prehospital phase of acute myocardial infarction.
• Patient receiving lidocaine I.M. will show a sevenfold increase in serum CPK level. Such CPK originates in skeletal muscle, not the heart. Test isoenzyme levels to confirm myocardial infarction, if using I.M. route.
• Solutions containing preservatives should not be used for spinal, epidural, or caudal block.
• With epidural use, a 2- to 5-ml test dose should be injected at least 5 minutes before giving total dose, to check for intravascular or subarachnoid injection. Motor paralysis and extensive sensory anesthesia indicate subarachnoid injection.
• Therapeutic serum levels range from 2 to 5 mcg/ml.
• Discard partially used vials containing no preservatives.
• Drug has been used investigationally to treat refractory status epilepticus.
• Xylocaine Viscous can interfere with the gag reflex.
• Oral absorption can lead to CNS or cardiovascular adverse effects.

Information for parents and patient

• Explain the need for frequent monitoring.
• Tell parents and patient drug should not be used on abraded skin.

---

lindane
Kwell, Kwildane, Scabene

• Classification: scabicide, pediculicide (chlorinated hydrocarbon insecticide)

How supplied

Available by prescription only
Cream: 1%
Lotion: 1%
Shampoo: 1%

Indications, route, and dosage
Scabies

Children over age 10 and adults: After bathing with soap and water, apply a thin layer of cream or lotion and gently massage it on all skin surfaces, moving from the neck to the toes. After 8 to 12 hours, remove drug by bathing and scrubbing well. Treatment may be repeated after 1 week.

Pediculosis

Children over age 10 and adults: After bathing with soap and water, apply lotion or cream to affected hairy areas and adjacent areas. After 8 to 12 hours, wash drug off with soap and water. Alternatively, apply shampoo to affected area, lather for 4 to 5 minutes, then rinse thoroughly. Comb hair thoroughly with a very fine-tooth comb to remove nits. Treatment may be repeated after 1 week.

Action and kinetics
• *Scabicide and pediculicide action:* Lindane is toxic to the parasitic arthropod *Sarcoptes scabiei* and its eggs, and to *Pediculus capitis, Pediculus corporis,* and *Phthirus pubis.* The drug is absorbed through the organism's exoskeleton and causes its death.
• *Kinetics in adults:* Ten percent of topical dose may be absorbed in 24 hours. Lindane is stored in body fat. Metabolism occurs in the liver. Lindane is excreted in urine and feces.

Contraindications and precautions
Lindane is contraindicated in patients with sensitivity to the drug. It should be used with caution in pregnancy because it can be absorbed systemically. Avoid contact with face, eyes, mucous membranes, and urethral meatus. Because lindane can be absorbed through the skin, the potential for CNS toxicity should be considered when the drug is used.

Interactions
None reported.

Effects on diagnostic tests
None reported.

Adverse reactions
• Local: irritation, contact dermatitis.
  Note: Drug should be discontinued if sensitization develops.

Overdose and treatment
Accidental ingestion may cause extreme CNS toxicity; reported symptoms include CNS stimulation, dizziness, and convulsions. To treat lindane ingestion, empty stomach by appropriate measures (emesis or lavage); follow with saline catharsis (do not use oil laxative). Treat seizures with pentobarbital, phenobarbital, or diazepam, as needed.

▶ Special considerations
• Warn patient that itching may continue for several weeks, even if treatment is effective, especially in scabies infestation.
• Patient's body should be clean (scrubbed well) and dry before application.
• If drug accidentally contacts eyes, patient should flush with water and call for further instructions. Patient should avoid inhaling vapor.
• Avoid applying drug to acutely inflamed skin, or raw, weeping surfaces.
• Place hospitalized patient in isolation with linen-handling precautions.

Information for parents and patient
• Drug should be used with caution, especially in infants and small children, who are much more susceptible to CNS toxicity. Discourage thumb-sucking in children using lindane, to prevent ingestion of the drug. The Centers for Disease Control recommend other scabicide therapies for children under age 10.
• Explain correct use of drug.
• Explain that reapplication usually is not necessary unless live mites are found; advise reapplication if drug is accidentally washed off, but discourage re-

peated use, which may irritate skin and cause systemic toxicity.
• Tell parents they may use lindane to clean combs and brushes, but should wash them thoroughly afterward; advise parents that all clothing and bed linen that patient used within the past 2 days should be washed in hot water and dried in hot dryer or dry-cleaned to avoid reinfestation or transmission of the organism.
• Caution parents or patient to avoid concomitant use of other oils or ointments.
• Explain that family and close contacts, including sexual contacts, should be treated concurrently.

---

liothyronine sodium (T₃)
Cytomel

• Classification: thyroid hormone

How supplied
Available by prescription only
Tablets: 5 mcg, 25 mcg, 50 mcg

Indications, route, and dosage
Cretinism
Children under age 3: 5 mcg P.O. daily, increased by 5 mcg q 3 to 4 days until desired response occurs.
Children age 3 and older: 50 to 100 mcg P.O. daily.
Myxedema
Adults: Initially, 5 mcg daily, increased by 5 to 10 mcg q 1 to 2 weeks. Maintenance dosage is 50 to 100 mcg daily.
Nontoxic goiter
Children: Initially, 5 mcg P.O. daily, increased by 5-mcg increments at weekly intervals until desired response is achieved.
Adults: Initially, 5 mcg P.O. daily; may be increased by 12.5 to 25 mcg daily q 1 to 2 weeks. Usual maintenance dosage is 75 mcg daily.
Thyroid hormone replacement
Adults: Initially, 25 mcg P.O. daily, increased by 12.5 to 25 mcg q 1 to 2 weeks until satisfactory response is achieved. Usual maintenance dosage is 25 to 75 mcg daily.
Liothyronine suppression test to differentiate hyperthyroidism from euthyroidism
Adults: 75 to 100 mcg daily for 7 days.

Action and kinetics
• *Thyroid hormone replacement:* Liothyronine is used to treat hypothyroidism, myxedema, and cretinism. This component of thyroid hormone affects protein and carbohydrate metabolism, promotes gluconeogenesis, increases the utilization and mobilization of glycogen stores, stimulates protein synthesis, and regulates cell growth and differentiation. The major effect of liothyronine is to increase the metabolic rate of tissue.
• *Kinetics in adults:* Liothyronine is 95% absorbed from the GI tract. Peak effect occurs within 24 to 72 hours. Liothyronine is highly protein-bound. Its distribution has not been fully described. The metabolism

---

*Canada only   †Unlabeled clinical use   Italicized adverse reactions have been observed in children.

of liothyronine is not fully understood. Half-life is 1 to 2 days.

Contraindications and precautions

Liothyronine is contraindicated in patients with thyrotoxicosis, acute myocardial infarction, and uncorrected adrenal insufficiency because the drug increases tissue metabolic demands. Liothyronine also is contraindicated to treat obesity because it is ineffective and can cause life-threatening adverse reactions.

Liothyronine should be used cautiously in patients with angina or other cardiovascular disease because of the risk of increased metabolic demands; in patients with diabetes mellitus because of reduced glucose tolerance; in patients with malabsorption states caused by decreased absorption; and in patients with long-standing hypothyroidism or myxedema because these patients may be more sensitive to the drug's effects.

Interactions

Concomitant use of liothyronine with adrenocorticoids or corticotropin alters thyroid status. Changes in liothyronine dosages may require dosage changes in the adrenocorticoid or corticotropin as well.

Concomitant use of liothyronine with anticoagulants may impair the latter's effects; an increase in liothyronine dosage may require a lower dosage of the anticoagulant. Concomitant use of liothyronine with tricyclic antidepressants or sympathomimetics may increase the effects of any or all of these medications, causing coronary insufficiency or cardiac dysrhythmias. Concomitant use of liothyronine with insulin may affect dosage requirements of insulin. Estrogens, which increase serum thyroxine-binding globulin levels, increase liothyronine requirements.

Effects on diagnostic tests

Liothyronine therapy alters radioactive iodine (^{131}I) uptake, protein-bound iodine levels, and liothyronine uptake.

Adverse reactions

• CNS: nervousness, insomnia, tremor.
• CV: tachycardia, palpitations, dysrhythmias, angina pectoris, hypertension, widened pulse pressure, cardiac arrest.
• GI: change in appetite, nausea, diarrhea.
• Other: headache, leg cramps, weight loss, sweating, heat intolerance, allergic skin reactions, fever, menstrual irregularities, hyperhidrosis.

Note: Drug should be discontinued if allergic reactions or signs of hyperthyroidism occur.

Overdose and treatment

Clinical manifestations of overdose include signs and symptoms of hyperthyroidism, including weight loss, increased appetite, palpitations, diarrhea, nervousness, abdominal cramps, sweating, headache, tachycardia, increased blood pressure, widened pulse pressure, angina, cardiac dysrhythmias, tremor, insomnia, heat intolerance, fever, and menstrual irregularities.

Treatment of overdose reduces GI absorption and

counteracts central and peripheral effects, primarily sympathetic activity. Use gastric lavage or induce emesis (followed by activated charcoal up to 4 hours after ingestion). If the patient is comatose or having seizures, inflate the cuff on an endotracheal tube to prevent aspiration. Treatment may include oxygen and ventilation to maintain respiration. It also should include appropriate measures to treat congestive heart failure and to control fever, hypoglycemia, and fluid loss. Propranolol (or another beta blocker) may be used to counteract many of the effects of increased sympathetic activity. Liothyronine should be withdrawn gradually over 2 to 6 days, then resumed at a lower dose.

▶ Special considerations

• During first few months of therapy, children may suffer partial hair loss. Reassure child and parents that this is temporary.
• Drug dosage varies widely among patients. Treatment should start at the lowest level, titrating to higher doses according to patient's symptoms and laboratory data, until euthyroid state is reached.
• Drug should be administered at the same time each day. Morning dosage is preferred to prevent insomnia.
• Monitor pulse rate and blood pressure.
• Monitor prothrombin time; patients taking anticoagulants usually require lower doses.
• Monitor for signs of overdose or hypothyroidism, including changes in menstrual periods, coldness, constipation, dry puffy skin, headache, listlessness, muscle aches, nausea, vomiting, weakness, fatigue, and unusual weight gain.
• Signs and symptoms of thyrotoxicosis or inadequate dosage include diarrhea, fever, irritability, listlessness, rapid heartbeat, vomiting, or weakness.
• Infants and children may experience an accelerated rate of bone maturation.
• Liothyronine may be preferred when rapid effect is desired or when GI absorption or peripheral conversion of levothyroxine to liothyronine is impaired.
• Oral absorption may be reduced in patients with congestive heart failure.
• When switching from levothyroxine to liothyronine, levothyroxine should be discontinued and liothyronine started at low dosage, increasing in small increments after residual effects of levothyroxine have disappeared. When switching from liothyronine to levothyroxine, levothyroxine should be started several days before withdrawing liothyronine to avoid relapse.
• Patients taking liothyronine who require radioactive iodine uptake studies must discontinue drug 7 to 10 days before test.
• A parenteral formulation is available by special request for investigational use to treat myxedema coma. The usual initial dose is 200 mcg I.V., followed by 10 to 25 mcg I.V. q 8 to 12 hours until the P.O. form of the drug can be used.
• Use with caution in patients with heart disease.

Information for parents and patient

• Tell parents to watch patient for and promptly report signs of excessive dosage (headache, diarrhea, nervousness, excessive sweating, heat intolerance, chest pain, increased pulse rate, or palpitations).

‡May contain sulfites   ◆May contain tartrazine   ◆◆ May contain benzyl alcohol

• Advise parents not to store liothyronine in warm, humid areas, such as the bathroom, to prevent drug deterioration.
• Patient should take the drug at the same time each day, preferably in the morning, to avoid insomnia.

---

liotrix
Euthroid, Thyrolar

• Classification: thyroid hormone

How supplied
Available by prescription only
Tablets: Euthroid-½ — levothyroxine sodium 30 mcg and liothyronine sodium 7.5 mcg
Euthroid-1 — levothyroxine sodium 60 mcg and liothyronine sodium 15 mcg
Euthroid-2 — levothyroxine sodium 120 mcg and liothyronine sodium 30 mcg
Euthroid-3 — levothyroxine sodium 180 mcg and liothyronine sodium 45 mcg
Thyrolar-¼ — levothyroxine sodium 12.5 mcg and liothyronine sodium 3.1 mcg
Thyrolar-½ — levothyroxine sodium 25 mcg and liothyronine sodium 6.25 mcg
Thyrolar-1 — levothyroxine sodium 50 mcg and liothyronine sodium 12.5 mcg
Thyrolar-2 — levothyroxine sodium 100 mcg and liothyronine sodium 25 mcg
Thyrolar-3 — levothyroxine sodium 150 mcg and liothyronine sodium 37.5 mcg

Indications, route, and dosage
Hypothyroidism
Dosages must be individualized to approximate the deficit in the patient's thyroid secretion.
Children and adults: Initially, 15 to 30 mg thyroid equivalent P.O. daily, increased by 15 to 30 mg thyroid equivalent q 1 to 2 weeks until desired response is achieved; increments in children's dosage q 2 weeks.

Action and kinetics
• *Thyroid stimulant and replacement:* Liotrix affects protein and carbohydrate metabolism, promotes gluconeogenesis, increases the utilization and mobilization of glycogen stores, stimulates protein synthesis, and regulates cell growth and differentiation. The major effect of liotrix is to increase the metabolic rate of tissue. It is used to treat hypothyroidism (myxedema, cretinism, and thyroid hormone deficiency).

Liotrix is a synthetic preparation combining levothyroxine sodium and liothyronine sodium. Such combination products were developed because circulating liothyronine was assumed to result from direct release from the thyroid gland. About 80% of liothyronine is now known to be derived from deiodination of levothyroxine in peripheral tissues, and patients receiving only levothyroxine have normal serum liothyronine and levothyroxine levels. *Therefore, there is no clinical advantage to combining thyroid agents; actually, it could result in excessive liothyronine concentration.*
• *Kinetics in adults:* About 50% to 95% of liotrix is

absorbed from the GI tract. Distribution is not fully understood. Liotrix is metabolized partially in peripheral tissues (liver, kidneys, and intestines) and is excreted partially in feces.

Contraindications and precautions
Liotrix is contraindicated in patients with thyrotoxicosis, acute myocardial infarction, and uncorrected adrenal insufficiency because liotrix increases tissue demands for adrenal hormones and may precipitate an acute adrenal crisis. Liotrix also is contraindicated to treat obesity because it is ineffective and can cause life-threatening adverse effects.

Liotrix should be used cautiously in patients with angina or other cardiovascular disease because of the risk of increased metabolic demands; in patients with diabetes mellitus because of reduced glucose tolerance; in patients with malabsorption states because of decreased absorption; and in patients with longstanding hypothyroidism or myxedema because these patients may be more sensitive to the drug's effects.

Interactions
Concomitant use of liotrix with corticotropin or an adrenocorticoid alters thyroid status; changes in liotrix dosage may require adrenocorticoid or corticotropin dosage changes as well. Concomitant use with an anticoagulant may alter anticoagulant effect; an increase in liotrix dosage may require a lower anticoagulant dose. Concomitant use of liotrix with tricyclic antidepressants or sympathomimetics may increase the effects of any or all of these drugs and may lead to coronary insufficiency or cardiac dysrhythmias. Concomitant use with insulin may affect dosage requirements of these agents. Beta blockers may decrease the conversion of thyroxine (T_4) to liothyroxine (T_3). Estrogens, which increase serum thyroxine-binding globulin levels, may increase liotrix dosage requirements. Cholestyramine may delay absorption of T_4. Hepatic enzyme inducers (such as phenytoin) may increase hepatic degradation of T_4, resulting in increased requirements of T_4. Concomitant use with somatrem may accelerate epiphyseal maturation.

Effects on diagnostic tests
Liotrix therapy alters radioactive iodine (^{131}I) thyroid uptake, protein-bound iodine levels, and T_3 uptake.

Adverse reactions
• CNS: nervousness, insomnia, tremor.
• CV: tachycardia, palpitations, dysrhythmias, angina pectoris, hypertension, widened pulse pressure, cardiovascular collapse, cardiac arrest.
• GI: change in appetite, nausea, diarrhea.
• Other: headache, leg cramps, weight loss, sweating, heat intolerance, allergic skin reactions, fever, and menstrual irregularities. Hypersensitivity to the drug or tartrazine (a dye contained in Euthroid-½, -1 and -3) has also been reported.
Note: Drug should be discontinued if allergic reaction or signs of hyperthyroidism occur.

Overdose and treatment
Clinical manifestations of overdose include signs and symptoms of hyperthyroidism, including weight loss,

---

increased appetite, palpitations, nervousness, diarrhea, abdominal cramps, sweating, tachycardia, increased pulse rate and blood pressure, angina, cardiac dysrhythmias, tremor, headache, insomnia, heat intolerance, fever, and menstrual irregularities.

Treatment of overdose requires reduction of GI absorption and efforts to counteract central and peripheral effects, primarily sympathetic activity. Use gastric lavage or induce emesis, then follow with activated charcoal, if less than 4 hours since ingestion. If the patient is comatose or having seizures, inflate the cuff on an endotracheal tube to prevent aspiration. Treatment may include oxygen and artificial ventilation as needed to maintain respiration. It should also include appropriate measures to treat congestive heart failure and to control fever, hypoglycemia, and fluid loss. Propranolol (or atenolol, metoprolol, acebutolol, nadolol, or timolol) may be used to combat many of the effects of increased sympathetic activity. Thyroid therapy should be withdrawn gradually over 2 to 6 days, then resumed at a lower dosage.

▶ Special considerations
• During first few months of therapy, children may suffer partial hair loss. Reassure child and parents that this is temporary.
• Drug dosage varies widely among patients. Treatment should start at the lowest level, titrating to higher doses according to patient's symptoms and laboratory data, until euthyroid state is reached.
• Drug should be administered at the same time each day. Morning dosage is preferred to prevent insomnia.
• Monitor prothrombin time; patients taking anticoagulants usually require lower doses.
• Monitor for signs of overdose or hypothyroidism, including changes in menstrual periods, coldness, constipation, dry puffy skin, headache, listlessness, muscle aches, nausea, vomiting, weakness, fatigue, and unusual weight gain.
• Signs and symptoms of thyrotoxicosis or inadequate dosage therapy include diarrhea, fever, irritability, listlessness, rapid heartbeat, vomiting, or weakness.
• Infants and children may experience accelerated rate of bone maturation.
• The two commercially prepared liotrix brands contain different amounts of each ingredient; do not change from one brand to the other without considering the differences in potency.
• Monitor the patient's pulse rate and blood pressure.
• Protect liotrix from heat and moisture.

Information for parents and patient
• Explain that drug usually must be taken for life. Warn against changing dosage or discontinuing the drug.
• Tell parents to watch patient for and promptly report signs of excessive dosage (headache, diarrhea, nervousness, excessive sweating, heat intolerance, chest pain, increased pulse rate, or palpitations).
• Advise parents not to store liotrix in warm and humid areas, such as the bathroom.
• Patient should take a single daily dose in the morning to avoid insomnia.
• Parents or patient should inform new physician or dentist that patient is taking this drug.

---

lithium carbonate
Carbolith★, Duoralith★, Eskalith, Eskalith CR, Lithane, Lithizine★, Lithobid, Lithonate, Lithotabs

lithium citrate
Cibalith-S

• Classification: antimanic, antipsychotic (alkali metal)

How supplied
Available by prescription only
Capsules: 300 mg
Tablets: 300 mg (300 mg = 8.12 mEq lithium)
Tablets (sustained-release): 300 mg, 450 mg
Syrup (sugarless): 300 mg/5 ml (0.3% alcohol)

Indications, route, and dosage
Prevention or control of mania; prevention of depression in patients with bipolar illness
†*Children:* 15 to 60 mg/kg/day in divided doses, or 0.4 to 1.6 mg/kg. May continue same dosage for maintenance or use 4.1 to 8.12 mEq daily titrated to individual need.
Adults: 300 to 600 mg or 5 to 10 ml lithium citrate (each 5 ml contains 8 mEq lithium, equivalent to 300 mg lithium carbonate) P.O. up to four times daily, increasing on the basis of blood levels and clinical response to achieve optimal dosage. Dosages to a maximum of 2.4 g daily divided t.i.d. or q.i.d. may be required in the acute manic phase of bipolar illness. Recommended therapeutic lithium blood levels: 1 to 1.5 mEq/liter for acute mania; 0.6 to 1.2 mEq/liter for maintenance therapy; and 2 mEq/liter as maximum. Dosage should be decreased rapidly when the acute attack has subsided.

Action and kinetics
• *Antipsychotic action:* Lithium is thought to exert its antipsychotic and antimanic effects by competing with other cations for exchange at the sodium-potassium ionic pump, thus altering cationic exchange at the tissue level.
• *Kinetics in adults:* Rate and extent of absorption vary with dosage form: absorption is complete within 6 hours of oral administration.

Lithium is distributed widely into the body, including breast milk; concentrations in thyroid gland, bone, and brain tissue exceed serum levels. Peak effects occur at 30 minutes to 3 hours; liquid peaks at 15 minutes to 1 hour. Steady-state serum level is achieved in 12 hours, at which time trough levels should be drawn: therapeutic effect begins in 5 to 10 days and is maximal within 3 weeks. Therapeutic and toxic serum levels and therapeutic effects show good correlation. Therapeutic range is 0.6 to 1.2 mEq/liter; adverse reactions increase as level reaches 1.5 to 2 mEq/liter – such concentrations may be necessary in acute mania. Toxicity usually occurs at levels above 2 mEq/liter.

Lithium is not metabolized. It is excreted 95% un-

---

changed in urine; about 50% to 80% of a given dose is excreted within 24 hours. Level of renal function determines elimination rate.

Contraindications and precautions
Lithium is contraindicated in patients with known hypersensitivity to lithium.

Lithium should be used cautiously in patients with cardiovascular disease because drug causes ECG changes (including T wave depression in 20% to 30% of patients), heart block, and premature ventricular contractions; in patients with renal dysfunction, because delayed elimination may induce lithium toxicity and diabetes insipidus (characterized by extreme thirst and excessive urination in 30% to 50% of patients); in patients with hypovolemia, sodium depletion, or dehydration, which increase drug's effects; in patients with hypothyroidism because of risk of disease exacerbation or goiter formation; in patients with psoriasis, because lithium may exacerbate condition; and in patients with epilepsy and other seizure disorders, because drug may induce seizures. Many oral lithium products contain tartrazine, which may exacerbate asthma or respiratory disorders in aspirin-allergic patients.

Interactions
Concomitant use of lithium with thiazide diuretics may decrease renal excretion and enhance lithium toxicity; diuretic dosage may need to be reduced by 30%. Indomethacin, phenylbutazone, piroxicam, and other nonsteroidal anti-inflammatory agents also decrease renal excretion of lithium and may require a 30% reduction in lithium dosage.

Mazindol, tetracyclines, phenytoin, carbamazepine, and methyldopa may increase lithium toxicity. Antacids and other drugs containing sodium, calcium, theophylline, aminophylline, or caffeine may increase lithium excretion by renal competition for elimination, thus decreasing lithium's therapeutic effect.

Lithium may interfere with pressor effects of sympathomimetic agents, especially norepinephrine; may potentiate the effects of neuromuscular blocking agents (such as succinylcholine, pancuronium, and atracurium); and may decrease the effects of chlorpromazine.

Concomitant use with haloperidol may result in severe encephalopathy characterized by confusion, tremors, extrapyramidal effects, and weakness. Use this combination with caution.

Effects on diagnostic tests
Lithium causes false-positive test results for thyroid function tests; drug also elevates white blood cell count.

Adverse reactions
• CNS: tremors, drowsiness, headache, confusion, restlessness, dizziness, psychomotor retardation, stupor, lethargy, coma, blackouts, epileptiform seizures, EEG changes, worsened organic brain syndrome, impaired speech, ataxia, muscle weakness, incoordination, hyperexcitability, exacerbation of psychotic symptoms.
• CV: reversible ECG changes, dysrhythmias, hypotension, peripheral circulatory collapse, allergic vasculitis, ankle and wrist edema, bradycardia.
• DERM: pruritus, rash, diminished or lost sensation, drying and thinning of hair.
• EENT: tinnitus, impaired vision.
• GI: nausea, vomiting, anorexia, diarrhea, dry mouth, thirst, metallic taste.
• GU: polyuria, glycosuria, incontinence, nephrotoxicity with long-term use, decreased renal concentrating capacity.
• Metabolic: transient hyperglycemia, goiter, hypothyroidism (lowered triiodothyronine, thyroxine, and protein-bound iodine levels; elevated ^{131}I uptake), hyponatremia.
• Other: weight gain (25%).

The severity of lithium toxicity parallels serum concentration:

Less than 1.5 mEq/liter: thirst, nausea, vomiting, diarrhea, polyuria, slurred speech, hand tremors, weakness.

1.5 to 2 mEq/liter: GI distress, hand tremors, confusion, muscle twitching, ECG changes, incoordination.

2 to 2.5 mEq/liter: ataxia, polyuria, large volume of dilute urine, ECG changes, seizures, abnormal motor activity, tinnitus, hypotension, coma.

Note: Drug should be discontinued if any of the following occurs: hypersensitivity, severe hypothyroidism or goiter, slurred speech, ataxia, incoordination, dysrhythmias, seizures, decreased renal function, or rash.

Overdose and treatment
Vomiting and diarrhea occur within 1 hour of acute ingestion (induce vomiting in noncomatose patients if it is not spontaneous). Death has occurred in patients ingesting 10 to 60 g of lithium; patients have ingested 6 g with minimal toxic effects. Serum lithium levels above 3.4 mEq/liter are potentially fatal.

Overdose with chronic lithium ingestion may follow altered pharmacokinetics, drug interactions, or volume or sodium depletion: sedation, confusion, hand tremors, joint pain, ataxia, muscle stiffness, increased deep tendon reflexes, visual changes, and nystagmus may occur. Symptoms may progress to coma, movement abnormalities, tremors, seizures, and cardiovascular collapse.

Treatment is symptomatic and supportive; if emesis is not feasible, treat with gastric lavage. Monitor fluid and electrolyte balance; correct sodium depletion with normal saline solution. Institute hemodialysis if serum level is above 3 mEq/liter, and in severely symptomatic patients unresponsive to fluid and electrolyte correction, or if urine output decreases significantly. Serum rebound of tissue lithium stores (from high volume distribution) commonly occurs after dialysis and may necessitate prolonged or repeated hemodialysis. Peritoneal dialysis may help but is less effective.

▶ Special considerations
• Lithium is not recommended for use in children under age 12.
• Shake syrup formulation before administration.
• Patient should take drug with food or milk to reduce GI upset.

• Use cautiously with haloperidol, other antipsychotics, neuromuscular blocking agents, and diuretics; in elderly or debilitated persons; and in thyroid disease, brain damage, severe debilitation or dehydration, and sodium depletion.

• Monitor baseline ECG, thyroid, and renal studies, and electrolyte levels. Monitor lithium blood levels 8 to 12 hours after first dose, usually before morning dose, two or three times weekly first month, then weekly to monthly on maintenance therapy.

• Determination of lithium blood concentration is crucial to the safe use of the drug. Lithium shouldn't be used in patients who can't have regular lithium blood level checks. Be sure patient or responsible family member can comply with instructions.

• When lithium blood levels are below 1.5 mEq/liter, adverse reactions usually remain mild.

• Monitor fluid intake and output, especially when surgery is scheduled.

• Expect lag of 1 to 3 weeks before drug's beneficial effects are noticed. Other psychotropic medications (for example, chlorpromazine) may be necessary during this interim period.

• Monitor for signs of edema or sudden weight gain.

• Adjust fluid and salt ingestion to compensate if excessive loss occurs through protracted sweating or diarrhea. Under normal conditions, patients should have adequate fluid intake daily and a balanced diet with adequate salt intake.

• Arrange for outpatient follow-up of thyroid and renal functions every 6 to 12 months. Thyroid should be palpated to check for enlargement.

• Patient should carry identification/instruction card (available from pharmacy) with toxicity and emergency information.

• Administer lithium with plenty of water and after meals to minimize GI upset.

• Check urine for specific gravity level below 1.015, which may indicate diabetes insipidus.

• Lithium may alter glucose tolerance in diabetic patients. Monitor blood glucose levels closely.

• Lithium is used investigationally to increase white blood cell count in patients undergoing cancer chemotherapy.

• Lithium is also used investigationally to treat cluster headaches, aggression, organic brain syndrome, and tardive dyskinesia. It has been used to treat syndrome of inappropriate secretion of antidiuretic hormone.

• Monitor serum levels and signs of impending toxicity.

• Lithane tablets contain tartrazine, a dye that may precipitate an allergic reaction in certain individuals, particularly asthmatics sensitive to aspirin.

Information for parents and patient

• Explain to patient that lithium has a narrow therapeutic margin of safety. A blood level that is even slightly too high can be dangerous.

• Warn patient and family to watch for signs of toxicity (diarrhea, vomiting, dehydration, drowsiness, muscle weakness, tremor, fever, and ataxia) and to expect transient nausea, polyuria, thirst, and discomfort during first few days. If toxic symptoms occur, patient should withhold one dose and call physician promptly.

• Warn ambulatory patient to avoid activities that require alertness and good psychomotor coordination until CNS response to drug is determined.

• Advise patient to maintain adequate water intake and adequate—but not excessive—salt in diet.

• Explain importance of regular follow-up visits to measure lithium serum levels.

• Tell patient to avoid large amounts of caffeine, which will interfere with drug's effectiveness.

• Advise patient to seek medical approval before initiating weight-loss program.

• Tell patient not to switch brands of lithium or take other drugs (prescription or nonprescription) without medical approval. Different brands may not provide equivalent effect.

• Warn patient against stopping drug abruptly.

• Tell patient to explain to close friend or family members the signs of lithium overdose, in case emergency aid is needed.

lomustine (CCNU)
CeeNU

Classification: antineoplastic (alkylating agent, nitrosourea [cell cycle-phase nonspecific])

How supplied
Available by prescription only
Capsules: 10 mg, 40 mg, 100 mg

Indications, route, and dosage
Dosage and indications may vary. Check current literature for recommended protocol.
†Brain, †colon, †lung, and †renal cell cancer; Hodgkin's disease; †lymphomas; †melanomas; †multiple myeloma
Children and adults: 130 mg/m² P.O. as single dose q 6 weeks. Reduce dose to 100 mg/m³ or less according to bone marrow depression. Repeat doses should not be given until WBC count is more than 4,000/mm³ and platelet count is more than 100,000/mm³.

If leukocyte count is over 3,000/mm³ and platelet count is over 75,000/mm³, reduce subsequent doses by 25%; if leukocyte count is over 2,000/mm³ and platelet count is over 50,000/mm³, reduce subsequent doses by 50%; if leukocyte count is under 2,000/mm³ and platelet count is under 25,000/mm³, do not repeat dosage.

Action and kinetics
• *Antineoplastic action:* Lomustine exerts its cytotoxic activity through alkylation, resulting in the inhibition of DNA and RNA synthesis. Like other nitrosourea compounds, lomustine is known to modify cellular proteins and alkylate proteins, resulting in an inhibition of protein synthesis. Cross-resistance exists between lomustine and carmustine.

• *Kinetics in adults:* Lomustine is rapidly and well absorbed across the GI tract after oral administration and is distributed widely into body tissues. Because of its high lipid solubility, the drug and its metabolites cross the blood-brain barrier to a significant extent.

Lomustine is metabolized rapidly and extensively

in the liver. Some of the metabolites have cytotoxic activity.

Metabolites of lomustine are excreted primarily in urine, with smaller amounts excreted in feces and through the lungs. The plasma elimination of lomustine is described as biphasic, with an initial phase half-life of 6 hours and a terminal phase of 1 to 2 days. The extended half-life of the terminal phase is thought to be caused by enterohepatic circulation and protein-binding.

Contraindications and precautions

Lomustine is contraindicated in patients with a history of hypersensitivity to the drug.

Drug should be used cautiously in patients with renal and hepatic dysfunction because drug accumulation may occur; and in patients with hematologic compromise and those who have recently received cytotoxic or radiation therapy because the drug's adverse hematologic effects may be exacerbated. Administer with caution in patients with infection because the drug is myelosuppressive and may exacerbate infections.

Interactions

None reported.

Effects on diagnostic tests

Lomustine therapy may cause transient increases in liver function tests.

Adverse reactions

• CNS: lethargy, ataxia, dysarthria.
• GI: nausea and vomiting, beginning within 4 to 5 hours and lasting 24 hours; stomatitis.
• GU: nephrotoxicity, progressive azotemia.
• HEMA: bone marrow depression (dose-limiting); leukopenia, delayed up to 6 weeks, lasting 1 to 2 weeks; thrombocytopenia, delayed up to 4 weeks, lasting 1 to 2 weeks.
• Other: hepatotoxicity, alopecia.

Overdose and treatment

Clinical manifestations of overdose include myelosuppression, nausea, and vomiting.

Treatment is usually supportive and includes antiemetics and transfusion of blood components.

▶ Special considerations

• Give 2 to 4 hours after meals. Lomustine will be more completely absorbed if taken when the stomach is empty. To avoid nausea, give antiemetic before administering.
• Anorexia may persist for 2 to 3 days after a given dose.
• Alcoholic beverages and alcohol-containing elixirs should be avoided for a short period after a dose of lomustine.
• Dose modification may be required in patients with decreased platelets, leukocytes, or erythrocytes.
• Monitor CBC weekly. Drug is usually not administered more often than every 6 weeks; bone marrow toxicity is cumulative and delayed.
• Frequently assess renal and hepatic status.

• Avoid all I.M. injections when platelet count is below 100,000/mm³.
• Use anticoagulants cautiously. Watch closely for signs of bleeding.
• Because lomustine crosses the blood-brain barrier, it may be used to treat primary brain tumors.
• Has been used to treat psoriasis and mycosis fungoides; however, systemic absorption and subsequent toxicity limit the drug's usefulness.
• Monitor weight, intake and output, BUN, hematocrit, platelet count, ALT (SGPT), AST (SGOT), LDH, serum bilirubin, serum creatinine, uric acid total and differential leukocyte.

Information for parents and patient

• Emphasize to the parents and child the importance of taking the exact dose prescribed and of continuing medication despite nausea and vomiting. Tell them that giving this drug at bedtime may minimize this reaction.
• Total dose should be taken at once.
• Tell parents to call immediately if vomiting occurs shortly after a dose is taken.
• Advise parents to avoid administering nonprescription products containing aspirin and to avoid acetaminophen preparations that contain alcohol.
• Advise parents to avoid patient's exposure to persons with bacterial or viral infections because chemotherapy can increase susceptibility to infection. Parents should watch for and report any signs of infection promptly.
• Advise parents that immunizations should be avoided if possible. Patient should avoid contact with persons who have received live virus immunizations (polio, measles/mumps/rubella).
• Explain importance of promptly reporting susceptible patient's exposure to chicken pox.
• Advise parents that the patient should complete dental work before therapy whenever possible, or delay it until blood counts are normal.
• Warn parents that patient may bruise easily because of drug's effect on blood count.
• Teach parents and patient to check for signs of bleeding and bruising. Parents may need to restrict child's participation in contact sports. Such activity is dangerous when patient's platelets are low.
• Tell patient to promptly report a sore throat, fever, or any unusual bruising or bleeding.
• Stress importance of keeping follow-up appointments for monitoring hematologic status.
• Instruct parents to monitor neutropenic patient's temperature every 4 hours (not rectally) and to report fever, cough, and other signs of infection *promptly.*
• Instruct patient to avoid foods that are spicy and extremely hot or cold. Topical anesthetics administered before meals (swish and spit) may relieve mouth discomfort.
• Premedicating with an antiemetic may prevent nausea and vomiting. If vomiting occurs, administer antiemetics p.r.n.
• Patients who have received drugs with strong emetic properties may experience anticipatory nausea and vomiting at subsequent treatments. They may benefit from treatment with an anxiolytic drug.
• Instruct patient to clean teeth with toothettes,

---

gauze, or soft toothbrush when platelets are low. Patient should perform frequent oral hygiene and should avoid using commercial mouthwashes which may contain alcohol and have an irritating effect. Solutions of sodium bicarbonate or hydrogen peroxide are more appropriate rinses.

loperamide hydrochloride
Imodium A-D liquid, Imodium capsules

• Classification: antidiarrheal (piperadine derivative)

How supplied
Available by prescription only
Capsules: 2 mg

Available without prescription.
Solution: 1 mg/5 ml

Indications, route, and dosage
Acute, nonspecific diarrhea
Children age 2 to 5: 1 mg t.i.d. on first day.
Children age 6 to 8: 2 mg t.i.d. on first day.
Children age 9 to 11: 2 mg t.i.d. on first day.
Children over age 12 and adults: Initially, 4 mg P.O., then 2 mg after each unformed stool. Maximum dosage is 16 mg daily.
Maintenance dose is ⅓ to ½ the initial dose.
Chronic diarrhea
Adults: Initially, 4 mg P.O., then 2 mg after each unformed stool until diarrhea subsides. Adjust dose to individual response.
Directions for patient self-medication (liquid)
Children age 2 to 5 (24-47 lb): 1 teaspoonfuls after first loose bowel movement, followed by 1 teaspoonful after each subsequent loose bowel movement. Do not exceed 3 teaspoonfuls a day.
Children age 6 to 8 (48-59 lb): 2 teaspoonfuls after first loose bowel movement, followed by 1 teaspoonful after each subsequent loose bowel movement. Do not exceed 4 teaspoonfuls a day.
Children age 9 to 11 (60-95 lb): 2 teaspoonfuls after first loose bowel movement, followed by 1 teaspoonful after each subsequent loose bowel movement. Do not exceed 6 teaspoonfuls a day.
Adults: 4 teaspoonfuls after the first loose bowel movement, followed by 2 teaspoonfuls after each subsequent loose bowel movement, but no more than 8 teaspoonfuls a day for no more than 2 days.

Action and kinetics
• *Antidiarrheal action:* Loperamide reduces intestinal motility by acting directly on intestinal mucosal nerve endings; tolerance to antiperistaltic effect does not develop. The drug also may inhibit fluid and electrolyte secretion by an unknown mechanism. Although it is chemically related to opiates, it has not shown any physical dependance characteristics in humans, and it possesses no analgesic activity.
• *Kinetics in adults:* Loperamide is absorbed poorly from the GI tract. Absorbed loperamide is metabolized

in the liver. Drug is excreted primarily in feces; less than 2% is excreted in urine.

Contraindications and precautions
Loperamide is contraindicated in patients with diarrhea from pseudomembranous colitis or ulcerative colitis because it may precipitate toxic megacolon; in patients with diarrhea resulting from poisoning or infection by microbes that can penetrate the intestinal mucosa, because expulsion of intestinal contents may be a protective mechanism; and in patients with known hypersensitivity to the drug.
Loperamide should be used cautiously in patients with hepatic disease because the drug may worsen the symptoms of this disorder.

Interactions
Concomitant use with an opioid analgesic may cause severe constipation.

Effects on diagnostic tests
None reported.

Adverse reactions
• CNS: drowsiness, fatigue, dizziness.
• GI: dry mouth, nausea, vomiting, abdominal cramps, abdominal distention, constipation.
• Other: rash.
Note: Drug should be discontinued if bowel sounds are absent, if abdominal distention occurs, or if patient does not improve within 48 hours (acute diarrhea) or 10 days (chronic diarrhea).

Overdose and treatment
Clinical effects of overdose include constipation, GI irritation, and CNS depression.
Treat with activated charcoal if ingestion was recent. If patient is vomiting, activated charcoal may be given in a slurry when patient can retain fluids. Alternately, gastric lavage may be performed, followed by administration of activated charcoal slurry. Monitor for CNS depression; treat respiratory depression with naloxone.

▶ Special considerations
• Drug is approved for use in children age 2 and older; however, children may be more susceptible to untoward CNS effects.
• After administration via nasogastric tube, tube should be flushed to clear it and ensure drug's passage to stomach.

Information for parents and patient
• Tell parents to give drug only as directed and not to exceed recommended dose.
• Patient should avoid hazardous activities requiring alertness because drug may cause drowsiness and dizziness.
• Instruct parents to call physician if no improvement occurs in 48 hours or if fever develops.

lymphocyte immune globulin (antithymocyte globulin [equine])
Atgam

• Classification: immunosuppressive agent (immunoglobulin)

How supplied
Available by prescription only
Injection: 50 mg of equine IgG per ml, 5-ml ampules

Indications, route, and dosage
Prevention of acute renal allograft rejection
Children over age 3 months and adults: 15 mg/kg/day I.V. for 14 days, then same dosage every other day for the next 14 days (to a total of 21 doses in 28 days). The first dose of ATG should be administered within 24 hours before or after transplantation.
Treatment of acute renal allograft rejection
Children over age 3 months and adults: 10 to 15 mg/kg/day for 14 days; if necessary, the same dosage may be given every other day for another 14 days (to a total of 21 doses in 28 days). Therapy with ATG should begin at the first sign of acute rejection.
Aplastic anemia
Children over age 3 months and adults: 10 to 20 mg/kg daily for 8 to 14 consecutive days, followed by alternate day therapy for up to another 14 days if necessary (up to 21 doses in 28 days).

Action and kinetics
• *Immunosuppressive action:* The exact mechanism has not been fully defined but may involve elimination of antigen-reactive T cells (T-lymphocytes) in peripheral blood or alteration of T-cell function. The effects of antilymphocyte preparations, including ATG, on T cells are variable and complex. Whether the effects of ATG are mediated through a specific subset of T cells has not been determined.
• *Kinetics in adults:* Peak plasma levels of equine IgG after I.V. administration of ATG vary, depending on the patient's ability to catabolize foreign IgG.

Since antilymphocyte serum reportedly is poorly distributed into lymphoid tissues (for example, spleen, lymph nodes), it is likely that ATG is also poorly distributed into these tissues.

Transplacental distribution of ATG is likely because other immunoglobulins cross the placenta. Virtually all transplacental passage of immunoglobulins occurs during the last 4 weeks of pregnancy. Metabolism of drug is unknown.

The plasma half-life of equine IgG reportedly averages about 6 days (range: 1.5 to 12 days). Approximately 1% of a dose of ATG is excreted in urine, principally as unchanged equine IgG. In one report, mean urinary concentration of equine IgG was approximately 4 mcg/ml after approximately 21 doses of ATG over 28 days.

Contraindications and precautions
ATG is contraindicated in patients who have had a severe systemic reaction during therapy with this drug or with another equine immunoglobulin G preparation. Anaphylaxis occurs in less than 1% of patients receiving ATG.

Serum sickness reactions have occurred in patients receiving ATG. The incidence of serum sickness reactions to ATG in renal allograft recipients is unknown, in part because of the difficulty in diagnosing the reaction in these patients; but serum sickness reactions have occurred in a high percentage (85% to 100%) of patients receiving this drug for the treatment of aplastic anemia. Fever, nausea and vomiting, cutaneous lesions, and lymphadenopathy are common signs of serum sickness. Corticosteroids may be used to treat these reactions.

Interactions
Concomitant use of ATG with other immunosuppressive therapy (azathioprine, corticosteroids, graft irradiation), may intensify immunosuppression, an effect that can be used to therapeutic advantage; however, such therapy may increase vulnerability to infection and possibly the risk of lymphoma or lymphoproliferative disorders.

Effects on diagnostic tests
Elevations of hepatic serum enzymes have been reported.

Adverse reactions
• CV: hypertension, hypotension, tachycardia, chest pain, edema, pulmonary edema, iliac vein obstruction, renal artery stenosis.
• CNS: arthralgia, malaise, weakness, faintness, seizures, night sweats.
• DERM: rash, pruritus, erythema.
• GI: nausea, vomiting, diarrhea, stomatitis, hiccups, epigastric pain, abdominal distention.
• Other: anaphylaxis, serum sickness, fever, chills, arthralgia, back pain, leukopenia, thrombocytopenia.
Note: Drug should be discontinued if signs and symptoms of anaphylaxis occur.

Overdose and treatment
No information available.

▶ Special considerations
• Safety and efficacy not established. Drug has had limited use in children age 3 months to 19 years.
• Dilute ATG concentrate for injection before I.V. infusion. Dilute the required dose of ATG in 0.45 or 0.9% sodium chloride injection (usually 250 to 1,000 ml); the final concentration preferably should not exceed 1 mg of equine IgG per ml.
• Infusion in dextrose or highly acidic solutions is not recommended.
• Invert the I.V. infusion solution container into which ATG concentrate is added to prevent contact of undiluted ATG with air inside the container. Diluted solutions of ATG should be refrigerated at 2° to 8° C. if administration is delayed. Reconstituted solutions should not be used after 12 hours (including actual infusion time), even if stored at 2° to 8° C.

• Because of the risk of a severe systemic reaction (anaphylaxis), the manufacturer recommends an intradermal skin test before administration of the initial dose of ATG. The skin test procedure consists of intradermal injection of 0.1 ml of a 1:1,000 dilution of ATG concentrate for injection in 0.9% sodium chloride injection (5 mcg of equine IgG). A control test using 0.9% sodium chloride injection should be administered in the other arm to facilitate interpretation of the results. If a wheal or area of erythema greater than 10 mm in diameter (with or without pseudopod formation) and itching or marked local swelling develops, infusion of ATG requires extreme caution; severe and potentially fatal systemic reactions can occur in patients with a positive skin test. A systemic reaction to the skin test such as generalized rash, tachycardia, dyspnea, hypotension, or anaphylaxis rules out further administration of ATG. The predictive value of the ATG skin test has not been clearly established, and an allergic reaction may occur despite a negative skin test.

• Anaphylaxis may occur at any time during ATG therapy and may be indicated by hypotension, respiratory distress, or pain in the chest, flank, or back. Monitor vital signs during and after infusion. Keep emergency drugs and oxygen set-up available in patient's room.

• The manufacturer has not yet determined the total number of ATG doses (10 to 20 mg/kg per dose) that can be administered safely to an individual patient. Some renal allograft recipients have received up to 50 doses in 4 months; others, up to four 28-day courses of 21 doses each without an increased incidence of adverse effects.

• ATG has been used to treat aplastic anemia, and as an adjunct in bone marrow and skin allotransplantation.

• Patients receiving ATG should be closely observed for signs of leukopenia, thrombocytopenia, and concurrent infection. To minimize the risks of leukopenia and infection, some clinicians recommend that azathioprine and corticosteroid dosages be reduced by 50% when ATG is used concomitantly with these drugs for the prevention or treatment of renal allograft rejection.

Information for parents and patient
• Warn parents and patient that a febrile reaction is likely. Instruct them about potential adverse reactions.

---

lypressin
Diapid

• Classification: antidiuretic hormone (posterior pituitary hormone)

How supplied
Available by prescription only
Nasal spray: 8-ml bottle, 0.185 mg/ml

Indications, route, and dosage
Nonnephrogenic diabetes insipidus
Children and adults: 1 or 2 sprays (approximately 2 USP posterior pituitary pressor units/spray) in either or both nostrils q.i.d. and an additional dose h.s., if needed, to prevent nocturia. If usual dosage is inadequate, increase frequency rather than number of sprays.

Action and kinetics
• *Antidiuretic action:* Lypressin is used to control or prevent signs and complications of neurogenic diabetes insipidus. Acting primarily at the renal tubular level, lypressin increases cyclic 3',5'-adenosine monophosphate, which increases water permeability at the renal tubule and collecting duct, resulting in increased urine osmolality and decreased urinary flow rate.

• *Kinetics in adults:* Lypressin is destroyed by trypsin in the GI tract; therefore, it is given intranasally. Absorption is rapid from the nasal mucosa. Onset of effect is rapid after intranasal application and peaks within ½ to 2 hours. Lypressin is distributed into the extracellular fluid and is metabolized by the kidneys and liver. A small amount of active drug and its inactive metabolites are excreted in urine. Duration of action is 3 to 8 hours. Half-life is about 15 minutes.

Contraindications and precautions
Lypressin is contraindicated in patients with known hypersensitivity to the drug. Large doses should be used with caution in patients with coronary artery disease because lypressin may cause coronary artery constriction. Although lypressin's pressor effects are minimal, the drug should be used with caution in patients in whom blood pressure elevation is hazardous.

Interactions
Concomitant use of lypressin with carbamazepine, chlorpropamide, or clofibrate may potentiate lypressin's antidiuretic effect; use with demeclocycline, lithium, norepinephrine, epinephrine, heparin, or alcohol may decrease the antidiuretic effect.

Effects on diagnostic tests
None reported.

Adverse reactions
• CNS: headache, dizziness, seizures, coma.
• DERM: hypersensitivity reaction.
• EENT: nasal congestion or ulceration, irritation, pruritus of nasal passages, rhinorrhea, conjunctivitis, perioribital edema.
• GI: heartburn from drip of excess spray into pharynx, abdominal cramps, frequent bowel movements.
• GU: possible transient fluid retention from overdose.
• Other: substernal tightness from inadvertent inhalation.
  Note: Drug should be discontinued if signs or symptoms of anaphylaxis, hypersensitivity, or water intoxication occur.

---

‡May contain sulfites   ◆May contain tartrazine   ◆◆May contain benzyl alcohol

Overdose and treatment

Clinical manifestations of overdose include drowsiness, listlessness, headache, confusion, anuria, and weight gain (water intoxication). Treatment requires water restriction and temporary withdrawal of lypressin until polyuria occurs. Severe water intoxication may require osmotic diuresis with mannitol, hypertonic dextrose, or urea, either alone or with furosemide.

▶ Special considerations

• Observe for signs and symptoms of early water intoxication – drowsiness, listlessness, headache, confusion, anuria, and weight gain – to prevent seizures, coma, and death.
• Adjust fluid intake to reduce risk of water intoxication and sodium depletion, especially in young patients.
• Overdose may cause oxytocic or vasopressor activity. If patient develops uterine cramps, increased GI activity, fluid retention, or hypertension, withhold drug until effects subside. Furosemide may be used if fluid retention is excessive.
• Some patients may have difficulty measuring and instilling drug into nostrils. Teach correct method of administration. Emphasize that drug should *not* be inhaled.

Information for parents and patient

• Instruct parents and patient about proper use: blow nose gently before using; hold bottle in an upright position; hold head upright and spray the medicine into each nostril by squeezing the bottle quickly and firmly; rinse the tip of the bottle with hot water and replace the cap after use; and do not allow water to enter bottle when rinsing.
• Instruct patient to carry medication at all times because of its fairly short duration of action.
• Tell parents to check the drug's expiration date.
• Tell parents to call physician if a cold or an allergy develops because inflammation of the nasal mucosa will diminish the drug's absorption.

---

mafenide acetate
Sulfamylon Acetate

• Classification: topical antibacterial (synthetic anti-infective)

How supplied
Available by prescription only
Cream: 8.5%

Indications, route, and dosage
Adjunctive treatment of second- and third-degree burns
Children and adults: Apply ¹⁄₁₆″ (16 mm) daily or b.i.d. to cleansed, debrided wounds. Reapply as needed to keep burned area covered.

Action and kinetics
• *Antibacterial action:* Mechanism of action of mafenide is undetermined; however, it appears that the drug interferes with bacterial cellular metabolism. Mafenide has a wide spectrum of activity and is bacteriostatic against many gram-negative and gram-positive organisms and several strains of anaerobes.
• *Kinetics in adults:* Drug diffuses through devascularized areas and is absorbed quickly. It is distributed rapidly after topical application. Mafenide is metabolized rapidly to a weak carbonic anhydrase inhibitor metabolite. The metabolite is excreted in urine.

Contraindications and precautions
Mafenide acetate is contraindicated in patients with known hypersensitivity to mafenide acetate or to other sulfonamide derivatives and in patients of childbearing age, unless benefit outweighs risk of hazard to fetus. Drug should be used with caution in patients with renal failure.

Drug is intended for topical use only; avoid contact with eyes and mucous membranes; use of mafenide may be followed by fungal colonization in and below eschar.

Interactions
None reported.

Effects on diagnostic tests
None reported.

Adverse reactions
• HEMA: *bone marrow suppression, fatal hemolytic anemia.*
• Metabolic: hyperchloremia, metabolic acidosis, porphyria.
• Pulmonary: hyperventilation, tachypnea.
• Local: pain, burning sensation, erythema, blisters, bleeding of new skin, excoriation.

• Other: hypersensitivity (rash, pruritus, itching, facial edema, urticaria, inflammation, eosinophilia).
Note: Drug should be discontinued if sensitization develops.

Overdose and treatment
Accidental ingestion may cause diarrhea. To treat local overapplication, discontinue drug and clean skin thoroughly.

▶ Special considerations
• Apply to clean, debrided wound with sterile gloved hand, covering wound to approximately ¹⁄₁₆″ (16 mm); reapply to areas if removed. Keep burned areas covered with cream at all times. Dressings usually are not required; if necessary, apply only a thin layer of dressing.
• Patient should be bathed daily to aid debridement; prior layer of cream should be removed before reapplication; whirlpool baths are no longer recommended because they increase the risk of infection.
• Continue treatment until site is healed or ready for grafting.
• Monitor patient for overgrowth of nonsusceptible organisms; severe prolonged pain may indicate allergy.
• Monitor acid-base balance closely, especially in patients with pulmonary or renal dysfunction; if metabolic acidosis develops, discontinue drug for 24 to 48 hours.
• Application of drug is extremely painful and should be used only on areas such as ear cartilage, where use of silvadene is inappropriate.

Information for parents and patient
Teach proper care of burn sites; stress importance of calling physician promptly if condition worsens or adverse reactions occur.

magnesium sulfate

• Classification: anticonvulsant (mineral/electrolyte)

How supplied
Injectable solutions: 10%, 12.5%, 25%, 50% in 2-ml, 5-ml, 10-ml, 20-ml, and 30-ml ampules, vials, and prefilled syringes

Indications, route, and dosage
Hypomagnesemic seizures
Neonates: 125 to 500 mg (1 to 4 mEq).
Infants and children: 50 to 100 mg/kg I.M. (0.4 to 0.8 mEq/kg) q 4 to 6 hours, as needed. May be given I.M., 20 to 40 mg/kg or 0.1 to 0.2 ml/kg of 20% solution.
Children and adults: 1 to 2 g (as 10% solution) I.V.

---

‡May contain sulfites   ◆May contain tartrazine   ◆◆May contain benzyl alcohol

over 15 minutes, then 1 g I.M. q 4 to 6 hours, based on patient's response and magnesium blood levels.
Seizures secondary to hypomagnesemia in acute nephritis
Children: 0.2 ml/kg of 50% solution I.M. q 4 to 6 hours, p.r.n., or 100 mg/kg of 10% solution I.V. given slowly. Titrate dosage according to magnesium blood levels and seizure response. Maintenance, 0.25 to 0.5 mEq/kg/day.

Action and kinetics
• *Anticonvulsant action:* Magnesium sulfate has CNS and respiratory depressant effects. It acts peripherally, causing vasodilation; moderate doses cause flushing and sweating, whereas high doses cause hypotension. It prevents or controls seizures by blocking neuromuscular transmission.

Magnesium sulfate is used primarily in pregnant patients to prevent or control preeclamptic or eclamptic seizures; it also is used to treat hypomagnesemic seizures in adults, and in children with acute nephritis.
• *Kinetics in adults:* I.V. magnesium sulfate acts immediately; effects last about 30 minutes. After I.M. injection, it acts within 60 minutes and lasts for 3 to 4 hours. Effective anticonvulsant serum levels are 2.5 to 7.5 mEq/liter. Magnesium sulfate is distributed widely throughout the body. Magnesium sulfate is excreted unchanged in urine; some is excreted in breast milk.

Contraindications and precautions
Magnesium sulfate is contraindicated in patients with known heart block, myocardial damage, respiratory depression, or renal failure; and in patients with eclampsia, for 2 hours preceding induced delivery, to prevent toxicity and respiratory and CNS depression in the newborn.

Patient's urine output should be maintained at 100 ml/4 hours; magnesium sulfate should be used with caution in patients with decreased renal function.

Interactions
Concomitant use with alcohol, narcotics, anxiolytics, barbiturates, antidepressants, hypnotics, antipsychotics, or general anesthetics may increase CNS depressant effects; reduced dosages may be required. Concomitant use of magnesium sulfate with succinylcholine or tubocurarine potentiates and prolongs neuromuscular blocking action of these drugs; use with caution.

Extreme caution should be used when magnesium sulfate is used concomitantly with cardiac glycosides; changes in cardiac conduction in digitalized patients may lead to heart block if calcium is administered I.V., especially by I.V. push.

Effects on diagnostic tests
None reported.

Adverse reactions
• CNS: sweating, drowsiness, depressed reflexes, flaccid paralysis, hypothermia.
• CV: hypotension, flushing, circulatory collapse, depressed cardiac function, heart block.

• Other: respiratory paralysis, hypocalcemia, pain at infusion site.
Note: Drug should be discontinued if signs of hypersensitivity, anuria, toxic symptoms, or toxic serum levels occur.

Overdose and treatment
Clinical manifestations of overdose with magnesium sulfate include a sharp drop in blood pressure and respiratory paralysis, ECG changes (increased PR, QRS, and QT intervals), heart block, and asystole.

Treatment requires artificial ventilation and I.V. calcium salt to reverse respiratory depression and heart block. Usual dosage is 5 to 10 mEq of calcium (10 to 20 ml of a 10% calcium gluconate solution).

▶ Special considerations
• I.V. bolus *must* be injected slowly (to avoid respiratory or cardiac arrest).
• If available, administer by constant infusion pump; maximum infusion rate is 150 mg/minute. Rapid drip causes feeling of heat.
• Discontinue drug as soon as needed effect is achieved.
• When giving repeated doses, test knee jerk reflex before each dose; if absent, discontinue magnesium. Use of magnesium sulfate beyond this point risks respiratory center failure.
• Respiratory rate must be 16 breaths per minute or more before each dose. Keep I.V. calcium salts on hand.
• To calculate grams of magnesium in a percentage of solution: $X\% = X$ g/100 ml (for example, 25% = 25 g/100 ml = 250 mg/ml).
• Monitor serum magnesium load and clinical status to avoid overdose.
• After use in toxemic women within 24 hours before delivery, watch newborn for signs of magnesium toxicity, including neuromuscular and respiratory depression.

mannitol
Osmitrol

• Classification: osmotic diuretic (hexahydric alcohol derivative)

How supplied
Available by prescription only
Injection: 5%, 10%, 15%, 20%, 25%

Indications, route, and dosage
Test dose for marked oliguria or suspected inadequate renal function
Children: test dose of 200 mg/kg or 6 g/m² as a 15% or 20% solution I.V. over 3 to 5 minutes. Response is adequate if 30 to 50 ml urine/hour is excreted over 2 to 3 hours. Therapeutic dose is 2 g/kg or 60 g/m².
To reduce intraocular pressure or intracranial pressure
Children over age 12 and adults: 250 mg/kg as a 15% to 25% solution I.V. over 30 to 60 minutes. Alternatively, may be administered with furosemide 1 mg/kg

---

*Canada only　　　†Unlabeled clinical use　　　Italicized adverse reactions have been observed in children.

I.V. concurrently. Dosage may be gradually increased to 1 g/kg per dose.

To promote diuresis in drug intoxication
Children over age 12 and adults: Use a 5% to 10% solution I.V. continuously, while maintaining 100 to 500 ml urine output/hour and positive fluid balance.

Action and kinetics
• *Diuretic action:* Mannitol increases the osmotic pressure of glomerular filtrate, inhibiting tubular reabsorption of water and electrolytes, thus promoting diuresis. This action also promotes urinary elimination of certain drugs. This effect is useful for prevention and management of acute renal failure or oliguria. This action is also useful for reduction of intracranial or intraocular pressure because mannitol elevates plasma osmolality, enhancing flow of water into extracellular fluid.
• *Kinetics in adults:* Mannitol is not absorbed from the GI tract. I.V. mannitol lowers intracranial pressure in 15 minutes and intraocular pressure in 30 to 60 minutes; it produces diuresis in 1 to 3 hours. Mannitol remains in the extracellular compartment. It does not cross the blood-brain barrier. Mannitol is metabolized minimally to glycogen in the liver. It is filtered by the glomeruli; half-life in adults with normal renal function is about 100 minutes.

Contraindications and precautions
Mannitol is contraindicated in patients with established anuria who do not respond to a test dose and in patients with severe pulmonary congestion, pulmonary edema, severe CHF, or severe dehydration, because of the risk of circulatory overload.

Do not administer mannitol until adequate renal function and urine flow are determined by a test dose. Evaluate patient's cardiovascular status before and during drug administration; sudden expansion of extracellular fluid may precipitate CHF.

Interactions
Mannitol may enhance renal excretion of lithium and lower serum lithium levels.

Effects on diagnostic tests
Mannitol therapy alters electrolyte balance. It also may interfere with tests for inorganic phosphorus concentration or blood ethylene glycol.

Adverse reactions
• CNS: rebound increase in intracranial pressure 8 to 12 hours after diuresis, headache, confusion.
• CV: transient expansion of plasma volume during infusion, causing circulatory overload, CHF, or pulmonary edema; tachycardia; angina-like chest pain; orthostatic hypotension.
• EENT: blurred vision, rhinitis.
• GI: thirst, nausea, vomiting.
• GU: urinary retention.
• Metabolic: fluid and electrolyte imbalance, water intoxication, cellular dehydration.

Note: Drug should be discontinued if patient's urine output continues to decline, if central venous pressure (CVP) rises, or if signs of tissue dehydration or circulatory overload occur.

Overdose and treatment
Clinical manifestations of overdose include polyuria, dehydration, hypotension, and cardiovascular collapse.

Discontinue infusion and institute supportive measures. Hemodialysis removes mannitol and decreases serum osmolality.

▶ Special considerations
• Maintain adequate hydration. Monitor fluid and electrolyte balance.
• Monitor I.V. infusion carefully for inflammation at the infusion site.
• Patient should have frequent mouth care or fluids as appropriate to relieve thirst.
• In patients with urethral catheter, an hourly urometer collection bag should be used to facilitate accurate measurement of urine output.
• Use with extreme caution in patients with compromised renal function; monitor vital signs (including CVP) hourly and input and output, weight, renal function, fluid balance, and serum and urinary sodium and potassium levels daily.
• For hyperosmolar therapy, serum osmolarity should be kept at 310 to 320 mOsm/kg.
• For maximum pressure reduction during surgery, give drug 1 to 1½ hours preoperatively.
• Mannitol should be administered I.V. via an in-line filter.
• Do not administer with whole blood; agglutination will occur.
• Mannitol solutions commonly crystallize at low temperatures; place crystallized solutions in a hot water bath, shake vigorously to dissolve crystals, and cool to body temperature before use. Do not use solutions with undissolved crystals.

Information for parents and patient
• Tell parents and patient that the patient may feel thirsty or experience mouth dryness, and emphasize importance of drinking only the amount of fluids provided, as ordered.
• With initial doses, warn patient to change position slowly, especially when rising to an upright position, to prevent dizziness from orthostatic hypotension.
• Instruct parents to watch for signs of chest, back, or leg pain or shortness of breath, and to report them immediately.

mebendazole
Vermox

• Classification: anthelmintic (benzimidazole)

How supplied
Available by prescription only
Tablets (chewable): 100 mg

Indications, route, and dosage
Pinworm infections
Children over age 2 and adults: 100 mg P.O. as a single dose. If infection persists 3 weeks later, repeat treatment.
Roundworm, whipworm, and hookworm infections
Children over age 2 and adults: 100 mg P.O. b.i.d. for 3 days. If infection persists 3 weeks later, repeat treatment.
†Trichinosis
Adults: 200 to 400 mg t.i.d. for 3 days, then 400 to 500 mg t.i.d. for 10 days.
†Hydatid disease
Adults: Limited use because of severe toxicity. 40 to 50 mg/kg/day for 3 to 8 months has been used to shrink cysts. Some clinicians maintain blood levels of 80 ng/ml with 100 mg/kg/day in four divided doses.

Action and kinetics
• *Anthelmintic action:* Mebendazole inhibits uptake of glucose and other low-molecular weight nutrients in susceptible helminths, depleting the glycogen stores they need for survival and reproduction. It has a broad spectrum and may be useful in mixed infections. It is considered a drug of choice in the treatment of ascariasis, enterobiasis, trichuriasis, and uncinariasis; it has been used investigationally to treat echinococciasis, onchocerciasis, and trichinosis.
• *Kinetics in adults:* About 5% to 10% of an administered dose of mebendazole is absorbed; peak plasma concentrations occur at 2 to 4 hours. Absorption varies widely among patients.

Mebendazole is highly bound to plasma proteins; it crosses the placenta. It is metabolized to inactive 2-amino-5(6)-benzimidazolyl phenylketone. Most of a mebendazole dose is excreted in feces; 2% to 10% is excreted in urine in 48 hours as either unchanged drug or the 2-amine metabolite. Mebendazole's half-life is 3 to 9 hours. It is unknown if mebendazole is excreted in breast milk.

Contraindications and precautions
Mebendazole is contraindicated in patients with hypersensitivity to the drug.

Interactions
None reported.

Effects on diagnostic tests
None reported.

Adverse reactions
• GI: *occasional, transient abdominal pain and diarrhea in massive infection.*
• HEMA: reversible neutropenia.
• Other: fever, dizziness.
Note: Drug should be discontinued if signs of hypersensitivity or toxicity occur.

Overdose and treatment
Signs and symtpoms of overdose may include GI disturbances and altered mental status. No specific recommendations exist; treatment is supportive. After recent ingestion (within 4 hours), empty stomach by induced emesis or gastric lavage. Follow with activated charcoal to decrease absorption.

▶ Special considerations
• Mebendazole should be given to children under age 2 only when potential benefits justify risks.
• Tablets may be chewed, swallowed whole, or crushed and mixed with food.
• Laxatives, enemas, or dietary restrictions are unnecessary.
• Collect stool specimens in a clean, dry container and transfer to a properly labeled container to send to laboratory; ova may be destroyed by toilet bowl water, urine, and some drugs.
• Encourage patient's family and contacts to be checked for infestation and treated, if necessary.
• High dose treatment of hydatid disease and trichinosis is investigational. Frequently monitor white blood cell counts to detect drug toxicity, especially during initial therapy.

Information for parents and patient
• If patient has a pinworm infection, advise parents and patient how to prevent reinfection by: washing perianal area and changing undergarments and bedclothes daily; washing hands and cleaning fingernails before meals and after defecation; and sanitary disposal of feces.
• Advise parents that patient should bathe often, by showering, if possible. Patient should keep hands away from mouth, keep fingernails short, and wear shoes to avoid hookworm; explain that ova are easily transmitted directly and indirectly by hands, food, or contaminated articles. Washing clothes in household washing machine will destroy ova.

---

mechlorethamine hydrochloride (nitrogen mustard)
Mustargen

• Classification: antineoplastic (alkylating agent [cell cycle-phase nonspecific])

How supplied
Available by prescription only
Injection: 10-mg vials
Topical solution: 10 mg in 5 to 10 ml normal saline solution (must be prepared just before administration)
Ointment: 0.01% to 0.04%
Must be compounded: not commercially available in the United States or Canada

Indications, route, and dosage
Dosage and indications may vary. Check current literature for recommended protocols.
Hodgkin's disease; non-Hodgkin's lymphomas; breast, lung, and ovarian cancer; diffuse lymphocytic lymphoma; multiple myeloma; chronic lymphocytic leukemia; mycosis fungoides
Children and adults: 0.4 mg/kg I.V. as a single dose or 0.1 mg/kg on 4 successive days q 3 to 6 weeks.

---

*Canada only   †Unlabeled clinical use   Italicized adverse reactions have been observed in children.

Give through running I.V. infusion. Dose reduced in prior radiation or chemotherapy to 0.2 to 0.4 mg/kg. Dose based on ideal or actual body weight, whichever is less.

Intracavitary doses for neoplastic effusions
Children and adults: 0.2 to 0.4 mg/kg.

Action and kinetics
• *Antineoplastic action:* Mechlorethamine exerts its cytotoxic activity through the basic processes of alkylation. The drug causes cross-linking of DNA strands, single-strand breakage of DNA, abnormal base pairing, and interruption of other intracellular processes, resulting in cell death.
• *Kinetics in adults:* Mechlorethamine is well absorbed after oral administration; however, because the drug is very irritating to tissue, it must be administered intravenously. After intracavitary administration, it is absorbed incompletely, probably from deactivation by body fluids in the cavity. Mechlorethamine does not cross the blood-brain barrier. Mechlorethamine is converted rapidly to its active form, which reacts quickly with various cellular components before being deactivated. Metabolites of mechlorethamine are excreted in urine. Less than 0.01% of an I.V. dose is excreted unchanged in urine.

Contraindications and precautions
Because of the potential of the drug to cause extensive and rapid development of amyloidosis, mechlorethamine is contraindicated in patients with foci of chronic or suppurative inflammation.

It may be necessary to adjust dosage or discontinue therapy in patients with infections, hematologic compromise, or bone marrow infiltration with malignant cells because of the drug's adverse hematologic effects.

Interactions
None reported.

Effects on diagnostic tests
Mechlorethamine therapy may increase blood and urine uric acid levels and may decrease serum pseudocholinesterase concentrations.

Adverse reactions
• EENT: tinnitus, metallic taste (immediately after dose), deafness (with high doses).
• GI: nausea, vomiting, and anorexia begin within 1 hour and last 8 to 24 hours.
• GU: oligomenorrhea, amenorrhea, azoospermia, delayed spermatogenesis.
• HEMA: *bone marrow depression* (dose-limiting) occurs by days 4 to 10, lasting 10 to 21 days; mild anemia begins in 2 to 3 weeks, possibly lasting 7 weeks.
• Metabolic: hyperuricemia.
• Local: thrombophlebitis, sloughing, severe irritation if drug extravasates or touches skin.
• Other: alopecia, herpes zoster.

Overdose and treatment
Clinical manifestations of overdose include lymphopenia and precipitation of uric acid crystals.

Treatment is usually supportive and includes transfusion of blood components, hydration, and allopurinol.

▶ Special considerations
• Follow established procedures for safe handling, administration, and disposal.
• Vital signs and patency of catheter or I.V. line should be monitored throughout administration.
• Drug is a vesicant. Avoid placement of I.V. site at or near a joint that may become immobilized if extravasation occurs. During I.V. administration, monitor continuously for extravasation. If it occurs, stop infusion, remove I.V., and treat promptly according to institutional policy.
• Monitor BUN, CBC, hematocrit, platelet count, ALT (SGPT), AST (SGOT), LDH, serum bilirubin, serum creatinine, uric acid total and differential leukocyte.
• To reconstitute powder, use 10 ml of sterile water for injection or normal saline solution to give a concentration of 1 mg/ml.
• Solution is very unstable. It should be prepared immediately before infusion and used within 20 minutes. Discard unused solution.
• Drug may be administered I.V. push over a few minutes into the tubing of a freely flowing I.V. infusion.
• Dilution of mechlorethamine into a large volume of I.V. solution is not recommended, because the drug may react with the diluent and is not stable for a prolonged period.
• Treatment of extravasation includes local injections of a 1/6 M sodium thiosulfate solution. Prepare solution by mixing 4 ml of sodium thiosulfate 10% with 6 ml of sterile water for injection. Also, apply ice packs constantly for first 24 hours to minimize local reactions.
• During intracavitary administration, patient should be turned from side to side every 15 minutes to 1 hour to distribute drug.
• Avoid contact with skin or mucous membranes. Wear gloves when preparing solution and during administration to prevent accidental skin contact. If contact occurs, wash with copious amounts of water, then irrigate with 2% sodium thiosulfate solution.
• Use cautiously in the presence of severe anemia and depressed neutrophil or platelet count and in patients recently treated with radiation or chemotherapy.
• To prevent hyperuricemia with resulting uric acid nephropathy, allopurinol may be given; keep patient well hydrated.
• Anticoagulants should be used cautiously. Watch closely for signs of bleeding.
• Avoid all I.M. injections when platelet count is low.
• Premedicating with an antiemetic may prevent nausea and vomiting. If vomiting occurs, administer antiemetics p.r.n.
• Patients who have received drugs with strong emetic properties may experience anticipatory nausea and vomiting at subsequent treatments. They may benefit from treatment with an anxiolytic drug.

Information for parents and patient
• Advise parents to have patient avoid exposure to persons with bacterial or viral infections because chemotherapy can increase susceptibility to infection.

Parents should watch for and report any signs of infection promptly.

• Advise parents that patient's dental work should be completed before therapy whenever possible, or delayed until blood counts are normal.

• Stress importance of keeping follow-up appointments for monitoring hematologic status.

• Teach parents and patient to check for signs of bleeding and bruising and report them promptly. Parents may need to restrict child's participation in contact sports. Such activity is dangerous when patient's platelets are low.

• Instruct parents to monitor neutropenic patient's temperature every 4 hours (not rectally) and to report fever, cough, and other signs of infection *promptly.*

• Patient should avoid contact with persons who have received live immunizations (polio, measles/mumps/rubella). Explain importance of promptly reporting susceptible patient's exposure to chicken pox.

• Instruct patient to clean teeth with toothettes, gauze, or soft toothbrush when platelets are low. Patient should perform frequent oral hygiene and should avoid using commercial mouthwashes which may contain alcohol and have an irritating effect. Solutions of sodium bicarbonate or hydrogen peroxide are more appropriate rinses.

• Advise parents that adequate fluid intake is very important to facilitate patient's excretion of uric acid.

• Reassure parents and patient's that hair should grow back after treatment has ended.

• Explain drug's effect on the reproductive system (amenorrhea, delayed spermatogenesis). Sexually active adolescents should practice contraception to avoid potential risk to fetus.

---

medium-chain triglycerides
M.C.T. Oil

• Classification: enteral nutrition supplement

How supplied
Available without prescription
Oil: 960 ml (115 calories/15 ml)

Indications, route, and dosage
Calorie supplementation
Neonates and small infants: 0.5 to 1 ml per feeding, added to formula or appropriate foods.
Older infants: 2 ml per feeding, added to formula or appropriate foods.
Children: Start at 5 ml per feeding, added to formula or appropriate foods, and increase as tolerated.
Adults: 15 ml P.O. t.i.d. or q.i.d. Maximum of 100 ml/day.

Action and kinetics
• *Metabolic action:* Medium-chain triglycerides are indicated as a supplementary fat source when conventional fats are not tolerated. Medium-chain triglycerides are more rapidly hydrolyzed than conventional food fat, require less bile for digestion, are carried by the portal circulation, and are not depen-

dent on chylomicron formation or lymphatic transport. Medium-chain triglycerides are a useful energy source in malabsorption patients but do not provide essential fatty acids.

• *Kinetics in adults:* Medium-chain triglycerides are absorbed by the portal circulation; they are not dependant upon chylomicron formation or lymphatic transport for absorption. As compared to dietary fat, they require less bile acid for digestion. Triglycerides are transported by lipoproteins to storage sites in adipose tissue. They are broken down by lipase to three fatty acids and glycerol. The three fatty acids are used to produce energy through the fatty acid cycle. Excess fat is excreted in feces; ketone bodies may appear in urine.

Contraindications and precautions
Medium-chain triglycerides are contraindicated in patients with advanced hepatic cirrhosis. Large amounts may elevate blood and spinal fluid levels of medium-chain fatty acids because of impaired hepatic clearance. These elevated levels have caused reversible coma and precoma in patients with advanced cirrhosis. Use cautiously in patients with hepatic cirrhosis, encephalopathy, or other precipitating factors.

Interactions
No information available.

Effects on diagnostic tests
None reported.

Adverse reactions
• CNS: reversible coma in susceptible patients with advanced cirrhosis.
• GI: nausea, vomiting, diarrhea, abdominal distention, cramps.

Overdose and treatment
No information available.

▶ Special considerations
• Medium-chaim triglycerides provide 7.7 calories/ml.
• Dosage should not provide more than 60% of total daily calories.
• To minimize GI adverse effects, give smaller doses more frequently with meals, or mixed with salad dressing or chilled fruit juice.
• Use metal, glass, or ceramic containers and utensils. Plastic may soften or break.

Information for parents and patient
• Provide counseling with the dietitian so parents can learn how to incorporate this substance into patient's diet.
• Advise parents to have patient take drug with meals or mix with salad dressing or chilled fruit juice.
• Advise parents to use metal, glass, or ceramic containers when giving drug to patient.

---

medrysone
HMS Liquifilm Ophthalmic

• Classification: ophthalmic anti-inflammatory agent (corticosteroid)

How supplied
Available by prescription only
Suspension: 1%

Indications, route, and dosage
Allergic conjunctivitis, vernal conjunctivitis, episcleritis, ophthalmic epinephrine sensitivity reaction
Children and adults: Instill 1 drop in conjunctival sac b.i.d. to q.i.d. May use q hour during first 1 to 2 days if needed.

Action and kinetics
• *Anti-inflammatory action:* Medrysone, a synthetic corticosteroid, stimulates the synthesis of enzymes needed to decrease the inflammatory response. Conjunctival administration of medrysone effectively reduces local inflammation. Because medrysone has not been proven to be effective in iritis and uveitis, it is not recommended for treatment of these conditions.
• *Kinetics in adults:* After ophthalmic administration, medrysone is absorbed through the aqueous humor. Because of the low doses used, very little drug is absorbed systemically. Medrysone is distributed through the local tissue layers and primarily metabolized locally. Any absorbed drug is distributed rapidly into muscle, liver, skin, intestines, and kidneys. It is metabolized primarily in the liver to inactive compounds. Inactive metabolites are excreted by the kidneys, primarily as glucuronides and sulfates, but also as unconjugated products. Small amounts of the metabolites are also excreted in feces.

Contraindications and precautions
Medrysone is contraindicated in patients who are hypersensitive to any component of the preparation; in patients with fungal infections of the eye; and in patients with acute, untreated purulent bacterial, viral, or fungal ocular infections. It should be used cautiously in patients with corneal abrasions. If a bacterial infection does not respond promptly to appropriate anti-infective therapy, the corticosteroid should be discontinued and another therapy applied.

Intraocular pressure should be measured every 2 to 4 weeks for the first 2 months of ophthalmic corticosteroid therapy and then, if no increase in pressure has occurred, about every 1 to 2 months thereafter.

Interactions
None reported.

Effects on diagnostic tests
None reported.

Adverse reactions
• Eye: transient burning or stinging on administration; mydriasis, ptosis, epithelial punctate keratitis, and corneal or scleral malacia (rare); increased intraocular pressure, thinning of the cornea, interference with corneal wound healing, increased susceptibility to viral or fungal corneal infection, corneal ulceration; glaucoma, cataracts, defects in visual acuity and visual field with (long-term use).
• Systemic: rare, but may occur with excessive doses or long-term use.
  Note: Drug should be discontinued if topical application results in local irritation, infection, significant systemic absorption, or hypersensitivity reaction; if visual acuity decreases or visual field is diminished; or if burning, stinging, or watering of eyes does not quickly resolve after administration.

Overdose and treatment
No information available.

▶ Special considerations
• Because of their greater ratio of skin surface area to body weight, children may be more susceptible than adults to topical corticosteroid-induced hypothalamic-pituitary-adrenal axis suppression and Cushing's syndrome. Although such reactions occur extremely rarely with ophthalmic therapy, it is still advisable to limit corticosteroid therapy in children to the minimum amount necessary for therapeutic efficacy.
• Ophthalmic products may initially cause sensitivity to bright light. This may be minimized by wearing sunglasses.
• Monitor the patient's response by observing the area of inflammation and eliciting patient comments concerning pruritus and vision. Inspect the eye and surrounding tissues for infection and additional irritation.
• Discontinue the drug if the patient develops signs of systemic absorption (including Cushing's syndrome, hyperglycemia, or glucosuria), skin irritation or ulceration, hypersensitivity, or infection (If antivirals or antibiotics are being used with corticosteroids and the infection does not respond immediately, corticosteroids should be stopped until the infection is controlled.)

Information for parents and patient
• Instruct parents to observe for adverse effects. They should call if no improvement occurs after 7 to 8 days; if the condition worsens; or if pain, itching, or swelling of the eye occurs.
• Warn parents to avoid administering any nonprescription opthalmic preparations that have not been specifically recommended. Nonprescription ophthalmic solutions should not be used for more than 7 days in children under age 2.
• Warn parents not to use leftover medication for a new eye inflammation and never to share eye medication with others.
• Parents should call for specific instructions before discontinuing therapy.
Method for administering eye drops
Advise the parents and patient to use the following steps when administering eye drops:
• Wash hands well.

• Shake solution or suspension well.
• Tilt head back or lie down.
• Lightly pull lower eyelid down by applying gentle pressure at the lid base in the bony rim of orbit.
• Approach the eye from below with the dropper, do not touch dropper to any tissue.
• Holding dropper no more than 1" above the eye, drop medication inside lower lid while looking up.
• Try to keep eye open for 30 seconds.
• Apply light finger pressure inward and down to the side of the bridge of the nose (the lacrimal canaliculi) of solution into nasal passages, where more of the drug is absorbed systemically.
• If using more than one drug at the same time, wait at least 5 minutes before applying the second drug.

Method for administering ophthalmic ointments
• Advise the parents and patient to use the following steps when administering ophthalmic ointments:
• Wash hands well. Hold the tube in your hand several minutes before use to warm it and impove flow of ointment.
• When opening the ointment tube for the first time, squeeze out the first ¼" of ointment and discard (using sterile gauze) because it may be too dry.
• Apply a small "ribbon" or strip of ointment (¼" to ½") to the inside of the lower eyelid. Do not touch any part of the eye with the tip of the tube. Close the eye gently and roll the eyeball in all directions to spread the ointment.
• If using a second eye ointment, wait at least 10 minutes before applying it.

---

melphalan (phenylalanine mustard)
Alkeran

• Classification: antineoplastic (alkylating agent [cell cycle-phase nonspecific)]

How supplied
Available by prescription only
Tablets: 2 mg

Indications, route, and dosage
Dosage and indications may vary. Check current literature for recommended dosage.
Multiple myeloma, †ovarian carcinoma, †malignant melanoma, †testicular seminoma, †non-Hodgkin's lymphoma, †osteogenic sarcoma, †breast cancer
Children over age 12 and adults: 0.15 mg/kg/day P.O. for 7 days, followed by a 3-week rest period. When leukocyte counts begin to rise, give maintenance dose of 50 mcg/kg. Alternatively, 100 to 500 mcg/kg/day P.O. for 2 to 3 weeks or 250 mcg/kg/day for 4 days, followed by a 2- to 4-week rest period. When leukocyte counts begin to rise above 3,000/mm³ and platelet counts are greater than 100,000/mm³, give maintenance dose of 2 to 4 mg/day. Or 250 mcg/kg/day P.O. or 7 mg/m²/day P.O. for 5 days every 5 to 6 weeks. Adjust dose to maintain mild leukopenia and thrombocytopenia.

Nonresectable advanced ovarian cancer
Adults: 200 mcg/kg/day P.O. for 5 days, repeated q 4 to 6 weeks if blood counts return to normal.

Action and kinetics
• *Antineoplastic action:* Melphalan exerts its cytotoxic activity by forming cross-links of strands of DNA and RNA and inhibiting protein synthesis.
• *Kinetics in adults:* The absorption of melphalan from the GI tract is incomplete and variable. One study found that absorption ranged from 25% to 89% after an oral dose of 0.6 mg/kg. Melphalan distributes rapidly and widely into total body water. The drug initially is 50% to 60% bound to plasma proteins and eventually increases to 80% to 90% over time. Melphalan is extensively deactivated by the process of hydrolysis. The elimination of melphalan has been described as biphasic, with an initial half-life of 8 minutes and a terminal half-life of 2 hours. Melphalan and its metabolites are excreted primarily in urine, with 10% of an oral dose excreted as unchanged drug.

Contraindications and precautions
Melphalan is contraindicated in patients with a history of hypersensitivity to the drug or resistance to previous therapy with it. A cross-sensitivity, which manifests as a rash, may occur between melphalan and chlorambucil.
Drug should be used with caution in patients with hematologic compromise or recent exposure to cytotoxic or radiation therapy because of the drug's myelosuppressive effects; and in patients with renal dysfunction because accumulation and excessive toxicity may occur.

Interactions
No clinically significant drug interactions have been reported with melphalan.

Effects on diagnostic tests
Melphalan therapy may increase blood and urine levels of uric acid.

Adverse reactions
• DERM: dermatitis.
• GI: mild nausea and vomiting, diarrhea, stomatitis.
• HEMA: *bone marrow depression* (dose-limiting); *leukopenia, thrombocytopenia, agranulocytosis;* acute nonlymphocytic leukemia may develop with chronic use.
• Other: alopecia, pneumonitis, *pulmonary fibrosis.*
Note: Drug should be discontinued at the first signs of bone marrow depression.

Overdose and treatment
Clinical manifestations of overdose include myelosuppression and hypocalcemia.
Treatment is usually supportive and includes transfusion of blood components.

▶ Special considerations
• Attempt to alleviate or reduce anxiety in parents and patient and family before treatment.
• Monitor BUN, hematocrit, platelet count, ALT

(SGPT), AST (SGOT), LDH, serum bilirubin, serum creatinine, uric acid total and differential leukocyte.
• Oral dose may be taken all at one time.
• Administer melphalan with meals to minimize nausea and vomiting.
• Premedicating with an antiemetic may prevent nausea and vomiting. If vomiting occurs, administer antiemetics p.r.n.
• Patients who have received drugs with strong emetic properties may experience anticipatory nausea and vomiting at subsequent treatments. They may benefit from treatment with an anxiolytic drug.
• Frequent hematologic monitoring, including a CBC, is necessary for accurate dosage adjustments and prevention of toxicity.
• Discontinue therapy temporarily or reduce dosage if leukocyte count falls below 3,000/mm³ or platelet count falls below 100,000/mm³.
• Avoid I.M. injections when platelet count is below 100,000/mm³.
• Anticoagulants, aspirin, and aspirin-containing products should be used cautiously.

Information for parents and patient
• Advise parents to have patient avoid exposure to persons with bacterial or viral infections because chemotherapy can increase susceptibility to infection. Parents should watch for and report any signs of infection promptly.
• Advise parents that patient should complete dental work before therapy whenever possible, or delay it until blood counts are normal.
• Advise parents that immunizations should be postponed during therapy if possible.
• Tell parents and patient that it is vital to continue drug despite nausea and vomiting. Parents should call immediately if vomiting occurs shortly after taking a dose.
• Explain that adequate fluid intake is important to facilitate excretion of uric acid.
• Reassure parents and patient that hair should grow back after treatment has ended.
• Warn parents that patient may bruise easily because of drug's effect on blood count.
• Teach parents and patient to check for signs of bleeding and bruising. Parents may need to restrict child's participation in contact sports. Such activity is dangerous when patient's platelets are low.
• Stress importance of keeping follow-up appointments for monitoring hematologic status.
• Instruct parents to monitor neutropenic patient's temperature every 4 hours (not rectally) and to report fever, cough, and other signs of infection *promptly*.
• Patient should avoid contact with persons who have received live virus immunizations (polio, measles/mumps/rubella). Explain importance of promptly reporting susceptible patient's exposure to chicken pox.
• Instruct patient to clean teeth with toothettes, gauze, or soft toothbrush when platelets are low. Patient should perform frequent oral hygiene and should avoid using commercial mouthwashes which may contain alcohol and have an irritating effect. Solutions of sodium bicarbonate or hydrogen peroxide are more appropriate rinses.
• Instruct patient to avoid foods that are spicy and

extremely hot or cold. Topical anesthetics administered before meals (swish and spit) may relieve mouth discomfort.
• Inform adolescents that they may develop amenorrhea. Emphasize to sexually active adolescents the importance of continuing effective contraception.

meperidine hydrochloride (pethidine hydrochloride)
Demerol

• Classification: analgesic, adjunct to anesthesia (opioid)
• Controlled substance schedule II

How supplied
Available by prescription only
Tablets: 50 mg, 100 mg
Liquid: 50 mg/ml
Injection: 10 mg/ml, 25 mg/ml, 50 mg/ml, 75 mg/ml, 100 mg/ml

Indications, route, and dosage
Moderate to severe pain
Children: 1.1. to 1.8 mg/kg P.O., I.M., or S.C. q 4 to 6 hours or 175 mg/m² daily in 6 divided doses. Maximum single dose for children should not exceed 100 mg. May also be given I.V. by slow intermittent or continuous infusion.
Adults: 50 to 150 mg P.O., I.M., or S.C. q 3 to 4 hours. Continuous I.V. infusion: 15 to 35 mg/hour p.r.n. or around the clock. May also be given I.V. by slow intermittent or continuous infusion.
Preoperatively
Children: 1 to 2.2 mg/kg I.M. or S.C. 30 to 90 minutes before surgery. Do not exceed adult dose.
Adults: 50 to 100 mg I.M. or S.C. 30 to 90 minutes before surgery. Do not exceed adult dose.

Action and kinetics
• *Analgesic action:* Meperidine is a narcotic agonist with actions and potency similar to those of morphine, with principle actions at the opiate receptors. It is recommended for the relief of moderate to severe pain.
• *Kinetics in adults:* Meperidine given orally is only half as effective as it is parenterally. Onset of analgesia occurs within 10 to 45 minutes. Duration of action is 2 to 4 hours.
  Meperidine is distributed widely throughout the body and is metabolized primarily by hydrolysis in the liver. About 30% of a dose of meperidine is excreted in the urine as the N-demethylated derivative; about 5% is excreted unchanged. Excretion is enhanced by acidifying the urine.

Contraindications and precautions
Meperidine is contraindicated in patients with known hypersensitivity to the drug or any phenylpiperidine opioid (meperidine or its analogs).
  Administer meperidine with extreme caution to patients with supraventricular dysrhythmias; avoid, or administer drug with extreme caution to patients with

head injury or increased intracranial pressure, because drug obscures neurologic parameters; and during pregnancy and labor, because drug readily crosses placenta (premature infants are especially sensitive to respiratory and CNS depressant effects of narcotic agonists). Administer meperidine cautiously to patients with renal or hepatic dysfunction, because drug accumulation or prolonged duration of action may occur; to patients with pulmonary disease (asthma, chronic obstructive pulmonary disease), because drug depresses respiration and suppresses cough reflex; to patients undergoing biliary tract surgery, because drug may cause biliary spasm; to patients with convulsive disorders, because drug may precipitate seizures; in debilitated patients, who are more sensitive to both therapeutic and adverse drug effects; and to patients prone to physical or psychic addiction, because of the high risk of addiction to this drug.

Meperidine has atropine-like effects. Administer cautiously to patients with glaucoma.

Interactions

Concomitant use with other CNS depressants (narcotic analgesics, general anesthetics, antihistamines, phenothiazines, barbiturates, benzodiazepines, sedative-hypnotics, tricyclic antidepressants, alcohol, and muscle relaxants) potentiates drug's respiratory and CNS depression, sedation and hypotensive effects. Concomitant use with cimetidine may also increase respiratory and CNS depression, causing confusion, disorientation, apnea, or seizures; such use requires reduced dosage of meperidine.

Drug accumulation and enhanced effects may result from concomitant use with other drugs that are extensively metabolized in the liver (rifampin, phenytoin, and digitoxin); combined use with anticholinergics may cause paralytic ileus.

Patients who become physically dependent on this drug may experience acute withdrawal syndrome if given a narcotic antagonist.

Severe cardiovascular depression may result from concomitant use with general anesthetics; meperidine can potentiate the adverse effects of isoniazid.

Concomitant use with monoamine oxidase (MAO) inhibitors may precipitate unpredictable and occasionally fatal reactions, even in patients who may receive MAO inhibitors within 14 days of receiving meperidine. Some reactions have been characterized by coma, respiratory depression, cyanosis, and hypotension; in others, hyperexcitability, convulsions, tachycardia, hyperpyrexia, and hypertension have occurred.

Effects on diagnostic tests

Meperidine increases plasma amylase or lipase levels through increased biliary tract pressure; levels may be unreliable for 24 hours after meperidine administration.

Adverse reactions

• CNS: *sedation, somnolence, clouded sensorium,* lightheadedness, dizziness, paradoxical excitement, euphoria, insomnia, agitation, confusion, headache, tremor, miosis, seizures, *psychic dependence,* convulsions (at high doses); inadvertent injection about a nerve trunk may result in sensory-motor paralysis which is usually but not always temporary.
• CV: *tachycardia, asystole, bradycardia,* palpitations, *hypotension,* syncope.
• DERM: sweating, flushing, *urticaria, rash, pruritus, pain at injection site,* local irritation and induration after subcutaneous injection (especially when repeated).
• GI: dry mouth, anorexia, *biliary spasms (colic),* ileus, nausea, vomiting, *constipation.*
• GU: urinary retention or hesitancy.
• Other: *respiratory depression, phlebitis.*
Note: Drug should be discontinued if hypersensitivity, seizures, or cardiac dysrhythmias occur.

Overdose and treatment

The most common signs and symptoms of meperidine overdose are CNS depression, respiratory depression, skeletal muscle flaccidity, cold and clammy skin, mydriasis, bradycardia, and hypotension. Other acute toxic effects include hypothermia, shock, apnea, cardiopulmonary arrest, circulatory collapse, pulmonary edema, and convulsions.

To treat acute overdose, first establish adequate respiratory exchange via a patent airway and ventilation as needed; administer a narcotic antagonist (naloxone) to reverse respiratory depression. (Because the duration of action of meperidine is longer than that of naloxone, repeated dosing is necessary.) Naloxone should not be given unless the patient has clinically significant respiratory or cardiovascular depression. Monitor vital signs closely.

If the patient presents within 2 hours of ingestion of an oral overdose, empty the stomach immediately by inducing emesis (ipecac syrup) or using gastric lavage. Use caution to avoid any risk of aspiration. Administer activated charcoal via nasogastric tube for further removal of meperidine, and acidify urine to help remove meperidine.

Provide symptomatic and supportive treatment (continued respiratory support, correction of fluid or electrolyte imbalance). Monitor laboratory parameters, vital signs, and neurologic status closely.

▶ Special considerations

• Meperidine should not be administered to infants under age 6 months.
• Administer with extreme caution to patients with head injury, increased intracranial pressure, seizures, asthma, chronic obstructive pulmonary disease, alcoholism, severe hepatic or renal disease, acute abdominal conditions, cardiac dysrhythmias, hypovolemia, or psychiatric disorders, and to debilitated patients. Reduced doses may be necessary.
• Consider possible interactions with other drugs the patient is taking.
• Keep resuscitative equipment and a narcotic antagonist (naloxone) available. Be prepared to provide support of ventilation and gastric lavage.
• Parenteral administration of opiates provides better analgesia than oral administration. Intravenous administration should be given by slow injection, preferably in diluted solution. Rapid I.V. injection increases the incidence of adverse effects.
• Parenteral injections by I.M. or S.C. route should be

given cautiously to patients who are chilled, hypovolemic, or in shock, because decreased perfusion may
lead to accumulation of the drug and toxic effects.
Rotate I.M. or S.C. injection sites to avoid induration.
• Before administration, visually inspect all parenteral products for particulate matter and discoloration.
• A regular dosage schedule (rather than "p.r.n. pain")
is preferred to alleviate the symptoms and anxiety
that accompany pain.
• The duration of respiratory depression may be longer
than the analgesic effect. Monitor the patient closely
with repeated dosing.
• With chronic administration, evaluate the patient's
respiratory status before each dose. Because severe
respiratory depression may occur (especially with accumulation from chronic dosing), watch for respiratory
rate below the patient's baseline level. Evaluate the
patient for restlessness, which may be a sign of compensatory response for hypoxia.
• Opiates or agonist-antagonists may cause orthostatic hypotension in ambulatory patients. Have the
patient sit or lie down to relieve dizziness or fainting.
• Since opiates depress respiration when they are used
postoperatively, encourage patient turning, coughing,
and deep-breathing to avoid atelectases.
• If gastric irritation occurs, give oral products with
food; food delays absorption and onset of analgesia.
• Opiates may obscure the signs and symptoms of an
acute abdominal condition or worsen gallbladder pain.
• The antitussive activity of opiates is used to control
persistent, exhausting cough or dry, non-productive
cough.
• The first sign of tolerance to the therapeutic effect
of opioid agonists or agonist-antagonists is usually a
shortened duration of effect.
• Meperidine may be administered to some patients
who are allergic to morphine.
• Meperidine and its active metabolite normeperidine
accumulate. This metabolite can cause seizures in
patients with poor renal function and in patients who
are receiving high dosage. Monitor for toxic effects.
• Because meperidine toxicity commonly appears after several days of treatment, this drug is not recommended for treatment of chronic pain.
• Meperidine may be given slow I.V., preferably as a
diluted solution. S.C. injection is very painful. During
I.V. administration, tachycardia may occur, possibly
as a result of the drug's atropine-like effects.
• Oral dose is less than half as effective as parenteral
dose. Give I.M. if possible. When changing from parenteral to oral route, dosage should be increased.
• Syrup has local anesthetic effect. Give with water.
• Alternating meperidine with a peripherally active
non-narcotic analgesic (aspirin, acetaminophen,
NSAIDs) may improve pain control while allowing
lower narcotic dosages. Also, utilize comfort measures to decrease pain stimuli.
• Injectable meperidine is compatible with saline and
dextrose 5% solutions and their combinations, and
with lactated Ringer's and sodium lactate solution.

Information for parents and patient
• Drug may produce drowsiness and sedation. Tell
parents to have patient use drug with caution and to

avoid hazardous activities that require full alertness
and coordination.
• Tell parents that patient should avoid ingestion of
alcoholic beverages or cough and cold preparations
containing alcohol when taking drug, because it will
cause additive CNS depression.
• Explain that constipation may result from taking
drug. Suggest measures to increase dietary fiber content, or recommend a stool softener.
• If patient's condition allows, instruct patient to
breathe deeply, cough, and change position every 2
hours to avoid respiratory complications.
• Patient should void at least every 4 hours to prevent
urinary retention.
• Tell the parents to have the patient take the medication as prescribed and to call the physician if significant adverse effects occur.
• Parents should not increase dosage if patient is not
experiencing the desired effect, but call for prescribed
dosage adjustment.
• Instruct the parents not to double the dose. Tell
them to have patient take a missed dose as soon as
he remembers unless it's almost time for the next
dose. If this is so, the patient should skip the missed
dose and go back to the regular dosage schedule.
• Tell the parents to call the physician immediately
for emergency help if they think the patient or someone
else has taken an overdose.
• Explain the signs of overdose to the parents and the
patient.

mephenytoin
Mesantoin

• Classification: anticonvulsant (hydantoin derivative)

How supplied
Available by prescription only
Tablets: 100 mg

Indications, route, and dosage
*Generalized tonic-clonic (grand mal) or com-
plex-partial (psychomotor) seizures*
Children: Initial dosage is 50 to 100 mg P.O. daily
(3 to 15 mg/kg/day or 100 to 450 mg/m²) in three
divided doses. May increase slowly by 50 to 100 mg
at weekly intervals up to 200 mg P.O. t.i.d., divided
q 8 hours. Dosage must be adjusted individually. Usual
maintenance dosage in children is 100 to 400 mg/day
divided q 8 hours.
Adults: 50 to 100 mg P.O. daily; may increase by 50
to 100 mg at weekly intervals, up to 200 mg P.O. q
8 hours. Dosages up to 800 mg/day may be required.

Action and kinetics
• *Anticonvulsant action:* Like other hydantoin derivatives, mephenytoin stabilizes the neuronal membranes and limits seizure activity either by increasing
efflux or by decreasing influx of sodium ions across
cell membranes in the motor cortex during generation

of nerve impulses. Like phenytoin, mephenytoin appears to have antiarrhythmic effects.

Mephenytoin is used for prophylaxis of tonic-clonic (grand mal), psychomotor, focal, and jacksonian-type partial seizures in patients refractory to less toxic agents. It usually is combined with phenytoin, phenobarbital, or primidone; phenytoin is preferred because it causes less sedation than barbiturates. Mephenytoin also is used with succinimides to control combined absence and tonic-clonic disorders; combined use with oxazolidines is not recommended because of the increased hazard of blood dyscrasias.

• *Kinetics in adults:* Mephenytoin is absorbed from the GI tract. Onset of action occurs in 30 minutes and persists for 24 to 48 hours.

Mephenytoin is distributed widely throughout the body; good seizure control without toxicity occurs when serum concentrations of drug and major metabolite reach 25 to 40 mcg/ml.

Mephenytoin is metabolized by the liver. Mephenytoin is excreted in urine.

Contraindications and precautions

Mephenytoin is contraindicated in patients with hypersensitivity to hydantoins. It should be used with caution, and patients should be monitored carefully for toxic reactions, including potentially fatal blood dyscrasias and mucocutaneous syndromes. Such reactions have occurred within 2 weeks to 2 years after initiation of therapy.

Interactions

Mephenytoin's therapeutic effects and toxicity may be increased by concomitant use with oral anticoagulants, antihistamines, chloramphenicol, cimetidine, diazepam, diazoxide, disulfiram, isoniazid, phenylbutazone, salicylates, sulfamethizole, or valproate. Mephenytoin's therapeutic effects may be decreased by concomitant use of alcohol or folic acid. Mephenytoin may decrease the effects of oral contraceptives.

Effects on diagnostic tests

Mephenytoin may elevate liver function test results.

Adverse reactions

• CNS: ataxia, drowsiness, fatigue, irritability, choreiform movements, depression, tremor, sleeplessness, dizziness, (usually transient).
• DERM: rashes, exfoliative dermatitis.
• EENT: photophobia, conjunctivitis, diplopia, nystagmus.
• GI: gingival hyperplasia, nausea and vomiting
• HEMA: leukopenia, neutropenia, agranulocytosis, thrombocytopenia, pancytopenia, eosinophilia.
• Other: alopecia, weight gain.
   Note: Drug should be discontinued if signs of hypersensitivity or hepatotoxicity occur; if neutrophil count decreases by 1,600 to 2,500/mm³ or other signs of hematological abnormalities occur; or if lymphadenopathy or rash occurs.

Overdose and treatment

Signs of acute mephenytoin toxicity may include restlessness, dizziness, drowsiness, nausea, vomiting, nystagmus, ataxia, dysarthria, tremor, and slurred speech; hypotension, respiratory depression, and coma may follow. Death may result from respiratory and circulatory depression.

Treat overdose with gastric lavage or emesis and follow with supportive treatment. Carefully monitor vital signs and fluid and electrolyte balance. Forced diuresis is of little or no value. Hemodialysis or peritoneal dialysis may be helpful.

▶ Special considerations

• Use of mephenytoin is reserved for pediatric patients who have not responded to less toxic anticonvulsants.
• Children usually require from 100 to 400 mg/day.
• Monitor baseline liver function and hematologic laboratory studies and repeat at monthly intervals.
• Observe patient closely during therapy for possible adverse effects, especially at start of therapy. Hydantoins may cause gingival hyperplasia; good oral hygiene and gum care are essential to minimize effects.
• Drug interactions are frequently a problem, primarily with hepatically cleared drugs, such as chloramphenicol, digitoxin, isoniazid, and griseofulvin; be especially alert for toxic symptoms or breakthrough seizures in patients taking any of these drugs.
• Carefully follow manufacturer's directions for reconstitution, storage, and administration of all preparations.
• Decreased alertness and coordination are most pronounced at start of treatment. Patient may need help with walking and other activities for first few days.
• Drug should not be discontinued abruptly. Transition from mephenytoin to other anticonvulsant drug should progress over 6 weeks.

Information for parents and patient

• Tell parents that patients should avoid alcohol-containing beverages or medications (elixirs) while taking drug, as it may decrease drug's effectiveness and may increase CNS adverse reactions.
• Advise parents that patient should avoid hazardous tasks that require mental alertness until degree of CNS sedative effect is determined.
• Tell parents and patient to take oral drug with food if GI distress occurs.
• Teach parents signs and symptoms of hypersensitivity, liver dysfunction, and blood dyscrasias and to call at once if any of the following occurs: sore throat, fever, bleeding, easy bruising, or rash.
• Explain to patient and her parents the importance of reporting suspected pregnancy immediately.
• Warn parents that patient should never discontinue drug suddenly or without medical supervision.
• Encourage parents to have patient wear a Medic Alert bracelet or necklace, indicating drug taken and seizure disorders, while taking anticonvulsants.
• Caution parents to consult pharmacist before changing brand or using generic drug; therapeutic effect may change.
• Explain that drug may increase gum growth and sensitivity (gingival hyperplasia); teach proper oral hygiene and urge parent or patient to establish good mouth care.
• Assure parents and patient that pink or reddish brown discoloration of urine is normal and harmless.

• Explain that follow-up laboratory tests are essential for safe use.

---

mephobarbital
Mebaral, Mentaban, Mephoral

• Classification: anticonvulsant, nonspecific CNS depressant (barbiturate)
• Controlled substance schedule IV

How supplied
Available by prescription only
Tablets: 32 mg, 50 mg, 100 mg

Indications, route, and dosage
Generalized tonic-clonic (grand mal) or absence (petit mal) seizures
Children: 6 to 12 mg/kg P.O. daily, divided q 6 to 8 hours (smaller doses are given initially and increased over 4 to 5 days as needed).
Adults: 400 to 600 mg P.O. daily or in divided doses.

Action and kinetics
• *Anticonvulsant action:* Mephobarbital increases seizure threshold in the motor cortex. It is indicated to treat generalized tonic-clonic (grand mal), absence (petit mal), myoclonic, and mixed-type seizures and, as a sedative, to relieve anxiety and tension. It is used chiefly to replace phenobarbital when less sedation is needed (no data support this rationale) and in children with hyperexcitability states or other mood disturbances.
• *Kinetics in adults:* About 50% of an oral dose of mephobarbital is absorbed from the GI tract; action begins within 30 to 60 minutes and lasts 10 to 16 hours.
Mephobarbital is distributed widely throughout the body.
Mephobarbital is metabolized by the liver to phenobarbital; about 75% of a given dose is converted in 24 hours. Therapeutic blood levels of phenobarbital are 15 to 40 mcg/ml.
Mephobarbital is excreted primarily in urine; small amounts are excreted in breast milk.

Contraindications and precautions
Mephobarbital is contraindicated in patients with known hypersensitivity to barbiturates; in suspected pregnancy and pregnancy near term because of the hazard of respiratory depression and neonatal coagulation defects; in patients with severe respiratory disease or status asthmaticus because it may cause respiratory depression; or in patients with a history of porphyria or marked hepatic impairment because it may exacerbate porphyria. Drug should be used with caution in patients taking alcohol, CNS depressants, monoamine oxidase (MAO) inhibitors, narcotic analgesics, or anticoagulants.

Interactions
Alcohol and other CNS depressants, including narcotic analgesics, cause excessive depression in patients taking mephobarbital. Although concrete data are lacking, mephobarbital is assumed to be an enzyme inducer (like phenobarbital); therefore all cautions for phenobarbital drug interactions apply. Barbiturates can induce hepatic metabolism of oral anticoagulants, combination oral contraceptives, and doxycycline. Concomitant use with MAO inhibitors potentiates CNS depressant effects of barbiturates; rifampin may decrease barbiturate levels and thereby decrease efficacy.

Effects on diagnostic tests
Mephobarbital may elevate liver function test results.

Adverse reactions
• CNS: dizziness, headache, hangover, confusion, paradoxical excitation, exacerbation of existing pain, drowsiness, nightmares, hallucinations.
• CV: hypotension.
• DERM: urticaria, morbilliform rash, blisters, purpura, erythema multiforme, Stevens-Johnson syndrome.
• GI: nausea, vomiting, epigastric pain, constipation.
• HEMA: megaloblastic anemia, agranulocytosis, thrombocytopenia.
• Other: allergic reactions (facial edema).
Note: Drug should be discontinued if signs of hypersensitivity or hepatic dysfunction occur.

Overdose and treatment
Symptoms of acute overdose include CNS and respiratory depression, areflexia, oliguria, tachycardia, hypotension, hypothermia, and coma. Shock may occur. In massive overdose, ECG may be flat, even if patient is not clinically dead.
Treat overdose symptomatically and supportively: in conscious patient with intact gag reflex, induce emesis with ipecac; follow in 30 minutes with repeated doses of activated charcoal. Forced diuresis and alkalinization of urine may hasten excretion. Hemodialysis may be necessary. Monitor vital signs and fluid and electrolyte balance.

▶ Special considerations
• Mephobarbital is not recommended for children under age 6.
• Premature infants are more susceptible to the depressant effects of barbiturates because of immature hepatic metabolism. Children receiving barbiturates may experience hyperactivity, excitement, or hyperalgia.
• Dosage of barbiturates must be individualized for each patient, because different rates of metabolism and enzyme induction occur.
• Assess level of consciousness before and frequently during therapy to evaluate effectiveness of drug. Monitor neurologic status for possible alterations or deteriorations. Monitor seizure character, frequency, and duration for changes. Institute seizure precautions, as necessary.
• Assess patient's sleeping patterns before and during therapy to ensure effectiveness of drug.
• Institute safety measures—side rails, assistance when out of bed, call light within reach—to prevent falls and injury.

---

‡May contain sulfites ◆May contain tartrazine ◆◆May contain benzyl alcohol

• Anticipate possible rebound confusion and excitatory reactions in patient.
• Assess bowel elimination patterns; monitor for complaints of constipation. Advise diet high in fiber, if indicated.
• Monitor prothrombin time carefully in patients taking anticoagulants; dosage of anticoagulant may require adjustment to counteract possible interaction.
• Observe patient to prevent hoarding or self-dosing, especially in depressed or suicidal patients, or those who are or have a history of being drug-dependent.
• Death is common with an overdose of 2 to 10 g; it may occur at much smaller doses if alcohol is also ingested.
• Avoid administering mephobarbital to patients with status asthmaticus.
• Monitor for signs of bleeding if patient is on stable anticoagulant regimen.
• Do not withdraw drug abruptly; after long-term use, lower dosage gradually.
• Mephobarbital impairs ability to perform tasks requiring mental alertness.

Information for parents and patient

• Warn parents that patient should avoid concurrent use of other drugs with CNS depressant effects, such as antihistamines, analgesics, and alcohol, because they will have additive effects and result in increased drowsiness. They should seek medical approval before giving patient any nonprescription cold or allergy preparations.
• Caution parents and patient not to increase or decrease dose or frequency without medical approval; abrupt discontinuation of medication may trigger rebound insomnia, with increased dreaming, nightmares, or seizures.
• Advise parents that patient should avoid hazardous tasks that require alertness while taking drug.
• Be sure parents and patient understand that mephobarbital can cause physical or psychological dependence (addiction), and that these effects may be transmitted to the fetus; withdrawal symptoms can occur in neonates whose mothers took barbiturates in the third trimester.
• Instruct parents to report any skin eruption or other marked adverse effect.
• Explain that a morning hangover is common after therapeutic use of barbiturates.
• Teach parents and patient how to recognize signs and symptoms of adverse reactions and what to do if they occur.
• Explain to sexually active adolescents that mephobarbital may render oral contraceptives ineffective and advise different birth control method.

meprobamate
Apo-Meprobomate*, Equanil, Meditran*, Meprospan, Miltown, Neo-Tran*, Neuramate, Neurate, Novomepro*, Sedabamate, SK-Bamate, Tranmep

• Classification: antianxiety agent (carbamate)
• Controlled substance schedule IV

How supplied
Available by prescription only
Tablets: 200 mg, 400 mg, 600 mg
Capsules: 200 mg, 400 mg
Capsules (sustained-release): 200 mg, 400 mg

Indications, route, and dosage
Anxiety and tension
Children age 6 to 12: 100 to 200 mg P.O. b.i.d. or t.i.d.; or 25 mg/kg/day in two or three divided doses. Not recommended for children under age 6.
Adults: 1.2 to 1.6 g P.O. in three or four equally divided doses. Maximum dosage is 2.4 g daily.

Action and kinetics
• *Anxiolytic action:* While the cellular mechanism of meprobamate is unknown, the drug causes nonselective CNS depression similar to that seen with use of barbiturates. Meprobamate acts at multiple sites in the CNS, including the thalamus, hypothalamus, limbic system, and spinal cord, but not the medulla or reticular activating system.
• *Kinetics in adults:* After oral administration, meprobamate is well absorbed; peak serum levels occur in 1 to 3 hours. Sedation usually occurs within 1 hour.
Meprobamate is distributed throughout the body; 20% is protein-bound. The drug occurs in breast milk at two to four times the serum concentration; meprobamate crosses the placenta.
Meprobamate is metabolized rapidly in the liver to inactive glucuronide conjugates.
The metabolites of meprobamate and 10% to 20% of a single dose as unchanged drug are excreted in urine.

Contraindications and precautions
Meprobamate is contraindicated in patients with known hypersensitivity to the drug or other carbamates and in patients with intermittent porphyria. Some formulations contain tartrazine, which is contraindicated in patients allergic to aspirin (because significant cross-reactivity has been demonstrated).
Meprobamate should be used cautiously in patients with impaired renal or hepatic function; and in patients with depression, suicidal tendencies, or a history of drug abuse or addiction.
Meprobamate may precipitate seizures or lower seizure threshold. Use cautiously, if at all, in patients with a history of seizures or an active seizure disorder.

Interactions

Meprobamate may add to or potentiate the effects of alcohol, barbiturates, antihistamines, tranquilizers, narcotics, or other CNS depressants.

Effects on diagnostic tests

Meprobamate therapy may falsely elevate urinary 17-ketosteroids, 17-ketogenic steroids (as determined by the Zimmerman reaction), and 17-hydroxycorticosteroid levels (as determined by the Glenn-Nelson technique).

Adverse reactions

• CNS: dizziness, drowsiness, ataxia, slurred speech, headache, vertigo, weakness, euphoria, paradoxical excitation.
• CV: palpitations, dysrhythmias, syncope, hypotension, tachycardia.
• DERM: pruritus, urticaria, dermatitis, erythematous maculopapular rash, exfoliative dermatitis, erythema multiforme.
• EENT: blurred vision.
• GI: anorexia, nausea, vomiting, diarrhea, stomatitis.
• HEMA: agranulocytosis, thrombocytopenic purpura, aplastic anemia, pancytopenia (rare).
• Other: hypersensitivity (eosinophilia, hyperpyrexia, chills, bronchospasm, angioedema, Stevens-Johnson syndrome, anaphylaxis).
  Note: Drug should be discontinued if hypersensitivity, paradoxical excitation with EEG changes, severe prolonged hypotension, skin rash, sore throat, or unusual bleeding or bruising occurs.

Overdose and treatment

Clinical manifestations of overdose include drowsiness, lethargy, ataxia, coma, hypotension, shock, and respiratory depression.

Treatment of overdose is supportive and symptomatic including maintaining adequate ventilation and a patent airway, with mechanical ventilation if needed.

Treat hypotension with fluids and vasopressors as needed. Empty gastric contents by emesis or lavage if ingestion was recent, followed by activated charcoal and a cathartic. Treat seizures with parenteral diazepam. Peritoneal and hemodialysis may effectively remove the drug. Serum levels greater than 100 mcg/ml may be fatal.

Contact local or regional poison control center for further information.

▶ Special considerations

• Safety has not been established in children under age 6. This drug is rarely used in children.
• Assess level of consciousness and vital signs frequently.
• Impose safety precautions, such as raised side rails.
• Periodic evaluation of complete blood count is recommended during long-term therapy.
• The possibility of abuse and addiction exists.
• Withdraw drug gradually; otherwise, withdrawal symptoms may occur if patient has been taking the drug for a long time.

Information for parents and patient

• Tell parents that patient should avoid other CNS depressants, such as antihistamines, narcotics, and tranquilizers and any ingestion of alcohol while taking this drug, unless prescribed.
• Advise parents not to increase the dose or frequency and not to abruptly discontinue or decrease the dose unless prescribed.
• Tell parents that patient should avoid tasks that require mental alertness or physical coordination until the drug's CNS effects are known.
• Advise parents and patient that sugarless candy or gum, or ice chips can help relieve dry mouth.
• Advise parents to report any sore throat, fever, or unusual bleeding or bruising.
• Advise parents of the potential for physical or psychological dependence with chronic use.

---

mercaptopurine (6-MP)
Purinethol

• Classification: antineoplastic (antimetabolite [cell cycle-phase specific, S phase])

How supplied

Available by prescription only
Tablets: 50 mg

Indications, route, and dosage

Dosage and indications may vary. Check current literature for recommended protocols.
Acute lymphoblastic leukemia (in children), acute myeloblastic leukemia, chronic myelocytic leukemia
Children age 5 and over: 1.5 mg/kg or 75 mg/m² P.O. daily. Maintenance dosage is 1.5 to 2.5 mg/kg daily.
Adults: 2.5 mg/kg or 80 to 100 mg/m² P.O. daily as a single dose, up to 5 mg/kg daily. Maintenance dosage is 1.5 to 2.5 mg/kg daily.

Action and kinetics

• *Antineoplastic action:* Mercaptopurine is converted intracellularly to its active form, which exerts its cytotoxic antimetabolic effects by competing for an enzyme required for purine synthesis. This results in inhibition of DNA and RNA synthesis. Cross-resistance exists between mercaptopurine and thioguanine.
• *Kinetics in adults:* The absorption of mercaptopurine after an oral dose is incomplete and variable; approximately 50% of a dose is absorbed. Peak serum levels occur 2 hours after a dose. Mercaptopurine distributes widely into total body water. The drug crosses the blood-brain barrier, but the cerebrospinal fluid concentration is too low for treatment of meningeal leukemias. Mercaptopurine is extensively metabolized in the liver. The drug appears to undergo extensive first-pass metabolism, contributing to its low bioavailability. Mercaptopurine and its metabolites are excreted in urine.

---

‡May contain sulfites   ◆May contain tartrazine   ◆◆May contain benzyl alcohol

Contraindications and precautions

Mercaptopurine is contraindicated in patients whose disease has shown resistance to therapy with this drug.

Interactions

When used concomitantly, allopurinol, at doses of 300 to 600 mg/day, increases the toxic effects of mercaptopurine, especially myelosuppression. This interaction is due to the inhibition of mercaptopurine metabolism by allopurinol. Reduce dosage of mercaptopurine by 25% to 30% when administering concomitantly with allopurinol.

Concomitant use with mercaptopurine decreases the anticoagulant activity of warfarin. The mechanism of this interaction is unknown.

Mercaptopurine should be used cautiously with other hepatotoxic drugs because of the increased potential for hepatotoxicity.

Effects on diagnostic tests

Mercaptopurine therapy may also cause falsely elevated serum glucose and uric acid values when sequential multiple analyzer is used.

Adverse reactions

• GI: *nausea, vomiting,* and anorexia in 25% of patients; *oral and intestinal ulcers, diarrhea.*
• HEMA: *bone marrow depression* (dose-limiting), decreased RBC count, leukopenia, *thrombocytopenia,* anemia (all may persist several days after drug is stopped).
• Hepatic: jaundice, *cholestatsis, hepatic necrosis.*
• Metabolic: hyperuricemia.
Note: Drug should be discontinued if signs of bone marrow toxicity or toxic hepatitis are evident.

Overdose and treatment

Clinical manifestations of overdose include myelosuppression, nausea, vomiting, and hepatic necrosis.

Treatment is usually supportive and includes transfusion of blood components and antiemetics. Mercaptopurine is dialyzable.

▶ Special considerations

• Follow established procedures for safe handling, administration and disposal.
• Warn patient that improvement may take 2 to 4 weeks or longer.
• Monitor weekly blood counts; watch for precipitous fall.
• Store tablets at room temperature and protect from light.
• Dose modifications may be required following chemotherapy or radiation therapy, in depressed neutrophil or platelet count, and in impaired hepatic or renal function.
• Monitor intake and output. Push fluids (3 liters daily).
• Drug is sometimes called 6-mercaptopurine or 6-MP.
• Monitor hepatic function and hematologic values weekly during therapy. Dosage is commonly adjusted according to severity of myelosuppression and liver toxicity.

• Premedicating with an antiemetic may prevent nausea and vomiting. If vomiting occurs, administer antiemetics p.r.n.
• Patients who have received drugs with strong emetic properties may experience anticipatory nausea and vomiting at subsequent treatments. They may benefit from treatment with an anxiolytic drug.
• Monitor serum uric acid levels. If allopurinol is necessary, use very cautiously.
• Observe for signs of bleeding and infection.
• Hepatic dysfunction is reversible when drug is stopped. Watch for jaundice, clay-colored stools, and frothy dark urine. Drug should be stopped if hepatic tenderness occurs.
• Avoid all I.M. injections when platelet count is below 100,000/mm³.
• Mercaptopurine has been used to treat regional enteritis (Crohn's disease) and ulcerative colitis. Usual dosage is 1.5 mg/kg/day, gradually increased to 2.5 mg/kg/day if tolerated.

Information for parents and patient

• Instruct parents how to achieve correct dosage. Tell them to administer oral dosage 1 hour before or 2 hours after meals for optimum absorption.
• Tell parents that patient's dental work should be completed before therapy whenever possible, or delayed until blood counts are normal.
• Teach parents how to recognize symptoms of hepatotoxicity and emphasize importance of reporting them promptly.
• Warn patient that he may bruise easily because of drug's effect on platelets.
• Stress importance of keeping follow-up appointments for monitoring hematologic status.
• Teach parents and patient to check for signs of bleeding and bruising. Parents may need to restrict child's participation in contact sports. Such activity is dangerous when patient's platelets are low.
• Warn patient to avoid close contact with persons who have taken live virus (polio, rubella, measles) vaccine and to avoid exposure to persons with bacterial or viral infection, because chemotherapy may increase susceptibility to infection. Instruct him to report signs of infection immediately. Explain importance of promptly reporting exposure to chicken pox in susceptible patient.
• Advise parents that patient should not receive live-virus immunizations during therapy and for several weeks after therapy. Members of the same household should not receive immunizations during the same period.
• Advise parents and patient the importance of continuing medication despite nausea and vomiting.
• Parents should call immediately if vomiting occurs shortly after taking a dose.
• Warn parents to check liquid medications for alcohol content (for example acetaminophen elixirs). Patient should avoid alcohol while taking this medication.
• Urge parents to encourage adequate fluid intake, to increase urine output and facilitate the excretion of uric acid.
• Instruct parents to monitor neutropenic patient's temperature every 4 hours (not rectally) and to report fever, cough and other signs of infection *promptly.*

• Instruct patient to clean teeth with toothettes, gauze, or soft toothbrush when platelets are low. Patient should perform frequent oral hygiene and should avoid using commercial mouthwashes which may contain alcohol and have an irritating effect. Solutions of sodium bicarbonate or hydrogen peroxide are more appropriate rinses.

• Instruct patient to avoid foods that are spicy and extremely hot or cold. Topical anesthetics administered before meals (swish and spit) may relieve mouth discomfort.

---

metaproterenol sulfate
Alupent, Metaprel

• Classification: bronchodilator (adrenergic)

How supplied
Available by prescription only
Tablets: 10 mg, 20 mg
Solution: 10 mg/5 ml
Aerosol inhaler: 0.65 mg/metered spray
Nebulizer inhaler: 0.6%, 5% solution

Indications, route, and dosage
Bronchial asthma and reversible broncho-spasm
Children age 6 to 9 or weighing less than 60 lb (27.3 kg): 10 mg P.O. t.i.d. or q.i.d.
Children age 9 to 12 or weighing more than 60 lb and adults: 20 mg P.O. t.i.d. or q.i.d.
Children age 12 and older and adults: Administered by metered aerosol, 2 or 3 inhalations, with at least 2 minutes between inhalations; no more than 12 inhalations in 24 hours. Administered by hand-bulb nebulizer, 10 inhalations of an undiluted 5% solution or alternatively, administered by IPPB, 0.3 ml (range 0.2 to 0.3 ml) of a 5% diluted solution or 2.5 ml of a 0.6% solution. These doses need not be repeated more often than every 4 hours for an acute attack. For chronic therapy, these doses may be administered t.i.d. or q.i.d.

Action and kinetics
• *Bronchodilator action:* Metaproterenol relaxes bronchial smooth muscle and peripheral vasculature by stimulating beta$_2$-adrenergic receptors, thus decreasing airway resistance via bronchodilation. It has lesser effect on beta$_1$ receptors and has little or no effect on alpha-adrenergic receptors. In high doses, it may cause CNS and cardiac stimulation, resulting in tachycardia, hypertension, or tremors.
• *Kinetics in adults:* Metaproterenol is well absorbed from the GI tract. Onset of action occurs within 1 minute after oral inhalation, 5 to 30 minutes after nebulization, and 15 to 30 minutes after oral administration, with peak effects seen in about 1 hour. Duration of action after oral inhalation is 1 to 4 hours after single dose; 1 to 2½ hours after multiple doses; after nebulization, 2 to 6 hours after single dose, 4 to 6 hours after repeated doses; after oral administration, 1 to 4 hours. Metaproterenol is widely distributed throughout the body. It is extensively

metabolized on first pass through the liver and is excreted in urine, mainly as glucuronic acid conjugates.

Contraindications and precautions
Metaproterenol is contraindicated in patients with pre-existing cardiac dysrhythmias associated with tachycardia, because of the drug's cardiac stimulant effects, and in those with hypersensitivity to the drug or ingredients in formulation.

Administer with extreme caution to patients with hypertension, coronary artery disease, CHF, hyperthyroidism, or diabetes, because the drug may worsen these conditions, or to patients who are sensitive to the effects of other sympathomimetics.

Administer cautiously to patients with sulfite sensitivity, because some preparations contain sulfite preservatives.

Interactions
Concomitant use with other sympathomimetics may produce additive effects and toxicity. Use of metaproterenol with general anesthetics (especially chloroform, cyclopropane, halothane, and trichlorethylene), theophylline derivatives, digitalis glycosides, levodopa, other sympathomimetics, or thyroid hormones may increase the potential for cardiac effects, including severe ventricular tachycardia, cardiac dysrhythmias, and coronary insufficiency.

Beta-adrenergic blockers, especially propranolol, antagonize metaproterenol's bronchodilating effects.

Increased CNS stimulation may result from concomitant use with xanthines, other sympathomimetics, and other CNS stimulating drugs.

Effects on diagnostic tests
None reported.

Adverse reactions
• CNS: weakness, drowsiness, *tremors*, nervousness, headache, dizziness, *muscle cramps.*
• CV: *tachycardia, palpitations, hypertension; with excessive use, cardiac arrest, dysrhythmias.*
• GI: *nausea, vomiting,* bad taste in mouth.
• Other: *paradoxical bronchoconstriction with excessive use,* muscle cramps in legs, hypersensitivity reactions.
Note: Drug should be discontinued if bronchoconstriction or hypersensitivity to drug or sulfite preservatives occurs.

Overdose and treatment
Clinical manifestations of overdose include exaggeration of common adverse reactions, particularly nausea and vomiting, cardiac dysrhythmias, angina, hypertension, and seizures.

Treatment includes supportive and symptomatic measures. Monitor vital signs closely. Support cardiovascular status. Use cardioselective beta$_1$-adrenergic blockers (acebutolol, atenolol, metoprolol) to treat symptoms with extreme caution; they may induce severe bronchospasm or asthmatic attack.

---

‡May contain sulfites   ◆May contain tartrazine   ◆◆May contain benzyl alcohol

► **Special considerations**
• The preservative sodium bisulfite is present in many adrenergic formulations. Patients with a history of allergy to sulfites should avoid preparations that contain this preservative.
• Therapy should be administered when patient arises in morning and before meals to reduce fatigue by improving lung ventilation.
• Adrenergic inhalation may be alternated with other adrenergics if necessary, but should not be administered simultaneously because of danger of excessive tachycardia.
• Do not use discolored or precipitated solutions.
• Protect solutions from light, freezing, and heat. Store at controlled room temperature.
• Adverse reactions are dose-related, characteristic of sympathomimetics, and may persist a long time because of the long duration of action of metaproterenol.
• Excessive or prolonged use may lead to decreased effectiveness.
• Avoid simultaneous administration of adrenocorticoid inhalation aerosol. Allow at least 5 minutes to lapse between using the two aerosols.
• Monitor patient for signs and symptoms of toxic effects (nausea and vomiting, tremors, and cardiac dysrhythmias).
• Aerosol treatments may be used with oral tablet dosing.
• Safety and efficacy of oral inhalation in children under age 12 not established. Safety and efficacy of oral preparations in children under age 6 not established.

Information for parents and patient
• Treatment should start with first symptoms of bronchospasm.
• Instruct patient to shake container, exhale through nose as completely as possible, then administer aerosol while inhaling deeply through mouth, and hold breath for 10 seconds before exhaling slowly. Patient should wait 1 to 2 minutes before repeating inhalations. Tell the patient that he may experience bad taste in mouth after using oral inhaler.
• Caution patient to keep spray away from eyes.
• Teach parents and patient that a single aerosol treatment is usually enough to control an asthma attack and to call promptly if the patient requires more than three aerosol treatments in 24 hours. Explain that overuse of adrenergic bronchodilators may cause tachycardia, palpitations, headache, nausea and dizziness, loss of effectiveness, possible paradoxical reaction, and cardiac arrest.
• Instruct parents to have patient use only as directed and to take no more than two inhalations at one time with 1- to 2-minute intervals between. Remind parents to save applicator; refills may be available.
• Warn parents that patient should avoid simultaneous use of adrenocorticoid aerosol, and to allow at least 5 minutes to lapse between using the two aerosols.
• Tell parents and patient that drug may have shorter duration of action after prolonged use. Advise parents to report failure to respond to usual dose.
• Warn parents that patient should not increase dose

or frequency unless prescribed; serious adverse reactions are possible.
• Tell parents to call if bronchodilator causes dizziness, chest pain, or lack of therapeutic response to usual dose.
• Patient should avoid other adrenergic medications unless they are prescribed.
• Tell parents that patient may take missed dose if remembered within 1 hour. If beyond 1 hour, patient should skip dose and resume regular schedule. The patient should *not* double dose.
• Inform parents and patient that saliva and sputum may appear pink after inhalation treatment.
• Tell parents and patient that increased fluid intake facilitates clearing of secretions.
• Teach parents and patient how to accomplish postural drainage, to cough productively, and to clap and vibrate to promote good respiratory hygiene.
• Information and instructions are furnished with the aerosol forms of these drugs. Urge parents and patient to read them carefully and ask questions if necessary.
• Tell parents to store drug away from heat and light, and safely out of small children's reach.

metaraminol bitartrate
Aramine

• Classification: vasopressor (adrenergic)

How supplied
Available by prescription only
Injection: 10 mg/ml parenteral

Indications, route, and dosage
Hypotension
Children: 0.1 mg/kg or 3 mg/m² S.C. or I.M.
Adults: 2 to 10 mg I.M. or S.C.
Hypotension in severe shock
Children: 0.01 mg/kg or 0.03 mg/m² direct I.V. followed by I.V. infusion, if necessary, of 0.4 mg/kg or 12 mg/m² diluted and titrated to maintain desired blood pressure.
Adults: 0.5 to 5 mg direct I.V. followed by I.V. infusion. If necessary, mix 15 to 100 mg in 500 ml normal saline solution or dextrose 5% in water; titrate infusion based on blood pressure response.

Action and kinetics
• *Vasopressor action:* Metaraminol acts predominantly by direct stimulation of alpha-adrenergic receptors, which constrict both capacitance and resistance blood vessels, resulting in increased total peripheral resistance; increased systolic and diastolic blood pressure; decreased blood flow to vital organs, skin, and skeletal muscle; and constriction of renal blood vessels, which reduces renal blood flow. It also has a direct stimulating effect on beta₁ receptors of the heart, producing a positive inotropic response, and an indirect effect, releasing norepinephrine from its storage sites, which, with repeated use, may result in tachyphylaxis. Metaraminol also acts as a weak or false neurotransmitter by replacing norepinephrine

in sympathetic nerve endings. Its main effects are vasoconstriction and cardiac stimulation. It does not usually cause CNS stimulation but may cause contraction of pregnant uterus and uterine blood vessels because of its alpha-adrenergic effects.

• *Kinetics in adults:* Onset of action after I.M. injection occurs within 10 minutes; after I.V. injection, within 1 to 2 minutes; after S.C. injection, 5 to 20 minutes. Pressor effects may persist 20 to 90 minutes, depending on route of administration and patient variability. Distribution is not completely known. In vitro tests suggest that metaraminol is not metabolized. Effects appear to be terminated by uptake of drug into tissues and by urinary excretion. Metaraminol is excreted in urine; may be accelerated by acidifying urine.

Contraindications and precautions

Metaraminol is contraindicated in patients with peripheral or mesenteric vascular thrombosis (may increase ischemia and extend area of infarction), in patients with profound hypoxia or hypercapnea, and in those undergoing general anesthesia with cyclopropane and other inhalation hydrocarbon anesthetics (risk of inducing cardiac dysrhythmias).

Administer cautiously to hypertensive or hyperthyroid patients (increased adverse reaction) and to those with diabetes, heart disease, cirrhosis, peripheral vascular disease, acidosis, or history of malaria (relapse may occur). Also administer cautiously in patients with known sensitivity to sulfites because commercially available formulations contain sulfites.

Interactions

Concomitant use may prolong and intensify cardiac stimulant and vasopressor effects of MAO inhibitors. Do not administer metaraminol until 14 days after MAO inhibitors have been discontinued.

Increased cardiac effects may result when metaraminol is used with general anesthetics, maprotiline, digitalis glycosides, levodopa, other sympathomimetics, or thyroid hormones.

When metaraminol is used with the alpha-adrenergic blocking agents, pressor effects may be decreased (but not completely blocked). When metaraminol is used with doxapram, trimethaphan, mazindol, methylphenidate, or ergot alkaloids, pressor effects may be increased.

Concomitant use of beta blockers with metaraminol may result in mutual inhibition of therapeutic effects, with increased potential for hypertension, and excessive bradycardia with possible heart block.

Metaraminol may also decrease the hypotensive effects of guanadrel, guanethidine, rauwolfia alkaloids, and diuretics used as antihypertensives. Concomitant use with atropine blocks the reflex bradycardia caused by metaraminol and enhances its pressor response.

Effects on diagnostic tests

None reported.

Adverse reactions

• CNS: apprehension, anxiety, tremor, restlessness, weakness, faintness, dizziness, headache, convulsions (excessive use).
• CV: precordial pain, peripheral and visceral vasoconstriction, palpitations, dysrhythmias, sinus or ventricular tachycardia, bradycardia, hypotension, hypertension.
• GI: nausea, vomiting.
• GU: decreased urine output.
• Other: hyperglycemia, pallor, sweating, respiratory distress, fever.
   Note: Drug should be discontinued if patient is hypersensitive to drugs or sulfites, or if infiltration or thrombosis occurs during I.V. administration.

Overdose and treatment

Clinical manifestations of overdose include severe hypertension, dysrhythmias, seizures, cerebral hemorrhage, acute pulmonary edema, and cardiac arrest.

Treatment requires discontinuation of drug followed by supportive and symptomatic measures. Monitor vital signs closely. Use atropine for reflex bradycardia and propranolol for dysrhythmias.

▶ Special considerations

• Use with caution in pediatric patients. Solutions for I.V. infusion can be prepared to contain 1 mg of metaraminol per 25 ml of diluent.
• Monitor blood pressure and heart rate and rhythm during and after metaraminol administration until patient is stable.
• Correct blood volume depletion before administration. Metaraminol is not a substitute for blood, plasma, fluids, or electrolyte replacement.
• Drug must be diluted before use. Preferred solutions for dilution are normal saline solution or dextrose 5% injection. Select injection site carefully. I.V. route is preferred, using large veins. Avoid extravasation. Monitor infusion rate; use of infusion controlling device preferred. Withdraw drug gradually; recurrent hypotension may follow abrupt withdrawal.
• Allow at least 10 minutes to elapse before administering additional doses because maximum effect is not immediately apparent.
• To treat extravasation, infiltrate site promptly with 10 to 15 ml normal saline solution containing 5 to 10 mg phentolamine, using fine needle.
• Cumulative effect possible after prolonged use. Excessive vasopressor response may persist after drug is withdrawn.
• Keep emergency drugs on hand to reverse effect of metaraminol: atropine for reflex bradycardia, phentolamine for extravasation, and propranolol for dysrhythmias.
• Monitor diabetic patients closely. Insulin adjustments may be needed.
• Closely monitor fluid and electrolyte status.
• Do not mix in bag or syringe with other medications.
• Tachyphylaxis (tolerance) may develop after prolonged or excessive use.

Information for parents and patient

• Ask parents and patient about allergy to sulfites before administering.

• Inform parents and patient that he'll need frequent assessment of vital signs.
• Tell parents and patient to report any adverse reactions.

metaxalone
Skelaxin

• Classification: skeletal muscle relaxant (oxazolidinone derivative)

How supplied
Available by prescription only
Tablets (scored): 400 mg

Indications, route, and dosage
Skeletal muscle relaxant; adjunct for relief of acute musculoskeletal conditions
Children over age 12 and adults: 800 mg P.O. t.i.d. or q.i.d.

Action and kinetics
• *Skeletal muscle relaxant action:* Metaxalone is a CNS depressant, which produces skeletal muscle relaxant effects through an unknown mechanism. Its effects may be related to its sedative actions.
• *Kinetics in adults:* Onset of action occurs within 1 hour and persists for 4 to 6 hours. Peak serum concentrations occur in 2 hours. Metaxalone is metabolized in the liver. Metaxalone is excreted in urine as metabolites; plasma half-life is 2 to 3 hours.

Contraindications and precautions
Metaxalone is contraindicated in patients with impaired hepatic or renal function because of the potential for accumulation of drug after repeated doses, in patients with known hypersensitivity to the drug or history of drug-induced hemolytic anemias or in patients with other anemias, because the drug may induce hemolytic anemia.

Administer cautiously to patients with history of hepatic disease.

Interactions
Concomitant use of metaxalone with other CNS depressants, including alcohol, narcotics, anxiolytics, antipsychotics, or tricyclic antidepressants, may produce additive CNS depression.

Effects on diagnostic tests
Metaxalone therapy alters cupric sulfate urine glucose test results (false-positive results with Benedict's solution, Clinitest, and Fehling's solution), but does not interfere with glucose tests using glucose oxidase (Clinistix, Diastix, Tes-Tape). Patients receiving metaxalone may develop abnormalities in liver function tests.

Adverse reactions
• CNS: drowsiness, dizziness, headache, nervousness, confusion, irritability.
• GI: nausea, anorexia, dry mouth, vomiting, GI upset.

• Other: urinary retention, exacerbation of tonic-clonic seizures, hypersensitivity reactions, rash, pruritus, leukopenia, hemolytic anemias, jaundice.
   Note: Drug should be discontinued if patient develops hypersensitivity, rash, elevated liver enzyme levels, or signs of hepatotoxicity.

Overdose and treatment
Clinical manifestations of overdose include exaggerated adverse reactions, particularly nausea and vomiting, seizures, and extreme drowsiness. Treat with gastric lavage and other supportive measures as needed. Monitor vital signs closely.

▶ Special considerations
• Liver function tests should be performed periodically throughout therapy.
• Safety has not been established in children under age 12.

Information for parents and patient
• Tell parents drug may cause drowsiness. Advise parents that patient should avoid hazardous activities that require alertness until degree of CNS depression can be determined.
• Advise parents that patient should avoid alcoholic beverages and to use care with cough and cold preparations because some may contain alcohol.
• Tell parent that patient may take missed dose if remembered within 1 hour. If beyond 1 hour, patient should skip dose and return to regular schedule. Warn parents not to double the dose.

metharbital
Gemonil

• Classification: anticonvulsant (barbiturate)
• Controlled substance schedule III

How supplied
Available by prescription only
Tablets: 100 mg

Indications, route, and dosage
Generalized toxic-clonic (grand mal), absence (petite mal), myoclonic, and mixed seizure patterns
Children: Recommended dosage is 5 to 15 mg/kg/day, or 50 mg once daily to t.i.d.
Adults: Usual starting dose is 100 mg once daily to t.i.d. In some patients, smaller doses may be effective; others may require from 600 to 800 mg/day.

Action and kinetics
• *Anticonvulsant action:* Metharbital is a nonspecific CNS depressant that depresses monosynaptic and polysynaptic transmission in the CNS and increases seizure threshold in the motor cortex. Metharbital usually is used in patients who cannot tolerate phenobarbital or mephobarbital; it may be more effective in the treatment of Lennox-Gestaut syndrome (petit mal variant epilepsy).

---

*Canada only   †Unlabeled clinical use   Italicized adverse reactions have been observed in children.

• *Kinetics in adults:* Metharbital is absorbed readily from the GI tract. Metharbital is distributed widely throughout the body. Metharbital is at least partially demethylated in the liver to barbital. Metharbital is excreted in urine.

Contraindications and precautions

Metharbital is contraindicated in patients with known hypersensitivity to barbiturates; in suspected pregnancy and pregnancy near term because of hazard of respiratory depression and neonatal coagulation defects; and in patients with respiratory disease, status asthmaticus, or a history of porphyria or impaired hepatic function. It should be used with caution in patients taking alcohol, CNS depressants, monoamine oxidase (MAO) inhibitors, narcotic analgesics, or anticoagulants.

Interactions

Alcohol and other CNS depressants, including narcotic analgesics, may cause excessive depression in patients taking metharbital. Barbiturates can induce hepatic metabolism of oral anticoagulants and increase metabolism of combination oral contraceptives. MAO inhibitors also potentiate CNS depressant effects of barbiturates; rifampin may decrease barbiturate levels and thereby decrease efficacy.

Effects on diagnostic tests

Metharbital may elevate liver function test results.

Adverse reactions

• CNS: dizziness, irritability, *drowsiness,* headache, confusion, excitation.
• CV: hypotension.
• DERM: rash, urticaria, purpura, erythema multiforme.
• GI: nausea, vomiting, discomfort.
• HEMA: megaloblastic anemia, agranulocytosis, thrombocytopenia.

 Note: Drug should be discontinued if signs of hypersensitivity or hepatic dysfunction occur.

Overdose and treatment

Symptoms of overdose include drowsiness, irritability, dizziness, and GI distress; high dosage may cause unconsciousness. Treat overdose symptomatically and supportively: in conscious patient with intact gag reflex, induce emesis with ipecac; follow in 30 minutes with repeated doses of activated charcoal to decrease absorption. Forced diuresis and alkalinization of urine may hasten excretion. Hemodialysis may be necessary. Monitor vital signs and fluid and electrolyte balance.

▶ Special considerations

• Metharbital is not recommended for young children.
• Premature infants are more susceptible to the depressant effects of barbiturates because of immature hepatic metabolism. Children receiving barbiturates may experience hyperactivity, excitement, or hyperalgia.
• Dosage of barbiturates must be individualized for each patient, because different rates of metabolism and enzyme induction occur.

• Assess level of consciousness before and frequently during therapy to evaluate effectiveness of drug. Monitor neurologic status for possible alterations or deteriorations. Monitor seizure character, frequency, and duration for changes. Institute seizure precautions, as necessary.
• Assess patient's sleeping patterns before and during therapy to ensure effectiveness of drug.
• Institute safety measures – side rails, assistance when out of bed, call light within reach – to prevent falls and injury.
• Anticipate possible rebound confusion and excitatory reactions in patient.
• Assess bowel elimination patterns; monitor for complaints of constipation. Advise diet high in fiber, if indicated.
• Monitor prothrombin time carefully in patients taking anticoagulants; dosage of anticoagulant may require adjustment to counteract possible interaction.
• Observe patient to prevent hoarding or self-dosing, especially in depressed or suicidal patients, or those who are or have a history of being drug-dependent.
• Death is common with an overdose of 2 to 10 g; it may occur at much smaller doses if alcohol is also ingested.
• Barbiturate dependence may be transmitted to the fetus; withdrawal symptoms can occur in neonates whose mothers took barbiturates in the third trimester.
• Avoid administering barbiturates to patients with status asthmaticus.
• Monitor for signs of bleeding if patient is on stable anticoagulant regimen.
• Do not withdraw drug abruptly; after long-term use, lower dosage gradually.
• Barbiturates impair ability to perform tasks requiring mental alertness, such as driving a car.

Information for parents and patient

• Warn parents that patient should avoid concurrent use of other drugs with CNS depressant effects, such as antihistamines, analgesics, and alcohol, because they will have additive effects and result in increased drowsiness. Instruct parents to seek medical approval before giving patient any nonprescription cold or allergy preparations.
• Caution parents and patient not to increase or decrease dose or frequency without medical approval; abrupt discontinuation may trigger rebound insomnia, with increased dreaming, nightmares, or seizures.
• Advise parents that patient should avoid hazardous activities that require alertness while taking barbiturates.
• Be sure parents and patient understand that barbiturates can cause physical or psychological dependence (addiction).
• Instruct parents to report any skin eruption or other marked adverse effect.
• Explain that a morning hangover is common after therapeutic use of barbiturates.
• Teach parents and patient signs and symptoms of adverse reactions and tell them to report them.
• Explain that barbiturates may render oral contraceptives ineffective; advise sexually active female patients to consider a different birth control method.

methdilazine
Dilysyn*

methdilazine hydrochloride
Tacaryl

- Classification: antihistamine, H₁-receptor antagonist, antipruritic (phenothiazine derivative)

How supplied
Available by prescription only
Tablets: 8 mg methdilazine hydrochloride
Tablets (chewable): 3.6 mg methdilazine (equal to 4 mg methdilazine hydrochloride)
Syrup: 4 mg/5 ml methdilazine hydrochloride

Indications, route, and dosage
Pruritus
Children over age 3: 4 mg P.O. b.i.d. to q.i.d. or (chewable tablets) 3.6 mg P.O. b.i.d. to q.i.d.
Adults: 8 mg P.O. b.i.d. to q.i.d. or (chewable tablets) 7.2 mg P.O. b.i.d. to q.i.d.

Action and kinetics
- *Antihistamine action:* Antihistamines compete with histamine for histamine H₁-receptor sites on the smooth muscle of the bronchi, GI tract, uterus, and large blood vessels; by binding to cellular receptors, they prevent access of histamine and suppress histamine-induced allergic symptoms, even though they do not prevent its release.
- *Kinetics in adults:* Absorption, distribution, metabolism, and excretion have not been reported.

Contraindications and precautions
Methdilazine is contraindicated in patients with known hypersensitivity to this medication or other antihistamines or phenothiazines with a similar chemical structure, such as promethazine or trimeprazine; during acute asthmatic attack, because it thickens bronchial secretions; in acutely ill or dehydrated children, because they are at increased risk of developing dystonias; and in patients who have taken MAO inhibitors within the preceding 2 weeks.

Methdilazine should be used with caution in children with a history of sleep apnea, a family history of sudden infant death syndrome, or Reye's syndrome; or in patients with acute or chronic respiratory dysfunction, because methdilazine may suppress the cough reflex.

Methdilazine should be used with caution in patients with narrow-angle glaucoma; in patients with pyloroduodenal obstruction or urinary bladder obstruction from narrowing of the bladder neck, because of its significant anticholinergic effects; or in patients with cardiovascular disease or hypertension, because of risks of palpitations and tachycardia.

Interactions
MAO inhibitors interfere with the detoxification of methdilazine and thus prolong and intensify its central depressant and anticholinergic effects; added sedation and CNS depression may occur when methdilazine is used concomitantly with other antihistamines, alcohol, barbiturates, tranquilizers, sleeping aids, or antianxiety agents.

Phenothiazines potentiate the CNS depressant and analgesic effect of narcotics; the phenothiazine activity of methdilazine is potentiated by oral contraceptives, progesterone, reserpine, and nylidrin hydrochloride.

Do not give epinephrine to reverse methdilazine-induced hypotension; partial adrenergic blockade may cause a further fall in blood pressure.

Effects on diagnostic tests
Methdilazine should be discontinued 4 days before diagnostic skin tests, to avoid preventing, reducing, or masking positive test response.

Adverse reactions
- CNS: extrapyramidal symptoms (especially at high doses), dizziness, drowsiness, headache, tinnitus, insomnia, euphoria, tremors, excitation, tonic-clonic convulsions, catatonia, increased appetite.
- CV: postural hypotension, reflex tachycardia, ECG changes.
- DERM: photosensitivity, rash, systemic lupus erythematosus-like symptoms.
- GI: anorexia, constipation, cholestatic jaundice.
- GU: urinary frequency and retention, dysuria.
- HEMA: leukopenia, agranulocytosis.
- Respiratory: thickened bronchial secretions.
- Chronic use: skin pigmentation, corneal opacities, impaired vision.

Overdose and treatment
Clinical manifestations of overdose may include either CNS depression (sedation, reduced mental alertness, apnea, and cardiovascular collapse) or CNS stimulation (insomnia, hallucinations, tremors, or convulsions). Atropine-like symptoms, such as dry mouth, flushed skin, fixed and dilated pupils, and GI symptoms, are common, especially in children.

Treat overdose by inducing emesis with ipecac syrup (in conscious patient), followed by activated charcoal to reduce further drug absorption. Use gastric lavage if patient is unconscious or ipecac fails. Treat hypotension with vasopressors, and control seizures with diazepam or phenytoin. *Do not give stimulants.*

▶ Special considerations
- Drug should be used with caution in children. Methdilazine is not indicated for use in premature infants or neonates. Children, especially those under age 6, may experience paradoxical hyperexcitability with restlessness, insomnia, nervousness, euphoria, tremors, and seizures.
- Drug is contraindicated during an acute asthma attack, because it may not alleviate the symptoms and because antimuscarinic effects can cause thickening of secretions.
- Monitor blood counts during long-term therapy; watch for signs of blood dyscrasias.
- Reduce GI distress by giving drug with food. Give sugarless gum, candy, or ice chips to relieve dry

---

mouth; increase fluid intake (if allowed) or humidify air to decrease adverse effect of thickened secretions.

Information for parents and patient
• Advise parents that patient should chew and swallow chewable tablets promptly, because local anesthetic effect may cause choking.
• Advise parents that patient should take drug with meals or snack to prevent gastric upset and to use any of the following measures to relieve dry mouth: warm water rinses, artifical saliva, ice chips, or sugarless gum or candy. Patient should avoid overusing mouthwash, which may add to dryness (alcohol content) and destroy normal flora.
• Warn parents that patient should avoid hazardous activities requiring mental alertness until extent of CNS effects are known and should not take tranquilizers, sedatives, pain relievers, or sleeping medications without medical approval.
• Advise parents to discontinue methdilazine 4 days before diagnostic skin tests, to preserve accuracy of tests.

---

methenamine hippurate
Hiprex, Urex

methenamine mandelate
Mandameth, Mandelamine

• Classification: urinary tract antiseptic (formaldehyde pro-drug)

How supplied
Available by prescription only
Methenamine hippurate
Tablets: 1 g
Methenamine mandelate
Tablets: 500 mg, 1 g
Tablets (enteric-coated): 250 mg, 500 mg, 1 g
Tablets (film-coated): 500 mg, 1 g
Suspension: 250 mg/5 ml
Granules: 500 mg, 1 g

Indications, route, and dosage
Long-term prophylaxis or suppression of chronic urinary tract infections
Methenamine hippurate
Children age 6 to 12: 500 mg to 1 g P.O. q 12 hours.
Children over age 12 and adults: 1 g P.O. q 12 hours.
Urinary tract infections, infected residual urine in patients with neurogenic bladder
Methenamine mandelate
Children under age 6: 50 mg/kg divided in four doses after meals.
Children age 6 to 12: 500 mg P.O. q.i.d. after meals.
Adults: 1 g P.O. q.i.d. after meals.

Action and kinetics
• *Antibacterial action:* Methenamine is hydrolyzed to formaldehyde and ammonia in the urine. Formaldehyde acts as a nonspecific antibacterial agent.
• *Kinetics in adults:* Methenamine is absorbed well

and rapidly (however, enteric coating decreases absorption by 30%). It crosses the placenta and enters breast milk; about 10% to 25% is metabolized in the liver. Most of dose is excreted by the kidneys via glomerular filtration and tubular secretion. In the urine, methenamine is converted to formaldehyde. Peak formaldehyde concentrations occur in approximately 2 hours. Plasma half-life of parent drug is 3 to 6 hours.

Contraindications and precautions
Methenamine is contraindicated in patients with severe renal or hepatic dysfunction because the drug may worsen these conditions; in patients who are severely dehydrated because crystalluria may occur in patients with reduced urine flow rates; and in patients with known hypersensitivity to the drug.

Interactions
When used concomitantly, urine alkalinizing agents, such as sodium bicarbonate and acetazolamide, reduce methenamine's effectiveness by elevating urine pH and inhibiting methenamine's conversion to its active agent, formaldehyde. Concomitant use with sulfonamides causes formaldehyde to form an insoluble precipitate in acidic urine.

Effects on diagnostic tests
Formaldehyde formation from methenamine may cause false elevations in catecholamine and 17-hydroxycorticosteroid levels and false decreases in 5-hydroxyindoleacetic acid and estriol levels.

Liver function test results may become abnormal during methenamine therapy.

Adverse reactions
• DERM: rashes.
• GI: nausea, vomiting, diarrhea.
• GU: urinary tract irritation, dysuria, urinary frequency, hematuria, albuminuria (all with high doses).
Note: Drug should be discontinued if patient develops hypersensitivity reaction.

Overdose and treatment
No information available.

▶ Special considerations
• Obtain a clean-catch urine specimen for culture and sensitivity tests before starting therapy and repeat as needed.
• Do not administer methenamine concomitantly with sulfonamides.
• Drug is ineffective against *Candida* infection.
• Oral suspension contains vegetable oil. Use cautiously in debilitated patients because aspiration may cause lipid pneumonia.
• Monitor fluid intake and output. Maintain fluid intake of 1,500 to 2,000 ml daily.
• For best results, maintain urine pH at 5.5 or less. Use Nitrazine paper to check pH. To effectively acidify urine, large doses of ascorbic acid (6 to 12 g/day) may be necessary.
• Obtain liver function studies periodically during long-term therapy.
• *Proteus* and *Pseudomonas* infections tend to raise

urine pH; urinary acidifiers are usually necessary when treating these infections.
• If rash appears, discontinue drug and re-evaluate therapy.
• Some products (such as Hiprex) may contain tartrazine dye, which may induce allergic reactions in certain individuals.

Information for parents and patient
• Instruct parents to limit patient's intake of alkaline foods, such as vegetables, milk, and peanuts and to encourage the intake of cranberry, plum, and prune juices; which may be used to acidify urine.
• Warn parents that patient should not take antacids, including Alka-Seltzer and sodium bicarbonate.
• Instruct parents to give drug after meals to minimize GI upset.

---

methicillin sodium
Staphcillin

• Classification: antibiotic (penicillinase-resistant penicillin)

How supplied
Available by prescription only
Injection: 1 g, 4 g, 6 g
Pharmacy bulk package: 10 g
I.V. infusions piggyback: 1 g, 4 g

Indications, route, and dosage
Systemic infections caused by susceptible organisms
Neonates age 0 to 7 days weighing < 2 kg: 25 mg/kg I.M. or I.V. q 12 hours.
Neonates age 0 to 7 days weighing ≥ 2 kg: 25 mg/kg I.M. or I.V. q 8 hours.
Neonates over age 7 days weighing < 2 kg: 25 mg/kg I.M. or I.V. q 8 hours.
Neonates over age 7 days weighing ≥ 2 kg: 25 mg/kg I.M. or I.V. q 6 hours.
Children older than age 1 month weighing < 40 kg: 100 to 200 mg/kg I.M. or I.V. daily, divided into doses given q 4 to 6 hours.
Adults and children 40 kg and over: 4 to 12 g I.M. or I.V. daily, divided into doses given q 4 to 6 hours.

Action and kinetics
• *Antibiotic action:* Methicillin is bactericidal; it adheres to bacterial penicillin-binding proteins, thus inhibiting bacterial cell wall synthesis. Methicillin resists the effects of penicillinases—enzymes that inactivate penicillin—and is thus active against many strains of penicillinase-producing bacteria. Its activity is most important against penicillinase-producing staphylococci; some strains may remain resistant. Methicillin is also active against a few gram-positive aerobic and anaerobic bacilli but has no significant effect on gram-negative bacilli.
• *Kinetics in adults:* Methicillin is inactivated by gastric secretions and must be given parenterally. Peak plasma concentrations occur 30 to 60 minutes after I.M. injection. Methicillin is distributed widely. CSF penetration is poor but enhanced by meningeal inflammation. Methicillin crosses the placenta; it is 30% to 50% protein-bound. Methicillin is metabolized only partially. Methicillin and metabolites are excreted in urine by renal tubular secretion and glomerular filtration. They are also excreted in breast milk and in bile. Elimination half-life in adults is about ½ hour, prolonged to 2½ hours in severe renal impairment; it is prolonged to 4 to 6 hours in anuric patients.
• *Kinetics in children:* Serum levels are usually higher and half-life is longer in neonates than in older children.

Contraindications and precautions
Methicillin is contraindicated in patients with known hypersensitivity to any other penicillin or to cephalosporins.

Interactions
Concomitant use of methicillin with aminoglycosides produces synergistic bactericidal effects against *Staphylococcus aureus.* However, the drugs are physically and chemically incompatible and are inactivated when mixed or given together.
Probenecid blocks renal tubular secretion of penicillin, raising its serum concentrations.

Effects on diagnostic tests
Methicillin falsely shows increases in serum uric acid concentration levels (copper-chelate method); it interferes with measurement of 17-hydroxycorticosteroids (Porter-Silber test) measurements. Positive Coombs' tests have been reported. Methicillin may cause transient reductions in red blood cell, white blood cell, and platelet counts. Abnormal urinalysis result may indicate drug-induced interstitial nephritis. Methicillin may falsely decrease serum aminoglycoside concentrations.

Adverse reactions
• CNS: neuropathy, seizures (with high doses).
• GI: glossitis, stomatitis, pseudomembranous colitis, intrahepatic cholestasis, diarrhea.
• GU: interstitial nephritis.
• HEMA: eosinophilia, hemolytic anemia, transient neutropenia, thrombocytopenia, agranulocytosis.
• Local: vein irritation, thrombophlebitis.
• Other: hypersensitivity reactions (chills, fever, edema, rash, urticaria, anaphylaxis), bacterial or fungal superinfection.
Note: Drug should be discontinued if immediate hypersensitivity reactions occur or if signs of acute interstitial nephritis or pseudomembranous colitis occur. Patient may require alternate therapy if any of the following occurs: drug fever, eosinophilia, hematuria, neutropenia, or unexplained elevations in serum creatinine or BUN levels.

Overdose and treatment
Clinical signs of overdose include neuromuscular irritability or seizures. Methicillin can be removed by gastric lavage, but is not appreciably removed by hemodialysis or peritoneal dialysis.

▶ Special considerations

• Assess patient's history of allergies; do not give methicillin to any patient with a history of hypersensitivity reactions to either penicillins or cephalosporins. Try to ascertain whether previous reactions were true hypersensitivity reactions or another reaction, such as GI distress, which the patient has interpreted as allergy.

• Keep in mind that a negative history for pencillin hypersensitivity does not preclude future allergic reactions; monitor patient continously for possible allergic reactions or other untoward effects.

• In patients with renal impairment, dosage should be reduced if creatinine clearance is below 10ml/minute.

• Assess level of consciousness, neurologic status, and renal function when high doses are used, because excessive blood levels can cause CNS toxicity.

• Obtain results of cultures and sensitivity tests before first dose; however, therapy may begin before test results are complete. Repeat tests periodically to assess drug efficacy.

• Monitor vital signs, electrolytes, and renal function studies, monitor body weight for fluid retention with extended-spectrum penicillins for possible hypokalemia or hypernatremia.

• Coagulation abnormalities, even frank bleeding, can follow high doses, especially of extended-spectrum penicillins; monitor prothrombin times and platelet counts, and assess patient for signs of occult or frank bleeding.

• Monitor patients on long-term therapy for possible superinfection, especially debilitated patients and others receiving immunosuppressants or radiation therapy; monitor closely, especially for fever.

Parenteral administration

• Give penicillins at least 1 hour before giving bacteriostatic antibiotics (tetracyclines, erythromycins, and chloramphenicol); these drugs inhibit bacterial cell growth, decreasing rate of penicillin uptake by bacterial cell walls.

• Always consult manufacturer's directions for reconstitution, dilution, and storage of drugs, check expiration dates.

• Administer I.M. dose deep into muscle mass (gluteal or midlateral thigh); rotate injection sites to minimize tissue injury; do not inject more than 2 g of drug or 2 cc per injection site. Apply ice to injection site for pain.

• Do not add or mix other drugs with I.V. infusions — particularly aminoglycosides, which will be inactivated if mixed with pencillins; they are chemically and physically incompatible. If other drugs must be given I.V., temporarily stop infusion of primary drug.

• Infuse I.V. drug continuously or intermittently (over 30 minutes) and assess I.V. site frequently to prevent infiltration or phlebitis; rotate infusion site q 48 hours; intermittent I.V. infusion may be diluted in 50 to 100 ml sterile water, 0.9% sodium chloride, dextrose 5% in water, dextrose 5% in water and half normal saline, or lactated Ringer's solution. Smaller volume may be appropriate depending on child's weight.

• Solutions should always be clear, colorless to pale yellow, and free of particles; do not give solutions containing precipitates or other foreign matter.

• Schedule for administration around the clock to maintain adequate plasma levels. Monitor serum drug levels frequently in infants because their urinary excretion of drug is slower.

• Frequently monitor results of urinalysis for signs of adverse renal effects.

• Monitor neurologic status. High blood concentrations may cause seizures.

• Periodically check renal, hepatic, and hematopoietic function during prolonged therapy.

• Because methicillin is dialyzable, patients undergoing hemodialysis or peritoneal dialysis may need dosage adjustments.

Information for the parents and patient

• Teach signs and symptoms of hypersensitivity and other adverse reactions, and emphasize need to report any unusual reactions.

• Teach parents and patient how to recognize signs of superinfection, and how to prevent it by practicing meticulous oral and anogenital hygiene. Parents of infants and toddlers should keep diaper area clean and dry and avoid using plastic pants.

---

methimazole
Tapazole

• Classification: antihyperthyroid agent (thyroid hormone antagonist)

How supplied

Available by prescription only
Tablets: 5 mg, 10 mg

Indications, route, and dosage
Hyperthyroidism

Children: 0.4 mg/kg/day divided q 8 hours. Continue until patient is euthyroid, then start maintenance dosage of 0.2 mg/kg/day divided q 8 hours.

Adults: 15 mg P.O. daily if mild; 30 to 40 mg P.O. daily if moderately severe; 60 mg P.O. daily if severe. Continue until patient is euthyroid, then start maintenance dosage of 5 mg daily to b.i.d. Maximum dosage is 150 mg daily.

Note: Dosage may be given in single daily dose or in divided daily doses q 8 hours.

Preparation for thyroidectomy

Children and adults: Same dosages as for hyperthyroidism until patient is euthyroid; then iodine may be added for 10 days before surgery.

Thyrotoxic crisis

Children and adults: Same dosages as for hyperthyroidism, with concomitant iodine therapy and propranolol. Propylthiouracil (PTU) is preferred for thyroid storm.

Action and kinetics

• *Antithyroid action:* In treating hyperthyroidism, methimazole inhibits synthesis of thyroid hormone by interfering with the incorporation of iodide into tyrosine. Methimazole also inhibits the formation of iodothyronine. As preparation for thyroidectomy, me-

---

thimazole inhibits synthesis of the thyroid hormone and causes a euthyroid state, reducing surgical problems during thyroidectomy; as a result, the mortality for a single-stage thyroidectomy is low. Iodide reduces the vascularity of the gland, making it less friable. For treating thyrotoxic crisis (thyrotoxicosis), PTU theoretically is preferred over methimazole because it inhibits peripheral deiodination of thyroxine to tri-iodothyronine.

• *Kinetics in adults:* Methimazole is absorbed rapidly from the GI tract (70% to 80% bioavailable). Peak plasma levels are reached within 1 hour. Methimazole readily crosses the placenta and is distributed into breast milk. It is concentrated in the thyroid. Drug is not protein-bound. Methimazole undergoes hepatic metabolism. About 80% of the drug and its metabolites are excreted renally; 7% is excreted unchanged. Half-life is between 5 and 13 hours.

Contraindications and precautions
Methimazole is contraindicated in patients with hypersensitivity to the drug and in breast-feeding patients. It should be used with caution at dosages greater than 40 mg/day because of increased risk of agranulocytosis; in patients receiving other agents known to cause agranulocytosis; and in patients with infection or hepatic dysfunction.

Interactions
Concomitant use of methimazole with PTU and adrenocorticoids or adrenocorticotropic hormone may require a dosage adjustment of the steroid when thyroid status changes. Concomitant use with other bone marrow depressant agents causes an increased risk of agranulocytosis. Concomitant use with other hepatotoxic agents increases the risk of hepatotoxicity. Concurrent use with iodinated glycerol, lithium, or potassium iodide may potentiate hypothyroid and goitrogenic effects.

Effects on diagnostic tests
Methimazole therapy alters selenomethionine (^{75}Se) uptake by the pancreas and radioactive iodine (^{123}I or ^{131}I) uptake by the thyroid. Hepatotoxicity may be evident by elevations of prothrombin time and of serum alanine aminotransferase, serum aspartate aminotransferase, bilirubin, alkaline phosphatase, and lactic dehydrogenase levels.

Adverse reactions
• CNS: *headache, drowsiness, vertigo, depression, paresthesias.*
• DERM: rash, urticaria, skin discoloration, pruritus, lupus-like syndrome, *exfoliative dermatitis.*
• GI: diarrhea, nausea, vomiting, epigastric distress, sialadenopathy (appear to be dose-related).
• HEMA: *agranulocytosis, leukopenia, granulocytopenia, thrombocytopenia* (appear to be dose-related).
• Hepatic: *jaundice, hepatitis.*
• Renal: nephritis.
• Other: *arthralgia,* myalgia, salivary gland enlargement, loss of taste, drug fever, lymphadenopathy, hair loss, edema, *hypothyroidism.*
Note: Drug should be discontinued at the first sign of hepatotoxicity or if the patient develops agranu-

locytosis, pancytopenia, hepatitis (fever, swelling of cervical lymph nodes), or exfoliative dermatitis.

Overdose and treatment
Clinical manifestations of overdose include nausea, vomiting, epigastric distress, fever, headache, arthralgia, pruritus, edema, and pancytopenia. Treatment is supportive; gastric lavage should be performed or emesis should be induced if possible. If bone marrow depression develops, fresh whole blood, corticosteroids, and anti-infectives may be required.

▶ Special considerations
• Signs and symptoms of overdose or hypothyroidism include mental depression; changes in menstrual periods; cold intolerance; constipation; dry, puffy skin; headache; listlessness; muscle aches; nausea; vomiting; weakness; fatigue; hard, nonpitting edema; and unusual weight gain.
• Watch for signs of hypothyroidism. Monitor serum levels of thyroid-stimulating hormone as a sensitive indicator of thyroid hormone levels. Dosage adjustment may be required.
• Signs and symptoms of thyrotoxicosis or inadequate thyroid suppression include diarrhea, fever, irritability, listlessnesss, rapid heartbeat, vomiting, and weakness.
• Treatment with methimazole requires complete blood counts periodically to detect impending leukopenia, thrombocytopenia, or agranulocytosis.
• Drug should be discontinued if patient develops severe rash or enlarged cervical lymph nodes.
• Best response occurs if dosage is administered around the clock and given at the same time each day in respect to meals.
• Dosages of over 40 mg/day increase the risk of agranulocytosis.
• A beta blocker, usually propranolol, usually is given to manage the peripheral signs of hyperthyroidism, primarily tachycardia.
• Euthyroid state may take several months to develop.

Information for parents and patient
• Advise parents to call physician immediately if patient develops sore throat, fever, or mouth sores (possible signs of developing agranulocytosis, which may not be detected by periodic blood cell counts because it can develop so rapidly). Parents should also report immediately any skin eruptions (sign of hypersensitivity).
• Suggest to parents and patient that patient take the drug with meals to reduce GI side effects.
• Tell parents and patient that patient should take drug at regular intervals around the clock and take it at the same time each day in relation to meals.
• Advise parents not to store drug in bathroom; heat and humidity cause it to deteriorate.
• Tell parents to inform all other physicians and dentists of methimazole therapy.
• Teach parents and patient how to recognize the signs and symptoms of hyperthyroidism and hypothyroidism and what to do if they occur.

---

*Canada only   †Unlabeled clinical use   Italicized adverse reactions have been observed in children.

methocarbamol
Delaxin, Robamol, Robaxin

• Classification: skeletal muscle relaxant (carbonate derivative of guaifenesin)

How supplied
Available by prescription only
Tablets: 500 mg, 750 mg
Injection: 100 mg/ml parenteral

Indications, route, and dosage
Adjunct in acute, painful musculoskeletal conditions
Adults: 1.5 g P.O. q.i.d. for 2 to 3 days. Maintenance dosage, 4 to 4.5 g P.O. daily in three to six divided doses. Alternatively, 1 g I.M. or I.V. Maximum dosage, 3 g daily I.M. or I.V. for 3 consecutive days.
Supportive therapy in tetanus management
Children: 15 mg/kg or 500 mg/m² I.V. May be repeated q 6 hours if necessary.
Adolescents: 500 to 750 mg P.O. q.i.d., increasing as needed to maximum 3 g/day I.M. or I.V. for 3 consecutive days.
Adults: 1 to 2 g direct I.V. at a rate of 300 mg/minute. Additional 1 to 2 g dose may be administered. Total initial I.V. dosage, 3 g. Repeat I.V. infusion of 1 to 2 g q 6 hours until nasogastric tube can be inserted. Total P.O. dosage, 24 g daily.

Action and kinetics
• *Skeletal muscle relaxant action:* Methocarbamol does not relax skeletal muscle directly. Its effects appear to be related to its sedative action; however, the exact mechanism of action is unknown.
• *Kinetics in adults:* Methocarbamol is rapidly and completely absorbed from the GI tract. Onset of action after single oral dose is within ½ hour. Onset of action after single I.V. dose is achieved immediately.
Methocarbamol is widely distributed throughout the body.
Methocarbamol is extensively metabolized in liver via dealkylation and hydroxylation.
Methocarbamol is rapidly and almost completely excreted in urine, mainly as its glucuronide and sulfate metabolites (40% to 50%), as unchanged drug (10% to 15%), and the rest as unidentified metabolites.

Contraindications and precautions
Methocarbamol is contraindicated in patients with known hypersensitivity to the drug.
Administer injectable methocarbamol with caution, if at all, to patients with known or suspected epilepsy, because of the potential for seizures; and to those with impaired renal function (propylene glycol vehicle may irritate the kidneys).

Interactions
Concomitant use of methocarbamol with other CNS depressant drugs, including alcohol, narcotics, anxiolytics, tricyclic antidepressants, and psychotics, may cause additive CNS depression. When used with other depressants, exercise care to avoid overdose. Patients with myasthenia gravis who receive anticholinesterase agents may experience severe weakness if given methocarbamol.

Effects on diagnostic tests
Methocarbamol therapy alters results of laboratory tests for urine 5-hydroxyindoleacetic acid (5-HIAA) using quantitative method of Udenfriend (false-positive) and for urine vanillylmandelic acid (false-positive when Gitlow screening test used; no problem when quantitative method of Sunderman used).

Adverse reactions
• CNS: drowsiness, dizziness, light-headedness, headache, vertigo, mild muscular incoordination, syncope, *seizures.*
• CV: hypotension, bradycardia.
• EENT: blurred vision, nystagmus, diplopia, conjunctivitis with nasal congestion.
• GI: nausea, adynamic ileus, metallic taste, GI upset, anorexia.
• Other: fever, allergic reactions, rash, pruritus, urticaria, flushing.
After I.M. or I.V. administration, anaphylaxis, thrombophlebitis, sloughing, pain at injection site, hemolysis, increased hemoglobin and red blood cells in urine, seizures.
Note: Drug should be discontinued if patient develops hypersensitivity, rash, or seizures.

Overdose and treatment
Clinical manifestations of overdose include extreme drowsiness, nausea and vomiting, and cardiac dysrhythmias.
Treatment includes symptomatic and supportive measures. If ingestion is recent, empty stomach by emesis or gastric lavage (may reduce absorption). Maintain adequate airway; monitor urine output and vital signs; and administer I.V. fluids if needed.

▶ Special considerations
• For children under age 12, use only as recommended for tetanus.
• Do not administer subcutaneously. Give I.V. undiluted at a rate not exceeding 300 mg per minute. May also be given by I.V. infusion after diluting in D₅W or normal saline solution.
• Patient should be supine during and for at least 10 to 15 minutes after I.V. injection.
• To give via nasogastric tube, crush tablets and suspend in water or normal saline solution.
• When used in tetanus, follow manufacturer's instructions.
• Patient's urine may turn black, blue, brown, or green on standing.
• Patient needs assistance in walking after parenteral administration.
• Extravasation of I.V. solution may cause thrombophlebitis and sloughing from hypertonic solution.

Information for parents and patient
• Tell parents and patient that drug may turn patient's urine black, blue, green or brown.

• Warn parents drug may cause drowsiness. Advise parents that child should avoid hazardous activities that require alertness until degree of CNS depression can be determined.
• Advise parents that child should make position changes slowly, particularly from recumbent to upright position, and to dangle legs before standing to prevent orthostatic hypotension.

methotrexate, methotrexate sodium
Folex, Mexate

• Classification: antineoplastic (antimetabolite [cell cycle-phase specific, S phase])

How supplied
Available by prescription only
Tablets (scored): 2.5 mg
Injection: 20-mg, 25-mg, 50-mg, 100-mg, 250-mg vials, lyophilized powder, preservative-free; 25-mg/ml vials, preservative-free solution; 2.5-mg/ml, 25-mg/ml vials lyophilized powder, preserved

Indications, route, and dosage
Dosage and indications may vary. Check current literature for recommended protocols.
Trophoblastic tumors (choriocarcinoma, hydatidiform mole)
Adults: 15 to 30 mg P.O. or I.M. daily for 5 days. Repeat after 1 or more weeks, according to response or toxicity.
Osteosarcoma
High dose methotrexate with leucovorin 'rescue' is used as part of a combination regimen that may include bleomycin, cisplastin, dactinomycin, cytoxan, and doxorubicin. Methotrexate is administered on weeks 4, 5, 6, 7, 11, 12, 15, 16, 28, 30, 44, and 45 after surgery.
Children and adults: 12 g/m² I.V. by infusion over 4 hours.
Dosage may be increased as necessary to achieve a peak serum methotrexate level of 1 millomolar (1 × 10 − 3 mol/L). Leucovorin rescue is initiated at 15 mg P.O. q 6 hours for 10 doses, beginning 24 hours after the methotrexate infusion is started. If the patient is vomiting, or cannot take oral medication, the leucovorin may be administered I.M. or I.V. at the same dosage.
Note: High dose methotrexate regimens should not be initiated unless adequate leucovorin is present and readily available for administration, since rescue is critical for patient survival.
Tumors of head and neck, refractory lymphomas
Children and adults: High-dose methotrexate—up to 6 gm/m² as an infusion over 6 to 12 hours.
Acute lymphoblastic and lymphatic leukemia
Children and adults: 3.3 mg/m² P.O., I.M., or I.V. daily for 4 to 6 weeks or until remission occurs; then 20 to 30 mg/m² P.O. or I.M. twice weekly or 2.5 mg/kg I.V. q 14 days.

Meningeal leukemia
Children and adults: 12 mg/m² intrathecally to a maximum dose of 15 mg q 2 to 5 days until cerebrospinal fluid is normal. Alternatively, base dosage on child's age, since CSF volume is based upon age, not body surface area:
Up to age 1: 6 mg
Age 1: 8 mg
Age 2: 10 mg
Age 3 and over: 12 mg
Use only vials of powder with no preservatives; dilute using normal saline solution injection *without* preservatives or Elliot's B solution. Use only new vials of drug and diluent. Use immediately after reconstitution.
Burkitt's lymphoma (Stage I or Stage II)
Adults: 10 to 25 mg P.O. daily for 4 to 8 days with 1-week rest intervals.
Lymphosarcoma (Stage III)(non-Hodgkin's lymphoma)
Adults: 0.625 to 2.5 mg/kg daily P.O., I.M., or I.V.
Breast Cancer
Adults: 40 to 60 mg/m² I.V. as a single dose. Usually used in combination with other agents.
Mycosis fungoides (advanced)
Adults: 2.5 to 10 mg P.O. daily or 50 mg I.M. weekly; or 25 mg I.M. twice weekly.
Psoriasis (severe)
Adults: 10 to 25 mg P.O., I.M., or I.V. as single weekly dose.
Rheumatoid arthritis (severe, refractory)
Adults: 7.5 to 15 mg/week in divided doses.

Action and kinetics
• *Antineoplastic action:* Methotrexate exerts its cytotoxic activity by tightly binding with an enzyme crucial to purine metabolism, resulting in an inhibition of DNA, RNA, and protein synthesis.
• *Kinetics in adults:* The absorption of methotrexate across the GI tract appears to be dose related. Lower doses are essentially completely absorbed, while absorption of larger doses is incomplete and variable. Intramuscular doses are absorbed completely. Peak serum levels are achieved 30 minutes to 2 hours after an intramuscular dose and 1 to 4 hours after an oral dose.
Methotrexate is distributed widely throughout the body, with the highest concentrations found in the kidneys, gallbladder, spleen, liver, and skin. The drug crosses the blood-brain barrier but does not achieve therapeutic levels in the CSF. Approximately 50% of the drug is bound to plasma protein.
Methotrexate is metabolized only slightly in the liver and is excreted primarily into urine as unchanged drug. The elimination has been described as biphasic, with a first-phase half-life of 45 minutes and a terminal phase half-life of 4 hours.

Contraindications and precautions
Methotrexate is contraindicated in patients with impaired renal, hepatic, or hematologic status because of the drug's adverse hematologic effects; and in pregnant patients because the drug may be fetotoxic.

---

*Canada only   †Unlabeled clinical use   Italicized adverse reactions have been observed in children.

Interactions

Concomitant use with probenecid increases the therapeutic and toxic effects of methotrexate by inhibiting the renal tubular secretion of methotrexate; salicylates also increase the therapeutic and toxic effects of methotrexate by the same mechanism. Combined use of these agents requires a lower dosage of methotrexate.

Chloramphenicol, sulfonamides, salicylates, sulfonylureas, phenytoin, phenylbutazone, and tetracycline may increase the therapeutic and toxic effects of methotrexate by displacing methotrexate from plasma proteins, increasing the concentrations of free methotrexate. Concurrent use of these agents with methotrexate should be avoided if possible. Vinca alkaloids are thought to increase the effects of methotrexate by increasing the cellular uptake of methotrexate by an unknown mechanism.

Effects on diagnostic tests

Methotrexate therapy may increase blood and urine concentrations of uric acid. Methotrexate may alter results of the laboratory assay for folate by inhibiting the organism used in the assay, thus interfering with the detection of folic acid deficiency.

Adverse reactions

• CNS: arachnoiditis within hours of intrathecal use; subacute neurotoxicity may begin a few weeks later; *necrotizing demyelinating leukoencephalopathy* a few years later.
• DERM: exposure to sun may aggravate psoriatic lesions, rash, photosensitivity, *depigmentation.*
• GI: stomatitis; *diarrhea* leading to hemorrhagic enteritis and intestinal perforation; *nausea; vomiting, oral and GI ulceration.*
• GU: *tubular necrosis.*
• HEMA: *bone marrow depression* (dose-limiting); leukopenia and thrombocytopenia (nadir occurring on day 7), anemia.
• Hepatic: *hepatic dysfunction leading to cirrhosis* or hepatic fibrosis.
• Metabolic: hyperuricemia.
• Other: alopecia, *pulmonary interstitial infiltrates and fibrosis;* long-term use in children may cause *osteoporosis, fever, anaphylaxis.*
Note: Drug should be discontinued if diarrhea or ulcerative stomatitis occurs.

Overdose and treatment

Clinical manifestations of overdose include myelosuppression, anemia, nausea, vomiting, dermatitis, alopecia, and melena.

The antidote for the hematopoietic toxicity of methotrexate is calcium leucovorin, started within 1 hour after the administration of methotrexate. The dosage of leucovorin should be high enough to produce plasma concentrations higher than those of methotrexate.

▶ Special considerations

• Follow established procedures for safe handling, administration, and disposal.
• Administer drug for *exactly* the time ordered because toxicity depends on duration of exposure to the drug.

• Monitor vital signs and patency of catheter or I.V. line throughout administration.
• Extravasations should be treated promptly.
• Monitor BUN, hematocrit, platelet count, ALT (SGPT), AST (SGOT), LDH, serum bilirubin, serum creatinine, uric acid, total and differential leukocyte.
• Methotrexate may be given undiluted by I.V. push injection.
• Drug can be diluted to a higher volume with normal saline solution for I.V. infusion.
• Use reconstituted solutions of preservative-free drug within 24 hours after mixing.
• For intrathecal administration, use preservative-free formulations only. Dilute with unpreserved normal saline and further dilute with either lactated Ringer's or Elliott's B solution, to a final concentration of 1 mg/ml.
• Dose modification may be required in impaired hepatic or renal function, bone marrow depression, aplasia, leukopenia, thrombocytopenia, or anemia. Use cautiously in infection, peptic ulcer, ulcerative colitis, and in very young, old, or debilitated patients.
• Premedicating with an antiemetic may prevent nausea and vomiting. If vomiting occurs, administer antiemetics p.r.n.
• Patients who have received drugs with strong emetic properties may experience anticipatory nausea and vomiting at subsequent treatments. They may benefit from treatment with an anxiolytic drug.
• GI adverse reactions may require stopping drug.
• Rash, redness, or ulcerations in mouth or pulmonary adverse reactions may signal serious complications.
• Monitor uric acid levels.
• Monitor intake and output daily. Force fluids (2 to 3 liters daily).
• Alkalinize urine by giving sodium bicarbonate tablets to prevent precipitation of drug, especially with high doses. Maintain urine pH at more than 6.5. Reduce dose if BUN level is 20 to 30 mg/dl or serum creatinine level is 1.2 to 2 mg/dl. Stop drug if BUN level is more than 30 mg/dl or serum creatinine level is more than 2 mg/dl.
• Watch for increases in AST (SGOT), ALT (SGPT), and alkaline phosphatase levels, which may signal hepatic dysfunction. Methotrexate should not be used when the potential for "third spacing" exists.
• Watch for bleeding (especially GI) and infection.
• Monitor temperature daily, and watch for cough, dyspnea, and cyanosis.
• Avoid all I.M. injections in patients with thrombocytopenia.
• Leucovorin rescue is necessary with high-dose protocols (doses greater than 100 mg). Precise timing of leucovorin dosage is critical to prevent toxicity.

Information for parents and patient

• For optimum absorption, parents should give oral drug 1 hour before or 2 hours after meals.
• Tell parents that patient's dental work should be completed before therapy whenever possible, or delayed until blood counts are normal.
• Stress importance of keeping follow-up appointments for monitoring hematologic status.
• Teach parents and patient to check for signs of bleeding and bruising. Parents may need to restrict child's

participation in contact sports. Such activity is dangerous when patient's platelets are low.
• Instruct parents to monitor neutropenic patient's temperature every 4 hours (not rectally) and to report fever, cough, and other signs of infection *promptly*.
• Patient should avoid contact with persons who have received live virus immunizations (polio, measles/mumps/rubella). Explain importance of promptly reporting susceptible patient's exposure to chicken pox.
• Patient should avoid exposure to persons with bacterial or viral infection, because chemotherapy may increase susceptibility to infection.
• Advise parents that patient should not receive immunizations during therapy and for several weeks after therapy. Members of the same household should not receive live-virus immunizations during the same period.
• Instruct patient to clean teeth with toothettes, gauze, or soft toothbrush when platelets are low. Patient should perform frequent oral hygiene and should avoid using commercial mouthwashes which may contain alcohol and have an irritating effect. Solutions of sodium bicarbonate or hydrogen peroxide are more appropriate rinses.
• Instruct patient to avoid foods that are spicy and extremely hot or cold. Topical anesthetics administered before meals (swish and spit) may relieve mouth discomfort.
• Emphasize to the parents and patient the importance of continuing drug despite nausea and vomiting. Advise parents to call immediately if vomiting occurs shortly after a dose.
• Tell patient to report immediately if any redness, pain, or swelling occurs at injection site. Local tissue injury and scarring may result from tissue infiltration at the infusion site.
• Encourage adequate fluid intake to increase urine output, to prevent nephrotoxicity, and to facilitate excretion of uric acid.
• Warn parents that patient should avoid alcohol during therapy with methotrexate. Parents should check liquid medications (for example, liquid forms of acetominophen) for alcohol content.
• Patient of childbearing age should avoid conception during and immediately after therapy because of possible abortion or congenital anomalies.
• Advise parents that after high I.V. dosage, patient's urine may be bright yellow.
• Patient should avoid prolonged exposure to sunlight and use a highly protective sunscreen when exposed to sunlight.
• Advise parents and patient that hair should grow back after treatment has ended.
• Recommend salicylate-free analgesics for pain relief or fever reduction.
• Instruct parents to report signs of CNS toxicity or arachnoiditis after intrathecal administration.
• Warn parents that patient should not take vitamins containing folic acid because drug is a folic acid antagonist.

methotrimeprazine hydrochloride
Levoprome, Nozinan★

• Classification: sedative, analgesic agent, antipruritic (propylamino phenothiazine)

How supplied
Available by prescription only
Injection: 20 mg/ml in 10-ml vial, 25 mg/ml★
Tablets★: 2 mg, 5 mg, 25 mg, 50 mg
Drops ★: 40 mg/ml
Solution★: 20 mg/ml

Indications, route, and dosage
Postoperative analgesia
Children over age 12 and adults: Initially, 2.5 to 7.5 mg I.M. q 4 to 6 hours, then adjust dose.
Preanesthetic medication
Children over age 12 and adults: 2 to 20 mg I.M. 45 minutes to 3 hours before surgery.
Sedation, analgesia
Children over age 12 and adults: 10 to 20 mg deep I.M. q 4 to 6 hours as required.

Action and kinetics
• *Sedative and analgesic actions:* Methotrimeprazine depresses the subcortical area of the brain at the levels of the thalamus, hypothalamus, and reticular and limbic systems. The resulting suppression of sensory impulses causes the marked sedation seen with the drug. Studies have not shown methotrimeprazine's analgesic effects to be independent of the sedative effects.
• *Kinetics in adults:* After I.M. injection, peak serum levels are attained in 30 to 90 minutes; maximum analgesic effects occur in 20 to 40 minutes.
Methotrimeprazine is distributed throughout the body, including the CNS. The drug also crosses the placenta into umbilical cord blood.
Methotrimeprazine is metabolized in the liver to less active metabolites. The metabolites of methotrimeprazine are excreted unchanged. Duration of sedation or analgesia is only 4 hours.

Contraindications and precautions
Methotrimeprazine is contraindicated in patients with known phenothiazine hypersensitivity; in patients hypersensitive to sulfites because the parenteral form of the drug contains sodium metabisulfite; in patients with severe renal or hepatic disease, because drug accumulation may occur; in patients with cardiac disease, because the drug may exacerbate the disease; and in patients with seizure disorders, because it may lower the seizure threshold.
Methotrimeprazine should be used cautiously debilitated patients with cardiovascular disease or in any patient in whom a sudden decrease in blood pressure might lead to serious complications. Use drug with great caution in patients with clinically significant hypotension or those who are receiving antihypertensives, because excessive hypotension may

occur; or in those receiving monoamine oxidase (MAO) inhibitors, because it may prolong sedative effects.

Interactions
Methotrimeprazine may add to or potentiate the effects of other CNS depressants such as opiates, benzodiazepines, antihistamines, tranquilizers, barbiturates, alcohol, and general anesthetics.

The drug may potentiate the anticholinergic effects of a number of drugs, including succinylcholine, atropine, and scopolamine. Increased CNS stimulation, including delirium and hallucinations, may occur.

Use of methotrimeprazine in patients receiving antihypertensives may cause a profound decrease in blood pressure.

Do not treat methotrimeprazine-induced hypotension with mixed alpha- and beta-adrenergic agonists such as epinephrine; that would cause an even greater decrease in blood pressure.

Effects on diagnostic tests
Methotrimeprazine therapy alters provocative and blocking tests for pheochromocytoma by producing sedation and orthostatic hypotension.

Adverse reactions
• CNS: disorientation, drowsiness, dizziness, euphoria, excessive sedation, headache, fainting, weakness, slurred speech, amnesia.
• CV: orthostatic hypotension, tachycardia, palpitations.
• DERM: local inflammation, swelling at injection site.
• EENT: blurred vision, dry mouth, nasal congestion.
• GI: nausea, vomiting, abdominal discomfort, constipation.
• GU: urinary retention.
• HEMA: agranulocytosis and other blood dyscrasias (with prolonged use).
• Hepatic: cholestatic jaundice with prolonged use.
• Other: phenothiazine adverse effects (neuroleptic malignant syndrome characterized by fever, leukocytosis, catatonia, and rigidity), dystonic reactions, akathisia, altered temperature regulation, pain and swelling at injection site.

Note: Drug should be discontinued if hypersensitivity, paradoxical euphoria, dystonic reactions, or severe prolonged hypotension occur.

Overdose and treatment
Clinical manifestations of overdose include excessive sedation, stupor, coma, hypotension, extrapyramidal reactions, and seizures.

Treat supportively. Maintain patent airway and adequate ventilation; maintain cardiovascular function with fluids and alpha-adrenergic agonists such as phenylephrine or norepinephrine. Do not use epinephrine for blood pressure control, because it may exacerbate hypotension. Treat seizures with parenteral diazepam, and extrapyramidal reactions with parenteral benztropine or diphenhydramine.

▶ Special considerations
• Safe use in children under age 12 has not been established.

• Observe patient for mood changes to monitor progress; benefits may not be apparent for several weeks.
• Monitor for involuntary movements. Check patient receiving prolonged treatment at least once every 6 months.
• Do not withdraw drug abruptly; although physical dependence does not occur with antipsychotic drugs, rebound exacerbation of psychotic symptoms may occur, and many drug effects persist.
• Carefully follow manufacturer's instructions for reconstitution, dilution, administration, and storage of drugs; slightly discolored liquids may or may not be all right to use. Check with pharmacist.
• Administer the drug deep I.M. into a large muscle mass and rotate sites. Do not give I.V.
• Methotrimeprazine may be mixed in the same syringe with scopolamine or atropine; do not mix with other drugs.
• Monitor level of consciousness and vital signs frequently.
• Check blood pressure frequently when first starting the drug or increasing the dose; blood pressure will fall within 10 to 20 minutes after injection; fainting, weakness, or dizziness may occur.
• Patient should be in bed and observed closely for 6 to 12 hours after administration.
• As necessary, institute safety measures – raise side rails, assistance when out of bed – to prevent injury.
• Monitor complete blood count and liver function tests during long-term use.
• Do not administer methotrimeprazine for longer than 30 days, except in terminal illness, or when narcotics are contraindicated.
• Store drug in a cool, dry place away from direct light.

Information for parents and patient
• Tell parents and patient drug may cause dizziness. Advise patient to stay in bed after drug administration, or to arise slowly, first to the sitting position, then pause before standing to prevent falls and injury.

methoxamine
Vasoxyl

• Classification: vasopressor, antiarrhythmic (synthetic sympathomimetic amine)

How supplied
Available by prescription only
Injection: 20 mg/ml

Indications, route, and dosage
Prophylaxis and treatment of acute hypotension during general anesthesia
Children: 250 mg/kg or 7.5 mg/m² I.M.; or 80 mcg/kg or 2.5 mg/m² I.V.
Adults: 10 to 15 mg I.M. or 3 to 5 mg I.V., administered slowly. Maximum dosage, 20 mg I.M. or 10 mg I.V. as single injection, or total of 60 mg daily.

Action and kinetics

• *Vasopressor action:* Methoxamine, primarily a direct-acting sympathomimetic amine, acts on alpha-adrenergic receptors of the peripheral vasculature to produce vasoconstriction and thus increase systolic and diastolic blood pressure.

• *Antiarrhythmic action:* Methoxamine produces bradycardia, probably by a carotid sinus reflex mediated over the vagus nerve as a result of increased arterial blood pressure.

• *Kinetics in adults:* Methoxamine is ineffective after oral administration and must be administered parenterally. After I.V. administration, pressor effect occurs immediately, peaks within 0.5 to 2 minutes, and persists for 5 to 15 minutes. After I.M. administration, pressor effect peaks within 15 to 20 minutes and effects persist for 60 to 90 minutes. Metabolic fate and the route and rate of excretion are unknown.

Contraindications and precautions

Methoxamine is contraindicated in patients with severe hypertension and in those who are hypersensitive to the drug. It should be used with caution in patients with hypothyroidism, bradycardia, partial heart block, myocardial disease, or severe arteriosclerosis, because it may worsen these conditions. Overdosage must be carefully avoided, because it may cause bradycardia and hypertension.

Methoxamine must not be used as sole therapy in hypovolemic patients and should be administered after replacement of depleted blood volume.

Hypoxia and acidosis must be identified and corrected before or during therapy, because they may impair the effectiveness of methoxamine. Drug should be used with caution in patients with sensitivity to sulfites, because the injection may contain potassium or sodium metabisulfite as a preservative.

Interactions

Administration with phentolamine or other alpha-adrenergic blocking agents (or other drugs that have alpha-adrenergic blocking effects, such as phenothiazines) may reduce the effectiveness and duration of pressor action of methoxamine. Administration with furosemide or other diuretics may also decrease arterial pressor response. Administration with propranolol or other beta-adrenergic agents may potentiate the vasoconstricting effects of methoxamine; use with atropine blocks reflex bradycardia and enhances the pressor response; administration with MAO inhibitors, tricyclic antidepressants, vasopressin, or ergot alkaloids (ergotamine, ergonovine, methylergonovine) may markedly potentiate the pressor effect and require particular caution and reduced dosage of methoxamine.

Concurrent use with alpha-adrenergic agents (such as labetalol, phenoxybenzamine, phentolamine, prazosin, or tolazoline) or with drugs that have alpha-adrenergic blocking action (haloperidol, loxapine, phenothiazines, thioxanthenes) may block the pressor response to methoxamine and lead to severe hypotension or may reduce the duration of methoxamine's pressor action; with antihypertensives or diuretics (furosemide), may reduce their antihypertensive effects; with propranolol or other beta-adrenergic block-

ing agents, may potentiate the vasoconstricting effects of methoxamine; with atropine, blocks reflex bradycardia and enhances the pressor response; with MAO inhibitors, tricyclic antidepressants, vasopressors, or ergot alkaloids (dihydroergotamine, ergonovine, methylergonovine, methysergide), may markedly potentiate the pressor effects and requires particularly cautious use and reduced dosage of methoxamine; with ergoloid mesylates or ergotamine, may cause peripheral vascular ischemia and gangrene and is not recommended; with ergonovine, ergotamine, methylergonovine, or oxytocin, may lead to severe hypertension and rupture of cerebral blood vessels; with atropine, blocks reflex bradycardia and enhances the pressor response. Concurrent use with guanadrel, guanethidine, mecamylamine, methyldopa, trimethaphan, or rauwolfia alkaloids may decrease the hypotensive effects of these drugs; with digitalis glycosides or levodopa, may increase the risk of cardiac dysrhythmias; with nitrates, may reduce their antianginal effects; with methylphenidate or mazindol, may potentiate the pressor effect of methoxamine; with doxapram, may increase the pressor effects of both drugs; with another sympathomimetic or cocaine, may increase the cardiovascular effects of either drug; with thyroid hormones, may increase the effects of either drug and may enhance the risk of coronary insufficiency when sympathomimetic drugs are given to patients with coronary artery disease; with maprotiline, may potentiate cardiovascular effects of methoxamine and may cause dysrhythmias, tachycardia, severe hypertension, or hyperpyrexia.

Effects on diagnostic tests

Methoxamine may increase plasma cortisol and corticotropin (ACTH) concentrations. It may increase the neurologic effects (including paraplegia) of diatrizoates, iothalamate, or ioxaglate during aortography.

Adverse reactions

• CNS: restlessness, anxiety, nervousness, weakness, dizziness, tremors, headache (with large doses); seizures, cerebral hemorrhage.

• CV: precordial pain, hypertension (with large doses), ventricular ectopic beats, bradycardia, decreased cardiac output, hypotension; may induce or exacerbate heart failure.

• GI: nausea and vomiting (often projectile) with high doses.

• Other: respiratory distress, sweating, pallor; desire to void or pilomotor response (with high dose), peripheral and visceral vasoconstriction; paresthesia in the extremities or a feeling of coldness, metabolic acidosis; reduced urine output; plasma volume depletion.

Overdose and treatment

Clinical effects of methoxamine overdosage may include bradycardia and an undesirable elevation in blood pressure. Treatment of bradycardia includes administration of atropine. Severe hypertension may be immediately reversed with an alpha-adrenergic blocking agent (such as phentolamine).

---

*Canada only　　　　†Unlabeled clinical use　　　　Italicized adverse reactions have been observed in children.

Special considerations
- Safety and efficacy of methoxamine in children has not been established.
- Methoxamine has no apparent stimulant effect on the heart or CNS.
- Methoxamine hydrochloride is administered by I.M. or I.V. injection or by I.V. infusion depending on individual needs. Patients who are in shock may require I.V. administration to ensure absorption of the drug.
- Methoxamine is not a substitute for replacement of blood, plasma, fluids, or electrolytes, which preferably should be accomplished before administration of the vasopressor.
- To prevent hypotension during spinal anesthesia, methoxamine should be administered by I.M. injection shortly before or at the time of spinal anesthetic administration. Hypertensive patients are more likely to experience a greater reduction in blood pressure during spinal anesthesia than patients with normal blood pressure range. Higher levels of anesthesia will usually cause a greater drop in blood pressure, which in turn will require an increased dose of methoxamine for control.
- When it is necessary to repeat I.M. doses of methoxamine, allow adequate time (about 15 minute) for the previous I.M. dose to elicit its effect before administering additional doses.
- Methoxamine is administered by slow, intravenous injection when the systolic blood pressure falls to 60 mm Hg or less, or when an emergency situation occurs. When methoxamine is administered I.V. during emergencies, supplemental doses may be given I.M. for prolonged effect.
- Avoid rapid administration of methoxamine because it produces added stress on the myocardium from markedly increased peripheral resistance during a reduction in stroke volume and cardiac output.
- Monitor cardiac rhythm and blood pressure carefully during therapy. Blood pressure should be increased to slightly less than patient's normal blood pressure. In previously normotensive patients, maintain systolic blood pressure at 80 to 100 mm Hg; in previously hypertensive patients, maintain systolic blood pressure at 30 to 40 mm Hg below usual blood pressure. Blood pressure should be checked frequently during methoxamine therapy, especially when the drug is given I.V. Patients receiving methoxamine by I.V. infusion should not be left unattended; the infusion flow rate must be closely monitored. When I.V. infusions are discontinued, the infusion rate should be decreased gradually. Avoid abrupt withdrawal.
- Methoxamine has also been used to produce vasoconstriction as an adjunct to correct hemodynamic imbalances in the treatment of shock that persists after adequate fluid volume replacement and (†) to raise blood pressure as an aid in the diagnosis of heart murmurs.

methoxsalen
Oxsoralen, Oxsoralen-Ultra

- Classification: pigmenting, antipsoriatic agent (psoralen derivative)

How supplied
Available by prescription only
Capsules: 10 mg
Lotion: 1%

Indications, route, and dosage
Induce repigmentation in vitiligo
Adults and children over age 12: 20 mg P.O. 2 to 4 hours before measured periods of sunlight or ultraviolet light exposive on alternate days. Alternatively, small well-defined lesions, apply lotion 1 to 2 hours before exposure to ultraviolet light, no more than once weekly.
Psoriasis
Adults: 10 to 70 mg P.O. 1.5 to 2 hours before exposure to high intensity ultraviolet A light, 2 to 3 times weekly, at least 48 hours apart. Dosage is based upon patient's weight.

Action and kinetics
- *Pigmenting action:* The exact mechanism of action of methoxsalen is not known; it is dependent on the presence of functioning melanocytes and UV light. Methoxsalen may stimulate the enzymes that catalyze melanin precursors. Also, the inflammatory response generated may stimulate melanin production.
- *Antipsoriatic action:* Methoxsalen probably exerts its antipsoriatic effects by inhibiting DNA synthesis and decreasing cell proliferation. Cell-regulating, leukocyte, and vascular effects may also be involved in this action.

The oral dosage form produces greater erythemic and melanogenic effects, while the topical preparation causes a more intense photosensitizing response.
- *Kinetics in adults:* After oral administration, methoxsalen is absorbed well but variably, with peak serum concentrations in 1½ to 3 hours. Food increases both absorption and peak concentration. The extent of topical absorption has not been determined. Skin sensitivity to UV light occurs in about 1 to 2 hours, reaches a maximum effect in 1 to 4 hours, and persists for 3 to 8 hours. Topical administration yields a UV sensitivity in 1 to 2 hours, which may persist for several days.

Methoxsalen is distributed throughout the body, with epidermal cells preferentially taking up the drug. It is 75% to 91% bound to serum proteins, most commonly albumin. Distribution across the placenta or in breast milk is unknown.

Drug is activated by long-wavelength UV light and is metabolized in the liver. It is excreted almost entirely as metabolites in the urine, with 80% to 90% eliminated within the first 8 hours.

---

‡May contain sulfites   ◆May contain tartrazine   ◆◆May contain benzyl alcohol

Contraindications and precautions

Methoxsalen is contraindicated in patients hypersensitive to psoralens and in those with diseases associated with photosensitivity because of the drug's photosensitization. Do not use in patients with melanoma, history of melanoma, or invasive squamous cell carcinoma, because the drug may be a photocarcinogen. Oral methoxsalen is contraindicated in patients with aphakia, because increased retinal damage may occur.

Oxsoralen capsules contain tartarazine; therefore, use cautiously in patients with tartrazine or asprin sensitivity.

Interactions

Methoxsalen reacts with other photosensitizing drugs and foods including sulfonamides, tetracyclines, phenothiazines, thiazides, griseofulvin, nalidixic acid, trioxsalen, and coal tar products to yield an additive photosensitizing effect. The ingestion of foods such as carrots, limes, figs, celery, mustard, parsley, and parsnips should be avoided. These foods contain furocoumarin, which may cause an additive effect. No serious reactions have been reported with these foods, but caution should be exercised.

Effects on diagnostic tests

Abnormal liver function test results have been reported, but the exact relationship is unknown.

Adverse reactions

• CNS: dizziness, headache, depression, nervousness, trouble sleeping.
• DERM: blistering, peeling, swelling of extremities, itching, erythema, photosensitivity.
• GI: nausea, abdominal discomfort, diarrhea.
• Other: cataracts, toxic hepatitis, leg cramps.
   Note: Drug should be discontinued if signs of overexposure to sunlight occur.

Overdose and treatment

Clinical manifestations of overdose include serious burning and blistering of skin, which may occur from overdose of drug or overexposure to UV light. Treat acute oral overdose with gastric lavage, which, however, is effective only in the first 2 to 3 hours. Place patient in a darkened room for 8 to 24 hours or until cutaneous reactions subside. Treat burns as necessary.

▶ Special considerations

• Use in children under age 12 is not recommended.
• Wear gloves when applying lotion.
• Temporary withdrawal of therapy is the recommended procedure in case of burning or blistering of the skin.

Information for parents and patient

• Teach parents and patient how and when to use product; tell patient to wear gloves to avoid photosensitization and possible burns. Stress adherence to correct dosage schedule. If a dose is missed, patient should not increase the next dose. If more than one dose is missed, a proportionately lower dose should be given when therapy is resumed.

• Advise taking with food and milk to reduce GI irritation and, possibly, increase absorption.
• Advise protective precautions, including sunglasses and sunscreens. However, sunscreens may be only partially effective. Patient should protect skin for 8 hours after oral administration.
• Explain that drug may take several months to work. Tell parents and patient *not* to increase the dose or UV light exposure during this time.

methsuximide
Celontin Kapseals, Celontin Half Strength Kapseals

• Classification: anticonvulsant (succinimide derivative)

How supplied

Available by prescription only
Capsules: 150 mg, 300 mg

Indications, route, and dosage
Refractory absence (petit mal) seizures

Children and adults: Initially, 300 mg P.O. daily; may increase by 300 mg weekly. Maximum daily dosage is 1.2 g in divided doses.

Action and kinetics

• *Anticonvulsant action:* Methsuximide raises the seizure threshold; it suppresses characteristic spike-and-wave pattern by depressing neuronal transmission in the motor cortex and basal ganglia. It is indicated for absence (petit mal) seizures refractory to other drugs.
• *Kinetics in adults:* Methsuximide is absorbed from the GI tract; peak plasma concentrations occur in 1 to 4 hours. Methsuximide is distributed widely throughout the body. Therapeutic plasma concentration levels appear to be 10 to 40 mcg/ml. Methsuximide is metabolized in the liver to several metabolites; N-demethyl methsuximide is a potent CNS depressant and may be the active metabolite. Methsuximide is excreted in urine.

Contraindications and precautions

Methsuximide is contraindicated in patients with known hypersensitivity to succinimides; and in patients with mixed forms of epilepsy, because it may precipitate grand mal seizures.

Methsuximide should be used with caution in patients with hepatic or renal disease and in patients taking other CNS depressants or anticonvulsants. Abrupt withdrawal may precipitate petit mal seizures. Use of anticonvulsants during pregnancy has been associated with increased incidence of birth defects.

Interactions

Concomitant use of methsuximide with other CNS depressants (alcohol, narcotics, anxiolytics, antidepressants, antipsychotics, and other anticonvulsants) causes additive sedative and CNS depressant effects.

Effects on diagnostic tests

Methsuximide may elevate liver enzymes and cause abnormal renal function test results.

Adverse reactions

• CNS: *drowsiness, ataxia, dizziness, irritability, nervousness, headache, insomnia, confusion, depression, aggressiveness, psychosis.*
• DERM: urticaria, pruritic and erythematous rashes, Stevens-Johnson syndrome, systemic lupus erythematosus.
• EENT: blurred vision, photophobia, periorbital edema.
• GI: *nausea, vomiting, anorexia, diarrhea,* weight loss, abdominal or epigastric pain, constipation.
• HEMA: *eosinophilia, leukopenia, monocytosis, pancytopenia.*
   Note: Drug should be discontinued if signs of hypersensitivity, rash or unusual skin lesions, or any of the following signs of blood dyscrasia occur: joint pain, fever, sore throat, or unusual bleeding or bruising.

Overdose and treatment

Symptoms of overdose may include dizziness and ataxia (beginning within 1 hour after overdose); condition may progress to stupor and coma.

   Treat overdose supportively. Monitor vital signs and fluid and electrolyte balance carefully. Charcoal hemo-perfusion or hemodialysis may be used for severe cases. Contact local or regional poison control center for more information.

▶ Special considerations

• Methsuximide may be hemodialyzable. Dosage adjustments may be necessary in patients undergoing hemodialysis.
• Never change or withdraw drug suddenly. Abrupt withdrawal may precipitate petit mal seizures.
• Obtain CBC every 3 months; urinalysis and liver function tests every 6 months.
• Protect capsules from excessive heat (104° F. or 40° C.).
• Drug produces greater renal and hepatic toxicity than ethosuximide.
• Observe patient closely for dermatologic reactions at initiation of therapy.
• Monitor closely for signs of hypersensitivity or adverse reactions: skin rash, sore throat, joint pain, unexplained fever, or unusual bleeding or bruising.
• Drug should not be discontinued abruptly.
• Drug adds to CNS depressant effects of alcohol, narcotics, anxiolytics, antidepressants, and tranquilizers.

Information for parents and patient

• Advise storing drug away from excessive heat and humidity to maintain effectiveness of drug.
• Warn parents that patient should avoid activities that require alertness and good psychomotor coordination until CNS response to drug has been determined.
• Tell parents that patient should not use alcohol while taking drug; it may decrease drug's effectiveness and increase CNS adverse effects.

• Tell patient to take oral drug with food if GI distress occurs.
• Teach parents and patient signs and symptoms of hypersensitivity, liver dysfunction, and blood dyscrasias, and advise patient to report them promptly.
• Explain to parents of adolescents the importance of reporting suspected pregnancy immediately.
• Warn parents and patient never to discontinue drug or to change dosage without medical approval.
• Encourage parents to have patient wear a Medic Alert bracelet or necklace, listing drug and seizure disorder.

methyclothiazide
Aquatensen, Enduron, Ethon

• Classification: diuretic, antihypertensive (thiazide)

How supplied

Available by prescription only
Tablets: 2.5 mg, 5 mg

Indications, route, and dosage
Edema, hypertension

Children: 0.05 to 0.2 mg/kg or 1.5 to 6 mg/m² P.O. daily in a single dose.
Adults: 2.5 to 10 mg P.O daily.

Action and kinetics

• *Diuretic action:* Methyclothiazide increases urinary excretion of sodium and water by inhibiting sodium reabsorption in the cortical diluting tubule of the nephron, thus relieving edema.
• *Antihypertensive action:* The exact mechanism of methyclothiazide's antihypertensive effect is unknown. It may partially result from direct arteriolar vasodilatation and a decrease in total peripheral resistance.
• *Kinetics in adults:* Methyclothiazide is absorbed rapidly from the GI tract. Methyclothiazide is thought to be distributed into extracellular space and is excreted unchanged in urine.

Contraindications and precautions

Methyclothiazide is contraindicated in patients with anuria and in those with known sensitivity to the drug or to other sulfonamide derivatives. Methyclothiazide should be used with caution in patients with severe renal disease, because it may decrease glomerular filtration rate and precipitate azotemia; in patients with impaired hepatic function or liver disease, because electrolyte changes may precipitate coma; and in patients taking digoxin, because hypokalemia may predispose them to digitalis toxicity.

Interactions

Methyclothiazide potentiates the hypotensive effects of most other antihypertensive drugs; this may be used to therapeutic advantage.

   Methyclothiazide may potentiate hyperglycemic, hypotensive, and hyperuricemic effects of diazoxide, and its hyperglycemic effect may increase insulin requirements in diabetic patients.

Methyclothiazide may reduce renal clearance of lithium, elevating serum lithium levels, and may necessitate a 50% reduction in lithium dosage.

Methyclothiazide turns urine slightly more alkaline and may decrease urinary excretion of some amines, such as amphetamine and quinidine; alkaline urine may also decrease therapeutic efficacy of methenamine compounds, such as methenamine mandelate.

Cholestyramine and colestipol may bind methyclothiazide, preventing its absorption; give drugs 1 hour apart.

Effects on diagnostic tests

Methyclothiazide therapy may alter serum electrolyte levels and may increase serum urate, glucose, cholesterol, and triglyceride levels. It also may interfere with tests for parathyroid function and should be discontinued before such tests.

Adverse reactions

• CV: volume depletion and dehydration, orthostatic hypotension, hypercholesterolemia, hypertriglyceridemia.
• DERM: dermatitis, photosensitivity.
• GI: anorexia, nausea, pancreatitis.
• HEMA: aplastic anemia, agranulocytosis, leukopenia, thrombocytopenia.
• Hepatic: hepatic encephalopathy.
• Metabolic: asymptomatic hyperuricemia; gout; hyperglycemia and impairment of glucose tolerance; fluid and electrolyte imbalances, including dilutional hyponatremia and hypochloremia, hypokalemia, and hypercalcemia; metabolic alkalosis.
• Other: hypersensitivity reactions, such as pneumonitis and vasculitis.

Note: Drug should be discontinued if rising BUN and serum creatinine levels indicate renal impairment or if patient shows signs of impending coma.

Overdose and treatment

Clinical signs of overdose include GI irritation, hypermotility, diuresis, and lethargy, which may progress to coma.

Treatment is mainly supportive; monitor and assist respiratory, cardiovascular, and renal function as indicated. Monitor fluid and electrolyte balance. Induce vomiting with ipecac in conscious patient; otherwise, use gastric lavage to avoid aspiration. Do not give cathartics; these promote additional loss of fluids and electrolytes.

▶ Special considerations

• Monitor weight and serum electrolyte levels regularly.
• Monitor serum potassium levels; encourage high-potassium diet. Foods rich in potassium include citrus fruits, tomatoes, bananas, dates, and apricots. Watch for signs of hypokalemia (for example, muscle weakness or cramps). Patients also taking digitalis have an increased risk of digitalis toxicity from the potassium-depleting effect of the drug.

• Methyclothiazide may be used with potassium-sparing diuretics to attenuate potassium loss.
• Check insulin requirements in patients with diabetes.
• Monitor serum creatinine and BUN levels regularly. Drug is not as effective if these levels are more than twice normal.
• Monitor blood uric acid levels.
• A.M. administration is recommended to prevent nocturia.
• Antihypertensive effects persist for approximately 1 week after discontinuation of the drug.
• Instruct parents to observe and to report any joint swelling, pain, or redness; these signs may indicate hyperuricemia.

Information for parents and patient

• Explain rationale of therapy and diuretic effects of drug.
• Advise parents to watch for and promptly report signs of electrolyte imbalance: weakness, fatigue, muscle cramps, paresthesias, confusion, nausea, vomiting, diarrhea, headache, dizziness, and palpitations.
• Tell parents to report any increased edema or weight or excess diuresis (more than 2%); advise parents to record child's weight each morning after voiding and before breakfast on the same scale and wearing the same type of clothing.
• Advise parents to give drug with food to minimize gastric irritation; to encourage child to eat potassium-rich foods, such as citrus fruits, potatoes, dates, raisins, and bananas; and to restrict child's access to salt and high-sodium foods, such as lunch meat, smoked meats, and processed cheeses.
• Tell parents to seek medical approval before giving patient nonprescription drugs; many contain sodium and potassium and can cause electrolyte imbalances.
• Explain photosensitivity reactions. In thiazide-related photosensitivity, ultraviolet radiation alters drug structure, causing allergic reactions in some persons; such reactions occur 10 days to 2 weeks after initial sun exposure.
• Warn parents to supervise the child's activities closely to prevent falls and other injuries that may result from dizziness, especially at beginning of therapy.
• Caution patient to change position slowly, especially when rising to upright position, to prevent dizziness from orthostatic hypotension.
• Advise parents to watch patient closely for chest, back, or leg pain or shortness of breath and to call immediately if they occur.
• Advise parents to administer drug only as prescribed and at the same time each day, to prevent nighttime diuresis and interrupted sleep.
• Emphasize importance of regular medical follow-up to monitor effectiveness of diuretic therapy.

methyldopa
Aldomet, Amodopa Tabs, Apo-
Methyldopa*, Dopamet*,
Novomedopa*

- Classification: antihypertensive (centrally acting antiadrenergic agent)

How supplied
Available by prescription only
Tablets: 125 mg, 250 mg, 500 mg
Oral suspension: 250 mg/5 ml
Injection (as methyldopate hydrochloride): 250 mg/5 ml in 5-ml vials

Indications, route, and dosage
Moderate to severe hypertension
Children: Initially, 10 mg/kg P.O. daily or 300 mg/m² P.O. daily in two to four divided doses; or 20 to 40 mg/kg I.V. daily or 0.6 to 1.2 g/m² I.V. daily in four divided doses. Increase dosage at least every 2 days until desired response occurs. Maximum daily dosage is 65 mg/kg, 2 g/m², or 3 g, whichever is least.
Adults: Initially, 250 mg P.O. b.i.d. or t.i.d. in first 48 hours, then increased or decreased as needed every 2 days. Entire daily dose may be given in the evening or at bedtime. Dosages may need adjustment if other antihypertensive drugs are added to or deleted from therapy.
Maintenance dosage: 500 mg to 2 g daily in two to four divided doses. Maximum recommended daily dosage is 3 g. I.V. infusion dosage is 250 to 500 mg given over 30 to 60 minutes q 6 hours. Maximum I.V. dosage is 1 g q 6 hours.

Action and kinetics
- *Antihypertensive action:* The exact mechanism of methyldopa's antihypertensive effect is unknown; it is thought to be caused by methyldopa's metabolite, alpha-methylnorepinephrine, which stimulates central inhibitory alpha-adrenergic receptors, decreasing total peripheral resistance; drug may also act as a false neurotransmitter.
- *Kinetics in adults:* Methyldopa is absorbed partially from the GI tract. Absorption varies, but usually about 50% of an oral dose is absorbed. After oral administration, maximal decline in blood pressure occurs in 3 to 6 hours; however, full effect is not evident for 2 to 3 days. No correlation exists between plasma concentration and antihypertensive effect. After I.V. administration, blood pressure usually begins to fall in 4 to 6 hours. Methyldopa is distributed throughout the body and is bound weakly to plasma proteins. Methyldopa is metabolized extensively in the liver and intestinal cells. The drug and its metabolites are excreted in urine; unabsorbed drug is excreted unchanged in feces. Elimination half-life is approximately 2 hours. Antihypertensive activity usually persists up to 24 hours after oral administration and 10 to 16 hours after I.V. administration.

Contraindications and precautions
Methyldopa is contraindicated in patients with known hypersensitivity to the drug and in patients with active hepatic disease, such as hepatitis or cirrhosis. Drug is also contraindicated in patients who developed hepatic dysfunction during previous methyldopa therapy; such patients may have impaired drug metabolism and may be predisposed to methyldopa-induced hepatic dysfunction.

Methyldopa should be used cautiously in patients taking diuretics and other antihypertensive drugs; in patients with renal failure, because accumulation of active metabolites may lead to prolonged hypotension; in patients with previous hepatic dysfunction, who may be predisposed to methyldopa-induced hepatic dysfunction; and in patients taking levodopa, because an additive antihypertensive effect may occur.

Interactions
Methyldopa may potentiate the antihypertensive effects of other antihypertensive agents and the pressor effects of sympathomimetic amines, such as phenylpropanolamine.

Concomitant use with phenothiazines or tricyclic antidepressants may cause a reduction in antihypertensive effects; use with haloperidol may produce dementia and sedation; use with phenoxybenzamine may cause reversible urinary incontinence.

Fenfluramine and verapamil may potentiate the effects of methyldopa.

Methyldopa may impair tolbutamide metabolism, enhancing tolbutamide's hypoglycemic effect.

Patients undergoing surgery may require reduced dosages of anesthetics.

Effects on diagnostic tests
Methyldopa alters urine uric acid, serum creatinine, and AST (SGOT) levels; it may also cause falsely high levels of urine catecholamines, interfering with the diagnosis of pheochromocytoma. A positive direct antiglobulin (Coombs') test may also occur.

Adverse reactions
- CNS: sedation, headache, weakness, dizziness, decreased mental acuity, involuntary choreoathetoid movements, psychic disturbances, depression, nightmares, *sedation.*
- CV: bradycardia, orthostatic hypotension, aggravated angina, myocarditis, edema, weight gain.
- EENT: dry mouth, nasal stuffiness.
- GI: diarrhea, pancreatitis, *GI upset.*
- HEMA: *hemolytic anemia,* reversible granulocytopenia, thrombocytopenia, *leukopenia.*
- Hepatic: hepatic necrosis (rare), abnormal liver function test results.
- Other: gynecomastia, lactation, rash, drug-induced *fever,* impotence.

Note: Drug should be discontinued if any of the following occur: abnormalities in liver function tests results, jaundice, positive Coombs' test, or choreoathetoid movements.

Overdose and treatment
Clinical signs of overdose include sedation, hypotension, impaired atrioventricular conduction, and coma.

After recent (within 4 hours) ingestion, empty stomach by induced emesis or gastric lavage. Give activated charcoal to reduce absorption; then treat symptomatically and supportively. In severe cases, hemodialysis may be considered.

▶ **Special considerations**
• Patients with impaired renal function may require smaller maintenance dosages of the drug.
• Methyldopate hydrochloride is administered I.V.; I.M. or S.C. administration is not recommended because of unpredictable absorption.
• Patients receiving methyldopa may become hypertensive after dialysis because drug is dialyzable.
• At the initiation of, and periodically throughout therapy, monitor hemoglobin, hematocrit, and RBC count for hemolytic anemia; also monitor liver function tests.
• Take blood pressure in supine, sitting, and standing positions during dosage adjustment; take blood pressure at least every 30 minutes during I.V. infusion until patient is stable.
• Sedation and drowsiness usually disappear with continued therapy; bedtime dosage will minimize this effect. Orthostatic hypotension may indicate a need for dosage reduction.
• Monitor intake and output and daily weight to detect sodium and water retention; voided urine exposed to air may darken because of the breakdown of methyldopa or its metabolites.
• Tolerance may develop after 2 to 3 weeks.
• Signs of hepatotoxicity may occur 2 to 4 weeks after therapy begins.
• Monitor for signs and symptoms of drug-induced depression.

Information for parents and patient
• Teach parents and patient signs and symptoms of adverse effects, such as "jerky" movements, and about the need to report them; parents should also report excessive weight gain (5 lb [2.25 kg] or more per week), signs of infection, or fever.
• Teach parents that patient can minimize adverse effects by taking drug at bedtime until tolerance develops to sedation, drowsiness, and other CNS effects; by avoiding sudden position changes to minimize orthostatic hypotension; and by using ice chips, hard candy, or gum to relieve dry mouth.
• Warn parents that patient should avoid hazardous activities that require mental alertness until sedative effects subside.
• Warn parents to call for instructions before giving patient nonprescription cold preparations.

methylphenidate hydrochloride
Methidate, Ritalin, Ritalin SR

• Classification: CNS stimulant (analeptic [piperidine CNS stimulant])
• Controlled substance schedule II

How supplied
Available by prescription only
Tablets: 5 mg, 10 mg, 20 mg
Tablets (sustained-release): 20 mg

Indications, route, and dosage
Attention deficit disorder with hyperactivity (ADDH)
Children age 6 and older: Initially, 5 to 10 mg P.O. daily before breakfast and lunch, with 5- to 10-mg increments weekly as needed until an optimum daily dosage of 2 mg/kg is reached, not to exceed 60 mg/day. The usual effective dosage is 10 to 20 mg/day.
Narcolepsy
Children age 6 and older and adults: 10 mg P.O. b.i.d. or t.i.d., ½ hour before meals. Dosage varies with patient needs, ranging from 5 mg to 60 mg daily.

Action and kinetics
• *Analeptic action:* The cerebral cortex and reticular activating system appear to be the primary sites of activity; methylphenidate releases nerve terminal stores of norepinephrine, promoting nerve impulse transmission. At high doses, effects are mediated by dopamine.
    Methylphenidate is used to treat narcolepsy and as an adjunctive to psychosocial measures in ADDH. Like amphetamine, it has a paradoxical calming effect in hyperactive children.
• *Kinetics in adults:* Methylphenidate is absorbed rapidly and completely after oral administration; peak plasma concentrations occur at 1 to 2 hours. Duration of action is usually 4 to 6 hours (with considerable individual variation); sustained-release tablets may act for up to 8 hours.
    The distribution of methylphenidate is unknown. Methylphenidate is metabolized by the liver and is excreted in urine.

Contraindications and precautions
Methylphenidate is contraindicated in patients with known hypersensitivity to sympathomimetic amines; in patients with symptomatic cardiovascular disease, hyperthyroidism, angina pectoris, moderate to severe hypertension, or advanced arteriosclerosis because it may cause dangerous dysrhythmias and blood pressure changes; in patients with severe exogenous or endogenous depression, glaucoma, parkinsonism, or agitated states; in patients with a history of marked anxiety, tension, or agitation because it can exacerbate such conditions; or in patients with a history of substance abuse.
    Methylphenidate should be used with caution in patients with a history of diabetes mellitus, cardiovascular disease, motor tics, seizures, or Gilles de la

Tourette's syndrome (drug may precipitate disorder); and in elderly, debilitated or hyperexcitable patients.

Interactions

Concomitant use with caffeine may decrease efficacy of methylphenidate in ADDH; use with monoamine oxidase (MAO) inhibitors (or drugs with MAO-inhibiting activity) or within 14 days of such therapy may cause severe hypertension.

Methylphenidate may inhibit metabolism and increase the serum levels of anticonvulsants (phenytoin, phenobarbital, primidone), coumarin anticoagulants, phenylbutazone, and tricyclic antidepressants; it also may decrease the hypotensive effects of guanethidine and bretylium.

Effects on diagnostic tests

None reported.

Adverse reactions

• CNS: *nervousness, insomnia*, dizziness, headache, akathisia, dyskinesia, *Gilles de la Tourette's syndrome, seizures*.
• CV: palpitations, angina, tachycardia, *changes in blood pressure* and pulse rate, dysrhythmias.
• EENT: difficulty with accommodation, blurring of vision.
• GI: nausea, dry throat, abdominal pain, anorexia, weight loss.
• Skin: rash, urticaria, exfoliative dermatitis, erythema multiforme.
• Other: *growth suppression, altered insulin requirements*.
Note: Drug should be discontinued if signs of hypersensitivity or seizures occur or if no improvement is noticed within 1 month at maintenance dosage level.

Overdose and treatment

Symptoms of overdose may include euphoria, confusion, delirium, coma, toxic psychosis, agitation, headache, vomiting, dry mouth, mydriasis, self-injury, fever, diaphoresis, tremors, hyperreflexia, muscle twitching, seizures, flushing, hypertension, tachycardia, palpitations, and dysrhythmias.

Treat overdose symptomatically and supportively: use gastric lavage or emesis in patients with intact gag reflex. Closely monitor vital signs and fluid and electrolyte balance. Maintain patient in cool room, monitor temperature, minimize external stimulation, and protect him against self-injury. External cooling blankets may be needed.

▶ Special considerations

• Methylphenidate is the drug of choice for ADDH. Therapy is usually discontinued after puberty.
• Methylphenidate is not recommended for ADDH in children under age 6. Drug has been associated with growth suppression; all patients should be monitored.
• Monitor initiation of therapy closely; drug may precipitate Gilles de la Tourette's syndrome.
• Check vital signs regularly for increased blood pressure or other signs of excessive stimulation; avoid late-day or evening dosing, especially of long-acting dosage forms, to minimize insomnia.

• Monitor blood and urine glucose levels in diabetic patients; drug may alter insulin requirements.
• Drug may decrease seizure threshold in seizure disorders.
• Monitor complete blood count, differential, and platelet counts when patient is taking drug long-term.
• Intermittent drug-free periods when stress is least evident (weekends, school holidays) may help prevent development of tolerance and permit decreased dosage when drug is resumed. Sustained-release form allows convenience of single, at-home dosing for school children.
• Abrupt withdrawal may unmask severe depression; after long-term use, lower dosage gradually to prevent acute rebound depression.
• Methylphenidate impairs ability to perform tasks requiring mental alertness.
• Be sure patient obtains adequate rest; fatigue may result as drug wears off.
• Regularly monitor height and weight; drug has been associated with growth suppression, which is reversible when drug is discontinued.

Information for parents and patient

• Explain rationale for therapy and the potential risks and benefits.
• Tell patient to avoid drinks containing caffeine to prevent added CNS stimulation and not to alter dosage unless prescribed.
• Advise parents of ADDH patient to give last dose early in the day to avoid insomnia.
• Tell patient not to chew or crush sustained-release dosage forms.
• Warn patient not to use drug to mask fatigue, to be sure to obtain adequate rest, and to call if excessive CNS stimulation occurs.
• Advise diabetic patients to monitor blood glucose levels, as drug may alter insulin needs.
• Advise patient to avoid hazardous activities that require mental alertness until degree of sedative effect is determined.

methylprednisolone
Systemic: Medrol, Medrone★

methylprednisolone acetate
Systemic: dep-Medalone, Depoject, Depo-Medrone★, Depo-Medrol, Depopred, Depo-Predate, Duralone, Durameth, Medralone, Medrone, M-Prednisol, Rep-Pred

Topical: Medrol

methylprednisolone sodium succinate
Systemic: A-methaPred, Solu-Medrane★, Solu-Medrol

• Classification: anti-inflammatory, immunosuppressant (glucocorticoid)

How supplied
Available by prescription only
Methylprednisolone
Tablets: 2 mg, 4 mg, 8 mg, 16 mg, 24 mg, 32 mg
Methylprednisolone acetate
Injection: 20 mg/ml, 40 mg/ml, 80 mg/ml suspension
Ointment: 0.25%, 1%
Methylprednisolone sodium succinate
Injection: 40 mg, 125 mg, 500 mg, 1,000 mg, 2,000 mg/vial

Indications, route, and dosage
Severe inflammation or immunosuppression
Children: 117 mcg/kg/day to 1.66 mg/kg/day P.O. in three or four divided doses. Alternatively (pulse therapy), 30 mg/kg I.V. as a single dose, or 10 mg/kg I.V. daily for 6 days, or 15 to 30 mg/kg or 600 mg/m² daily for 3 days.
Adults: 4 to 48 mg P.O. daily in a single dose or in divided doses.
Methylprednisolone acetate
Children: 117 mcg/kg I.M. q 3 days; or 140 to 835 mcg/kg I.M. q 12 to 24 hours.
Adults: 10 to 80 mg I.M. daily; or 4 to 80 mg into joints and soft tissue p.r.n. q 1 to 5 weeks; or 20 to 60 mg intralesionally.
Inflammation of corticosteroid-responsive dermatoses
Children: Apply sparingly to affected area once or twice a day.
Adults: Apply ointment sparingly in a thin film once daily to q.i.d. (Occlusive dressings may be used for severe or resistant dermatoses.) Rub gently into affected area.
Severe asthma
Methylprednisolone sodium succinate
Children: 1 to 2 mg/kg I.V.; then 1 to 2 mg/kg daily divided q 6 hours.
Adults: 10 to 250 mg I.M. or I.V. q 4 hours.

Action and kinetics
• *Anti-inflammatory action:* Methylprednisolone stimulates the synthesis of enzymes needed to decrease the inflammatory response. It suppresses the immune system by reducing activity and volume of the lymphatic system, thus producing lymphocytopenia (primarily of T-lymphocytes), decreasing immunoglobulin and complement concentrations, decreasing passage of immune complexes through basement membranes, and possibly by depressing reactivity of tissue to antigen-antibody interactions.

Methylprednisolone is an intermediate-acting glucocorticoid. It has essentially no mineralocorticoid activity but is a potent glucocorticoid, with five times the potency of an equal weight of hydrocortisone. It is used primarily as an anti-inflammatory agent and immunosuppressant.

Methylprednisolone may be administered orally. Methylprednisolone sodium succinate may be administered by I.M. or I.V. injection or by I.V. infusion, usually at 4- to 6-hour intervals. Methylprednisolone acetate suspension may be administered by intra-articular, intrasynovial, intrabursal, intralesional, or soft tissue injection. It has a slow onset but a long duration of action. The injectable forms are usually used only when the oral dosage forms cannot be used. Topical methylprednisolone ointment is classified as a group VI potency corticosteroid.
• *Kinetics in adults:* Methylprednisolone is absorbed readily after oral administration. After oral and I.V. administration, peak effects occur in about 1 to 2 hours. The acetate suspension for injection has a variable absorption over 24 to 48 hours, depending on whether it is injected into an intra-articular space or a muscle, and on the blood supply to that muscle.

Absorption after topical application depends on concentration, the amount applied, and the application site. It ranges from about 1% in areas with a thick stratum corneum (such as the palms, soles, elbows, and knees) to as high as 36% in areas of the thinnest stratum corneum (face, eyelids, and genitals). Absorption increases in areas that are damaged, inflamed, or under occlusion. Some systemic absorption of topical steroids occurs, especially through the oral mucosa.

Methylprednisolone is distributed rapidly to muscle, liver, skin, intestines, and kidneys. After topical application, methylprednisolone is distributed throughout the local skin and metabolized primarily locally. Any drug absorbed is distributed rapidly into muscle, liver, skin, intestines, and kidneys, and metabolized primarily in the liver to inactive compounds. Inactive metabolites are excreted by the kidneys, primarily as glucuronides and sulfates, but also as unconjugated products. Small amounts of the metabolites are also excreted in feces. The biological half-life of methylprednisolone is 18 to 36 hours.

Contraindications and precautions
Methylprednisolone is contraindicated in patients with hypersensitivity to ingredients of adrenocorticoid preparations and in patients with systemic fungal infections (except in adrenal insufficiency); topical use is contraindicated in those with viral, fungal, or tubercular skin lesions. Patients who are receiving

methylprednisolone should not be given live virus vaccines because methylprednisolone suppresses the immune response.

Methylprednisolone should be used with extreme caution in patients with GI ulceration, renal disease, hypertension, osteoporosis, diabetes mellitus, thromboembolic disorders, seizures, myasthenia gravis, CHF, tuberculosis, hypoalbuminemia, hypothyroidism, cirrhosis of the liver, emotional instability, psychotic tendencies, hyperlipidemias, glaucoma, or cataracts, because the drug may exacerbate these conditions. Topical forms should be used with extreme caution in patients with impaired circulation because it may increase the risk of skin ulceration.

Because adrenocorticoids increase the susceptibility to and mask symptoms of infection, methylprednisolone should not be used (except in life-threatening situations) in patients with viral or bacterial infections not controlled by anti-infective agents.

Interactions

When used concomitantly, adrenocorticoids may decrease the effects of oral anticoagulants by unknown mechanisms.

Glucocorticoids increase the metabolism of isoniazid and salicylates; cause hyperglycemia, requiring dosage adjustment of insulin in diabetic patients; and may enhance hypokalemia associated with diuretic or amphotericin B therapy. The hypokalemia may increase the risk of toxicity in patients concurrently receiving digitalis glycosides.

Barbiturates, phenytoin, and rifampin may cause decreased corticosteroid effects because of increased hepatic metabolism. Cholestyramine, colestipol, and antacids decrease the corticosteroid effect by adsorbing the corticosteroid, decreasing the amount absorbed.

Concomitant use with estrogens may reduce the metabolism of corticosteroids by increasing the concentration of transcortin. The half-life of the corticosteroid is then prolonged because of increased protein binding. Concomitant administration of ulcerogenic drugs such as nonsteroidal anti-inflammatory agents may increase the risk of GI ulceration.

Effects on diagnostic tests

Methylprednisolone suppresses reactions to skin tests; causes false-negative results in the nitroblue tetrazolium test for systemic bacterial infections; decreases ^{131}I uptake and protein-bound iodine concentrations in thyroid function tests; may increase glucose and cholesterol levels; may decrease serum potassium, calcium, thyroxine, and triiodothyronine levels; and may increase urine glucose and calcium levels.

Adverse reactions

When administered in high doses or for prolonged therapy, methylprednisolone suppresses release of adrenocorticotropic hormone (ACTH) from the pituitary gland; in turn, the adrenal cortex stops secreting endogenous corticosteroids. The degree and duration of hypothalamic-pituitary-adrenal (HPA) axis suppression produced by the drug is highly variable among patients and depends on the dose, frequency and time of administration, and duration of glucocorticoid therapy.

• CNS: euphoria, insomnia, headache, psychotic behavior, pseudotumor cerebri, mental changes, nervousness, restlessness, *psychoses*.
• CV: CHF, *hypertension*, edema.
• DERM: delayed healing, *acne*, skin eruptions, striae.
• EENT: *cataracts*, glaucoma, thrush.
• GI: *peptic ulcer*, irritation, increased appetite.
• Immune: immunosuppression, *increased susceptibility to infection*.
• Metabolic: *hypokalemia*, sodium retention, fluid retention, weight gain, hyperglycemia, *osteoporosis*, growth suppression in children, *glycosuria*.
• Musculoskeletal: muscle atrophy, weakness, *myopathy*.
• Local: burning, itching, irritation, dryness, folliculitis, hypertrichosis, acneiform eruptions, hypopigmentation, perioral dermatitis, allergic contact dermatitis, maceration, secondary infection, atrophy, striae, miliaria.
• Other: pancreatitis, *hirsutism, cushingoid symptoms*, withdrawal syndrome (nausea, fatigue, anorexia, dyspnea, hypotension, hypoglycemia, myalgia, arthralgia, fever, dizziness, and fainting), *ecchymoses*. Sudden withdrawal may be fatal or may exacerbate the underlying disease. Acute adrenal insufficiency may occur with increased stress (infection, surgery, trauma) or abrupt withdrawal after long-term therapy. Topical application should be discontinued if local irritation, infection, systemic absorption, or hypersensitivity reaction occurs.

Overdose and treatment

Acute ingestion, even in massive doses, is rarely a clinical problem. Toxic signs and symptoms rarely occur if drug is used for less than 3 weeks, even at large doses. However, chronic use causes adverse physiologic effects, including suppression of the HPA axis, cushingoid appearance, muscle weakness, and osteoporosis.

▶ Special considerations

• Chronic use of adrenocorticoids in children and adolescents may delay growth and maturation.
• If possible, avoid long-term administration of pharmacologic dosages of glucocorticoids in children because these drugs may retard bone growth. Manifestations of adrenal suppression in children include retardation of linear growth, delayed weight gain, low plasma cortisol concentrations, and lack of response to corticotropin stimulation. In children who require prolonged therapy, closely monitor growth and development. Alternate-day therapy is recommended to minimize growth suppression.

Topical use

• Children may show greater susceptibilty to topical corticosteroid-induced HPA axis suppression and Cushing's syndrome than mature patients because of a higher ratio of skin surface area to body weight. Hypothalamic-pituitary-adrenal (HPA) axis suppression, Cushing's syndrome, and intracranial hypertension have been reported in children receiving topical corticosteroids. Signs of intracranial hypertension in-

---

‡May contain sulfites   ♦May contain tartrazine   ♦♦May contain benzyl alcohol

clude bulging fontanelles, headaches, and bilateral papilledema.
• Administration of topical corticosteroids to children should be limited to the least effective amount. Chronic corticosteroid therapy may interfere with growth and development.
• Stop drug if the patient develops signs of systemic absorption (including Cushing's syndrome, hyperglycemia, or glucosuria), skin irritation or ulceration, hypersensitivity, or infection. (If antifungals or antibiotics are being used with corticosteroids and the infection does not respond immediately, drug should be discontinued until infection is controlled.)
• Monitor patient response. Observe area of inflammation and elicit patient comments concerning pruritus. Inspect skin for infection, striae, and atrophy. Skin atrophy is common and may be clinically significant within 3 to 4 weeks of treatment with high-potency preparations; it also occurs more readily at sites where percutaneous absorption is high.
• Do not apply occlusive dressing over topical steroids because this may lead to secondary infection, maceration, atrophy, striae, or miliaria caused by increasing steroid penetration and potency.
• Establish baseline blood pressure, fluid intake and output, weight, and electrolyte status. Watch for any sudden patient weight gain, edema, change in blood pressure, or change in electrolyte status.
• During times of physiologic stress (trauma, surgery, infection), the patient may require additional steroids and may experience signs of steroid withdrawal; patients who were previously steroid-dependent may need systemic corticosteroids to prevent adrenal insufficiency.
• After long-term therapy, the drug should be reduced gradually. Acute withdrawal of drug may result in fever, myalgia, arthralgia, malaise, hypotension, or hypoglycemic shock.
• Be aware of the patient's psychological history and watch for any behavioral changes.
• Observe for signs of infection or delayed wound healing.

Information for parents and patient
• Be sure that the parents and patient understands the need to take methylprednisolone as prescribed. Give instructions on what to do if a dose is inadvertently missed.
• Patient may take drug with food or milk to minimize GI upset.
• Warn the parent and patient not to discontinue the drug abruptly or without medical approval, or to take any other medications without medical approval.
• Patient should reduce salt (sodium) intake and increase potassium intake.
• Inform the parents and patient of the possible therapeutic and adverse effects of the drug, so that they may report any complications promptly.
• Advise the parents that the patient should wear a Medic Alert bracelet or necklace indicating the need for supplemental adrenocorticoids during times of stress.
• Parents and patient should tell new physician or dentist that patient is taking this drug.

• Instruct parents and patient in application of the drug. Tell them the following:
Method for applying topical preparations
• Wash your hands before and after applying the drug. Gently cleanse the area of application. Washing or soaking the area before application may increase drug penetration. Then, apply sparingly in a light film; rub in lightly. Avoid contact with patient's eyes.
• Avoid prolonged application on the face, in skin folds, and in areas near the eyes, genitals and rectum. High-potency topical corticosteroids are more likely to cause striae in these areas because of their higher rates of absorption.
• If an occlusive dressing is necessary, minimize adverse reactions by using it intermittently. Do not leave it in place longer than 16 hours each day.
• Warn patient not to use nonprescription topical preparations other than those specifically recommended.
• Advise parents not to use tight-fitting diapers or plastic pants on a child being treated in the diaper area, because such garments may serve as occlusive dressing.

---

methyltestosterone
Android 5, Android 10, Android 25, Metandren, Metandren Linguets, Oreton-Methyl, Testred, Virilon

• Classification: androgen

How supplied
Available by prescription only
Tablets: 10 mg, 25 mg
Buccal tablets: 5 mg 10 mg
Capsules: 10 mg

Indications, route, and dosage
Delayed puberty in males
Adolescents: 5 to 25 mg P.O. daily (oral capsules) or 2.5 to 12.5 mg daily (buccal tablets) for up to 6 months.
Male hypogonadism
Adolescents and adults: 10 to 50 mg P.O. daily, or 5 to 25 mg buccal daily.
Postpubertal cryptorchidism
Adults: 30 mg P.O. daily, or 15 mg buccal daily.

Action and kinetics
• *Androgenic action:* Methyltestosterone mimics the action of the endogenous androgen testosterone by stimulating receptors in androgen-responsive organs and tissues. It exerts inhibitory, antiestrogenic effects on hormone-responsive breast tumors and metastases.
• *Kinetics in adults:* Methyltestosterone is eliminated primarily by hepatic metabolism. Its pharmacokinetics are otherwise poorly described.

Contraindications and precautions
Methyltestosterone is contraindicated in patients with known sensitivity to the drug; and in patients with severe renal or cardiac disease, which may be aggravated by fluid and electrolyte retention caused by this drug; in patients with hepatic disease because im-

---

paired elimination may cause toxic accumulation of drug; in male patients with prostatic or breast cancer or benign prostatic hypertrophy with obstruction because this drug can stimulate the growth of cancerous breast or prostate tissue in males; in pregnant and breast-feeding patients because administration of androgens during pregnancy causes masculinization of the fetus; and in patients with undiagnosed abnormal genital bleeding, as this drug can stimulate the growth of malignant neoplasms. Metandren 10 mg linguets and 25 mg tablets contain tartrazine which may cause allergic reactions in sensitive patients. Use with caution.

Interactions
In patients with diabetes, decreased blood glucose levels may require adjustment of insulin dosage.

Methyltestosterone may potentiate the effects of warfarin-type anticoagulants, resulting in increased prothrombin time. Use with adrenocorticosteroids or ACTH increases potential for fluid and electrolyte accumulation. Concurrent administration with oxyphenbutazone may increase serum oxyphenbutazone concentrations.

Effects on diagnostic tests
Methyltestosterone may cause abnormal results of fasting plasma glucose (FBS), glucose tolerance (GTT), and metyrapone tests. Sulfobromophthalein (BSP) retention may be increased. Thyroid function test results (protein-bound iodine, radioactive iodine uptake, thyroid-binding capacity) and 17-ketosteroid levels may decrease. Liver function test results, prothrombin time (especially in patients on anticoagulant therapy), and serum creatinine may be elevated. Because of this agent's anabolic activity, serum sodium, potassium, calcium, phosphate, and cholesterol levels may all rise.

Adverse reactions
• Androgenic: *in males:* prepubertal — premature epiphyseal closure, priapism, phallic enlargement; postpubertal — testicular atrophy, oligospermia, decreased ejaculatory volume, impotence, gynecomastia, epididymitis.
• CNS: headache, anxiety, mental depression, generalized paresthesia.
• CV: edema.
• DERM: acne, oily skin, hirsutism, flushing, sweating, male pattern baldness.
• GI: gastroenteritis, constipation, nausea, vomiting, diarrhea, change in appetite, weight gain.
• GU: bladder irritability.
• HEMA: polycythemia, suppression of clotting factors II, V, VII, and X.
• Hepatic: cholestatic hepatitis or jaundice.
• Local: irritation of oral mucosa with buccal administration.
• Other: hypercalcemia, hepatocellular cancer (long-term use).

Note: Drug should be discontinued if hypercalcemia, edema, hypersensitivity reaction, priapism, or excessive sexual stimulation occurs.

Overdose and treatment
No information available.

▶ Special considerations
• Children receiving androgens must be observed carefully for excessive virilization and precocious puberty. Androgen therapy may cause premature epiphyseal closure and short stature. Regular X-ray examinations of hand bones may be used to monitor skeletal maturation during therapy.
• Do not administer androgens to males with breast or prostatic cancer, or symptomatic hypertrophy; to patients with severe cardiac, renal, or hepatic disease; or to patients with undiagnosed abnormal genital bleeding.
• Hypercalcemia symptoms may be difficult to distinguish from symptoms of the condition being treated unless anticipated and thought of as a cluster.
• Priapism in males indicates that dosage is excessive. Serious acute toxicities from large overdoses have not been reported.
• Yellowing of the sclera of the eyes, or of the skin, may indicate hepatic dysfunction resulting from administration of androgens.
• Androgens do not improve athletic performance, but they are abused for this purpose by some athletes. Risks associated with their use for this purpose far outweigh any possible benefits.
• Observe for signs and symptoms of hypoglycemia in patients with diabetes, and for signs and symptoms of bleeding such as ecchymoses or petechiae in patients receiving oral anticoagulants.

Information parents and patient
• Tell parents and patient to promptly report GI upset, which may be caused by the drug.
• Tell patient to place buccal tablets in upper or lower buccal pouch between cheek and gum and to allow 30 to 60 minutes to dissolve. The patient should not eat, drink, or smoke until drug is absorbed; should not chew or swallow the tablets; and should change absorption site with each buccal dose to minimize risk of buccal irritation.
• Discuss side effects that alter body image.
• Tell parents and patient to report inflamed or painful oral membranes or any discomfort. Emphasize good oral hygiene.
• Advise parents to report patient's too frequent or persistent erections immediately.

---

metoclopramide hydrochloride
Clopra, Emex*, Maxeran*, Maxolon, Reclomide, Reglan

• Classification: antiemetic, gastrointestinal stimulant (para-aminobenzoic acid [PABA] derivative)

How supplied
Available by prescription only
Tablets: 5 mg, 10 mg
Syrup: 5 mg/5 ml
Injection: 5 mg/5 ml

Indications, route, and dosage
To prevent or reduce nausea and vomiting induced by cisplatin and other chemotherapy
Children: 1 mg/kg I.V. per dose for maximum four doses.
Adults: 2 mg/kg I.V. q 2 hours for 5 doses, beginning 30 minutes before cisplatin administration.
To facilitate small-bowel intubation and to aid in radiologic examinations
Children under age 6: 0.1 mg/kg I.V.
Children age 6 to 14: 2.5 to 5 mg I.V.
Adults: 10 mg I.V. as a single dose over 1 to 2 minutes.
Delayed gastric emptying secondary to diabetic gastroparesis
Adults: 10 mg P.O. 30 minutes before meals and h.s. for 2 to 8 weeks, depending on response.
† *Gastroesophageal reflux*
Children age 1 to 6: 0.1 mg/kg I.V. or P.O. q.i.d. 30 minutes before meals.
Children age 7 to 12: 2.5 to 9 mg I.V. or P.O. q.i.d. 30 minutes before meals.
Children over age 12 and adults: 10 to 15 mg P.O. q.i.d., p.r.n. Take 30 minutes before meals.

Action and kinetics
• *Antiemetic action:* Metoclopramide inhibits dopamine receptors in the brain's chemoreceptor trigger zone to inhibit or reduce nausea and vomiting.
• *Gastrointestinal stimulant action:* Metoclopramide relieves gastric stasis by increasing lower esophageal sphincter tone and stimulates motility of the upper GI tract, thus shortening gastric emptying time.
• *Kinetics in adults:* After oral administration, metoclopramide is absorbed rapidly and thoroughly from the G.I. tract; action begins in 30 to 60 minutes. After I.M. administration, about 74% to 96% of the drug is bioavailable; action begins in 10 to 15 minutes. After I.V. administration, onset of action occurs in 1 to 3 minutes. Metoclopramide is distributed to most body tissues and fluids, including the brain. It crosses the placenta and is distributed in breast milk. Drug is not metabolized extensively; a small amount is metabolized in the liver. Most metoclopramide is excreted in urine and feces. Hemodialysis and renal dialysis remove minimal amounts. Duration of effect is 1 to 2 hours.

Contraindications and precautions
Metoclopramide is contraindicated in patients with known hypersensitivity to the drug or to sulfonamides; in patients with pheochromocytoma because it may induce hypertensive crisis; and in patients with seizure disorders, renal failure, liver failure, Parkinson's disease, GI hemorrhage, or intestinal obstruction or perforation, because the drug may exacerbate symptoms of these disorders.
Metoclopramide should be used cautiously in children because they may have a higher incidence of CNS adverse effects and in patients with a history of breast cancer because the drug stimulates prolactin secretion.
Do not use the drug for more than 12 weeks.

Interactions
Metoclopramide may increase or decrease absorption of other drugs, depending on changes in transit time through intestinal tract; it may increase absorption of aspirin, acetaminophen, diazepam, ethanol, levodopa, lithium, and tetracycline and may decrease absorption of digoxin.
Anticholinergics and opiates may antagonize metoclopramide's effect on GI motility. Concomitant use with antihypertensives and CNS depressants (such as alcohol, sedatives, and tricyclic antidepressants) may lead to increased CNS depression.

Effects on diagnostic tests
Metoclopramide may increase serum aldosterone and prolactin levels.

Adverse reactions
• CNS: *restlessness, anxiety, drowsiness, fatigue,* lassitude, insomnia, headache, dizziness, *extrapyramidal symptoms, tardive dyskinesia, dystonic reactions,* sedation, *agitation.*
• CV: transient hypertension, *hypotension, dysrhythmias.*
• DERM: rash.
• Endocrine: prolactin secretion, loss of libido.
• GI: *nausea,* bowel disturbances, *vomiting, diarrhea.*
• Other: fever, *oculogyric crisis, periorbital edema.*
Note: Drug should be discontinued if extrapyramidal effects occur.

Overdose and treatment
Clinical effects of overdose (which is rare) include drowsiness, dystonia, seizures, and extrapyramidal effects.
Treatment includes administration of antimuscarinics, antiparkinsonian agents, or antihistamines with antimuscarinic activity (for example, 50 mg diphenhydramine, given I.M.).

▶ Special considerations
• Children have an increased incidence of adverse CNS effects, especially extrapyramidal dystonic reactions.
• For I.V. *push* administration, use undiluted and inject over a 1- to 2-minute period. For I.V. *infusion,* dilute with 50 ml of dextrose 5% in water, dextrose 5% in 0.45% sodium chloride, sodium chloride injection, Ringer's injection, or lactated Ringer's injection, and infuse over at least 15 minutes.
• Administer by I.V. infusion 30 minutes before chemotherapy.
• Drug may be used to facilitate nasoduodenal tube placement.
• Diphenhydramine may be used to counteract extrapyramidal effects of high-dose metoclopramide.
• Drug is not recommended for long-term use.
• Metoclopramide has been used investigationally to treat anorexia nervosa, dizziness, migraine, and intractable hiccups; oral dose form is being used investigationally to treat nausea and vomiting.

Information for parents and patient
• Tell parents to report any twitching or involuntary movement.

metronidazole
Femazole, Flagyl, Metric 21, Metronid, Metryl, Protostat, Satric, Apo-metronidazole*, Neo-metric*, Novonidazol*, PMS metronidazole*

metronidazole hydrochloride
Flagyl I.V., Flagyl I.V. RTU, Metro I.V., Metronidazole Redi-Infusion

• Classification: antibacterial, antiprotozoal, amebicide (nitroimidazole)

How supplied
Available by prescription only
Tablets: 250 mg, 500 mg
Powder for injection: 500-mg single-dose vials
Injection: 500 mg/dl ready to use

Indications, route, and dosage
Amebic hepatic abscess
Children: 35 to 50 mg/kg daily (in three doses) for 10 days.
Adults: 500 to 750 mg P.O. t.i.d. for 5 to 10 days.
Intestinal amebiasis
Children: 35 to 50 mg/kg daily (in three doses) for 10 days. Follow this therapy with oral iodoquinol.
Adults: 750 mg P.O. t.i.d. for 5 to 10 days. Centers for Disease Control recommends addition of iodoquinol 650 mg P.O. t.i.d. for 20 days.
Trichomoniasis
Children: 5 mg/1 kg P.O. t.i.d. for 7 days.
Adults (men and women concurrently): 250 mg P.O. t.i.d. for 7 days or 2 g P.O. as a single dose; 4 to 6 weeks should elapse between courses of therapy.
Refractory trichomoniasis
Adults (women): 250 mg P.O. b.i.d. for 10 days.
Bacterial infections caused by anaerobic microorganisms
Neonates: Loading dose is 15 mg/kg I.V., followed by 7.5 mg/kg q 12 hours in neonates less than 7 days old, 7.5 mg/kg q 8 hours in neonates older than 7 days.
Children and adults: Loading dose is 15 mg/kg I.V. infused over 1 hour (approximately 1 g for a 70-kg adult). Maintenance dose is 7.5 mg/kg I.V. or P.O. q 6 hours (approximately 500 mg for a 70-kg adult). The first maintenance dose should be administered 6 hours after the loading dose. Maximum dosage should not exceed 4 g daily.
Giardiasis
Children: 5 mg/kg P.O. t.i.d. for 7 to 10 days.
Adults: 250 mg P.O. t.i.d. for 5 days.
Prevention of postoperative infection in contaminated or potentially contaminated colorectal surgery
Adults: 15 mg/kg infused over 30 to 60 minutes and completed approximately 1 hour before surgery. Then 7.5 mg/kg infused over 30 to 60 minutes at 6 and 12 hours after the initial dose.

Action and kinetics
• *Bactericidal, amebicidal, and trichomonicidal action:* The nitro group of metronidazole is reduced inside the infecting organism; this reduction product disrupts DNA and inhibits nucleic acid synthesis. The drug is active in intestinal and extraintestinal sites. It is active against most anaerobic bacteria and protozoa, including *Bacteroides fragilis, B. melaninogenicus, Fusobacterium, Veillonella, Clostridium, Peptococcus, Peptostreptococcus, Entamoeba histolytica, Trichomonas vaginalis, Giardia lamblia,* and *Balantidium coli.*
• *Kinetics in adults:* About 80% of an oral dose is absorbed, with peak serum concentrations occurring at about 1 hour; food delays peak concentrations to about 2 hours. Metronidazole is distributed into most body tissues and fluids, including cerebrospinal fluid (CSF), bone, bile, saliva, pleural and peritoneal fluids, vaginal secretions, seminal fluids, middle ear fluid, and hepatic and cerebral abscesses. CSF levels approach serum levels in patients with inflamed meninges; they reach about 50% of serum levels in patients with uninflamed meninges. Less than 20% of metronidazole is bound to plasma proteins. It readily crosses the placenta.

Metronidazole is metabolized to an active 2-hydroxymethyl metabolite and also to other metabolites. About 60% to 80% of the dose is excreted as the parent compound or its metabolites. About 20% of a metronidazole dose is excreted unchanged in urine; about 6% to 15% is excreted in feces. Metronidazole's half-life is 6 to 8 hours in adults with normal renal function; the half-life may be prolonged in patients with impaired hepatic function. It is secreted into breast milk.

Contraindications and precautions
Metronidazole is contraindicated in patients with hypersensitivity to nitroimidazole derivatives.

Metronidazole should be used with caution in patients with a history of blood dyscrasia, because the drug can cause leukopenia; in patients receiving corticosteroids; and in those with edema from the sodium content of the injection.

It should be used with extreme caution (at lower than recommended doses) in patients with severe hepatic impairment because metronidazole and its metabolites accumulate in the plasma. Metronidazole should not be used indiscriminately because animal studies suggest carcinogenicity. Because of this potential, some clinicians prefer other agents (such as quinacrine) for giardiasis.

Interactions
Concomitant use of metronidazole with oral anticoagulants prolongs prothrombin time. Concomitant use with alcohol inhibits alcohol dehydrogenase activity, causing a disulfiram-like reaction (nausea, vomiting, headache, cramps, and flushing) in some patients; it is not recommended. Concomitant use with disulfiram may precipitate psychosis and confusion and should be avoided.

Concomitant use with barbiturates and phenytoin may diminish the antimicrobial effectiveness of metronidazole by increasing its metabolism and may require higher doses of metronidazole.

Concomitant use with cimetidine may decrease the clearance of metronidazole, thereby increasing its potential for causing adverse effects.

Effects on diagnostic tests
Metronidazole may interfere with the chemical analyses of aminotransferases and triglyceride, leading to falsely decreased values. Rarely, it has been reported to flatten the T waves on ECG.

Adverse reactions
• CNS: *vertigo,* headache, ataxia, incoordination, confusion, irritability, depression, restlessness, weakness, fatigue, drowsiness, insomnia, sensory neuropathy, paresthesias of extremities, psychic stimulation, neuromyopathy, and seizures.
• CV: ECG changes, (flattened T wave), edema (with I.V. RTU preparation).
• DERM: pruritus, flushing, *urticaria.*
• GI: abdominal cramping, stomatitis, *nausea,* vomiting, anorexia, *diarrhea,* constipation, proctitis, dry mouth, pseudomembranous colitis.
• GU: darkened urine, polyuria, dysuria, pyuria, incontinence, cystitis, decreased libido, dyspareunia, dryness of vagina and vulva, sense of pelvic pressure.
• HEMA: *transient leukopenia,* neutropenia.
• Local: thrombophlebitis after I.V. infusion.
• Other: *bacterial and fungal superinfection, especially Candida* (glossitis, furry tongue), metallic taste, fever, gynecomastia, nasal congestion.

Overdose and treatment
Clinical signs of overdose include nausea, vomiting, ataxia, seizures, and peripheral neuropathy.

There is no known antidote for metronidazole; treatment is supportive. If patient does not vomit spontaneously, induced emesis or gastric lavage is indicated for an oral overdose; activated charcoal and a cathartic may be used. Diazepam or phenytoin may be used to control seizures.

▶ Special considerations
• Trichomoniasis should be confirmed by wet smear and amebiasis by culture before giving metronidazole.
• If indicated during pregnancy for trichomoniasis, the 7-day regimen is preferred over the single-dose regimen. Treatment with metronidazole should be avoided during the first trimester.
• The I.V. form should be administered by slow infusion only; if used with a primary I.V. fluid system, discontinue the primary fluid during the infusion; *do not give by I.V. push.*
• Monitor patient on I.V. metronidazole for candidiasis.
• A 1% solution may be effective topically to treat decubitus ulcers.
• When treating amebiasis, monitor number and character of stools; send fecal specimens to laboratory promptly; infestation is detectable only in warm specimens. Repeat fecal examinations at 3-month intervals to ensure elimination of amebae.
• When preparing powder for injection, follow manufacturer's instructions carefully; use solution prepared from powder within 24 hours.

Information for parents and patient
• Tell parents and patient that drug may cause metallic taste and discolored (red-brown) urine.
• Patient should take tablets with meals to minimize GI distress. Tablets may be crushed to facilitate swallowing.
• Advise parents to report any adverse effects.
• Tell parents that patient should avoid alcohol and alcohol-containing medications during therapy and for at least 48 hours after the last dose.
• Explain the need for medical follow-up after discharge.
• Patients treated for amebiasis should have follow-up examinations of stool specimens for 3 months after treatment is discontinued, to ensure elimination of amebae. To help prevent reinfection, they should practice proper hygiene, including hand washing after defecation and before handling, preparing, or eating food. Emphasize the risk of eating raw food and the control of contamination by flies. Encourage other household members and suspected contacts to be tested and, if necessary, treated.
• Teach patients treated for trichomoniasis correct personal hygiene, including perineal care. Explain that asymptomatic sexual partners of patients being treated for trichomoniasis should be treated simultaneously to prevent reinfection; patient should refrain from intercourse during therapy or have partner use condom.

---

mexiletine hydrochloride
Mexitil

• Classification: ventricular antiarrhythmic (lidocaine analogue, sodium channel antagonist)

How supplied
Available by prescription only
Capsules: 150 mg, 200 mg, 250 mg

Indications, route, and dosage
Refractory ventricular dysrhythmias, including ventricular tachycardia and premature ventricular contractions
†*Children:* 2 to 4 mg/kg P.O. q 8 hours.
Adults: 200 to 400 mg P.O. followed by 200 mg q 8 hours. May increase dose to 400 mg q 8 hours if satisfactory control is not obtained. Some patients may respond well to 450 mg q 12 hours.

Action and kinetics
• *Antiarrhythmic action:* Mexiletine is structurally similar to lidocaine and exerts similar electrophysiologic and hemodynamic effects. A Class IB antiarrhythmic, it suppresses automaticity and shortens the effective refractory period and action potential duration of His-Purkinje fibers and suppresses spontaneous ventricular depolarization during diastole. At therapeutic serum levels, the drug does not affect conductive atrial tissue or AV conduction.

Unlike quinidine and procainamide, mexiletine does not significantly alter hemodynamics when given in

---

usual doses. Its effects on the conduction system inhibit reentry mechanisms and halt ventricular dysrhythmias. The drug does not have a significant negative inotropic effect.

• *Kinetics in adults:* About 90% of drug is absorbed from the GI tract; peak serum levels occur in 2 to 3 hours. Absorption rate decreases with conditions that speed gastric emptying. Mexiletine is distributed widely throughout the body. Distribution volume declines in patients with liver or hepatic disease, resulting in toxic serum drug levels with usual doses. About 50% to 60% of circulating drug is bound to plasma proteins. Usual therapeutic drug level is 0.5 to 2 mcg/ml. Although toxicity may occur within this range, levels above 2 mcg/ml are considered toxic and are associated with an increased frequency of adverse CNS effects, warranting dosage reduction. Mexiletine is metabolized in the liver to relatively inactive metabolites. Less than 10% of a parenteral dose escapes metabolism and reaches the kidneys unchanged. Metabolism is affected by hepatic blood flow, which may be reduced in patients who are recovering from myocardial infarction and in those with CHF. Liver disease also limits metabolism. In healthy patients, drug's half-life is 10 to 12 hours. Elimination half-life may be prolonged in patients with CHF or liver disease. Urinary excretion increases with urine acidification and slows with urine alkalinization.

Contraindications and precautions

Mexiletine is contraindicated in patients with cardiogenic shock, because the drug has a mild negative inotropic effect and may increase systemic vascular resistance slightly, thereby exacerbating this condition; in patients with preexisting second- or third-degree heart block without an artificial pacemaker, because the drug may further depress cardiac conduction; and in patients with hypersensitivity to the drug.

Mexiletine should be used with caution in patients with severe degrees of SA, AV, or intraventricular heart block who do not have an artificial pacemaker, because the drug may worsen these conditions; in patients with hepatic or myocardial failure, because the drug may accumulate and cause toxicity; in patients with seizure disorders, because the drug may induce seizures; and in patients with bradycardia or hypotension, because the drug may worsen these conditions.

Interactions

Concomitant use of mexiletine with drugs that alter gastric emptying time (such as narcotics, antacids containing aluminum-magnesium hydroxide, and atropine) may delay mexiletine absorption; concomitant use with metoclopramide may increase absorption.

Concomitant use with drugs that alter hepatic enzyme function (such as rifampin, phenobarbital, and phenytoin) may induce hepatic metabolism of mexiletine and thus reduce serum drug levels. Concomitant use with cimetidine may decrease mexiletine metabolism, resulting in increased serum levels. Concomitant use with drugs that acidify the urine (such as ammonium chloride) enhances mexiletine excretion; concomitant use with drugs that alkalinize urine

(such as high-dose antacids, carbonic anhydrase inhibitors, and sodium bicarbonate) decreases mexiletine excretion.

Effects on diagnostic tests

Liver function test results may be transiently altered during mexiletine therapy.

Adverse reactions

• CNS: *tremors, dizziness,* blurred vision, ataxia, diplopia, confusion, nystagmus, nervousness, headache.
• CV: hypotension, bradycardia, *dysrhythmias,* angina.
• DERM: rash.
• GI: *nausea, vomiting, anorexia, diarrhea, constipation.*
• Respiratory: dyspnea.
• Other: elevation of liver function test values.

Overdose and treatment

Clinical effects of overdose are primarily extensions of adverse CNS effects. Convulsions are the most serious effect.

Treatment usually involves symptomatic and supportive measures. In acute overdose, emesis induction or gastric lavage should be performed. Urine acidification may accelerate drug elimination. If patient has bradycardia and hypotension, atropine may be given.

▶ Special considerations

• Dosage should be administered with meals, if possible.
• Avoid administering drug within 1 hour of antacids containing aluminum-magnesium hydroxide.
• When changing from lidocaine to mexiletine, stop infusion when first mexiletine dose is given. Keep infusion line open, however, until dysrhythmia appears to be satisfactorily controlled.
• Patients who are not controlled by dosing every 8 hours may respond to dosing every 6 hours.
• Many patients who respond well to mexiletine can be maintained on an every-12-hour schedule. Twice-daily doses improve patient compliance.
• Monitor blood pressure and heart rate and rhythm for significant change.
• Tremors (usually a fine hand tremor) are commonly evident in patients taking high doses of mexiletine.
• Therapeutic serum drug levels range from 0.75 to 2 mcg/ml.

Information for parents and patient

• Instruct parents to have patient take drug with food to reduce risk of nausea.
• Instruct parents to watch for and report any of the following: unusual bleeding or bruising, signs of infection (such as fever, sore throat, stomatitis, or chills), or fatigue.

mezlocillin sodium
Mezlin

• Classification: antibiotic (extended-spectrum penicillin, acyclaminopenicillin)

How supplied
Available by prescription only
Injection: 1 g, 2 g, 3 g, 4 g

Indications, route, and dosage
Infections caused by susceptible organisms
Neonates age 0 to 7 days: 75 mg/kg q 12 hours.
Neonates age 8 days and older weighing 2 kg and less: 75 mg/kg I.V. or I.M. q 8 hours.
Neonates age 8 days and older weighing more than 2 kg: 75 mg/kg I.V. or I.M. q 6 hours.
Children age 1 month to 12 years: 50 mg/kg I.V. or I.M. q 4 hours.
Adults: 100 to 300 mg/kg I.V. or I.M. daily given in four to six divided doses. Usual dose is 3 g q 4 hours or 4 g q 6 hours. For serious infections, up to 24 g daily may be administered.
Dosage in renal failure
Adults: If creatinine clearance is 10 to 30 ml/min, give 3 g q 8 hours. If creatinine clearance is < 10 ml/min, give 2 g q 8 hours. (If the infection is life-threatening, the above doses may be given every 6 hours.) Patients on hemodialysis should be given 3 to 4 g after each dialysis session, then every 12 hours. Patients on peritoneal dialysis may receive 3 g q 12 hours.

Action and kinetics
• *Antibiotic action:* Mezlocillin is bactericidal; it adheres to bacterial penicillin-binding proteins, thereby inhibiting bacterial cell wall synthesis.

Extended-spectrum penicillins are more resistant to inactivation by certain beta-lactamases, especially those produced by gram-negative organisms, but are still liable to inactivation by certain others.

Mezlocillin's spectrum of activity includes many gram-negative aerobic and anaerobic bacilli, many gram-positive and gram-negative aerobic cocci, and some gram-positive aerobic and anaerobic bacilli, but a large number of these organisms are resistant to mezlocillin. Mezlocillin may be effective against some strains of carbenicillin-resistant and ticarcillin-resistant gram-negative bacilli, but should not be used as sole therapy because of the rapid development of resistance. Some clinicians feel that there is no evidence that it has any advantages over ticarcillin or carbenicillin, at least with respect to cure rates. Mezlocillin is less active against *Pseudomonas aeruginosa* than other members of this class, such as azlocillin and piperacillin; however, both mezlocillin and piperacillin are more effective against *Enterobacteriaceae* than is azlocillin.

• *Kinetics in adults:* After an I.M. dose, peak plasma concentrations occur at ¾ to 1½ hours.

Mezlocillin is distributed widely. It penetrates minimally into CSF with uninflamed meninges. It crosses the placenta and is 16% to 42% protein-bound.

Mezlocillin is metabolized partially; about 15% of a dose is metabolized to inactive metabolites.

Mezlocillin is excreted primarily (39% to 72%) in urine by glomerular filtration and renal tubular secretion; up to 30% of a dose is excreted in bile, and some is excreted in breast milk. Elimination half-life in adults is about ¾ to 1½ hours; in extensive renal impairment, half-life is extended to 2 to 14 hours.

Mezlocillin is removed by hemodialysis but not by peritoneal dialysis.

• *Kinetics in children:* Serum half-life is 3.7 to 4.4 hours in neonates younger than age 7 days and 2.4 and 2.6 hours in neonates over 7 days old.

Contraindications and precautions
Mezlocillin is contraindicated in patients with known hypersensitivity to any other penicillin or to cephalosporins.

Mezlocillin should be used cautiously in patients with renal impairment because it is excreted in urine; decreased dosage is required in moderate to severe renal failure.

Interactions
Concomitant use with aminoglycoside antibiotics results in a synergistic bactericidal effect against *Pseudomonas aeruginosa, Escherichia coli, Klebsiella, Citrobacter, Enterobacter, Serratia,* and *Proteus mirabilis.* However, the drugs are physically and chemically incompatible and are inactivated when mixed or given together.

Concomitant use of mezlocillin (and other extended-spectrum penicillins) with clavulanic acid also produces a synergistic bactericidal effect against certain beta-lactamase producing bacteria.

Probenecid blocks tubular secretion of penicillins, raising their serum concentrations.

Large doses of penicillins may interfere with renal tubular secretion of methotrexate, thus delaying elimination and elevating serum concentrations of methotrexate.

Effects on diagnostic tests
Mezlocillin alters tests for urinary or serum proteins; it interferes with turbidimetric methods that use sulfosalicylic acid, trichloroacetic acid, acetic acid, or nitric acid.

Mezlocillin does not interfere with tests using bromo-phenol blue (Albustix, Albutest, MultiStix).

Positive Coombs' tests have been reported in patients taking carbenicillin disodium.

Mezlocillin may falsely decrease serum aminoglycoside concentrations. Mezlocillin may cause hypokalemia and hypernatremia and prolong prothrombin times; it may also cause transient elevations in liver function studies and transient reductions in red blood cell, white blood cell, and platelet counts.

Adverse reactions
• CNS: neuromuscular irritability, seizures.
• GI: nausea, diarrhea, vomiting, *pseudomembranous colitis.*
• GU: acute interstitial nephritis.

• HEMA: *bleeding with high doses,* neutropenia, eosinophilia, leukopenia, *thrombocytopenia.*
• Metabolic: hypokalemia.
• Local: pain at injection site, vein irritation, phlebitis.
• Other: hypersensitivity reactions, (edema, fever, chills, rash, pruritus, urticaria, anaphylaxis), bacterial and fungal superinfection.

Note: Drug should be discontinued if immediate hypersensitivity reactions occur; if bleeding complications occur; or if severe diarrhea occurs, as this may indicate pseudomembranous colitis.

Overdose and treatment
Clinical signs of overdose include neuromuscular sensitivity or seizures; a 4- to 6-hour hemodialysis will remove 20% to 30% of mezlocillin.

▶ Special considerations
• Assess patient's history of allergies; do not give mezlocillin to any patient with a history of hypersensitivity reactions to either penicillins or cephalosporins. Try to determine whether previous reactions were true hypersensitivity reactions or another reaction, such as GI distress, which the patient has interpreted as allergy.
• Keep in mind that a negative history for penicillin hypersensitivity does not preclude future allergic reactions; monitor patient continuously for possible allergic reactions or other untoward effects.
• In patients with renal impairment, dosage should be reduced if creatinine clearance is below 10 ml/minute.
• Assess level of consciousness, neurologic status, and renal function when high doses are used, because excessive blood levels can cause CNS toxicity.
• Obtain results of cultures and sensitivity tests before first dose; however, therapy may begin before test results are complete. Repeat test periodically to assess drug efficacy.
• Monitor vital signs, electrolytes, and renal function studies; monitor body weight for fluid retention with extended-spectrum penicillins for possible hypokalemia or hypernatremia.
• Coagulation abnormalities, even frank bleeding, can follow high doses, especially of extended-spectrum penicillins; monitor prothrombin times and platelet counts, and assess patient for signs of occult or frank bleeding.
• Monitor patients on long-term therapy for possible superinfection, especially debilitated patients and others receiving immunosuppressants or radiation therapy; monitor closely, especially for fever.
Parenteral administration
• Give penicillins at least 1 hour before giving bacteriostatic antibiotics (tetracyclines, erythromycins, and chloramphenicol); these drugs inhibit bacterial cell growth, decreasing rate of penicillin uptake by bacterial cell walls.
• Always consult manufacturer's directions for reconstitution, dilution, and storage of drugs; check expiration dates.
• Administer I.M. dose deep into large muscle mass (gluteal or midlateral thigh); rotate injection sites to minimize tissue injury; do not inject more than 2 g

or 2 cc of drug per injection site. Apply ice to injection site for pain.
• Do not add or mix other drugs with I.V. infusions—particulary aminioglycosides, which will be inactivated if mixed with penicillins; they are chemically and physically incompatible. If other drugs must be given I.V., temporarily stop infusion of primary drug.
• Infuse I.V. drug continuously or intermittently (over 30 minutes) and assess I.V. site frequently to prevent infiltration or phlebitis; rotate infusion site q 48 hours; intermittent I.V. infusion may be diluted in 50 to 100ml sterile water, 0.9% sodium chloride, dextrose 5% in water, dextrose 5% in water and half normal saline, or lactated Ringer's solution. Adjust dilution as appropriate for patient's weight.
• Solutions should always be clear, colorless to pale yellow, and free of particles; do not give solutions containing precipitates or other foreign matter.
• Mezlocillin may be more suitable than carbenicillin or ticarcillin for patients on salt-free diets; mezlocillin contains only 2.17 mEq of sodium per gram.
• Monitor serum potassium level and liver function studies.
• Patient with high serum concentrations may have seizures.
• This drug is almost always used with another antibiotic, such as an aminoglycoside, in life-threatening infections.
• Inject I.M. dose slowly over 12 to 15 seconds to minimize pain. Do not exceed 2 g per site.
• If precipitate forms during refrigerated storage, warm to 98.6° F. (37° C.) in warm water bath and shake well. Solution should be clear.
• Because mezlocillin is partially dialyzable, patients undergoing hemodialysis may need dosage adjustments.

Information for parents and patient
• Teach signs and symptoms of hypersensitivity and other adverse reactions and emphasize need to report any unusual reactions.
• Teach signs and symptoms of bacterial and fungal superinfection to parents and patients, especially debilitated patients and others with low resistance from immunosuppressants or irradiation; emphasize need to report signs of infection.

miconazole
Monistat I.V.

miconazole nitrate
Micatin, Monistat 3, Monistat 7, Monistat-Derm

• Classification: antifungal (imidazole derivative)

How supplied
Available by prescription only
Injection: 10 mg/ml
Vaginal suppositories: 100 mg, 200 mg
Vaginal cream: 2%

Available without prescription
Cream: 2%
Lotion: 2%
Powder: 2%
Spray: 2%

Indications, route, and dosage
Systemic fungal infections caused by susceptible organisms
Neonates: 5 to 15 mg/kg I.V. q 8 to 24 hours.
Infants and children: 20 to 60 mg/kg/day I.V., divided q 8 hours. Do not exceed 60 mg/kg per infusion.
Adults: 200 to 3,600 mg daily. I.V. dosages may vary with diagnosis and with infective agent. May divide daily dosage over three infusions, 200 to 1,200 mg per infusion. Dilute in at least 200 ml of 0.9% sodium chloride. Repeated courses may be needed because of relapse or reinfection.
Bladder instillation: 200 mg diluted and instilled into the bladder b.i.d. to q.i.d. or by continuous irrigation.
Fungal meningitis
Children and adults: 20 mg intrathecally as an adjunct to intravenous administration.
Cutaneous or mucocutaneous fungal infections caused by susceptible organisms
Topical use
Children and adults: Cover affected areas twice daily for 2 to 4 weeks.
Vaginal use
Children and adults: Insert 200-mg suppository at bedtime for 3 days, or 100-mg suppository or cream at bedtime for 7 days.
Note: Adjust dosage in patients with hepatic dysfunctions.

Action and kinetics
• *Antifungal action:* Miconazole is both fungistatic and fungicidal, depending on drug concentration. In *Coccidioides immitus, Candida albicans, Cryptococcus neoformans, Histoplasma capsulatum, Candida tropicalis, Candida parapsilosis, Paracoccidioides brasiliensis, Sporothrix schenckii, Aspergillus flavus, A. ustus, Microsporum canis, Curvularia, Petriellidium boydii,* dermatophytes, and some gram-positive bacteria. Miconazole causes thickening of the fungal cell wall, altering membrane permeability; it also may kill the cell by interference with peroxisomal enzymes, causing accumulation of peroxide within the cell wall. It attacks virtually all pathogenic fungi.
In clinical use, miconazole is considered an alternative to amphotericin B to treat coccidiomycosis, but ketoconazole is preferred. Its clinical effectiveness in blastomycosis and histoplasmosis is highly variable. Its broad spectrum of activity makes it useful in treating superficial cutaneous infections and vaginal candidal infections.
• *Kinetics in adults:* About 50% of an oral miconazole dose is absorbed; however, no oral dosage form is currently available. A small amount of drug is systemically absorbed after vaginal administration. Drug penetrates well into inflamed joints, vitreous humor, and the peritoneal cavity. Distribution into sputum and saliva is poor, and CSF penetration is unpredictable. Miconazole is over 90% bound to plasma proteins.

Miconazole is metabolized in the liver, predominantly to inactive metabolites. Miconazole elimination is triphasic; terminal half-life is about 24 hours. Between 10% and 14% of an oral dose is excreted in urine; 50%, in feces. Up to 1% of a vaginal dose is excreted in urine; 14% to 22% of an I.V. dose is excreted in urine. It is unknown whether it is excreted in breast milk.

Contraindications and precautions
Miconazole is contraindicated in patients with known hypersensitivity to the drug. It should be used with caution in patients with hepatic disease.

Interactions
Miconazole enhances the anticoagulant effect of warfarin. It may antagonize the effects of amphotericin B.

Effects on diagnostic tests
Miconazole may cause a transient decrease in hematocrit levels and an increase or decrease in platelet counts; it frequently causes erythrocyte aggregation. Miconazole also may cause hyponatremia, hyperlipidemia, and hypertriglyceridemia; abnormalities in lipoprotein and immunoelectrophoretic patterns are from the polyoxyl 35 castor oil vehicle.

Adverse reactions
• CNS: dizziness, *drowsiness.*
• DERM: *pruritic rash,* irritation, contact dermatitis.
• GI: *nausea, vomiting, diarrhea, anorexia.*
• HEMA: transient decreases in hematocrit levels, thrombocytopenia, erythrocyte aggregation.
• Metabolic: transient decrease in serum sodium levels, hyperlipidemia.
• Local: *phlebitis at injection site.*
• Other: *fever, flushing.*
Note: Drug should be discontinued if condition worsens or irritation or signs of toxicity occur.

Overdose and treatment
Symptoms of overdose include GI complaints and altered mental status. Treatment after recent oral ingestion (within 4 hours) includes emesis or lavage followed by activated charcoal and an osmotic cathartic; subsequent care is supportive, as needed.

▶ Special considerations
• Safe use in children under age 1 has not been established.
• Identify causative organism by culture and sensitivity studies before I.V. or topical therapy is started.
• Initial I.V. therapy requires direct medical supervision; cardiorespiratory arrest has occurred with first dose.
• Check for possible hypersensitivity to drug before I.V. infusion; be prepared for anaphylaxis.
• Infuse over 30 to 60 minutes; rapid injection of undiluted miconazole may cause dysrhythmias.
• Premedication with an antiemetic may lessen nausea and vomiting.
• Monitor CBC and electrolyte, triglyceride, and cholesterol levels before and frequently throughout therapy to detect adverse effects.

• Pruritic rash may persist for weeks after drug is discontinued; it may be controlled with oral or I.V. diphenhydramine.
• Cleanse affected area before applying cream or lotion. After application, massage area gently until cream disappears. Use lotion rather than cream in intertriginous areas to prevent maceration.
• Continue topical therapy for at least 1 month; improvement should begin in 1 to 2 weeks. If no improvement occurs by 4 weeks, reevaluate diagnosis.
• Insert vaginal applicator high into vagina.
• Fungal meningitis requires both I.V. and intrathecal therapy.
• Miconazole has the advantage of causing fewer and less severe adverse reactions than amphotericin B.

Information for parents and patient
• Teach parents and patient the symptoms of fungal infection, and explain treatment rationale.
• Explain importance of following prescribed regimen, follow-up visits and reporting adverse effects.
• Teach patient correct procedure for intravaginal or topical applications.
• To prevent vaginal reinfection, teach correct perineal hygiene and recommend that adolescent patients abstain from sexual intercourse during therapy.

minocycline hydrochloride
Minocin

• Classification: antibiotic (tetracycline)

How supplied
Available by prescription only
Capsules: 50 mg, 100 mg
Tablets: 50 mg, 100 mg
Suspension: 50 mg/5 ml

Indications, route, and dosage
Infections caused by sensitive organisms
Children over age 8: Initially, 4 mg/kg P.O., then 4 mg/kg P.O. daily, divided q 12 hours.
Adults: Initially, 200 mg P.O., I.V.; then 100 mg q 12 hours or 50 mg P.O. q 6 hours.

Action and kinetics
• *Antibacterial action:* Minocycline is bacteriostatic; it binds reversibly to ribosomal units, thus inhibiting bacterial protein synthesis.
   Minocycline is active against many gram-negative and gram-positive organisms, *Mycoplasma, Rickettsia, Chlamydia,* and spirochetes; it may be more active against staphylococci than other tetracyclines.
   The potential vestibular toxicity particulary in children and cost of minocycline limits its usefulness. It may be more active than other tetracyclines against *Nocardia asteroides;* it is also effective against *Mycobacterium marinum* infections. It has been used for meningococcal meningitis prophylaxis because of its activity against *Neisseria meningitidis.*
• *Kinetics in adults:* Minocycline is 90% to 100% absorbed after oral administration and is distributed

widely into body tissues and fluids, including synovial, pleural, prostatic, and seminal fluids, bronchial secretions, saliva, and aqueous humor; CSF penetration is poor. Minocycline crosses the placenta; it is 55% to 88% protein-bound. Minocycline is metabolized partially and excreted primarily unchanged in urine by glomerular filtration. Plasma half-life is 11 to 26 hours in adults with normal renal function. Some drug is excreted in breast milk.
• *Kinetics in children:* Tetracyclines form a stable complex in bone-forming tissue, and may cause permanent enamel hypoplasia or yellow-gray discoloration of teeth in children under age 8.

Contraindications and precautions
Minocycline is contraindicated in children with known hypersensitivity to any tetracycline; and in children under age 8 because of the risk of permanent discoloration of teeth, enamel defects, and retardation of bone growth.
   Use drug with caution in children likely to be exposed to direct sunlight or ultraviolet light because of the risk of photosensitivity reactions.

Interactions
Concomitant use of minocycline with antacids containing aluminum, calcium, or magnesium or with laxatives containing magnesium decreases oral absorption of minocycline (because of chelation); concomitant use with oral iron products or sodium bicarbonate also decreases absorption. Foods and milk and other dairy products may also decrease absorption of minocycline, but less so than with other tetracyclines.
   Tetracyclines may antagonize bactericidal effects of penicillin, inhibiting cell growth through bacteriostatic action; administer penicillin 2 to 3 hours before tetracycline.
   Concomitant use of tetracycline necessitates lowered dosage of oral anticoagulants due to enhanced effects, and lowered dose of digoxin due to increased bioavailability.

Effects on diagnostic tests
Minocycline causes false-negative results in urine glucose tests using glucose oxidase reagent (Clinistix or Tes-Tape).
   Minocycline causes false elevations in fluorometric test results for urinary catecholamines.

Adverse reactions
• CNS: light-headedness, *dizziness from vestibular toxicity.*
• CV: pericarditis.
• DERM: maculopapular and erythematous rashes, photosensitivity, increased pigmentation, urticaria, discolored nails and teeth.
• EENT: dysphagia, glossitis.
• GI: anorexia, epigastric distress, nausea, vomiting, diarrhea, enterocolitis, inflammatory lesions in anogenital region.
• GU: reversible nephrotoxicity (Fanconi's syndrome) from *outdated* tetracyclines.
• HEMA: neutropenia, eosinophilia.
• Metabolic: increased BUN level.

---

‡May contain sulfites   ♦May contain tartrazine   ♦♦May contain benzyl alcohol

• Local: thrombophlebitis.
• Other: hypersensitivity, bacterial and fungal super-infection.

Note: Drug should be discontinued if signs of toxicity, hypersensitivity, or superinfection occur; if erythema follows exposure to sunlight or ultraviolet light; or if severe diarrhea indicates pseudomembranous colitis.

Overdose and treatment

Clinical signs of overdose are usually limited to GI tract; give antacids or empty stomach by gastric lavage if ingestion occurred within the preceding 4 hours.

▶ Special considerations

• Assess child's allergic history; do not give minocycline to a patient with a history of hypersensitivity reactions to any other tetracycline. Monitor continuously for this and other adverse reactions.
• Obtain results of cultures and sensitivity tests before first dose; but do not delay therapy; check cultures periodically to assess drug efficacy.
• Monitor vital signs, electrolytes, and renal function studies before and during therapy.
• Check expiration dates. Outdated tetracyclines may cause nephrotoxicity.
• Monitor for bacterial and fungal superinfection, especially in debilitated children and those who are receiving immunosuppressants or radiation therapy, watch especially for oral candidasis. If symptoms occur, discontinue drug.
• Children age 8 and under should not receive tetracyclines unless there is no alterative. Tetracyclines can cause permanent discoloration of teeth, enamel hypoplasia, and a reversible decrease in bone calcification.
• Reversible decreases in bone calcification have been reported in infants.

Administration

• Give water with and after oral drug to facilitate passage to stomach, because incomplete swallowing can cause severe esophageal irritation; do not administer witin 1 hour of bedtime, to prevent esophageal reflux.

Information for parents and patient

• Teach parents how to recognize signs and symptoms of adverse reactions, and emphasize need to report these promptly, urge parents to report any unusual effects.
• Teach parents of children with low resistance from immunosuppressants or irradiation how to recognize signs and symptoms of bacterial and fungal super-infections.
• Patient should avoid direct exposure to sunlight and use a sunscreen to help prevent photosensitivity reactions.
• Patient should take drug with enough water to facilitate passage to the stomach, 1 hour before or 2 hours after meals for maximum absorption, and not less than 1 hour before bedtime (to prevent irritation from esophageal reflux).
• Patient should avoid hazardous activities that require coordination because drug may cause dizziness.

• Emphasize that taking the drug with food, milk or other dairy products, sodium bicarbonate, or iron compounds may interfere with absorption. Patients who need antacids should take them 3 hours after minocycline.
• Emphasize importance of completing prescribed regimen exactly as ordered and keeping follow-up appointments.
• Tell parents to check expiration dates and discard any expired drug.

minoxidil (systemic)
Loniten

• Classification: antihypertensive (peripheral vasodilator)

How supplied

Available by prescription only
Tablets: 2.5 mg, 10 mg

Indications, route, and dosage
Severe hypertension

Children under age 12: 0.2 mg/kg (maximum 5 mg) as a single daily dose. Effective dosage range is usually 0.25 to 1 mg/kg daily in one or two doses. Maximum dosage is 50 mg/day.
Children older than age 12 and adults: Initially, 5 mg P.O. as a single daily dose. Effective dosage range is usually 10 to 40 mg daily. Maximum dosage is 100 mg/day.

Action and kinetics

• *Antihypertensive action:* Minoxidil produces its antihypertensive effect by a direct vasodilating effect on vascular smooth muscle; the effect on resistance vessels (arterioles and arteries) is greater than that on capacitance vessels (venules and veins).
• *Kinetics in adults:* Minoxidil is absorbed rapidly from the GI tract; antihypertensive effect occurs in 30 minutes, peaking at 2 to 8 hours. Minoxidil is distributed widely into body tissues; it is not bound to plasma proteins. Approximately 90% of a given dose is metabolized. Drug and metabolites are excreted primarily in urine. Antihypertensive action persists for 2 to 5 days.

Contraindications and precautions

Minoxidil is contraindicated in patients with known hypersensitivity to the drug, and in patients with pheochromocytoma because it may stimulate catecholamine secretion from the tumor.

Minoxidil should be used cautiously in patients with recent myocardial infarction, because vasodilation may increase myocardial oxygen demand via reflex tachycardia; and in patients with pulmonary hypertension, CHF, or significant renal impairment, because pulmonary artery pressure may increase.

Interactions

Minoxidil may potentiate the effects of diuretics or other antihypertensive drugs; concomitant use with

---

*Canada only   †Unlabeled clinical use   Italicized adverse reactions have been observed in children.

guanethidine may cause profound orthostatic hypotension.

Effects on diagnostic tests
Minoxidil may elevate serum alkaline phosphatase, serum creatinine, and BUN levels as well as antinuclear antibody titers; drug may transiently decrease hemoglobin and hematocrit levels. Minoxidil may also alter direction and magnitude of T waves on ECG.

Adverse reactions
• CV: edema, tachycardia, pericardial effusion and cardiac tamponade, CHF, ECG changes.
• DERM: rash, Stevens-Johnson syndrome.
• HEMA: thrombocytopenia and leukopenia (rare).
• Other: reversible hypertrichosis (elongation, thickening, and enhanced pigmentation of fine body hair), breast tenderness.
   Note: Drug should be discontinued if pericardial effusion develops.

Overdose and treatment
Clinical signs of overdose include hypotension, tachycardia, headache, and skin flushing.
   After acute ingestion, empty stomach by induced emesis or gastric lavage, and give activated charcoal to reduce absorption. Further treatment is usually symptomatic and supportive.

▶ Special considerations
• Because of limited experience in children, use with caution. Cautious drug titration is necessary.
• Minoxidil therapy is usually given concomitantly with two or more other antihypertensive drugs, such as diuretics, beta blockers, or sympathetic nervous system suppressants.
• Monitor blood pressure and pulse after administration, and report significant changes; assess intake, output, and body weight for sodium and water retention.
• Monitor for CHF, pericardial effusion, and cardiac tamponade; have phenylephrine, dopamine, and vasopressin on hand to treat hypotension.
• Patients with renal failure or on dialysis may require smaller maintenance doses of minoxidil. Because minoxidil is removed by dialysis, on the day of dialysis, the drug should be administered immediately after dialysis if dialysis is at 9 a.m.; if dialysis is after 3 p.m., the daily dose should be given at 7 a.m. (8 hours before dialysis).

Information for parents and patient
• Explain that minoxidil is usually taken with other antihypertensive medications; emphasize importance of taking medication as prescribed.
• Caution parents or patient to report the following cardiac symptoms promptly: increased heart rate (20 beats/minute over normal), rapid weight gain, shortness of breath, chest pain, severe indigestion, dizziness, light-headedness, or fainting.
• Tell parents to call for instructions before giving patient nonprescription cold preparations.
• Advise parents and patient that hypertrichosis will disappear 1 to 6 months after stopping drug.

mitomycin
Mutamycin

• Classification: antineoplastic (antineoplastic antibiotic [cell cycle-phase nonspecific])

How supplied
Available by prescription only
Injection: 5-mg, 20-mg vials

Indications, route, and dosage
Dosage and indications may vary. Check current literature for recommended protocol.
Stomach, pancreatic, †breast, †colon, †head, †neck, †lung, and †hepatic cancer
†*Children and adults:* 2 mg/m² I.V. daily for 5 days. Stop drug for 2 days, then repeat dose for 5 more days; or 10 to 20 mg/m² as a single dose. Repeat cycle q 6 to 8 weeks. Stop drug if WBC count is below 3,000/mm³ or platelet count is below 75,000/mm³.

Action and kinetics
• *Antineoplastic action:* Mitomycin exerts its cytotoxic activity by a mechanism similar to that of the alkylating agents. The drug is converted to an active compound which forms cross-links between strands of DNA, inhibiting DNA synthesis. Mitomycin also inhibits RNA and protein synthesis to a lesser extent.
• *Kinetics in adults:* Because it is a vesicant, mitomycin must be administered intravenously. Mitomycin distributes widely into body tissues; animal studies show that the highest concentrations are found in the muscle, eyes, lungs, intestines, and stomach. The drug does not cross the blood-brain barrier. Mitomycin is metabolized by hepatic microsomal enzymes and is also deactivated in the kidneys, spleen, brain, and heart. Mitomycin and its metabolites are excreted in urine. A small portion is eliminated in bile and feces.

Contraindications and precautions
Mitomycin is contraindicated in patients with a history of hypersensitivity to the drug; in patients with a WBC count below 3,000/mm³, platelet count below 75,000/mm³, or serum creatinine level above 1.7 mg/100 ml; and in those with coagulation disorders, prolonged prothrombin time, or serious infections, because of the potential for adverse effects.

Interactions
Concomitant use with dextran and urokinase enhances the cytotoxic activity of mitomycin. Through a series of enzymatic processes, these agents increase autolysis of cells, adding to the cell death caused by mitomycin.

Effects on diagnostic tests
Mitomycin therapy, through drug-induced renal toxicity, may increase serum creatinine and BUN concentrations.

---

‡May contain sulfites .   ◆May contain tartrazine   ◆◆May contain benzyl alcohol

Adverse reactions
- CNS: paresthesias.
- GI: nausea, vomiting, anorexia, stomatitis.
- HEMA: bone marrow depression (dose-limiting), thrombocytopenia, leukopenia (may be delayed up to 8 weeks and may be cumulative with successive doses).
- Local: desquamation, induration, pruritus, pain at site of injection; with extravasation, cellulitis, ulceration, sloughing.
- Other: reversible alopecia; purple coloration of nail beds; fever; syndrome characterized by microangiopathic hemolytic anemia, thrombocytopenia, renal toxicity, and hypertension.

Note: Drug should be discontinued if WBC count is below 3,000/mm³ or platelet count is below 75,000/mm³.

Overdose and treatment
Clinical manifestations of overdose include myelosuppression, nausea, vomiting, and alopecia.

Treatment is usually supportive and includes transfusion of blood components, antiemetics, and antibiotics for infections that may develop.

▶ Special considerations
- Vital signs and patency of catheter or I.V. line should be monitored throughout administration.
- Carefully follow established procedures for safe handling, administration, and disposal.
- Drug is a vesicant. Avoid placement of I.V. site at or near a joint that may become immobilized if extravasation occurs. During I.V. administration, monitor continuously for extravasation. If it occurs, stop infusion, remove I.V. and treat promptly according to institutional policy. Administer prolonged infusion only via central venous catheter.
- Treat extravasation promptly.
- Ulcers caused by extravasation develop late and dorsal to the extravasation site. Apply cold compresses for at least 12 hours.
- Premedicating with an antiemetic may prevent nausea and vomiting. If vomiting occurs, administer antiemetics p.r.n.
- Patients who have received drugs with strong emetic properties may experience anticipatory nausea and vomiting at subsequent treatments. They may benefit from treatment with an anxiolytic drug.
- Monitor patient's intake, output, and weight.
- Continue I.V. hydration until patient resumes sufficient oral intake.
- Monitor BUN, hematocrit, platelet count, ALT (SGPT), AST (SGOT), LDH, serum bilirubin, serum creatinine, uric acid, and total and differential leukocytes.
- To reconstitute 5-mg vial, use 10 ml of sterile water for injection; to reconstitute 20-mg vial, use 40 ml of sterile water for injection, to give a concentration of 0.5 mg/ml.
- Drug may be administered by I.V. push injection slowly over 5 to 10 minutes into the tubing of a freely flowing I.V. infusion.
- Drug can be further diluted to 100 to 150 ml with normal saline solution or dextrose 5% in water for I.V. infusion (over 30 to 60 minutes or longer).

- Reconstituted solution remains stable for 1 week at room temperature and for 2 weeks if refrigerated.
- Mitomycin has been used intraarterially to treat certain tumors, for example, into hepatic artery for colon cancer. It has also been given as a continuous daily infusion.
- An unlabeled use of this drug is to treat small bladder papillomas. It is instilled directly into the bladder in a concentration of 20 mg/20 ml sterile water.
- Continue CBC and blood studies at least 7 weeks after therapy is stopped. Monitor for signs of bleeding.

Information for parents and patient
- Stress importance of keeping follow-up appointments for monitoring hematologic status.
- Teach parents and patient to check for signs of bleeding and bruising. Parents may need to restrict child's participation in contact sports. Such activity is dangerous when patient's platelets are low.
- Instruct parents to monitor neutropenic patient's temperature every 4 hours (not rectally) and to report fever, cough and other signs of infection *promptly.*
- Patient should avoid contact with persons who have received live virus immunizations (polio, measles/mumps/rubella). Explain importance of promptly reporting susceptible patient's exposure to chicken pox.
- Instruct patient to clean teeth with toothettes, gauze, or soft toothbrush when platelets are low. Patient should perform frequent oral hygiene and should avoid using commercial mouthwashes which may contain alcohol and have an irritating effect. Solutions of sodium bicarbonate or hydrogen peroxide are more appropriate rinses.
- Instruct patient to avoid foods that are spicy and extremely hot or cold. Topical anesthetics administered before meals (swish and spit) may relieve mouth discomfort.
- Tell parents that patient's dental work should be completed before therapy whenever possible, or delayed until blood counts are normal.
- Tell parents and patient to immediately report redness, pain, or swelling at injection site. Local tissue injury and scarring may result if I.V. infiltrates.
- Explain that fever may be a reaction to the drug. Advise parents to report fever that persists for more than 24 hours after the drug is administered.
- Patient should not receive immunizations during therapy and for several weeks afterward. Members of the same household should not receive live-virus immunizations during the same pereiod.
- Reassure parents and patient that hair should grow back after treatment has been discontinued.
- Tell parents to call promptly if the patient develops a sore throat or fever or notices any unusual bruising or bleeding.

---

*Canada only   †Unlabeled clinical use   Italicized adverse reactions have been observed in children.

morphine hydrochloride*
M.O.S.*, Morphitec*

morphine sulfate
Astramorph, Duramorph, Epimorph*, MS Contin, RMS Uniserts, Roxanol, Statex*

- Classification: narcotic analgesic (opioid)
- Controlled substance schedule II

How supplied
Available by prescription only
Morphine hydrochloride*
Tablets: 10 mg, 20 mg, 40 mg, 60 mg
Oral solution: 1 mg/ml, 5 mg/ml, 10 mg/ml, 20 mg/ml, and 50 mg/ml
Syrup: 1 mg/ml, 5 mg/ml
Suppositories: 20 mg, 30 mg
Morphine sulfate
Tablets: 10 mg, 15 mg, 30 mg
Tablets (extended release): 30 mg
Oral solution: 10 mg/5 ml, 20 mg/5 ml, 20 mg/ml
Syrup: 1 mg/ml, 5 mg/ml
Injection (with preservative): 2 mg/ml, 4 mg/ml, 8 mg/ml, 10 mg/ml and 15 mg/ml
Injection (without preservative): 500 mcg/ml, 1 mg/ml
Soluble tablets: 10 mg, 15 mg, 30 mg
Suppositories: 5 mg, 10 mg, 20 mg

Indications, route, and dosage
Severe pain
Children: 0.1 to 0.2 mg/kg S.C. Maximum dose: 15 mg.
In some situations, morphine may be administered by continuous I.V. infusion or by intraspinal and intrathecal injection.
Adults: 4 to 15 mg S.C. or I.M., or 30 to 60 mg P.O. or by rectum q 4 hours, p.r.n. or around the clock. May be injected slow I.V. (over 4 to 5 minutes) diluted in 4 to 5 ml water for injection. May also administer controlled-release tablets q 8 to 12 hours. As an epidural injection, 5 mg via an epidural catheter every 24 hours.
Tetralogy of Fallot; adjunct in pulmonary edema; to reduce preload
Infants and children: Initially 0.05 mg/kg to 1 mg/kg S.C., increasing to 0.1 to 0.2 mg/kg S.C. Maximum dose, 15 mg.

Drug is also used for preoperative sedation, as an adjunct to induction of anesthesia, and to control pain of myocardial infarction and pulmonary dyspnea or edema.

Action and kinetics
- *Analgesic action:* Morphine is the principal opium alkaloid, the standard for opiate agonist analgesic activity. The mechanism of action is thought to be via the opiate receptors, altering the patient's perception of pain. Morphine is particularly useful in severe, acute pain or severe, chronic pain. Morphine also has a central depressant effect on respiration and on the cough reflex center.
- *Kinetics in adults:* Morphine is absorbed variably from the GI tract. Onset of analgesia occurs within 15 to 60 minutes. Peak analgesia occurs ½ to 1 hour after dosing. Morphine is distributed widely through the body and is metabolized primarily in the liver. Duration of action is 3 to 7 hours. Morphine is excreted in the urine and bile.

Contraindications and precautions
Morphine is contraindicated in patients with known hypersensitivity to the drug or other phenanthrene opioids (codeine, hydrocodone, hydromorphone, oxycodone, oxymorphone).

Administer morphine with extreme caution to patients with supraventricular dysrhythmias; avoid, or administer drug with extreme caution to patients with head injury or increased intracranial pressure, because it obscures neurologic parameters; and during pregnancy and labor, because drug readily crosses placenta (premature infants are especially sensitive to respiratory and CNS depressant effects).

Administer morphine cautiously to patients with renal or hepatic dysfunction, because drug accumulation or prolonged duration of action may occur; to patients with pulmonary disease (asthma, chronic obstructive pulmonary disease), because drug depresses respiration and suppresses cough reflex; to patients undergoing biliary tract surgery, because drug may cause biliary spasm; to patients with convulsive disorders, because drug may precipitate seizures; to debilitated patients, who are more sensitive to both therapeutic and adverse drug effects; and to patients prone to physical or psychic addiction, because of the high risk of addiction to this drug.

Interactions
Concomitant use with other CNS depressants (narcotic analgesics, general anesthetics, antihistamines, monoamine oxidase inhibitors, phenothiazines, barbiturates, benzodiazepines, sedative-hypnotics, tricyclic antidepressants, alcohol, and muscle relaxants) potentiates drug's respiratory and CNS depression, sedation, and hypotensive effects. Concomitant use with cimetidine also may increase respiratory and CNS depression, causing confusion, disorientation, apnea, or seizures. Reduced dosage of morphine is usually necessary.

Drug accumulation and enhanced effects may result from concomitant use with other drugs that are extensively metabolized in the liver (rifampin, phenytoin, and digitoxin); combined use with anticholinergics may cause paralytic ileus.

Patients who become physically dependent on this drug may experience acute withdrawal syndrome if given a narcotic antagonist.

Severe cardiovascular depression may result from concomitant use with general anesthetics.

Effects on diagnostic tests
Morphine increases plasma amylase levels.

---

‡May contain sulfites ◆May contain tartrazine ◆◆May contain benzyl alcohol

Adverse reactions

• CNS: sedation, somnolence, clouded sensorium, euphoria, insomnia, agitation, confusion, *headache,* tremor, miosis, seizures, *psychic dependence,* nightmares (with long-acting dosage form).
• CV: *tachycardia,* asystole, *bradycardia,* palpitations, chest wall rigidity, hypertension, *hypotension,* syncope, edema.
• DERM: flushing (with epidural use), rashes, pruritus, pain at injection site.
• GI: dry mouth, anorexia, biliary spasms (colic), ileus, nausea, vomiting, *constipation.*
• GU: *urinary retention* or hesitancy, decreased libido.
• Other: *respiratory depression, physiologic dependence, muscule rigidity.*
Note: Drug should be discontinued if hypersensitivity, seizures, or cardiac dysrhythmias occur.

Overdose and treatment

Rapid I.V. administration may result in overdose because of the delay in maximum CNS effect (30 minutes). The most common signs and symptoms of morphine overdose is respiratory depression with or without CNS depression, respiratory depression, and miosis (pinpoint pupils). Other acute toxic effects include hypotension, bradycardia, hypothermia, shock, apnea, cardiopulmonary arrest, circulatory collapse, pulmonary edema, and convulsions.

To treat acute overdose, first establish adequate respiratory exchange via a patent airway and ventilation as needed; administer a narcotic antagonist (naloxone) to reverse respiratory depression. (Because the duration of action of morphine is longer than that of naloxone, repeated naloxone dosing is necessary.) Naloxone should not be given in the absence of clinically significant respiratory or cardiovascular depression. Monitor vital signs closely.

If the patient presents within 2 hours of ingestion of an oral overdose, empty the stomach immediately by inducing emesis (ipecac syrup) or using gastric lavage. Use caution to avoid any risk of aspiration. Administer activated charcoal via nasogastric tube for further removal of the drug in an oral overdose.

Provide symptomatic and supportive treatment (continued respiratory support, correction of fluid or electrolyte imbalance). Monitor laboratory parameters, vital signs, and neurologic status.

▶ Special considerations

• Administer with extreme caution to patients with head injury, increased intracranial pressure, seizures, asthma, chronic obstructive pulmonary disease, alcoholism, severe hepatic or renal disease, acute abdominal conditions, cardiac dysrhythmias, hypovolemia, or psychiatric disorders, or to elderly or debilitated patients. Reduced doses may be necessary.
• Consider possible interactions with other drugs the patient is taking.
• Keep resuscitative equipment and a narcotic antagonist (naloxone) available. Be prepared to provide support of ventilation and gastric lavage.
• Parenteral administration of opiates provides better analgesia than oral administration. Intravenous administration should be given by slow injection, preferably in diluted solution. Rapid I.V. injection increases the incidence of adverse effects.
• Parenteral injections by I.M. or S.C. route should be given cautiously to patients who are chilled, hypovolemic, or in shock, because decreased perfusion may lead to accumulation of the drug and toxic effects. Rotate I.M. or S.C. injection sites to avoid induration.
• Before administration, visually inspect all parenteral products for particulate matter and discoloration.
• Oral solutions of varying concentrations are available. Carefully note the strength of the solution.
• A regular dosage schedule (rather than "p.r.n. pain") is preferred to alleviate the symptoms and anxiety that accompany pain.
• The duration of respiratory depression may be longer than the analgesic effect. Monitor the patient closely with repeated dosing.
• Provide comfort measures.
• With chronic administration, evaluate the patient's respiratory status before each dose. Because severe respiratory depression may occur (especially with accumulation from chronic dosing), watch for respiratory rate below the patient's baseline level. Evaluate the patient for restlessness, which may be a sign of compensatory response for hypoxia.
• Opiates or agonist-antagonists may cause orthostatic hypotension in ambulatory patients. Have the patient sit or lie down to relieve dizziness or fainting.
• Since opiates depress respiration when they are used postoperatively, encourage patient turning, coughing, and deep breathing to avoid atelectases.
• If gastric irritation occurs, give oral products with food; food delays absorption and onset of analgesia.
• The antitussive activity of opiates is used to control persistent, exhausting cough or dry, non-productive cough.
• The first sign of tolerance to the therapeutic effect of opioid agonists or agonist-antagonists is usually a shortened duration of effect.
• Morphine is the drug of choice in relieving pain of myocardial infarction; may cause transient decrease in blood pressure.
• Regimented scheduling (around the clock) is beneficial in severe, chronic pain.
• Oral solutions of various concentrations are available, as well as a new intensified oral solution.
• For sublingual administration, measure out oral solution with tuberculin syringe, and administer dose a few drops at a time to allow maximal sublingual absorption and to minimize swallowing.
• Refrigeration of rectal suppositories is not necessary. Note that in some patients, rectal and oral absorption may not be equivalent.
• Preservative-free morphine (Astramorph, Duramorph) is now available for epidural or intrathecal use.
• Epidural morphine has proven to be an excellent analgesic for patients with postoperative pain. After epidural administration, monitor closely for respiratory depression up to 24 hours after the injection. Check respiratory rate and depth according to protocol (for example, every 15 minutes for 2 hours, followed by every hour for 18 hours). Some clinicians advocate a dilute naloxone infusion (5 to 10 mcg/kg/hr) during

the first 12 hours to minimize respiratory depression without altering pain relief.
• Morphine may worsen or mask gallbladder pain.

Information for parents and patient
• Drug may produce drowsiness and sedation. Tell parents to have patient use drug with caution and to avoid hazardous activities that require full alertness and coordination.
• Tell parents that patient should avoid ingestion of alcohol-containing beverages or elixirs when taking drug, because it will cause additive CNS depression.
• Explain that constipation may result from taking drug. Suggest measures to increase dietary fiber content, or recommend a stool softener.
• If patient's condition allows, instruct patient to breathe deeply, cough, and change position every 2 hours to avoid respiratory complications.
• Patient should void at least every 4 hours to prevent urinary retention.
• Tell parents to have the patient take the medication as prescribed and to call the physician if significant adverse effects occur.
• Tell parents not to increase dosage if patient is not experiencing the desired effect, but to call the physician for prescribed dosage adjustment.
• Instruct the parents and patient not to double the dose. Tell the patient to take a missed dose as soon as he remembers unless it's almost time for the next dose. If this is so, the patient should skip the missed dose and go back to the regular dosage schedule.
• Tell the parents to call immediately for emergency help if they think the patient or someone else has taken an overdose.
• Explain the signs of overdose to the parents and patient.
• Tell parents that oral liquid form of morphine may be mixed with a glass of fruit juice immediately before giving it to the patient, if desired, to improve the taste.
• Tell parents and patient taking long-acting morphine tablets to swallow them whole. Patient should not break, crush, or chew the tablets before swallowing them.

---

moxalactam
Moxam

• Classification: antibiotic (third-generation cephalosporin)

How supplied
Available by prescription only
Parenteral: 1 g, 2 g

Indications, route, and dosage
Serious respiratory, urinary, CNS, intraabdominal, gynecologic, and skin infections; bacteremia; and septicemia
Neonates age 1 to 7 days weighing ≤ 2000 g: 50 mg/kg divided q 12 hours
Neonates age 8 days to 4 weeks: 50 mg/kg divided q 8 hours

Neonates over age 4 weeks: 50 mg/kg I.M. or I.V., divided q 6 hours
Children: 50 mg/kg I.M. or I.V. q 6 to 8 hours.
Adults: Usual daily dose is 2 to 6 g I.M. or I.V. administered in divided doses q 8 hours for 5 to 10 days, or up to 14 days. Up to 12 g/day may be needed in life-threatening infections or in infections caused by less susceptible organisms.

For treatment of meningitis or other severe infection, therapy may begin with single loading dose: 100 mg/kg.

Total daily dosage is same for I.M. or I.V. administration and depends on susceptibility of organism and severity of infection. In patients with impaired renal function, doses or frequency of administration must be modified according to degree of impairment, severity of infection, and susceptibility of organism. Moxalactam should be injected deep I.M. into the gluteus or lateral aspect of the thigh. I.V. infusion should be given over 3 to 5 minutes.

Action and kinetics
• *Antibacterial action:* Moxalactam is 1-oxa-beta-lactam and has a mechanism of action similar to other cephalosporins. Moxalactam is primarily bactericidal; however, it may be bacteriostatic. Activity depends on the organism, tissue penetration, drug dosage, and rate of organism multiplication. It acts by adhering to penicillin-binding enzymes, thus inhibiting bacterial protein synthesis. Third-generation cephalosporins appear more active against some beta-lactamase-producing gram-negative organisms.

Moxalactam is active against some gram-positive organisms and many enteric gram-negative bacilli and some strains of *Pseudomonas aeruginosa, Bacteroides,* and other anaerobes. *Acinetobacter* and *Listeria* are usually resistant to moxalactam.
• *Kinetics in adults:* Moxalactam is not absorbed from the GI tract and must be given parenterally; peak serum levels occur ½ to 1 hour after an I.M. dose. Moxalactam is distributed widely into most body tissues and fluids, including the gallbladder, liver, kidneys, bone, sputum, bile, and pleural and synovial fluids; unlike most other cephalosporins, it has good CSF penetration. Moxalactam crosses the placenta; it is 45% to 60% protein-bound. Moxalactam is not metabolized. It is excreted primarily in urine by glomerular filtration; small amounts of drug are excreted in breast milk. Elimination half-life is 2 to 3½ hours in normal adults; severe renal disease prolongs half-life to about 5 to 10 hours. Hemodialysis removes moxalactam, but peritoneal dialysis does not.
• *Kinetics in children:* Serum half-life is prolonged in neonates and in infants up to age 1.

Contraindications and precautions
Moxalactam is contraindicated in patients with known hypersensitivity to any cephalosporin.

Use moxalactam with caution in patients with penicillin allergy, who are usually more susceptible to such reactions; and in patients with coagulopathy and elderly, debilitated, or malnourished patients, who are usually at greater risk of bleeding complications.

---

‡May contain sulfites   ◆May contain tartrazine   ◆◆May contain benzyl alcohol

Interactions

Concomitant use with aminoglycosides results in synergistic activity against *Pseudomonas aeruginosa* and *Serratia marcescens;* such combined use slightly increases risk of nephrotoxicity.

Concomitant use with alcohol may cause disulfiram-type reactions (flushing, sweating, tachycardia, headache, abdominal cramping).

Effects on diagnostic tests

Moxalactam causes positive Coombs' tests and may elevate liver function test results and prothrombin times.

Adverse reactions

- CNS: headache, malaise, paresthesias, dizziness, seizures.
- DERM: maculopapular and erythematous rashes, *urticaria.*
- GI: *pseudomembranous colitis,* nausea, anorexia, vomiting, *diarrhea,* glossitis, dyspepsia, abdominal cramps, tenesmus, pruritus ani.
- GU: genital pruritus.
- HEMA: transient neutropenia, eosinophilia, hemolytic anemia, hypoprothrombinemia, *bleeding.*
- Local: *pain at injection site,* induration, sterile abscesses, tissue sloughing; *phlebitis* and thrombophlebitis with I.V. injection.
- Other: *hypersensitivity,* dyspnea, fever, bacterial and fungal *superinfection.*

Note: Drug should be discontinued if signs of toxicity, immediate hypersensitivity reaction, or hypoprothrombinemia occur or if severe diarrhea indicates pseudomembranous colitis; alternative therapy should be considered if the patient develops fever, eosinophilia, hematuria, or neutropenia.

Overdose and treatment

Clinical signs of overdose include neuromuscular hypersensitivity. Seizure may follow high CNS concentrations. Hypoprothrombinemia and bleeding may occur and may require treatment with vitamin K or blood products. Moxalactam may be removed by hemodialysis.

▶ Special considerations

- For patients on sodium restriction, note that moxalactam injection contains 3.8 mEq of sodium chloride per gram of drug.
- Obtain results of cultures and sensitivity tests before first dose; but do not delay therapy; check test results periodically to assess drug efficacy.
- Moxalactam does not interfere with urine glucose determinations.
- Dilute I.M. dose with sterile or bacteriostatic water, 0.9% NaCl, or 0.5% or 1% lidocaine HCl injection.
- Administer deep I.M. into large muscle mass to prevent tissue damage. Aspirate before injection to avoid inadvertent entry into blood vessel. Rotate injection sites to prevent tissue damage. Apply ice to site to minimize pain.
- For direct intermittent I.V. administration, add 10 ml of sterile water for injection, dextrose 5% injection, or 0.9% NaCl injection per gram of moxalactam. Administer slowly over 3 to 5 minutes or through tubing of free-flowing compatible I.V. solution.
- Adequate dilution of I.V. infusion and frequent rotation of the site help minimize local vein irritation, use of small-guage needle in larger available vein may be helpful.
- Monitor for signs and symptoms of overt or occult bleeding. Monitor complete blood count, platelet count, and prothrombin time for abnormalities.
- Bleeding associated with hypoprothrombinemia can be prevented with vitamin K, 10 mg per week, to be given prophylactically. Bleeding can be promptly reversed with the administration of vitamin K.
- Because moxalactam is hemodialyzable, patients undergoing treatment with hemodialysis may require dosage adjustments.
- Review patient's history of allergies; do not give moxalactam to any patient with a history of hypersensitivity reactions to cephalosporins; administer cautiously to patients with penicillin allergy.
- Try to determine whether previous reactions were true hypersensitivity reactions and not another reaction that the patient has interpreted as allergy.
- Monitor continuously for possible hypersensitivity reactions or other untoward effects.
- Monitor renal function studies; dosages of certain cephalosporins must be lowered in patients with severe renal impairment. In decreased renal function, monitor BUN levels, serum creatinine levels, and urine output for significant changes.
- Monitor patients on long-term therapy for possible bacterial and fungal superinfection, especially debilitated patients, and others receiving immunosuppressants or radiation therapy.
- Cephalosporins cause false-positive results in urine glucose tests utilizing cupric sulfate solutions (Benedict's reagent or Clinitest); glucose oxidase tests (Clinistix or Tes-Tape) are not affected.
- Administer cephalosporins at least 1 hour before bacteriostatic antibiotics (tetracyclines, erythromycins, and chloramphenicol); these drugs inhibit bacterial cell growth, decreasing cephalosporin uptake by bacterial cell walls.

Information for parents and patient

- Teach parents how to recognize signs and symptoms of hypersensitivity, bacterial and fungal superinfection and other adverse reactions; urge them to report any unusual effects.
- Patient should not ingest alcohol in any form within 72 hours of cephalosporin dose. Warn parents that some liquid forms of acetaminophen contain alcohol.
- Advise parents to add live-culture yogurt or buttermilk to child's diet to prevent intestinal superinfection resulting from suppression of normal intestinal flora.
- Teach parents how to prevent superinfection by practicing meticulous oral and anogenital hygiene. Parents of infants and toddlers should keep diaper area clean and dry and avoid using plastic pants.

---

mumps skin test antigen
MSTA

• Classification: skin test antigen (viral)

How supplied
Available by prescription only
Injection: 20 complement-fixing units/ml suspension; 10 tests/1-ml vial

Indications, route, and dosage
To assess cell-mediated immunity
Children and adults: 0.1 ml intradermally into the volar surface of the forearm.

Action and kinetics
• *Antigenic action:* Mumps skin test is not indicated for the immunization, diagnosis, or treatment of mumps virus infection.
   The status of cell-mediated immunity can be determined from use of mumps with other antigens. In vitro tests (such as lymphocyte stimulation and assays for T and B cells) are necessary to diagnose a specific disorder.
• *Kinetics in adults:* After intradermal injection of mumps skin test antigen, the test site should be examined in 48 to 72 hours. Injection must be given intradermally; subcutaneous injection invalidates the test.

Contraindications and precautions
Mumps skin test antigen is contraindicated in persons sensitive to avian protein (chicken, eggs, or feathers) and in those hypersensitive to thimerosal.

Interactions
None reported.

Effects on diagnostic tests
None reported.

Adverse reactions
• Systemic: nausea, headache, anorexia, drowsiness.
• Local: tenderness, pruritus, and rash occur at injection site. Occasionally, a severe delayed-hypersensitivity reaction will produce vesiculation, local tissue necrosis, abscess, and scar formation.
• Other: anaphylaxis, Arthus reaction, urticaria, angioedema, shortness of breath, excessive perspiration.

Overdose and treatment
Administer epinephrine 1:1,000 if anaphylaxis occurs.

▶ Special considerations
• Obtain history of allergies and reactions to skin tests. In patients hypersensitive to feathers, eggs, or chicken, a severe reaction may follow administration of mumps skin test antigen.
• Before injection, assess patient's history of immunization or mumps infection.
• After injection of mumps skin test antigen, observe the patient for 15 minutes for possible immediate-type

systemic allergic reaction. Keep epinephrine 1:1,000 available.
• Accurate dosage (0.1 ml) and administration are essential with the use of mumps skin test antigen.
• Examine injection site within 48 to 72 hours, interpreting as follows:
Positive reaction: An area of erythema 1.5 cm or more in diameter, with or without induration, indicates sensitivity.
Negative reaction: Erythema of less than 1.5 cm or induration less than 5 mm means the individual has not been sensitized to mumps or is anergic.
• Reactivity to this test may be depressed or suppressed for as long as 6 weeks in individuals who have received concurrent virus vaccines, in those who are receiving a corticosteroid or other immunosuppressive agents, in those who have had viral infections, and in malnourished patients.
• Mumps skin test antigen is not used to assess exposure to mumps. It is used in assessing T cell function for immunocompetence since most normal individuals will exhibit a positive reaction.
• Cold packs or topical steroids relieve pain, pruritus, and discomfort if a local reaction occurs.
• Store vial in refrigerator.

Information for parents and patient
• Have parents report any unusual side effects.
• Explain that the induration will disappear in a few days.

muromonab-CD3
Orthoclone OKT3

• Classification: immunosuppressive agent (monoclonal antibody)

How supplied
Injection: 5 mg/5 ml in 5-ml ampules

Indications, route, and dosage
Treatment of acute allograft rejection in renal transplant patients
Children younger than age 12: 2.5 mg/day rapid I.V. for 10 to 14 days or 100 mcg (0.1 mg) per kg of body weight for 10 to 14 days.
Adults: 5 mg/day, for 10 to 14 days. Begin treatment once acute renal rejection is diagnosed.

Action and kinetics
• *Immunosuppressive action:* Muromonab-CD3 reverses graft rejection, probably by interfering with T cell function that promotes acute renal rejection. It interacts with, and prevents the function of, a T cell molecule (CD3) in the cellular membrane that influences antigen recognition and is essential for signal transduction. Muromonab-CD3 reacts with most peripheral T cells in blood and in body tissues, and blocks all known T cell functions.
• *Kinetics in adults:* Absorption is immediate after I.V. administration. Distribution, metabolism, and excretion are unknown.

Contraindications and precautions

Contraindicated in patients allergic to muromonab-CD3. Use with extreme caution in patients allergic to products of murine origin.

This drug contains polysorbate 80 and should not be used for the in vitro treatment of bone marrow. Because this drug is a heterologous protein, it induces antibodies, which could limit its efficacy and may cause serious reactions upon readministration. A second course should be administered with caution.

Monitor patient closely for 48 hours after the first dose. Administration of methylprednisolone sodium succinate 1 mg/kg I.V. before muromonab-CD3 and I.V. hydrocortisone sodium succinate 100 mg given 30 minutes after is strongly recommended to minimize the first-dose reaction. Acetaminophen and antihistamines, given concomitantly, may reduce early reactions.

The most serious first-dose reaction, potentially fatal severe pulmonary edema, has occurred infrequently (in fewer than 5% of the first 107 patients and in none of the subsequent 311 patients treated with first-dose restrictions). In every patient who developed pulmonary edema, fluid overload was present before treatment. Therefore, carefully evaluate patients for fluid overload by chest X-ray or weight gain of > 3%. The patient's weight should be less than 3% above minimum weight the week before treatment begins.

Interactions

Muromonab-CD3 may potentiate immunosuppressive effects of other immunosuppressant drugs (azathioprine, cyclosporine).

Effects on diagnostic tests

None reported.

Adverse reactions

- CNS: pyrexia, chills, tremor.
- CV: chest pain, severe pulmonary edema.
- EENT: wheezing.
- GI: nausea, vomiting, diarrhea.
- Other: dyspnea, infections, anaphylaxis, serum sickness.

Overdose and treatment

No information available.

▶ Special considerations

- Safety and efficacy for use in children have not been established. Patients as young as age 2 have had no unexpected adverse effects.
- Preparation of solution: Draw solution into a syringe through a low protein-binding 0.2 or 0.22 micrometer (mcm) filter. Discard filter and attach needle for I.V. bolus injection.
- Because this drug is a protein solution, it may develop a few fine translucent particles, which do not affect its potency.
- Administer as an I.V. bolus in less than 1 minute. Do not give by I.V. infusion or combined with other drug solutions.
- Have emergency drugs and equipment available in patient's room when administering this drug.

- The manufacturer recommends if the patient's temperature exceeds 37.8° C. (100° F.), lower it with antipyretics before muromonab-CD3 administration.
- Chest X-ray taken within 24 hours before treatment must be clear of fluid; monitor WBCs and differentials at intervals during treatment. Monitor the drug's effect on circulating T cells expressing the CD3 antigen by in vitro assay.
- Immunosuppressive therapy increases susceptibility to infection and to lymphoproliferative disorders. Occurrence of lymphomas seems related to the intensity and duration of immunosuppression rather than the use of specific agents since most patients receive a combination of treatments.
- A "first-dose" reaction is common within ½ to 6 hours after the first dose, consisting of significant fever, chills, dyspnea, and malaise. Pulmonary edema may occur if patient is not pretreated with a corticosteroid. Maintain I.V. access after drug administeration in case of emergency.
- Concomitant immunosuppressive therapy should be reduced to a daily dose of prednisone 0.5 mg/kg and azathioprine 25 mg. Cyclosporine should be reduced or discontinued. Maintenance immmuosuppression can resume 3 days before discontinuation of muromonab-CD3.
- Storage and stability: Refrigerate at 2° to 8° C. (36° to 46° F.). Do not freeze or shake.

Information for parents and patient

- Inform parents and patient of expected first-dose effects (fever, chills, dyspnea, chest pain, nausea, and vomiting).

---

nafcillin sodium
Nafcil, Nallpen, Unipen

• Classification: antibiotic (penicillinase-resistant penicillin)

How supplied
Available by prescription only
Capsules: 250 mg
Solution: 250 mg/5 ml (after reconstitution)
Tablets: 500 mg
Injection: 500 mg, 1 g, 2 g
Pharmacy bulk package: 10 g
I.V. infusion piggyback: 1 g, 1.5 g, 2 g, 4 g

Indications, route, and dosage
Systemic infections caused by susceptible organisms (methicillin-sensitive S. aureus)
†*Neonates:* 30 to 40 mg/kg/day P.O. three or four divided doses.

†*Neonates younger than 7 days:* 40 to 100 mg/kg daily I.M. in equally divided doses q 12 hours; or 50 to 100 mg/kg/day I.V. divided q 12 hours.

†*Neonates 7 to 28 days:* 60 to 200 mg/kg I.M. daily in equally divided doses q 8 hours, or 100 to 200 mg/kg/day I.V. divided doses q 6 to 8 hours.

†*Children over 1 month:* 50 mg/kg/day I.M. in two equally divided doses, or 50 to 100 mg/kg/day I.M., I.V., or P.O. in equal doses q 6 hours for mild to moderate infections and 100 to 200 mg/kg/day I.M., I.V., or P.O. in equally divided doses q 4 to 6 hours for severe infections.

Adults: 2 to 4 g P.O. daily, divided into doses given q 6 hours; 2 to 12 g I.M. or I.V. daily, divided into doses given q 4 to 6 hours.

Action and kinetics
• *Antibiotic action:* Nafcillin is bactericidal; it adheres to bacterial penicillin-binding proteins, thus inhibiting bacterial cell wall synthesis.

Nafcillin resists the effects of penicillinases — enzymes that inactivate penicillin — and is thus active against many strains of penicillinase-producing bacteria; this activity is most important against penicillinase-producing staphylococci; some strains may remain resistant. Nafcillin is also active against a few gram-positive aerobic and anaerobic bacilli but has no significant effect on gram-negative bacilli.
• *Kinetics in adults:* Nafcillin is absorbed erratically and poorly from the GI tract; peak serum levels occur at ½ to 2 hours after an oral dose and 30 to 60 minutes after an I.M. dose. Food decreases absorption.

Nafcillin is distributed widely; CSF penetration is poor but enhanced by meningeal inflammation. Nafcillin crosses the placenta and is 70% to 90% protein-bound.

Nafcillin is metabolized primarily in the liver; it undergoes enterohepatic circulation. No dosage adjustment is necessary for patients in renal failure.

Nafcillin and metabolites are excreted primarily in bile; about 25% to 30% is excreted in urine unchanged. It may also be excreted in breast milk. Elimination half-life in adults is ½ to 1½ hours.
• *Kinetics in children:* Serum levels are higher and serum half-life is longer in neonates than in older children.

Contraindications and precautions
Nafcillin is contraindicated in patients with known hypersensitivity to any other penicillin or to cephalosporins. I.V. nafcillin should be used with caution in neonates and infants.

Interactions
Concomitant use of nafcillin with aminoglycosides produces synergistic bactericidal effects against *Staphylococcus aureus.* However, the drugs are physically and chemically incompatible and are inactivated when mixed or given together.

Probenecid blocks renal tubular secretion of penicillin, raising its serum concentrations.

Effects on diagnostic tests
Nafcillin alters tests for urinary and serum proteins; turbidimetric urine and serum proteins are often falsely positive or elevated in tests using sulfosalicylic acid or trichloroacetic acid.

Nafcillin may cause transient reductions in red blood cell, white blood cell, and platelet counts. Abnormal urinalysis results may indicate drug-induced interstitial nephritis.

Adverse reactions
• GI: nausea, vomiting, diarrhea, pseudomembranous colitis.
• GU: hematuria, acute interstitial nephritis.
• HEMA: transient leukopenia, neutropenia, granulocytopenia, thrombocytopenia with high doses.
• Local: vein irritation, thrombophlebitis.
• Other: hypersensitivity reactions (chills, fever, rash, pruritus, urticaria, anaphylaxis), bacterial or fungal superinfection.
Note: Drug should be discontinued if immediate hypersensitivity reactions occur or if signs of interstitial nephritis or pseudomembranous colitis occur. Patient may require alternate therapy if any of the following occurs: drug fever, eosinophilia, hematuria, neutropenia, or unexplained elevations in serum creatinine concentrations, BUN levels, or liver function studies.

Overdose and treatment
Clinical signs of overdose include neuromuscular irritability or seizures. No specific recommendations. Treatment is supportive. After recent ingestion (4

---

‡May contain sulfites   ◆May contain tartrazine   ◆◆May contain benzyl alcohol

hours or less), empty stomach by induced emesis or gastric lavage; follow with activated charcoal to reduce absorption. Nafcillin is not appreciably removed by hemodialysis.

▶ **Special considerations**
• Nafcillin that has been reconstituted with bacteriostatic water for injection with benzyl alcohol should not be used in neonates because of *toxicity*.
• Assess patient's history of allergies; do not give nafcillin to any patient with a history of hypersensitivity reactions to either penicillins or cephalosporins. Try to ascertain whether previous reactions were true hypersensitivity reactions or another reaction, such as GI distress, which the patient has interpreted as allergy.
• Keep in mind that a negative history for penicillin hypersensitivity does not preclude future allergic reactions; monitor patient continuously for possible allergic reactions or other untoward effects.
• In patients with renal impairment, dosage should be reduced if creatinine clearance is below 10 ml/minute.
• Assess level of consciousness, neurologic status, and renal function when high doses are used, because excessive blood levels can cause CNS toxicity.
• Obtain results of cultures and sensitivity tests before first dose; however, therapy may begin before test results are complete. Repeat test periodically to assess drug efficacy.
• Monitor intake and output, vital signs, electrolytes, and renal function studies; monitor body weight for fluid retention with extended-spectrum penicillins for possible hypokalemia or hypernatremia.
• Coagulation abnormalities, even frank bleeding, can follow high doses, especially of extended-spectrum penicillins; monitor prothrombin times and platelet counts, and assess patient for signs of occult or frank bleeding. Check for hematuria.
• Monitor patients on long-term therapy for possible superinfection, especially debilitated patients and others receiving immunosuppressants or radiation therapy; monitor closely, especially for fever.

Oral and parenteral administration
• Give penicillins at least 1 hour before giving bacteriostatic antibiotics (tetracyclines, erythromycins, and chloramphenicol); these drugs inhibit bacterial cell growth, decreasing rate of penicillin uptake by bacterial cell walls.
• Always consult manufacturer's directions for reconstitution, dilution, and storage of drugs; check expiration dates.
• Give oral penicillin at least 1 hour before or 2 hours after meals to enhance gastric absorption; food may or may not decrease absorption.
• Administer I.M. dose deep into large muscle mass (gluteal or midlateral thigh); rotate injection sites to minimize tissue injury; do not inject more than 2 g of drug per injection site. Apply ice to injection site for pain.
• Do not add or mix other drugs with I.V. infusions—particulary aminoglycosides, which will be inactivated if mixed with penicillins; they are chemically and physically incompatible. If other drugs must be given I.V., temporarily stop infusion of primary drug.

• Infuse I.V. drug continuously or intermittently (over 30 minutes) and assess I.V. site frequently to prevent infiltration or phlebitis; rotate infusion site q 48 hours; intermittent I.V. infusion may be diluted in 50 to 100 ml sterile water, 0.9% sodium chloride, dextrose 5% in water, dextrose 5% in water and half normal saline, or lactated Ringer's solution.
• Solutions should always be clear, colorless to pale yellow, and free of particles; do not give solutions containing precipitates or other foreign matter.

Information for parents and patient
• Tell parents to report severe diarrhea or allergic reactions promptly.
• Teach signs and symptoms of hypersensitivity and other adverse reactions, and emphasize need to report any unusual reactions.
• Teach signs and symptoms of bacterial and fungal superinfection to parents and patients, especially for debilitated patients and others with low resistance from immunosuppressants or irradiation; emphasize need to report signs of infection. Explain the importance of practicing meticulous oral and anogenital hygiene. Parents of infants and toddlers should keep diaper area clean and dry and avoid using plastic pants.
• Be sure parents understand how and when to administer drugs; urge them to complete entire prescribed regimen, to comply with instructions for around-the-clock dosage, and to keep follow-up appointments.
• Counsel parents to check expiration date of drug and to discard unused drug and not give it to family member or friends.

---

nalidixic acid
NegGram

• Classification: urinary tract antiseptic (quinolone antibiotic)

How supplied
Available by prescription only
Tablets: 250 mg, 500 mg, 1 g
Suspension: 250 mg/5 ml

Indications, route, and dosage
Acute and chronic urinary tract infections caused by susceptible gram-negative organisms
Children over age 3 months: 55 mg/kg P.O. daily divided q.i.d. for 7 to 14 days; 33 mg/kg P.O. daily divided q.i.d. for long-term use.
Adults: 1 g P.O. q.i.d. for 7 to 14 days; 2 g P.O. daily for long-term use.

Action and kinetics
• *Antimicrobial action:* Drug inhibits microbial synthesis of deoxyribonucleic acid (DNA). Spectrum of action includes most gram-negative organisms except *Pseudomonas.* (Approximately 10% of patients de-

velop nalidixic acid-resistant organisms during therapy.)

• *Kinetics in adults:* Nalidixic acid is well absorbed from the GI tract; peak concentrations occur in 1 to 2 hours. Nalidixic acid concentrates in renal tissue and seminal fluid; it does not penetrate prostatic tissue and only minimal amounts appear in CSF and the placenta. The drug is highly protein-bound. It is metabolized to hydroxynalidixic acid and inactive conjugates in the liver. Metabolites and 2% to 3% of unchanged drug are excreted via the kidneys. In patients with normal renal function, plasma half-life is 1 to 2½ hours.

Contraindications and precautions
Nalidixic acid is contraindicated in children with a history of seizure disorders because the drug may induce seizures; in patients with glucose-6-phosphate dehydrogenase deficiency because drug may induce hemolytic anemia; and in patients with known hypersensitivity to the drug.

Nalidixic acid should be administered cautiously to children with renal or hepatic dysfunction because of potential for drug accumulation.

Interactions
When used concomitantly with warfarin or dicumarol, nalidixic acid may displace clinically significant amounts of these anticoagulants from serum albumin binding sites, possibly causing excessive anticoagulation. When taken with other photosensitizing drugs, additive effects may occur.

Effects on diagnostic tests
False-positive reactions may occur in urine glucose tests using cupric sulfate reagents (such as Benedict's test, Fehling's test, and Clinitest), from reaction between glucuronic acid (liberated by urinary metabolites of nalidixic acid) and cupric sulfate. Urine 17-ketosteroid and urine 17-ketogenic steroid levels may be falsely elevated because nalidixic acid interacts with *m*-dinitrobenzene, used to measure these urine metabolites. Urinary vanillylmandelic acid levels may also be falsely elevated.

Circulating erythrocyte, platelet, and leukocyte counts may decrease transiently during nalidixic acid therapy.

Adverse reactions
• CNS: drowsiness, weakness, headache, dizziness, vertigo, convulsions in epileptic patients, confusion, hallucinations.
• DERM: pruritus, photosensitivity, urticaria, rash.
• EENT: sensitivity to light, change in color perception, diplopia, blurred vision.
• GI: abdominal pain, nausea, vomiting, diarrhea.
• HEMA: eosinophilia, thrombocytopenia, leukopenia, hemolytic anemia.
• Other: angioedema, fever, chills, increased intracranial pressure (ICP), and bulging fontanelles in infants and children.
Note: Drug should be discontinued if patient develops hypersensitivity reaction, seizures, toxic psychosis, evidence of increased ICP, or photosensitivity reaction.

Overdose and treatment
Clinical effects of overdose include toxic psychosis, seizures, increased ICP, metabolic acidosis, lethargy, nausea, and vomiting. However, because nalidixic acid is rapidly excreted, such reactions usually resolve in 2 to 3 hours.

Gastric lavage may be performed after recent ingestion. However, if drug absorption has occurred, supportive measures, including increased fluid administration, should be initiated. Anticonvulsants may be used to treat nalidixic acid-induced seizures; however, this measure is rarely required.

▶ Special considerations
• Use very cautiously in prepubertal children because the drug may be toxic to cartilage in weight-bearing joints. Arthropathy has been reported in inmature animals.
• Obtain culture and sensitivity tests before starting therapy, and repeat as needed.
• Obtain CBC and renal and liver function studies periodically during long-term therapy.
• Drug is ineffective against *Pseudomonas* infection or infection found outside urinary tract.
• Resistant bacteria may emerge after first 48 hours of therapy (especially after inadequate dosage).
• Although CNS toxicity is rare, brief convulsions, increased ICP, and toxic psychosis may occur in infants and children.

Information for parents and patient
• Teach parents how to recognize signs of hypersensitivity and rising ICP.
• Instruct them to report visual disturbances; these usually disappear with dosage reduction.
• Warn parents and child that exposure to sunlight may cause photosensitivity. Inform them that photosensitivity may persist for up to 3 months after drug therapy ends. Also warn that bullae may continue to follow subsequent exposure to sunlight or mild skin trauma for up to 3 months after drug therapy ends.
• Advise parents to give the drug with food or milk to avoid GI upset.

---

naloxone hydrochloride
Narcan

• Classification: narcotic antagonist (opioid)

How supplied
Available by prescription only
Injection: 0.4 mg/ml, 1 mg/ml, 0.02 mg/ml, 0.4 mg/ml (paraben free)

Indications, route, and dosage
Postoperative narcotic depression
Children: 0.01 mg/kg dose I.M., I.V., or S.C., repeated q 2 to 3 minutes p.r.n. Note: If initial dose does not result in clinical improvement, up to 10 times this dose (0.1 mg/kg) may be needed to be effective.

Neonatal opiate depression (asphyxia neonatorium):

Neonates: 0.01 mg/kg I.V. into umbilical vein repeated q 2 to 3 minutes for three doses. Concentration for use in neonates and children is 0.02 mg/ml.

Adults: 0.1 to 0.2 mg I.V. q 2 to 3 minutes, p.r.n. Adult concentration is 0.4 mg/ml. Some clinicians advocate much smaller doses: dilute to 40 mcg/ml and administer in 40 mcg doses. These small doses are used to reverse respiratory depression while maintaining analgesia.

Action and kinetics

• *Narcotic (opioid) antagonism:* Naloxone is essentially a pure antagonist. In patients who have received an opioid agonist or other analgesic with narcotic-like effects, naloxone antagonizes most of the opioid effects, especially respiratory depression, sedation, and hypotension. Because the duration of action of naloxone in most cases is shorter than that of the opioid, opiate effects may return as those of naloxone dissipate. Naloxone does not produce tolerance or physical or psychological dependence. The precise mechanism of action is unknown, but is thought to involve competitive antagonism of more than one opiate receptor in the CNS.

• *Kinetics in adults:* Naloxone is rapidly inactivated after oral administration; therefore, it is given parenterally. Its onset of action is 1 to 2 minutes after I.V. administration, and 2 to 5 minutes after I.M. or S.C. administration. The duration of action is longer after I.M. use and higher doses, when compared to I.V. use and lower doses.

Naloxone is rapidly distributed into body tissues and fluids.

Naloxone is rapidly metabolized in the liver, primarily by conjugation.

Duration of action is approximately 45 minutes, depending on route and dose. Drug is excreted in urine. The plasma half-life has been reported to be from 30 to 90 minutes in adults, and 3 hours in neonates.

Contraindications and precautions

Naloxone is contraindicated in patients with known hypersensitivity to the drug.

Administer naloxone with extreme caution to patients with supraventricular dysrhythmias; avoid or administer drug with extreme caution to patients with a head injury or increased intracranial pressure, because drug obscures neurologic parameters.

Administer cautiously to patients with convulsive disorders, because naloxone can precipitate seizures; and to elderly or debilitated patients, who are more sensitive to the drug's therapeutic and adverse effects.

Naloxone should be administered cautiously to narcotic addicts, including newborns of women with narcotic dependence, in whom it may produce an acute abstinence syndrome.

Because the duration of action of naloxone is shorter than that of most opiates, continued surveillance of the patient is mandatory, and repeated naloxone doses are often necessary. Other supportive therapy, with attention to maintenance of adequate respiratory and cardiovascular function, is imperative.

Interactions

When given to a narcotic addict, naloxone may produce an acute abstinence syndrome. Use with caution, and monitor closely.

Effects on diagnostic tests

None reported.

Adverse reactions

• CV: *tachycardia, increased blood pressure.*
• GI: *nausea and vomiting* (with high doses).
• Other: *tremors,* sweating, pulmonary edema (postoperatively), *tachypnea, lethargy, elevated PTT.*

   Note: Drug should be discontinued if signs of a severe acute abstinence syndrome appear.

Overdose and treatment

No serious adverse reactions to naloxone overdose are known, except those of acute abstinence syndrome in narcotic dependent persons.

▶ Special considerations

• Administer with extreme caution to children. Adult concentration (0.4 mg/ml) may be diluted by mixing 0.5 ml with 9.5 ml sterile water or saline solution for injection to make neonatal concentration (0.02 mg/ml).

• Use with extreme caution in patients with head injury, increased intracranial pressure, seizures, asthma, alcoholism, severe hepatic or renal disease, acute abdominal conditions, cardiac dysrhythmias, hypovolemia, or psychiatric disorders; and in debilitated patients. Reduced doses may be necessary.

• Opioid antagonists should not be used in narcotic addicts, including newborns of mothers with narcotic dependence, in whom they may produce an acute abstinence syndrome.

• Keep resuscitative equipment available. Be prepared to provide supported ventilation and gastric lavage.

• Maintain airway and monitor circulatory status.

• Before administration, visually inspect all parenteral products for particulate matter and discoloration.

• Take a careful drug history to rule out possible narcotic addiction, to avoid inducing withdrawal symptoms (apply cautions also to the baby of an addicted woman).

• Avoid relying on the drug too much, that is, do not neglect attention to the ABCs (airway, breathing, and circulation). Maintain adequate respiratory and cardiovascular status at all times. Respiratory "overshoot" may occur; monitor for respiratory rate higher than before respiratory depression. Respiratory rate increases in 1 to 2 minutes, and effect lasts 1 to 4 hours.

• Naloxone is not effective in treating respiratory depression caused by nonopioid drugs.

• Naloxone can be diluted in dextrose 5% or normal saline solution. Use within 24 hours after mixing.

• Naloxone is the safest drug to use when cause of respiratory depression is uncertain.

• Naloxone may be administered by continuous I.V. infusion, which is necessary in many cases to control the adverse effects of epidurally administered morphine.

---

*Canada only   †Unlabeled clinical use   Italicized adverse reactions have been observed in children.

• Naloxone has been shown to improve circulation in refractory shock, and has been used by some researchers to relieve certain cases of chronic constipation.

nandrolone decanoate
Anabolin LA-100, Androlone-D 100, Deca-Durabolin, Hybolin Decanoate, Kabolin, Nandrobolic L.A., Neo-Durabolic

• Classification: anabolic steroid, erythropoietic agent

How supplied
Available by prescription only
Injection: 50 mg/ml, 100 mg/ml, and 200 mg/ml (in oil)

Indications, route, and dosage
Anemia associated with renal insufficiency
Decanoate
Children age 2 to 13: 25 to 50 mg I.M. every 3 to 4 weeks.
Children over age 14 and adults: 100 mg to 200 mg I.M. weekly in males; 50 to 100 mg/week in females.

Action and kinetics
• *Androgenic action:* Nandrolone exerts inhibitory effects on hormone-responsive breast tumors and metastases.
• *Erythropoietic action:* Nandrolone stimulates the kidneys' production of erythropoietin, leading to increases in red blood cell mass and volume.
• *Anabolic action:* Nandrolone may reverse corticosteroid-induced catabolism and promote tissue development in severely debilitated patients.
• *Kinetics in adults:* Nandrolone is metabolized by the liver. Its pharmacokinetics are otherwise poorly described.

Contraindications and precautions
Nandrolone is contraindicated in patients with severe renal or cardiac disease because fluid and electrolyte retention caused by this agent may aggravate these disorders; in patients with hepatic disease because impaired elimination of the drug may cause toxic accumulation; in male patients with prostatic or breast cancer or benign prostatic hypertrophy with obstruction and in patients with undiagnosed abnormal genital bleeding because this drug can stimulate the growth of cancerous breast or prostate tissue in males; and in pregnant or breast-feeding patients because animal studies have shown that administration of anabolic steroids during pregnancy causes masculinization of the female fetus. Administer nandrolone decanoate cautiously in patients with a history of coronary artery disease because the drug has hypercholesterolemic effects.

Interactions
In patients with diabetes, decreased blood glucose levels may require adjustment of insulin dosage.
Nandrolone decanoate may potentiate the effects of warfarin-type anticoagulants, causing increases in prothrombin time. Use with adrenocorticosteroids or adrenocorticotropic hormone increases the potential for fluid and electrolyte retention.

Effects on diagnostic tests
Nandrolone may cause abnormal results of fasting plasma glucose, glucose tolerance, and metyrapone tests. It may increase sulfobromophthalein retention. Thyroid function test results (protein-bound iodine, radioactive iodine uptake, thyroid-binding capacity) and 17-ketosteroid levels may decrease. Liver function test results, prothrombin time (especially in patients receiving anticoagulant therapy), and serum creatinine levels may be elevated. Because of this agent's anabolic activity, serum sodium, potassium, calcium, phosphate, and cholesterol levels may all rise.

Adverse reactions
• Androgenic: *in females:* deepening of voice, clitoral enlargement, decreased or increased libido; *in males:* prepubertal — premature epiphyseal closure, priapism, phallic enlargement; postpubertal — testicular atrophy, oligospermia, decreased ejaculatory volume, impotence, gynecomastia, epididymitis.
• CNS: headache, mental depression.
• CV: edema.
• DERM: acne, oily skin, hirsutism, flushing, sweating.
• GI: gastroenteritis, nausea, vomiting, diarrhea, change in appetite, weight gain.
• GU: bladder irritability, vaginitis, menstrual irregularities.
• Hepatic: reversible jaundice, hepatotoxicity.
• Local: pain at injection site, induration.
• Other: hypercalcemia, hypercalciuria.
Note: Drug should be discontinued if hypercalcemia, edema, hypersensitivity reaction, priapism, or excessive sexual stimulation occurs or if virilization occurs in females.

Overdose and treatment
No information available.

▶ Special considerations
• Anabolic steroids should be used with caution in prepubertal children. Boys should be closely observed for precocious development of male sexual characteristics.
• In children, X-rays of wrist bones should establish level of bone maturation before therapy is initiated. During treatment, bone maturation may proceed more rapidly than linear growth. Intermittent dosage and periodic X-rays are recommended to monitor skeletal effects.
• Watch female patients for signs of virilization. If possible, discontinue therapy when virilization first becomes apparent because some adverse effects (deepening of voice, clitoral enlargement) are irreversable.
• Anabolic steroids do not improve athletic performance. Risks associated with their use for this pur-

pose far outweigh any possible benefits. Proof of anabolic steroid use is grounds for disqualification in many athletic events.

• Hypercalcemia symptoms may be difficult to distinguish from symptoms of condition being treated unless anticipated and thought of as a cluster. Hypercalcemia is most likely to occur in metastatic breast cancer and may indicate bone metastases.

• Edema usually is controllable with salt restriction diuretics, or both. Monitor weight routinely.

• Watch for symptoms of jaundice. Dosage adjustment may reverse condition. Periodic liver function tests are recommended.

• Observe patient on concomitant anticoagulant therapy for ecchymotic areas, petechia, or abnormal bleeding. Monitor prothrombin time.

• Watch for symptoms of hypoglycemia in patients with diabetes. Change of antihypoglycemic drug dosage may be required.

• Anabolic steroids may alter many laboratory studies during therapy and for 2 to 3 weeks after therapy is stopped.

• Use with diet high in calories and protein unless contraindicated. Give small, frequent meals.

• Nandrolone injections should be administered deeply into the gluteal muscle.

• An adequate iron intake is necessary for maximum response when patient is receiving nandrolone decanoate injections. Patient may need iron supplement.

Information for parents and patient

• Advise parents to administer drug with foods or meals if it causes GI upset.

• Instruct parents and patient regarding iron-rich foods.

• Tell parents and female patient to report menstrual irregularities; therapy should be discontinued until their cause is determined.

• Discuss potential changes in body image with adolescent patients.

---

naproxen
Naprosyn

naproxen sodium
Anaprox

• Classification: nonnarcotic analgesic, antipyretic, nonsteroidal anti-inflammatory propionic acid derivative

---

How supplied
Available by prescription only
Naproxen
Tablets: 250 mg, 375 mg, 500 mg
Suspension: 125 mg/5 ml
Naproxen sodium
Tablets (film-coated): 275 mg, 500 mg
   Note: 275 mg naproxen sodium = 250 mg naproxen.

Indications, route, and dosage
Mild to moderately severe musculoskeletal or soft tissue irritation
Naproxen
Adults: 250 to 375 mg b.i.d.
Naproxen sodium
Adults: 275 mg in the morning and 375 mg in the evening.
Mild to moderate pain; primary dysmenorrhea
Naproxen sodium
Adolescents and adults: 500 to 550 mg P.O. to start, followed by 250 to 275 mg q 6 to 8 hours p.r.n. Maximum daily dose should not exceed 1.25 g of naproxen of 1.375 g of naproxen sodium.
Acute gout
Naproxen
Adults: 750 mg initially, then 250 mg q 8 hours until episode subsides.
Naproxen sodium
Adults: 825 mg initially, then 275 mg q 8 hours until attack has subsided.
Juvenile rheumatoid arthritis
Naproxen
Children over age 2: 10 mg/kg/day in two divided doses.

Action and kinetics
• *Analgesic, antipyretic, and anti-inflammatory actions:* Mechanisms of action are unknown; naproxen is thought to inhibit prostaglandin synthesis.
• *Kinetics in adults:* Naproxen is absorbed rapidly and completely from the GI tract. Effect peaks at 2 to 4 hours. Naproxen is highly protein-bound, and is metabolized in the liver. Naproxen is excreted in urine.

Contraindications and precautions
Naproxen and naproxen sodium are contraindicated in patients with known hypersensitivity and in patients in whom aspirin or other nonsteroidal anti-inflammatory drugs (NSAIDs) induce symptoms of asthma, urticaria, or rhinitis.

Naproxen should be used cautiously in patients with a history of angioedema or of GI disease, peptic ulcer, or renal or cardiovascular disease, because the drug may worsen these conditions. Avoid use during pregnancy (especially the third trimester) because these drugs may prolong labor.

Patients with known "triad" symptoms (aspirin hypersensitivity, rhinitis/nasal polyps, and asthma) are at high risk of cross-sensitivity to naproxen with precipitation of bronchospasm.

The signs and symptoms of acute infection (fever, myalgias, erythema) may be masked by the use of naproxen. Carefully evaluate patients with high infection risk (such as diabetic patients).

Interactions
Concomitant use of naproxen with anticoagulants and thrombolytic drugs (coumarin derivatives, heparin, streptokinase, or urokinase) may potentiate anticoagulant effects. Bleeding problems may occur if used with other drugs that inhibit platelet aggregation, such as azlocillin, parenteral carbenicillin, dextran, dipyridamole, mezlocillin, piperacillin, sulfinpyrazone, ticarcillin, valproic acid, cefamandole, cefoper-

---

azone, moxalactam, plicamycin, aspirin, salicylates, or other anti-inflammatory agents. Concomitant use with salicylates, anti-inflammatory agents, alcohol, corticotropin, or steroids may cause increased GI adverse reactions, including ulceration and hemorrhage. Aspirin may decrease the bioavailability of naproxen.

Because of the influence of prostaglandins on glucose metabolism, concomitant use with insulin or oral hypoglycemic agents may potentiate hypoglycemic effects. Naproxen may displace highly protein-bound drugs from binding sites. Toxicity may occur with coumarin derivatives, phenytoin, verapamil, or nifedipine. Increased nephrotoxicity may occur with gold compounds, other anti-inflammatory agents, or acetaminophen. Naproxen may decrease the renal clearance of methotrexate and lithium. Naproxen may decrease the clinical effectiveness of antihypertensive agents and diuretics. Concomitant use may increase risk of nephrotoxicity.

Effects on diagnostic tests
Naproxen and its metabolites may interfere with urinary 5-hydroxyindoleacetic acid (5-HIAA) and 17-hydroxy-corticosteroid determinations. The physiologic effects of naproxen may lead to an increase in bleeding time (may persist for 4 days after withdrawal of drug); serum creatinine, potassium, and BUN serum transaminase levels may also increase.

Adverse reactions
• CNS: headache, drowsiness, pulmonary infiltrates, light-headedness, vertigo, excitation, dizziness.
• CV: peripheral edema, CHF, hypotension, palpitations.
• DERM: pruritus, rash, urticaria.
• EENT: visual disturbances.
• GI: nausea, epigastric pain, dyspepsia, vomiting, constipation, GI bleeding or perforation, occult blood loss.
• GU: hematuria, cystitis, nocturia, nephrotoxicity.
• HEMA: prolonged bleeding time, aplastic anemia, neutropenia.
• Other: elevated liver enzymes.
Note: Drug should be discontinued if hypersensitivity or signs and symptoms of hepatotoxicity occur.

Overdose and treatment
Clinical manifestations of overdose include drowsiness, heartburn, indigestion, nausea, and vomiting.

To treat overdose of naproxen, empty stomach immediately by inducing emesis with ipecac syrup or by gastric lavage. Administer activated charcoal via nasogastric tube. Provide symptomatic and supportive measures (respiratory support and correction of fluid and electrolyte imbalances). Monitor laboratory parameters and vital signs closely. Hemodialysis is ineffective in naproxen removal.

▶ Special considerations
• Naproxen is approved by the FDA for use in juvenile rheumatoid arthritis at a dose of 10 mg/kg/day. It is also now available in a suspension.
• Use drug cautiously in patients with a history of GI disease, increased risk of GI bleeding, or decreased renal function.

• Patients with known "triad" symptoms (aspirin hypersensitivity, rhinitis/nasal polyps, and asthma) are at high risk of bronchospasm.
• Drug may mask the signs and symptoms of acute infection (fever, myalgia, erythema); carefully evaluate patients at high risk for infection (for example, those with diabetes).
• Administer drug with enough water to ensure passage into stomach. Have patient sit up for 15 to 30 minutes after taking the drug to prevent lodging in the esophagus.
• Tablets may be crushed and mixed with food or fluids to aid swallowing, and with antacids to minimize gastric upset.
• Assess level of pain and inflammation before start of therapy. Evaluate patient for relief or reduction of these symptoms.
• Monitor for signs and symptoms of bleeding.
• Monitor ophthalmic and auditory function before and periodically during therapy to prevent toxicity.
• Monitor CBC, platelets, prothrombin times, and hepatic and renal function studies periodically to detect abnormalities.
• Use of naproxen with an opioid analgesic has an additive effect and may allow use of lower doses of the opioid analgesic.
• Use lowest possible effective dose; 250 mg of naproxen is equivalent to 275 mg of naproxen sodium.
• Relief usually begins within 2 weeks after beginning therapy with naproxen.
• Institute safety measures to prevent injury resulting from possible CNS effects.
• Monitor fluid balance. Monitor for signs and symptoms of fluid retention, especially significant weight gain.
• Avoid combining naproxen (Naprosyn) with naproxen sodium (Anaprox) because both circulate in the blood as naproxen anion.

Information for parents and patient
• Tell parents to have patient take medication with adequate amount of water 30 minutes before or 2 hours after meals, or with food or milk if gastric irritation occurs.
• Explain that taking the drug as directed is necessary to achieve the desired effect; 2 to 4 weeks of treatment may be needed before benefit is seen.
• Advise parents of patients on chronic therapy that follow-up laboratory tests may be necessary.
• Warn parents and patient that use of alcoholic beverages while taking drug may cause increased GI irritation and, possibly, GI bleeding.
• Caution parents to avoid concomitant administration of nonprescription drugs to patients.
• Reinforce signs and symptoms of possible adverse reactions. Instruct parents to report them to physician promptly.
• Instruct parents to check patient's weight every 2 to 3 days and to report any weight gain of 3 pounds or more within 1 week.
• Instruct parents in safety measures; patient should avoid hazardous activities that require alertness until CNS effects are known.

neomycin sulfate
Mycifradin Sulfate, Myciguent

• Classification: antibiotic (aminoglycoside)

How supplied
Available by prescription only
Oral solution: 125 mg/ml
Tablets: 500 mg
Otic: with hydrocortisone and polymyxin B

Available without prescription
Ointment: 0.5%
Cream: 0.5%

Indications, route, and dosage
Infectious diarrhea caused by enteropatho-genic Escherichia coli
Premature infants age 1 to 7 days: 12.5 mg/kg P.O. q 6 hours
Full-term neonates: 25 mg/kg P.O. q 6 hours
Children: 50 to 100 mg/kg P.O. daily divided q 4 to 6 hours for 2 to 3 days.
Adults: 50 mg/kg P.O. daily in 4 divided doses for 2 to 3 days.
Suppression of intestinal bacteria preoperatively
Neonates age 8 days or older: 50 mg/kg P.O. daily in divided doses q 6 hours.
Children: 40 to 100 mg/kg P.O. daily divided q 4 to 6 hours for 3 days. First dose should be preceded by saline cathartic.
Adults: 1 g P.O. q 1 hour for 4 doses, then 1 g q 4 hours for the balance of the 24 hours. A saline cathartic should precede therapy.
Adjunctive treatment in hepatic coma
Children: In acute stage, 2.5 to 7 g/m²/day P.O. divided q 6 hours for 5 to 7 days; in chronic stage, 2.5 g/m²/day P.O., q.i.d.
Adults: 1 to 3 g P.O. q.i.d. for 5 to 6 days; 200 ml of 1% or 100 ml of 2% solution as enema retained for 20 to 60 minutes q 6 hours.
External ear canal infection
Children and adults: Two to five drops into ear canal t.i.d. or q.i.d.
Topical bacterial infections, burns, wounds, skin grafts, following surgical procedure, lesions, pruritus, trophic ulcerations, and edema
Children and adults: Rub in small amount gently b.i.d., t.i.d.

Action and kinetics
• *Antibiotic action:* Neomycin is bactericidal; it binds directly to the 30S ribosomal subunit, thus inhibiting bacterial protein synthesis. Its spectrum of action includes many aerobic gram-negative organisms and some aerobic gram-positive organisms. Generally, neomycin is far less active against many gram-negative organisms than are tobramycin, gentamicin, amikacin, and netilmicin. Given orally or as retention enema, neomycin inhibits ammonia-forming bacteria

in the GI tract, reducing ammonia and improving neurologic status of patients with hepatic encephalopathy. It is rarely given systemically because of its high potential for ototoxicity and nephrotoxicity. The FDA recently revoked licensing of the parenteral preparation for this reason.
• *Kinetics in adults:* Neomycin is absorbed poorly (about 3%) after oral administration, although oral administration is enhanced in patients with impaired GI motility or mucosal intestinal ulcerations. After oral administration, peak serum levels occur at 1 to 4 hours. Neomycin is not absorbed through intact skin; it may be absorbed from wounds, burns, or skin ulcers.

Neomycin is distributed widely after parenteral administration into synovial, pleural, peritoneal, pericardial, ascitic, and abscess fluids, and bile. Intraocular penetration is poor; CSF penetration is low even in patients with inflamed meninges. Protein binding is minimal. Neomycin crosses the placenta. Oral administration restricts distribution to the GI tract.

Neomycin is excreted primarily in urine by glomerular filteration. Elimination half-life in adults is 2 to 3 hours; in severe renal damage, half-life may extend to 24 hours. After oral administration, neomycin is excreted primarily unchanged in feces.

Contraindications and precautions
Neomycin is contraindicated in patients with known hypersensitivity to neomycin or any other aminoglycoside and, when given orally, in patients with intestinal obstruction or ulcerative bowel disease. Otic preparation is contraindicated in perforated eardrum.

Neomycin should be used cautiously in neonates and other infants; in patients with intestinal mucosal ulcerations or large skin wounds; with decreased renal function; with tinnitus, vertigo, and high frequency hearing loss who are susceptible to ototoxicity; and in patients with dehydration, myasthenia gravis, parkinsonism, and hypocalcemia.

Chronic application to inflamed skin increases hazard of sensitization to neomycin.

Interactions
Concomitant use with the following drugs may increase the hazard of nephrotoxicity, ototoxicity, and neurotoxicity: methoxyflurane, polymyxin B, vancomycin, amphotericin B, cisplatin, cephalosporins, and other aminoglycosides; hazard of ototoxicity is also increased during use with ethacrynic acid, furosemide, bumetanide, urea, or mannitol. Dimenhydrinate and other antiemetics and antivertigo drugs may mask neomycin-induced ototoxicity.

Concomitant use with penicillins results in a synergestric bactericidal effect against *Pseudomonas aeruginosa, Escherichia coli, Klebsiella, Citrobacter, Enterobacter, Serratia,* and *Proteus mirabilis.* However, the drugs are physically and chemically incompatible and are inactivated when mixed or given together.

Neomycin may potentiate neuromuscular blockade from general anesthetics or neuromuscular blocking agents such as succinylcholine and tubocurarine.

Oral neomycin inhibits vitamin K-producing bac-

---

teria in GI tract and may potentiate action of oral anticoagulants; dosage adjustment of anticoagulants may be necessary.

Effects on diagnostic tests
Neomycin-induced nephrotoxicity may elevate levels of BUN, nonprotein nitrogen, or serum creatinine; it may increase urinary excretion of casts, if systemic absorption occurs.

Adverse reactions
• CNS: headache, lethargy, *neuromuscular blockade with respiratory depression.*
• DERM: rash, urticaria, contact dermatitis. Systemic absorption possible when used on extensive areas.
• EENT: *ototoxicity (tinnitus, vertigo, hearing loss); if used in ear, burning, erythema, vesicular dermatitis.*
• GI: nausea, vomiting, *diarrhea,* pseudomembranous colitis.
• GU: *nephrotoxicity (cells or casts in the urine, oliguria, proteinuria, decreased creatinine clearance, increased BUN, serum creatinine, and nonprotein nitrogen levels).*
• Other: *hypersensitivity reactions* (eosinophilia, fever, rash, urticaria, pruritus), bacterial or fungal superinfection.
  Note: Drug should be discontinued if signs of ototoxicity, nephrotoxicity, or hypersensitivity occur; if severe diarrhea indicates pseudomembranous colitis; or if intestinal obstruction develops. Drug should be discontinued or serum concentrations monitored if intestinal ulcerations develop, especially in renal impairment.

Overdose and treatment
Clinical signs of overdose include ototoxicity, nephrotoxicity, and neuromuscular toxicity. Remove drug by hemodialysis or peritoneal dialysis; treatment with calcium salts or anticholinesterases reverses neuromuscular blockade. After recent ingestion (4 hours or less), empty the stomach by induced emesis or gastric lavage; follow with activated charcoal to reduce absorption.

▶ Special considerations
• Assess patient's allergic history; do not give neomycin to a patient with a history of hypersensitivity reactions to any aminoglycoside; monitor patient continuously for this and other adverse reactions.
• Obtain results of culture and sensitivity tests before first dose; however, therapy may begin before tests are completed. Repeat tests periodically to assess drug efficacy.
• Monitor vital signs, intake and output, weight, electrolyte levels, and renal function studies before and during therapy; be sure patient is well hydrated to minimize chemical irritation of renal tubules; watch for signs of declining renal function.
• Keep peak serum levels and trough serum levels at recommended concentrations, especially in patients with decreased renal function.
• Evaluate patient's hearing before and during therapy; monitor for complaints of tinnitus, vertigo, or hearing loss.

• Avoid concomitant use with other ototoxic or nephrotoxic drugs.
• Usual duration of therapy is 7 to 10 days; if no response occurs in 3 to 5 days, drug should be discontinued and cultures repeated for reevaluation of therapy.
• Closely monitor patients on long-term therapy – especially debilitated patients and others receiving immunosuppressants or radiation therapy – for possible bacterial or fungal superinfection; monitor especially for fever.
• Oral aminoglycoside may be absorbed systemically in patients with ulcerative GI lesions; significant absorption may endanger patients with decreased renal function.

Preoperative bowel contamination
• Provide low-residue diet and cathartic immediately before administration of oral neomycin; follow-up enemas may be necessary to completely empty bowel.

Topical therapy
• Do not apply to more than 20% of body surface.
• Do not apply to any body surface of patient with decreased renal function without considering risk/benefit ratio.
• Monitor patient for hypersensitivity or contact dermatitis.

Otic therapy
• Reculture persistent drainage.
• Drug best used in combination with other antibiotics.
• Avoid touching ear with dropper.

Information for parents and patient
• Wash hands before and after topical administration. Contact physician if topical use causes irritation or dermatitis.
• During otic use, avoid getting water in patient's ears.
• Teach parents and patients how to recognize signs of superinfection, and how to prevent it by practicing meticulous oral and anogenital hygiene. Parents of infants and toddlers should keep diaper area clean and dry and avoid using plastic pants.

---

neostigmine bromide
neostigmine methylsulfate
Prostigmin

• Classification: muscle stimulant (cholinesterase inhibitor)

How supplied
Available by prescription only
Tablets: 15 mg
Injection: 0.25 mg/ml, 0.5 mg/ml, 1 mg/ml

Indications, route, and dosage
Antidote for tubocurarine
Children: 0.07 to 0.08 mg/kg I.V. after pretreatment with an anticholinergic.
Adults: 0.5 to 2.5 mg slow I.V. Repeat p.r.n. Give 0.6 to 1.2 mg atropine sulfate I.V. before antidote dose.

Myasthenia gravis
Children: 0.01 to 0.04 mg/kg I.M., I.V. or S.C. q 2 to 3 hours prn; or 2 mg/kg/day P.O. in divided doses every 3 to 4 hours.
Adults: 15 to 30 mg t.i.d. (range 15 to 375 mg daily); or 0.5 to 2 mg I.M. or I.V. q 1 to 3 hours. Dosage must be individualized, depending on response and tolerance of adverse effects. Therapy may be required day and night.

Action and kinetics
• *Muscle stimulant action:* Neostigmine blocks acetylcholine's hydrolysis by cholinesterase, resulting in acetylcholine accumulation at cholinergic synapses. That leads to increased cholinergic receptor stimulation at the myoneural junction.
• *Kinetics in adults:* Neostigmine is poorly absorbed (1% to 2%) from GI tract after oral administration. Action usually begins 2 to 4 hours after oral administration and 10 to 30 minutes after injection.

About 15% to 25% of dose binds to plasma proteins.

Drug is hydrolyzed by cholinesterases and metabolized by microsomal liver enzymes. Duration of effect varies considerably, depending on patient's physical and emotional status and on disease severity.

About 80% of dose is excreted in urine as unchanged drug and metabolites in the first 24 hours after administration.

Contraindications and precautions
Neostigmine is contraindicated in patients with mechanical obstruction of the urinary or intestinal tract, because of its stimulatory effect on smooth muscle; in patients with bradycardia or hypotension, because the drug may exacerbate these conditions; and in patients with known hypersensitivity to cholinergics or bromides.

Administer neostigmine with extreme caution to patients with bronchial asthma, because the drug may precipitate bronchospasm. Administer cautiously to patients with epilepsy, because it may stimulate the CNS; to patients with peritonitis, vagotonia, hyperthyroidism, or cardiac dysrhythmias, because it may exacerbate these conditions; to patients with peptic ulcer disease, because it may increase gastric acid secretion; and to patients with recent coronary occlusion, because drug stimulates the cardiovascular system.

Interactions
Concomitant use with procainamide or quinidine may reverse neostigmine's cholinergic effect on muscle. Corticosteroids may also decrease cholinergic effects; when corticosteroids are stopped, however, neostigmine's cholinergic effects may increase, possibly affecting muscle strength.

Concomitant use with succinylcholine may result in prolonged respiratory depression from plasma esterase inhibition, causing delayed succinylcholine hydrolysis; use with other cholinergic drugs may cause additive toxicity. Use with ganglionic blockers, such as mecamylamine, may critically decrease blood pressure; effect is usually preceded by abdominal symptoms.

Magnesium has a direct depressant effect on skeletal muscle and may antagonize neostigmine's beneficial effects.

Effects on diagnostic tests
None reported.

Adverse reactions
• CNS: headache, dizziness, muscle weakness, confusion, nervousness, sweating.
• CV: dysrhythmias, bradycardia, hypotension.
• DERM: rash (bromide).
• EENT: miosis, lacrimation, spasm of accommodation, diplopia, conjunctival hyperemia.
• GI: nausea, vomiting, diarrhea, abdominal cramps, excessive salivation.
• Other: bronchospasm, bronchoconstriction, respiratory depression, muscle cramps.
Note: Drug should be discontinued if hypersensitivity, skin rash, or difficulty breathing occurs.

Overdose and treatment
Clinical signs of overdose include headache, nausea, vomiting, diarrhea, blurred vision, miosis, excessive tearing, bronchospasm, increased bronchial secretions, hypotension, incoordination, excessive sweating, muscle weakness, cramps, fasciculations, paralysis, bradycardia or tachycardia, excessive salivation, and restlessness or agitation.

Support respiration; bronchial suctioning may be performed. The drug should be discontinued immediately. Atropine should be given to block neostigmine's muscarinic effects but will not counter the drug's paralytic effects on skeletal muscle. Avoid atropine overdose, because it may lead to bronchial plug formation.

▶ Special considerations
• Observe patients closely for cholinergic reactions, especially with parenteral forms.
• Have atropine available to reduce or reverse hypersensitivity reactions.
• Dosage must be individualized according to severity of disease and patient response.
• Myasthenic patients may become refractory to this drug after prolonged use; however, responsiveness may be restored by reducing the dose or discontinuing the drug for a few days.
• Monitor patient's vital signs, particularly pulse.
• If muscle weakness is severe, determine if this stems from drug toxicity or from exacerbation of myasthenia gravis. A test dose of edrophonium I.V. will aggravate drug-induced weakness but will temporarily relieve weakness resulting from the disease.
• Give neostigmine with food or milk to reduce the chance for GI adverse effects.
• When administering drug to patient with myasthenia gravis, schedule largest dose before anticipated periods of fatigue. For example, if patient has dysphagia, schedule this dose 30 minutes before each meal.
• All other cholinergic drugs should be discontinued during neostigmine therapy because of the risk of additive toxicity.
• When administering neostigmine to prevent abdom-

inal distention and GI distress, insertion of a rectal tube may be indicated to help passage of gas.

• Administering atropine concomitantly with neostigmine can relieve or eliminate adverse reactions; these symptoms which may indicate neostigmine overdose, will be masked by atropine.

• Patients may develop resistance to this drug.

Information for parents and patient

• Instruct parents and patient to observe and record changes in muscle strength.

• Tell parents to have patient take dose with food or milk to reduce adverse effects.

• Advise parents to keep daily record of dose and effects during initial phase of therapy to help identify an optimum therapeutic regimen.

• Warn parents to have patient take drug exactly as prescribed, and to take missed dose as soon as possible. If almost time for next dose, patient should skip the missed dose and return to prescribed schedule. Patient should not double the dose.

• Advise parents to store drug away from children, and from direct heat and light.

---

netilmicin sulfate
Netromycin

• Classification: antibiotic (aminoglycoside)

How supplied
Available by prescription only
Injection: 10 mg/ml, 25 mg/ml, 100 mg/ml

Indications, route, and dosage
Serious infections caused by aerobic gram negative bacilli (P. aeruginosa, and some enterobacteriaceae) resistant to gentamicin or tobramycin

Neonates under 6 weeks: 4 to 6.5 mg/kg/day by I.M. injection or I.V. infusion given as 2 to 3.25 mg/kg q 12 hours.

Children age 6 weeks to 12 years: 5.5 to 8 mg/kg/day by I.M. injection or I.V. infusion given either as 1.8 to 2.7 mg/kg q 8 hours or as 2.7 to 4 mg/kg q 12 hours.

Children over age 12 and adults: 3 to 6.5 mg/kg/day by I.M. injection or I.V. infusion. May be given q 12 hours to treat serious urinary tract infections and q 8 to 12 hours to treat serious systemic infections.

Dosage in renal failure
In all patients, monitor serum blood levels to keep peak serum concentrations between 6 and 12 mcg/ml and trough serum concentrations between 0.5 and 2 mcg/ml. Several methods are available for calculating dosage in renal failure. One source recommends decreasing both dose and interval:

DOSAGE IN ADULTS		
Creatinine clearance (ml/min/ 1.73 m²)	Percentage of usual dose	Interval
> 50	50 to 90	q 8 to 12 hours
10 to 50	20 to 60	q 12 hours
< 10	10 to 20	q 24 to 48 hours

Action and kinetics
• *Antibiotic action:* Netilmicin is bactericidal; it binds directly to the 30S ribosomal subunit, thus inhibiting bacterial protein synthesis. Its spectrum of activity includes many aerobic gram-negative organisms (including most strains of *P. aeruginosa*) and some aerobic gram-positive organisms and generally is similar to gentamicin and tobramycin in spectrum. Netilmicin may act against some bacterial strains resistant to other aminoglycosides but generally amikacin is preferred.

• *Kinetics in adults:* Netilmicin is absorbed poorly after oral administration and is given parenterally; peak serum concentrations occur 30 to 60 minutes after I.M. administration.

Netilmicin is distributed widely after parenteral administration; intraocular penetration is poor. CSF penetration is low, even in patients with inflamed meninges. Protein binding is minimal. Netilmicin crosses the placenta.

Netilmicin is excreted unmetabolized, primarily in urine by glomerular filtration; small amounts may be excreted in bile and breast milk. Elimination half-life in adults is 2 to 2½ hours. In severe renal damage, half-life may extend beyond 30 hours.

• *Kinetics in children:* Plasma half-life inversely related to postnatal or gestational age and birth weight. Neonates less than 7 days of age weighing 1.5 to 2 kg exhibited increased netilmicin half-life of about 8 hours, while infants weighing 3 to 4 kg exhibited a plasma elimination half-life of about 4.5 hours. Infants 6 weeks of age and older exhibit a plasma elimination half-life of 1.5 to 2 hours.

Contraindications and precautions
Netilmicin is contraindicated in patients with known hypersensitivity to netilmicin or any other aminoglycoside, or bisulfites.

Netilmicin should be used cautiously in neonates and other infants; in patients with decreased renal function; in patients with tinnitus, vertigo, and high-frequency hearing loss who are susceptible to ototoxicity; and in patients with dehydration, myasthenia gravis, parkinsonism, and hypocalcemia.

Interactions
Concomitant use of netilmicin with the following drugs may increase the hazard of nephrotoxicity, ototoxicity,

---

‡May contain sulfites ◆May contain tartrazine ◆◆May contain benzyl alcohol

and neurotoxicity: methoxyflurane, polymyxin B, vancomycin, capreomycin, cisplatin, cephalosporins, amphotericin B, and other aminoglycosides; hazard of ototoxicity is also increased during use with ethacrynic acid, furosemide, bumetanide, urea, or mannitol. Dimenhydrinate or other antiemetic and antivertigo drugs may mask netilmicin-induced ototoxicity.

Concomitant use with penicillins results in a synergistic bactericidal effect against *P. aeruginosa, E. coli, Klebsiella, Citrobacter, Enterobacter, Serratia,* and *Proteus mirabilis.* However, the drugs are physically and chemically incompatible and are inactivated when mixed or given together. In vivo inactivation has been reported when aminoglycosides and penicillins are used concomitantly.

Netilmicin may potentiate neuromuscular blockade due to general anesthetics or neuromuscular blocking agents such as succinylcholine and tubocurarine.

Effects on diagnostic tests

Netilmicin-induced nephrotoxicity may elevate levels of blood urea nitrogen (BUN), nonprotein nitrogen, or serum creatinine and increase urinary excretion of casts.

Adverse reactions

• CNS: headache, lethargy, *neuromuscular blockade with respiratory depression.*
• EENT: ototoxicity (tinnitus, vertigo, hearing loss).
• GI: diarrhea, *pseudomembranous colitis.*
• GU: *nephrotoxicity* (cells or casts in the urine; oliguria; proteinuria; decreased creatinine clearance; increased BUN, nonprotein nitrogen, and serum creatinine levels).
• Other: hypersensitivity reactions (eosinophilia, fever, rash, urticaria, pruritus), bacterial or fungal superinfection.

Note: Drug should be discontinued if signs of ototoxicity or nephrotoxicity occur or if severe diarrhea indicates pseudomembranous colitis.

Overdose and treatment

Clinical signs of overdose include ototoxicity, nephrotoxicity, and neuromuscular blockade. Remove drug by hemodialysis or peritoneal dialysis. Treatment with calcium salts or anticholinesterases reverses neuromuscular blockade.

▶ Special considerations

• Netilmicin is the newest aminoglycoside; animal data suggest that it may be less ototoxic than other aminoglycosides.
• Because netilmicin is dialyzable, patients undergoing hemodialysis or peritoneal dialysis may need dosage adjustment.
• Assess patient's allergic history; do not give netilmicin to a patient with a history of hypersensitivity reactions to any aminoglycosides; monitor patient continuously for this and other adverse reactions.
• Obtain results of culture and sensitivity tests before first dose; however, therapy may begin before test results are completed. Repeat tests periodically to assess drug efficacy.
• Monitor vital signs, intake and output, weight, electrolyte levels, and renal function studies before and during therapy; be sure patient is well hydrated to minimize chemical irritation of renal tubules; watch for signs of declining renal function.
• Keep peak serum levels and trough serum levels at recommended concentrations, especially in patients with decreased renal function. Draw blood for peak level 1 hour after I.M. injection (30 minutes to 1 hour after I.V. infusion); for trough level, draw sample just before the next dose. Time and date all blood samples. Do not use heparinized tube to collect blood samples; it interferes with results.
• Evaluate patient's hearing before and during therapy; monitor for complaints of tinnitus, vertigo, or hearing loss.
• Avoid concomitant use of aminoglycosides with other ototoxic or nephrotoxic drugs.
• Usual duration of therapy is 7 to 10 days; if no response occurs in 3 to 5 days, drug should be discontinued and cultures repeated for reevaluation of therapy.
• Closely monitor patients on long-term therapy — especially debilitated patients and others receiving immunosuppressants or radiation therapy — for possible bacterial or fungal superinfection; monitor especially for fever.
• Do not add or mix other drugs with I.V. infusions — particularly penicillins, which will be inactivated by aminoglycoside; the two groups are chemically and physically incompatible. If other drugs must be given I.V., temporarily stop infusion of primary drug.
• Too-rapid I.V. administration may cause neuromuscular blockade. Infuse I.V. drug continuously or intermittently over 30 to 60 minutes for adults, 1 to 2 hours for infants; dilution volume for children is determined individually.
• Solutions should always be clear, colorless to pale yellow, and free of particles; do not give solutions containing precipitates or other foreign matter.
• Administer I.M. dose deep into large muscle mass (gluteal or midlateral thigh); rotate injection sites to minimize tissue injury; do not inject more than 2 g or 2 cc of drug per injection site. Apply ice to injection site for pain.

Information for parents and patient

• Instruct parents and patient regarding adverse reactions and which ones should be reported promptly.
• Teach parents and patients how to recognize signs of superinfection, and how to prevent it by practicing meticulous oral and anogenital hygiene. Parents of infants and toddlers should keep diaper area clean and dry and avoid using plastic pants.

---

*Canada only   †Unlabeled clinical use   Italicized adverse reactions have been observed in children.

niacin (vitamin B₃, nicotinic acid)
Niac, Nico-400, Nicobid, Nicolar,
Nicotinex, Span-Niacin, Vitamin B-3

• Classification: (vitamin) antilipemic, peripheral
vasodilator

How supplied
Available without prescription
Tablets: 20 mg, 25 mg, 50 mg, 100 mg
Capsules (timed-release): 125 mg, 300 mg, 400 mg
Elixir: 50 mg/5 ml

Available by prescription only
Tablets: 500 mg
Tablets (timed-release): 150 mg
Capsules (timed-release): 125 mg, 250 mg, 500 mg
Injection: 30-ml vials, 100 mg/ml

Indications, route, and dosage
Pellagra
Children: Up to 300 mg P.O. or 100 mg I.V. infusion
daily, depending on severity of niacin deficiency.
Adults: 10 to 20 mg P.O., S.C., I.M., or I.V. infusion
daily, depending on severity of niacin deficiency. Maximum recommended daily dosage is 500 mg; should
be divided into 10 doses, 50 mg each.

To prevent recurrence after symptoms subside, advise adequate nutrition and adequate supplements to
meet recommended daily allowance (RDA).

Action and kinetics
• *Vitamin replacement:* As a vitamin, niacin functions
as a coenzyme essential to tissue respiration, lipid
metabolism, and glycogenolysis. Niacin deficiency
causes pellagra, which manifests as dermatitis, diarrhea, and dementia; administration of niacin cures
pellagra. Niacin lowers cholesterol and triglyceride
levels by an unknown mechanism.
• *Vasodilating action:* Niacin acts directly on peripheral vessels, dilating cutaneous vessels and increasing blood flow, predominantly in the face, neck, and
chest.
• *Kinetics in adults:* Niacin is absorbed rapidly from
the GI tract. Peak plasma levels occur in 45 minutes.
Cholesterol and triglyceride levels decrease after several days. Niacin coenzymes are distributed widely
in body tissues; niacin is distributed in breast milk.
Niacin is metabolized by the liver and is excreted in
urine.

Contraindications and precautions
Niacin is contraindicated in patients with known hypersensitivity to the drug and with liver disease because large doses may cause liver damage; in patients
with peptic ulcer, which niacin may activate; and in
patients with arterial hemorrhage, severe hypotension, or niacin hypersensitivity.

Use niacin cautiously in patients with gout, diabetes mellitus, or gallbladder disease because it may
exacerbate the symptoms associated with these disorders.

Interactions
Concomitant use with sympathetic blocking agents
may cause added vasodilation and hypotension.

Effects on diagnostic tests
Niacin therapy alters fluorometric test results for urine
catecholamines and results for urine glucose tests
using cupric sulfate (Benedict's reagent).

Adverse reactions
Most adverse reactions are dose-dependent.
• CNS: dizziness, syncope, transient headache.
• CV: tachycardia, hypotension, excessive peripheral
vasodilation.
• DERM: flushing, warmth, burning, tingling, rash,
dryness.
• GI: nausea, stomach pain, vomiting, diarrhea, bloat-
ing, flatulence, activation of peptic ulcer, hepatotox-
icity.
• Metabolic: hyperglycemia, hyperuricemia.
• Other: blurred vision.
Note: Drug should be discontinued if abnormal liver
function tests signal hepatotoxicity.

Overdose and treatment
Niacin is a water-soluble vitamin; these seldom cause
toxicity in children with normal renal function.

▶ Special considerations
• RDA of niacin in children is 6 to 16 mg; in adult
males, 18 mg; and in adult females, 13 mg.
• For I.V. infusion in patients of adult size, use concentration of 10 mg/ml or dilute in 500 ml normal
saline solution; give slowly, no faster than 2 mg/min-
ute. To avoid fluid overload in children, give undiluted
injection I.V.
• I.V. administration of niacin may cause fibrinolysis,
metallic taste in mouth, and anaphylactic shock.
• Megadoses of niacin are not usually recommended.
• Monitor hepatic function and blood glucose levels
during initial therapy.
• Aspirin may reduce flushing response.
• Correction of niacin deficiency requires correction of
tryptophan as well.

Information for parents and patient
• Explain disease process and rationale for therapy;
emphasize that use of niacin to treat hyperlipidemia
or to dilate peripheral vessels is not "just taking a
vitamin," but serious medicine. Emphasize importance of complying with therapy.
• Explain that cutaneous flushing and warmth commonly occur in the first 2 hours; they will cease on
continued therapy.
• Advise parents that patient should not make sudden
postural changes to minimize effects of postural hypotension.
• Instruct parents that patient should avoid hot liquids
when taking drug initially to reduce flushing response. Recommend taking niacin with meals to minimize GI irritation.

niacinamide (nicotinamide)

• Classification: vitamin B_3

How supplied
Available by prescription only
Injection: 30-ml vials, 100 mg/ml

Available without prescription
Tablets: 50 mg, 100 mg, 500 mg
Tablets (timed-release): 1,000 mg

Indications, route, and dosage
Pellagra
Children: Up to 300 mg P.O. or 100 mg I.V. infusion daily, depending on severity of niacin deficiency.
Adults: 10 to 20 mg P.O., S.C., I.M., or I.V. infusion daily, depending on severity of niacin deficiency. Maximum daily dose recommended, 500 mg; should be divided into 10 doses, 50 mg each.

To prevent recurrence after symptoms subside, advise adequate nutrition and supplements to meet recommended daily allowance.

Action and kinetics
• *Vitamin replacement:* Niacinamide is used by the body as a source of niacin; it is essential for tissue respiration, lipid metabolism, and glycogenolysis, but lacks the vasodilating and antilipemic effects of niacin.
• *Kinetics in adults:* Niacinamide is absorbed readily from the GI tract and is distributed widely in body tissues. It is metabolized in the liver and is excreted in urine.

Contraindications and precautions
Niacinamide is contraindicated in patients with known hypersensitivity to the drug or liver disease because the drug may be hepatotoxic; or in patients with active peptic ulcer because niacinamide may exacerbate peptic ulcer disease.

Interactions
None reported.

Effects on diagnostic tests
Niacinamide alters liver function and serum bilirubin test results.

Adverse reactions
• CNS: mild headache, dizziness.
• GI: activation of peptic ulcer, vomiting, stomach pain, bloating, flatulence, diarrhea, hepatotoxicity.
Note: Drug should be discontinued if liver function tests indicate abnormalities.

Overdose and treatment
Niacinamide is a water-soluble vitamin; these seldom cause toxicity in patients with normal renal function.

▶ Special considerations
• When giving I.V. infusion, use a concentration of 10 mg/ml or, as an infusion, in an appropriate volume of normal saline solution. Inject slowly, no faster than 2 mg/minute.
• Megadoses of niacinamide are not usually recommended.
• Monitor hepatic function and blood glucose levels during initial therapy.

Information for parents and patient
Recommend taking niacinamide with meals to minimize GI irritation.

niclosamide
Niclocide

• Classification: anthelmintic (salicylanilide)

How supplied
Available by prescription only
Tablets (chewable): 500 mg

Indications, route, and dosage
Tapeworms (fish, beef and pork)
Children weighing 11 to 34 kg: 2 tablets (1 g) chewed thoroughly as a single dose.
Children weighing more than 34 kg: 3 tablets (1.5 g) chewed thoroughly as a single dose.
Adults: 4 tablets (2 g) chewed thoroughly as a single dose.
Dwarf tapeworm
Children weighing 11 to 34 kg: 2 tablets chewed thoroughly on the 1st day, then 1 tablet daily for the next 6 days.
Children weighing more than 34 kg: 3 tablets chewed thoroughly on the 1st day, then 2 tablets for the next 6 days.
Adults: 4 tablets chewed thoroughly as a single daily dose for 7 days.

Action and kinetics
• *Anthelmintic action:* Niclosamide inhibits mitochondrial oxidative phosphorylation in tapeworms; it also decreases uptake of glucose, decreasing anaerobic generation of adenosine triphosphate needed for cell function. Niclosamide is active against *Diphyllobothrium latum, Dipylidium caninum, Hymenolepis diminuta, H. nana, Taenia saginata, T. solium,* and *Enterobius vermicularis.*
• *Kinetics in adults:* An oral dose of niclosamide is absorbed poorly. Distribution of the small amount of drug absorbed has not been studied. Niclosamide is not appreciably metabolized by the mammalian host but may be metabolized in the GI tract by the worm. Niclosamide is excreted in feces. It is unknown if it is excreted in breast milk.

Contraindications and precautions
Niclosamide is contraindicated in patients who are hypersensitive to the drug.

Interactions
None reported.

Effects on diagnostic tests
Transient elevation of AST (SGOT) levels was reported in an I.V. narcotics addict taking niclosamide. No other effects have been reported.

Adverse reactions
• CNS: drowsiness, dizziness, headache.
• DERM: rash, pruritus ani, alopecia.
• EENT: oral irritation, bad taste in mouth.
• GI: nausea, vomiting, anorexia, diarrhea, constipation, rectal bleeding.
• Other: fever, sweating, palpitations, backache.
   Note: Drug should be discontinued if signs of hypersensitivity or toxicity occur.

Overdose and treatment
Treat overdose by giving a fast-acting laxative and an enema. Do not induce vomiting.

▶ Special considerations
• Safety and efficacy in children under age 2 have not been established.
• Tablets should be taken as a single dose after breakfast; they can be crushed and mixed with water or applesauce for small children.
• A mild laxative is indicated in constipated children to cleanse bowel before starting drug.
• Persistent tapeworm segments or ova excreted on or after the 7th day of therapy indicate failure; repeat course of treatment.
• Protect drug from light.

Information for parents and patient
• Inform parents about sources of tapeworm and means to avoid them.
• Teach parents and patient proper hygiene measures to prevent reinfection, including daily bathing of perianal area, washing hands after defecation and before eating, and sanitary disposal of feces.
• Explain importance of keeping follow-up appointments for repeat stool examinations 1 and 3 months after drug is discontinued, to ensure that worms and ova are completely eliminated.
• Urge patient with dwarf tapeworms to drink fruit juices; this helps eliminate accumulated intestinal mucus that harbors them.

---

nifedipine
Adalat, Procardia

• Classification: antianginal (calcium channel blocker)

How supplied
Available by prescription only
Capsules: 10 mg, 20 mg

Indications, route, and dosage
† *Essential hypertension*
Children: 0.25 to 0.5 mg/kg P.O. q 6 to 8 hours. Do not exceed 30 mg per dose or 180 mg daily.

Action and kinetics
• *Antianginal action:* Nifedipine dilates systemic arteries, resulting in decreased total peripheral resistance, and modestly decreased systemic blood pressure with a slightly increased heart rate, decreased afterload, and increased cardiac index. Reduced afterload and the subsequent decrease in myocardial oxygen consumption probably account for nifedipine's value in treating chronic stable angina. In Prinzmetal's angina, nifedipine inhibits coronary artery spasm, increasing myocardial oxygen delivery.
• *Kinetics in adults:* Nifedipine is absorbed rapidly from the GI tract; however, only about 65% to 70% of drug reaches the systemic circulation because of a significant first-pass effect in the liver. Peak serum levels occur in about 30 minutes to 2 hours. Hypotensive effects may occur 5 minutes after sublingual administration. About 92% to 98% of circulating nifedipine is bound to plasma proteins. Nifedipine is metabolized in the liver and excreted in the urine and feces as inactive metabolites. Elimination half-life is 2 to 5 hours. Duration of effect ranges from 4 to 12 hours.

Contraindications and precautions
Nifedipine is contraindicated in patients with known hypersensitivity to the drug. It should be used with caution when administered to patients with CHF or aortic stenosis (especially if they are receiving concomitant beta blockers), because the drug may precipitate or worsen heart failure and cause excessive hypotension (from its peripheral vasodilatory effects), possibly exacerbating angina symptoms when therapy begins or dosage is increased.

Interactions
Concomitant use of nifedipine with beta blockers may exacerbate angina, CHF, hypotension, and dysrhythmias. Concomitant use with fentanyl may cause excessive hypotension. Concomitant use with digoxin may cause increased serum digoxin levels. Use with hypotensive agents may precipitate excessive hypotension.

Effects on diagnostic tests
Mild to moderate increase in serum concentrations of alkaline phosphate, lactic dehydrogenase, AST (SGOT), and ALT (SGPT) have been noted.

Adverse reactions
• CNS: *dizziness, light-headedness, flushing, headache,* weakness, *syncope.*
• CV: *peripheral edema, hypotension, palpitations, tachycardia,* worsening of angina, myocardial infarction, CHF.
• EENT: nasal congestion.
• GI: *nausea,* heartburn, diarrhea.
• Other: muscle cramps, dyspnea.

---

‡May contain sulfites   ◆May contain tartrazine   ◆◆May contain benzyl alcohol

3

Overdose and treatment

Clinical effects of overdose are extensions of the drug's pharmacologic effects, primarily peripheral vasodilation and hypotension.

Treatment includes such basic support measures as hemodynamic and respiratory monitoring. If patient requires blood pressure support by a vasoconstrictor, norepinephrine may be administered. Extremities should be elevated and any fluid deficit corrected.

▶ Special considerations

• Initial doses or dosage increase may exacerbate angina briefly. Reassure patient that this symptom is temporary.
• Nifedipine is not available in sublingual form. However, liquid in oral capsule may be withdrawn by puncturing capsule with needle, and the drug may be instilled into the buccal pouch. Or, a punctured capsule may be chewed.
• Monitor cardiac rate and rhythm and blood pressure regularly, especially if patient is also taking beta blockers or antihypertensives.
• Although rebound effect has not been observed when drug is withdrawn, dosage should be reduced slowly under medical supervision.

Information for parents and patient

• Instruct parents that patient should swallow capsules whole without breaking, crushing, or chewing them.
• Advise parents that patient may experience annoying hypotensive effects during titration of dose. Urge compliance.
• Tell parents that patient should not abruptly discontinue the drug; gradual dosage reduction may be necessary.
• Instruct parents to report any of the following: irregular heartbeat, shortness of breath, swelling of hands and feet, pronounced dizziness, constipation, nausea, or hypotension.
• Advise parents that patient who misses a dose should take the dose as soon as possible, but not if almost time for next dose. Warn parents not to double the dose.

---

nitrofurantoin
Furadantin, Furalan, Furan, Furanite, Furantoin, Nitrofan

nitrofurantoin macrocrystals
Macrodantin

• Classification: urinary tract antiseptic (nitrofuran)

How supplied
Available by prescription only
Microcrystals
Tablets: 50 mg, 100 mg
Capsules: 50 mg, 100 mg
Suspension: 25 mg/5 ml

Macrocrystals
Capsules: 25 mg, 50 mg, 100 mg
Suspension: 25 mg/5 ml

Indications, route, and dosage
Pyelonephritis, pyelitis, and cystitis caused by susceptible organisms
Children age 1 month to 12 years: 5 to 7 mg/kg P.O. daily, divided q.i.d.
Children over age 12 and adults: 50 to 100 mg P.O. q.i.d., with meals. Or 180 mg I.V. b.i.d. in patients over 54 kg; 6.6 mg/kg daily I.V. in two divided doses in patients under 54 kg.
Long-term suppression therapy
Children: As low as 1 mg/kg/day in two divided doses.
Adults: 50 to 100 mg P.O. daily h.s. or in four divided doses.

Action and kinetics
• *Antibacterial action:* Nitrofurantoin has bacteriostatic action in low concentrations and possible bactericidal action in high concentrations. Although its exact mechanism of action is unknown, it may inhibit bacterial enzyme systems. Drug is most active at an acidic pH.

Drug's spectrum of activity includes many common gram-positive and gram-negative urinary pathogens, including *Escherichia coli, Staphylococcus aureus,* enterococci, and certain strains of *Klebsiella, Proteus,* and *Enterobacter.* Organisms that usually resist nitrofurantoin include *Pseudomonas, Acinetobacter, Serratia,* and *Providencia.*
• *Kinetics in adults:* When administered orally, nitrofurantoin is well absorbed (mainly by the small intestine) from the GI tract. Presence of food aids drug's dissolution and speeds absorption. The macrocrystal form exhibits slower dissolution and absorption; it causes less GI distress. Nitrofurantoin crosses into bile and placenta. From 20% to 60% binds to plasma proteins. Plasma half-life is approximately 20 minutes. Peak urine concentrations occur in about 30 minutes when drug is given as microcrystals, somewhat later when given as macrocrystals. Nitrofurantoin is metabolized partially in the liver. About 30% to 50% of dose is eliminated by glomerular filtration and tubular excretion into urine as unchanged drug within 24 hours. Some drug may be excreted in breast milk.

Contraindications and precautions
Nitrofurantoin is contraindicated in patients with severe renal dysfunction (creatinine clearance below 40 ml/minute) because urine concentrations of the drug will be ineffective and toxicity may occur; in infants under age 1 month, in pregnant patients, and in patients with glucose-6-phosphate dehydrogenase (G6PD) deficiency because of the potential for hemolytic anemias; and in patients with known hypersensitivity to the drug.

Nitrofurantoin should be administered cautiously to patients with diabetes mellitus, asthma, anemia, vitamin B deficiency, or electrolyte imbalance, because it increases the risk of peripheral neuropathy.

Interactions

When used concomitantly, probenecid and sulfinpyrazone reduce renal excretion of nitrofurantoin, leading to increased serum and decreased urine nitrofurantoin concentrations. Increased serum concentration may lead to increased toxicity; decreased urine concentration may reduce drug's antibacterial effectiveness.

Concomitant use with magnesium-containing antacids may decrease nitrofurantoin absorption. Concomitant use with nalidixic acid antagonizes nalidixic acid's antibacterial activity.

Anticholinergic drugs and foods enhance nitrofurantoin's bioavailability by slowing GI motility, thereby increasing the drug's dissolution and absorption.

Effects on diagnostic tests

Nitrofurantoin may cause false-positive results in urine glucose tests using cupric sulfate reagents (such as Benedict's test, Fehling's test, or Clinitest) because it reacts with these reagents.

Anemia and abnormal results of liver function tests may occur during nitrofurantoin therapy.

Adverse reactions

- CNS: peripheral neuropathy, headache, dizziness, drowsiness, ascending polyneuropathy with high doses or renal impairment.
- DERM: maculopapular, erythematous, or eczematous eruption; pruritus; urticaria; exfoliative dermatitis; Stevens-Johnson syndrome.
- GI: anorexia, nausea, vomiting, abdominal pain, diarrhea, hepatitis.
- HEMA: hemolysis in patients with G6PD deficiency, agranulocytosis, thrombocytopenia.
- Other: asthma attacks in patients with history of asthma, anaphylaxis, *hypersensitivity*, transient alopecia, drug fever, overgrowth of nonsusceptible organisms in urinary tract, pulmonary sensitivity reactions (cough, chest pains, fever, chills, dyspnea).
  Note: Drug should be discontinued if patient develops hypersensitivity, hemolysis, peripheral neuropathy, or pulmonary reaction.

Overdose and treatment

No information available.

▶ Special considerations

- Drug is contraindicated in infants under age 1 month because their immature enzyme systems increase the risk of hemolytic anemia.
- Obtain culture and sensitivity tests before starting therapy, and repeat as needed. This drug is associated with a relatively high rate of development of resistance.
- Give oral preparations 1 hour apart from magnesium-containing antacids. Oral suspension may be mixed with water, milk, fruit juice, and formulas.
- Dilute I.V. nitrofurantoin in 500 ml of I.V. solution before administering. Infuse at 50 to 60 drops/minute.
- For I.V. infusion, reconstitute in 20 ml of dextrose 5% solution or sterile water without preservatives.
- Monitor CBC regularly.
- Monitor fluid intake and output and pulmonary status.

- Drug may turn urine brown or rust-yellow.
- Avoid administering drug with nalidixic acid.
- Continue treatment for at least 3 days after sterile urine specimens have been obtained.
- Long-term therapy may cause hypersensitivity.
- Drug may cause growth of nonsusceptible organisms, especially *Pseudomonas*.

Information for parents and patient

- Instruct parents to give drug with food or milk to minimize GI distress.
- Caution parents that drug may cause false-positive results in urine glucose tests using cupric sulfate reduction method (Clinitest) but not in glucose oxidase test (Tes-Tape, Diastix, Clinistix).
- Warn parents and the patient that drug may turn urine brown or rust-yellow.
- Warn parents and patient that oral suspension may temporarily discolor or stain teeth. To avoid this, patient should rinse mouth with water after swallowing medication.
- Instruct parents to store drug in original container.

nitrofurazone
Furacin

- Classification: topical antibacterial (synthetic antibacterial nitrofuran derivative)

How supplied

Available by prescription only
Topical solution: 0.2%
Ointment: 0.2% soluble dressing
Cream: 0.2%

Indications, route, and dosage
Adjunct for major burns (especially when resistance to other anti-infectives occurs); prevention of skin graft infection before or after surgery
Children and adults: Apply directly to lesion or to dressings used to cover the affected area daily or as indicated, depending on severity of burn.

Action and kinetics

- *Antibacterial action:* The exact mechanism of action is unknown. However, it appears that the drug inhibits bacterial enzymes involved in carbohydrate metabolism. Nitrofurazone has a broad spectrum of activity.
- *Kinetics in adults:* Absorption is limited with topical use.

Contraindications and precautions

Use may result in bacterial or fungal overgrowth of nonsusceptible organisms, which may lead to secondary infections. Drug should be used with caution in patients with renal impairment. Nitrofurazone is contraindicated in patients with hypersensitivity to the drug.

Interactions

None reported.

Effects on diagnostic tests
None reported.

Adverse reactions
• Local: allergic contact dermatitis.
  Note: Drug should be discontinued if sensitization, superinfection, or irritation develops.

Overdose and treatment
Discontinue use and cleanse area with mild soap and water.

▶ Special considerations
• Avoid contact with eyes and mucous membranes.
• Monitor patient for overgrowth of nonsusceptible organisms, including fungi.
• Use diluted solutions within 24 hours after preparation; discard diluted solution that becomes cloudy.

Information for parents and patient
• Teach parents and patient proper application of drug. Apply directly on lesion or place on gauze.
• Tell parents or patient to avoid exposing drug to direct sunlight, excessive heat, strong fluorescent lighting, and alkaline materials.

nitroglycerin (glyceryl trinitrate)
Tridil, Nitrol IV, Nitrostat IV, Nitrobid IV

• Classification: antianginal, vasodilator (nitrate)

How supplied
Available by prescription only
I.V.: 0.5 mg/ml, 0.8 mg/ml, 5 mg/ml

Indications, route, and dosage
Hypertension, CHF, angina
†*Children:* 0.5 to 20 mcg/kg/minute by continuous I.V. infusion.
Adults: Initial infusion rate is 5 mcg/minute. May be increased by 5 mcg/minute q 3 to 5 minutes until a response is noted. If a 20 mcg/minute rate doesn't produce desired response, dosage may be increased by as much as 20 mcg/minute q 3 to 5 minutes.

Action and kinetics
• *Vasodilating action:* Nitroglycerin dilates peripheral vessels, making it useful (in I.V. form) in producing controlled hypotension during surgical procedures and in controlling blood pressure in perioperative hypertension. Because peripheral vasodilation decreases venous return to the heart (preload), nitroglycerin also helps to treat pulmonary edema and CHF. Arterial vasodilation decreases arterial impedance (afterload), thereby decreasing left ventricular work and aiding the failing heart. These combined effects may prove valuable in treating some patients with acute myocardial infarction.
• *Kinetics in adults:* Nitroglycerin is well absorbed from the GI tract. However, because it undergoes first-pass metabolism in the liver, the drug is incompletely absorbed into the systemic circulation. Onset of action

for oral preparations is slow (except for sublingual tablets). After sublingual administration, absorption from the oral mucosa is relatively complete. Nitroglycerin also is well absorbed after topical administration as an ointment or transdermal system. Onset of action for various preparations is as follows: I.V., 1 to 2 minutes; sublingual, 1 to 3 minutes; translingual spray, 2 minutes; transmucosal tablet, 3 minutes; ointment, 20 to 60 minutes; oral (sustained-release), 40 minutes; transdermal, 40 to 60 minutes. Nitroglycerin is distributed widely throughout the body. About 60% of circulating drug is bound to plasma proteins.
Nitroglycerin is metabolized in the liver and serum to 1,3 glyceryl dinitrate, 1,2 glyceryl dinitrate, and glyceryl mononitrate. Dinitrate metabolites have slight vasodilatory effect. Nitroglycerin metabolites are excreted in the urine; elimination half-life is about 1 to 4 minutes. Duration of effect for various preparations is as follows: I.V., 30 minutes; sublingual, up to 30 minutes; translingual spray, 30 to 60 minutes; transmucosal tablet, 5 hours; ointment, 3 to 6 hours; oral (sustained-release), 4 to 8 hours; transdermal, 18 to 24 hours.

Contraindications and precautions
Nitroglycerin is contraindicated in patients with head trauma or cerebral hemorrhage, because of potential for increased intracranial pressure; in patients with severe anemia, because nitrate ions can readily oxidize hemoglobin to methemoglobin; and in patients with a history of hypersensitivity or idiosyncratic reaction to nitrates.
I.V. nitroglycerin is contraindicated in patients with hypotension or uncorrected hypovolemia, because the drug may cause severe hypotension and shock; and in patients with constrictive pericarditis and pericardial tamponade, because the drug may cause hypotension, reduce preload, and decrease cardiac output.
Nitroglycerin should be used with caution in patients with increased intracranial pressure, because the drug dilates meningeal vessels; in patients with open- or closed-angle glaucoma, although intraocular pressure is increased only briefly and drainage of aqueous humor from the eye is unimpeded; in patients with diuretic-induced fluid depletion or low systolic blood pressure (less than 90 mm Hg), because of the drug's hypotensive effect; and during the initial days after acute myocardial infarction, because the drug may cause excessive hypotension and tachycardia. (However, nitroglycerin has been used with some success to decrease myocardial ischemia and possibly reduce the extent of infarction.)

Interactions
Concomitant use of nitroglycerin with alcohol, antihypertensive drugs, or phenothiazines may cause additive hypotensive effects. Concomitant use with ergot alkaloids may precipitate angina. Oral nitroglycerin may increase the bioavailability of ergot alkaloids.

---

*Canada only   †Unlabeled clinical use   Italicized adverse reactions have been observed in children

Effects on diagnostic tests

Nitroglycerin may interfere with serum cholesterol determination tests using the Zlatkis-Zak color reaction, resulting in falsely decreased values.

Adverse reactions

• CNS: *headache* (sometimes throbbing), dizziness, weakness, *blurred vision.*
• CV: orthostatic hypotension, tachycardia, *flushing,* palpitations, fainting.
• DERM: cutaneous vasodilation, skin irritation (topical form).
• GI: *nausea, vomiting.*
• Local: sublingual burning, dry mouth.
• Other: hypersensitivity reactions (rash, dermatitis), methemoglobinemia.
   Note: Drug should be discontinued if rash, dermatitis, blurred vision, or dry mouth occurs.

Overdose and treatment

Clinical effects of overdose result primarily from vasodilation and methemoglobinemia and include hypotension, persistent throbbing headache, palpitations, visual disturbances, flushing of the skin, sweating (with skin later becoming cold and cyanotic), nausea and vomiting, colic, bloody diarrhea, orthostasis, initial hyperpnea, dyspnea, slow respiratory rate, bradycardia, heart block, increased intracranial pressure with confusion, fever, paralysis, tissue hypoxia (from methemoglobinemia) leading to cyanosis, metabolic acidosis, coma, clonic convulsions, and circulatory collapse. Death may result from circulatory collapse or asphyxia.

   After oral overdose, treatment includes gastric lavage followed by administration of activated charcoal to remove remaining gastric contents. Blood gas measurements and methemoglobin levels should be monitored, as indicated. Supportive care includes respiratory support and oxygen administration, passive movement of the extremities to aid venous return, and recumbent positioning.

▶ Special considerations

• Oral, sublingual, and topical preparations are available for use in adults. These dosage forms are not routinely used in children.
• Administration as I.V. infusion requires special nonabsorbent tubing supplied by manufacturer, because regular plastic tubing may absorb up to 80% of drug. Infusion should be prepared in glass bottle or container.
• If drug causes headache (especially likely with initial doses), aspirin or acetaminophen may be indicated. Dosage may need to be reduced temporarily.
• Sublingual dose may be administered before anticipated stress or at bedtime if angina is nocturnal.
• Drug may cause orthostatic hypotension. To minimize this, patient should change to upright position slowly, go up and down stairs carefully, and lie down at the first sign of dizziness.
• When administering drug to patients during initial days after acute myocardial infarction, monitor hemodynamic and clinical status carefully.
• Monitor blood pressure and intensity and duration of patient's response to drug.

Information for parents and patient

• Methemoglobinemia may occur in infants receiving large doses of nitroglycerin.
• Warn parents and patient that headache may follow initial doses but that this symptom may respond to usual headache remedies or dosage reduction. Assure patient that headache usually subsides gradually with continued treatment.
• Tell patient to report blurred vision, dry mouth, or persistent headache.
• Explain that patient should avoid alcohol while taking this drug because severe hypotension and cardiovascular collapse may occur.
• Because drug may cause dizziness, advise patient to move to an upright position slowly.

nitroprusside sodium
Nipride, Nitropress

• Classification: antihypertensive (vasodilator)

How supplied

Available by prescription only
Injection: 50 mg/5-ml vial

Indications, route, and dosage
Hypertensive emergencies

Children and adults: Initially, 1 mcg/kg/minute by I.V. infusion. Titrate according to blood pressure; average dose is 3 mcg/kg/minute, with a range of 0.5 to 10 mcg/kg/minute. Maximum infusion rate is 10 mcg/kg/minute.

Action and kinetics

• *Antihypertensive action:* Nitroprusside acts directly on vascular smooth muscle, causing peripheral vasodilation.
• *Kinetics in adults:* Drug is administered by I.V. route and, therefore, is not absorbed. I.V. infusion of nitroprusside reduces blood pressure almost immediately. Distribution is unknown. Nitroprusside is metabolized rapidly in erythrocytes and tissues and is converted to thiocyanate in the liver. Nitroprusside is excreted primarily in urine, entirely as metabolites. Blood pressure returns to pretreatment level 1 to 10 minutes after completion of infusion.

Contraindications and precautions

Nitroprusside is contraindicated in patients with known hypersensitivity to the drug and in patients with compensatory hypertension secondary to arteriovenous shunt or coarctation of the aorta, because a decrease in blood pressure may be harmful to these patients.

   Nitroprusside should be used cautiously in patients with renal insufficiency because thiocyanate, one of the metabolic products of nitroprusside, is excreted by the kidney, and may accumulate; in patients with hepatic insufficiency because drug metabolism may be impaired; in patients with hypothyroidism because thiocyanate inhibits iodine uptake and binding; and in patients with low vitamin B_{12} concentrations because the drug may interfere with vitamin B_{12} distribution and metabolism.

Interactions
Nitroprusside may potentiate antihypertensive effects of other antihypertensive medications; its antihypertensive effects may be potentiated by general anesthetics, particularly halothane and enflurane, and by ganglionic blocking agents. Pressor agents, such as epinephrine, may cause an increase in blood pressure during nitroprusside therapy.

Effects on diagnostic tests
An increase in serum creatinine concentration may occur during therapy.

Adverse reactions
The following adverse reactions usually indicate overdose:
• CNS: headache, dizziness, agitation, ataxia, loss of consciousness, coma, absent reflexes, widely dilated pupils, *restlessness, muscle twitching,* diaphoresis.
• CV: distant heart sounds, palpitations, dyspnea, weak pulse, shallow breathing, *hypotension.*
• DERM: pink color, *rash.*
• GI: *vomiting,* nausea, abdominal pain.
• GU: may aggravate renal insufficiency.
• Metabolic: acidosis.
• Respiratory: pulmonary shunting.
   Note: Drug should be discontinued if metabolic acidosis occurs; it may indicate cyanide toxicity.

Overdose and treatment
Clinical manifestations of overdose include the adverse reactions listed above and increased tolerance to the drug's antihypertensive effects.
   Treat overdose by giving nitrites to induce methemoglobin formation. Discontinue the nitroprusside and administer amyl nitrite inhalations for 15 to 30 seconds each minute until a 3% sodium nitrite solution can be prepared. Administer amyl nitrite cautiously to minimize risk of additional hypotension secondary to vasodilation. Then administer the sodium nitrite solution by I.V. infusion at a rate not exceeding 2.5 to 5 ml/minute up to a total dose of 10 to 15 ml. Follow with I.V. sodium thiosulfate infusion (12.5 g in 50 ml of dextrose 5% in water) over 10 minutes. If necessary, repeat infusions of sodium nitrite and sodium thiosulfate at half the initial doses. Further treatment involves symptomatic and supportive care.

▶ Special considerations
• Blood pressure should be checked at least every 5 minutes at the start of the infusion and at least every 15 minutes thereafter during infusion.
• Monitor intake and output.
• Prepare solution using dextrose 5% in water; do not use bacteriostatic water for injection or sterile saline solution for reconstitution. Because of light sensitivity, foil-wrap I.V. solution (but not tubing). Fresh solutions have faint brownish tint; discard after 24 hours.
• Infuse drug with infusion pump.
• This drug is best run piggyback through a peripheral line with no other medications; do not adjust rate of main I.V. line while drug is running because even small boluses can cause severe hypotension.
• Nitroprusside can cause cyanide toxicity; therefore, check serum thiocyanate levels every 72 hours. Levels above 100 mcg/ml are associated with cyanide toxicity, which can produce profound hypotension, metabolic acidosis, dyspnea, ataxia, and vomiting. If such symptoms occur, discontinue infusion and re-evaluate therapy.
• Nitroprusside also may be used to produce controlled hypotension during anesthesia, to reduce bleeding from the surgical procedure.
• Hypertensive patients are more sensitive to nitroprusside than normotensive patients. Also, patients taking other antihypertensive drugs are extremely sensitive to nitroprusside. Nitroprusside has been used in patients with acute myocardial infarction, refractory heart failure, and severe mitral regurgitation. It has also been used orally as an antihypertensive.

Information for parents and patient
Ask parents and patient to report any CNS symptoms (such as headache or dizziness) promptly.

---

norepinephrine bitartrate (formerly levarterenol bitartrate)
Levophed

• Classification: vasopressor (direct-acting adrenergic)

How supplied
Available by prescription only
Injection: 1 mg/ml parenteral

Indications, route, and dosage
To maintain blood pressure in acute hypotensive states
Children: Initially, 2 mcg/minute or 2 mcg/m²/minute I.V. infusion, then titrated to maintain desired blood pressure. For advanced cardiac life support, initial infusion rate is 0.1 mcg/kg/minute.
Adults: Initially, 8 to 12 mcg/minute I.V. infusion, then titrated to maintain desired blood pressure; maintenance dosage, 2 to 4 mcg/minute.

Action and kinetics
• *Vasopressor action:* Norepinephrine acts predominantly by direct stimulation of alpha-adrenergic receptors, constricting both capacitance and resistance blood vessels. That results in increased total peripheral resistance; increased systolic and diastolic blood pressure; decreased blood flow to vital organs, skin, and skeletal muscle; and constriction of renal blood vessels, which reduces renal blood flow. It also has a direct stimulating effect on beta₁ receptors of the heart, producing a positive inotropic response. Its main therapeutic effects are vasoconstriction and cardiac stimulation.
• *Kinetics in adults:* Pressor effect occurs rapidly after infusion, is of short duration, and stops 1 to 2 minutes after infusion is stopped. Norepinephrine localizes in

sympathetic nerve tissues. It is metabolized in the liver and other tissues to inactive compounds and excreted in urine primarily as sulfate and glucuronide conjugates. Small amounts are excreted unchanged in urine.

Contraindications and precautions

Norepinephrine is contraindicated in patients with peripheral or mesenteric vascular thrombosis (may increase ischemia and extend area of infarction), profound hypoxia or hypercapnea, hypovolemia, and in those undergoing general anesthesia with cyclopropane and other inhalation hydrocarbon anesthetics (risk of inducing cardiac dysrhythmias). Norepinephrine is also contraindicated for use with local anesthetics in fingers, toes, ears, nose, or genitalia.

Administer cautiously to hypertensive or hyperthyroid patients (increased risk of adverse reactions). Also administer cautiously to patients with known hypersensitivity to sulfites; commercially available formulation contains sodium metabisulfite.

Interactions

When used concomitantly with general anesthetics, norepinephrine may cause increased cardiac dysrhythmias; when used with tricyclic antidepressants, MAO inhibitors, some antihistamines, parenteral ergot alkaloids, guanethidine, and methyldopa, norepinephrine may cause severe, prolonged hypertension.

Use with beta blockers may result in an increased potential for hypertension. (Propranolol may be used to treat cardiac dysrhythmias occurring during norepinephrine administration.) Use with furosemide or other diuretics may decrease arterial responsiveness.

Concomitant use with atropine blocks the reflex bradycardia caused by norepinephrine and enhances its pressor effects.

Effects on diagnostic tests

None reported.

Adverse reactions

- CNS: headache, *weakness,* dizziness, *restlessness,* anxiety, insomnia, *tremors.*
- CV: precordial pain, *severe hypertension,* severe peripheral and visceral vasoconstriction, *dysrhythmias, bradycardia.*
- GI: nausea, vomiting.
- GU: *decreased urine output.*
- Local: *severe irritation and necrosis with extravasation.*
- Other: respiratory difficulty, apnea, pallor, swelling and engorgement of thyroid, photophobia, sweating, cerebral hemorrhage, convulsions, metabolic acidosis, hyperglycemia, hyperthermia.
  Note: Drug should be discontinued if hypersensitivity, infiltration, or thrombosis occurs.

Overdose and treatment

Clinical manifestations of overdose include severe hypertension, photophobia, retrosternal or pharyngeal pain, intense sweating, vomiting, cerebral hemorrhage, convulsions, and cardiac dysrhythmias. Monitor vital signs closely.

Treatment includes supportive and symptomatic measures. Use atropine for reflex bradycardia, phentolamine for extravasation, and propranolol for dysrhythmias.

▶ Special considerations

- Correct blood volume depletion before administration. Norepinephrine is not a substitute for blood, plasma, fluid, or electrolyte replacement.
- Select injection site carefully. Administration by I.V. infusion requires an infusion pump or other device to control flow rate. If possible, infuse into antecubital vein of the arm or the femoral vein. Change injection sites for prolonged therapy. Must be diluted before use with 5% dextrose with or without normal saline solution. (Dilution with normal saline solution alone not recommended.) Monitor infusion rate. Withdraw drug gradually; recurrent hypotension may follow abrupt withdrawal.
- Prepare infusion solution by adding 4 mg norepinephrine to 1 liter of 5% dextrose. The resultant solution contains 4 mcg/ml.
- To treat extravasation, infiltrate site promptly with 10 to 15 ml of normal saline solution containing 5 to 10 mg phentolamine, using a fine needle.
- Monitor intake and output. Norepinephrine reduces renal blood flow, which may cause decreased urine output initially.
- Patient should be attended constantly during administration of norepinephrine. Baseline blood pressure and pulse should be taken before therapy, then repeated every 2 minutes until stabilization; then repeated every 5 minutes during drug administration.
- Monitor blood pressure, pulse, and respirations carefully during therapy. In addition to vital signs, monitor patient's mental state, skin temperature of extremities, and skin color (especially earlobes, lips, and nail beds).
- In patients with previously normal blood pressure, adjust flow rate to maintain blood pressure at low normal (usually 80 to 100 mm Hg systolic); in hypertensive patients, maintain systolic no higher than 40 mm Hg below preexisting pressure level.
- Tachyphylaxis (tolerance) may develop after prolonged or excessive use.
- Protect solution from light. Discard solution that is discolored or contains a precipitate.
- Norepinephrine has been used to control upper GI hemorrhage with instillation of 8 mg of norepinephrine in 100 ml of normal saline solution through a nasogastric tube q hour for 6 to 8 hours, then q 2 hours for 4 to 6 hours, then gradually reduced until drug is discontinued. Alternatively, 8 mg of norepinephrine in 250 ml of normal saline solution may be administered intraperitoneally.

Information for parents and patient

- Inform parents and patient that frequent monitoring of vital signs will be required.
- Tell parents and patient to report any adverse reactions.

nystatin
Korostatin, Mycostatin, Mykinac,
Nilstat, Nystex, O-V Statin

- Classification: antifungal (polyene macrolide)

How supplied
Available by prescription only
Tablets: 500,000 units
Suspension: 100,000 units/ml
Vaginal suppositories: 100,000 units
Cream: 100,000 units/g
Ointment: 100,000 units/g
Powder: 100,000 units/g

Indications, route, and dosage
Oral, vaginal, and intestinal infections caused by susceptible organisms
Newborn and premature infants: 100,000 units of oral suspension q.i.d.
Children and infants over age 3 months: 250,000 to 500,000 units of oral suspension q.i.d.
Adults: 400,000 to 600,000 units of oral suspension q.i.d. for oral candidiasis.
Gastrointestinal infections
Adults: 500,000 to 1 million units as oral tablets, t.i.d.
Cutaneous or mucocutaneous candidal infections
Children and adults (topical use): Apply to affected areas two or three times daily until healing is complete.
Children and adults (vaginal use): 100,000 units, as vaginal tablets, inserted high into vagina daily or b.i.d. for 14 days.

Action and kinetics
- *Antifungal action:* Nystatin is both fungistatic and fungicidal. It binds to sterols in the fungal cell membrane, altering its permeability and allowing leakage of intracellular components. Is is active against a variety of pathogenic and nonpathogenic yeasts and fungi, including *Candida albicans* and *C. guilliermondii.*
- *Kinetics in adults:* Nystatin is not appreciably absorbed from the GI tract, nor through the intact skin or mucous membranes. No detectable amount of the drug is available for tissue distribution. Nystatin is excreted almost entirely unchanged in feces.

Contraindications and precautions
Nystatin is contraindicated in patients with known hypersensitivity to the drug.

Interactions
None reported.

Effects on diagnostic tests
None reported.

Adverse reactions
- GI: *transient nausea, vomiting, diarrhea* (usually with large oral dosage).

Note: Drug should be discontinued if skin irritation or signs of toxicity occur.

Overdose and treatment
Nystatin overdose may result in nausea, vomiting, and diarrhea. Treatment is unnecessary because toxicity is negligible.

▶ Special considerations
- Avoid hand contact with drug; hypersensitivity is rare but can occur.
- For treatment of oral candidiasis, patient should have mouth free of food debris, and should hold suspension in mouth for several minutes before swallowing; for infant thrush, medication should be swabbed on oral mucosa.
- Immunosuppressed patient may be given vaginal tablets (100,000 units) by mouth to provide prolonged drug contact with oral mucosa.
- For candidiasis of the feet, patient should dust powder on shoes and stockings as well as feet for maximal contact and effectiveness.
- Avoid occlusive dressings or applying ointment to most covered body areas that favor yeast growth.
- Use cream rather than ointment for intertriginous areas, and powder for moist lesions, to prevent maceration.
- Cleanse affected skin gently before topical application; cool, moist compresses applied for 15 minutes between applications help soothe and dry skin.
- Cleansing douches may be used by nonpregnant adolescent patients for aesthetic reasons; they should use preparations that do not contain antibacterials, which may alter flora and promote reinfection.
- Protect drug from light, air, and heat.
- Nystatin is ineffective in systemic fungal infection.

Information for parents and patient
- Teach parents and patient signs and symptoms of candidal infection. Tell them about predisposing agents: use of antibiotics, oral contraceptives, and corticosteroids; diabetes; infected sexual partners; and tight-fitting jeans, pantyhose, and undergarments.
- Teach patient good oral hygiene techniques. Explain that overuse of mouthwash may alter flora and promote infection.
- Tell patient to continue using vaginal cream through menstruation; emphasize importance of washing applicator thoroughly after each use.
- Advise patient to wear cotton underpants and to change stockings and undergarments daily; teach good skin care.
- Teach parents and patient correct way to administer each dosage form prescribed. Advise them to continue drug for 1 to 2 weeks after symptoms clear, to prevent reinfection.

---

*Canada only   †Unlabeled clinical use   Italicized adverse reactions have been observed in children.

opium tincture, camphorated
Paregoric

• Classification: antidiarrheal (opiate)
• Controlled substance schedule II

How supplied
Available by prescription only
Alcoholic solution: Each 5 ml contains morphine, 2 mg; anise oil, 0.2 ml; benzoic acid, 20 mg; camphor, 20 mg; glycerin, 0.2 ml; and ethanol to make 5 ml

Indications, route, and dosage
Acute, nonspecific diarrhea
Children: 0.25 to 0.5 ml/kg daily, b.i.d., t.i.d., or q.i.d. until diarrhea subsides.
Adults: 5 to 10 ml daily, b.i.d., t.i.d., or q.i.d. until diarrhea subsides.

Action and kinetics
• *Antidiarrheal action:* Opium, derived from the opium poppy, contains several ingredients. The most active ingredient, morphine, increases GI smooth muscle tone, inhibits motility and propulsion, and diminishes secretions. By inhibiting peristalsis, the drug delays passage of intestinal contents, increasing water resorption and relieving diarrhea.
• *Kinetics in adults:* Morphine is absorbed variably from the gut. Although opium alkaloids are distributed widely in the body, the low doses used to treat diarrhea act primarily in the GI tract. Camphor crosses the placenta. Opium is metabolized in the liver. It is excreted in urine; opium alkaloids (especially morphine) enter breast milk. Drug effect persists 4 to 5 hours.

Contraindications and precautions
Camphorated opium tincture is contraindicated in patients with known hypersensitivity to morphine alkaloids; in patients with acute respiratory depression because it may worsen this condition; in patients with diarrhea resulting from pseudomembranous colitis or ulcerative colitis because of the potential for toxic megacolon; and in patients with diarrhea resulting from poisoning or from certain bacterial or parasitic infections because expulsion of intestinal contents may be beneficial.

Camphorated opium tincture should be used cautiously in patients with asthma because the drug may exacerbate symptoms associated with this disorder; in patients with hepatic disease because of the potential for drug accumulation; and in patients with narcotic or alcohol dependence because the drug contains alcohol and opiates.

Interactions
When used concomitantly with other CNS depressants, opium tincture and camphorated opium tincture result in an additive effect. Concomitant use with metoclopramide may antagonize the effects of metoclopramide.

Effects on diagnostic tests
Camphorated opium tincture may prevent delivery of technetium-99m disofenin to the small intestine during hepatobiliary imaging tests; delay test until 24 hours after last dose. The drugs also may increase serum amylase and lipase levels by inducing contractions of the sphincter of Oddi and increasing biliary tract pressure.

Adverse reactions
• CNS: sedation, dizziness, *lethargy,* euphoria.
• GI: nausea, vomiting, abdominal cramps, dry mouth, anorexia, *constipation.*
• Other: physical dependence in long-term use.
  Note: Drug should be discontinued if signs of CNS or respiratory depression occur.

Overdose and treatment
Overdose is particularly hazardous in children. Clinical effects of overdose include drowsiness, hypotension, seizures, and apnea. Empty stomach by induced emesis or gastric lavage; maintain patent airway. Use naloxone to treat respiratory depression. Monitor patient for signs and symptoms of CNS or respiratory depression.

▶ Special considerations
• Uncomplicated diarrhea in children is often better left untreated. Especially in young children, inhibition of peristalsis can cause retention of fluid in the bowel, exacerbating dehydration and electrolyte depletion; it may also change response to the drug.
• Mix drug with sufficient water to ensure passage to stomach.
• Monitor patient's vital signs and bowel function.
• Risk of physical dependence on drug increases with long-term use.
• Do not refrigerate drug.

Information for parents and patient
• Warn parents that physical dependence may result from long-term use.
• Patient should avoid hazardous activities requiring alertness because drug may cause drowsiness, dizziness, and blurred vision.
• Because drug is indicated only for short-term use, instruct parents to report diarrhea that persists longer than 48 hours.
• Patient should take drug with food if it causes nausea, vomiting, or constipation.
• Instruct parents to call physician immediately if patient has difficulty breathing or shortness of breath.

• Patient should drink adequate fluids while diarrhea persists.

oxacillin sodium
Bactocill, Prostaphlin

• Classification: antibiotic (penicillinase-resistant penicillin)

How supplied
Available by prescription only
Capsules: 250 mg, 500 mg
Oral solution: 250 mg/5 ml (after reconstitution)
Injection: 250 mg, 500 mg, 1 g, 2 g, 4 g, 10 g
Pharmacy bulk package: 4 g, 10 g
I.V. infusion: 1 g, 2 g, 4 g

Indications, route, and dosage
Systemic infections caused by susceptible strains of staphylococci
Neonates age 0 to 7 days weighing < 2 kg: 25 mg/kg I.V. q 12 hours.
Neonates age 0 to 7 days weighing > 2 kg: 25 mg/kg I.V. q 8 hours.
Neonates over 7 days weighing < 2 kg: 25 mg/kg I.V. q 8 hours.
Neonates over 7 days weighing > 2 kg: 25 mg/kg I.V. q 6 hours.
Children and adults 40 kg and over: 2 to 4 g P.O. daily, divided into doses give q 6 hours; or 2 to 12 g I.M. or I.V. daily, divided 4 to 6 hours.
Children over 1 month of age weighing < 40 kg: 50 to 100 mg/kg P.O.
Meningitis
Neonates age 0 to 7 days weighing < 2 kg: 50 mg/kg I.V. q 12 hours.
Neonates age 0 to 7 days weighing > 2 kg: 50 mg/kg I.V. q 8 hours.
Neonates over 7 days weighing < 2 kg: 50mg/kg I.V. q 8 hours.
Neonates over 7 days weighing > 2 kg: 50 mg/kg I.V. q 6 hours.

Action and kinetics
• *Antibiotic action:* Oxacillin is bactericidal; it adheres to bacterial penicillin-binding proteins, thus inhibiting bacterial cell wall synthesis. Oxacillin resists the effects of penicillinases – enzymes that inactivate penicillin – and is thus active against many strains of penicillinase-producing bacteria; this activity is most important against penicillinase-producing staphylococci; some strains may remain resistant. Oxacillin is also active against a few gram-positive aerobic and anaerobic bacilli but has no significant effect on gram-negative bacilli.
• *Kinetics in adults:* Oxacillin is absorbed rapidly but incompletely from the GI tract; it is stable in an acid environment. Peak serum concentrations occur within ½ to 2 hours after an oral dose and 30 minutes after an I.M. dose. Food decreases absorption.

Oxacillin is distributed widely. CSF penetration is poor but enhanced by meningeal inflammation. Oxacillin crosses the placenta; it is 89% to 94% protein-bound.

Oxacillin is metabolized partially.

Oxacillin and metabolites are excreted primarily in urine by renal tubular secretion and glomerular filtration; it is also excreted in breast milk and in small amounts in bile. Elimination half-life in adults is ½ to 1 hour, extended to 2 hours in severe renal impairment. Serum levels are generally higher, and serum half-life is longer in neonates rather than older children. Dosage adjustments are not usually required in patients with renal impairment.

Contraindications and precautions
Oxacillin is contraindicated in patients with known hypersensitivity to any other penicillin or to cephalosporins.

Interactions
Concomitant use of oxacillin with aminoglycosides produces synergistic bactericidal effects against *Staphylococcus aureus.* However, the drugs are physically and chemically incompatible and are inactivated when mixed or given together. In vivo inactivation has been reported when aminoglycosides and penicillins are used concomitantly.

Probenecid blocks renal tubular secretion of penicillins, raising their serum levels.

Effects on diagnostic tests
Oxacillin alters tests for urinary and serum proteins; turbidimetric urine and serum proteins are often falsely positive or elevated in tests using sulfosalicylic acid or trichloroacetic acid.

Oxacillin may cause transient reductions in red blood cell, white blood cell, and platelet counts. Elevations in liver function tests may indicate drug-induced hepatitis or cholestasis. Abnormal urinalysis results may indicate drug-induced interstitial nephritis.

Oxacillin may falsely decrease serum aminoglycoside concentrations.

Adverse reactions
• CNS: neuropathy, neuromuscular irritability, seizures.
• GI: oral lesions, diarrhea, pseudomembranous colitis, intrahepatic cholestasis.
• GU: interstitial nephritis, transient hematuria, proteinuria.
• HEMA: granulocytopenia, thrombocytopenia, eosinophilia, hemolytic anemia, transient neutropenia.
• Hepatic: hepatitis, elevated enzymes.
• Local: thrombophlebitis.
• Other: hypersensitivity reactions (fever, chills, rash, urticaria, anaphylaxis), bacterial or fungal superinfection.

Note: Drug should be discontinued if immediate hypersensitivity reactions occur or if signs of interstitial nephritis or pseudomembranous colitis occur. Patient may require alternate therapy if any of the following occurs: drug fever, eosinophilia, hematuria, neutropenia, or unexplained elevations in serum creatinine concentration, BUN levels, or liver function studies.

Overdose and treatment
Clinical signs of overdose include neuromuscular sensitivity or seizures. No specific recommendations. Treatment is supportive. After recent ingestion (within 4 hours), empty the stomach by induced emesis or gastric lavage; follow with activated charcoal to reduce absorption. Oxacillin is not appreciably removed by peritoneal or hemodialysis.

▶ Special considerations
• Assess patient's history of allergies; do not give oxacillin to any patient with a history of hypersensitivity reactions to either penicillins or cephalosporins. Try to ascertain whether previous reactions were true hypersensitivity reactions or another reaction, such as GI distress, which the patient has interpreted as allergy.
• Keep in mind that a negative history for penicillin hypersensitivity does not preclude future allergic reactions; monitor patient continuously for possible allergic reactions or other untoward effects.
• In patients with severe renal impairment, dosage should be reduced if creatinine clearance is below 10 ml/minute.
• Assess level of consciousness, neurologic status, and renal function when high doses are used, because excessive bloodlevels can cause CNS toxicity.
• Obtain results of cultures and sensitivity tests before first dose; however, therapy may begin before test results are complete. Repeat tests periodically to assess drug efficacy.
• Monitor vital signs, electrolytes, and renal function studies; monitor body weight for fluid retention with extended-spectrum penicillins for possible hypokalemia or hypernatremia.
• Coagulation abnormalities, even frank bleeding, can follow high doses, especially of extended-spectrum penicllins; monitor prothrombin times and platelet counts and assess patient for signs of occult or frank bleeding.
• Monitor patients on long-term therapy for possible superinfection, especially debilitated patients and others receiving immunosuppressants or radiation therapy; monitor closely, especially for fever.

Oral and parenteral administration
• Give penicillins at least 1 hour before giving bacteriostatic antibiotics (tetracyclines, erythromycins, and chloramphenicol); these drugs inhibit bacterial cell growth, decreasing rate of penicillin uptake by bacterial cell walls.
• Give oral penicillin at least 1 hour before or 2 hours after meals to enhance gastric absorption. Give oral drug with water only; acid in fruit juice or carbonated beverage may inactivate drug.
• Administer I.M. dose deep into large muscle mass (gluteal or midlateral thigh); rotate injection sites to minimize tissue injury; do not inject more than 2 g of drug per injection site. Apply ice to injection site for pain.
• Do not add or mix other drugs with I.V. infusions — particularly aminoglycosides, which will be inactivated if mixed with pencillins; they are chemically and physically incompatible. If other drugs must be given I.V., temporarily stop infusion of primary drug.
• Infuse I.V. drug continuously or intermittenly (over 30 minutes) and assess I.V. site frequently to prevent infiltration or phlebitis; intermittent I.V. infusion may be diluted in sterile water, 0.9% sodium chloride dextrose 5% in water, dextrose 5% in water and half normal saline, or lactated Ringer's solution. Oxacillin may be diluted in less fluid as long as the final concentration does not exceed 100 mg/ml.
• Solutions should always be clear, colorless to pale yellow, and free of particles; do not give solutions containing precipitates or other foreign matter.
• Elimination of oxacillin is reduced in neonates. Transient hematuria, azotemia, and albuminuria have occurred in some neonates receiving oxacillin; monitor renal function closely. Frequently check urine for protein.
• Assess renal and hepatic function; watch for elevated AST (SGOT) and ALT (SGPT) and report significant changes.

Information for parents and patient
• Explain need to take oral preparations without food and to follow with water only because of acid content of fruit juice or carbonated beverages.
• Tell parents to report any allergic reactions or severe diarrhea promptly.
• Teach signs and symptoms of hypersensitivity and other adverse reactions, and emphasize need to report any unusual reactions.
• Teach signs and symptoms of bacterial and fungal superinfection to parents and patient, especially for debilitated patients and others with low resistance from immunosuppressants or irradiation; emphasize need to report signs of infection. Teach how to prevent infection by practicing meticulous oral and anogenital hygiene. Parents of infants and toddlers should keep diaper area clean and dry and avoid using plastic pants.
• Be sure parents understand how to administer drug; urge them to complete entire prescribed regimen, to comply with instructions for around-the-clock dosage, and to keep follow-up appointments.
• Counsel parents to check expiration date of drug and to discard unused drug.

oxamniquine
Vansil

• Classification: anthelmintic (tetrahydroquinoline)

How supplied
Available by prescription only
Capsules: 250 mg

Indications, route, and dosage
Schistosomiasis caused by Schistosoma mansoni, *Western Hemisphere strains*
Children < 30 kg: 10 mg/kg P.O., followed by 10 mg/kg P.O. in 2 to 8 hours on the same day.
Children > 30 kg and adults: 12 to 15 mg/kg P.O. as a single dose.

Action and kinetics
• *Anthelmintic action:* Oxamniquine paralyzes worm musculature; worms subsequently are dislodged from mesenteric veins and killed by host tissue reactions. Female worms cease to lay eggs after treatment. Oxamniquine is active against *Schistosoma mansoni.*
• *Kinetics in adults:* Oxamniquine is well absorbed, with peak plasma concentrations reached at 1 to 3 hours. Food decreases the rate and extent of absorption. The distribution of oxamniquine is not clearly defined. Oxamniquine is metabolized extensively to inactive acid metabolites in the GI lumen and mucosa. Oxamniquine and its metabolites are excreted primarily in urine; plasma half-life is 1 to 2½ hours. It is unknown if oxamniquine is excreted in breast milk.

Contraindications and precautions
Oxamniquine should be used with caution in patients with seizure disorders because it may cause seizures.

Interactions
Concomitant use of oxamniquine and praziquantel may result in synergistic antischistosomal activity; the clinical significance of such action is unknown.

Effects on diagnostic tests
Oxamniquine therapy may interfere with spectometric urinalysis; it also may cause transient elevation of liver enzyme levels. It may increase erythrocyte sedimentation rate and the reticulocyte count and may increase or decrease the leukocyte count. Rarely, electroencephalogram changes and minor ECG and pulmonary X-ray changes have been reported.

Adverse reactions
• CNS: seizures, dizziness, drowsiness, headache, excitation, hallucinations, insomnia.
• DERM: urticaria, rash, pruritus.
• GI: nausea, vomiting, abdominal pain, anorexia.
• Renal: proteinuria, hematuria, bilirubinuria.
• Other: joint pain, malaise, fever (usually occurs 5 to 7 days after treatment).
   Note: Drug should be discontinued if signs of hypersensitivity or toxicity occur.

Overdose and treatment
Treatment of overdose is largely supportive, particularly of cardiovascular and respiratory functions. After recent ingestion (within 4 hours), empty stomach by induced emesis or gastric lavage. Follow with activated charcoal to decrease absorption. Osmotic cathartics may be helpful.

▶ Special considerations
• Give drug after meals or with food to minimize GI distress.
• Monitor neurologic function; if patient has history of seizures, be alert to possible drug-induced recurrences.

Information for parents and patient
• Tell parents that patient should take drug with food to decrease the incidence of adverse reactions, especially dizziness, drowsiness, and nausea.
• Tell parents that child should avoid hazardous activities that require alertness and coordination because drug causes dizziness or drowsiness.
• Tell parents and patient that oxamniquine may cause orange-red discoloration of urine.

---

oxandrolone
Anavar

• Classification: anabolic, antiosteoporotic (anabolic steroid)

How supplied
Available by prescription only
Tablets: 2.5 mg

Indications, route, and dosage
To combat catabolic effects of corticosteroid therapy, osteoporosis, prolonged immobilization, and debilitated states
Children: 0.25 mg/kg P.O. daily for 2 to 4 weeks. Continuous therapy should not exceed 3 months.
Adults: 2.5 mg P.O. b.i.d., t.i.d., or q.i.d.; up to 20 mg/day for 2 to 4 weeks.
†**Turner's syndrome**
Children: 0.05 to 0.125 mcg/kg daily. Initiate and maintain lowest possible effective dosage.

Action and kinetics
• *Anabolic action:* Oxandrolone may reverse corticosteroid-induced catabolism and promote tissue development in severely debilitated patients. It causes calcium and phosphate retention and may relieve bone pain in severe osteoporosis.
• *Kinetics in adults:* The pharmacokinetics of oxandrolone are not well described.

Contraindications and precautions
Oxandrolone is contraindicated in patients with severe renal or cardiac disease, which may be worsened by the fluid and electrolyte retention caused by this drug; in patients with hepatic disease because impaired elimination of the drug may cause toxic accumulation; in patients with prostatic hypertrophy with obstruction or with undiagnosed abnormal genital bleeding because this drug can stimulate the growth of cancerous breast or prostate tissue in males; and in pregnant or breast-feeding patients because administration of anabolic steroids during pregnancy causes masculinization of the female fetus. Because of its hypercholesterolemic effects, oxandrolone should be administered cautiously in patients with a history of coronary artery disease. Because it may elevate serum calcium, use with caution (if at all) in patients with hypercalcemia.

Interactions
In patients with diabetes, decreased blood glucose levels may require adjustment of insulin or oral hypoglycemic drug dosage.
   Oxandrolone may potentiate the effect of warfarin-type anticoagulants, prolonging prothrombin time. Use with adrenocorticosteroids or adrenocorticotropic

---

hormone results in increased potential for fluid and electrolyte retention.

Effects on diagnostic tests

Oxandrolone may cause abnormal results of fasting plasma glucose, glucose tolerance, and metyrapone tests. It may increase sulfobromophthalein retention. Thyroid function test results (protein-bound iodine, radioactive iodine uptake, thyroid-binding capacity) and 17-ketosteroid levels may decrease. Liver function test results, prothrombin time (especially in patients receiving anticoagulant therapy), and serum creatinine levels may be elevated. Because of this agent's anabolic activity, serum sodium, potassium, calcium, phosphate, and cholesterol levels may all rise.

Adverse reactions

• Androgenic: *in females:* deepening of voice, clitoral enlargement, changes in libido; *in males:* prepubertal—premature epiphyseal closure, priapism, phallic enlargement; postpubertal—testicular atrophy, oligospermia, decreased ejaculatory volume, impotence, gynecomastia, epididymitis.
• CNS: headache, mental depression.
• CV: edema.
• DERM: acne, oily skin, hirsutism, flushing, sweating.
• GI: gastroenteritis, nausea, vomiting, constipation or diarrhea, change in appetite, weight gain.
• GU: bladder irritability, vaginitis, menstrual irregularities.
• Hepatic: reversible jaundice, hepatotoxicity.
• Other: hypercalcemia, hypersensitivity.

Note: Drug should be discontinued if hypercalcemia, edema, hypersensitivity reaction, priapism, or excessive sexual stimulation occurs or if virilization occurs in females.

Overdose and treatment

No information available.

▶ Special considerations

• Anabolic steroids should be used with caution in prepubertal children. Boys should be closely observed for precocious development of male sexual characteristics.
• In children, X-rays of wrist bones should establish level of bone maturation before therapy is initiated. During treatment, bone maturation may proceed more rapidly than linear growth, intermittent dosage and periodic X-rays are recommended to monitor skeletal effects.
• Watch female patients for signs of virilization. If possible, discontinue therapy when virilization first becomes apparent because some adverse effects (deepening of voice, clitoral enlargement) are irreversible.
• Anabolic steroids do not improve athletic performance. Risks associated with their use for this purpose far outweigh any possible benefits. Proof of anabolic steroid use is grounds for disqualification in many athletic events.
• Hypercalcemia symptoms may be difficult to distinguish from symptoms of condition being treated unless anticipated and thought of as a cluster.

• Edema usually is controllable with salt restriction, diuretics or both. Monitor weight routinely.
• Watch for symptoms of jaundice. Dosage adjustment may reverse condition. Periodic liver function tests are recommended.
• Observe patient on concomitant anticoagulation therapy for ecchymotic areas, petechiae, or abnormal bleeding. Monitor prothrombin time.
• Watch for symptoms of hypoglycemia in patients with diabetes. Change of antihypoglycemic drug dosage may be required.
• Anabolic steroids may alter many laboratory studies during therapy and for 2 to 3 weeks after therapy is stopped.
• Use with diet high in calories and protein unless contraindicated. Give small, frequent meals.

Information for parents and patient

• Advise parents to administer drug with foods or meals if it causes GI upset.
• Tell parents and female patient to report menstrual irregularities and to discontinue therapy until the cause is determined.
• Sexually active patients should practice contraception while taking this drug.
• Discuss reactions that alter body image with adolescent patients.
• Explain appropriate nutrition to facilitate therapeutic effect.

---

oxtriphylline
Apo-Oxtriphylline*, Choledyl, Novotriphyl*

• Classification: bronchodilator (xanthine derivative)

How supplied

Available by prescription only
Tablets: 100 mg, 200 mg
Tablets (sustained-release): 400 mg, 600 mg
Syrup: 50 mg/5 ml
Elixir: 100 mg/5 ml

Indications, route, and dosage
Chronic asthma

Children under age 9 years: 37.5 mg/kg/day P.O.
Children age 9 to 12 years: 31 mg/kg/day P.O.
Adolescents over age 12 to 16 years: 28 mg/kg/day P.O.
Adolescents over age 16 years: 20 mg/kg/day or 1400 mg/day P.O. (whichever is less).

Acute asthmatic attack (in patients not receiving theophylline)

Children age 6 months to 9 years: Loading dose 9.4 mg/kg, followed by 6.2 mg/kg q 4 hours for next 12 hours; then, 6.2 mg/kg q 6 hours.
Children over age 9 to 16 years and young adult smokers: Loading dose 9.4 mg/kg followed by 4.7 mg/kg q 4 hours for next 12 hours; then, 4.7 mg/kg q 6 hours.
Otherwise healthy, non-smoking young adults: Load-

ing dose 9.4 mg/kg, followed by 4.7 mg/kg q 6 hours for next 12 hours; then, 4.7 mg/kg q 8 hours.

Patients with cor pulmonale: Loading dose, 9.4 mg/kg, followed by 3.1 mg/kg q 6 hours for next 12 hours; then, 3.1 mg/kg q 12 hours.

Patients with CHF: Loading dose, 9.4 mg/kg, followed by 3.1 mg/kg q 8 hours for next 12 hours; then 1.6 to 3.1 mg/kg q 12 hours. Increase as needed to maintain therapeutic levels of theophylline (generally regarded as 10 to 20 mcg/ml, but some patients may respond to lower plasma levels).

Action and kinetics
• *Bronchodilating action:* Oxtriphylline exerts its bronchodilating action after it is converted to theophylline. (Oxtriphylline is 64% anhydrous theophylline.) Theophylline antagonizes adenosine receptors in the bronchi, and may inhibit phosphodiesterase and increase levels of cyclic adenosine monophosphate (CAMP), thus relaxing smooth muscle of the respiratory tract.
• *Kinetics in adults:* Drug is well absorbed; rate of absorption and onset of action depend on dosage form. Drug is distributed rapidly throughout body fluids and tissues. Oxtriphylline, the choline salt of theophylline, is converted to theophylline, then metabolized to inactive compounds. Drug is excreted in the urine as theophylline (10%) and theophyllic metabolites.

Contraindications and precautions
Oxtriphylline is contraindicated in patients with hypersensitivity to xanthines. Use cautiously in patients with compromised cardiac or circulatory function, diabetes, glaucoma, hypertension, hyperthyroidism, peptic ulcer, or gastroesophageal reflux, because drug may worsen these symptoms or conditions.

Interactions
When used concomitantly, oxtriphylline increases the excretion of lithium. Cimetidine, allopurinol (high dose), propranolol, erythromycin, and troleandomycin may increase serum concentration of oxtriphylline by decreasing hepatic clearance. Barbiturates, nicotine, marijuana, and aminoglutethimide decrease effects of oxtriphylline by enhancing its metabolism. Beta blockers exert antagonistic pharmacologic effects.

Effects on diagnostic tests
Oxtriphylline may falsely elevate serum uric acid levels measured by colorimetric methods. Theophylline levels may be falsely elevated in patients using furosemide, phenylbutazone, probenecid, some cephalosporins, sulfa medications, theobromine, caffeine, tea, chocolate, cola beverages, and acetaminophen, depending on assay method used.

Adverse reactions
• CNS: *irritability, restlessness,* headache, insomnia, dizziness, *seizures,* depression, light-headedness, *muscle twitching.*
• CV: palpitations, marked flushing, *hypotension, sinus tachycardia, ventricular tachycardia* and other life-threatening dysrhythmias, extrasystoles, circulatory failure.

• GI: *nausea, vomiting,* epigastric pain, loss of appetite, *diarrhea.*
• Respiratory: tachypnea, respiratory arrest.
• Other: fever, urinary retention, *hyperglycemia.*

Note: Drug should be discontinued if any adverse reaction intensifies; this signals impending overdose.

Overdose and treatment
Clinical manifestations of overdose include nausea, vomiting, insomnia, irritability, tachycardia, extrasystoles, tachypnea, or tonic/clonic seizures. The onset of toxicity may be sudden and severe, with dysrhythmias and seizures as the first signs. Induce emesis except in convulsing patients; follow with activated charcoal and cathartics. Treat dysrhythmias with lidocaine and seizures with I.V. diazepam; support cardiovascular and respiratory systems.

▶ Special considerations
• Use with caution in neonates.
• Many dosage forms and agents are available; it is important to select the form that offers maximum potential for patient compliance and minimal toxicity to the individual. Timed-release preparations may not be crushed or chewed.
• Dosage should be calculated from lean body weight, because theophylline does not distribute into fatty tissue.
• Administer drug with food to reduce GI upset.
• Observe for dysrhythmias.
• In infants, do not use liquid forms, which contain alcohol.
• Individuals metabolize theophylline at different rates, and metabolism is influenced by many factors, including age and life-style (smoking).
• Daily dosage may need to be adjusted in patients with CHF or hepatic disease. Monitor carefully, using blood levels.
• Oxtriphylline releases theophylline in the blood; theophylline blood levels are used to monitor therapy.
• Do not crush sustained-release tablets.
• Monitor vital signs and intake and output. Observe for CNS stimulation and CV adverse reactions.
• Store at 59° to 86° F. (15° to 30° C.) away from direct heat and light.

Information for parents and patient
• Patient may take drug with food to reduce GI upset.
• Instruct parents and patient about the drug and dosage schedule; if a dose is missed, patient should take it as soon as possible but never double the dose.
• Warn parents not to crush timed-release forms of drug.
• Advise parents of the adverse effects and possible signs of toxicity, and to report sign of excessive CNS stimulation (nervousness, tremors, akathisia).
• Warn parents to have patient avoid consuming large quantities of xanthine-containing foods and beverages.
• Patient should not take any other drug without medical approval.

---

oxybutynin chloride
Ditropan

• Classification: antispasmodic (synthetic tertiary amine)

How supplied
Available by prescription only
Tablets: 5 mg
Syrup: 5 mg/5 ml

Indications, route, and dosage
Antispasmodic for neurogenic bladder
Children over age 5: 5 mg P.O. b.i.d. to maximum of 5 mg t.i.d.
Adults: 5 mg P.O. b.i.d. to t.i.d. to maximum of 5 mg q.i.d.

Action and kinetics
• *Antispasmodic action:* Oxybutynin reduces the urge to void, increases bladder capacity, and reduces the frequency of contractions to the detrusor muscle. The drug exerts a direct spasmolytic action and an antimuscarinic action on smooth muscle.
• *Kinetics in adults:* Oxybutynin is absorbed rapidly, with peak levels occurring in 3 to 6 hours. Action begins in 30 to 60 minutes and persists for 6 to 10 hours. Drug is metabolized by the liver and is excreted principally in urine.

Contraindications and precautions
Oxybutynin is contraindicated in patients with partial or complete GI tract obstruction, glaucoma, myasthenia gravis, adynamic ileus, megacolon, or severe or ulcerative colitis, because it may worsen these symptoms or disorders; in debilitated patients with intestinal atony; in hemorrhaging patients with unstable cardiovascular status; and in patients with obstructive uropathy.

Oxybutynin should be used with caution in patients with autonomic neuropathy or hepatic or renal disease, and in patients with reflux esophagitis because drug may aggravate these conditions.

Interactions
Oxybutynin intensifies the antimuscarinic effects of atropine and related compounds. There is a possibility of an additive sedative effect with other CNS depressants.

Effects on diagnostic tests
None reported.

Adverse reactions
• CNS: drowsiness, dizziness, insomnia, flushing.
• CV: palpitations, tachycardia.
• DERM: urticaria, rash, severe allergic reactions in patients sensitive to anticholinergics.
• EENT: transient blurred vision; mydriasis; cycloplegia; dry mouth, nose, and throat; increased intraocular pressure.
• GI: nausea, vomiting, constipation, bloated feeling.
• GU: impotence, urinary hesitance or retention.
• Other: decreased sweating, fever, suppression of lactation.
Note: Drug should be discontinued if a hypersensitivity reaction occurs or if signs and symptoms of circulatory or respiratory distress or CNS excitation occur.

Overdose and treatment
Clinical manifestations of overdose include restlessness, excitement, psychotic behavior, flushing, hypotension, circulatory failure, and fever. In severe cases, paralysis, respiratory failure, and coma may occur. Treatment requires gastric lavage followed by physostigmine 0.5 to 2 mg slow I.V. push repeated up to 5 mg if necessary. Use ice packs, alcohol sponges, or a cooling blanket to control fever. Counteract CNS excitation, if necessary, with a slow I.V. drip of 2% thiopental or 2% chloral hydrate rectal suspension (100 to 200 ml). Maintain artificial respiration if paralysis of respiratory muscles occurs.

▶ Special considerations
• Dosage guidelines have not been established for children under age 5.
• Oxybutynin may cause gastric irritation when taken on an empty stomach. Food or milk may relieve the symptoms.
• Cystometry and other appropriate urologic procedures are performed prior to starting therapy and periodically to evaluate patient response.
• Store in tightly closed containers between 59° and 86° F. (15° and 30° C.).

Information for parents and patient
• Instruct parents and patient regarding medication and dosage schedule; patient should take a missed dose as soon as possible but should not double-dose.
• Warn parents about the possibility of decreased mental alertness or visual changes.
• Inform parents how to minimize the patient's risk of heatstroke.

oxymetazoline hydrochloride
Afrin, Allerest 12-Hour Nasal, Coricidin Nasal Mist, Dristan Long Lasting Nasal Mist, Duramist Plus, Duration, 4-Way Long-Acting Nasal Spray, Nafrine★, Neo-Synephrine 12 Hour Nasal Spray, Nōstrilla Long Acting Nasal Decongestant, NTZ Long Acting Nasal, Sinarest 12-Hour, Sinex Long-Lasting

• Classification: decongestant, vasoconstrictor (sympathomimetic agent)

How supplied
Available without prescription
Nasal solution: 0.025% (drops) for children
Nasal drops or spray: 0.05%

Indications, route, and dosage
Nasal congestion

Children age 2 to 6: Apply 2 to 3 drops of 0.025% solution to nasal mucosa b.i.d. Use no longer than 3 to 5 days. Dosage for younger children has not been established.

Children over age 6 and adults: Apply 2 to 4 drops or sprays of 0.05% solution to nasal mucosa b.i.d.

Action and kinetics
• *Decongestant action:* Produces local vasoconstriction of arterioles through alpha receptors to reduce blood flow and nasal congestion.
• *Kinetics in adults:* Unknown.

Contraindications and precautions
Oxymetazoline hydrochloride is contraindicated in patients with narrow-angle glaucoma or hypersensitivity to any components of the preparation.

It should be used with caution in patients with hyperthyroidism, cardiac disease, hypertension, diabetes mellitus, and advanced arteriosclerosis.

Interactions
Oxymetazoline hydrochloride may potentiate the pressor effects of tricyclic antidepressants from significant systemic absorption of the decongestant.

Effects on diagnostic tests
None reported.

Adverse reactions
• CNS: headache, drowsiness, dizziness, insomnia, tremor, psychological disturbances, seizures, CNS depression, weakness, hallucinations, prolonged psychosis.
• CV: palpitations, hypotension with cardiovascular collapse, tachycardia, precordial pain.
• EENT: rebound nasal congestion or irritation (with excessive or long-term use), dryness of nose and throat, increased nasal discharge, stinging, sneezing, blurred vision, ocular irritation, tearing, photophobia.
• Other: dysuria, orofacial dystonia, pallor, sweating.
Note: Drug should be discontinued if symptoms of systemic toxicity occur.

Overdose and treatment
Clinical manifestations of overdose include somnolence, sedation, sweating, CNS depression with hypertension, bradycardia, decreased cardiac output, rebound hypotension, cardiovascular collapse, depressed respirations, coma.

Because of rapid onset of sedation, emesis is not recommended unless given early. Activated charcoal or gastric lavage may be utilized initially. Monitor vital signs and ECG. Treat seizures with I.V. diazepam.

▶ Special considerations
• Children may exhibit increased side effects from systemic absorption.
• Monitor carefully for adverse reactions in patients with cardiovascular disease or diabetes mellitus, because systemic absorption can occur.

Information for parents and patient
• Emphasize that only one person should use dropper bottle or nasal spray.
• Advise parents and patient not to exceed recommended dosage and to use drug only when needed.
• Tell parents and patient that nasal mucosa may sting, burn, or become dry.
• Warn parents that excessive use may cause bradycardia, hypotension, dizziness, and weakness.
• Show parents and patient how to apply: have patient bend head forward and sniff spray briskly.

---

oxymetholone
Anadrol, Anapolon

• Classification: antianemic (anabolic steroid)

How supplied
Available by prescription only
Tablets: 50 mg

Indications, route, and dosage
Aplastic anemia
Premature infants and neonates: 0.175 mg/kg of body weight, or 5 mg/m² of body surface area, daily, as a single dose.

Children and adults: 1 to 5 mg/kg P.O. daily. Dose highly individualized; response not immediate. Trial of 3 to 6 months required. Although the maximum dosage is 5 mg/kg/day, most patients respond to 1 to 2 mg/kg/day.

Action and kinetics
• *Erythropoietic action:* Oxymetholone stimulates the kidneys' production of erythropoietin, leading to increases in red blood cell number, mass, and volume.
• *Kinetics in adults:* Oxymetholone is metabolized by the liver. Its pharmacokinetics are otherwise poorly described.

Contraindications and precautions
Oxymetholone is contraindicated in patients with severe renal or cardiac disease which may be worsened by the fluid and electrolyte retention this drug may cause; in patients with hepatic disease, because impaired elimination may cause toxic accumulation of the drug; in male patients with prostatic or breast cancer, benign prostatic hypertrophy with obstruction, or undiagnosed abnormal genital bleeding because this drug can stimulate the growth of cancerous breast or prostate tissue in males; and in pregnant and breast-feeding patients because administration of anabolic steroids during pregnancy causes masculinization of the female fetus.

Because of its hypercholesterolemic effects, this drug should be administered cautiously in patients with a history of coronary artery disease.

Interactions
In patients with diabetes, decreased blood glucose levels may require adjustment of insulin dosage.

Oxymetholone may potentiate the effects of warfarin-type anticoagulants, prolonging prothrombin time. Use with adrenocorticosteroids or adrenocorticotropin results in increased potential for fluid and electrolyte retention.

Effects on diagnostic tests
Oxymetholone may cause abnormal results of fasting plasma glucose, glucose tolerance, and metyrapone tests. It may increase sulfobromophthalein retention. Thyroid function test results (protein-bound iodine, radioactive iodine uptake, thyroid-binding capacity) and 17-ketosteroid levels may decrease. Liver function test results, prothrombin time (especially in patients receiving anticoagulant therapy), and serum creatinine levels may be elevated. Because of this agent's anabolic activity, serum sodium, potassium, calcium, phosphate, and cholesterol levels may all rise.

Adverse reactions
• Androgenic: *in females:* deepening of voice, clitoral enlargement, changes in libido; *in males:* prepubertal—premature epiphyseal closure, priapism, phallic enlargement; postpubertal—testicular atrophy, oligospermia, decreased ejaculatory volume, impotence, gynecomastia, epididymitis.
• CNS: headache, mental depression.
• CV: edema.
• DERM: acne, oily skin, hirsutism, flushing, sweating.
• GI: gastroenteritis, nausea, vomiting, constipation, diarrhea, change in appetite, weight gain.
• GU: bladder irritability, vaginitis, menstrual irregularities.
• Hepatic: reversible jaundice, hepatotoxicity.
• Other: hypercalcemia.
  Note: Drug should be discontinued if hypercalcemia, edema, hypersensitivity reaction, priapism, or excessive sexual stimulation occurs or if virilization occurs in females.

Overdose and treatment
No information available.

▶ Special considerations
• Anabolic steroids should be used with caution in prepubertal children. Boys should be closely observed for precocious development of male sexual characteristics.
• In children, X-rays of wrist bones should establish level of bone maturation before therapy is initiated. During treatment, bone maturation may proceed more rapidly than linear growth, intermittent dosage and periodic X-rays are recommended to monitor skeletal effects.
• Watch female patients for signs of virilization. If possible, discontinue therapy when virilization first becomes apparent because some adverse effects (deepening of voice, clitoral enlargement) are irreversible.
• Anabolic steroids do not improve athletic performance. Risks associated with their use for this purpose far outweigh any possible benefits. Proof of anabolic steroid use is grounds for disqualification in many athletic events.
• Hypercalcemia symptoms may be difficult to distinguish from symptoms of condition being treated unless anticipated and thought of as a cluster.
• Edema usually is controllable with salt restriction, diuretics or both. Monitor weight routinely.
• Watch for symptoms of jaundice. Dosage adjustment may reverse condition. Periodic liver function tests are recommended.
• Observe patient on concomitant anticoagulation therapy for ecchymotic areas, petechiae, or abnormal bleeding. Monitor prothrombin time.
• Watch for symptoms of hypoglycemia in patients with diabetes. Change of antihypoglycemic drug dosage may be required.
• Anabolic steroids may alter many laboratory studies during therapy and for 2 to 3 weeks after therapy is stopped.
• Patient should have diet high in calories and protein unless contraindicated. Give small, frequent meals.

Information for parents and patient
• Advise parents to administer drug with foods or meals if it causes GI upset.
• Tell parents and female patient to report menstrual irregularities and to discontinue therapy until the cause is determined.
• Sexually active patients should practice contraception while taking this drug.
• Discuss reactions that alter body image with adolescent patients.

---

oxytetracycline hydrochloride
Dalimycin, E.P. Mycin, Oxlopar, Oxy-Kesso-Tetra, Oxymycin, Oxytetrachlor, Terramycin, Uri-Tet

• Classification: antibiotic (tetracycline)

How supplied
Available by prescription only
Capsules: 250 mg
Tablets: 250 mg
Injectable: (I.V.) 250 mg, 500 mg; (I.M.) 500 mg/ml, 125 mg/ml with lidocaine 2%

Indications, route, and dosage
Infections caused by sensitive organisms
Children over age 8: 25 to 50 mg/kg P.O. daily, divided q 6 hours; 15 to 25 mg/kg I.M. daily, divided q 8 to 12 hours; or 10 to 20 mg/kg I.V. daily, divided q 12 hours.
Adults: 250 mg P.O. q 6 hours; 100 mg I.M. q 8 to 12 hours; 250 mg I.M. as a single dose.
Dosage in renal failure
Specific recommendations are unavailable. Decreased dosage and/or increased intervals between doses is recommended by the manufacturer for children with significant renal impairment.

Action and kinetics
• *Antibacterial action:* Oxytetracycline is bacteriostatic; it binds reversibly to ribosomal units, thereby inhibiting bacterial protein synthesis.

Oxytetracycline is active against many gram-negative and gram-positive organisms, *Mycoplasma, Rickettsia, Chlamydia,* and spirochetes. Its spectrum of antibiotic action is similar to other tetracyclines, and many clinicians feel it offers no advantages over less expensive tetracycline alternatives.

Tetracyclines are drugs of choice in Brucellosis, glanders, cholera, relapsing fever, melioidosis, leptospirosis, and early stages of Lyme disease. They are preferred drugs for chlamydial infections, granuloma inguinale, and urethritis due to ureaplasma urealyticum (but some clinicians prefer erythromycin).

• *Kinetics in adults:* Oxytetracycline is absorbed from the GI tract after oral administration. Absorption is significantly reduced by food and/or milk and other dairy products. I.M. absorption is erratic and incomplete.

Oxytetracycline is distributed widely into body tissues and fluids, including synovial, pleural, prostatic, and seminal fluids, bronchial secretions, saliva, and aqueous humor; CSF penetration is poor. Oxytetracycline crosses the placenta; Oxytetracycline is not metabolized.It is excreted primarily unchanged in urine by glomerular filtration.

• *Kinetics in children:* Tetracyclines form a stable complex in bone-forming tissue, and may cause permanent enamel hypoplasia or yellow-gray discoloration of teeth in children under age 8.

Contraindications and precautions
Oxytetracycline is contraindicated in children with known hypersensitivity to any tetracycline; and in children under age 8 because of the risk of permanent discoloration of teeth, enamel defects, and retardation of bone growth.

Use drug with caution in children with decreased renal function because drug may elevate BUN levels and exacerbate dysfunction; and in children apt to be exposed to sunlight or ultraviolet light because of the risk of photosensitivity reactions.

Interactions
Concomitant use of oxytetracycline with antacids containing aluminum, calcium, or magnesium or with laxatives containing magnesium decreases absorption of oxytetracycline (because of chelation); concomitant use with food, milk and other dairy products, oral iron products, or sodium bicarbonate also impairs oral absorption.

Tetracyclines may antagonize bactericidal effects of penicillin, inhibiting cell growth through bacteriostatic action; administer penicillin 2 to 3 hours before oxytetracycline.

Oxytetracycline enhances the risk of nephrotoxicity from methoxyflurane; it also necessitates lowered dosage of oral anticoagulants because of enhanced effects, and lowered dosage of digoxin because of increased bioavailability.

Effects on diagnostic tests
Oxytetracycline causes false-negative results in urine glucose tests utilizing glucose oxidase reagent (Clinistix, or Tes-Tape); parenteral dosage form may cause false-negative results on Clinitest.

Oxytetracycline causes false elevations in fluorometric tests for urinary catecholamines.

Oxytetracycline may elevate BUN level in patients with decreased renal function.

Adverse reactions
• CNS: intracranial hypertension.
• CV: pericarditis.
• DERM: maculopapular and erythematous rashes, urticaria, photosensitivity, increased pigmentation, discolored nails and teeth.
• EENT: dysphagia, glossitis.
• GI: anorexia, nausea, vomiting, diarrhea, enterocolitis, anogenital inflammation.
• GU: reversible nephrotoxicity (Fanconi's syndrome) with *outdated* tetracyclines.
• HEMA: neutropenia, eosinophilia.
• Metabolic: increased BUN levels.
• Local: irritation after I.M. injection, thrombophlebitis.
• Other: hypersensitivity, bacterial and fungal superinfection.
Note: Drug should be discontinued if signs of toxicity, hypersensitivity, progressive renal dysfunction, or superinfection occur; if erythema follows exposure to sunlight or ultraviolet light; or if severe diarrhea indicates pseudomembranous colitis.

Overdose and treatment
Clinical signs of overdose are usually limited to GI tract; give antacids or empty stomach by gastric lavage if ingestion occurred within the preceding 4 hours.

▶ Special considerations
• Assess child's allergic history; do not give oxytetracycline to a patient with a history of hypersensitivity reactions to any other tetracycline; monitor continuously for this and other adverse reactions.
• Obtain results of cultures and sensitivity tests before first dose, but do not delay therapy; check cultures periodically to assess drug efficacy.
• Monitor vital signs, electrolytes, and renal function studies before and during therapy.
• Monitor for bacterial and fungal superinfection, especially in debilitated children and those who are receiving immunosuppressants or radiation therapy; watch especially for oral candidiasis. If symptoms occur, discontinue drug.
• I.V. use may cause thrombophlebitis. Monitor carefully to avoid extravasation.
• Children age 8 and under should not receive tetracyclines unless there is no alternative. Tetracyclines can cause permanent discoloration of teeth, enamel hypoplasia, and a reversible decrease in bone calcification.
• Reversible decreases in bone calcification have been reported in infants.
Administration
• Give oral tetracyclines 1 hour before or 2 hours after meals for maximum absorption; do not give with food, milk, or other dairy products, sodium bicarbonate, iron compounds, or antacids, which may impair absorption.
• Give water with and after oral drug to facilitate

---

passage to stomach, because incomplete swallowing can cause severe esophageal irritation; do not administer within 1 hour of bedtime, to prevent esophageal influx.
• For I.V. use, reconstitute 250 mg and 500 mg of powder for injection with 10 ml of sterile water. Dilute in dextrose 5% in water, normal saline solution, or Ringer's solution in volume appropriate to patient's weight. Do not mix with any other drug.
• Reconstituted solution is stable for 48 hours in refrigerator.
• Monitor I.V. injection sites and rotate routinely to minimize local irritation. I.V. administration may cause severe phlebitis.
• Inject I.M. dose deeply into large muscle mass to reduce pain. Rotate injection sites. Because I.M. preparations contain a local anesthetic, rule out hypersensitivity to local anesthetics before injecting.
• Avoid I.V. use in children with decreased renal function. I.V. use of tetracyclines in children with renal impairment, especially when dosage exceeds 2 g/day can cause hepatic failure.
• Store dry powder at room temperature; store syrup in cool place, protected from light.

Information for parents and patient
• Teach signs and symptoms of adverse reactions, and emphasize need to report these promptly; urge parents to report any unusual effects.
• Teach signs and symptoms of bacterial and fungal superinfections to parents of children with low resistance from immunosuppressants or irradiation. Teach them how to prevent it by practicing meticulous oral and anogenital hygiene. Parents of infants and toddlers should keep diaper area clean and dry and avoid using plastic pants.
• Advise parents to prevent child's direct exposure to sunlight and of the need to use a sunscreen to help prevent photosensitivity reactions.
• Patient should take oral tetracyclines with enough water to facilitate passage to the stomach, 1 hour before or 2 hours after meals for maximum absorption and not less than 1 hour before bedtime (to prevent irritation from esophageal reflux).
• Emphasize that taking the drug with food, milk, or other dairy products, sodium bicarbonate, or iron compounds may interfere with absorption. Tell patient to take antacids 3 hours after tetracycline.
• Emphasize importance of completing prescribed regimen exactly as ordered and keeping follow-up appointments.
• Tell parents to check expiration dates and discard any expired drug.

pancreatin
Dizymes, Hi-Vegi-Lip, Pancreatin
Enseals, Pancreatin Tablets

• Classification: digestant (pancreatic enzyme)

How supplied
Available without prescription
Dizymes
Tablets (enteric-coated): 250 mg pancreatin, 6,750 units lipase, 41,250 units protease, 43,750 units amylase
Hi-Vegi-Lip
Tablets (enteric-coated): 2,400 mg pancreatin, 12,000 units lipase, 60,000 units protease, and 60,000 units amylase
Pancreatin Enseals
Tablets (enteric-coated): 1,000 mg pancreatin, 2,000 units lipase, 25,000 units protease, 25,000 units amylase
Pancreatin Tablets
Tablets (enteric-coated): 325 mg pancreatin, 650 units lipase, 8,125 units protease, 8,125 units amylase

Indications, route, and dosage
Exocrine pancreatic secretion insufficiency, digestive aid in cystic fibrosis, steatorrhea and other disorders of fat metabolism secondary to insufficient pancreatic enzymes
Children and adults: 1 to 3 tablets P.O. with meals.

Action and kinetics
• *Digestive action:* The proteolytic, amylolytic, and lipolytic enzymes enhance the digestion of proteins, starches, and fats. This agent is sensitive to acids and is more active in neutral or slightly alkaline environments.
• *Kinetics in adults:* Drug is not absorbed; it acts locally in the GI tract. Drug is excreted in feces.

Contraindications and precautions
Pancreatin is contraindicated in patients with hypersensitivity to hog protein.

Interactions
Pancreatin activity may be reduced by calcium- or magnesium-containing antacids; however, antacids or H₂ blockers (such as cimetidine) may reduce the inactivation of the enzymes by gastric acid. Pancreatin decreases absorption of iron-containing products.

Effects on diagnostic tests
Pancreatin, particularly in large doses, increases serum uric acid concentrations.

Adverse reactions
There are usually no reactions to standard doses.
• GI: nausea, vomiting, diarrhea, stomach cramps.
  Note: Drug should be discontinued if an allergic reaction occurs.

Overdose and treatment
Clinical manifestations of overdose include hyperuricosuria and hyperuricemia.

▶ Special considerations
• Contraindicated in patients with severe pork hypersensitivity.
• Antacids or H₂ blockers, such as cimetidine or ranitidine, may be administered concurrently to prevent inactivation of non-enteric-coated drug products; enteric coating on some products may reduce availability of enzyme in upper portion of jejunum.
• For young children, mix powders (including contents of capsule) with applesauce and give at mealtime. Avoid inhalation of powder. Older children may swallow capsules with food.
• For maximal effect, administer dose just before or during a meal.
• Tablets may not be crushed or chewed. They also should not be held in mouth before swallowing to prevent irritation of oral mucosa.
• Diet should balance fat, protein, and starch intake properly to avoid indigestion. Dosage varies according to degree of maldigestion and malabsorption, amount of fat in diet, and enzyme activity of individual preparations.
• Adequate replacement decreases number of bowel movements and improves stool consistency.
• Use only after confirmed diagnosis of exocrine pancreatic insufficiency. Not effective in GI disorders unrelated to pancreatic enzyme deficiency.

Information for parents and patient
• Explain use of drug, and advise storing it away from heat and light.
• Be sure parents understand special dietary instructions.
• Advise parents and patient that adequate replacement decreases number of bowel movements and improves stool consistency.
• Advise parents and patient that preparations are coated to protect the enzymes from gastric juices; patient should not crush or chew.

---

pancrelipase
Cotazym, Cotazym-S, Festal II,
Ilozyme, Ku-Zyme HP, Pancrease,
Viokase

• Classification: digestant (pancreatic enzyme)

How supplied
Available by prescription only
Cotazym
Capsules: 8,000 units lipase, 30,000 units protease,
30,000 units amylase
Cotazym-S
Capsules: 5,000 units lipase, 20,000 units protease,
20,000 units amylase
Ilozyme
Tablets: 11,000 units lipase, 30,000 units protease,
30,000 units amylase
Available without prescription
Festal II
Tablets: 6,000 units lipase, 20,000 units protease,
30,000 units amylase
Ku-Zyme HP
Capsules: 8,000 units lipase, 30,000 units protease,
30,000 units amylase
Pancrease
Capsules: 4,000 units lipase, 25,000 units protease,
20,000 units amylase
Viokase
Powder: 16,800 units lipase, 70,000 units protease,
70,000 units amylase

Indications, route, and dosage
***Exocrine pancreatic secretion insufficiency,
cystic fibrosis in adults and children, steatorrhea and other disorders of fat metabolism
secondary to insufficient pancreatic enzymes***
Children and adults: Dosage range is 1 to 3 capsules
or tablets P.O. before or with meals and 1 capsule or
tablet with snack; or 1 to 2 powder packets before
meals or snacks. Dose must be titrated to patient's
response.

Action and kinetics
• *Digestive action:* The proteolytic, amylolytic, and
lipolytic enzymes enhance the digestion of proteins,
starches, and fats. This agent is sensitive to acids
and is more active in neutral or slightly alkaline environments.
• *Kinetics in adults:* Drug is not absorbed and acts
locally in the GI tract. Drug is excreted in feces.

Contraindications and precautions
Pancrelipase is contraindicated in patients with hypersensitivity to pork or pork derivatives. The powder
is extremely irritating if inhaled.

Interactions
When used concomitantly, pancrelipase activity may
be reduced by calcium- or magnesium-containing antacids; however, antacids or H_2 blockers (such as cimetidine), may reduce inactivation of the enzymes by

gastric acid. Pancrelipase decreases absorption of iron-
containing products.

Effects on diagnostic tests
Pancrelipase therapy increases serum uric acid concentrations, particularly with large doses.

Adverse reactions
There are usually no reactions to standard doses.
• GI: nausea, vomiting, diarrhea, stomach cramps, oc-
cult bleeding (with high doses).
• Other: hyperuricemia, hyperuricosuria (with high
doses).
  Note: Drug should be discontinued if an allergic
reaction occurs.

Overdose and treatment
Clinical manifestations of overdose include hyperuricosuria and hyperuricemia.

▶ Special considerations
• Contraindicated in patients with severe pork hypersensitivity.
• Antacids or H_2 blockers, such as cimetidine or ranitidine, may be administered concurrently to prevent
inactivation of non-enteric-coated drug products; enteric coating on some products may reduce availability
of enzyme in upper portion of jejunum.
• For maximal effect, administer dose just before or
during a meal.
• Preparations may not be crushed or chewed.
• Microspheres may be mixed with each feeding for
infants.
• Use only after confirmed diagnosis of exocrine pancreatic insufficiency. Not effective in GI disorders unrelated to enzyme deficiency.
• Dosage varies with degree of maldigestion and malabsorption, amount of fat in diet, and enzyme activity
of individual preparations.
• Adequate replacement decreases number of bowel
movements and improves stool consistency.

Information for parents and patient
• Teach parents and patient proper use of drug, and
advise storing it away from heat and light.
• Be sure parents understand special dietary instruc-
tions.
• For young children, mix powders (including content
of capsules) with applesauce and give at mealtime.
Avoid inhalation of powder. Older children may swallow capsules with food.
• Capsules may be opened to facilitate swallowing.
They may be sprinkled on food, but a pH of 5.5 or
greater is necessary to ensure stability.
• Advise parents and patient that adequate replacement decreases number of bowel movements and improves stool consistency.
• Advise parents and patient that the preparations
are coated to protect the enzymes from gastric juices;
patient should not crush or chew.

papaverine hydrochloride
Cerebid, Cerespan, Delapav, Myobid, Papacon, Pavabid, Pavacap, Pavacen, Pavadur, Pavadyl, Pavagen, Pava-Par, Pava-Rx, Pavased, Pavasule, Pavatine, Paverolan, P-200, Vasal

• Classification: peripheral vasodilator (benzylisoquinoline derivative, opiate alkaloid)

How supplied
Available by prescription only
Tablets: 30 mg, 60 mg, 100 mg, 200 mg, 300 mg
Tablets (sustained-release): 200 mg
Capsules (sustained-release): 150 mg
Injection: 2-ml ampules – 30 mg/ml; 10-ml ampules – 30 mg/ml

Indications, route, and dosage
Ischemic states and smooth muscle spasm
Drug is indicated for relief of cerebral and peripheral ischemia associated with arterial spasm and myocardial ischemia, and for treatment of coronary occlusion, angina pectoris, and certain cerebral angiospastic states.
Children: 6 mg/kg I.M.or I.V. q.i.d.
Adults: 75 to 300 mg P.O. one to five times daily or 150 to 300 mg sustained-release preparations q 8 to 12 hours; 30 to 120 mg I.M. or I.V. q 3 hours, as indicated.

Action and kinetics
• *Vasodilating action:* Papaverine relaxes smooth muscle directly by inhibiting phosphodiesterase, thus increasing concentration of cyclic adenosine monophosphate. There is considerable controversy regarding the clinical effectiveness of of papaverine. Some clinicians find little objective evidence of any clinical value.
• *Kinetics in adults:* 54% of orally administered papaverine is bioavailable. Peak plasma levels occur 1 to 2 hours after an oral dose; half-life varies from ½ to 24 hours, but levels can be maintained by giving drug at 6-hour intervals. Sustained-release forms are sometimes absorbed poorly and erratically. Papaverine tends to localize in adipose tissue and in the liver; the remainder is distributed throughout the body. About 90% of the drug is protein-bound. It is metabolized by the liver and excreted in urine as metabolites.

Contraindications and precautions
Papaverine is contraindicated in patients with complete AV heart block because large doses may depress AV and intraventricular conduction, causing serious dysrhythmias.
Use drug cautiously in patients with glaucoma.

Interactions
Papaverine may decrease the antiparkinsonian effects of levodopa and exacerbate such symptoms as rigidity and tremors. Heavy tobacco smoking may interfere with the therapeutic effect of papaverine because nicotine constricts the blood vessels. Papaverine's effects may be potentiated by CNS depressants and may have a synergic response with morphine.

Effects on diagnostic tests
Papaverine therapy alters serum concentrations of eosinophils, ALT (SGPT), alkaline phosphatase, and bilirubin. Elevated serum bilirubin levels signal hepatic hypersensitivity to papaverine.

Adverse reactions
• CNS: headache, drowsiness, dizziness, depression, sedation, or lethargy.
• CV: increased heart rate, hypertension (with parenteral use), depressed AV and intraventricular conduction, dysrhythmias.
• GI: nausea, constipation, diarrhea, abdominal distress, anorexia.
• Other: hepatic hypersensitivity, sweating, flushing, increased depth of respiration.
Note: Drug should be discontinued if signs of hepatic hypersensitivity occur (jaundice, eosinophilia, and altered liver function test results).

Overdose and treatment
Clinical signs of overdose include drowsiness, weakness, nystagmus, diplopia, incoordination, and lassitude, progressing to coma with cyanosis and respiratory depression.
To slow drug absorption, give activated charcoal, tap water, or milk, then evacuate stomach contents by gastric lavage or emesis, and follow with catharsis. If coma and respiratory depression occur, take appropriate measures; maintain blood pressure. Hemodialysis may be helpful.

▶ Special considerations
• Papaverine is an opiate; however, it has strikingly different pharmacologic properties.
• Children's doses are administered parenterally.
• Inject I.V. slowly over 1 to 2 minutes; dysrhythmias and fatal apnea may follow rapid injection.
• Papaverine injection is incompatible with lactated Ringer's injection; a precipitate will form.

Information for parents and patient
• Advise parents to have patient to avoid sudden postural changes to minimize possible orthostatic hypotension.
• Instruct parents to watch patient for and report nausea, abdominal distress, anorexia, constipation, diarrhea, jaundice, rash, sweating, tiredness, or headache.

---

paramethadione
Paradione

• Classification: anticonvulsant (oxazolidinedione derivative)

How supplied
Available by prescription only
Capsules: 150 mg, 300 mg
Solution: 300 mg/ml (65% alcohol) with dropper

Indications, route, and dosage
Refractory absence (petit mal) seizures
Children under age 2: 300 mg P.O. daily in divided doses b.i.d.
Children age 2 to 6: 600 mg P.O. daily in divided doses t.i.d. or q.i.d.
Children over age 6: 900 mg P.O. daily in divided doses t.i.d. or q.i.d.
Adults: Initially, 300 mg P.O. t.i.d; may increase by 300 mg weekly, up to 600 mg q.i.d., if needed.

Action and kinetics
• *Anticonvulsant action:* Paramethadione raises the threshold for cortical seizures but does not modify the seizure pattern. It decreases projection of focal activity and reduces both repetitive spinal cord transmission and spike-and-wave patterns of absence (petit mal) seizures.
• *Kinetics in adults:* Paramethadione is absorbed from the GI tract and is distributed widely throughout the body. Paramethadione is demethylated in the liver to active metabolites. Drug is excreted in urine; it is unknown whether drug is excreted in breast milk.

Contraindications and precautions
Paramethadione is contraindicated during pregnancy and in patients with known hypersensitivity to oxazolidinedione derivatives; use paramethadione with extreme caution in patients with severe hepatic or renal disease, severe blood dyscrasias, or diseases of the retina or optic nerve because the drug may exacerbate diseases of the optic nerve. Preparation contains tartrazine; use with caution in patients with asthma or aspirin allergy because of possible allergic reactions.

Interactions
Concomitant use of paramethadione and mephenytoin or phenacemide may result in a high incidence of toxicity; such combinations should be avoided.

Effects on diagnostic tests
Paramethadione may cause abnormalities in liver function test results.

Adverse reactions
• CNS: drowsiness, fatigue, vertigo, headache, paresthesias, irritability.
• CV: hypertension, hypotension.
• DERM: acneiform or morbilliform rash, exfoliative dermatitis, erythema multiforme, petechiae, alopecia.
• EENT: hemeralopia, photophobia, diplopia, epistaxis, retinal hemorrhage.
• GI: nausea, vomiting, abdominal pain, weight loss, bleeding gums.
• GU: albuminuria, vaginal bleeding.
• HEMA: neutropenia, leukopenia, eosinophilia, thrombocytopenia, pancytopenia, agranulocytosis, hypoplastic and aplastic anemia.
• Hepatic: abnormal liver function test results.
• Other: lymphadenopathy, lupus erythematosus.
   Note: Drug should be discontinued if signs of hypersensitivity, any rash (even acneiform), or unusual skin lesions occur; if scotomata occur; if neutrophil count falls below 2,500/mm³; if any of the following signs of blood dyscrasia occur: joint pain, fever, sore throat, or unusual bleeding or bruising; if patient has persistent or increasing albuminuria; if jaundice or other signs of hepatic dysfunction occur; or if syndromes resembling systemic lupus erythematosus, malignant lymphoma, or myasthenia gravis occur.

Overdose and treatment
Symptoms of overdose include nausea, drowsiness, ataxia, and visual disturbances; coma may follow massive overdose.
   Treat overdose with immediate gastric lavage or emesis, and with supportive measures. Monitor vital signs and fluid and electrolyte balance carefully. Alkalinization of urine may hasten renal excretion. Monitor blood counts and hepatic and renal function after recovery.

▶ Special considerations
• Drug is extremely toxic and is not considered drug of choice for absence seizures.
• For pediatric patients, dilute oral solution with water because of 65% alcohol content.
• Monitor baseline liver and renal function and CBC at beginning of therapy and monthly during therapy.
• Drug should be discontinued if neutrophil count falls below 2,500/mm³ or if any of the following occur: hypersensitivity, scotomata, hepatitis, systemic lupus erythematosus, lymphadenopathy, rash, nephrosis, alopecia, or grand mal seizures.

Information for parents and patient
• Emphasize need for close medical supervision.
• Explain to parents of adolescents the importance of reporting suspected pregnancy immediately.
• Tell parents and patient that patient should take drug with food or milk to prevent GI distress.
• Urge parents to report the following reactions promptly: visual disturbance, excessive dizziness or drowsiness, sore throat, fever, bleeding or bruising, or skin rash.
• Inform parents and patient that hemeralopia (day blindness) may be relieved with dark glasses.
• Warn parents and patients never to discontinue drug without medical supervision.
• Patient should avoid alcohol while taking drug because it may decrease drug's effectiveness and increase CNS effects.
• Advise parents that patient should avoid hazardous activities that require mental alertness until degree

of sedative effect is determined. Drug may cause dizziness, drowsiness, or blurred vision.
• Encourage parents to have patient wear a Medic Alert bracelet or necklace, listing the drug and seizure disorder, while taking paramethadione.

---

paramethasone acetate
Haldrone

• Classification: anti-inflammatory, immunosuppressant (glucocorticoid)

How supplied
Available by prescription only
Tablets: 1 mg, 2 mg

Indications, route, and dosage
Inflammatory conditions
Children: 58 to 800 mcg/kg daily divided t.i.d. or q.i.d.
Adults: 0.5 to 6 mg P.O. t.i.d. or q.i.d.

Action and kinetics
• *Immunosuppressant action:* Paramethasone stimulates the synthesis of enzymes needed to decrease the inflammatory response. It suppresses the immune system by reducing activity and volume of the lymphatic system, thus producing lymphocytopenia (primarily of T-lymphocytes), decreasing passage of immune complexes through basement membranes, and possibly by depressing reactivity of tissue to antigen-antibody interactions.
• *Anti-inflammatory action:* Paramethasone is a long-acting steroid with anti-inflammatory potency 10 times that of an equal weight of hydrocortisone. It has essentially no mineralocorticoid activity. Paramethasone tablets are used as oral anti-inflammatory agents.
• *Kinetics in adults:* Paramethasone is absorbed readily after oral administration. Peak effects occur within 1 to 2 hours.
Paramethasone is distributed rapidly to muscle, liver, skin, intestines, and kidneys. Paramethasone is bound weakly to plasma proteins (transcortin and albumin). Only the unbound portion is active. Adrenocorticoids are distributed into breast milk and through the placenta.
Paramethasone is metabolized in the liver to inactive glucuronide and sulfate metabolites.
The inactive metabolites and small amounts of unmetabolized drug are excreted by the kidneys. Insignificant quantities of drug are excreted in feces. The biological half-life of paramethasone is 36 to 54 hours.

Contraindications and precautions
Paramethasone is contraindicated in patients with systemic fungal infections (except in adrenal insufficiency) or a hypersensitivity to ingredients of adrenocorticoid preparations. Patients receiving paramethasone should not be given live virus vaccines because paramethasone suppresses the immune response.
Paramethasone should be used with extreme cau-

tion in patients with GI ulceration, renal disease, hypertension, osteoporosis, diabetes mellitus, thromboembolic disorders, seizures, myasthenia gravis, CHF, tuberculosis, hypoalbuminemia, hypothyroidism, cirrhosis of the liver, emotional instability, psychotic tendencies, hyperlipidemias, glaucoma, or cataracts, because the drug may exacerbate these conditions.
Because adrenocorticoids increase the susceptibility to and mask symptoms of infection, paramethasone should not be used (except in life-threatening situations) in patients with viral or bacterial infections not controlled by anti-infective agents.

Interactions
When used concomitantly, paramethasone rarely may decrease the effects of oral anticoagulants by unknown mechanisms.
Glucocorticoids increase the metabolism of isoniazid and salicylates; they cause hyperglycemia, requiring dosage adjustment of insulin in diabetic patients; and may enhance hypokalemia associated with diuretic or amphotericin B therapy. The hypokalemia may increase the risk of toxicity in patients concurrently receiving digitalis glycosides.
Barbiturates, phenytoin, and rifampin may cause decreased paramethasone effects because of increased hepatic metabolism. Cholestyramine, colestipol, and antacids decrease the corticosteroid effect by adsorbing the corticosteroid, decreasing the amount absorbed.
Concomitant use with estrogens may reduce the metabolism of paramethasone by increasing the concentration of transcortin. The half-life of paramethasone is then prolonged because of increased protein binding. Concomitant administration of ulcerogenic drugs, such as nonsteroidal anti-inflammatory drug, may increase the risk of GI ulceration.

Effects on diagnostic tests
Paramethasone suppresses reactions to skin tests; causes false-negative results in the nitroblue tetrazolium test for systemic bacterial infections; decreases ^{131}I uptake and protein-bound iodine concentrations in thyroid function tests; may increase glucose and cholesterol levels; may decrease serum potassium, calcium, thyroxine, and triiodothyronine levels; and may increase urine glucose and calcium levels.

Adverse reactions
When administered in high doses or for prolonged therapy, the glucocorticoids suppress release of adrenocorticotropic hormone (ACTH) from the pituitary gland; in turn, the adrenal cortex stops secreting endogenous corticosteroids. The degree and duration of hypothalamic-pituitary-adrenal (HPA) axis suppression produced by the drugs is highly variable among patients and depends on the dose, frequency and time of administration, and duration of glucocorticoid therapy.
• CNS: euphoria, insomnia, headache, psychotic behavior, pseudotumor cerebri, mental changes, nervousness, restlessness, *psychoses*.
• CV: CHF, *hypertension*, edema.

---

*Canada only   †Unlabeled clinical use   Italicized adverse reactions have been observed in children.

- DERM: delayed healing, *acne,* skin eruptions, striae.
- EENT: *cataracts,* glaucoma, thrush.
- GI: *peptic ulcer,* irritation, increased appetite.
- Immune: immunosuppression, *increased susceptibility to infection.*
- Metabolic: *hypokalemia,* sodium retention, fluid retention, weight gain, hyperglycemia, *osteoporosis,* growth suppression in children, glycosuria.
- Musculoskeletal: muscle atrophy, weakness, *myopathy*
- Other: pancreatitis, *hirsutism, cushingoid symptoms,* withdrawal syndrome (nausea, fatigue, anorexia, dyspnea, hypotension, hypoglycemia, myalgia, arthralgia, fever, dizziness, and fainting), *ecchymoses.* Sudden withdrawal may be fatal or may exacerbate the underlying disease. Acute adrenal insufficiency may occur with increased stress (infection, surgery, trauma) or abrupt withdrawal after long-term therapy.

Overdose and treatment
Acute ingestion, even in massive doses, is rarely a clinical problem. Toxic signs and symptoms rarely occur if drug is used for less than 3 weeks, even at large dosage ranges. However, chronic use causes adverse physiologic effects, including suppression of the HPA axis, cushingoid appearance, muscle weakness, and osteoporosis.

▶ **Special considerations**
- Long-acting glucocorticoids such as paramethasone are likely to inhibit maturation and growth in adolescents and children. Long-term use in children is not recommended.
- If possible, avoid long-term administration of pharmacologic dosages of glucocorticoids in children because these drugs may retard bone growth. Manifestations of adrenal suppression in children include retardation of linear growth, delayed weight gain, low plasma cortisol concentrations, and lack of response to corticotropin stimulation. In children who require prolonged therapy, closely monitor growth and development. Alternate-day therapy is recommended to minimize growth suppression.
- Establish baseline blood pressure, fluid intake, and output, weight, and electrolyte status. Watch for any sudden patient weight gain, edema, change in blood pressure, or change in eletrolyte status.
- During times of physiologic stress (trauma, surgery, infection), the patient may require additional steroids and may experience signs of steroid withdrawal; patients who were previously steroid-dependent may need systemic corticosteroids to prevent adrenal insufficiency.
- After long-term therapy, the drug should be reduced gradually. Rapid reduction may cause withdrawal symptoms.
- Acute withdrawal of drug may result in fever, myalgia, arthralgia, malaise, hypotension, hypoglycemic shock.
- Be aware of the patient's psychological history and watch for any behavioral changes.
- Observe for key signs of infection or delayed wound healing.

Information for parents and patient
- Be sure that the parents and patient understand the need to take the adrenocorticosteroid as prescribed. Give instructions on what to do if a dose is inadvertently missed.
- Warn parents and patient not to discontinue the drug abruptly.
- Inform the parents and patient of the possible therapeutic and adverse effects of the drug, so they may report any complications as soon as possible.
- Advise the parents that the patient should wear a Medic Alert bracelet or necklace indicating the need for supplemental adrenocorticoids during times of stress.

███████████████████████

paromomycin sulfate
Humatin

- Classification: antibacterial, amebicide (aminoglycoside)

How supplied
Available by prescription only
Capsules: 250 mg

Indications, route, and dosage
Intestinal amebiasis (acute and chronic)
Children: 750 mg/m² P.O. daily, divided q 8 hours for 5 days.
Children and adults: May receive 25 to 35 mg/kg P.O. daily in three doses for 5 to 10 days after meals.
Tapeworm (fish, beef, pork, and dog) infections
Children: 11 mg/kg P.O. q 15 minutes for four doses.
Adults: 1 g P.O. q 15 minutes for four doses.
Adjunct in hepatic coma: 4 g daily in two to four divided doses for 5 to 6 days.

Action and kinetics
- *Amebicidal action:* Paromomycin acts on contact in the intestinal lumen by an unknown mechanism. It is effective against the trophozoite and encysted forms of *Entamoeba histolytica* and against *Diphyllobothrium latum* (fish tapeworm), *Dipylidium caninum* (dog and cat tapeworm), *Hymenolepis nanal* (dwarf tapeworm), *Taenia saginata* (beef tapeworm), and *T. solium* (pork tapeworm).
- *Adjunct in hepatic coma:* Paromomycin inhibits nitrogen-forming bacteria in the GI tract by inhibiting protein synthesis at the 30S subunit of the ribosome.
- *Kinetics in adults:* Very small amounts of an oral dose of paromomycin are absorbed by the intact GI tract; however, larger amounts may be absorbed in patients with ulcerative intestinal disorders or renal insufficiency. Distribution of paromomycin has not been characterized adequately. No metabolites have been detected. Almost 100% of paromomycin is excreted unchanged in the feces; systemically absorbed drug is excreted in urine and may accumulate in patients with renal dysfunction. It is unknown if paromomycin is excreted in breast milk.

---

‡May contain sulfites   ♦May contain tartrazine   ♦♦May contain benzyl alcohol

Contraindications and precautions

Paromomycin is contraindicated in patients with impaired renal function because of its potential for nephrotoxicity; in patients with intestinal obstruction; and in patients with known hypersensitivity to the drug.

Paromomycin should be administered cautiously to patients with ulcerative intestinal lesions because of potential absorption that could exaggerate the risk of ototoxicity and nephrotoxicity. Some clinicians prefer other agents for cestodiasis because of this drug's potential for toxic effects.

Interactions

None reported.

Effects on diagnostic tests

None reported.

Adverse reactions

• CNS: headache, vertigo.
• DERM: rash, exanthema, pruritus.
• EENT: ototoxicity.
• GI: anorexia, nausea, vomiting, epigastric pain and burning, abdominal cramps, diarrhea, constipation, increased motility, steatorrhea, pruritus ani, malabsorption syndrome.
• GU: hematuria, nephrotoxicity.
• HEMA: eosinophilia.
• Other: bacterial and fungal superinfection.
    Note: Drug should be discontinued if signs of hypersensitivity or toxicity occur.

Overdose and treatment

Paromomycin overdose may affect cardiovascular and respiratory function. Treatment is largely supportive. After recent ingestion (within 4 hours), empty stomach by induced emesis or gastric lavage. Follow with activated charcoal to decrease absorption. Osmotic cathartics also may help.

▶ Special considerations

• Administer paromomycin after meals to prevent GI upset.
• Watch for signs of bacterial or fungal superinfection.
• Monitor patients with GI ulceration or renal dysfunction; drug absorption may impair renal clearance.
• Criterion of cure is absence of fecal amebae in specimen examined weekly for 6 weeks after discontinuation of treatment and thereafter monthly for 2 years.
• Isolating patient is unnecessary.

Information for parents and patient

• Emphasize need for medical follow-up after discharge.
• Advise parents to report any adverse effects.
• Explain how disease is transmitted.
• To help prevent reinfection, instruct parents and patient in proper hygiene, including disposal of feces and hand washing after defecation and before eating, and about the risks of eating raw food and the control of contamination by flies. Patient should not prepare, process, or serve food until treatment is completed.
• Advise use of liquid soap or reserved bar of soap to prevent cross contamination.

• Other household members and suspected contacts should be tested and, if necessary, treated.

---

pemoline
Cylert

• Classification: analeptic (oxazolidinedione derivative, CNS stimulant)
• Controlled substance schedule IV

How supplied

Available by prescription only
Tablets: 18.75 mg, 37.5 mg, 75 mg
Tablets (chewable and containing povidine): 37.5 mg

Indications, route, and dosage
Attention deficit disorder (ADD)

Children age 6 and older: Initially, 37.5 mg P.O. given in the morning. Daily dosage can be raised by 18.75 mg weekly. Effective dosage range is 56.25 to 75 mg daily; maximum is 112.5 mg daily.

Action and kinetics

• *Analeptic action:* Pemoline differs structurally from methylphenidate and amphetamines; however, like those drugs, pemoline has a paradoxical calming effect in children with ADD.

Pemoline's mechanism of action is unknown; it may be mediated by enhanced cerebral neurotransmission.

Pemoline is used primarily to treat ADD in children age 6 and over.

• *Kinetics in adults:* Pemoline is well absorbed after oral administration. Peak therapeutic effects occur at 4 hours and persist about 8 hours. Distribution is unknown. Drug is 50% protein-bound. Pemoline is metabolized by the liver to active and inactive metabolites. Pemoline and its metabolites are excreted in urine; 75% of an oral dose is excreted within 24 hours.

Contraindications and precautions

Pemoline is contraindicated in patients with hypersensitivity to pemoline; in those with impaired hepatic function because it may have an adverse effect on liver function; and in children under age 6. It should be used with caution in patients with decreased renal function and in patients with a history of Gilles de la Tourette's syndrome because it may precipitate this disorder.

Interactions

Concomitant use with caffeine may decrease efficacy of pemoline in ADD; concomitant use with anticonvulsants may decrease the seizure threshold.

Effects on diagnostic tests

Pemoline may cause abnormalities in liver function test results.

Adverse reactions

• CNS: *insomnia,* malaise, irritability, fatigue, mild depression, dizziness, headache, drowsiness, hallu-

---

cinations, nervousness (large doses), seizures, nystagmus, oculogyric crisis, unusual facial movement, Gilles de la Tourette's syndrome, psychosis.
• CV: tachycardia (with large doses).
• DERM: rash.
• GI: *anorexia,* abdominal pain, nausea, diarrhea.
• Hepatic: liver enzyme elevations, jaundice.
• Other: weight loss on initial therapy, weight gain after 3 to 6 months, *hypersensitivity,* growth suppression.

Note: Drug should be discontinued if signs of hypersensitivity occur or if markedly elevated liver function test results and jaundice occur concurrently.

Overdose and treatment
Symptoms of overdose may include restlessness, tachycardia, hallucinations, excitement, and agitation.

Treat overdose symptomatically and supportively: use gastric lavage if symptoms are not severe (hyperexcitability or coma). Monitor vital signs and fluid and electrolyte balance. Maintain patient in a cool room, monitor temperature, and minimize external stimulation; protect patient from self-injury. Chlorpromazine or haloperidol usually can reverse CNS stimulation. Hemodialysis may help. Contact local or regional poison control center for more information.

▶ **Special considerations**
• Pemoline is not recommended for ADD in children under age 6.
• Monitor initiation of therapy closely; drug may precipitate Gilles de la Tourette's syndrome.
• Check vital signs regularly for increased blood pressure or other signs of excessive stimulation.
• Monitor blood and urine glucose levels in diabetic patients; drug may alter insulin requirement.
• Monitor CBCs, differential, and platelet counts while patient is on long-term therapy.
• Monitor height and weight; long-term use of drug has been associated with growth suppression.
• Abrupt withdrawal after high-dose, long-term use may unmask severe depression. Lower dosage gradually to prevent acute rebound depression.
• Pemoline impairs ability to perform tasks requiring mental alertness.
• Be sure patient obtains adequate rest; fatigue may result as drug wears off.
• Discourage pemoline use for analeptic effect because drug has abuse potential; CNS stimulation superimposed on CNS depression may cause neuronal instability and seizures.
• Carefully follow manufacturer's directions for reconstitution, storage, and administration of all preparations. Pemoline has been used to treat narcolepsy in adults as well as depression and schizophrenia, but these uses are controversial.

Information for parents and patient
• Explain rationale for therapy and the anticipated risks and benefits; teach signs and symptoms of adverse reactions and need to report these.
• Explain that therapeutic effects may not appear for 3 to 4 weeks and that intermittent drug-free periods when stress is least evident (weekends, school holidays) may help prevent development of tolerance and permit decreased dosage when drug is resumed.
• Give drug in a single morning dose for maximum daytime benefit and to minimize insomnia.
• Patient should avoid drinks containing caffeine, to prevent added CNS stimulation and should not alter dosage without medical approval.
• Teach parents and patient how and when to use drug; tell patient not to chew or crush sustained-release dosage form.
• Warn patient not to use drug to mask fatigue, to be sure to obtain adequate rest, and to report excessive CNS stimulation.
• Advise parents of diabetic children to monitor blood glucose levels because drug may alter insulin needs.
• Advise parents that patient should avoid hazardous activities that require mental alertness until degree of sedative effect is determined.

---

penicillamine
Cuprimine, Depen

• Classification: heavy metal antagonist, antirheumatic agent (chelating agent)

How supplied
Available by prescription only
Capsules: 125 mg, 250 mg
Tablets: 250 mg

Indications, route, and dosage
Wilson's disease
Children: 20 mg/kg P.O. daily divided q.i.d. 30 to 60 minutes before meals and at least 2 hours after the evening meal. Adjust dosage to achieve urinary copper excretion of 0.5 to 1 mg daily.
Adults: 250 mg P.O. q.i.d. 30 to 60 minutes before meals and at least 2 hours after the evening meal. Adjust dosage to achieve urinary copper excretion of 0.5 to 1 mg daily.
Cystinuria
Children: 30 mg/kg daily P.O. divided q.i.d. 30 to 60 minutes before meals and at least 2 hours after the evening meal. Adjust dosage to achieve urinary cystine excretion of less than 100 mg daily when renal calculi are present, or 100 to 200 mg daily when no calculi are present.
Adults: 250 mg P.O. daily in 4 divided doses, then gradually increasing dosage. Usual dosage is 2 g daily (range is 1 to 4 g daily). Adjust dosage to achieve urinary cystine excretion of less than 100 mg daily when renal calculi are present, or 100 to 200 mg daily when no calculi are present.
Rheumatoid arthritis, †Felty's syndrome
Adults: Initially, 125 to 250 mg P.O. daily, with increases of 125 to 250 mg daily at 1- to 3-month intervals if necessary. Maximum dosage is 1 g daily.
†Adjunctive treatment of heavy metal poisoning
Children: 30 to 40 mg/kg or 600 to 750 mg/m² P.O. daily for 1 to 6 months.
Adults: 500 to 1,500 mg P.O. daily for 1 to 2 months.

Action and kinetics

• *Antirheumatic action:* Mechanism of action in rheumatoid arthritis is unknown; penicillamine depresses circulating IgM rheumatoid factor (but not total circulating immunoglobulin levels) and depresses T-cell but not B-cell activity. It also depolymerizes some macroglobulins (for example, rheumatoid factors).

• *Chelating agent:* Penicillamine forms stable, soluble complexes with copper, iron, mercury, lead, and other heavy metals that are excreted in urine; it is particularly useful in chelating copper in patients with Wilson's disease. Penicillamine also combines with cystine to form a complex more soluble than cystine alone, thereby reducing free cystine below the level of urinary stone formation.

• *Kinetics in adults:* Drug is well absorbed after oral administration; peak serum levels occur at 1 hour. Food and mineral supplements, especially those containing iron, decrease absorption by complexing in the gut. Uncomplexed penicillamine is metabolized in the liver to inactive disulfides. Only small amounts of penicillamine are excreted unchanged; after 24 hours, 50% of the drug is excreted in urine, 20% in feces, and 30% is unaccounted for.

Contraindications and precautions

Penicillamine is contraindicated in patients with known hypersensitivity to the drug; in patients with a history of penicillamine-related aplastic anemia or agranulocytosis; in patients with significant renal or hepatic insufficiency; in pregnant patients with cystinuria; and in patients receiving gold salts, immunosuppressants, antimalarials, or phenylbutazone, because of the increased risk of serious hematologic effects.

Penicillamine should be used with caution in patients allergic to penicillin (cross reaction is rare); in patients who receive a second course of therapy and who may have become sensitized and are more likely to have allergic reactions; and in patients who develop proteinuria not associated with Goodpasture's syndrome.

Interactions

None reported.

Effects on diagnostic tests

Penicillamine therapy may cause positive test results for antinuclear antibody (ANA), with or without clinical systemic lupus erythematosus-like syndrome.

Penicillamine may (rarely) elevate lactic dehydrogenase, AST (SGOT), ALT (SGPT), and alkaline phosphatase levels. Such elevations do not necessarily indicate significant hepatotoxicity.

Adverse reactions

• DERM: pruritus; erythematous rash; intensely pruritic rash with scaly, macular lesions on trunk; pemphigoid reactions; urticaria; exfoliative dermatitis; increased skin friability; purpuric or vesicular ecchymoses; wrinkling.

• EENT: oral ulcerations, glossitis, cheilosis, *cataracts.*

• GI: anorexia, nausea, vomiting, dyspepsia, diarrhea, dysgeusia or hypogeusia.

• HEMA: eosinophilia, leukopenia, granulocytopenia, thrombocytopenia, thrombotic thrombocytopenia, purpura, hemolytic anemia or iron deficiency anemia, lupus-like syndrome.

• Hepatic: cholestatic jaundice, pancreatitis, hepatic dysfunction.

• Other: proteinuria, arthralgia, lymphadenopathy, pneumonitis, alteration in sense of taste (salty and sweet), metallic taste, Goodpasture's syndrome, alopecia, drug fever, myasthenia gravis (with prolonged use).

Note: Drug should be discontinued if patient has signs of hypersensitivity or drug fever, usually in conjunction with other allergic manifestations (if Wilson's disease, may rechallenge); or if any of the following occur: rash developing 6 months or more after start of therapy; pemphigoid reaction; hematuria or proteinuria with hemoptysis or pulmonary infiltrates; gross or persistent microscopic hematuria or proteinuria greater than 2 g/day in patients with rheumatoid arthritis; platelet count below 100,000/mm³ or leukocyte count below 3,500 mm³, or if either shows three consecutive decreases (even within normal range).

Overdose and treatment

There are no reports of significant overdose with penicillamine. To treat penicillamine overdose, induce emesis unless unconscious or gag reflex is absent; otherwise empty stomach by gastric lavage and then administer activated charcoal and sorbital. Thereafter, treat supportively. Treat seizures with diazepam (or pyridoxine if previously successful). Hemodialysis will remove penicillamine.

▶ Special considerations

• Check for possible iron deficiency resulting from chronic use.

• Perform urinalyses, CBC including differential blood count every 2 weeks for 4 to 6 months, then monthly; kidney and liver functions studies also should be performed, usually every 6 months. Report fever or allergic reactions (rash, joint pains, easy bruising) immediately. Check routinely for proteinuria, and handle patient carefully to avoid skin damage.

• About one-third of patients receiving penicillamine experience an allergic reaction. Monitor patient for signs and symptoms of allergic reaction.

• Patients with Wilson's disease or cystinuria may require daily pyridoxine (vitamin B₆) supplementation.

• Prescribe drug to be taken 1 hour before or 2 hours after meals or other medications to facilitate absorption.

• For the initial treatment of Wilson's disease, 10 to 40 mg of sulfurated potash should be administered with each meal during penicillamine therapy for 6 months to 1 year, then discontinued.

• Penicillamine also has been used to treat lead poisoning and primary biliary cirrhosis.

Information for parents and patient

• For parents and patients with Wilson's disease, rheumatoid arthritis, or cystinuria; explain disease pro-

---

cess, rationale for therapy and explain that clinical results may not be evident for 3 months.
• Encourage compliance with therapy and follow-up visits.
• Emphasize immediate reporting of any fever, chills, sore throat, bruising, bleeding, or allergic reaction.
• Patient should take the medication on an empty stomach, 30 minutes to 1 hour before meals, or 2 hours after ingesting food, antacids, mineral supplements, vitamins, or other medications, and should drink large amounts of water, especially at night.
• Explain to parents and patient receiving penicillamine for rheumatoid arthritis that exacerbation of the disease may occur during therapy. This usually can be controlled by the concomitant administration of nonsteroidal anti-inflammatory drugs.
• Advise parents and patient taking penicillamine for Wilson's disease to maintain a low-copper (less than 2 mg daily) diet by excluding foods with high copper content, such as chocolate, nuts, liver, and broccoli. Also, sulfurated potash may be administered with meals to minimize copper absorption.

penicillin G benzathine
Bicillin*, Bicillin L-A, Megacillin Suspension, Permapen

penicillin G potassium
Cryspen, Deltapen, Lanacillin, Parcillin, Pensorb, Pentids, Pentids syrup*, Pentids '400' syrup*, Pentids 800*, Pfizerpin

penicillin G procaine
Crysticillin A.S., Duracillin A.S., Pfizerpen A.S., Wycillin

penicillin G sodium
Crystapen*

• Classification: antibiotic (natural penicillin)

How supplied
Available by prescription only
Penicillin G benzathine
Tablets: 200,000 units
Injection: 300,000 units/ml, 600,000 units/ml
Penicillin G procaine
Injection: 300,000 units/ml, 500,000 units/ml, 600,000 units/ml
Penicillin G potassium
Tablets: 200,000 units, 250,000 units, 400,000 units, 500,000 units, 800,000 units
Oral suspension: 200,000 units/5 ml, 250,000 units/5 ml, 400,000 units/5 ml (after reconstitution) suspension
Injection: 200,000 units, 500,000 units, 1 million units, 5 million units, 10 million units, 20 million units
Penicillin G sodium
Injection: 5 million units

Indications, route, and dosage
Mild to moderate staphylococcal and streptococcal infections
Penicillin G benzathine
Children age 1 month and over weighing less than 27 kg: 300,000 to 600,000 U I.M.
Older children weighing 27 kg and over: 900,000 to 1.2 million U I.M. as a single dose.
Adults: 1.2 million U. I.M. as a single dose.
    Alternatively, penicillin G benzathine may be given orally—
Children under age 12: 25,000 to 90,000 U/kg P.O. daily in 3 to 6 divided doses. Alternatively, give 32,500 to 65,000 U/kg P.O. in 4 to 6 divided doses.
Children age 12 and over and adults: 400,000 to 600,000 U P.O. q 4 to 6 hours
Penicillin G potassium
Neonates age 0 to 7 days weighing less than 2 kg: 50,000 to 100,000 U/kg I.M. or I.V. daily divided q 12 hours.
Neonates age 0 to 7 days weighing more than 2 kg: 50,000 to 100,000 U/kg I.M. or I.V. daily divided q 8 hours.
Neonates over age 7 days weighing less than 2 kg: 75,000 to 200,000 U/kg daily I.M. or I.V. divided q 8 hours.
Neonates over age 7 days, weighing more than 2 kg: 75,000 to 200,000 U/kg I.M. or I.V. divided q 6 hours.
Infants and children younger than age 12: 25,000 to 90,000U/kg daily P.O. in 3 to 6 divided doses, or 25,000 to 50,000 U/kg I.M. or I.V. daily in divided doses q 6 hours.
Children and adults age 12 and over: 200,000 to 500,000 U P.O.q 6 to 8 hours.
Moderately severe penicillin-sensitive staphylococcal and streptococcal infections
Penicillin G potassium
Neonates age 0 to 7 days weighing less than 2 kg: 100,000 to 150,000 U/kg I.M. or I.V. daily divided q 12 hours.
Neonates age 0 to 7 days weighing more than 2 kg: 100,000 to 150,000 U/kg I.M. or I.V. daily divided q 8 hours.
Neonates over age 7 days weighing less than 2 kg: 150,000 U/kg daily I.M. or I.V. divided q 8 hours.
Neonates over age 7 days weighing more than 2 kg: 200,000 U/kg daily I.M. or I.V. divided q 6 hours.
Children age 1 month to 12 years: 100,000 to 400,000 U/kg I.V. in divided doses.
Adults: 15 million units I.V. daily in divided doses q 4 hours.
Penicillin G procaine
Neonates: Generally not used, but some clinicians recommend 50,000 U/kg daily as a single dose.
Children over 1 month: 25,000 to 50,000 U/kg or 500,000 to 1 million U/m² I.M. as a single daily dose. Do not exceed adult dosage.
Children age 12 and over and adults: 600,000 to 1.2 million U. I.M. daily as a single dose for 7 to 10 days.
Penicillin G benzathine
Children under age 6 weighing less than 30 kg.: 600,000 U I.M. as a single dose
Children age 6 and over and adults: 1.2 million U I.M. as a single dose

‡May contain sulfites　　◆May contain tartrazine　　◆◆May contain benzyl alcohol

†Treatment of diphtheria
Penicillin G procaine
Children 10 kg or less: 300,000 U I.M. daily for 14 days.

Children over 10 kg.: 600,000 U I.M. daily for 14 days.

Adults: 600,000 U I.M. q 12 hours for 14 days.

Should be used in conjunction with diphtheria antitoxin.

Diphtheria toxoid active immunization should also be administered. Patients who fail to respond should be given an additional 10 day course of erythromycin.

Prophylaxis of recurrent rheumatic fever
Penicillin G benzathine
Children and adults: 1.2 million U I.M. once every 4 weeks, or 600,000 U I.M. once every 2 weeks. Alternatively, give 200,000 U P.O. b.i.d. Some clinicians initiate therapy with I.M. injections and change to oral prophylaxis when the patient reaches adolescence and has remained free of rheumatic attacks for 5 years.

Penicillin G potassium
Children age 1 to 12: 200,000 U P.O. b.i.d.

Children over age 12 and adults: 200,000 to 250,000 U P.O b.i.d.

Prophylaxis of bacterial endocarditis in patients unable to take oral medication receiving dental or minor upper respiratory tract surgery
Penicillin G potassium
Children less than 27 kg.: 50,000 U/kg I.M. or I.V. 30 to 60 minutes before the procedure, and 25,000 to 50,000 U/kg I.M. or I.V. 6 hours after the procedure.

Children over 27 kg. and adults: 2 million units I.M. or I.V. 30 minutes to 1 hour prior to the procedure, and 1 million units I.M. or I.V. 6 hours after the procedure.

Treatment of congenital syphilis; primary, secondary, or latent syphilis of less than 1 year's duration
Penicillin G benzathine
Neonates and infants: 50,000 U/kg I.M. as a single dose. Maximum dose 2.4 million U.

Adults: 2.4 million U. I.M. as a single dose.

Penicillin G potassium
Children: 50,000 U/kg I.M or I.V. daily in 2 divided doses for a minimum of 10 days.

Penicillin G sodium
Children: 50,000 U/kg I.M. or I.V. daily in 2 divided doses for a minimum of 10 days.

Penicillin G procaine
Neonates and children: 50,000 U/kg I.M. daily for a minimum of 10 days.

Children age 12 and over and adults: 600,000 U. I.M. daily for 8 days.

Treatment of syphilis with greater than 1 year's duration (except neurosyphilis)
Penicillin G benzathine
Neonates and children: 50,000 U/kg I.M. once weekly for 3 weeks. Maximum single dose is 2.4 million U.

Adults: 2.4 million U I.M. once weekly for 3 weeks.

Penicillin G procaine
Children age 12 and over and adults: 600,000 U I.M. daily for 10 to 15 days.

Neurosyphilis
Penicillin G benzathine
Neonates and children under age 2: 50,000 U/kg I.M. as a single dose.

Older children: 2.4 million units weekly for 3 weeks.

Penicillin G procaine
Children age 12 and over and adults: 2.4 million U. I.M. daily for 10 days. Administer with probenicid 500 mg P.O. q 6 hours. Follow with penicillin G benzathine 2.4 million U I.M. weekly for 3 weeks.

Acute, uncomplicated gonorrhea caused by Neisseria gonorrhoeae
Penicillin G procaine
Children weighing 45 kg or more and adults: 4.8 million units (administered as 2 injections of 2.4 million units each) as a single I.M. dose. Should be given with probenicid 1 g. P.O.

Children under 45 kg.: 100,000 U/kg I.M. as a single dose. Administer probenicid 25 mg/kg (up to a maximum dose of 1 g.) P.O. 30 minutes prior to injection.

Dosage in renal failure

Creatinine clearance (ml/min/1.73 m²)	Dosage
10 to 50	50% of the usual dose every 4 to 5 hours; alternatively, give the usual dose every 8 to 12 hours.
< 10	50% of the usual dose every 8 to 12 hours; alternatively, give the usual dose every 12 to 18 hours.

Action and kinetics
• *Antibiotic action:* Penicillin G is bactericidal; it adheres to penicillin-binding proteins, thus inhibiting bacterial cell wall synthesis. Penicillin G's spectrum of activity includes most non-penicillinase-producing strains of gram-positive and gram-negative aerobic cocci; spirochetes; and some gram-positive aerobic and anaerobic bacilli.

• *Kinetics in adults:* Penicillin G is available as four salts, each having the same bactericidal action, but designed to offer greater oral stability (potassium salt) or to prolong duration of action by slowing absorption after I.M. injection (benzathine and procaine salts).

Oral — penicillins are hydrolyzed by gastric acids; only 15% to 30% of an oral dose of penicillin G potassium is absorbed; the remainder is hydrolyzed by gastric secretions. Peak serum concentrations of penicillin G potassium occur at 30 minutes. Food in stomach reduces rate and extent of absorption. Penicillin V is absorbed better after oral administration than penicillin G potassium.

Intramuscular — sodium and potassium salts of penicillin G are absorbed rapidly after I.M. injection; peak serum concentrations occur within 15 to 30 minutes. Absorption of other salts is slower in adults. Peak serum concentrations of penicillin G procaine occur at 1 to 4 hours, with drug detectable in serum for 1 to 2 days; peak serum concentrations of penicillin

G benzathine occur at 13 to 24 hours, with serum concentrations detectable for 1 to 4 weeks.

Penicillin G is distributed widely into synovial, pleural, pericardial, and ascitic fluids and bile, and into liver, skin, lungs, kidneys, muscle, intestines, tonsils, maxillary sinuses, saliva, and erythrocytes. CSF penetration is poor but is enhanced in patients with inflamed meninges. Penicillin G crosses the placenta; it is 45% to 68% protein-bound. Between 16% and 30% of an I.M. dose of penicillin G is metabolized to inactive compounds.

Penicillin G is excreted primarily in urine by tubular secretion; 20% to 60% of dose is recovered in 6 hours. Some drug is excreted in breast milk. Elimination half-life in adults is about ½ to 1 hour. Renal clearance is delayed in neonates and young infants. Serum half-life in neonates appears to be a function of age and is not affected by birth weight. The serum half-life in neonates 6 days of age and younger is 3.2 to 3.4 hours; neonates age 7 to 13 days, 1.2 to 2.2 hours, and in neonates 14 days and over, 0.9 to 1.9 hours. Severe renal impairment prolongs half-life; penicillin G is removed by hemodialysis and only minimally removed by peritoneal dialysis.

• *Kinetics in children:* Peak levels may be delayed for up to 24 hours in children.

Contraindications and precautions

Penicillin G is contraindicated in patients with known hypersensitivity to any other penicillin or to cephalosporins.

Penicillin G should be used cautiously in patients with renal impairment because it is excreted in urine; decreased dosage is required in patient with moderate to severe renal failure.

Interactions

Concomitant use with aminoglycosides produces synergistic therapeutic effects, chiefly against enterococci; this combination is most effective in enterococcal bacterial endocarditis. However, the drugs are physically and chemically incompatible and are inactivated when mixed or given together. In vivo inactivation has been reported when aminoglycosides and penicillins are used concomitantly.

Probenecid blocks tubular secretion of penicillin, raising its serum concentrations.

Concomitant use of penicillin G with clavulanate appears to enhance effect of penicillin G against certain beta-lactamase-producing bacteria.

Large doses of penicillin may interfere with renal tubular secretion of methotrexate, thus delaying elimination and elevating serum concentrations of methotrexate.

Concomitant use of penicillin G with some nonsteroidal anti-inflammatory drugs prolongs penicillin half-life by competition for urinary excretion or displacement of penicillin from protein-binding sites; similarly, concomitant use with sulfinpyrazone, which inhibits tubular secretion of penicillin G, also prolongs its half-life.

Concomitant use of parenteral penicillin G potassium with potassium-sparing diuretics may cause hyperkalemia; penicillin G potassium is contraindicated in patients with renal failure.

Effects on diagnostic tests

Penicillin G alters test results for urine and serum protein levels; it interferes with turbidimetric methods using sulfosalicylic acid, trichloracetic acid, acetic acid, and nitric acid. Penicillin G does not interfere with tests using bromophenol blue (Albustix, Albutest, Multistix).

Penicillin G alters urine glucose testing using cupric sulfate (Benedict's reagent); use Clinistix or Tes-Tape instead. Penicillin G may cause falsely elevated results of urine specific gravity tests in patients with low urine output and dehydration, and falsely elevated Norymberski and Zimmermann test results for 17-ketogenic steroids; it causes false-positive CSF protein test results (Folin-Ciocalteau method) and may cause positive Coombs' test results.

Penicillin G may falsely decrease serum aminoglycoside concentrations. Adding beta-lactamase to the sample inactivates the penicillin, rendering the assay more accurate. Alternatively, the sample can be spun down and frozen immediately after collection.

Adverse reactions

• CNS: neuropathy, seizures at high doses.
• CV: congestive heart failure with high doses (penicillin G sodium).
• GI: *diarrhea,* epigastric distress, vomiting, nausea.
• HEMA: hemolytic anemia, leukopenia, eosinophilia, thrombocytopenia.
• Metabolic: possible potassium poisoning (hyperreflexia, convulsions, coma).
• Local: vein pain and irritation, injection-site sterile abscess or thrombophlebitis.
• Other: *hypersensitivity (rash,* urticaria, maculopapular eruptions, exfoliative dermatitis, chills, fever, edema, *anaphylaxis*), arthralgia, bacterial or fungal superinfection, *serum sickness.*

Note: Drug should be discontinued if immediate hypersensitivity reactions occur or if severe diarrhea indicates pseudomembranous colitis.

Overdose and treatment

Clinical signs of overdose include neuromuscular irritability or seizures. No specific recommendations available. Treatment is supportive. After recent ingestion (within 4 hours), empty stomach by induced emesis or gastric lavage. Follow with activated charcoal to decrease absorption. Penicillin G can be removed by hemodialysis.

▶ Special considerations

• Assess patient's history of allergies; do not give penicillin G to any patient with a history of hypersensitivity reactions to either penicillins or cephalosporins. Try to determine whether previous reactions were true hypersensitivity reactions or another reaction, such as GI distress, which the patient has interpreted as allergy.

• Keep in mind that a negative history for penicillin hypersensitivity does not preclude future allergic reactions; monitor patient continuously for possible allergic reactions or othr untoward effects.

• In patients with renal impairment, dosage should be reduced if creatinine clearance is below 10 ml/minute.

• Assess level of consciousness, neurologic status, and renal function when high doses are used, because excessive blood levels can cause CNS toxicity.
• Obtain results of cultures and sensitivity tests before first dose; however, therapy may begin before test results are complete. Repeat tests periodically to assess drug efficacy.
• Monitor vital signs, electrolytes, and renal function studies; monitor body weight for fluid retention with extended-spectrum penicillins for possible hypokalemia, hyperkalemia, or hypernatremia.
• Coagulation abnormalities, even frank bleeding, can follow high doses, especially of extended-spectrum penicillins; monitor prothrombin times and platelet counts, and assess patient for signs of occult or frank bleeding.
• Monitor patients on long-term therapy for possible superinfection, especially debilitated patients and others receiving immunosuppressants or radiation therapy; monitor closely, especially for fever.

Oral and parenteral administration
• Give penicillins at least 1 hour before giving bacteriostatic antibiotics (tetracyclines, erythromycins, and chloramphenicol); these drugs inhibit bacterial cell growth, decreasing rate of penicillin uptake by bacterial cell walls.
• Give oral penicillin at least 1 hour before or 2 hours after meals to enhance gastric absorption; food may or may not decrease absorption. Follow drug only with water because acid in citrus juices and carbonated beverages impairs absorption.
• Refrigerate oral suspensions (stable for 14 days); shake well before administering to assure correct dosage.
• Administer I.M. dose deep into large muscle mass (gluteal or midlateral thigh); rotate injection sites to minimize tissue injury; do not inject more than 2 g of drug per injection site. Apply ice to injection site for pain.
• Do not add or mix other drugs with I.V. infusions—particularly aminoglycosides, which will be inactivated if mixed with penicillins; they are chemically and physically incompatible. If other drugs must be given I.V., temporarily stop infusion of primary drug.
• Infuse I.V. drug continuously or intermittently (over 30 minutes) and assess I.V. site frequently to prevent infiltration or phlebitis; rotate infusion site q 48 hours; intermittent I.V. infusion may be diluted in 0.9% sodium chloride, dextrose 5% in water, dextrose 5% in water and half normal saline, or lactated Ringer's solution to volumes appropriate for the patient's weight.
• Solutions should always be clear, colorless to pale yellow, and free of particles; do not give solutions containing precipitates or other foreign matter.

Information for parents and patient
• Teach signs and symptoms of hypersensitivity and other adverse reactions, and emphasize need to report any unusual reactions.
• Teach signs and symptoms of bacterial and fungal superinfection to parents and patients, especially for debilitated patients and others with low resistance from immunosuppressants or irradiation; emphasize need to report signs of infection. Teach them how to prevent infection by practicing meticulous oral and

anogenital hygiene. Parents of infants and toddlers should keep diaper area clean and dry and avoid using plastic pants.
• Be sure parents and patient understand how and when to administer penicillin; urge them to complete entire prescribed regimen, to comply with instructions for around-the-clock dosage, and to keep follow-up appointments.
• Tell parents to check expiration date of drug and to discard unused drug.

penicillin V

penicillin V potassium
Betapen-VK, Biotic-V Powder, Bopen V-K, Cocillin V-K, Lanacillin VK, Ledercillin VK, LV, Nadopen-V*, Novopen VK*, Penapar VK, Penbec-V*, Pen-Vee K, Pfizerpen VK, PVF K*, Robicillin-VK, Uticillin VK, V-Cillin K, Veetids, Veetids '125'* with tartrazine

• Classification: antibiotic (natural penicillin)

How supplied
Available by prescription only
Penicillin V
Suspension: 125 mg/5 ml, 250 mg/5 ml (after reconstitution)
Tablets: 250 mg, 500 mg
Penicillin V potassium
Suspension: 125 mg/5 ml, 250 mg/5 ml (after reconstitution)
Tablets: 125 mg, 250 mg, 500 mg
Tablets (film-coated): 250 mg, 500 mg

Indications, route, and dosage
Mild to moderate infections caused by penicillin-sensitive organisms
Children over age 1 month: 15 to 62.5 mg/kg or 0.5 to 1 g/m^2 P.O. daily in 3 to 6 divided doses.
Adults: 250 to 500 mg P.O. every 6 hours.
Endocarditis prophylaxis for dental sugery
Children under 27 kg: 1 g P.O. 1 hour prior to the procedure, and 500 mg 6 hours after as a single dose. Some clinicians recommend follow up dosage mg P.O. q 6 hours for 8 doses after the initial dose.
Children over 27 kg and adults: 2 g P.O. 30 to 60 minutes prior to procedure, then 1 g P.O. 6 hours after procedure.
Early stages of Lyme disease
Children under age 9: 50 mg/kg daily in divided doses for 10 to 20 days. Do not give less than 1 g. or more than 2 g. daily. Tetracycline is preferred in older children.
†*Prophylaxis of pneumococcal infections in children with anatomic asplenia or hypogammaglobulinemia*
Children under age 5: 125 mg P.O. b.i.d.
Children age 5 and over: 250 mg P.O. b.i.d.
Prophylaxis of recurrent rheumatic fever
Children and adults: 125 to 250 mg P.O. b.i.d.

---

*Canada only   †Unlabeled clinical use   Italicized adverse reactions have been observed in children.

Action and kinetics

• *Antibiotic action:* Penicillin V is bactericidal; it adheres to penicillin-binding proteins, thus inhibiting bacterial cell wall synthesis.

Penicillin V's spectrum of activity includes most nonpenicillinase-producing strains of gram-positive and gram-negative aerobic cocci; spirochetes; and some gram-positive aerobic and anaerobic bacilli.

• *Kinetics in adults:* Penicillin V has greater acid stability and is absorbed more completely than penicillin G after oral administration. About 60% to 75% of an oral dose of penicillin V is absorbed. Peak serum concentrations occur at 60 minutes in fasting subjects; food has no significant effect.

Penicillin V is distributed widely into synovial, pleural, pericardial, and ascitic fluids and bile, and into liver, skin, lungs, kidneys, muscle, intestines, tonsils, maxillary sinuses, saliva, and erythrocytes. CSF penetration is poor but is enhanced in patients with inflamed meninges. Penicillin V crosses the placenta; it is 75% to 89% protein-bound.

Between 35% and 70% of a Penicillin V dose is metabolized to inactive compounds.

Penicillin V is excreted primarily in urine by tubular secretion; 26% to 65% of dose is recovered in 6 hours. Some drug is excreted in breast milk. Elimination half-life in adults is ½ hour. Severe renal impairment prolongs half-life.

Contraindications and precautions

Penicillin V is contraindicated in patients with known hypersensitivity to any other penicillin or to cephalosporins.

Penicillin V should be used cautiously in patients with renal impairment because it is excreted in urine; decreased dosage is required in patients with moderate to severe renal failure.

Interactions

Penicillin V may decrease efficacy of estrogen-containing oral contraceptives; breakthrough bleeding may occur.

Concomitant use with aminoglycosides produces synergistic therapeutic effects, chiefly against enterococci; however, the drugs are physically and chemically incompatible and are inactivated when mixed or given together. In vivo inactivation has been reported when aminoglycosides and penicillins are used concomitantly.

Probenecid blocks tubular secretion of penicillin, resulting in higher serum concentrations of drug.

Concomitant use of penicillin V with sulfinpyrazone, which inhibits tubular secretion of penicillin V, prolongs its half-life.

Effects on diagnostic tests

Penicillin V alters test results for urine and serum protein levels; it interferes with turbidimetric methods using sulfosalicylic acid, trichloracetic acid, acetic acid, and nitric acid. Penicillin V does not interfere with tests using bromophenol blue (Albustix, Albutest, MultiStix). Penicillin V may falsely decrease serum aminoglycoside concentrations.

Adverse reactions

• CNS: neuropathy, seizures at high doses.
• GI: diarrhea, epigastric distress, vomiting, nausea.
• HEMA: hemolytic anemia, leukopenia, eosinophilia, thrombocytopenia.
• Other: hypersensitivity (rash, urticaria, maculopapular eruptions, exfoliative dermatitis, chills, fever, edema, anaphylaxis), arthralgia, bacterial or fungal superinfection.

Note: Drug should be discontinued if immediate hypersensitivity reactions occur or if severe diarrhea indicates pseudomembranous colitis.

Overdose and treatment

Clinical signs of overdose include neuromuscular sensitivity or seizures. No specific recommendations are available. Treatment is supportive. After recent ingestion (within 4 hours), empty stomach by induced emesis or gastric lavage; follow with activated charcoal to reduce absorption.

▶ Special considerations

• Assess patient's history of allergies; do not give penicillin V to any patient with a history of hypersensitivity reactions to either penicillins or cephalosporins. Try to ascertain whether previous reactions were true hypersensitivity reactions or another reaction, such as GI distress, which the patient has interpreted as allergy.
• Keep in mind that a negative history for penicillin hypersensitivity does not preclude future allergic reactions; monitor continuously for possible allergic reactions or other untoward effects.
• In patients with renal impairment, dosage should be reduced if creatinine clearance is below 10 ml/minute.
• Assess level of consciousness, neurologic status, and renal function when high doses are used, because excessive blood levels can cause CNS toxicity.
• Obtain results of cultures and sensitivity tests before first dose; however, therapy may begin before test results are complete. Repeat tests periodically to assess drug efficacy.
• Monitor vital signs, electrolytes, and renal function studies; monitor body weight for fluid retention with extended-spectrum penicillins for possible hypokalemia or hypernatremia.
• Coagulation abnormalities, even frank bleeding, can follow high doses, especially of extended-spectrum penicillins; monitor prothrombin times and platelet counts, and assess patient for signs of occult or frank bleeding.
• Monitor patients on long-term therapy for possible superinfection, especially debilitated patients and others receiving immunosuppressants or radiation therapy; monitor closely, especially for fever.

Oral and parenteral administration

• Give penicillins at least 1 hour before giving bacteriostatic antibiotics (tetracyclines, erythromycins, and chloramphenicol); these drugs inhibit bacterial cell growth, decreasing rate of penicillin uptake by bacterial cell walls.
• Drug may be given with food.
• Refrigerate oral suspensions (stable for 14 days);

shake well before administering to assure correct dosage.

Information for parents and patient
• Teach signs and symptoms of hypersensitivity and other adverse reactions, and emphasize need to report any unusual reactions.
• Teach signs and symptoms of bacterial and fungal superinfection to parents and patients, especially for debilitated patients and others with low resistance from immunosuppressants or irradiation; emphasize need to report signs of infection. Teach prevention of infection by practicing meticulous oral and anogenital hygiene. Parents of infants and toddlers should keep diaper area clean and dry and avoid using plastic pants.
• Be sure parents and patient understand how and when to administer drug; urge them to complete entire prescribed regimen, to comply with instructions for around-the-clock dosage, and to keep follow-up appointments.
• Patient should take oral dose 1 hour before or 2 hours after meals for maximum absorption.
• Tell parents to check expiration date of drug and to discard expired or unused drug.
• Instruct parents or patient to shake suspension before administration to ensure correct dosage.

---

pentamidine isethionate
Pentam 300

• Classification: antiprotozoal (diamidine derivative)

How supplied
Available by prescription only
Injection: 300-mg vials

Indications, route, and dosage
Pneumonia caused by Pneumocystis carinii
Children and adults: 4 mg/kg I.V. or I.M. once a day for 14 days. As alternate dose in children, 150 mg/m² daily for 5 days, then 100 mg/m² for duration of therapy.
Prophylaxis of Pneumocystis carinii pneumonia in patients with AIDS
Adults: 300 mg by aerosol inhalation (using Respigard II nebulizer) q 4 weeks.

Action and kinetics
• *Antiprotozoal action:* Mechanism is unknown. However, pentamidine may work by inhibiting synthesis of ribonucleic acid (RNA), deoxyribonucleic acid (DNA), proteins, or phospholipids. It may also interfere with several metabolic processes, particularly certain energy-yielding reactions and reactions involving folic acid. Drug's spectrum of activity includes *P. carinii* and *Trypanosoma* organisms.
• *Kinetics in adults:* Daily I.M. doses (4 mg/kg) produce surprisingly few plasma level fluctuations. Plasma levels usually increase slightly 1 hour after I.M. injection. Little information exists regarding pharmacokinetics with I.V. administration. Pentam-

idine appears to be extensively tissue-bound. CNS penetration is poor. Extent of plasma protein-binding is unknown. Pentamidine's metabolism is unknown. Most of drug is excreted unchanged in the urine. Drug's extensive tissue-binding may account for its appearance in urine 6 to 8 weeks after therapy ends.

Contraindications and precautions
Because of its potentially toxic effect, pentamidine is only used as a second-line agent for *P. carinii* pneumonia. Drug should be administered cautiously to patients with hypertension, hypotension, hyperglycemia, hypoglycemia, hypocalcemia, leukopenia, thrombocytopenia, anemia, or hepatic or renal dysfunction because of risk of serious adverse effects.

Interactions
When used concomitantly, pentamidine may have additive nephrotoxic effects with aminoglycosides, amphotericin B, capreomycin, colistin, cisplatin, methoxyflurane, polymyxin B, and vancomycin.

Effects on diagnostic tests
Blood urea nitrogen (BUN), serum creatinine, AST (SGOT), and ALT (SGPT) levels may increase during pentamidine therapy.

Other abnormal findings may include hyperkalemia and hypocalcemia. Hypoglycemia may occur initially (possibly from stimulation of endogenous insulin release); later, hyperglycemia may result from direct pancreatic cell damage.

Adverse reactions
• CNS: confusion, hallucinations, dizziness.
• CV: hypotension (possibly severe and fatal), dysrhythmias (*ventricular tachycardia*).
• DERM: flushing, rash, pruritus, toxic epidermal necrolysis, *Stevens-Johnson syndrome.*
• Endocrine: hypoglycemia within first 5 to 7 days (possibly severe and prolonged, requiring I.V. dextrose infusion); latent hyperglycemia (may occur several months after therapy, possibly causing insulin-dependent diabetes mellitus); hypocalcemia; hyperkalemia.
• GI: nausea, vomiting, diarrhea, anorexia, metallic taste, acute pancreatitis, elevated liver enzyme levels.
• GU: elevated BUN and serum creatinine levels, renal toxicity (usually reversible).
• HEMA: leukopenia, thrombocytopenia, neutropenia, anemia, megaloblastic changes (secondary to folate decrease).
• Local: pain, sterile abscess, induration at injection site, phlebitis (with I.V. infusion).
• Other: fever, *anaphylaxis.*

Overdose and treatment
No information available.

▶ Special considerations
• Make sure patient has adequate fluid status before administering drug; dehydration may lead to hypotension and renal toxicity.
• I.V. infusion avoids risk of local reactions and proves as safe as I.M. injection when given slowly, over at least 60 minutes. To prepare drug for I.V. infusion, add 3 to 5 ml of sterile water for injection or dextrose

---

5% in water (D_5W) to 300-mg vial to yield 100 mg/ml or 60 mg/ml, respectively. Withdraw desired dose and dilute further into 50 to 250 ml of D_5W; infuse over at least 60 minutes. Diluted solution remains stable for 5 days.

• To prepare drug for I.M. injection, add 3 ml of sterile water for injection to 300-mg vial to yield 100 mg/ml. Withdraw desired dose and inject deep I.M.
• Patient should be supine during administration to minimize hypotension risk. Monitor blood pressure frequently until patient is stable.
• Keep emergency drugs and equipment (including emergency airway, vasopressors, and I.V. fluids) on hand.
• Monitor ECG during I.V. infusion.
• Monitor daily blood glucose, BUN, and serum creatinine levels. Monitor periodic electrolyte levels, complete blood count, platelet count, and liver function tests.
• Observe patient for signs and symptoms of hypoglycemia.

Information for parents and patient
• Explain disease process and therapy, and need for restraints to maintain safety of I.V. infusion.
• Explain that patient must remain supine during I.V. administration.
• Encourage the parents and patient to report signs of hypoglycemia such as profuse sweating, confusion, tremors.
• If patient has AIDS, explain that treatment is suppressive, not curative.

pentobarbital sodium
Nembutal

• Classification: anticonvulsant, sedative-hypnotic (barbiturate)
• Controlled substance schedule II (suppositories schedule III)

How supplied
Available by prescription only
Elixir: 20 mg/5 ml
Capsules: 50 mg, 100 mg
Injection: 50 mg/ml, 1-ml and 2-ml disposable syringes; 2-ml, 20-ml, and 50-ml vials
Suppositories: 30 mg, 60 mg, 120 mg, 200 mg

Indications, route, and dosage
Sedation
Children: 2 to 6 mg/kg P.O. or I.M. daily in divided doses, to a maximum of 100 mg/dose.
Adults: 20 to 40 mg P.O. or I.M. b.i.d., t.i.d., or q.i.d.
Insomnia
Children: 2 to 6 mg/kg I.M., up to a maximum of 100 mg/dose. Or 30 mg rectally (age 2 months to 1 year), 30 to 60 mg rectally (age 1 to 4), 60 mg rectally (age 5 to 12), 60 to 120 mg rectally (age 12 to 14).
Adults: 100 to 200 mg P.O. h.s. or 150 to 200 mg deep I.M.; 120 to 200 mg rectally.

Preanesthetic medication
Infants and children to age 5: 5mg/kg, rectally.
Children over age 5: 5 mg/kg I.M.
Adults: 150 to 200 mg I.M. or P.O. in two divided doses.
Anticonvulsant
Children: Initially, 50 mg or 3 to 8 mg/kg I.M. or I.V.; after 1 minute additional doses may be given.
Children over age 5: 5 mg/kg I.M.
Adults: Initially, 100 mg I.V.; after 1 minute additional doses may be given. Maximum dosage is 500 mg.
†Elevated intracranial pressure
Children and adults: Loading dose, 3 to 35 mg/kg I.V. infused over 10 to 12 minutes; then maintenance with 1.5 mg to 3.5 mg/kg/hour. Adjust dosage in renal or hepatic dysfunction.

Action and kinetics
• *Sedative-hypnotic action:* The exact cellular site and mechanism(s) of action are unknown. Pentobarbital acts throughout the CNS as a nonselective depressant with a fast onset of action and short duration of action. Particularly sensitive to this drug is the reticular activating system, which controls CNS arousal. Pentobarbital decreases both presynaptic and postsynaptic membrane excitability by facilitating the action of gamma-aminobutyric acid (GABA).
• *Anticonvulsant action:* Pentobarbital suppresses the spread of seizure activity produced by epileptogenic foci in the cortex, thalamus, and limbic systems by enhancing the effect of GABA. Both presynaptic and postsynaptic excitability are decreased, and the seizure threshold is raised.
• *Kinetics in adults:* Pentobarbital is absorbed rapidly after oral or rectal administration, with an onset of action of 10 to 15 minutes. Peak serum concentrations occur between 30 and 60 minutes after oral administration. After I.M. injection, the onset of action occurs within 10 to 25 minutes. After I.V. administration, the onset of action occurs immediately. Serum concentrations needed for sedation and hypnosis are 1 to 5 mcg/ml and 5 to 15 mcg/ml, respectively. After oral or rectal administration, duration of hypnosis is 1 to 4 hours.

Pentobarbital is distributed widely throughout the body. Approximately 35% to 45% is protein-bound. Pentobarbital is metabolized in the liver by penultimate oxidation. Approximately 99% of pentobarbital is eliminated as glucuronide conjugates and other metabolites in the urine. Terminal half-life ranges from 35 to 50 hours. Duration of action is 3 to 4 hours.

Contraindications and precautions
Pentobarbital is contraindicated in patients with known hypersensitivity to barbiturates and in patients with bronchopneumonia, status asthmaticus, or severe respiratory distress, because of the potential for respiratory depression. Pentobarbital should not be used in patients who are depressed or have suicidal ideation because the drug can worsen depression; in patients with uncontrolled acute or chronic pain, because exacerbation of pain and paradoxical excitement can occur; or in patients with porphyria, because this drug can trigger symptoms of this disease.

Pentobarbital should be used cautiously in patients

who must perform hazardous tasks requiring mental alertness, because the drug causes drowsiness. Administer parenteral pentobarbital slowly and with extreme caution to patients with hypotension or severe pulmonary or cardiovascular disease because of potential adverse hemodynamic effects. Because tolerance and physical or psychological dependence may occur, prolonged use of high doses should be avoided. Pentobarbital capsules may contain tartrazine, which may cause an allergic reaction in certain individuals, especially those who are sensitive to aspirin.

Interactions

Pentobarbital may potentiate or add to CNS and respiratory depressant effects of other sedative-hypnotics, antihistamines, narcotics, antidepressants, tranquilizers, and alcohol.

Pentobarbital enhances the enzymatic degradation of warfarin and other oral anticoagulants; patients may require increased doses of the anticoagulants. Drug also enhances hepatic metabolism of some drugs, including digitoxin (not digoxin), corticosteroids, oral contraceptives and other estrogens, theophylline and other xanthines, and doxycycline. Pentobarbital impairs the effectiveness of griseofulvin by decreasing absorption from the GI tract.

Valproic acid, phenytoin, disulfiram, and monoamine oxidase inhibitors decrease the metabolism of pentobarbital and can increase its toxicity. Rifampin may decrease pentobarbital levels by increasing hepatic metabolism.

Effects on diagnostic tests

Pentobarbital may cause a false-positive phentolamine test. The drug's physiologic effects may impair the absorption of cyanocobalamin ^{57}Co; it may decrease serum bilirubin concentrations in neonates, epileptic patients, and in patients with congenital nonhemolytic unconjugated hyperbilirubinemia. EEG patterns show a change in low-voltage, fast activity; changes persist for a time after discontinuation of therapy.

Adverse reactions

• CNS: drowsiness, lethargy, vertigo, headache, CNS depression, rebound insomnia, increased dreams or nightmares, possibly seizures (after acute withdrawal or reduction in dosage), mental confusion, *paradoxical excitement*, confusion and agitation.
• CV: hypotension (after rapid I.V. administration), bradycardia, circulatory collapse.
• DERM: urticaria, rash, exfoliative dermatitis, Stevens-Johnson syndrome.
• EENT: miosis.
• GI: nausea, vomiting, diarrhea, constipation.
• Local: thrombophlebitis, pain and possible tissue damage at the site of extravascular injection.
• Other: laryngospasm, bronchospasm, respiratory depression, angioedema; vitamin K deficiency and bleeding have occurred in newborns of mothers treated during pregnancy. Hyperalgesia occurs in low doses or in patients with chronic pain.
  Note: Drug should be discontinued if hypersensitivity reaction, profound CNS or respiratory depression, or skin eruptions occur.

Overdose and treatment

Clinical manifestations of overdose include unsteady gait, slurred speech, sustained nystagmus, somnolence, confusion, respiratory depression, pulmonary edema, areflexia, and coma. Typical shock syndrome with tachycardia and hypotension may occur. Jaundice, hypothermia followed by fever, and oliguria also may occur. Serum concentrations greater than 10 mcg/ml may produce profound coma; concentrations greater than 30 mcg/ml may be fatal.

To treat, maintain and support ventilation and pulmonary function as necessary; support cardiac function and circulation with vasopressors and I.V. fluids, as needed. If patient is conscious and gag reflex is intact, induce emesis (if ingestion was recent) by administering ipecac syrup. If emesis is contraindicated, perform gastric lavage while a cuffed endotracheal tube is in place to prevent aspiration. Follow with administration of activated charcoal or saline cathartic. Measure intake and output, vital signs, and laboratory parameters. Maintain body temperature.

Alkalinization of urine may be helpful in removing drug from the body. Hemodialysis may be useful in severe overdose.

▶ Special considerations

• Drug has been used in treatment of cerebral ischemia or cerebral edema following stroke, head trauma, or Reye's syndrome (barbiturate coma).
• High dose therapy for elevated intracranial pressure may require mechanically assisted ventilation.
• Barbiturates may cause paradoxical excitement in children. Use with caution.
• Premature infants are more susceptible to the depressant effects of barbiturates because of immature hepatic metabolism. Children receiving pentobarbital may experience hyperactivity, excitement, or hyperalgesia.
• Dosage must be individualized for each patient, because different rates of metabolism and enzyme induction occur.
• May be given rectally if oral or parenteral route is inappropriate.
• Assess level of consciousness before and frequently during therapy to evaluate effectiveness of drug. Monitor neurologic status for possible alterations or deteriorations. Monitor seizure character, frequency, and duration for changes. Institute seizure precautions, as necessary.
• Assess patient's sleeping patterns before and during therapy to ensure effectiveness of drug.
• Institute safety measures—side rails, assistance when out of bed, call light within reach—to prevent falls and injury.
• Anticipate possible rebound confusion and excitatory reactions in patient.
• Assess bowel elimination patterns; monitor for complaints of constipation. Advise diet high in fiber, if indicated.
• Monitor prothrombin time carefully in patients taking anticoagulants; dosage of anticoagulant may require adjustment to counteract possible interaction.
• Observe patient to prevent hoarding or self-dosing,

---

especially in depressed or suicidal patients, or those who are or have a history of being drug-dependent.
• Abrupt discontinuation may cause withdrawal symptoms; discontinue slowly.
• Death is common with an overdose of 2 to 10 g; it may occur at much smaller doses if alcohol is also ingested.

---

phenacemide
Phenurone

• Classification: anticonvulsant (substituted acetylurea derivative, open-chain hydantoin)

How supplied
Available by prescription only
Tablets: 500 mg

Indications, route, and dosage
Refractory, complex-partial (psychomotor), generalized tonic-clonic (grand mal), absence (petit mal), and atypical absence seizures
Children age 5 to 10: 250 mg P.O. t.i.d.; may increase by 250 mg weekly, up to 1.5 g daily, p.r.n.
Adults: 500 mg P.O. t.i.d; may increase by 500 mg weekly up to 5 g daily, p.r.n.
  Satisfactory seizure control may occur with dosages as low as 250 mg t.i.d.

Action and kinetics
• *Anticonvulsant action:* Phenacemide elevates the seizure threshold by an unknown mechanism; it is extremely toxic and is usually reserved for patients with severe epilepsy (especially mixed forms) resistant to other anticonvulsants.
• *Kinetics in adults:* Phenacemide is absorbed well from the GI tract; duration of action is about 5 hours. Distribution is unknown. Phenacemide is metabolized by the liver. Phenacemide is excreted in urine. It is unknown whether drug is excreted in breast milk.

Contraindications and precautions
Phenacemide is contraindicated in patients with known hypersensitivity to phenacemide and in patients with jaundice or other signs of liver dysfunction because it may be hepatotoxic.
  Use phenacemide with caution in patients with a history of drug allergy, especially to anticonvulsants; and in patients with personality disorders, as suicide attempts have occurred. Use phenacemide with extreme caution in patients taking other anticonvulsants. Paranoid symptoms have developed in patients receiving phenacemide and ethotoin concurrently.

Interactions
Concomitant use of phenacemide with ethotoin may cause paranoid symptoms; use with other anticonvulsants (mephenytoin, trimethadione, or paramethadione) may markedly increase toxicity.

Effects on diagnostic tests
Phenacemide may cause abnormalities in liver enzyme test results.

Adverse reactions
• CNS: drowsiness, dizziness, insomnia, headaches, paresthesias, depression, suicidal tendencies, aggressiveness, psychic changes.
• DERM: rashes.
• GI: anorexia, weight loss.
• GU: nephritis with marked albuminuria.
• HEMA: aplastic anemia, agranulocytosis, leukopenia.
• Hepatic: hepatitis, jaundice.
  Note: Drug should be discontinued if signs of hypersensitivity, jaundice, or other hepatotoxicity occur; if marked depression of white blood cell (WBC) count (leukocyte level below 4,000/mm^3) occurs; if albumin, blood, casts, or leukocytes occur in urine; if rash occurs; or if patient shows new or exacerbated personality disorder.

Overdose and treatment
Symptoms of overdose include initial excitement followed by drowsiness, nausea, ataxia, and coma.
  Treat overdose with gastric lavage or emesis and follow with supportive treatment. Monitor vital signs and fluid and electrolyte balance carefully. Hemodialysis or total exchange transfusion has been used for severe cases and pediatric patients. Careful evaluation of renal, hepatic, and hematologic status is crucial after recovery.

▶ Special considerations
• Drug is reserved only for pediatric patients who have not responded to less toxic anticonvulsants.
• Safety is not established for children under 5.
• Observe patient closely during therapy for possible adverse effects, especially at start of therapy. Monitor for signs of hematologic toxicity (sore throat, fever, malaise).
• Drug should not be discontinued abruptly, but slowly over 6 weeks; abrupt discontinuation may cause status epilepticus.
• Drug interactions are frequently a problem, primarily with hepatically cleared drugs, such as chloramphenicol, digitoxin, isoniazid, and griseofluvin; be especially alert for toxic symptoms or breakthrough seizures in patients taking any of these drugs.
• Carefully follow manufacturer's directions for reconstitution, storage, and administration of all preparations.
• Obtain baseline liver function tests, complete blood counts, and urinalyses before and at monthly intervals during treatment; discontinue drug if a marked depression of blood count is observed.

Information for parents and patient
• Advise parents and patients of potential serious toxicity with phenacemide. Urge them to report any of the following immediately: pregnancy, jaundice, abdominal pain, pale stools, dark urine, fever, sore throat, mouth sores, rashes, unusual bleeding or bruising, or loss of appetite. All such reports mandate immediate review of laboratory studies.

---

‡May contain sulfites   ◆May contain tartrazine   ◆◆May contain benzyl alcohol

• Inform parents and patient about possible psychological reactions, and tell them to report immediately any changes in mood or affect, such as the patient's decreased interest in himself or his surroundings, depression, or aggression.
• Tell parents that patient should avoid alcohol while taking drug, as it may decrease drug's effectiveness and may increase CNS adverse reactions. Explain that some liquid medications contain alcohol.
• Advise parents that patient should avoid hazardous tasks that require mental alertness until degree of CNS sedative effect is determined.
• Tell patient to take oral drug with food if GI distress occurs.
• Explain to adolescent patient the need to report suspected pregnancy immediately.
• Warn parents that patient should never discontinue drug suddenly or without medical supervision.
• Encourage parents to have patients wear a Medic Alert bracelet or necklace, listing drug and seizure disorders, while taking anticonvulsants.
• Caution parents to consult pharmacist before changing brand or using generic drug; therapeutic effect may change.
• Assure parents and patient that pink or reddish brown discoloration of patient's urine is normal and harmless.

---

phenazopyridine hydrochloride
Azo-Standard, Baridium, Di-Azo, Diridone, Phenazo*, Phenazodine, Pyridiate, Pyridium, Pyronium*, Urodine

• Classification: urinary analgesic (azo dye)

How supplied
Available by prescription only
Tablets: 100 mg, 200 mg

Indications, route, and dosage
Pain with urinary tract irritation or infection
Children over age 6: 4 mg/kg t.i.d.; or 100 mg P.O. t.i.d.
Adults: 100 to 200 mg P.O. t.i.d.

Action and kinetics
• *Analgesic action:* Phenazopyridine has a local anesthetic effect on urinary tract mucosa via an unknown mechanism.
• *Kinetics in adults:* Absorption and distribution have not been described, although traces are thought to enter CSF and cross the placenta. Drug is metabolized in the liver and excreted in urine.

Contraindications and precautions
Drug is contraindicated in patients with known hypersensitivity to phenazopyridine and in patients with renal and hepatic insufficiency because of the potential for drug accumulation.

Interactions
None significant.

Effects on diagnostic tests
Drug may alter results of Clinistix, Tes-Tape, Acetest, and Ketostix. Clinitest should be used to obtain accurate urine glucose test results.
Phenazopyridine may also interfere with Ehrlich's test for urine urobilinogen; phenolsulfonphthalein (PSP) excretion tests of kidney function; sulfobromophthalein (BSP) excretion tests of liver function; and urine tests for protein, steroids, or bilirubin.

Adverse reactions
• CNS: headache, vertigo.
• DERM: rash.
• GI: nausea.
• GU: renal stones.
• Other: *hemolytic anemia, methemoglobinemia.*
Note: Drug should be discontinued if skin or sclera becomes yellow-tinged. This may indicate accumulation or hepatotoxicity from impaired renal excretion.

Overdose and treatment
Clinical manifestations of overdose include methemoglobinemia (most obvious as cyanosis), along with renal and hepatic impairment and failure.
To treat overdose of phenazopyridine, empty stomach immediately by inducing emesis with ipecac syrup or by gastric lavage. Administer methylene blue, 1 to 2 mg/kg I.V., or 100 to 200 mg ascorbic acid P.O. to reverse methemoglobinemia. Provide symptomatic and supportive measures (respiratory support and correction of fluid and electrolyte imbalances). Monitor laboratory parameters and vital signs closely.

▶ Special considerations
• Drug colors urine red or orange; it may stain fabrics.
• Use only as urinary analgesic.
• May be used with an antibiotic to treat urinary tract infections.
• Phenazopyridine should be discontinued in 2 days with concurrent antibiotic use.

Information for parents and patient
• Teach measures to prevent urinary tract infection.
• Advise parents and patient of possible adverse reactions; caution that drug colors urine red or orange and may stain clothing.
• Tell parents that stains on clothing may be removed with a 0.25% solution of sodium dithionate or hydrosulfite.
• Patient should take a missed dose as soon as possible and not double-dose.
• Instruct parents to report symptoms that persist or worsen.

---

phenobarbital
Barbita, Gardenal*, Solfoton

phenobarbital sodium
Luminal

- Classification: anticonvulsant, sedative-hypnotic (barbiturate)
- Controlled substance schedule IV

How supplied
Available by prescription only
Oral solution: 15 mg/5 ml; 20 mg/5 ml
Elixir: 20 mg/5 ml
Capsules: 16 mg
Tablets: 8 mg, 15 mg, 16 mg, 30 mg, 32 mg, 60 mg, 65 mg, 100 mg
Injection: 30 mg/ml, 60 mg/ml, 65 mg/ml, 130 mg/ml
Powder for injection: 120 mg/ampule

Indications, route, and dosage
All forms of epilepsy, febrile seizures in children
Children: 4 to 6 mg/kg P.O. or I.M. daily, usually divided q 12 hours. It can, however, be administered once daily.
Adults: 100 to 200 mg P.O. or I.M. daily, divided t.i.d. or given as single dose h.s.
Status epilepticus
Children: 5 to 10 mg/kg I.V. May repeat q 10 to 15 minutes up to total of 20 mg/kg. I.V. injection rate should not exceed 50 mg/minute. Alternatively, administer according to age:
—less than 1 month: 20 mg/kg I.V.
—1 month to 1 year: 15 mg/kg I.V.
—over 1 year: 10 mg/kg I.V.
Adults: 10 mg/kg as I.V. infusion no faster than 50 mg/minute. May give up to 20 mg/kg total. Administer in acute care or emergency area only.
Sedation
Children: 6 mg/kg P.O. divided t.i.d.
Adults: 30 to 120 mg P.O. daily in two or three divided doses.
Insomnia
Children: 3 to 6 mg/kg.
Adults: 100 to 320 mg P.O. or I.M.
Preoperative sedation
Children: 16 to 100 mg I.M. 60 to 90 minutes before surgery.
Adults: 100 to 200 mg I.M. 60 to 90 minutes before surgery.
†Hyperbilirubinemia
Neonates: 5 to 10 mg/kg P.O. daily or 5 to 10 mg/kg I.M. daily for the first few days after birth.
†Chronic cholestasis
Children under age 12: 3 to 12 mg/kg P.O. daily in two or three divided doses.
Adults: 90 to 180 mg P.O. daily in two or three divided doses.

Action and kinetics
- *Anticonvulsant action:* Phenobarbital suppresses the spread of seizure activity produced by epileptogenic foci in the cortex, thalamus, and limbic systems by enhancing the effect of gamma-aminobutyric acid (GABA). Both presynaptic and postsynaptic excitability are decreased; also, phenobarbital raises the seizure threshold.
- *Sedative-hypnotic action:* Phenobarbital acts throughout the CNS as a nonselective depressant with a slow onset of action and a long duration of action. Particularly sensitive to this drug is the reticular activating system, which controls CNS arousal. Phenobarbital decreases both presynaptic and postsynaptic membrane excitability by facilitating the action of GABA. The exact cellular site and mechanism(s) of action are unknown.
- *Kinetics in adults:* Phenobarbital is absorbed well after oral and rectal administration, with 70% to 90% reaching the bloodstream. Absorption after I.M. administration is 100%. After oral administration, peak serum levels are reached in 1 to 2 hours, and peak levels in the CNS are achieved at 1 to 3 hours. Onset of action occurs 1 hour or longer after oral dosing; onset after I.V. administration is about 5 minutes. A serum concentration of 10 mcg/ml is needed to produce sedation; 40 mcg/ml usually produces sleep. Concentrations of 20 to 40 mcg/ml are considered therapeutic for anticonvulsant therapy.
  Phenobarbital is distributed widely throughout the body and is approximately 25% to 30% protein-bound. Phenobarbital is metabolized by the hepatic microsomal enzyme system. Approximately 25% to 50% of a phenobarbital dose is eliminated unchanged in urine. The remainder is excreted as metabolites of glucuronic acid. Phenobarbital's half-life is 5 to 7 days.

Contraindications and precautions
Phenobarbital is contraindicated in patients with known hypersensitivity to barbiturates and in patients with bronchopneumonia, status asthmaticus, or other severe respiratory distress because of the potential for respiratory depression. Phenobarbital should not be used in patients who are depressed or have suicidal ideation, because the drug can worsen depression; in patients with uncontrolled acute or chronic pain, because exacerbation of pain or paradoxical excitement can occur; or in patients with porphyria, because this drug can trigger symptoms of this disease; or in treatment of seizures when level of consciousness is critical (as in head trauma) because of this drug's depressant effects on the CNS.
  Phenobarbital should be used cautiously in patients who must perform hazardous tasks requiring mental alertness, because the drug causes drowsiness; and in patients with impaired renal function, because up to 50% of phenobarbital is excreted in urine. Administer parenteral phenobarbital slowly and with extreme caution to patients with hypotension or severe pulmonary or cardiovascular disease because of potential adverse hemodynamic effects. Because tolerance and physical or psychological dependence may occur, prolonged use of high doses should be avoided.
  Prenatal exposure to barbiturates is associated with an increased incidence of fetal abnormalities and, pos-

sibly, brain tumors. Use of barbiturates in the third trimester may be associated with physical dependence in neonates. Risk-benefit must be considered.

Interactions

Phenobarbital may add to or potentiate CNS and respiratory depressant effects of other sedative-hypnotics, antihistamines, narcotics, phenothiazines, antidepressants, tranquilizers, and alcohol.

Phenobarbital enhances the enzymatic degradation of warfarin and other oral anticoagulants; patients may require increased doses of the anticoagulant. Drug also enhances hepatic metabolism of some drugs, including digitoxin (not digoxin), corticosteroids, oral contraceptives and other estrogens, theophylline and other xanthines, and doxycycline.

Phenobarbital impairs the effectiveness of griseofulvin by decreasing absorption from the GI tract.

Valproic acid, phenytoin, disulfiram, and monoamine oxidase inhibitors decrease the metabolism of phenobarbital and can increase its toxicity.

Rifampin may decrease phenobarbital levels by increasing hepatic metabolism.

Effects on diagnostic tests

Phenobarbital may cause a false-positive phentolamine test. The physiologic effects of the drug may impair the absorption of cyanocobalamin ^{57}Co; it may decrease serum bilirubin concentrations in neonates, epileptics, and in patients with congenital nonhemolytic unconjugated hyperbilirubinemia. Barbiturates may increase sulfobromophthalein retention. EEG patterns show a change in low-voltage, fast activity; changes persist for a time after discontinuation of therapy.

Adverse reactions

• CNS: *drowsiness, lethargy,* vertigo, headache, *CNS depression,* paradoxical excitement, confusion and *agitation; hyperexcitability* in children; rebound insomnia, increased dreams or nightmares, possibly seizures (after acute withdrawal or reduction in dosage).
• CV: *hypotension* (after rapid I.V. administration), bradycardia, circulatory collapse.
• DERM: urticaria, *rash,* exfoliative dermatitis, and Stevens-Johnson syndrome.
• EENT: miosis.
• GI: epigastric pain, nausea, vomiting, diarrhea, constipation.
• Local: thrombophlebitis, pain and possible tissue damage at site of extravascular injection.
• Other: *respiratory depression, laryngospasm, bronchospasm,* vitamin K deficiency and bleeding have occurred in newborns of mothers treated during pregnancy. Hyperalgesia may occur in low doses or in patients with chronic pain.

Note: Drug should be discontinued if hypersensitivity reaction, profound CNS or respiratory depression, or skin eruptions occur.

Overdose and treatment

Clinical manifestations of overdose include unsteady gait, slurred speech, sustained nystagmus, somnolence, confusion, respiratory depression, pulmonary edema, areflexia, and coma. Typical shock syndrome with tachycardia and hypotension along with jaundice, oliguria, and chills followed by fever may occur.

Treatment is aimed at the maintenance and support of ventilation and pulmonary function as necessary; support of cardiac function and circulation with vasopressors and I.V. fluids as needed. If patient is conscious and gag reflex is intact, induce emesis (if ingestion was recent) by administering ipecac syrup. If emesis is contraindicated, perform gastric lavage while a cuffed endotracheal tube is in place to prevent aspiration. Follow with administration of repeated doses of activated charcoal or saline cathartic. Measure intake and output, vital signs, and laboratory parameters. Maintain body temperature.

Alkalinization of urine may be helpful in removing drug from the body; hemodialysis may be useful in severe overdose. Oral activated charcoal may enhance phenobarbital elimination regardless of its route of administration.

▶ Special considerations

• Paradoxical hyperexcitability may occur in children. Use with caution. Use of phenobarbital extended-release capsules is not recommended in children under age 12.
• Premature infants are more susceptible to the depressant effects of barbiturates because of immature hepatic metabolism. Children receiving barbiturates may experience hyperactivity, excitement, or hyperalgia.
• Dosage of barbiturates must be individualized for each patient, because different rates of metabolism and enzyme induction occur.
• May be given rectally if oral or parenteral route is inappropriate.
• Assess level of consciousness before and frequently during therapy to evaluate effectiveness of drug. Monitor neurologic status for possible alterations or deteriorations. Monitor seizure character, frequency, and duration for changes. Institute seizure precautions, as necessary.
• Vital signs should be checked frequently, especially during I.V. administration.
• Assess patient's sleeping patterns before and during therapy to ensure effectiveness of drug.
• Institute safety measures—side rails, assistance when out of bed, call light within reach—to prevent falls and injury.
• Anticipate possible rebound confusion and excitatory reactions in patient.
• Assess bowel elimination patterns; monitor for complaints of constipation. Advise diet high in fiber, if indicated.
• Monitor prothrombin time carefully in patients taking anticoagulants; dosage of anticoagulant may require adjustment to counteract possible interaction.
• Observe patient to prevent hoarding or self-dosing, especially in depressed or suicidal patients, or those who are or have a history of being drug-dependent.
• Abrupt discontinuation may cause withdrawal symptoms; discontinue slowly.
• Death is common with an overdose of 2 to 10 g; it may occur at much smaller doses if alcohol is also ingested.

- Avoid administering barbiturates to patients with status asthmaticus.
- Oral solution may be mixed with water or juice to improve taste.
- Do not crush or break extended-release form; this will impair drug action.
- Reconstitute powder for injection with 2.5 to 5 ml sterile water for injection. Roll vial in hands; do not shake.
- Use a larger vein for I.V. administration to prevent extravasation.
- Avoid I.V. administration at a rate greater than 60 mg/minute to prevent hypotension and respiratory depression. It may take up to 30 minutes after I.V. administration to achieve maximum effect.
- Administer parenteral dose within 30 minutes of reconstitution because phenobarbital hydrolyzes in solution and on exposure to air.
- Keep emergency resuscitation equipment on hand when administering phenobarbital I.V.
- Administer I.M. dose deep into a large muscle mass to prevent tissue injury.
- Only parenteral solutions prepared from powder may be given S.C.; however, this route is not recommended.
- Do not use injectable solution if it contains a precipitate.
- Administration of full loading doses over short periods of time to treat status epilepticus will require ventilatory support in adults.
- Full therapeutic effects are not seen for 2 to 3 weeks, except when loading dose is used.

Information for parents and patient
- Advise parents of potential for physical and psychological dependence with prolonged use.
- Warn parents or patient to avoid concurrent use of other drugs with CNS depressant effects, such as antihistamines, analgesics, and alcohol, because they will have additive effects and result in increased drowsiness. Instruct parents to seek medical approval before giving patient any nonprescription cold or allergy preparations.
- Caution parents and patient not to increase or decrease dose or frequency without medical approval; abrupt discontinuation of drug may trigger rebound insomnia, with increased dreaming, nightmares, or seizures.
- Patient should avoid hazardous tasks that require alertness while taking phenobarbital.
- Be sure parents and patient understand that phenobarbital can cause physical or psychological dependence (addiction).
- Instruct parents or patient to report any skin eruption or other marked adverse effect.
- Explain that a morning hangover is common after therapeutic use of phenobarbital.

phenoxybenzamine hydrochloride
Dibenzyline

- Classification: antihypertensive for pheochromocytoma, cutaneous vasodilator (alpha-adrenergic blocking agent)

How supplied
Available by prescription only
Capsules: 10 mg

Indications, route, and dosage
To control or prevent paroxysmal hypertension and sweating in patients with pheochromocytoma
Children: Initially, 0.2 mg/kg or 6 mg/m² P.O. daily in a single dose. Maintenance dosage is 0.4 to 1.2 mg/kg or 12 to 36 mg/m² daily.
Adults: Initially, 10 mg P.O. b.i.d., then increased every other day until desired response is achieved. Usual maintenance dosage is 20 to 40 mg b.i.d or t.i.d daily.

Action and kinetics
- *Antihypertensive action:* Phenoxybenzamine noncompetitively blocks stimulation of alpha-adrenergic receptors, causing long-acting sympathetic blockade. The drug acts on vascular smooth muscle to block epinephrine- and norepinephrine-induced vasoconstriction, causing peripheral vasodilation and reflex tachycardia. Phenoxybenzamine reverses the pressor effect of epinephrine (epinephrine reversal) and blocks, but does not reverse, the vasoconstrictor effects of norepinephrine.
- *Cutaneous vasodilator action:* Phenoxybenzamine blocks epinephrine- and norepinephrine-induced vasodilation.
- *Kinetics in adults:* After oral administration, phenoxybenzamine is absorbed variably from the GI tract; its effects begin gradually over several hours. Phenoxybenzamine is highly lipid-soluble and may accumulate in fat after large doses. The drug's metabolism is unknown. Phenoxybenzamine is excreted in urine and bile; alpha-adrenergic blocking effects may persist for up to 7 days after therapy is discontinued.

Contraindications and precautions
Phenoxybenzamine is contraindicated in patients with known hypersensitivity to the drug.

The drug should be used cautiously in patients with cerebrovascular or coronary insufficiency, because decreased blood pressure may precipitate stroke or angina; in patients with CHF, coronary artery disease, or advanced renal disease, because hypotension may exacerbate these conditions; and in patients in shock, because additional fluid replacement will be needed.

Interactions
Phenoxybenzamine may antagonize the effects of alpha-adrenergic stimulating sympathomimetic agents.

Concomitant use with drugs that stimulate both alpha- and beta-adrenergic receptors — for example, epinephrine — may cause vasodilation, an increased hypotensive response, and tachycardia.

Effects on diagnostic tests
None reported.

Adverse reactions
- CNS: lethargy, drowsiness.
- CV: orthostatic hypotension, tachycardia, *shock*.
- EENT: nasal stuffiness, dry mouth, miosis.
- GI: vomiting, abdominal distress.

Note: Drug should be discontinued if patient shows signs of overdose.

Overdose and treatment
Clinical signs of overdose include postural hypotension, dizziness, tachycardia, vomiting, lethargy, and shock.

After acute ingestion, empty stomach by induced emesis or gastric lavage, and give activated charcoal to reduce absorption. Further treatment is usually symptomatic and supportive. Most vasopressors are ineffective; however, adequate doses of norepinephrine may overcome phenoxybenzamine-induced alpha blockade. Because drug effects are cumulative, extended monitoring of patient is necessary.

▶ Special considerations
- Administer cautiously to children.
- Administer dose at bedtime to reduce potential of dizziness or light-headedness.
- During dosage adjustment, monitor pulse rate and rhythm; check blood pressure in recumbent and standing positions.
- Monitor respiratory status carefully; symptoms of pneumonia and asthma may be aggravated.
- Place patient in Trendelenburg's position if faintness or dizziness occurs.
- Optimal effect may require several weeks; monitor patient closely for adverse effects.
- Nasal congestion and other adverse effects usually subside during continued therapy.
- Administer drug with milk or in divided doses to reduce GI irritation.
- Phenoxybenzamine has been used to establish adequacy of fluid volume replacement in patients in shock; to treat micturition disorders; and intravenously to treat hypertensive crisis caused by sympathomimetic amines, foods, or drugs in patients taking MAO inhibitors.

Information for parents and patient
- Teach parents and patient about disease and rationale for therapy; explain that the patient must continue drug even if he feels well, never discontinue it suddenly, and report any unusual symptoms or malaise.
- Explain that patient can minimize postural hypotension by rising slowly and avoiding sudden position changes; relieve dry mouth by chewing ice chips, hard candy, or sugarless gum; and minimize gastric irritation by taking drug in divided doses with milk.

- Tell parents to watch for and promptly report dizziness or irregular heart beat.
- Advise parents to have patient take dose at bedtime to reduce potential for dizziness or light-headedness.
- Warn parents that patient should avoid hazardous tasks that require mental alertness until effects of medication are established.
- Reassure parents and patient that adverse effects should subside after several doses.
- Tell parents and patient that the use of alcohol, excessive exercise, prolonged standing, and exposure to heat will intensify adverse effects. Emphasize that some liquid cough and cold medications contain alcohol.
- Advise parents against giving patient any other medication, including any that can be purchased without a prescription, unless medically approved.

---

phensuximide
Milontin

- Classification: anticonvulsant (succinimide derivative)

How supplied
Available by prescription only
Capsules: 500 mg

Indications, route, and dosage
Absence (petit mal) seizures
Children and adults: 500 mg to 1 g P.O. b.i.d. or t.i.d.

Action and kinetics
- *Anticonvulsant action:* Phensuximide raises the seizure threshold; it suppresses characteristic spike-and-wave pattern by depressing neuronal transmission in the motor cortex and basal ganglia. It is indicated for absence (petit mal) seizures refractory to other drugs.
- *Kinetics in adults:* Phensuximide is absorbed from the GI tract; peak plasma concentrations occur at 1 to 4 hours. Phensuximide is distributed widely throughout the body. Little is known about phensuximide's metabolism; hydroxy metabolite has been isolated. Excretion of phensuximide has not been studied; it is at least partially excreted in urine.

Contraindications and precautions
Phensuximide is contraindicated in patients with known hypersensitivity to succinimide derivatives. It should be use with caution in patients with hepatic or renal disease and in patients taking other CNS depressants or anticonvusants.

Phensuximide may increase the incidence of generalized tonic-clonic seizures if used alone to treat mixed seizures; abrupt withdrawal may precipitate petit mal seizures. Use of anticonvulsants during pregnancy has been associated with an increased incidence of birth defects.

Interactions
Concomitant use of phensuximide and other CNS depressants (alcohol, narcotics, anxiolytics, antide

---

pressants, antipsychotics, and other anticonvulsants) may increase sedative effects.

Effects on diagnostic tests
None reported.

Adverse reactions
• CNS: muscular weakness, drowsiness, dizziness, ataxia, headache, insomnia, confusion, psychosis.
• DERM: pruritus, eruptions, erythema, Stevens-Johnson syndrome.
• GI: nausea, vomiting, anorexia, abdominal pain, diarrhea.
• GU: urinary frequency, renal damage, hematuria.
• HEMA: transient leukopenia, pancytopenia, agranulocytosis, eosinophilia.
• Other: periorbital edema.
  Note: Drug should be discontinued if signs of hypersensitivity, rash, or unusual skin lesions occur; or if any of the following signs of blood dyscrasia occur: joint pain, fever, sore throat, or unusual bleeding or bruising.

Overdose and treatment
Symptoms of overdose may include dizziness and ataxia, which may progress to stupor and coma. Treat overdose supportively. Carefully monitor vital signs and fluid and electrolyte balance. Charcoal hemoperfusion or hemodialysis may be used for severe cases.

▶ Special considerations
• Observe patient closely for dermatologic reactions at initiation of therapy.
• Monitor closely for signs of hematologic reactions or other adverse reactions: skin rash, sore throat, joint pain, unexplained fever, or unusual bleeding or bruising.
• Drug should not be discontinued abruptly.
• Drug adds to CNS depressant effects of alcohol, narcotics, anxiolytics, antidepressants, and tranquilizers.
• Patient should have periodic tests for hematologic and liver function. Complete blood counts are recommended every 3 months; urinalysis and liver function tests, every 6 months.
• Phensuximide may be removed by hemodialysis. Dosage adjustments may be necessary in patients undergoing dialysis.

Information for parents and patient
• Tell parents and patient that drug may color urine pink, red, or brown. This is not harmful.
• Tell parents that patient should take drug with food or milk to avoid GI upset should avoid use of alcoholic beverages, and should not discontinue drug abruptly or change dose except as directed.
• Advise parents that patient should avoid hazardous tasks that require mental alertness until degree of sedative effect is determined.
• Teach parents and patient signs and symptoms of hypersensitivity, liver dysfunction, and blood dyscrasias, and advise patient to report them promptly. Also, explain to parents of adolescents the importance of reporting suspected pregnancy immediately.
• Encourage parents to have patient wear a Medic

Alert bracelet or necklace, listing drug and seizure disorder.
• Advise storing drug away from excessive heat to maintain effectiveness.

---

phentolamine mesylate
Regitine

• Classification: antihypertensive agent for pheochromocytoma, cutaneous vasodilator (alpha-adrenergic blocking agent)

How supplied
Available by prescription only
Injection: 5 mg/ml in 1-ml vials

Indications, route, and dosage
Aid for diagnosis of pheochromocytoma
Children: 1 mg I.V., 3 mg I.M., or 0.1 mg/kg or 3 mg/m^2 I.V.
Adults: 5 mg I.V. or I.M.
Control or prevention of paroxysmal hypertension immediately before or during pheochromocytomectomy
Children: 1 mg, 0.1 mg/kg, or 3 mg/m^2 I.M. or I.V. 1 to 2 hours preoperatively, repeated as necessary; 1 mg, 0.1 mg/kg, or 3 mg/m^2 I.V. during surgery if indicated.
Adults: 5 mg I.M. or I.V. 1 to 2 hours preoperatively, repeated as necessary; 5 mg I.V. during surgery if indicated.
Prevention of dermal necrosis and sloughing or extravasation after I.V. administration of norepinephrine
Children and adults: Inject 5 to 10 mg in 10 ml of normal saline solution into the affected area, or add 10 mg to each liter of I.V. fluids containing norepinephrine.
†Adjunctive treatment of CHF
Children and adults: 170 to 400 mcg/minute by I.V. infusion.

Action and kinetics
• *Antihypertensive action:* Phentolamine competitively antagonizes endogenous and exogenous amines at presynaptic and postsynaptic alpha-adrenergic receptors, decreasing both preload and afterload.
• *Cutaneous vasodilation:* Phentolamine blocks epinephrine- and norepinephrine-induced vasodilation.
• *Kinetics in adults:* Antihypertensive effect is immediate after I.V. administration. The drug's distribution and metabolism are unknown. About 10% of a given dose of phentolamine is excreted unchanged in urine; excretion of remainder is unknown. Phentolamine has a short duration of action; plasma half-life is 19 minutes after I.V. administration.

Contraindications and precautions
Phentolamine is contraindicated in patients with known hypersensitivity to the drug and in patients with coronary artery disease or recent myocardial

infarction, because the drug may exacerbate these conditions.

Drug should be given cautiously to patients with gastritis or peptic ulcer and to patients receiving other antihypertensives.

Interactions
Phentolamine antagonizes vasoconstrictor and hypertensive effects of epinephrine and ephedrine.

Effects on diagnostic tests
None reported.

Adverse reactions
• CNS: dizziness, lethargy, flushing.
• CV: *hypotension, shock, dysrhythmias,* palpitations, *tachycardia,* angina pectoris, *hypertension.*
• GI: diarrhea, abdominal pain, nausea, vomiting, hyperperistalsis, *increased secretions.*
• Other: nasal stuffiness, hypoglycemia, *tissue sloughing and necrosis at I.V. site.*
  Note: Drug should be discontinued if severe hypotension develops.

Overdose and treatment
Signs of overdose include hypotension, dizziness, fainting, tachycardia, vomiting, lethargy, and shock.

Treat supportively and symptomatically. Use norepinephrine if necessary to increase the blood pressure. *Do not use epinephrine;* it stimulates both alpha and beta receptors and will cause vasodilation and a further drop in blood pressure.

▶ Special considerations
• Usual doses of phentolamine have little effect on the blood pressure of normal individuals or patients with essential hypertension.
• Before test for pheochromocytoma, have the patient rest in supine position until blood pressure is stabilized. When phentolamine is administered I.V., inject dose rapidly after effects of the venipuncture on the blood pressure have passed. A marked decrease in blood pressure will be seen immediately, with the maximum effect seen within 2 minutes. Record blood pressure immediately after the injection, at 30-second intervals for the first 3 minutes, at 1-minute intervals for the next 7 minutes. When phentolamine is administered I.M., maximum effect occurs within 20 minutes. Record blood pressure every 5 minutes for 30 to 45 minutes after injection.
• A positive test response occurs when the patient's blood pressure decreases at least 35 mm Hg systolic and 25 mm Hg diastolic; a negative test response occurs when the patient's blood pressure remains unchanged, is elevated, or decreases less than 35 mm Hg systolic and 25 mm Hg diastolic.
• When possible, sedatives, analgesics, and all other medication should be withdrawn at least 24 hours (preferably 48 to 72 hours) before the phentolamine test; antihypertensive drugs should be withdrawn and test should not be performed until blood pressure returns to pretreatment levels; rauwolfia drugs should be withdrawn at least 4 weeks before test.
• Phentolamine has been used to treat hypertension resulting from clonidine withdrawal and to treat the reaction to sympathetic amines or other drugs or foods in patients taking MAO inhibitors.
• Phentolamine also has been used in patients with myocardial infarction associated with left ventricular failure in an attempt to reduce infarct size and decrease left ventricular ejection impedance. It also has been used to treat supraventricular premature contractions.
• Monitor for extravasation. If it occurs, discontinue I.V. immediately and elevate extremity.
• To administer drug for treatment of local tissue infiltration, inject drug locally S.C. or intradermally using a 25G or 27G needle; inject drug at edge of extravasation site, then wrap extremity loosely with sterile dressing for 2 hours to absorb drainage. Do not apply heat.
• Monitor vital signs, especially blood pressure.
• Administer dose at bedtime to reduce potential potential of dizziness or light-headedness.

Information for parents and patient
• Teach patient about phentolamine test, if appropriate.
• Tell parents to report adverse effects at once, especially dizziness or irregular heart beat.
• Tell parents that patient should not take sedatives or narcotics for at least 24 hours before phentolamine test.
• Warn parents and patient about postural hypotension. Patient should avoid sudden changes to upright position.
• Advise parents to have patient take dose at bedtime to reduce potential for dizziness or light-headedness.
• Warn parents that patient should avoid hazardous activities that require mental alertness until effects of medication are established.
• Reassure parents and patient that adverse effects should subside after several doses.
• Tell parents and patient that the use of alchohol, excessive exercise, prolonged standing, and exposure to heat will intensify adverse effects. Emphasize that some liquid cough and cold medications contain alcohol.
• Advise parents against giving patient any other medication, unless medically approved.

phenylephrine hydrochloride
Nasal products
Allerest, Neo-Synephrine, Sinex

Parenteral
Neo-Synephrine

Ophthalmic
Ak-Dilate, Ak-Nefrin, Isopto Frin,
Mydfrin, Neo-Synephrine, Prefin
Liquifilm

• Classification: vasoconstrictor (adrenergic)

How supplied
Available by prescription only
Injection: 10 mg/ml parenteral
Ophthalmic solution: 0.12%, 2.5%, 10%

Available without prescription
Nasal solution: 0.123%, 0.16%, 0.2%, 0.5%, 1%
Nasal spray: 0.2%, 0.25%, 0.5%

Indications, route, and dosage
Hypotensive emergencies during spinal anesthesia
Children: 0.044 to 0.088 mg/kg I.M. or S.C.
Adults: Initially, 0.1 to 0.2 mg I.V.; subsequent doses should also be low (0.1 mg).
Mild to moderate hypotension
Children: 0.1 mg/kg or 3 mg/m² I.M. or S.C. May repeat q 2 hours as needed.
Adults: 1 to 10 mg S.C. or I.M. (initial dose should not exceed 5 mg). Additional doses may be given in 1 to 2 hours if needed. Or, 0.1 to 0.5 mg slow I.V. injection (initial dose should not exceed 0.5 mg). Additional doses may be given q 10 to 15 minutes.
Paroxysmal supraventricular tachycardia
Children: 5 to 10 mcg/kg by I.V. push.
Adults: Initially, 0.5 mg rapid I.V.; subsequent doses may be increased in increments of 0.1 to 0.2 mg. Maximum dose should not exceed 1 mg.
Adjunct in the treatment of severe hypotension or shock
Children: 5 to 20 mcg/kg I.V. q 10 to 15 minutes as needed. Alternatively, give by I.V. infusion at a rate of 0.1 to 0.5 mcg/kg/minute.
Adults: 0.1 to 0.18 mg/minute I.V. infusion. After blood pressure stabilizes, maintain at 0.04 to 0.06 mg/minute, adjusted to patient response.
Mydriasis (without cycloplegia)
Adolescents and adults: Instill 1 or 2 drops 2.5% or 10% solution in eye before procedure. May be repeated in 10 to 60 minutes if needed.
Nasal, †sinus, or eustachian tube congestion
Children under age 6: Apply 2 to 3 drops or sprays of 0.125% or 0.16% solution in each nostril.
Children 6 to 12: Apply 2 to 3 drops or 1 to 2 sprays in each nostril.
Children over age 12 and adults: Apply 2 to 3 drops or 1 to 2 sprays of 0.25% to 1% solution instilled in each nostril; or a small quantity of 0.5% nasal jelly applied into each nostril. Apply jelly or spray to nasal mucosa.
Drops, spray, or jelly can be given q 4 hours, p.r.n.
Conjunctival congestion
Adolescents and adults: 1 to 2 drops of 0.12% to 0.25% solution applied to conjunctiva q 3 to 4 hours p.r.n.

Action and kinetics
• *Vasopressor action:* Phenylephrine acts predominantly by direct stimulation of alpha-adrenergic receptors, which constrict resistance and capacitance blood vessels, resulting in increased total peripheral resistance; increased systolic and diastolic blood pressure; decreased blood flow to vital organs, skin, and skeletal muscle; and constriction of renal blood vessels, reducing renal blood flow. Its main therapeutic effect is vasoconstriction.

It may also act indirectly by releasing norepinephrine from its storage sites. Phenylephrine does not stimulate beta receptors except in large doses (activates beta₁ receptors). Tachyphylaxis (tolerance) may follow repeated injections.

Other alpha-adrenergic effects include action on the dilator muscle of the pupil (producing contraction) and local decongestant action in the arterioles of the conjunctiva (producing constriction).

Phenylephrine acts directly on alpha-adrenergic receptors in the arterioles of conjunctiva nasal mucosa, producing constriction. Its vasoconstricting action on skin, mucous membranes, and viscera slows the vascular absorption rate of local anesthetics, which prolongs their action, localizes anesthesia, and decreases the risk of toxicity.

Phenylephrine may cause contraction of pregnant uterus and constriction of uterine blood vessels.
• *Kinetics in adults:* Pressor effects occur almost immediately after I.V. injection and persist 15 to 20 minutes; after I.M. injection, onset is within 10 to 15 minutes, persisting ½ to 2 hours; after S.C. injection, onset is within 10 to 15 minutes, with effects persisting 50 to 60 minutes. Nasal or conjunctival decongestant effects persist 30 minutes to 4 hours. Peak effects for mydriasis are 15 to 60 minutes for the 2.5% solution, 10 to 90 minutes for the 10% solution. Mydriasis recovery time is 3 hours for the 2.5% solution, 3 to 7 hours for the 10% solution. Distribution is unknown. Phenylephrine is metabolized in the liver and intestine by the enzyme monoamine oxidase. The drug's excretion is unknown.

Contraindications and precautions
Phenylephrine is contraindicated in patients with severe coronary disease, cardiovascular disease including myocardial infarction, or peripheral or mesenteric vascular thrombosis, because this may increase ischemia or extend area of infarction; in patients with severe hypertension or ventricular tachycardia; or for use with local anesthetics on fingers, toes, ears, nose, and genitalia.

Administer with extreme caution to debilitated patients and those with hyperthyroidism, bradycardia, partial heart block, myocardial disease, diabetes mellitus, narrow-angle glaucoma, severe arteriosclerosis, acute pancreatitis, or hepatitis (may increase ischemia in liver or pancreas).

---

‡May contain sulfites   ◆May contain tartrazine   ◆◆May contain benzyl alcohol

Also administer cautiously to patients with known hypersensitivity to sulfites because phenylephrine contains sulfite preservatives.

Interactions

Phenylephrine may increase risk of cardiac dysrhythmias, including tachycardia, when used concomitantly with epinephrine or other sympathomimetics, digitalis glycosides, levodopa, guanadrel or guanethidine, tricyclic antidepressants, MAO inhibitors, or general anesthetics (chloroform, cycloproprane, and halothane).

Pressor effects are potentiated when phenylephrine is used with oxytocics, doxapram, MAO inhibitors, methyldopa, trimethaphan, mecamylamine, mazindol, and ergot alkaloids.

Decreased pressor response (hypotension) may result when phenylephrine is used with alpha-adrenergic blockers, antihypertensives, diuretics used as antihypertensives, guanadrel or guanethidine, rauwolfia alkaloids, or nitrates.

Use of phenylephrine with thyroid hormones may increase effects of either drug; with nitrates, it may reduce antianginal effects.

The mydriatic response to phenylephrine is decreased in concomitant use of levodopa and increased in concomitant use with cycloplegic antimuscarinic drugs, such as atropine.

Effects on diagnostic tests

Phenylephrine may lower intraocular pressure in normal eyes or in open-angle glaucoma. The drug also may cause false-normal tonometry readings.

Adverse reactions

• CNS: restlessness, *insomnia,* anxiety, nervousness, light-headedness, weakness, dizziness, *tremors,* paresthesias in extremities and coolness in skin (after injection), headache, browache, seizures.
• CV: precordial pain or discomfort, peripheral and visceral vasoconstriction, bradycardia, tachycardia, decreased cardiac output, hypertension, *palpitations,* anginal pain.
• EENT: blurred vision; transient burning and stinging on instillation; increased sensitivity of eyes to light; iris floaters; glaucoma; rebound miosis; dermatitis; burning, stinging, and dryness of nasal mucosa; rebound nasal congestion.
• GI: vomiting.
• Local: tissue sloughing with extravasation.
• Other: respiratory distress, sweating, blanching of skin, tolerance with prolonged use.
  Note: Drug should be discontinued if hypersensitivity or cardiac dysrhythmias occur.

Overdose and treatment

Clinical manifestations of overdose include exaggeration of common adverse reactions, palpitations, paresthesia, vomiting, cardiac dysrhythmias, hypertension.

To treat, discontinue drug and provide symptomatic and supportive measures. Monitor vital signs closely. Use atropine sulfate to block reflex bradycardia; phentolamine to treat excessive hypertension; and propranolol to treat cardiac dysrhythmias, or levodopa

to reduce an excessive mydriatic effect of an ophthalmic preparation as necessary.

▶ Special considerations

• Infants and children may be more susceptible than adults to drug effects. Because of the risk of precipitating severe hypertension, only ophthalmic solutions containing 0.5% or less should be used in infants under age 1. The 10% ophthalmic solution is contraindicated in infants. Most manufacturers recommend that the 0.5% nasal solution not be used in children under age 12 and the 0.25% nasal solution should not be used in children under age 6 except under medical supervision.
• Tachyphylaxis (tolerance) may develop after prolonged or excessive use.
• Give I.V. through large veins, and monitor flow rate. To treat extravasation ischemia, infiltrate site promptly and liberally with 10 to 15 ml of normal saline solution containing 5 to 10 mg of phentolamine through fine needle. Topical nitroglycerin has also been used.
• During I.V. administration, pulse, blood pressure, and central venous pressure should be monitored (every 2 to 5 minutes). Control flow rate and dosage to prevent excessive increases. I.V. overdoses can induce ventricular dysrhythmias.
• Hypovolemic states should be corrected before administration of drug; phenylephrine should not be used in place of fluid, blood, plasma, and electrolyte replacement.
• Phenylephrine is chemically incompatible with butacaine, sulfate, alkalies, ferric salts, and oxidizing agents and metals.

Ophthalmic
• Apply digital pressure to lacrimal sac during and for 1 to 2 minutes after instillation to prevent systemic absorption.
• Prolonged exposure to air or strong light may cause oxidation and discoloration. Do not use if solution is brown or contains precipitate.
• To prevent contamination, do not touch applicator tip to any surface. Instruct patient in proper technique.

Nasal
• Prolonged or chronic use may result in rebound congestion and chronic swelling of nasal mucosa.
• To reduce risk of rebound congestion, use weakest effective dose.
• After use, rinse tip of spray bottle or dropper with hot water and dry with clean tissue. Wipe tip of nasal jelly container with clean, damp tissues.

Information for parents and patient

• Tell parents to store away from heat, light, and humidity (not in bathroom medicine cabinet) and out of small children's reach.
• Warn parents and patient to use only as directed. If using nonprescription product, the patient should follow directions on label and not use more often or in larger doses than prescribed or recommended.
• Caution parents and patient not to exceed recommended dosage regardless of formulation; patient should not double, decrease, or omit doses nor change dosage intervals unless so instructed.
• Tell parents to call if drug provides no relief in 2

days after using phenylephrine ophthalmic solution or 3 days after using the nasal solution.

• Explain that systemic absorption from nasal and conjunctival membranes can occur. Parents should report systemic reactions, such as dizziness and chest pain, and discontinue drug.

Ophthalmic

• Tell parents not to use if solution is brown or contains a precipitate.

• Tell parents or patient to wash hands before applying and to use finger to apply pressure to patient's lacrimal sac during and for 1 to 2 minutes after instillation to decrease systemic absorption.

• Tell parents and patient to avoid touching tip to any surface to prevent contamination.

• Tell parents and patient that after applying drops, patient's pupils will become unusually large. Patient should use sunglasses to protect eyes from sunlight and other bright lights. Parents should call if effects persist 12 hours or more.

Nasal

• After use, parents or patient should rinse tip of spray bottle or dropper with hot water and dry with clean tissue or wipe tip of nasal jelly container with clean, damp tissues.

• Instruct patient to blow nose gently (with both nostrils open) to clear nasal passages well, before using medication.

• Teach parents and patient correct instillation.

—Drops: tilt head back while sitting or standing up, or lie on bed and hang head over side. Stay in position a few minutes to permit medication to spread through nose.

—Spray: with head upright, squeeze bottle quickly and firmly to produce 1 or 2 sprays into each nostril; wait 3 to 5 minutes, blow nose and repeat dose.

—Jelly: place in each nostril and sniff it well back into nose.

• Tell parents and patient that increased fluid intake helps keep secretions liquid.

• Warn parents that patient should avoid using nonprescription medications with phenylephrine to prevent possible hazardous interactions.

---

phenytoin, phenytoin sodium, phenytoin sodium (extended)
Dilantin

phenytoin sodium (prompt)
Di-Phen, Diphenylan

• Classification: anticonvulsant (hydantoin derivative)

How supplied
Available by prescription only
Phenytoin
Tablets (chewable): 50 mg
Oral suspension: 30 mg/5 ml, 125 mg/5 ml
Phenytoin sodium
Capsules: 30 mg, 100 mg
Injection: 50 mg/ml

Phenytoin sodium, extended
Capsules: 30 mg, 100 mg
Phenytoin sodium, prompt
Capsules: 30 mg, 100 mg

Indications, route, and dosage
Generalized tonic-clonic (grand mal) seizures, status epilepticus, nonepileptic seizures (post-head trauma, Reye's syndrome)
Children: Loading dosage is 15 to 20 mg/kg I.V. at 50 mg/minute, or P.O. divided q 8 to 12 hours; then start maintenance dosage of 4 to 8 mg/kg P.O. or I.V. daily, divided q 12 hours.
Adults: Loading dosage is 15 to 20 mg/kg I.V. slowly, not to exceed 50 mg/minute; oral loading dosage consists of 1 g divided into three doses (400 mg, 300 mg, 300 mg) given at 2-hour intervals. Maintenance dosage is 300 mg P.O. daily (extended only) or divided t.i.d. (extended or prompt).
Seizures in patients who have been receiving phenytoin but have missed one or more doses and have subtherapeutic levels
Neonates: Loading dose 10 to 25 mg/kg I.V., in normal saline solution, infused slowly at a rate not to exceed 0.5 mg/kg/minute. Maintenance dosage, 4 to 8 mg/kg/day, divided q 8, 12, or 24 hours.
Children: 5 to 7 mg/kg I.V., not to exceed 50 mg/minute. May repeat lower dose in 30 minutes if needed.
Adults: 100 to 300 mg I.V., not to exceed 50 mg/minute.
†*Neuritic pain (migraine, trigeminal neuralgia, and Bell's palsy)*
Adults: 200 to 600 mg P.O. daily in divided doses.
†*Ventricular dysrhythmias unresponsive to lidocaine or procainamide, and dysrhythmias induced by cardiac glycosides*
Children: 3 to 8 mg/kg P.O. or slow I.V. daily, or 250 mg/m² daily given as single dose or divided in two doses.
Adults: Loading dosage is 1 g P.O. divided over first 24 hours, followed by 500 mg daily for 2 days, then maintenance dosage 300 mg P.O. daily; 250 mg I.V. over 5 minutes until dysrhythmias subside, adverse effects develop, or 1 g has been given. Infusion rate should never exceed 50 mg/minute (slow I.V. push). Alternate method: 100 mg I.V. q 15 minutes until adverse effects develop, dysrhythmias are controlled, or 1 g has been given. Also may administer entire loading dose of 1 g I.V. slowly at 25 mg/minute. Can be diluted in normal saline solution. I.M. dosage is not recommended because of pain and erratic absorption.
†*Treatment of recessive dystrophic epidermolysis bullosa*
Adults: Initially 2 to 3 mg/kg P.O. daily divided b.i.d. Increase dosage at 2 to 3 week intervals to a plasma level of 8 mcg/ml (usual dose: 100 to 300 mg daily).

Action and kinetics
• *Anticonvulsant action:* Like other hydantoin derivatives, phenytoin stabilizes neuronal membranes and limits seizure activity by either increasing efflux or decreasing influx of sodium ions across cell membranes in the motor cortex during generation of nerve impulses. Phenytoin exerts its antiarrhythmic effects

---

‡May contain sulfites   ♦May contain tartrazine   ♦♦May contain benzyl alcohol

by normalizing sodium influx to Purkinje's fibers in patients with digitalis-induced dysrhythmias. It is indicated for tonic-clonic (grand mal) and partial seizures.

• *Other actions:* Phenytoin inhibits excessive collagenase activity in patients will epidermolysis bullosa.

• *Kinetics in adults:* Phenytoin is absorbed slowly from the small intestine; absorption is formulation-dependent and bioavailability may differ among products. Extended-release capsules give peak serum concentrations at 4 to 12 hours; prompt-release products peak at 1½ to 3 hours. I.M. doses are absorbed erratically; about 50% to 75% of I.M. dose is absorbed in 24 hours.

Phenytoin is distributed widely throughout the body; therapeutic plasma levels are 10 to 20 mcg/ml, although in some patients, they occur at 5 to 10 mcg/ml. Lateral nystagmus may occur at levels above 20 mcg/ml; ataxia usually occurs at levels above 30 mcg/ml; significantly decreased mental capacity occurs at 40 mcg/ml. Phenytoin is about 90% protein-bound, less so in uremic patients.

Phenytoin is metabolized by the liver to inactive metabolites. It is excreted in urine and exhibits dose-dependent (zero-order) elimination kinetics; above a certain dosage level, small increases in dosage disproportionately increase serum levels.

Contraindications and precautions

Phenytoin is contraindicated in patients with hypersensitivity to hydantoins or phenacemide; I.V. phenytoin is contraindicated in patients with sinus bradycardia, sinoatrial or atrioventricular block, or Stokes-Adams syndrome.

Phenytoin should be used with caution in patients with acute intermittent porphyria, hepatic or renal dysfunction (especially in uremic patients, who have higher serum drug levels from decreased protein-binding), myocardial insufficiency, or respiratory depression; in debilitated patients; and in patients taking other hydantoin derivatives.

Interactions

Phenytoin interacts with many drugs. Diminished therapeutic effects and toxic reactions often are the result of recent changes in drug therapy. Phenytoin's therapeutic effects may be increased by concomitant use with allopurinol, chloramphenicol, cimetidine, diazepam, disulfiram, ethanol (acute), isoniazid, miconazole, phenacemide, phenylbutazone, succinimides, trimethoprim, valproic acid, salicylates, ibuprofen, chlorpheniramine, or imipramine.

Phenytoin's therapeutic effects may be decreased by barbiturates, carbamazepine, diazoxide, ethanol (chronic), folic acid, theophylline, antacids, antineoplastics, calcium gluconate, calcium, charcoal, loxapine, nitrofurantoin, or pyridoxine.

Phenytoin may decrease the effects of the following drugs by stimulating hepatic metabolism: corticosteroids, cyclosporine, dicumarol, digitoxin, meperidine, disopyramide, doxycycline, estrogens, haloperidol, methadone, metyrapone, quinidine, oral contraceptives, dopamine, furosemide, levodopa, or sulfonylureas.

Effects on diagnostic tests

Phenytoin may raise blood glucose levels by inhibiting pancreatic insulin release; it may decrease serum levels of protein-bound iodine and may interfere with the 1-mg dexamethasone suppression test.

Adverse reactions

• CNS: *ataxia,* slurred speech, confusion, dizziness, insomnia, nervousness, twitching, headache, *CNS depression, lethargy, drowsiness, irritability.*

• CV: *hypotension,* ventricular fibrillation, *ccardiovascular collapse and asystole* (with rapid I.V. administration.)

• DERM: *scarlatiniform or morbilliform rash; bullous, exfoliative, or purpuric dermatitis; Stevens-Johnson syndrome;* lupus erythematosus; *hirsutism;* toxic epidermal necrolysis; photosensitivity.

• EENT: *nystagmus,* diplopia, blurred vision.

• GI: *nausea, vomiting, gingival hyperplasia, constipation.*

• HEMA: thrombocytopenia, leukopenia, agranulocytosis, pancytopenia, macrocytosis, *megaloblastic anemia, blood dyscrasias, lymphoadenopathy.*

• Hepatic: toxic hepatitis, jaundice, *liver damage.*

• Local: *pain, necrosis, and inflammation at injection site;* purple glove syndrome.

• Other: *periarteritis nodosa, lymphadenopathy, hyperglycemia, osteomalacia,* hypertrichosis.

Note: Drug should be discontinued if signs of hypersensitivity, hepatotoxicity, or blood dyscrasias occur, or if lymphadenopathy or skin rash occurs.

Overdose and treatment

Early signs of overdose may include drowsiness, nausea, vomiting, nystagmus, ataxia, dysarthria, tremor, and slurred speech; hypotension, respiratory depression, and coma may follow. Death is caused by respiratory and circulatory depression. Estimated lethal dose in adults is 2 to 5 g.

Treat overdose with gastric lavage or emesis and follow with supportive treatment. Carefully monitor vital signs and fluid and electrolyte balance. Forced diuresis is of little or no value. Hemodialysis or peritoneal dialysis may be helpful.

▶ Special considerations

• Special pediatric-strength suspension is available (30 mg/5 ml). Take extreme care to use correct strength. Do not confuse with adult strength (125 mg/5 ml).

• Monitor baseline liver function and hematologic laboratory studies including blood glucose levels and repeat at monthly intervals.

• Observe patient closely during therapy for possible adverse effects, especially at start of therapy. Phenytoin may cause gingival hyperplasia; good oral hygiene and gum care are essential to minimize this effect.

• Drug should not be discontinued abruptly, but slowly over 6 weeks; abrupt discontinuation may cause status epilepticus.

• Drug interactions are frequently a problem, primarily with hepatically cleared drugs, such as chloramphenicol, digitoxin, isoniazid, and griseofulvin; be

especially alert for toxic symptoms or breakthrough seizures in patients taking any of these drugs.
• Carefully follow manufacturer's directions for reconstitution, storage, and administration of all preparations.
• Monitoring of serum levels is essential because of dose-dependent excretion.
• Only extended-release capsules are approved for once-daily dosing; all other forms are given in divided doses every 8 to 12 hours.
• Oral or nasogastric feeding may interfere with absorption of oral suspension; separate doses as much as possible from feedings. During continuous tube feeding, tube should be flushed before and after dose.
• If suspension is used, shake well.
• I.M. administration should be avoided; it is painful and drug absorption is erratic.
• Mix I.V. doses in normal saline solution and use within 1 hour; mixtures with dextrose 5% will precipitate. Do not refrigerate solution; do not mix with other drugs.
• When giving I.V., continuous monitoring of ECG, blood pressure, and respiratory status is essential.
• Abrupt withdrawal may precipitate status epilepticus.
• If using I.V. bolus, use slow (50 mg/minute) I.V. push or constant infusion; too-rapid I.V. injection may cause hypotension and circulatory collapse. Do not use I.V. push in veins on back of hand; larger veins are needed to prevent discoloration associated with purple glove syndrome.
• Phenytoin often is abbreviated as DPH (diphenylhydantoin), an older drug name.

Information for parents and patient
• Tell parents that patient should avoid alcohol-containing beverages or elixirs while taking drug, as it may decrease drug's effectiveness and may increase CNS adverse reactions.
• Advise parents that patient should avoid hazardous tasks that require mental alertness until degree of CNS sedative effect is determined.
• Tell patient to take oral drug with food if GI distress occurs.
• Teach parents and patient signs and symptoms of hypersensitivity, liver dysfunction, and blood dyscrasias and to call the physician at once if any of the following occurs: sore throat, fever, bleeding, easy bruising, lymphadenopathy, or rash.
• Explain to adolescent patient and her parents the need to report suspected pregnancy immediately.
• Warn parents that patient should never discontinue drug suddenly or without medical supervision.
• Encourage parents to have patient wear a Medic Alert bracelet or necklace, indicating drug taken and seizure disorders.
• Caution parents to consult pharmacist before changing brand or using generic drug; therapeutic effect may change.
• Explain that drug may increase gum growth and sensitivity (gingival hyperplasia); teach proper oral hygiene and urge parents and patient to establish good mouth care.
• Assure parents and patient that pink or reddish brown discoloration of urine is normal and harmless.

physostigmine salicylate
Antilirium

physostigmine sulfate
Eserine, Isopto Eserine

• Classification: antimuscarinic antidote, antiglaucoma agent (cholinesterase inhibitor)

How supplied
Available by prescription only
Injection: 1 mg/ml
Ophthalmic ointment: 0.25%
Ophthalmic solution: 0.25%, 0.5%

Indications, route, and dosage
Tricyclic antidepressant and anticholinergic poisoning
Children: Not more than 0.5 mg I.V. over at least 1 minute. Dosage may be repeated at 5- to 10-minute intervals to a maximum of 2 mg if no adverse cholinergic signs are present.
Adults: 0.5 to 2 mg I.M. or I.V. given slowly (not to exceed 1 mg/minute I.V.) Dosage individualized and repeated as necessary.
Open-angle glaucoma
Children and adults: Instill 2 drops into eye(s) up to q.i.d., or apply ointment to lower fornix up to t.i.d.

Action and kinetics
• *Antimuscarinic action:* Physostigmine competitively blocks acetylcholine hydrolysis by cholinesterase, resulting in acetylcholine accumulation at cholinergic synapses; that antagonizes the muscarinic effects of overdose with antidepressants and anticholinergics. With ophthalmic use, miosis and ciliary muscle contraction increase aqueous humor outflow and decrease intraocular pressure.
• *Kinetics in adults:* Physostigmine is well absorbed when given I.M. or I.V., with effects peaking within 5 minutes. After ophthalmic use, physostigmine may be absorbed orally after passage through the nasolacrimal duct.
  Physostigmine is distributed widely and crosses the blood-brain barrier.
  Cholinesterase hydrolyzes physostigmine relatively quickly. Duration of effect is 1 to 2 hours after I.V. administration, 12 to 36 hours after ophthalmic use.
  Only a small amount of physostigmine is excreted in urine. Exact mode of excretion is unknown.

Contraindications and precautions
Physostigmine is contraindicated in patients with narrow angle glaucoma becuase it may cause pupilary blockage, resulting in increased intraocular pressure; and in patients with known hypersensitivity to cholinesterase inhibitors. Administer cautiously to patients with vagotonia, because they may experience enhanced drug effects; to patients with diabetes, because it may change insulin requirements; to patients with mechanical obstruction of the intestine or urinary tract, because of the drug's stimulatory effect

on smooth muscle; to patients with bradycardia and hypotension, because the drug may exacerbate these conditions; and to patients receiving depolarizing neuromuscular blocking agents, because physostigmine may enhance and prolong the effects of such drugs.

Also administer the drug cautiously to patients with epilepsy, because of the drug's possible CNS stimulatory effects; to patients with recent coronary occlusion or cardiac dysrhythmias, because of the drug's stimulatory effects on the cardiovascular system; to patients with peptic ulcer disease, because the drug may stimulate gastric acid secretion; and to patients with bronchial asthma, because the drug may precipitate asthma attacks.

Interactions

Concomitant use with succinylcholine may prolong respiratory depression by inhibiting hydrolysis of succinylcholine by plasma esterases. Concomitant use with ganglionic blockers, such as mecamylamine, may critically decrease blood pressure; this effect is usually preceded by abdominal symptoms. Concomitant use with systemic cholinergic agents may cause additive toxicity.

Effects on diagnostic tests

None reported.

Adverse reactions

• CNS: headache, convulsions, confusion, restlessness, hallucinations, muscle twitching, muscle weakness, ataxia, excitability.
• CV: bradycardia, hypotension, cardiac irregularities.
• EENT: blurred vision, conjunctivitis, miosis, ocular burning or stinging, lacrimation, browache, accommodative spasm, eyelid twitching, myopia, retinal detachment, vitreous hemorrhage, conjunctival and ciliary erythema, lens opacities, obstructed nasolacrimal canals, paradoxical increased intraocular pressure, activation of latent iritis or uveitis, iris cysts (usually in children).
• GI: nausea, vomiting, increased gastric and intestinal secretions, epigastric pain, diarrhea, excessive salivation.
• GU: urinary urgency, incontinence.
• Respiratory: increased tracheobronchial secretions, bronchiolar constriction, bronchospasm.
• Other: allergic reaction, sweating.
  Note: Drug should be discontinued if hypersensitivity, difficulty breathing, incoordination, restlessness, agitation, or skin rash occurs.

Overdose and treatment

Clinical effects of overdose include headache, nausea, vomiting, diarrhea, blurred vision, miosis, myopia, excessive tearing, bronchospasm, increased bronchial secretions, hypotension, incoordination, excessive sweating, muscle weakness, bradycardia, excessive salivation, restlessness or agitation, and confusion.

Support respiration; bronchial suctioning may be performed. The drug should be discontinued immediately. Atropine may be given to block physostigmine's muscarinic effects. Avoid atropine overdose, because it may cause bronchial plug formation.

▶ Special considerations

• Observe patients closely for cholinergic reactions, especially with parenteral forms.
• Have atropine available to reduce or reverse hypersensitivity reactions.
• Administer atropine before or with large doses of parenteral anticholinesterases to counteract muscarinic side effects.
• Dosage must be individualized according to severity of disease and patient response.
• Observe solution for discoloration. Do not use if darkened; contact pharmacist.
• Physostigmine sulfate injection has been used to reverse CNS depression caused by general anesthesia and drug overdose. However, this is an experimental use.

Ophthalmic administration

• Have patient lie down or tilt his head back to facilitate administration of eye drops.
• Wait at least 5 minutes before administering any other eye drops.
• Gently pinch patient's nasal bridge for 1 to 2 minutes after administering each dose of eye drops to minimize systemic absorption.
• After applying ointment, have patient close eyelids and roll eye.

Information for parents and patient

• Teach parents how to administer ophthalmic ointment or solution.
• Instruct patient not to close his eyes tightly or blink unnecessarily after instilling the ophthalmic solution.
• Warn parents and patient that blurred vision may follow initial doses.
• Instruct parents to report abdominal cramps, diarrhea, or excessive salivation.
• Remind parents to wait 5 minutes (if using eye drops) or 10 minutes (if using ointment) before using another eye preparation.

pilocarpine hydrochloride
Adsorbocarpine, Akarpine, Almocarpine, I-Pilopine, Isopto Carpine, Minims Pilocarpine*, Miocarpine*, Ocusert Pilo, Pilocar, Pilokair, Pilopine HS

pilocarpine nitrate
P.V. Carpine Liquifilm

• Classification: miotic (cholinergic agonist)

How supplied

Available by prescription only
Pilocarpine hydrochloride
Solution: 0.25%, 0.5%, 1%, 2%, 3%, 4%, 5%, 6%, 8%, 10%
Gel: 4%
Releasing-system insert: 20 mcg/hr, 40 mcg/hr
Pilocarpine nitrate
Solution: 1%, 2%, 4%

Indications, route, and dosage
Chronic open-angle glaucoma
Children and adults: Instill 1 or 2 drops of 1% to 4% solution in eye daily b.i.d. to q.i.d.; or apply gel (Pilopine HS) once daily.

Alternatively, apply one Ocusert Pilo (20 or 40 mcg/hour) every 7 days.
Emergency treatment of acute angle-closure glaucoma
Children and adults: Instill 1 drop of 2% solution in affected eye q 5 to 10 minutes for three to six doses, followed by 1 drop q 1 to 3 hours until pressure is controlled.

Action and kinetics
• *Miotic action:* Pilocarpine stimulates cholinergic receptors of the sphincter muscles of the iris, resulting in miosis. It also produces ciliary muscle contraction, resulting in accommodation with deepening of the anterior chamber, and vasodilation of conjunctival vessels of the outflow tract.

• *Kinetics in adults:* Pilocarpine drops act within 10 to 30 minutes, with peak effect at 2 to 4 hours. With the Ocusert Pilo, 0.3 to 7 mg of pilocarpine are released during the initial 6-hour period; during the remainder of the 1-week insertion period, the release rate is within ± 20% of the rated value. Effect is seen in 1½ to 2 hours and is maintained for the 1-week life of the insertion. Duration of effect of pilocarpine drops is 4 to 6 hours.

Contraindications and precautions
Pilocarpine is contraindicated in patients with acute iritis or hypersensitivity to the drug or any of the preparation's components. It should be used cautiously in patients with acute cardiac failure, bronchial asthma, urinary tract obstruction, GI spasm, peptic ulcer, or hyperthyroidism.

Interactions
When used concomitantly, pilocarpine can enhance reductions in intraocular pressure caused by epinephrine derivatives and timolol.

Demecarium, echothiophate, and isoflurophate decrease the pharmacologic effects of pilocarpine.

Effects on diagnostic tests
None reported.

Adverse reactions
• CNS: headache, syncope, tremors.
• CV: flushing, sweating, hypotension, bradycardia, dysrhythmias.
• Eye: myopia, burning, itching, ciliary spasm, blurred vision, conjunctival irritation, lacrimation, changes in visual field, brow ache.
• GI: nausea, vomiting, epigastric distress, abdominal cramps, diarrhea, salivation.
• GU: bladder tightness.
• Respiratory: asthma, bronchospasm.
Note: Drug should be discontinued if signs of systemic toxicity appear.

Overdose and treatment
Clinical manifestations of overdose include flushing, vomiting, bradycardia, bronchospasm, increased bronchial secretion, sweating, tearing, involuntary urination, hypotension, and tremors. Vomiting is usually spontaneous with accidental ingestion; if not, induce emesis and follow with activated charcoal or a cathartic. Treat dermal exposure by washing the areas twice with water. Use epinephrine to treat the cardiovascular responses. Atropine sulfate is the antidote of choice. Flush the eye with water or saline to treat a local overdose. Doses up to 20 mg are generally considered nontoxic.

▶ Special considerations
Drug may be used alone or with mannitol, urea, glycerol, or acetazolamide. It also may be used to counteract effects of mydriatic and cycloplegic agents after surgery or ophthalmoscopic examination.

Information for parents and patient
• Warn parents and patient that vision will be temporarily blurred, that miotic pupil may make surroundings appear dim and reduce peripheral field of vision, and that transient brow ache and myopia are common at first; assure them that side effects subside 10 to 14 days after therapy begins.
• Instruct parents and patient that if the Ocusert Pilo falls out of the eye during sleep, patient should wash hands, then rinse Ocusert in cool tap water and reposition it in the eye.
• Tell parents that patient should use caution in activities in poor illumination because miotic pupil diminishes side vision and illumination.
• Stress importance of complying with prescribed medical regimen.
• Apply light finger pressure to patient's lacrimal sac for 1 minute after administration to minimize systemic absorption.

pimozide
Orap

• Classification: antipsychotic (diphenylbutylpiperidine)

How supplied
Available by prescription only
Tablets: 2 mg

Indications, route, and dosage
Suppression of severe motor and phonic tics in patients with Gilles de la Tourette's syndrome
Adolescents age 12 and over and adults: Initially, 1 to 2 mg/day in divided doses. Then, increase dosage as needed every other day.
Maintenance dose: From 7 to 16 mg/day. Maximum dosage is 20 mg/day.

Action and kinetics

• *Antipsychotic action:* Pimozide's mechanism of action in Gilles de la Tourette's syndrome is unknown: it is thought to exert its effects by postsynaptic and/or presynaptic blockade of CNS dopamine receptors, thus inhibiting dopamine-mediated effects. Pimozide also has anticholinergic, antiemetic, and anxiolytic effects and produces alpha blockade.

• *Kinetics in adults:* Pimozide is absorbed slowly and incompletely from the GI tract; bioavailability is about 50%. Peak plasma levels may occur from 4 to 12 hours (usually in 6 to 8 hours). Pimozide is distributed widely into the body. Pimozide is metabolized by the liver; a significant first-pass effect exists. About 40% of a given dose is excreted in urine as parent drug and metabolites in 3 to 4 days; about 15% is excreted in feces via the biliary tract within 3 to 6 days.

Contraindications and precautions

Pimozide is contraindicated in patients with known hypersensitivity to phenothiazines, thioxanthenes, haloperidol, and molindone; in patients with any form of mild or severe tic, including those induced by pemoline, methylphenidate, or amphetamines; in patients with dysrhythmias because drug may cause ventricular dysrhythmias or aggravate existing dysrhythmias; in patients with congenital long QT syndrome because drug may cause conduction defects and sudden death; and in comatose states and CNS depression because of the risk of additive effects.

Pimozide should be used with extreme caution in patients taking antiarrhythmic drugs, tricyclic antidepressants, or other antipsychotic agents because additive effect may further depress cardiac conduction and prolong QT interval, and may induce dysrhythmias. Use pimozide cautiously in patients with other cardiac disease (congestive heart failure, angina pectoris, valvular disease, or heart block), encephalitis, Reye's syndrome, hematologic disorders, epilepsy and other seizure disorders, glaucoma, prostatic hypertrophy, urinary retention, hepatic or renal dysfunction, and Parkinson's disease because drug may worsen these conditions.

Interactions

Concomitant use of pimozide with quinidine, procainamide, disopyramide and other antiarrhythmics, phenothiazines, other antipsychotics, and antidepressants may further depress cardiac conduction and prolong QT interval, resulting in serious dysrhythmias.

Concomitant use with anticonvulsants (phenytoin, carbamazepine, or phenobarbital) may induce seizures, even in patients previously stabilized on anticonvulsants; an anticonvulsant dosage increase may be required.

Concomitant use with amphetamines, methylphenidate, or pemoline may induce Tourette-like tic and may exacerbate existing tics.

Concomitant use with CNS depressants, including alcohol, analgesics, barbiturates, narcotics, anxiolytics, parenteral magnesium sulfate, tranquilizers, and general, spinal, or epidural anesthetics may cause over-sedation and respiratory depression because of additive CNS depressant effects.

Effects on diagnostic tests

Pimozide causes quinidine-like ECG effects (including prolongation of QT interval and flattened T waves).

Adverse reactions

• CNS: parkinsonian symptoms, other extrapyramidal symptoms (dystonia, akathisia, hyperreflexia, opisthotonos, oculogyric crisis), tardive dyskinesia, sedation, headache, neuroleptic malignant syndrome (dose-related; fatal respiratory failure in over 10% of patients if untreated), hyperpyrexia. Seizures and sudden death have occurred with doses above 20 mg/day.

• CV: ventricular dysrhythmias (rare), ECG changes (prolonged QT interval, hypotension).

• EENT: visual disturbances, photophobia.

• GI: dry mouth, constipation, nausea, vomiting, taste changes.

• GU: impotence.

• Other: muscle tightness.

Note: Drug should be discontinued immediately if hypersensitivity or neuroleptic malignant syndrome (marked hyperthermia, extrapyramidal effects, autonomic dysfunction) occurs; if severe extrapyramidal symptoms occur even after dose is lowered; if ventricular dysrhythmias occur; or if QT interval is prolonged as follows: beyond 0.52 second in adults, beyond 0.47 second in children, or over 25% of patient's original baseline.

When feasible, drug should be withdrawn slowly and gradually; many drug effects persist after withdrawal.

Overdose and treatment

Clinical signs of overdose include severe extrapyramidal reactions, hypotension, respiratory depression, coma, and ECG abnormalities, including prolongation of QT interval, inversion or flattening of T waves, and/or new appearance of U waves.

Treat with gastric lavage to remove unabsorbed drug. Maintain blood pressure with I.V. fluids, plasma expanders, or norepinephrine. *Do not use epinephrine.*

Do not induce vomiting because of the potential for aspiration.

Treat extrapyramidal symptoms with parenteral diphenhydramine. Monitor for adverse effects for at least 4 days because of prolonged half-life (55 hours) of drug.

▶ Special considerations

• Use and efficacy in children under age 12 are limited. Dosage should be kept at the lowest possible level. Use of the drug in children for any disorder other than Gilles de la Tourette's syndrome is not recommended.

• All patients should have have baseline ECGs before therapy begins and periodic ECGs thereafter to monitor cardiovascular effects.

• Patient's serum potassium level should be maintained within normal range at all times; decreased potassium concentrations increase risk of dysrhythmias. Monitor potassium level in patients with diarrhea and those who are taking diuretics.

• Extrapyramidal reactions develop in approximately 10% to 15% of patients at normal doses. They are especially likely to occur during early days of therapy.

---

*Canada only   †Unlabeled clinical use   Italicized adverse reactions have been observed in children.

• If excessive restlessness and agitation occur, therapy with a beta blocker, such as propranolol or metoprolol, may be helpful.

Information for parents and patient
• Advise parents to have child take pimozide exactly as prescribed, not to double the dose for missed doses, not to share drug with others, and not to stop taking it suddenly.
• Explain that pimozide's therapeutic effect may not be apparent for several weeks.
• Inform parents of the risks, signs, and symptoms of dystonic reactions and tardive dyskinesia. Urge them to report unusual effects promptly.
• Tell parents that patient should not take pimozide with alcohol, sleeping medications, or any other drugs that may cause drowsiness without medical approval.
• Suggest using sugarless hard candy or chewing gum to relieve dry mouth.
• To prevent dizziness at start of therapy, patient should lie down for 30 minutes after taking each dose and should avoid sudden changes in posture, especially when rising to upright position.
• To minimize daytime sedation, the patient may take the entire daily dose at bedtime.
• Warn parents that patient should avoid hazardous activities that require alertness until the drug's effects are known.

---

piperacillin sodium
Pipracil

• Classification: antibiotic (extended-spectrum penicillin, acyclaminopenicillin)

How supplied
Available by prescription only
Injection: 2 g, 3 g, 4 g
Pharmacy bulk package: 40 g

Indications, route, and dosage
Infections caused by susceptible organisms
†*Children age 1 month to 12 years:* 50 mg/kg or 1.5 g/m² q 4 hours by I.V. infusion.
†*Neonates less than 1 week old:* 75 mg/kg I.V. q 8 to 12 hours.
Neonates older than 1 week: 75 mg/kg I.V. q 6 to 8 hours.
†*Premature infants:* 100 to 200 mg/kg I.V. daily, divided every 12 hours.
†*Term infants:* 150 to 300 mg mg/kg I.V. daily, divided every 6 to 8 hours.
Children with cystic fibrosis: 350 to 500 mg/kg/day divided q 4 hours.
Children over age 12 and adults: 100 to 300 mg/kg/day divided q 4 to 6 hours I.V. or I.M. Usual dosage is 3 g q 4 hours (18 g/day) and it is usually administered with an aminoglycoside. Maximum daily dosage is usually 24 g. Dosage for children under age 12 has not been established.

Prophylaxis of surgical infections
Adults: 2 g I.V., given 30 to 60 minutes before surgery. Depending on type of surgery, dose may be repeated during surgery and once or twice more after surgery according to the manufacturer. However, clinicians strongly discourage this practice.

Dosage in renal failure

DOSAGE IN ADULTS			
Creatinine clearance (ml/min/1.73 m²)	Urinary tract infection		Serious systemic infection
	uncomplicated	complicated	
> 40	*	*	*
20 to 40	*	3g q 8 hr	4g q 8 hr
< 20	3g q 12 hr	3g q 12 hr	4g q 12 hr
*no dosage adjustment necessary			

Action and kinetics
• *Antibiotic action:* Piperacillin is bactericidal; it adheres to bacterial penicillin-binding proteins, thus inhibiting bacterial cell wall synthesis.

Extended-spectrum penicillins resist inactivation by certain beta-lactamases, especially those produced by gram-negative organisms, but are still liable to inactivation by certain others. Because of the potential for rapid development of bacterial resistance, drug should not be used as a sole agent in the treatment of an infection.

Piperacillin's spectrum of activity includes many gram-negative aerobic and anaerobic bacilli, many gram-positive and gram-negative aerobic cocci, and some gram-positive aerobic and anaerobic bacilli. Piperacillin may be effective against some strains of carbenicillin-resistant and ticarcillin-resistant gram-negative bacilli. Piperacillin is more active against *Pseudomonas aeruginosa* than is mezlocillin and more active against *Enterobacteriaceae* than is azlocillin.
• *Kinetics in adults:* Peak plasma concentrations occur 30 to 50 minutes after an I.M. dose.

Piperacillin is distributed widely after parenteral administration. It penetrates minimally into uninflamed meninges and slightly into bone and sputum. Piperacillin is 16% to 22% protein-bound; it crosses the placenta.

Piperacillin is probably not significantly metabolized.

It is excreted primarily (42% to 90%) in urine by renal tubular secretion and glomerular filtration; it is also excreted in bile and in breast milk. Elimination half-life in adults is about ½ to 1½ hours; in extensive renal impairment, half-life is extended to about 2 to 6 hours; in combined hepatorenal dysfunction, half-life may extend from 11 to 32 hours. Piperacillin is removed by hemodialysis but not by peritoneal dialysis.

Contraindications and precautions

Piperacillin is contraindicated in patients with known hypersensitivity to any other penicillin or to cephalosporins.

Piperacillin should be used cautiously in patients with renal impairment because it is excreted in urine; decreased dosage is required in moderate to severe renal failure. Use with caution in patients with bleeding tendencies, uremia, or hypokolemia.

Interactions

Concomitant use of piperacillin with aminoglycoside antibiotics results in synergistic bactericidal effects against *Pseudomonas aeruginosa, Escherichia coli, Klebsiella, Citrobacter, Enterobacter, Serratia,* and *Proteus mirabilis.* However, the drugs are physically and chemically incompatible and are inactivated when mixed or given together. In vivo inactivation has been reported when aminoglycosides and extended-spectrum penicillins are used concomitantly.

Concomitant use of piperacillin (and other extended-spectrum penicillins) with clavulanic acid also produces a synergistic bactericidal effect against certain beta-lactamase-producing bacteria.

Probenecid blocks tubular secretion of piperacillin, raising serum concentrations of drug.

Large doses of penicillins may interfere with renal tubular secretion of methotrexate, thus delaying elimination and elevating serum concentrations of methotrexate.

Effects on diagnostic tests

Piperacillin may falsely decrease serum aminoglycoside concentrations. Piperacillin may cause hypokalemia and hypernatremia and may prolong prothrombin times; it may also cause transient elevations in liver function studies and transient reductions in red blood cell, white blood cell, and platelet counts.

Piperacillin may cause positive Coombs' tests.

Adverse reactions

• CNS: neuromuscular irritability, headache, dizziness.
• GI: nausea, diarrhea, vomiting.
• GU: acute interstitial nephritis.
• HEMA: bleeding with high doses, neutropenia, eosinophilia, leukopenia, thrombocytopenia.
• Metabolic: hypokalemia.
• Local: pain at injection site, vein irritation, phlebitis.
• Other: hypersensitivity reactions (edema, fever, chills, rash, pruritus, urticaria, anaphylaxis), bacterial and fungal superinfections.

Note: Drug should be discontinued if immediate hypersensitivity reactions occur, if bleeding complications occur, or if severe diarrhea occurs, as this may indicate pseudomembranous colitis.

Overdose and treatment

Clinical signs of overdose include neuromuscular hypersensitivity or seizures resulting from CNS irritation by high drug concentrations. A 4- to 6-hour hemodialysis will remove 10% to 50% of piperacillin.

▶ Special considerations

• Assess patient's history of allergies; do not give piperacillin to any patient with a history of hypersensitivity reactions to either penicillins or cephalosporins. Try to determine whether previous reactions were true hypersensitivity reactions or another reaction, such as GI distress, which the patient has interpreted as allergy.
• Keep in mind that a negative history for penicillin hypersensitivity does not preclude future allergic reactions; monitor patient continuously for possible allergic reactions or other untoward effects.
• In patients with renal impairment, dosage should be reduced if creatinine clearance is below 10 ml/minute.
• Assess level of consciousness, neurologic status, and renal function when high doses are used, because excessive blood levels can cause CNS toxicity.
• Obtain results of cultures and sensitivity tests before first dose; however, therapy may begin before test results are complete. Repeat tests periodically to assess drug efficacy.
• Monitor vital signs, electrolytes, and renal function studies; monitor body weight for fluid retention with extended-spectrum penicillins for possible hypokalemia or hypernatremia.
• Coagulation abnormalities, even frank bleeding, can follow high doses, especially of extended-spectrum penicillins; monitor prothrombin times and platelet counts, and assess patient for signs of occult or frank bleeding.
• Monitor patients on long-term therapy for possible superinfection, especially debilitated patients and others receiving immunosuppressants or radiation therapy; monitor closely, especially for fever.

Oral and parenteral administration

• Piperacillin may be more suitable than carbenicillin or ticarcillin for patients on salt-free diets; piperacillin contains only 1.98 mEq of sodium per gram.
• Give penicillins at least 1 hour before giving bacteriostatic antibiotics (tetracyclines, erythromycins, and chloramphenicol); these drugs inhibit bacterial cell growth, decreasing rate of penicillin uptake by bacterial cell walls.
• Administer I.M. dose deep into large muscle mass (gluteal or midlateral thigh); rotate injection sites to minimize tissue injury; do not inject more than 2 g of drug per injection site. Apply ice to injection site for pain.
• Do not add or mix other drugs with I.V. infusions—particularly aminoglycosides, which will be inactivated if mixed with penicillins; they are chemically and physically incompatible. If other drugs must be given I.V., temporarily stop infusion of primary drug.
• Infuse I.V. drug continuously or intermittently (over 30 minutes) and assess I.V. site frequently to prevent infiltration or phlebitis; rotate infusion site q 48 hours; intermittent I.V. infusion may be diluted in sterile water, 0.9% sodium chloride, dextrose 5% in water, dextrose 5% in water and half normal saline, or lactated Ringer's solution to a volume appropriate for the patient's weight.
• Solutions should always be clear, colorless to pale yellow, and free of particles; do not give solutions containing precipitates or other foreign matter.

- Piperacillin is almost always used with another antibiotic, such as an aminoglycoside, in life-threatening situations.
- Piperacillin may be administered by direct I.V. injection, given slowly over at least 5 minutes; chest discomfort occurs if injection is given too rapidly.
- Patients with cystic fibrosis are most susceptible to fever or rash from piperacillin.
- Monitor serum electrolytes, especially potassium.
- Monitor neurologic status. High serum levels of this drug may cause seizures.
- Reduced dosage is necessary in patients with creatinine clearance below 40 ml/minute.
- Monitor complete blood count, differential, and platelets. Drug may cause thrombocytopenia. Observe patient carefully for signs of occult bleeding.
- Because piperacillin is dialyzable, patients undergoing hemodialysis may need dosage adjustments.

Information for parents and patient
- Teach signs and symptoms of hypersensitivity and other adverse reactions, and emphasize need to report any unusual reactions.
- Teach signs and symptoms of bacterial and fungal superinfection to parents and patients, especially for debilitated patients and others with low resistance from immunosuppressants or irradiation; emphasize need to report signs of infection. Teach that meticulous oral and anogenital hygiene helps prevent such infection. Parents of infants and toddlers should keep diaper area clean and dry and avoid using plastic pants.
- Be sure parents and patient understand how and when to administer drug; urge them to complete entire prescribed regimen, to comply with instructions for around-the-clock dosage, and to keep follow-up appointments.
- Tell parents to check expiration date of drug and to discard unused drug.

piperazine citrate
Antepar, Vermizine

- Classification: anthelmintic (piperazine)

How supplied
Available by prescription only
Tablets: 250 mg, 500 mg
Syrup: 500 mg/5 ml

Indications, route, and dosage
Pinworm infections
Children and adults: 65 mg/kg P.O. daily for 7 to 8 days. Maximum daily dosage is 2.5 g. Repeat treatment course after 1-week interval in severe infection.
Roundworm infections
Children: 75 mg/kg P.O. daily in single doses for 2 consecutive days. Maximum daily dosage is 3.5 g.
Adults: 3.5 g P.O. in single doses for 2 consecutive days.

Action and kinetics
- *Anthelmintic action:* Piperazine blocks the stimulatory effects of acetylcholine at the neuromuscular junction of *Ascaris lumbricoides* (roundworm); it also inhibits succinate production, causing paralysis in the parasite. The mechanism of action against *Enterobius vermicularis* (pinworm) is unknown.
- *Kinetics in adults:* Piperazine is absorbed readily from the GI tract. It is metabolized partially by the liver. Most of an administered dose is excreted unchanged in the urine within 24 hours. It is unknown if piperazine is excreted in breast milk.

Contraindications and precautions
Piperazine is contraindicated in children with known sensitivity to piperazine compounds; in patients with impaired renal or hepatic function; and in patients with seizure disorders because it can exacerbate seizures.
Piperazine should be used with caution in children with severe malnutrition anemia because it can cause anemia.

Interactions
Concomitant use with chlorpromazine or other tranquilizers may exaggerate extrapyramidal symptoms. Piperazine antagonizes the effects of pyrantel pamoate.

Effects on diagnostic tests
Piperazine may cause electroencephalogram (EEG) changes, particularly in children; it may also interfere with serum uric acid measurements, leading to falsely low values.

Adverse reactions
- CNS: ataxia, tremors, choreiform movements, *muscular weakness,* myoclonus, hyporeflexia, paresthesias, convulsions, sense of detachment, *EEG abnormalities,* memory defect, headache, vertigo, seizures.
- DERM: *urticaria,* photodermatitis, erythema multiforme, purpura, eczematous skin reactions.
- EENT: nystagmus, *blurred vision,* paralytic strabismus, cataracts with visual impairment, lacrimation, difficulty in focusing, rhinorrhea, cough.
- GI: nausea, *vomiting,* diarrhea, abdominal cramps.
- Other: arthralgia, fever, bronchospasm.
  Note: Drug should be discontinued if significant GI or hypersensitivity reactions occur.

Overdose and treatment
Overdose may cause nausea, vomiting, confusion, weakness, ataxia, seizures, and coma. Treatment includes gastric lavage, followed by activated charcoal and cathartics. Seizures should be managed initially with diazepam; phenytoin or phenobarbital should be reserved for refractory seizures. Monitor fluid and electrolyte balance.

▶ Special considerations
- Avoid prolonged treatment or repeated treatment in excess of recommended dosage because of hazard of neurotoxicity; therapeutic dosages have caused EEG changes in children.

---

‡May contain sulfites   ◆May contain tartrazine   ◆◆May contain benzyl alcohol

• Piperazine may be taken with food but is most effective when taken on an empty stomach.
• Worm specimens are best obtained in early morning on arising.
• Laxatives, enemas, or dietary restrictions are unnecessary.
• Protect drug from light, air, and moisture.

Information for parents and patient
• Warn parents and patient not to exceed recommended dosage because of hazard of neurotoxicity at high doses.
• Tell parents to discontinue drug and to report CNS, GI, or hypersensitivity reactions.
• Emphasize importance of personal hygiene to prevent reinfection: washing perianal area daily, changing undergarments and bedclothes daily, washing hands and cleaning fingernails before meals and after defecation.
• Explain that transmission can occur by direct or indirect transfer of ova by hands, food, or contaminated articles and that washing clothes in a household washing machine will destroy ova.

---

plasma protein fraction
Plasmanate, Plasma-Plex, Plasmatein, Protenate

• Classification: plasma volume expander (blood derivative)

How supplied
Available by prescription only
Injection: 5% solution in 50-ml, 250-ml, 500-ml vials

Indications, route, and dosage
Shock
Children: 22 to 33 ml/kg I.V. infused at rate of 5 to 10 ml/minute.
Adults: Varies with patient's condition and response, but usually 250 to 500 ml (12.5 to 25 g protein) I.V., not to exceed 10 ml/minute.
Hypoproteinemia
Adults: 1,000 to 1,500 ml I.V. daily. Maximum infusion rate: 8 ml/minute.

Action and kinetics
• *Plasma-expanding action:* Plasma protein fraction supplies colloid to the blood and expands plasma volume. It causes fluid to shift from interstitial spaces into the circulation, and slightly increases plasma protein concentration. It is comprised mostly of albumin, but may contain up to 17% alpha and beta globulins, and not more than 1% gamma globulin. The pharmacokinetics of plasma protein fraction (PPF) are similar to its chief constituent, albumin (approximately 83% to 90%).
• *Kinetics in adults:* Albumin is not adequately absorbed from the GI tract. Albumin accounts for approximately 50% of plasma proteins. It is distributed into the intravascular space and extravascular sites, including skin, muscle, and lungs. In patients with reduced circulating blood volumes, hemodilution secondary to albumin administration persists for many hours; in patients with normal blood volume, excess fluid and protein are lost from the intravascular space within a few hours. Although albumin is synthesized in the liver, the liver is not involved in clearance of albumin from the plasma in healthy individuals. Little is known about albumin excretion in healthy individuals. Administration of albumin decreases hepatic albumin synthesis and increases albumin clearance if plasma oncotic pressure is high. In certain pathologic states, the liver, kidneys, or intestines may provide elimination mechanisms.

Contraindications and precautions
Plasma protein fraction (PPF) is contraindicated in patients with severe anemia or heart failure, in patients undergoing cardiac bypass surgery, and in patients with increased blood volume.
Administer PPF cautiously to patients with hepatic or renal failure, low cardiac reserve, or restricted salt intake.

Interactions
None significant.

Effects on diagnostic tests
PPF slightly increases plasma protein levels.

Adverse reactions
• CNS: headache.
• CV: variable effects on blood pressure after rapid I.V. infusion or after intraarterial administration, vascular overload after rapid infusion.
• DERM: erythema, urticaria.
• GI: nausea, vomiting, hypersalivation.
• Other: hypersensitivity, (flushing, chills, fever, back pain, dyspnea, chest tightness, cyanosis, shock).

Overdose and treatment
Rapid infusion can cause circulatory overload and pulmonary edema. Watch patient for signs of hypervolemia; monitor blood pressure and central venous pressure. Treatment is symptomatic.

▶ Special considerations
• Do not use solution that is cloudy, contains sediment, or has been frozen. Store at room temperature; freezing may break bottle and allow bacterial contamination.
• Use opened solution promptly, discarding unused portion after 4 hours; solution contains no preservatives and becomes unstable.
• One "unit" is usually considered to be 250 ml of the 5% concentration.
• Avoid rapid I.V. infusion. Rate is individualized according to patient's age, condition, and diagnosis. Maximum dosage is 250 g/48 hours; do not give faster than 10 ml/minute. Decrease infusion rate to 5 to 8 ml/minute as plasma volume approaches normal.
• Monitor blood pressure frequently; slow or stop infusion if hypotension suddenly occurs. Vital signs should return to normal gradually.
• Observe patient for signs of vascular overload (heart failure, pulmonary edema, widening pulse pressure

indicating increased cardiac output) and signs of hemorrhage or shock (after surgery or trauma); be alert for bleeding sites not evident at lower blood pressure.
• Monitor intake and output (watch especially for decreased output), hemoglobin, hematocrit, and serum protein and electrolyte levels to help determine ongoing dosage.
• If patient is dehydrated, give additional fluids either P.O. or I.V.
• Each liter contains 130 to 160 mEq of sodium before dilution with any additional I.V. fluids; a 250-ml container of the 5% concentration contains approximately 33 to 40 mEq sodium.

Information for parents and patient
• Explain therapy to parents and patient. Advise parents to monitor for adverse reactions.
• Inform parents or patient that drug is derived from donated human blood; however, risk of infection (hepatitis, HIV) is relatively low.

---

plicamycin (formerly mithramycin)
Mithracin

• Classification: antineoplastic, hypocalcemic agent (antibiotic antineoplastic [cell cycle-phase nonspecific])

How supplied
Available by prescription only
Injection: 2.5-mg vials

Indications, route, and dosage
Dosage and indications may vary. Check current literature for recommended protocol.
Hypercalcemia
Children and adults: 25 mcg/kg/dose I.V. daily over a period of 4 to 6 hours for 3 to 4 days. Repeat at intervals of 1 week as needed.

Action and kinetics
• *Antineoplastic action:* Plicamycin exerts its cytotoxic activity by intercalating between DNA base pairs and also binding to the outside of the DNA molecule. The result is inhibition of DNA-dependent RNA synthesis.
• *Hypocalcemic action:* The exact mechanism by which plicamycin lowers serum calcium levels is unknown. Plicamycin may block the hypercalcemic effect of vitamin D or may inhibit the effect of parathyroid hormone upon osteoclasts, preventing osteolysis. Both mechanisms reduce serum calcium concentrations.
• *Kinetics in adults:* Plicamycin is not administered orally. Plicamycin distributes mainly into the Kupffer's cells of the liver, into renal tubular cells, and along formed bone surfaces. The drug also crosses the blood-brain barrier and achieves appreciable concentrations in the CSF. The metabolic fate of plicamycin is unclear. It is eliminated primarily through the kidneys.

Contraindications and precautions
Plicamycin is contraindicated in patients with impaired bone marrow function, thrombocytopenia, thrombocytopathy, coagulation disorders, or electrolyte imbalance because it may worsen the symptoms associated with these disorders.

Exercise caution in patients with hepatic and renal dysfunction and in those who have previously received abdominal or mediastinal radiation, because these patients may be more susceptible to the drug's toxic effects.

Interactions
None reported.

Effects on diagnostic tests
Because of drug-induced toxicity, plicamycin therapy may increase serum concentrations of alkaline phosphatase, AST (SGOT), ALT (SGPT), lactic dehydrogenase (LDH), and bilirubin; it may also increase serum creatinine and BUN levels through nephrotoxicity.

Adverse reactions
• CNS: severe headache, lethargy.
• DERM: periorbital pallor, usually the day before toxic symptoms occur.
• GI: nausea, vomiting, anorexia, diarrhea, stomatitis, metallic taste.
• GU: proteinuria; increased BUN and serum creatinine levels.
• HEMA: *bone marrow depression* (dose-limiting); thrombocytopenia; *bleeding syndrome,* from epistaxis to generalized hemorrhage; facial flushing; depression of clotting factors.
• Metabolic: *decreased serum calcium,* potassium, and phosphorus levels.
• Local: *extravasation causes irritation, cellulitis.*
• Other: *hepatotoxicity, renal toxicity.*

Overdose and treatment
Clinical manifestations of overdose include myelosuppression, electrolyte imbalance, and coagulation disorders.

Treatment is usually supportive and includes transfusion of blood components and appropriate symptomatic therapy. Patient's renal and hepatic status should be closely monitored.

▶ Special considerations
• Not a first-line drug. Commonly used after other therapeutic alternatives have failed.
• To reconstitute drug, use 4.9 ml of sterile water to give a concentration of 0.5 mg/ml. Reconstitute drug immediately before administration, and discard any unused solution.
• Drug may be further diluted with normal saline solution or dextrose 5% in water (D_5W) to a volume of 1,000 ml and administered as an I.V. infusion over 4 to 8 hours.
• Drug may be administered by I.V. push injection, except in children. However, this method is discouraged because of the higher incidence and greater severity of GI toxicity. Nausea and vomiting are greatly diminished as the infusion rate is decreased.

---

‡May contain sulfites   ◆May contain tartrazine   ◆◆May contain benzyl alcohol

• Infusions of plicamycin in 1,000 ml D₅W are stable for up to 24 hours.
• If I.V. infiltrates, infusion should be stopped immediately and ice packs applied before restarting an I.V. in other arm.
• Give antiemetics before administering drug, to reduce nausea.
• Monitor LDH, AST (SGOT), ALT (SGPT), alkaline phosphatase, BUN, creatinine, potassium, calcium, and phosphorus levels.
• Monitor platelet count and prothrombin time before and during therapy.
• Check serum calcium levels. Monitor patient for tetany, carpopedal spasm, Chvostek's sign, and muscle cramps, because a precipitous drop in calcium levels is possible.
• Observe for signs of bleeding. Facial flushing may be an early indicator.
• Therapeutic effect in hypercalcemia may not be seen for 24 to 48 hours; may last 3 to 15 days.
• Avoid drug contact with skin or mucous membranes.
• Store lyophilized powder in refrigerator.

Information for parents and patient
• Tell parents that patient should use salicylate-free medication for pain or fever.
• Tell parents that patient should avoid exposure to people with infections.
• Advise parents that patient and other members of the household should not receive immunizations during therapy and for several weeks after therapy.

polythiazide
Renese

• Classification: diuretic, antihypertensive (thiazide)

How supplied
Available by prescription only
Tablets: 1 mg, 2 mg, 4 mg

Indications, route, and dosage
Hypertension, edema
Children: 0.02 to 0.08 mg/kg or 2 mg/m² P.O. daily.
Adults: 1 to 4 mg P.O. daily.

Action and kinetics
• *Diuretic action:* Polythiazide increases urinary excretion of sodium and water by inhibiting sodium reabsorption in the cortical diluting tubule of the nephron, thus relieving edema.
• *Antihypertensive action:* The exact mechanism of polythiazide's antihypertensive effect is unknown. It may be partially from direct arteriolar vasodilatation and a decrease in total peripheral resistance.
• *Kinetics in adults:* Polythiazide is absorbed from the GI tract. Distribution is unknown. In dogs, about 30% of a polythiazide dose is metabolized by the liver; the percentage metabolized in humans is unknown. Between 60% and 90% of polythiazide and its metabolites are excreted in urine.

Contraindications and precautions
Polythiazide is contraindicated in patients with anuria and in those with known sensitivity to the drug or to other sulfonamide derivatives. Polythiazide should be used cautiously in patients with severe renal disease, because it may decrease glomerular filtration rate and precipitate azotemia; in patients with impaired hepatic function or liver disease, because electrolyte changes may precipitate coma; and in patients taking digoxin, because hypokalemia may predispose them to digitalis toxicity.

Interactions
Polythiazide potentiates the hypotensive effects of most other antihypertensive drugs; this may be used to therapeutic advantage.

Polythiazide may potentiate hyperglycemic, hypotensive, and hyperuricemic effects of diazoxide, and its hyperglycemic effect may increase insulin requirements in diabetic patients.

Polythiazide may reduce renal clearance of lithium, elevating serum lithium levels, and may necessitate a 50% reduction in lithium dosage.

Polythiazide turns urine slightly more alkaline and may decrease urinary excretion of some amines, such as amphetamine and quinidine; alkaline urine may also decrease therapeutic efficacy of methenamine compounds, such as methenamine mandelate.

Cholestyramine and colestipol may bind polythiazide, preventing its absorption; give drugs 1 hour apart.

Effects on diagnostic tests
Polythiazide therapy may alter serum electrolyte levels and may increase serum urate, glucose, cholesterol, and triglyceride levels. It also may interfere with tests for parathyroid function and should be discontinued before such tests.

Adverse reactions
• CV: volume depletion and dehydration, orthostatic hypotension, hypercholesterolemia, hypertriglyceridemia.
• DERM: dermatitis, photosensitivity, rash.
• GI: anorexia, nausea, pancreatitis.
• HEMA: *aplastic anemia, agranulocytosis, leukopenia, thrombocytopenia.*
• Hepatic: hepatic encephalopathy.
• Metabolic: asymptomatic hyperuricemia; gout; hyperglycemia and impairment of glucose tolerance; fluid and electrolyte imbalances, including dilutional hyponatremia and hypochloremia, hypercalcemia, and hypokalemia; metabolic alkalosis.
• Other: hypersensitivity reactions, such as pneumonitis and vasculitis.

Note: Drug should be discontinued if rising BUN and serum creatinine levels indicate renal impairment or if patient shows signs of impending coma.

Overdose and treatment
Clinical signs of overdose include GI irritation and hypermotility, diuresis, and lethargy, which may progress to coma.

Treatment is mainly supportive; monitor and assist respiratory, cardiovascular, and renal function as indicated. Monitor fluid and electrolyte balance. Induce vomiting with ipecac in conscious patient; otherwise, use gastric lavage to avoid aspiration. Do not give cathartics; these promote additional loss of fluids and electrolytes.

▶ Special considerations
• Monitor weight and serum electrolyte levels regularly.
• Monitor serum potassium levels; encourage high-potassium diet. Foods rich in potassium include citrus fruits, tomatoes, bananas, dates, and apricots. Watch for signs of hypokalemia (for example, muscle weakness or cramps). Patients also taking digitalis have an increased risk of digitalis toxicity from the potassium-depleting effect of the drug.
• Polythiazide may be used with potassium-sparing diuretics to attenuate potassium loss.
• Check insulin requirements in patients with diabetes.
• Monitor serum creatinine and BUN levels regularly. Drug is not as effective if these levels are more than twice normal.
• Monitor blood uric acid levels.
• A.M. administration is recommended to prevent nocturia.
• Antihypertensive effects persist for approximately 1 week after discontinuation of the drug.
• Instruct parents to observe for and to report any joint swelling, pain, or redness; these signs may indicate hyperuricemia.

Information for parents and patient
• Explain rationale of therapy and diuretic effects of drug (increased volume and frequency of urination).
• Advise parents to watch for and promptly report signs of electrolyte imbalance: weakness, fatigue, muscle cramps, paresthesias, confusion, nausea, vomiting, diarrhea, headache, dizziness, and palpitations.
• Tell parents to report any increased edema or weight or excess diuresis (more than a 2% weight loss or gain); advise patient to record the child's weight each morning after voiding and before breakfast, using the same scale and wearing the same type of clothing.
• Advise parents to give drug with food to minimize gastric irritation; to encourage child to eat potassium-rich foods, such as citrus fruits, potatoes, dates, raisins, and bananas; and to restrict child's access to salt and high-sodium foods, such as lunch meat, smoked meats, and processed cheeses.
• Tell parents to seek medical approval before giving patient nonprescription drugs; many contain sodium and potassium and can cause electrolyte imbalances.
• Explain photosensitivity reactions. In thiazide-related photosensitivity, ultraviolet radiation alters drug structure, causing allergic reactions in some persons; such reactions occur 10 days to 2 weeks after initial sun exposure.
• Warn parents to supervise the child's activities closely to prevent falls and other injuries that may result from dizziness, especially at beginning of therapy.
• Caution patient to change position slowly, especially when rising to upright position, to prevent dizziness from orthostatic hypotension.

• Advise parents to watch patient closely for chest, back, or leg pain or shortness of breath and to call immediately if they occur.
• Advise parents to administer drug only as prescribed and at the same time each day, to prevent nighttime diuresis and interrupted sleep.
• Emphasize importance of regular medical follow-up to monitor effectiveness of diuretic therapy.

potassium iodide (KI, SSKI)
Pima, Iosat, Thyro-Block

• Classification: antihyperthyroid agent (electrolyte)

How supplied
Available by prescription only
Tablets (enteric-coated): 300 mg
Syrup: 325 mg/5 ml
Solution: 500 mg/15 ml
Saturated solution (SSKI): 1 g/ml
Strong iodine solution (Lugol's solution): iodine 50 mg/ml and potassium iodide 100 mg/ml

Indications, route, and dosage
Expectorant
Children: 60 to 250 mg q.i.d.
Adults: 300 to 650 mg t.i.d. or q.i.d.
Thyrotoxicosis
Children: 200 to 300 mg/day divided b.i.d. or t.i.d.
Adults: 300 to 900 mg/day t.i.d.
Preoperative thyroidectomy
Children and adults: 50 to 250 mg (or one to five drops) SSKI t.i.d.; or 0.1 to 0.3 ml (or three to five drops) Lugol's solution t.i.d.; give drug for 10 to 14 days before surgery.
Nuclear radiation protection
Infants under age 1: Half the adult dosage.
Children and adults: 0.13 ml P.O. of SSKI (130 mg) immediately before or after initial exposure will block 90% of radioactive iodine. Same dosage given 3 to 4 hours after exposure will provide 50% block. Drug should be administered for up to 10 days under medical supervision.

Potassium iodide is used unofficially as an iodine replenisher (adults: 5 to 10 mg daily; children: 1 mg/day) and as an antifungal agent.

Actions and kinetics
• *Expectorant action:* The exact mechanism of potassium iodide's expectorant effect is unknown; it is believed that potassium iodide reduces viscosity of mucus by increasing respiratory tract secretions.
• *Antihyperthyroid agent action:* Potassium iodide acts directly on the thyroid gland to inhibit synthesis and release of thyroid hormone.
• *Kinetics in adults:* Absorption, distribution, metabolism, and excretion have not been reported.

Contraindications and precautions
Potassium iodide is contraindicated in patients hypersensitive to iodides or iodine, and during pregnancy, because abnormal thyroid and goiter may occur.

---

‡May contain sulfites   ◆May contain tartrazine   ◆◆May contain benzyl alcohol

Drug should be used with caution in patients with hyperkalemia, acute bronchitis, or tuberculosis; in children with cystic fibrosis, because they are especially susceptible to the goitrogenic effects of iodides; and in patients with thyroid disease. Prolonged use of potassium iodide may cause hypothyroidism; goiter may occur in iodide-sensitive hyperthyroid patients.

Interactions

Lithium potentiates both hypothyroid and goitrogenic effects of potassium iodide. Concomitant use with potassium-sparing diuretics or potassium-containing drugs may cause hyperkalemia and subsequent dysrhythmia or cardiac arrest.

Effects on diagnostic tests

Potassium iodide may alter the results of thyroid function tests.

Adverse reactions

• DERM: *rash.*
• GI: *nausea, vomiting, epigastric pain.*
• Metabolic: goiter, hyperthyroid adenoma, hypothyroidism (with excessive use), collagen disease-like syndrome.
• Other: *metallic taste, salivary gland inflammation, headache, lacrimation, rhinitis.*
• Prolonged use: chronic iodine poisoning, soreness of mouth, coryza, sneezing, swelling of eyelids.

Note: Drug should be discontinued if skin rash or signs of acute or chronic poisoning occur; or if patient has abdominal pain, distention, nausea, vomiting, or GI bleeding: enteric-coated tablets reportedly have caused bowel lesions, with possible obstruction, perforation, and hemorrhage.

Overdose and treatment

Acute overdose is rare; angioedema, laryngeal edema, and cutaneous hemorrhages may occur. Treat hyperkalemia immediately; salt and fluid intake help eliminate iodide.

Iodism (chronic iodine poisoning) may follow prolonged use; symptoms include metallic taste, sore mouth, swollen eyelids, sneezing, skin eruptions, nausea, vomiting, epigastric pain, and diarrhea. Discontinue drug and treat supportively.

▶ **Special considerations**

• Strong iodine solution is used for treating Graves' disease in neonates (1 drop q 8 hours).
• Monitor serum potassium levels before and during therapy; patients taking any diuretic, especially potassium-sparing diuretics, are at risk for hyperkalemia.
• Dilute with 180 ml of water, fruit juice, or broth to reduce GI distress and disguise strong, salty metallic taste; advise patient to use a straw to avoid teeth discoloration.
• Store in light-resistant container because exposure to light liberates traces of free iodine; if crystals develop in solution, dissolve them by placing container in warm water and carefully agitating it.
• Drug may cause flare-up of adolescent acne or other skin rash.

• Sudden withdrawal may precipitate thyroid storm.
• Maintain fluid intake when using drug as an expectorant; adequate hydration encourages optimal expectorant action.

Information for parents and patient

• When enteric-coated tablets are prescribed, tell parents to give tablet with small amount of water, and tell patient to swallow tablet whole (not crush or chew) and follow with a glass of water or juice.
• Advise parents and patient that patient should drink all of solution prepared and should use a straw to avoid discoloring teeth.
• Review symptoms of iodism with parents, and instruct them to report such symptoms, especially abdominal pain, distention, nausea, vomiting, or GI bleeding.
• Caution parents not to give patient OTC drugs without medical approval; many preparations contain iodides and could potentiate drug. For the same reason, discuss ingestion of iodized salt and shellfish.

potassium salts, oral

potassium acetate

potassium bicarbonate
Klor-Con, EF, K-Lyte, Quic-K

potassium chloride
Apo-K*, Cena-K, K-10*, Kalium Durules*, Kaochlor, Kaochlor S-F, Kaon-Cl, Kato, Kay Ciel, KCL*, K-Dur, K-Long*, K-Lor, Klor-10%, Klor-Con, Klor-Con/25, Klorvess, Klotrix, K-Lyte/Cl Powder, K-Tab, Micro-K, Novolente-K*, Potachlor, Potage, Potasalan, Potassine, Roychlor*, Rum-K, Slo-Pot*, Slow-K, Ten-K

potassium gluconate

• Classification: potassium supplement (electrolyte)

How supplied

Available by prescription only
Sustained-released tablets (chloride): 8 mEq, 10 mEq
Powder: 20 mEq/package
Liquid: 15 mEq/15 ml, 20 mEq/15 ml, 30 mEq/15 ml
Effervescent tablets: 20 mEq, 25 mEq, 50 mEq
Vial: 2 mEq/ml in 20, 50, and 100 ml vials (acetate); 2 mEq/ml in 5, 10, 15, 20, 30, and 100 ml vials (chloride)

Indications, route, and dosage
Hypokalemia

Children and adults: 25-mEq tablet of potassium bicarbonate dissolved in water daily to q.i.d. Use I.V. potassium phosphate when oral replacement is not feasible or when hypokalemia is life-threatening; dosage is up to 20 mEq/hour in concentration of 60 mEq/liter or less. Maximum rate of infusion in children

---

*Canada only   †Unlabeled clinical use   Italicized adverse reactions have been observed in children.

should not exceed 0.5 to 1 mEq/kg/hour. Further doses are based on individual requirements and serum potassium determinations. Total daily dose should not exceed 3 mEq/kg in children or 150 mEq in adults.

To treat, give 40 to 100 mEq potassium phosphate orally divided into three to four doses daily; further doses are based on serum potassium level and blood pH. Potassium replacement should be carried out only with ECG monitoring and frequent serum potassium determinations.

Prevention of hypokalemia
Children and adults: Initially, 20 mEq of potassium acetate P.O. daily, in divided doses if needed; or 10 to 15 mEq of potassium chloride three or four times a day.

Potassium replacement
Children and adults: Potassium chloride should be diluted in a suitable I.V. solution (not more than 40 mEq/liter) and administered at a rate no greater than 10 to 15 mEq/hour or 0.5 to 1 mEq/kg/hour in children. Total dosage should not exceed 400 mEq/day. Potassium replacement should be carried out only with ECG monitoring and frequent serum potassium determinations.

Action and kinetics
• *Potassium replacement action:* Potassium, the main cation in body tissue, is necessary for maintaining intracellular tonicity, maintaining a balance with sodium across cell membranes, transmitting nerve impulses, maintaining cellular metabolism, contracting cardiac and skeletal muscle, maintaining acid-base balance, and maintaining normal renal function.
• *Kinetics in adults:* Potassium is well absorbed from the GI tract. It should be taken with meals and sipped slowly over a 5- to 10-minute period to decrease irritation. Potassium bicarbonate does not correct hypochloremic alkalosis. The normal serum levels of potassium range from 3.8 to 5 mEq/liter. Up to 60 mEq/liter of potassium may be found in gastric secretions and diarrhea fluid. Potassium is excreted largely by the kidneys. Small amounts of potassium may be excreted via the skin and intestinal tract, but intestinal potassium usually is reabsorbed. A healthy patient on a potassium-free diet will excrete 40 to 50 mEq of potassium daily.

Contraindications and precautions
Potassium is contraindicated in patients with severe renal impairment, oliguria, anuria, or azotemia (unless patient is hypokalemic); hyperkalemia from any cause; untreated Addison's disease because of the potential for hyperkalemia; acute dehydration; or heat cramps because administration of potassium can worsen these conditions. Concomitant use of potassium-sparing diuretics is contraindicated, unless patients are routinely monitored.

Administer potassium (particularly I.V. potassium) cautiously in patients with cardiac disease, renal disease, or acidosis; conduct careful analysis of the acid-base balance, and monitor serum electrolyte levels, ECG, and clinical status of the patient. Acidosis can raise serum potassium levels to the normal range even when total body potassium is reduced.

Interactions
When used concomitantly with potassium, anticholinergics that slow GI motility may increase the chance of GI irritation and ulceration.

Concomitant administration with potassium-containing products may cause hyperkalemia within 1 to 2 days. Potassium should be used cautiously in digitalized patients with severe or complete heart block because of potential for dysrhythmias. Concomitant use with potassium-sparing diuretics or salt substitutes containing potassium salts can cause severe hyperkalemia.

Effects on diagnostic tests
None reported.

Adverse reactions
Signs of hyperkalemia:
• CNS: paresthesias of the extremities, headache, *listlessness*, mental confusion, *weakness* or heaviness of limbs, *flaccid paralysis*.
• CV: *hypotension*, peripheral vascular collapse with fall in blood pressure, *cardiac dysrhythmias*, heart block, possible cardiac arrest, ECG changes (prolonged PR interval; wide QRS complex; ST segment depression; tall, tented T waves). Extremely high plasma concentrations (8 to 11 mEq/liter) may cause death from cardiac depression, dysrhythmias, or arrest.
• DERM: cold skin, gray pallor.
• GI: *nausea, vomiting, abdominal pain, diarrhea, GI ulcerations* (possible stenosis, hemorrhage, obstruction, perforation), esophageal ulceration from wax matrix tablets (sustained-release) in patient with enlarged atrium.
• GU: oliguria.
• Local: postinfusion phlebitis.
• Other: soft tissue calcification.

Overdose and treatment
Clinical manifestations of overdose include increased serum potassium concentration and characteristic ECG changes. Late clinical signs include weakness, paralysis of voluntary muscles, respiratory distress, and dysphagia. These may precede severe or fatal cardiac toxicity. Hyperkalemia produces symptoms paradoxically similar to those of hypokalemia.

Treatment of potassium overdose includes discontinuation of the potassium supplement and, if necessary, lavage of the GI tract. In patients with a potassium concentration greater then 6.5 mEq/liter, supportive therapy may include the following interventions (with continuous ECG monitoring):

Infuse 40 to 160 mEq sodium bicarbonate I.V. over a 5-minute interval; repeat in 10 to 15 minutes if ECG abnormalities persist.

Infuse 300 to 500 ml of dextrose 10% to 25% over 1 hour. Insulin (5 to 10 units per 20 g of dextrose) should be added to the infusion or, ideally, administered as a separate injection.

Patients with absent P waves or broad QRS complex who are not receiving cardiotonic glycosides should immediately be given 0.5 g to 1 g of calcium gluconate or another calcium salt I.V. over a 2-minute period (with continuous ECG monitoring) to antagonize the cardiotoxic effect of the potassium. May be repeated in 1 to 2 minutes if ECG abnormalities persist.

To remove potassium from the body, use sodium polystyrene sulfonate resin, hemodialysis, or peritoneal dialysis. Administer potassium-free I.V. fluids when hyperkalemia is associated with water loss.

▶ **Special considerations**
• In patients receiving digitalis, removing potassium too rapidly may result in digitalis toxicity.
• Monitor serum potassium and other electrolyte, BUN, and serum creatinine levels; pH; intake and output; and ECG.
• Potassium should not be given during immediate postoperative period until urine flow is established.
• Give parenteral potassium by slow infusion only, never by I.V. push or I.M. Dilute I.V. potassium preparations with large volume of parenteral solutions.
• Give oral potassium supplements with extreme caution, because its many forms deliver varying amounts of potassium. Patient may tolerate one product better than another.
• Potassium gluconate does not correct hypokalemic hypochloremic alkalosis.
• Enteric-coated tablets are not recommended because of the potential for GI bleeding and small-bowel ulcerations.
• Tablets in wax matrix sometimes lodge in esophagus and cause ulceration in cardiac patients who have esophageal compression due to enlarged left atrium. In such patients and in those with esophageal or GI stasis or obstruction, use liquid form.
• Often used orally with diuretics that cause potassium excretion. Potassium chloride most useful since diuretics waste chloride ion. Hypokalemic alkalosis treated best with potassium chloride.
• Do not crush sustained-released potassium products.

Information for parents and patient
• Tell parents that potassium is available only with a prescription because the wrong amount may cause severe reactions.
• Suggest diluting liquid potassium product in at least 4 to 8 oz of water; taking it after meals; and sipping liquid potassium slowly, to minimize GI irritation.
• Tell parents to dissolve powder, soluble tablets, or granules completely in at least 4 oz of water or juice and to allow fizzing to finish before giving to patient.
• Sustained-release capsules should not be crushed or chewed, but the capsule contents can be opened and sprinkled onto applesauce or other soft food.
• Tell parents to discontinue drug immediately if patient develops any of the following reactions: confusion; irregular heartbeat; numbness of feet, fingers, or lips; shortness of breath; anxiety; excessive tiredness or weakness of legs; unexplained diarrhea; nausea and vomiting; stomach pain; or bloody or black stools. Such reactions should be reported promptly.
• Tell the parents that patient may expel a whole tablet in the stool (sustained-release tablet). The body eliminates the shell after absorbing the potassium.

pramoxine hydrochloride
Fleet relief, PrameGel, Prax, ProctoFoam, Tronolane, Tronothane

• Classification: topical anesthetic

How supplied
Available without a prescription
Cream: 1%
Lotion: 1%
Ointment: 1%
Suppositories: 1%
Aerosol: 1% foam suspension
Gel: 1% gel

Indications, route, and dosage
For temporary relief of pain and itching caused by dermatoses, minor burns
Children and adults: Apply cream, gel or lotion to affected area t.i.d or q.i.d. or as directed.
For temporary relief of pain and itching associated with anogenital pruritus or irritation
Children and adults: Apply aerosol foam to affected area as directed.
For temporary relief of pain and itching caused by hemorrhoids
Adults: Apply cream, ointment, or suppositories up to 5 times daily or as directed; or alternatively, one applicatorful of the foam rectally b.i.d. or q.i.d. and after bowel movements.

Action and kinetics
• *Anesthetic action:* Inhibits the conduction of nerve impulses by causing an alteration of cell membrane permeability to ions. This causes a specific anesthetic action on the local nerve cells.
• *Kinetics in adults:* Absorption is limited with topical use, unless skin tissue is abraded or drug is applied to mucous membranes.

Contraindications and precautions
Avoid use over large areas. Do not use in or near the eyes or nose. Pramoxine is contraindicated in patients with known hypersensitivity to the drug.

Interactions
None reported.

Effects on diagnostic tests
None reported.

Adverse reactions
• Local: burning, stinging.
   Note: Drug should be discontinued if sensitization, extreme irritation, or redness occurs.

Overdose and treatment
No information available.

▶ **Special considerations**
• Dosage should be adjusted to patient's age, size, and physical condition.

• Drug is not recommended for prolonged use. Drug should be discontinued after 4 consecutive weeks of use.

• Drug may be applied with gauze or sprayed directly on skin. Cleanse and thoroughly dry rectal area before applying.

Information for parents and patient

• Tell parents to wash hands thoroughly before and after use.

• Advise parents to apply drug sparingly, to minimize untoward effects.

---

praziquantel
Biltricide

• Classification: anthelmintic (pyrazinoisoquinoline)

How supplied
Available by prescription only
Tablets: 600 mg

Indications, route, and dosage
Schistosomiasis
Children age 4 and over and adults: 20 mg/kg P.O. t.i.d. as a 1-day treatment. The interval between doses should be between 4 and 6 hours, and all doses should be given on the same day.
Trematodiasis caused by Clonorchis sinesis, Fasciolopsis buski, Heterophyes heterophyes, Metagonimus yokagowai, or Opisthorchis viverinii
Children and adults: 25 mg/kg P.O. t.i.d. as a 1-day-treatment. The interval between the doses should be between 4 and 6 hours, and all doses should be given on the same day.
Trematodiasis caused by Fasciola hepatica
Children and adults: 25 mg/kg P.O. t.i.d. for 5 to 8 days
Trematodiasis caused by Clonorchis sinensis, Paragonimus westermani, or Paragonimus uterobilateralis
Children and adults: 25 mg/kg P.O. t.i.d. for 2 days.
Adult (intestinal stage) cestodiasis caused by Diphlobothrium latum, Dipylidium caninum, or Taenia saginata
Children and adults: 10 to 20 mg mg/kg P.O. as a single dose.
Adult (intestinal stage) cestodiasis caused by Hymenolepsis nana
Children and adults: 50 mg/kg/day P.O. in 3 divided doses for 14 days.
Neurocysticercosis
Children and adults: 50 mg/kg/day P.O. in 3 divided doses for 14 to 21 days. Usually administered with corticosteroids.

Action and kinetics
• *Anthelmintic action:* Praziquantel appears to increase cell permeability to calcium, causing paralysis of the worms' musculature, dislodgment from mesenteric and pelvic veins, and subsequent death by host tissue reaction. It is effective against all pathogenic *Schistosoma*, including *S. mekongi, S. japonica, S. mansoni,* and *S. haematobia,* and has some activity against tapeworms.
• *Kinetics in adults:* About 80% of praziquantel is absorbed; peak serum concentrations occur at 1 to 3 hours. Distribution of praziquantel is not well documented; however, CSF levels are approximately 14% to 20% of plasma levels. Praziquantel undergoes significant first-pass metabolism to hydroxylated metabolites in the liver. Drug and metabolites are excreted primarily in urine. Drug half-life is about 1 to 1 ½ hours; metabolite half-life is 4 to 5 hours. Drug is excreted in breast milk.

Contraindications and precautions
Praziquantel is contraindicated in patients with known hypersensitivity to the drug and in patients with ocular involvement of schistosomiasis, because destruction of parasites within eyes may cause irreversible ocular damage. Safety has not been established in children under age 4.

Interactions
None reported.

Effects on diagnostic tests
Praziquantel may increase CSF protein concentrations and serum liver enzyme concentrations.

Adverse reactions
• CNS: drowsiness, malaise, headache, dizziness, seizures.
• GI: abdominal discomfort, nausea, vomiting, anorexia, diarrhea.
• Hepatic: minimal increase in liver enzyme levels.
• Other: rise in body temperature, sweating.
  Note: Drug should be discontinued if signs of hypersensitivity or toxicity occur.

Overdose and treatment
Acute overdose has not been reported. Should it occur, a fast-acting laxative would be appropriate treatment.

▶ Special considerations
• Give drug during meals or with food, and follow with water to minimize GI discomfort; tablets are bitter and may cause gagging or vomiting if incompletely swallowed.
• Adverse effects may be more common and severe in patients with heavy infestation.
• When treating neurocysticercosis, most clinicians recommend the administration of corticosteroids to minimize the CSF reaction syndrome (seizures, increased CSF protein concentration, increased anticysteral IgG levels, intracranial hypertension) which may result from an intense inflammatory response to dead and dying larvae within the CNS.

Information for parents and patient
• Explain that drug may cause drowsiness; patient should avoid hazardous activities that require alertness on the day of and the day after treatment.
• Recommend post-treatment evaluation of stool specimens, to ensure destruction of parasites.

---

prazosin hydrochloride
Minipress

• Classification: antihypertensive (alpha-adrenergic blocking agent)

How supplied
Available by prescription only
Capsules: 1 mg, 2 mg, 5 mg

Indications, route, and dosage
Hypertension
†*Children:* 25 to 40 mcg/kg P.O. q 6 hours.
Adults: Initially, 1 mg P.O. b.i.d. or t.i.d.; gradually increased to a maximum of 20 mg daily. Usual maintenance dosage is 6 to 15 mg daily in divided doses. If other antihypertensive or diuretics are added to prazosin therapy, reduce dosage of prazosin to 1 or 2 mg t.i.d. and then gradually increase as necessary.

Action and kinetics
• *Antihypertensive action:* Prazosin selectively and competitively inhibits alpha-adrenergic receptors, causing arterial and venous dilation and reducing peripheral vascular resistance and blood pressure.
• *Kinetics in adults:* Absorption from the GI tract is variable; antihypertensive effect begins in about 2 hours, peaking in 2 to 4 hours. Full antihypertensive effect may not occur for 4 to 6 weeks. Prazosin is distributed throughout the body and is highly protein-bound (approximately 97%). Prazosin is metabolized extensively in the liver. Over 90% of a given dose is excreted in feces via bile; remainder is excreted in urine. Plasma half-life is 2 to 4 hours. Antihypertensive effect lasts less than 24 hours.

Contraindications and precautions
Prazosin is contraindicated in patients with known hypersensitivity to the drug.
Drug should be used cautiously in patients taking other antihypertensive drugs and those with chronic renal failure.

Interactions
Prazosin may potentiate the antihypertensive effects of other antihypertensive agents, including propranolol.
Concomitant use with propranolol and other beta blockers may cause severe hypotension.
Because prazosin is highly bound to plasma proteins, it may interact with other highly-protein bound drugs.

Effects on diagnostic tests
Prazosin alters results of screening tests for pheochromocytoma and causes increases in levels of the urinary metabolite of norepinephrine and vanillylmandelic acid; it may cause positive antinuclear antibody (ANA) titer and liver function test abnormalities. A transient fall in leukocyte count and increased serum uric acid and BUN levels may also occur.

Adverse reactions
• CNS: *dizziness, headache, drowsiness,* weakness, *fatigue, first-dose syncope,* depression.
• CV: *orthostatic hypotension,* palpitations, *tachycardia.*
• EENT: blurred vision, dry mouth.
• GI: vomiting, diarrhea, abdominal cramps, constipation, *nausea.*
• GU: priapism, impotence.

Overdose and treatment
Overdose is manifested by hypotension and drowsiness. After acute ingestion, empty stomach by induced emesis or gastric lavage, and give activated charcoal to reduce absorption. Further treatment is usually symptomatic and supportive. Prazosin is not dialyzable.

▶ Special considerations
• Safety and efficacy in children have not been established; use only when potential benefit outweighs risk.
• First-dose syncope — dizziness, light-headedness, and syncope — may occur within 30 minutes to 1 hour after the initial dose; it may be severe, with loss of consciousness, if initial dose is greater than 2 mg. The effect is transient and may be diminished by giving the drug at bedtime; it is more common during febrile illness and more severe if patient has hyponatremia. Always increase dosage gradually and have patient sit or lie down if he experiences dizziness.
• Prazosin's effect is most pronounced on diastolic blood pressure.
• Prazosin has been used to treat vasospasm associated with Raynaud's syndrome. It also has been used with diuretics and cardiac glycosides to treat severe CHF, to manage the signs and symptoms of pheochromocytoma preoperatively, and to treat ergotamine-induced peripheral ischemia.
• Monitor vital signs, especially blood pressure.

Information for parents and patient
• Teach parents and patient about the disease and therapy, and explain why the patient must take drug exactly as prescribed, even when feeling well; advise him never to discontinue drug suddenly, because severe rebound hypertension may occur, and to promptly report any malaise or any unusual adverse effects.
• Tell parents that patient should avoid hazardous activities that require mental alertness until tolerance develops to sedation, drowsiness, and other CNS effects; avoid sudden position changes to minimize orthostatic hypotension; and use ice chips, candy, or gum to relieve dry mouth.
• Warn parents to seek medical approval before giving patient nonprescription cold preparations.
• Warn parents and patient about postural hypotension. Tell patient to avoid sudden changes to upright position.
• Tell parents to promptly report dizziness or irregular heart beat.
• Advise parents to have patient take dose at bedtime to reduce potential for dizziness or light-headedness.
• Reassure parents and patient that adverse effects should subside after several doses.

• Tell parents and patient that the use of alcohol, excessive exercise, prolonged standing, and exposure to heat will intensify adverse effects.
• Advise parents against giving patient any other medication, including any that can be purchased without a prescription.

---

prednisolone
Systemic: Cortalone, Delta-Cortef, Novoprednisolone*, Prelone

prednisolone acetate
Systemic: Articulose, Deltastab*, Key-Pred, Predaject, Predate, Predcor

Ophthalmic: AK-Tate, Econopred Ophthalmic, I-Prednicet, Ocu-Pred-A, Predair-A, Pred Forte, Pred Mild Ophthalmic

prednisolone acetate and prednisolone sodium phosphate

prednisolone sodium phosphate
Systemic: Codelsol*, Hydeltrasol, Key-Pred SP, Pediapred, Predate-S

Ophthalmic: AK Pred, Inflamase, Inflamase Mild Ophthalmic, Inflamase Forte, I-Pred, Metreton, Ocu-Pred, Predair, Predsol*

prednisolone tebutate
Systemic: Hydeltra-T.B.A., Metalone T.B.A., Nor-Pred T.B.A., Predate T.B.A., Predcor T.B.A., Predisol T.B.A.

• Classification: anti-inflammatory, immunosuppressant (glucocorticoid, mineralocorticoid)

How supplied
Available by prescription only
Prednisolone
Tablets: 5 mg
Syrup: 15 mg/5 ml
Prednisolone acetate
Injection: 25 mg/ml, 50 mg/ml, 100 mg/ml suspension
Ophthalmic suspension: 0.12%, 0.125%, 0.25%, 1%
Prednisolone acetate and prednisolone sodium phosphate
Injection: 80 mg acetate and 20 mg sodium phosphate/ml suspension
Prednisolone sodium phosphate
Oral liquid: 6.7 mg (5 mg base)/5 ml
Injection: 20 mg/ml solution
Ophthalmic solution: 0.125%, 0.5%, 1%
Prednisolone tebutate
Injection: 20 mg/ml suspension

Indications, route, and dosage
Severe inflammation or immunosuppression
Adults: 2.5 to 15 mg P.O. b.i.d., t.i.d., or q.i.d.

Prednisolone acetate
Adults: 2 to 30 mg I.M. q 12 hours
Prednisolone sodium phosphate
Children: .04 to .25 mg/kg or 1.5 to 7.5mg/m² I.V. once or twice daily.
Adults: 2 to 30 mg I.M. or I.V. q 12 hours, or into joints, lesions and soft tissue, p.r.n.
Prednisolone tebutate
Adults: 4 to 40 mg into joints and lesions, p.r.n.
Prednisolone acetate and prednisolone sodium phosphate suspension
Adults: 0.25 to 1 ml into joints weekly, p.r.n.

Inflammation of palpebral and bulbar conjunctiva, cornea, and anterior seqment of globe
Predinsolone acetate, prednisolone sodium phosphate
Children and adults: Instill 1 or 2 drops in eye. In severe conditions, may be used hourly, tapering to discontinuation as inflammation subsides. In mild conditions, may be used four to six times daily.

Action and kinetics
• *Anti-inflammatory action:* Prednisolone stimulates the synthesis of enzymes needed to decrease the inflammatory response. It suppresses the immune system by reducing activity and volume of the lymphatic system, thus producing lymphocytopenia (primarily of T-lymphocytes), decreasing immunoglobulin and complement concentrations, decreasing passage of immune complexes through basement membranes, and possibly by depressing reactivity of tissue to antigen-antibody interactions.

The mineralocorticoids regulate electrolyte homeostasis by acting renally at the distal tubules to enhance the reabsorption of sodium ions (and thus water) from the tubular fluid into the plasma and enhance the excretion of both potassium and hydrogen ions.

Prednisolone is an adrenocorticoid with both glucocorticoid and mineralocorticoid properties. It is a weak mineralocorticoid with only half the potency of hydrocortisone but is a more potent glucocorticoid, having four times the potency of equal weight of hydrocortisone. It is used primarily as an anti-inflammatory agent and an immunosuppressant. It is not used for mineralocorticoid replacement therapy because of the availability of more specific and potent agents.

Prednisolone may be administered orally. Prednisolone sodium phosphate is highly soluble, has a rapid onset and a short duration of action, and may be given I.M. or I.V. Prednisolone acetate and tebutate are suspensions that may be administered by intra-articular, intrasynovial, intrabursal, intralesional, or soft tissue injection. They have a slow onset but a long duration of action. Prednisolone sodium phosphate and prednisolone acetate is a combination product of the rapid-acting phosphate salt and the slightly soluble, slowly released acetate salt. This product provides rapid anti-inflammatory effects with a sustained duration of action. It is a suspension and should not be given I.V. It is particularly useful as an anti-inflammatory agent in intra-articular, intradermal, and intralesional injections.

---

‡May contain sulfites   ◆May contain tartrazine   ◆◆May contain benzyl alcohol

• *Kinetics in adults:* Prednisolone is absorbed readily after oral administration. After oral and I.V. administration, peak effects occur in about 1 to 2 hours. The acetate and tebutate suspensions for injection have a variable absorption over 24 to 48 hours, depending on whether they are injected into an intra-articular space or a muscle, and on the blood supply to that muscle. Systemic absorption occurs slowly after intra-articular injection. After ophthalmic administration, prednisolone is absorbed through the aqueous humor and primarily metabolized locally, then distributed throughout the local tissue layers.

Absorbed prednisolone is removed rapidly from the blood and distributed to muscle, liver, skin, intestines, and kidneys. Prednisolone is extensively bound to plasma proteins (transcortin and albumin). Only the unbound portion is active. Adrenocorticoids are distributed into breast milk and through the placenta.

Prednisolone is metabolized in the liver to inactive glucuronide and sulfate metabolites. These inactive metabolites, and small amounts of unmetabolized drug, are excreted in urine. Insignificant quantities of drug are excreted in feces. The biological half-life of prednisolone is 18 to 36 hours.

Contraindications and precautions

Prednisolone is contraindicated in patients with hypersensitivity to ingredients of adrenocorticoid preparations or in those with systemic fungal infections (except in adrenal insufficiency). Patients who are receiving prednisolone should not receive live virus vaccines because prednisolone suppresses the immune response.

Prednisolone should be used with extreme caution in patients with GI ulceration, renal disease, hypertension, osteoporosis, diabetes mellitus, thromboembolic disorders, seizures, myasthenia gravis, CHF, tuberculosis, hypoalbuminemia, hypothyroidism, cirrhosis of the liver, emotional instability, psychotic tendencies, hyperlipidemias, glaucoma, or cataracts, because the drug may exacerbate these conditions.

Because adrenocorticoids increase the susceptibility to and mask symptoms of infection, prednisolone should not be used (except in life-threatening situations) in patients with viral or bacterial infections not controlled by anti-infective agents.

Interactions

When used concomitantly, prednisolone rarely may decrease the effects of oral anticoagulants by unknown mechanisms.

Glucocorticoids increase the metabolism of isoniazid and salicylates; they cause hyperglycemia, requiring dosage adjustment of insulin or in diabetic patients; and may enhance hypokalemia associated with diuretic or amphotericin B therapy. The hypokalemia may increase the risk of toxicity in patients concurrently receiving digitalis glycosides.

Barbiturates, phenytoin, and rifampin may cause decreased corticosteroid effects because of increased hepatic metabolism. Cholestyramine, colestipol, and antacids decrease prednisolone's effect by adsorbing the corticosteroid, decreasing the amount absorbed.

Concomitant use with estrogens may reduce the metabolism of prednisolone by increasing the concentration of transcortin. The half-life of the corticosteroid is then prolonged because of increased protein binding. Concomitant administration of ulcerogenic drugs such as nonsteroidal anti-inflammatory agents may increase the risk of GI ulceration.

Effects on diagnostic tests

Prednisolone suppresses reactions to skin tests; causes false-negative results in the nitroblue tetrazolium test for systemic bacterial infections; decreases ^{131}I uptake and protein-bound iodine concentrations in thyroid function tests; may increase glucose and cholesterol levels; may decrease serum potassium, calcium, thyroxine, and triiodothyronine levels; and may increase urine glucose and calcium levels.

Adverse reactions

When administered in high doses or for prolonged therapy, prednisolone suppresses release of adrenocorticotropic hormone (ACTH) from the pituitary gland; in turn, the adrenal cortex stops secreting endogenous corticosteroids. The degree and duration of hypothalamic-pituitary-adrenal (HPA) axis suppression produced by the drugs is highly variable among patients and depends on the dose, frequency, and time of administration, and duration of glucocorticoid therapy.

• CNS: euphoria, insomnia, headache, psychotic behavior, pseudotumor cerebri, mental changes, nervousness, restlessness, *psychoses.*
• CV: CHF, *hypertension,* edema.
• DERM: delayed healing, *acne,* skin eruptions, striae.
• ENT: *cataracts,* glaucoma, thrush.
• Eye: transient burning or stinging on administration, mydriasis, ptosis, epithelial punctate keratitis, possible corneal or scleral malacia (rare); increased intraocular pressure, thinning of the cornea, interference with corneal wound healing, increased susceptibility to viral or fungal corneal infection, corneal ulceration, glaucoma, cataracts, defects in visual acuity and visual field (with long-term use).
• GI: *peptic ulcer,* irritation, increased appetite.
• Immune: immunosuppression, *increased susceptibility to infection.*
• Metabolic: *hypokalemia,* sodium retention, fluid retention, weight gain, hyperglycemia, *osteoporosis,* growth suppression in children, *glycosuria.*
• Musculoskeletal: muscle atrophy, weakness, *myopathy.*
• Other: pancreatitis, *hirsutism, cushingoid symptoms,* withdrawal syndrome (nausea, fatigue, anorexia, dyspnea, hypotension, hypoglycemia, myalgia, arthralgia, fever, dizziness, and fainting) *ecchymoses.* Sudden withdrawal may be fatal or may exacerbate the underlying disease. Acute adrenal insufficiency may occur with increased stress (infection, surgery, trauma) or abrupt withdrawal after long-term therapy.

Note: Drug should be discontinued if topical application results in local irritation, infection, significant systemic absorption, or hypersensitivity reaction; if visual acuity decreases or visual field is diminished; or if burning, stinging, or watering of eyes does not resolve quickly after administration.

Overdose and treatment

Acute ingestion, even in massive doses, is rarely a clinical problem. Toxic signs and symptoms rarely occur if drug is used for less than 3 weeks, even at large dosage ranges. However, chronic use causes adverse physiologic effects, including suppression of the HPA axis, cushingoid appearance, muscle weakness, and osteoporosis.

▶ Special considerations

• If possible, avoid long-term administration of pharmacologic dosages of glucosteroids in children and adolescents because these drugs may retard bone growth. Manifestations of adrenal suppression in children include retardation of linear growth, delayed weight gain, low plasma cortisol concentrations, and lack of response to corticotropin stimulation. In children who require prolonged therapy, closely monitor growth and development. Alternate-day therapy is recommended to minimize growth suppression.
• Establish baseline blood pressure, fluid intake and output, weight, and electrolyte status. Watch for any sudden patient weight gain, edema, change in blood pressure, or change in electrolyte status.
• During times of physiologic stress (trauma, surgery, infection), the patient may require additional steroids and may experience signs of steroid withdrawal; patients who were previously steroid-dependent may need systemic corticosteroids to prevent withdrawal symptoms.
• Be aware of the patient's psychological history and watch for any behavioral changes.
• Observe for signs of infection or delayed wound healing.
• Sudden withdrawal of drug may result in fever, myalgia, arthralgia, malaise, hypotension, and hypoglycemic shock.

Ophthalmic administration

• Because of their greater ratio of skin surface area to body weight, children may be more susceptible than adults to topical corticosteroid-induced hypothalamic-pituitary-adrenal axis suppression and Cushing's syndrome. Although such reactions occur extremely rarely with ophthalmic therapy, it is still advisable to limit corticosteroid therapy in children to the minimum amount necessary for therapeutic efficacy.
• Ophthalmic products may initially cause sensitivity to bright light. This may be minimized by wearing sunglasses.
• Monitor the patient's response by observing the area of inflammation and eliciting patient comments concerning pruritus and vision. Inspect the eye and surrounding tissues for infection and additional irritation.
• Discontinue the drug if the patient develops signs of systemic absorption (including Cushing's syndrome, hyperglycemia, or glucosuria), skin irritation or ulceration, hypersensitivity, or infection (If antivirals or antibiotics are being used with corticosteroids and the infection does not respond immediately, prednisolone should be discontinued until the infection is controlled.)

Information for parents and patient

• Be sure that the parents and patient understand the need to take the adrenocorticosteroid as pre-scribed. Give the patient instructions on what to do if a dose is inadvertently missed.
• Warn the parents and patient not to discontinue the drug abruptly.
• Inform the parents and patient of the possible therapeutic and adverse effects of the drug, so that they may report any complications as soon as possible.
• Advise the parents that the patient should wear a Medic Alert bracelet or necklace indicating the need for supplemental adrenocorticoids during times of stress.

Ophthalmic administration

Advise the parents and patient to use the following steps when administering eye drops:

Method for applying eye drops
• Wash hands well. Shake solution or suspension well. Tilt head back or lie down and lightly pull lower eyelid down by applying gentle pressure at the lid base in the bony rim of orbit. Approach the eye from below with the dropper, do not touch dropper to any tissue. Holding dropper no more than 1" above the eye, drop medication inside lower lid while looking up. Try to keep eye open for 30 seconds. Finally, apply light finger pressure inward and down to the side of the bridge of the nose (the lacrimal canaliculi) of solution into nasal passages, where more of the drug is absorbed systemically.
• If using more than one kind of drug at the same time, wait at least 5 minutes before applying the second drug.

Method for applying ointments
• Advise following steps when administering ophthalmic ointments: Wash hands well. Hold the tube in your hand several minutes before use to warm it and impove flow of ointment. When opening the ointment tube for the first time, squeeze out the first ¼" of ointment and discard (using sterile gauze) because it may be too dry. Apply a small "ribbon" or strip of ointment (¼" to ½") to the inside of the lower eyelid. Do not touch any part of the eye with the tip of the tube. Close the eye gently and roll the eyeball in all directions to spread the ointment. If using a second eye ointment, wait at least 10 minutes before applying it.
• Instruct parents to observe for adverse effects and to call if no improvement occurs after 7 to 8 days. If the condition worsens, or if pain, itching, or swelling of the eye occurs.
• Warn parents not to administer nonprescription ophthalmic preparations other than those specifically recommended. Nonprescription ophthalmic solutions should not be used for more than 7 days in children under age 2.
• Warn parents not to use leftover medication for a new eye inflammation and never to share eye medication with others. Tell them to store all eye medications in original container.
• Parents should call for specific instructions before discontinuing therapy.
• Advise patient that drug may cause sensitivity to light. Recommend wearing sunglasses to minimize this effect.

---

‡May contain sulfites   ◆May contain tartrazine   ◆◆May contain benzyl alcohol

prednisone
Apo-Prednisone*, Meticorten,
Novoprednisone*, Orasone, Panasol,
Prednicen-M, SK-Prednisone,
Winpred*

- Classification: anti-inflammatory, immunosuppressant (adrenocorticoid)

How supplied
Available by prescription only
Tablets: 1 mg, 2.5 mg, 5 mg, 10 mg, 20 mg, 25 mg, 50 mg
Oral solution: 5 mg/ml; 5 mg/5 ml .
Syrup: 5 mg/5 ml

Indications, route, and dosage
Physiologic replacement
Children: 4 to 5 mg/2 daily in divided doses.
Severe inflammation or immunosuppression
Children: 0.5 mg/kg or 25 to 60 mg/m2 daily q 6 to 12 hours. Alternatively, adjust dosage based upon age:
Children age 18 months to 4 years: 7.5 to 10 mg P.O. q.i.d.
Children age 5 to 10: 15 mg P.O. q.i.d.
Children age 11 to 18: 20 mg P.O. q.i.d.
Adults: 5 to 60 mg P.O. daily in single dose or divided doses. (Maximum daily dose is 250 mg.) Maintenance dose given once daily or every other day. Dosage must be individualized.
Acute exacerbations of multiple sclerosis
Adults: 200 mg P.O. daily for 1 week, then 80 mg every other day for 1 month.
Nephrotic syndrome
Children: 2 mg/kg daily in divided doses t.i.d. or q.i.d. for a maximum of 23 days, or until urine is protein-free for 5 days. Maximum dose is 80 mg/day. Maintenance dose is 2 mg/kg every other day for 4 weeks. Then gradually taper over 4 to 6 weeks.
Asthma
Children: 0.5 to 1 mg/kg daily for 3 to 5 days. Maximum dose is 40 mg/kg daily.

Action and kinetics
- *Immunosuppressant action:* Prednisone stimulates the synthesis of enzymes needed to decrease the inflammatory response. It suppresses the immune system by reducing activity and volume of the lymphatic system, thus producing lymphocytopenia (primarily of T-lymphocytes), decreasing immunoglobulin and complement concentrations, decreasing passage of immune complexes through basement membranes, and possibly by depressing reactivity of tissue to antigen-antibody interactions.
- *Anti-inflammatory action:* Prednisone is one of the intermediate-acting glucocorticoids, with greater glucocorticoid activity than cortisone and hydrocortisone, but less anti-inflammatory activity than betamethasone, dexamethasone, and paramethasone. Prednisone is about four to five times more potent as an anti-inflammatory agent than hydrocortisone, but it has only half the mineralocorticoid activity of an

equal weight of hydrocortisone. Prednisone is the oral glucocorticoid of choice for anti-inflammatory or immunosuppressant effects. For those patients who cannot swallow tablets, liquid forms are available. The oral concentrate (5 mg/ml) may be diluted in juice or another flavored diluent or mixed in semisolid food (such as applesauce) before administration.
- *Kinetics in adults:* Prednisone is absorbed readily after oral administration, with peak effects occuring in about 1 to 2 hours.
    Prednisone is distributed rapidly to muscle, liver, skin, intestines, and kidneys. Prednisone is extensively bound to plasma proteins (transcortin and albumin). Only the unbound portion is active. Adrenocorticoids are distributed into breast milk and through the placenta.
    Prednisone is metabolized in the liver to the active metabolite prednisolone, which in turn is then metabolized to inactive glucuronide and sulfate metabolites
    The inactive metabolites and small amounts of unmetabolized drug are excreted by the kidneys. Insignificant quantities of drug are also excreted in feces. The biological half-life of prednisone is 18 to 36 hours.

Contraindications and precautions
Prednisone is contraindicated in patients with systemic fungal infections (except in adrenal insufficiency) and in those with hypersensitivity to ingredients of adrenocorticoid preparations. Patients receiving prednisone should not be given live-virus vaccines because prednisone suppresses the immune response.
    Prednisone should be used with extreme caution in patients with GI ulceration, renal disease, hypertension, osteoporosis, diabetes mellitus, thromboembolic disorders, seizures, myasthenia gravis, CHF, tuberculosis, hypoalbuminemia, hypothyroidism, cirrhosis of the liver, emotional instability, psychotic tendencies, hyperlipidemias, glaucoma, or cataracts because the drug may exacerbate these conditions.
    Because adrenocorticoids increase the susceptibility to and mask symptoms of infection, prednisone should not be used (except in life-threatening situations) in patients with viral or bacterial infections not controlled by anti-infective agents.

Interactions
Concomitant use of prednisone rarely may decrease the effects of oral anticoagulants by unknown mechanisms.
    Prednisone increases the metabolism of isoniazid and salicylates; causes hyperglycemia, requiring dosage adjustment of insulin in diabetic patients; and may enhance hypokalemia associated with diuretic or amphotericin B therapy. The hypokalemia may increase the risk of toxicity in patients concurrently receiving digitalis glycosides.
    Barbiturates, phenytoin, and rifampin may cause decreased effects because of increased hepatic metabolism. Cholestyramine, colestipol, and antacids decrease the effect of prednisone by adsorbing the corticosteroid, decreasing the amount absorbed.
    Concomitant use with estrogens may reduce the metabolism of prednisone by increasing the concen-

tration of transcortin. The half-life of prednisone is then prolonged because of increased protein binding.

Concomitant administration of ulcerogenic drugs, such as nonsteroidal anti-inflammatory agents, may increase the risk of GI ulceration.

Effects on diagnostic tests

Prednisone suppresses reactions to skin tests; causes false-negative results in the nitroblue tetrazolium test for systemic bacterial infections; decreases ^{131}I uptake and protein-bound iodine concentrations in thyroid function tests; may increase glucose and cholesterol levels; may decrease serum potassium, calcium, thyroxine, and triiodothyronine levels; and may increase urine glucose and calcium levels.

Adverse reactions

When administered in high doses or for prolonged therapy, prednisone suppresses release of adrenocorticotropic hormone (ACTH) from the pituitary gland. In turn, the adrenal cortex stops secreting endogenous corticosteroids. The degree and duration of hypothalamic-pituitary-adrenal (HPA) axis suppression produced by the drugs is highly variable among patients and depends on the dose, frequency and time of administration, and duration of glucocorticoid therapy.

• CNS: euphoria, insomnia, headache, psychotic behavior, pseudotumor cerebri, mental changes, nervousness, restlessness, *psychoses.*
• CV: CHF, *hypertension,* edema.
• DERM: delayed healing, *acne,* skin eruptions, striae.
• EENT: *cataracts,* glaucoma, thrush.
• GI: *peptic ulcer,* irritation, increased appetite.
• Immune: *increased susceptibility to infection.*
• Metabolic: *hypokalemia,* sodium retention, fluid retention, weight gain, hyperglycemia, *osteoporosis,* growth suppression in children, *glycosuria.*
• Musculoskeletal: muscle atrophy, weakness, *myopathy.*
• Other: pancreatitis, *hirsutism, cushingoid symptoms,* withdrawal syndrome (nausea, fatigue, anorexia, dyspnea, hypotension, hypoglycemia, myalgia, arthralgia, fever, dizziness, and fainting). Sudden withdrawal may be fatal or may exacerbate the underlying disease. Acute adrenal insufficiency may occur with increased stress (infection, surgery, trauma) or abrupt withdrawal after long-term therapy.

Overdose and treatment

Acute ingestion, even in massive doses, is rarely a clinical problem. Toxic signs and symptoms rarely occur if drug is used for less than 3 weeks, even at large dosage ranges. However, chronic use causes adverse physiologic effects, including suppression of the HPA axis, cushingoid appearance, muscle weakness, and osteoporosis.

▶ Special considerations

• Chronic use of prednisone in children or adolescents may delay growth and maturation.
• If possible, avoid long-term administration of pharmacologic dosages of glucosteroids in children because these drugs may retard bone growth. Manifestations of adrenal suppression in children in-

clude retardation of linear growth, delayed weight gain, low plasma cortisol concentrations, and lack of response to corticotropin stimulation. In children who require prolonged therapy, closely monitor growth and development. Alternate-day therapy is recommended to minimize growth suppression.
• Establish baseline blood pressure, fluid intake and output, weight, and electrolyte status. Watch for any sudden patient weight gain, edema, change in blood pressure, or change in electrolyte status.
• During times of physiologic stress (trauma, surgery, infection), the patient may require additional steroids and may experience signs of steroid withdrawal; patients who were previously steroid-dependent may need systemic corticosteroids to prevent adrenal insufficiency.
• After long-term therapy, the drug should be reduced gradually. Rapid reduction may cause withdrawal symptoms.
• Be aware of the patient's psychological history and watch for any behavioral changes.
• Observe for signs of infection or delayed wound healing.
• Acute withdrawal of drug may result in fever, myalgia, arthralgia, malaise, hypotension, or hypoglycemic shock.

Information for parents and patient

• Be sure that the parents and patient understand the need to take the adrenocorticosteroid as prescribed. Give instructions on what to do if a dose is inadvertently missed.
• Warn the parents and patient not to discontinue the drug abruptly.
• Inform the parents and patient of the possible therapeutic and adverse effects of the drug, so they may report any complications as soon as possible.
• Advise parents that the patient should wear a Medic Alert bracelet or necklace indicating the need for supplemental adrenocorticoids during times of stress.

---

primaquine phosphate

• Classification: antimalarial (8-aminoquinoline)

How supplied

Available by prescription only
Tablets: 26.3 mg (15-mg base)

Indications, route, and dosage
Radical cure of Plasmodium vivax and P. ovale malaria

Children: 0.3 mg (base)/kg/day for 14 days, or 0.9 mg (base)/kg/day once a week for 8 weeks.
Adults: 15 mg (base) P.O. daily for 14 days (26.3-mg tablet equals 15 mg of base), or 79 mg (45-mg base) once a week for 8 weeks.

Action and kinetics

• *Antimalarial action:* Primaquine disrupts the parasitic mitochondria, thereby interrupting metabolic processes requiring energy.

The spectrum of activity includes preerythrocytic and exoerythrocytic forms of *P. falciparum, P. malariae, P. ovale,* and *P. vivax.* Nifurtimox (Lampit), an investigational agent available from the Centers for Disease Control, is preferred for intracellular parasites.

• *Kinetics in adults:* Primaquine is well absorbed from the GI tract, with peak concentrations occurring at 2 to 6 hours. Primaquine is distributed widely into the liver, lungs, heart, brain, skeletal muscle, and other tissues. Drug is carboxylated rapidly in the liver. Only a small amount of primaquine is excreted unchanged in urine. The elimination half-life is 4 to 10 hours.

Contraindications and precautions
Primaquine is contraindicated in patients receiving quinacrine because of possible additive toxicity. It also is contraindicated in patients predisposed to granulocytopenia and in patients receiving other drugs that might cause hemolysis or bone marrow depression.

Primaquine should be used cautiously in patients who previously have had an idiosyncratic reaction to primaquine and in patients with a history of favism, glucose-6-phosphate dehydrogenase (G6PD) deficiency, or NADH methemoglobin reductase deficiency, because hemolytic reactions may occur in these groups. It is contraindicated in patients with lupus erythematosus or rheumatoid arthritis.

Interactions
Quinacrine may potentiate the toxic effects of primaquine. Concomitant use with magnesium and aluminum salts may decrease gastrointestinal absorption.

Effects on diagnostic tests
Decreases or increases in white blood cell counts and decreases in red blood cell counts may occur during primaquine therapy. Methemoglobinemia may occur.

Adverse reactions
• CNS: headache.
• DERM: urticaria.
• EENT: disturbances of visual accommodation.
• GI: nausea, vomiting, epigastric distress, abdominal cramps.
• HEMA: leukopenia, hemolytic anemia in G6PD deficiency, methemoglobinemia in NADH methemoglobin reductase deficiency, leukocytosis, mild anemia, *granulocytopenia,* agranulocytosis.
Note: Drug should be discontinued immediately if urine darkens or if hemoglobin or hematocrit levels fall.

Overdose and treatment
Symptoms of overdose include abdominal distress, vomiting, CNS and cardiovascular disturbances, cyanosis, methemoglobinemia, leukocytosis, leukopenia, and anemia. Treatment is symptomatic.

▶ Special considerations
• Children are especially susceptible to overdose with aminoquinolines and should not receive long-term therapy.
• Primaquine is often used with a fast-acting anti-

malarial, such as chloroquine, to prevent delayed malaria attacks or relapses.
• Before starting therapy, screen patients for possible G6PD deficiency.
• Administer drug with meals or antacids, if prescribed, to minimize gastric irritation.
• Light-skinned patients taking more than 30 mg daily, dark-skinned patients taking more than 15 mg daily, and patients with severe anemia or suspected sensitivity should have frequent blood studies and urine examinations. A sudden fall in hemoglobin concentrations or erythrocyte or leukocyte counts, or a marked darkening of the urine suggests impending hemolytic reaction.
• All patients should have periodic blood studies and urinalyses to monitor for impending hemolytic reactions.
• Obtain a baseline ECG, blood counts, and an ophthalmologic examination, and check periodically for changes.
• Monitor patient for signs of cumulative effects, such as blurred vision, increased sensitivity to light, muscle weakness, impaired hearing, tinnitus, fever, sore throat, unusual bleeding or bruising, unusual pigmentation of the oral mucous membranes, and jaundice. Maximal effects may not occur for 6 months.
• Muscle weakness and alterations of deep tendon reflexes may require discontinuing the drug.

Information for parents and patient
• Tell parents to report any visual or hearing changes, muscle weakness, or darkening of urine immediately.
• Patient should take drug after meals to help prevent GI distress and should report any pronounced GI distress. Tell parents to separate use of magnesium and kaolin compounds from drug by at least 4 hours.
• Advise parents that patient should wear sunglasses in bright light or sunlight to reduce risk of ocular damage and should avoid prolonged exposure to sunlight to avoid exacerbation of drug-induced dermatoses.
• Counsel parents to complete the entire prescribed course of therapy and to comply with follow-up blood tests and examinations.
• Warn parents to keep drug out of the reach of children.

primidone
Myidone, Mysoline, Sertan

• Classification: anticonvulsant (barbiturate analogue)

How supplied
Available by prescription only
Tablets: 50 mg, 250 mg
Suspension: 250 mg/5 ml

Indications, route, and dosage
Generalized tonic-clonic (grand mal) seizures, complex-partial (psychomotor) seizures
Neonates: Initially, 15 to 25 mg/kg as a single dose, then 12 to 20 mg/kg/day divided b.i.d. to q.i.d.

Children under age 8: 125 mg P.O. daily. Increase by 125 mg weekly, up to a maximum of 1 g daily, divided q.i.d.

Children age 8 and over and adults: 250 mg P.O. daily. Increase by 250 mg weekly, up to a maximum of 2 g daily, divided q.i.d.

Action and kinetics
• *Anticonvulsant action:* Primidone acts as a nonspecific CNS depressant used alone or with other anticonvulsants to control refractory grand mal seizures and to treat psychomotor or focal seizures. Mechanism of action is unknown; some activity may be from phenobarbital, an active metabolite.

• *Kinetics in adults:* Primidone is absorbed readily from the GI tract; serum concentrations peak at about 3 hours. Phenobarbital appears in plasma after several days of continuous therapy; most laboratory assays detect both phenobarbital and primidone. Therapeutic levels are 5 to 12 mcg/ml for primidone and 10 to 30 mcg/ml for phenobarbital.

Primidone is distributed widely throughout the body.

Primidone is metabolized slowly by the liver to phenylethylmalonamide (PEMA) and phenobarbital; PEMA is the major metabolite.

Primidone is excreted in urine; substantial amounts are excreted in breast milk.

Contraindications and precautions
Primidone is contraindicated in patients with known hypersensitivity to barbiturates; in pregnancy because of hazard of respiratory depression and neonatal coagulation defects; in patients with severe respiratory disease or status asthmaticus because of respiratory depressant effects; in patients with porphyria because of potential for adverse hematologic effects; and in patients with markedly impaired hepatic function because of potential for enhanced hepatic impairment. Use drug with caution in patients taking alcohol and other CNS depressants.

Interactions
Alcohol and other CNS depressants, including narcotic analgesics, cause excessive depression in patients taking primidone. Carbamazepine and phenytoin may decrease effects of primidone and increase its conversion to phenobarbital; monitor serum levels to prevent toxicity.

Effects on diagnostic tests
Primidone may cause abnormalities in liver function test results.

Adverse reactions
• CNS: *drowsiness,* ataxia, emotional disturbances, vertigo, hyperirritability, fatigue.
• DERM: morbilliform rash, alopecia.
• EENT: diplopia, nystagmus, edema of the eyelids.
• GI: anorexia, nausea, vomiting.
• GU: impotence, polyuria.

• HEMA: leukopenia, eosinophilia.
• Other: edema, thirst.

Note: Drug should be discontinued if signs of hypersensitivity or hepatic dysfunction occur.

Overdose and treatment
Symptoms of overdose resemble those of barbiturate intoxication; they include CNS and respiratory depression, areflexia, oliguria, tachycardia, hypotension, hypothermia, and coma. Shock may occur.

Treat overdose supportively: in conscious patient with intact gag reflex, induce emesis with ipecac; follow in 30 minutes with repeated doses of activated charcoal and sorbitol mixture. Use lavage if emesis is not feasible. Alkalinization of urine and forced diuresis may hasten excretion. Hemodialysis may be necessary. Monitor vital signs and fluid and electrolyte balance.

▶ Special considerations
• Premature infants are more susceptible to the depressant effects of barbiturates because of immature hepatic metabolism. Primidone may cause hyperexcitability in children under age 6.

• Dosage of primidone must be individualized for each patient, because different rates of metabolism and enzyme induction occur.

• Assess level of consciousness before and frequently during therapy to evaluate effectiveness of drug. Monitor neurologic status for possible alterations or deteriorations. Monitor seizure character, frequency, and duration for changes. Institute seizure precautions, as necessary.

• Assess patient's sleeping patterns before and during therapy to ensure effectiveness of drug.

• Institute safety measures—side rails, assistance when out of bed, call light within reach—to prevent falls and injury.

• Anticipate possible rebound confusion and excitatory reactions in patient.

• Assess bowel elimination patterns; monitor for complaints of constipation. Advise diet high in fiber, if indicated.

• Monitor prothrombin time carefully in patients taking anticoagulants; dosage of anticoagulant may require adjustment to counteract possible interaction.

• Observe patient to prevent hoarding or self-dosing, especially in depressed or suicidal patients, or those who are or have a history of being drug-dependent.

• Death is common with an overdose of 2 to 10 g; it may occur at much smaller doses if alcohol is also ingested.

• Barbiturate dependence may be transmitted to the fetus; withdrawal symptoms can occur in neonates whose mothers took barbiturates in the third trimester.

• Patient should have review of complete blood count and liver function tests every 6 months.

• Abrupt withdrawal of primidone may cause status epilepticus; dosage should be reduced gradually.

• Primidone impairs ability to perform tasks requiring mental alertness.

Information for parents and patient
• Warn parents or patient to avoid concurrent use of other drugs with CNS depressant effects, such as antihistamines, analgesics, and alcohol, because they will have additive effects and result in increased drowsiness. Instruct parents to seek medical approval before giving patient any nonprescription cold or allergy preparations.
• Caution parents and patient not to increase or decrease dose or frequency without medical approval; abrupt discontinuation may trigger rebound insomnia, with increased dreaming, nightmares, or seizures.
• Patient should avoid hazardous tasks that require alertness while taking barbiturates. Instruct patient in safety measures to prevent injury.
• Be sure parents or patient understand that primidone can cause physical or psychological dependence (addiction).
• Instruct parents to report any skin eruption or other marked adverse effect.
• Explain that a morning hangover is common after therapeutic use of barbiturates.
• Teach parents and patient signs and symptoms of adverse reactions.
• Explain to sexually active adolescents that primidone may render oral contraceptives ineffective; advise a different birth control method.
• Recommend to parents that patient wear a Medic Alert bracelet or necklace indicating the drug taken and seizure disorder.

---

probenecid
Benemid, Probalan

• Classification: uricosuric agent (sulfonamide-derivative uricosuric agent)

How supplied
Available by prescription only
Tablets: 500 mg

Indications, route, and dosage
Adjunct to penicillin therapy
Children age 2 to 14 or weighing less than 50 kg:
Initially, 25 mg/kg or 1.2 g/m² daily, then 40 mg/kg or 700 mg/m² divided q.i.d.
Children over age 14 or weighing more than 50 kg and adults: 500 mg P.O. q.i.d.
Single-dose penicillin treatment of gonorrhea
Adults: 1 g P.O. given together with penicillin treatment P.O., or 1 g P.O. 30 minutes before I.M. dose of penicillin.

Action and kinetics
• *Uricosuric action:* Probenecid competitively inhibits the active reabsorption of uric acid at the proximal convoluted tubule, thereby increasing urinary excretion of uric acid.
• *Adjunctive action in antibiotic therapy action:* Probenecid competitively inhibits secretion of weak organic acids, including penicillins, cephalosporins, and

other beta-lactam antibiotics, thereby increasing concentrations of these drugs.
• *Kinetics in adults:* Probenecid is completely absorbed after oral administration; peak serum levels are reached at 2 to 4 hours. It distributes throughout the body; drug is about 75% protein-bound. CSF levels are about 2% of serum levels. Probenecid is metabolized in the liver to active metabolites, with some uricosuric effect. Drug and metabolites are excreted in urine; probenecid (but not metabolites) is actively reabsorbed.

Contraindications and precautions
Probenecid is contraindicated in patients with hypersensitivity to the drug and in patients with acute gout, blood dyscrasias, or uric acid kidney stones because it may worsen these conditions.
Probenecid should be used cautiously in patients with a history of peptic ulcer disease; in patients with renal impairment (drug is ineffective if glomerular filtration rate is lower than 30 ml/minute).

Interactions
Probenecid significantly increases or prolongs effects of penicillins, cephalosporins, and other beta-lactam antibiotics, and possibly thiopental and ketamine; it increases serum levels (thus increasing risk of toxicity) of dapsone, aminosalicylic acid, methotrexate, and nitrofurantoin.
Probenecid inhibits urinary excretion of weak organic acids; it impairs natriuretic effects of ethacrynic acid, furosemide, and bumetanide; it also decreases excretion of indomethacin and naproxen, permitting use of lower doses.
Diuretics, alcohol, and pyrazinamide decrease uric acid levels of probenecid; increased doses of probenecid may be required. Salicylates inhibit the uricosuric effect of probenecid only in doses that achieve levels of 50 mcg/ml or more; occasional use of low-dose aspirin does not interfere.

Effects on diagnostic tests
Probenecid causes false-positive tests results for urinary glucose with tests using cupric sulfate reagent (Benedict's reagent, Clinitest, and Fehling's); perform tests with glucose oxidase reagent (Clinistix, Tes-Tape) instead.

Adverse reactions
• CNS: *headache,* dizziness.
• CV: hypotension.
• EENT: sore gums.
• GI: anorexia, *nausea, vomiting,* gastric distress.
• GU: urinary frequency, renal colic, hematuria, uric acid stones.
• HEMA: leukopenia, *hemolytic or aplastic anemia.*
• Other: hair loss, increased gouty arthritis attacks, fever, sweating, flushing, *hypersensitivity.*
Note: Drug should be discontinued if patient shows signs of hypersensitivity reaction, rash, leukopenia, hemolytic anemia, or aplastic anemia.

Overdose and treatment
Clinical signs include nausea, copious vomiting, stupor, coma, and tonic-clonic seizures. Treat support-

---

ively, using mechanical ventilation if needed; induce emesis or use gastric lavage, as appropriate. Control seizures with I.V. phenobarbital and phenytoin.

▶ Special considerations
• Drug is contraindicated in children younger than age 2.
• Monitor BUN and serum creatinine levels closely; drug is ineffective in severe renal insufficiency.
• Give with food, milk, or prescribed antacids to lessen GI upset.
• Maintain adequate hydration with high fluid intake to prevent formation of uric acid stones. Also maintain alkalinization of urine.
• Probenecid has been used in the diagnosis of parkinsonian syndrome and mental depression.

Information for parents and patient
• Advise parents that patient should not discontinue drug without medical approval.
• Warn parents and patient not to use drug for pain or inflammation and not to increase dose during gouty attack.
• Patient should drink 8 to 10 glasses of fluid daily and take drug with food to minimize GI upset.
• Explain that Tes-tape, Diastix, or Clinistix should be used for accurate urine glucose testing.

---

procainamide hydrochloride
Procan SR, Promine, Pronestyl, Pronestyl-SR, Rhythmin

• Classification: ventricular antiarrhythmic, supra-ventricular antiarrhythmic (procaine derivative)

How supplied
Available by prescription only
Tablets: 250 mg, 375 mg, 500 mg; 250 mg, 500 mg, 750 mg, 1 g (extended-release)
Capsules: 250 mg, 375 mg, 500 mg
Injection: 100 mg/ml, 500 mg/ml

Indications, route, and dosage
Premature ventricular contractions; ventricular tachycardia; atrial fibrillation and flutter unresponsive to quinidine; paroxysmal atrial tachycardia
Infants: Load with 1 mg/kg infused over 5 minutes; repeat as necessary to total of 10 to 15 mg/kg; then, 0.02 to 0.8 mg/kg I.V. by continuous drip.
Children: Load with 3 to 6 mg/kg repeated q 5 minutes to maximum of 500 mg; then infuse 15 mg/kg over 30 minutes.
Adults: 100 mg q 5 minutes by slow I.V. push, no faster than 25 to 50 mg/minute, until dysrhythmias disappear, adverse effects develop, or 1 g has been given. When dysrhythmias disappear, give continuous infusion of 2 to 6 mg/minute. Usual effective loading dose is 500 to 600 mg. If dysrhythmias recur, repeat bolus as above and increase infusion rate; alternatively, administer 0.5 to 1 g I.M. q 4 to 8 hours until oral therapy begins.

Loading dose for atrial fibrillation or paroxysmal atrial tachycardia
Children: 10 to 15 mg/kg I.V. over 30 minutes.
Adults: 1 to 1.25 g P.O. If dysrhythmias persist after 1 hour, give additional 750 mg. If no change occurs, give 500 mg to 1 g q 2 hours until dysrhythmias disappear or adverse effects occur.
Loading dose for ventricular tachycardia
Children: 15 to 50 mg P.O. daily in divided doses q 3 to 6 hours. Maximum dosage is 4 g daily.
Adults: 1 g P.O. Maintenance dosage is 50 mg/kg/day given at 3-hour intervals; average is 250 to 500 mg q 4 hours but may require 1 to 1.5 g q 4 to 6 hours.
Note: In adults, sustained-release tablets may be used for maintenance dosing when treating ventricular tachycardia, atrial fibrillation, and paroxysmal atrial tachycardia. Dosage is 500 mg to 1 g q 6 hours.

Action and kinetics
• *Antiarrhythmic action:* A Class IA antiarrhythmic agent, procainamide depresses phase 0 of the action potential. It is considered a myocardial depressant because it decreases myocardial excitability and conduction velocity and may depress myocardial contractility. It also possesses anticholinergic activity, which may modify its direct myocardial effects. In therapeutic doses, it reduces conduction velocity in the atria, ventricles, and His-Purkinje system. Its effectiveness in controlling atrial tachydysrhythmias stems from its ability to prolong the effective refractory period (ERP) and increase the action potential duration in the atria, ventricles, and His-Purkinje system. Because ERP prolongation exceeds action potential duration, tissue remains refractory even after returning to resting membrane potential (membrane-stabilizing effect). Procainamide shortens the effective refractory period of the AV node. The drug's anticholinergic action also may increase AV node conductivity. Suppression of automaticity in the His-Purkinje system and ectopic pacemakers accounts for the drug's effectiveness in treating ventricular premature beats. At therapeutic doses, procainamide prolongs the PR and QT intervals (this effect may be used as an index of drug effectiveness and toxicity.) The QRS interval usually is not prolonged beyond normal range; the QT interval is not prolonged to the extent achieved with quinidine.
Procainamide exerts a peripheral vasodilatory effect; with I.V. administration, it may cause hypotension, which limits the administration rate and amount of drug deliverable.
• *Kinetics in adults:* Rate and extent of drug's absorption from the intestines vary; usually, 75% to 90% of an orally administered dose is absorbed. With administration of tablets and capsules, peak plasma levels occur in approximately 1 hour. Extended-release tablets are formulated to provide a sustained and relatively constant rate of release and absorption throughout the small intestine. After the drug's release, extended wax matrix is not absorbed and may appear in feces after 15 minutes to 1 hour. With I.M. injection, onset of action occurs in about 10 to 30 minutes, with peak levels in about 1 hour.
Procainamide is distributed widely in most body

---

tissues, including CSF, liver, spleen, kidneys, lungs, muscles, brain, and heart. Only about 15% binds to plasma proteins. Usual therapeutic range for serum procainamide concentrations is 4 to 8 mcg/ml. Some experts suggest that a range of 10 to 30 mcg/ml for the sum of procainamide and N-acetylprocainamide (NAPA) serum concentrations are therapeutic.

Procainamide is acetylated in the liver to form NAPA. Acetylation rate is determined genetically and affects NAPA formation. (NAPA also exerts antiarrhythmic activity.) Procainamide and NAPA metabolite are excreted in the urine. Procainamide's half-life is about 2½ to 4¾ hours. NAPA's half-life is about 6 hours. In patients with CHF and/or renal dysfunction, half-life increases; therefore, in such patients, dosage reduction is required to avoid toxicity.

Contraindications and precautions
Procainamide is contraindicated in patients with complete AV block with AV junctional or idioventricular pacemaker without an operative artificial pacemaker, and in patients with prolonged QT interval or QRS duration, because of potential for heart block; in patients with digitalis toxicity, because the drug may further depress conduction, which may result in ventricular asystole or fibrillation; in patients with Torsades de Pointes, because the drug may exacerbate this dysrhythmia; in patients with myasthenia gravis, because the drug may exacerbate muscle weakness; and in patients with hypersensitivity to procainamide or related compounds (such as procaine).

Procainamide should be used with caution in patients with incomplete AV block or bundle branch block, because the drug may further depress conduction; in patients with CHF, because drug may worsen this condition; and in patients with renal or hepatic dysfunction, because the drug may accumulate, causing toxicity.

Interactions
Concomitant use of procainamide with neuromuscular blocking agents (such as pancuronium bromide, succinylcholine chloride, tubocurarine chloride, gallium triethiodide, metocurine iodide, and decamethonium bromide) may potentiate procainamide drug effects. Concomitant use with anticholinergic agents (such as diphenhydramine, atropine, and tricyclic antidepressants) may cause additive anticholinergic effects.

Concomitant use with cholinergic agents (such as neostigmine and pyridostigmine, which are used to treat myasthenia gravis) may negate the effects of these agents, requiring increased dosage.

Concomitant use with antihypertensives may cause additive hypotensive effects (most common with I.V. procainamide). Concomitant use with other antiarrhythmics may result in additive or antagonistic cardiac effects and with possible additive toxic effects. Concomitant use with cimetidine may result in impaired renal clearance of procainamide and NAPA, with elevated serum drug concentrations. Concomitant use with captopril may cause additive immunosuppression.

Effects on diagnostic tests
Procainamide will invalidate bentiromide test results; discontinue at least 3 days before bentiromide test. Procainamide may alter edrophonium test results; positive ANA titers, positive direct antiglobulin (Coombs') tests, and EKG changes may be seen. The physiologic effects of the drug may result in decreased leukocytes and platelets, and increased bilirubin, lactic dehydrogenase, alkaline phosphatase, ALT (SGPT), and AST (SGOT).

Adverse reactions
• CNS: hallucinations, confusion, convulsions, depression.
• CV: severe hypotension, bradycardia, AV block, ventricular fibrillation (with parenteral administration).
• DERM: maculopapular rash.
• GI: nausea, vomiting, anorexia, diarrhea, bitter taste.
• HEMA: thrombocytopenia, neutropenia (especially with sustained-release forms), agranulocytosis, hemolytic anemia, increased antinuclear antibody (ANA) titer.
• Other: fever, lupus erythematosus syndrome (especially after prolonged administration).
Note: Drug should be discontinued if granulocytopenia or lupus erythematosus syndrome occur, unless drug's benefits outweigh risks.

Overdose and treatment
Clinical effects of overdose include severe hypotension, widening QRS complex, junctional tachycardia, intraventricular conduction delay, ventricular fibrillation, oliguria, confusion and lethargy, and nausea and vomiting.

Treatment involves general supportive measures (including respiratory and cardiovascular support) with hemodynamic and ECG monitoring. After recent ingestion of oral form, gastric lavage, emesis, and activated charcoal may be used to decrease absorption. Phenylephrine or norepinephrine may be used to treat hypotension after adequate hydration has been ensured. Hemodialysis may be effective in removing procainamide and NAPA. A ⅙ molar solution of sodium lactate may reduce procainamide's cardiotoxic effect.

▶ Special considerations
• Manufacturer has not established dosage guidelines for pediatric patients. For treating dysrhythmias, the suggested dosage is 40 to 60 mg/kg of standard tablets or capsules, P.O. daily, given in 4 to 6 divided doses; or 3 to 6 mg/kg I.V. over 5 minutes, followed by a drip of 0.02 to 0.08 mg/kg/minute.
• In treating atrial fibrillation and flutter, ventricular rate may accelerate due to vagolytic effects on the AV node; to prevent this effect, digitalis may be administered before procainamide therapy begins.
• Patients receiving infusions must be attended at all times.
• Infusion pump or microdrip system and timer should be used to monitor infusion precisely.
• Monitor blood pressure and ECG continuously during I.V. administration. Watch for prolonged QT and QRS intervals, heart block, or increased dysrhythmias.
• Monitor therapeutic serum levels of procainamide:

3 to 10 mcg/ml (most patients are controlled at 4 to 8 mcg/ml); may exhibit toxicity at levels greater than 16 mcg/ml. Monitor NAPA levels as well; some clinicians feel that procainamide and NAPA levels should be 10 to 30 mcg/ml.

• Baseline and periodic determinations of ANA titers, lupus erythematosus (LE) cell preparations, and CBCs may be indicated, because procainamide therapy (usually long-term) has been associated with syndrome resembling systemic lupus erythematosus.

• I.V. drug form is more likely to cause adverse cardiac effects, possibly resulting in severe hypotension.

• In prolonged use of oral form, ECGs should be performed occasionally to determine continued need for the drug.

Information for parents and patient
• Inform parents and patient about the purpose of drug therapy and the need for frequent monitoring.

• Patient should take drug as directed and should not crush sustained-release tablets.

• Explain that laboratory tests may be required to measure blood levels of drug.

• Parents or patient should report palpitations or other adverse reactions.

---

procarbazine hydrochloride
Matulane, Natulan*

• Classification: antineoplastic (antibiotic antineoplastic [cell cycle-phase specific, S phase])

How supplied
Available by prescription only
Capsules: 50 mg

Indications, route, and dosage
Dosage and indications may vary. Check current literature for recommended protocol.
Hodgkin's disease; lymphomas; brain and lung cancer
Children: 50 mg P.O. daily for first week, then 100 mg/m² until response or toxicity occurs. Maintenance dosage is 50 mg P.O. daily after bone marrow recovery.

Adults: 2 to 4 mg/kg/day P.O. in single or divided doses for the first week, followed by 4 to 6 mg/kg/day until response or toxicity occurs. Maintenance dosage is 1 to 2 mg/kg/day.

Action and kinetics
• *Antineoplastic action:* The exact mechanism of procarbazine's cytotoxic activity is unknown. The drug appears to have several sites of action; the result is inhibition of DNA, RNA, and protein synthesis. Procarbazine has also been reported to damage DNA directly and to inhibit the mitotic S phase of cell division.

• *Kinetics in adults:* Procarbazine is rapidly and completely absorbed following oral administration. Procarbazine distributes widely into body tissues, with the highest concentrations found in the liver, kidneys, intestinal wall, and skin. The drug crosses the blood-brain barrier. Procarbazine is extensively metabolized in the liver. Some of the metabolites have cytotoxic activity. Procarbazine and its metabolites are excreted primarily in urine.

Contraindications and precautions
Procarbazine is contraindicated in patients with a history of hypersensitivity to the drug and in patients with poor bone marrow reserve because of potential for serious toxicity.

Drug should be used cautiously in patients with hepatic or renal impairment because of potential for drug accumulation; in those with infections because of decreased immune response; and in those taking concurrent CNS antidepressants or MAO inhibitors because the drug has MAO-inhibiting activity.

Interactions
Concomitant use of procarbazine with alcohol can cause a disulfiram-like reaction. The mechanism of this interaction is poorly defined. Concomitant use with CNS depressants enhances CNS depression through an additive mechanism; concomitant use with sympathomimetics, tricyclic antidepressants, MAO inhibitors, or tyramine-rich foods can cause a hypertensive crisis, tremors, excitation, and cardiac palpitations through inhibition of MAO by procarbazine.

Effects on diagnostic tests
None reported.

Adverse reactions
• CNS: paresthesias, myalgias, arthralgias, fatigue, lethargy, nervousness, depression, insomnia, nightmares, hallucinations, confusion.

• DERM: dermatitis, pruritus, flushing, hyperpigmentation, photosensitivity.

• EENT: retinal hemorrhage, nystagmus, photophobia, diplopia, papilledema, altered hearing abilities.

• GI: nausea, vomiting, anorexia, stomatitis, dry mouth, dysphagia, diarrhea, constipation.

• GU: decreased spermatogenesis, infertility.

• HEMA: bone marrow depression (dose-limiting), pancytopenia, hemolysis, bleeding tendency, thrombocytopenia, leukopenia, anemia.

• Other: chills, fever, pneumonitis, hypotension, reversible alopecia, pleural effusion.

Note: Drug should be discontinued if the following occur: bleeding or bleeding tendencies, stomatitis, diarrhea, paresthesias, neuropathies, confusion, or hypersensitivity.

Overdose and treatment
Clinical manifestations of overdose include myalgia, arthralgia, fever, weakness, dermatitis, alopecia, paresthesias, hallucinations, tremors, convulsions, coma, myelosuppression, nausea, and vomiting.

Treatment is usually supportive and includes transfusion of blood components, antiemetics, antipyretics, and appropriate antianxiety agents.

---

‡May contain sulfites   ♦May contain tartrazine   ♦♦May contain benzyl alcohol

▶ Special considerations

• Use in children requires close monitoring and individualized dosages because of potential for toxicity that may include tremors, seizures, and comas.
• Monitor BUN, hematocrit, platelet count, ALT (SGPT), AST (SGOT), LDH, serum bilirubin, serum creatinine, uric acid, and total and differential leukocytes.
• Severe reactions, such as tremors, seizures, and coma, have occurred after administration of procarbazine to children.
• Nausea and vomiting may be decreased if taken at bedtime and in divided doses.
• Procarbazine inhibits MAO. Use procarbazine cautiously with MAO inhibitors, tricyclic antidepressants, or tyramine-rich foods.
• Use cautiously in inadequate bone marrow reserve, leukopenia, thrombocytopenia, anemia, and impaired hepatic or renal function.
• Observe for signs of bleeding.
• Store capsules in dry environment.

Information for parents and patient

• Tell parents to avoid patient's exposure to persons with bacterial or viral infections as chemotherapy can make the patient more susceptible to infection. Urge parents to report infection immediately.
• Advise parents that patient should not receive live virus immunizations during therapy and for several weeks after therapy. Members of the same household should not receive live-virus immunizations during the same period.
• Patient should avoid contact with persons who have received live virus immunizations (polio, measles/mumps/rubella). Explain importance of promptly reporting susceptible patient's exposure to chicken pox.
• Tell parents that patient's dental work should be completed before therapy whenever possible, or delayed until blood counts are normal.
• Tell parents which foods are high in tyramine content and should be avoided.
• Warn parents and patient that bruising may easily occur because of drug's effect on blood count. Teach parents and patient to check for signs of bleeding and bruising. Parents may need to restrict child's participation in contact sports. Such activity is dangerous when patient's platelets are low.
• Stress importance of keeping follow-up appointments for monitoring hematologic status. Bone marrow toxicity may develop 2 to 5 weeks after therapy.
• Instruct parents to monitor neutropenic patient's temperature every 4 hours (not rectally) and to report fever, cough, and other signs of infection *promptly*.
• Instruct patient to clean teeth with toothettes, gauze, or soft toothbrush when platelets are low. Patient should perform frequent oral hygiene and should avoid using commercial mouthwashes, which may contain alcohol and have an irritating effect. Solutions of sodium bicarbonate or hydrogen peroxide are more appropriate rinses.
• Instruct patient to avoid foods that are spicy and extremely hot or cold. Topical anesthetics administered before meals (swish and spit) may relieve mouth discomfort.
• Emphasize to the parents and patient the importance

of continuing medication despite nausea and vomiting. Advise parents to call immediately if vomiting occurs shortly after taking dose.
• Premedicating with an antiemetic may prevent nausea and vomiting. If vomiting occurs, administer antiemetics p.r.n.
• Patients who have received drugs with strong emetic properties may experience anticipatory nausea and vomiting at subsequent treatments. They may benefit from treatment with an anxiolytic drug.
• Tell parents and patient to immediately report redness, pain, or swelling at injection site. Local tissue injury and scarring may result if I.V. infiltrates.
• Warn parents and patient that drowsiness may occur, so patient should avoid hazardous activities that require alertness until drug's effect is established.
• Advise parents that patient should avoid alcoholic beverages or medications containing alcohol (for example, acetaminophen elixirs) while taking this drug. They should stop medication and call immediately if patient experiences a disulfiram-like reaction (chest pains, rapid or irregular heartbeat, severe headache, stiff neck).
• Explain that orthostatic hypotension may occur. Advise patient to avoid abrupt changes in position.
• Warn parents that patient should avoid prolonged exposure to the sun because photosensitivity occurs during therapy.
• Tell parents to report rash or fever, which may indicate an allergic reaction.
• Sexually active patients should practice contraception while taking this drug.

---

prochlorperazine
Compazine, Stemetil∗

prochlorperazine edisylate
Compazine

prochlorpazine maleate
Chlorazine, Compazine, Compazine Spansule, Stemetil∗

• Classification: antipsychotic, antiemetic, antianxiety agent (phenothiazine [piperazine derivative])

How supplied
Available by prescription only
Prochlorperazine maleate
Tablets: 5 mg, 10 mg, 25 mg
Prochlorperazine edisylate
Spansules (sustained-release): 10 mg, 15 mg, 30 mg
Syrup: 1 mg/ml
Injection: 5 mg/ml
Suppositories: 2.5 mg, 5 mg, 25 mg

Indications, route, and dosage
Preoperative nausea control
Adults: 5 to 10 mg I.M. 1 to 2 hours before induction of anesthesia, repeated once in 30 minutes if necessary; or 5 to 10 mg I.V. 15 to 30 minutes before induction of anesthesia, repeated once if necessary;

---

or 20 mg/liter dextrose 5% and sodium chloride 0.9% solution by I.V. infusion, added to infusion 15 to 30 minutes before induction. Maximum parenteral dosage is 40 mg daily.

Severe nausea, vomiting of known origin
Children weighing 9 to 13 kg: 2.5 mg P.O. or rectally daily or b.i.d.; or 0.132 mg/kg deep I.M. injection. (Control usually is obtained with one dose.) Maximum dosage is 7.5 mg daily.

Children weighing 14 to 17 kg: 2.5 mg P.O. or rectally b.i.d. or t.i.d.; or 0.132 mg/kg deep I.M. injection. (Control usually is obtained with one dose.) Maximum dosage is 10 mg daily.

Children weighing 18 to 39 kg: 2.5 mg P.O. or rectally t.i.d.; or 5 mg P.O. or rectally b.i.d.; or 0.132 mg/kg deep I.M. injection. (Control usually obtained with one dose.) Maximum dosage is 15 mg daily.

Adults: 5 to 10 mg P.O. t.i.d. or q.i.d.; or 15 mg of sustained-release form P.O. on arising; or 10 to 30 mg of sustained-release form P.O. q 12 hours; or 25 mg rectally b.i.d.; or 5 to 10 mg I.M. injected deeply into upper outer quadrant of gluteal region. Repeat q 3 to 4 hours, p.r.n. May be given I.V. Maximum parenteral dosage is 40 mg daily.

Symptomatic relief of psychotic symptoms
Children age 2 to 12: 2.5 mg P.O. b.i.d. or t.i.d. Total dosage on the first day should not exceed 10 mg. Increase dosage as needed and tolerated to the following maximum: 20 mg daily in children age 2 to 5 years; 25 mg daily in children age 6 to 12 years. Dosage is not established for infants younger than age 2 years, or weighing less than 9 kg.

Action and kinetics
• *Antipsychotic action:* Prochlorperazine is thought to exert its antipsychotic effects by postsynaptic blockade of CNS dopamine receptors, thus inhibiting dopamine-mediated effects.

• *Antiemetic action:* Antiemetic effects are attributed to dopamine receptor blockade in the medullary chemoreceptor trigger zone.

Prochlorperazine has many other central and peripheral effects: it produces alpha and ganglionic blockade and counteracts histamine- and serotonin-mediated activity. Its most prevalent adverse reactions are extrapyramidal. It is used primarily as an antiemetic; it is ineffective against motion sickness.

• *Kinetics in adults:* Rate and extent of absorption vary with administration route: oral tablet absorption is erratic and variable, with onset of action ranging from ½ to 1 hour; oral concentrate absorption is more predictable. I.M. drug is absorbed rapidly.

Prochlorperazine is distributed widely into the body, including breast milk. Drug is 91% to 99% protein-bound. Peak effect occurs at 2 to 4 hours; steady-state serum levels are achieved within 4 to 7 days.

Prochlorperazine is metabolized extensively by the liver, but no active metabolites are formed; duration of action is about 4 to 6 hours.

Most of drug is excreted in urine via the kidneys; some is excreted in feces via the biliary tract.

Contraindications and precautions
Procholorperazine is contraindicated in patients with known hypersensitivity to phenothiazines and related compounds, including allergic reactions involving hepatic function; in patients with blood dyscrasias and bone marrow depression; and in patients with disorders accompanied by coma, brain damage, CNS depression, circulatory collapse, or cerebrovascular disease, because of adverse effects on blood pressure and possible additive CNS depression. It also is contraindicated for use with adrenergic-blocking agents or spinal or epidural anesthetics.

Prochlorperazine should be used cautiously in patients with cardiac disease (dysrhythmias, congestive heart failure, angina pectoris, valvular disease, or heart block) because of additive dysrhythmic effects; in patients with encephalitis; in patients with Reye's syndrome, head injury, or respiratory disease, because of additive CNS and respiratory depression; in patients with epilepsy and other seizure disorders because of lowered seizure threshold; in patients with glaucoma because of increased intraocular pressure; in patients with prostatic hypertrophy; in patients with urinary retention; in patients with hepatic or renal dysfunction; in patients with Parkinson's disease; in patients with pheochromocytoma because excessive buildup of neurotransmitters may have adverse cardiovascular effects; and in patients with hypocalcemia, which increases the risk of extrapyramidal symptoms. Drug therapy of uncomplicated nausea and vomiting in children should be avoided to prevent masking symptoms of serious underlying disease such as Reye's syndrome.

Interactions
Concomitant use of prochlorperazine with sympathomimetics, including epinephrine, phenylephrine, phenylpropanolamine, and ephedrine (often found in nasal sprays), and with appetite suppressants may decrease their stimulatory and pressor effects and may cause epinephrine reversal (hypotensive response to epinephrine).

Prochlorperazine may inhibit blood pressure response to centrally acting antihypertensive drugs, such as guanethidine, guanabenz, guanadrel, clonidine, methyldopa, and reserpine. Additive effects are likely after concomitant use of prochlorperazine with CNS depressants, including alcohol, analgesics, barbiturates, narcotics, tranquilizers, and anesthetics (general, spinal, or epidural), and parenteral magnesium sulfate (oversedation, respiratory depression, and hypotension); antiarrhythmic agents, quinidine, disopyramide, and procainamide (increased incidence of cardiac dysrhythmias and conduction defects); atropine and other anticholinergic drugs, including antidepressants, monoamine oxidase inhibitors, phenothiazines, antihistamines, meperidine, and antiparkinsonian agents (oversedation, paralytic ileus, visual changes, and severe constipation); nitrates (hypotension); and metrizamide (increased risk of convulsions).

Beta-blocking agents may inhibit prochlorperazine metabolism, increasing plasma levels and toxicity.

Concomitant use with propylthiouracil increases risk of agranulocytosis; concomitant use with lithium may result in severe neurologic toxicity with an encephalitis-like syndrome, and in decreased therapeutic response to prochlorperazine.

‡May contain sulfites ◆May contain tartrazine ◆◆May contain benzyl alcohol

Pharmacokinetic alterations and subsequent decreased therapeutic response to prochlorperazine may follow concomitant use with phenobarbital (enhanced renal excretion); aluminum- and magnesium-containing antacids and antidiarrheals (decreased absorption); caffeine; or heavy smoking (increased metabolism).

Prochlorperazine may antagonize therapeutic effect of bromocriptine on prolactin secretion; it also may decrease the vasoconstricting effects of high-dose dopamine and may decrease effectiveness and increase toxicity of levodopa (by dopamine blockade). Prochlorperazine may inhibit metabolism and increase toxicity of phenytoin.

Effects on diagnostic tests

Prochlorperazine causes false-positive test results for urinary porphyrins, urobilinogen, amylase, and 5-HIAA, because of darkening of urine by metabolites; it also causes false-positive urine pregnancy results in tests using human chorionic gonadotropin as the indicator.

Prochlorperazine elevates test results for liver enzymes and protein-bound iodine and causes quinidine-like ECG effects.

Adverse reactions

• CNS: *extrapyramidal symptoms—dystonia, akathisia, torticollis, tardive dyskinesia (dose-related, long-term therapy),* pseudoparkinsonism, neuroleptic malignant syndrome (dose-related; fatal respiratory failure in over 10% of patients if untreated), dizziness, drowsiness, sedation, headache, exacerbation of psychotic symptoms.
• CV: asystole, orthostatic hypotension, tachycardia, dizziness or fainting, dysrhythmias, ECG changes, increased anginal pain after I.M. injection.
• EENT: blurred vision, tinnitus, mydriasis, increased intraocular pressure, ocular changes (retinal pigmentary change with long-term use).
• GI: dry mouth, constipation, nausea, vomiting, anorexia, diarrhea.
• GU: urinary retention, gynecomastia, hypermenorrhea, inhibited ejaculation.
• HEMA: transient leukopenia, agranulocytosis, thrombocytopenia, anemia (within 30 to 90 days).
• Local: contact dermatitis from concentrate or injectable form, muscle necrosis from I.M. injection.
• Other: hyperprolactinemia, photosensitivity, increased appetite (weight gain), hypersensitivity (rash, urticaria, drug fever, edema, cholestatic jaundice [in 2% to 4% of patients within first 30 days]).

After abrupt withdrawal of long-term therapy, gastritis, nausea, vomiting, dizziness, tremors, feeling of heat or cold, sweating, tachycardia, headache, or insomnia may occur.

Note: Drug should be discontinued if hypersensitivity, jaundice, agranulocytosis, neuroleptic malignant syndrome (marked hyperthermia, extrapyramidal effects, autonomic dysfunction) occurs or if severe extrapyramidal symptoms occur even after dose is lowered. Drug should be discontinued 48 hours before and 24 hours after myelography using metrizamide, because of the risk of convulsions. When feasible, drug should be withdrawn slowly and gradually; many drug effects persist after withdrawal.

Overdose and treatment

CNS depression is characterized by deep, unarousable sleep and possible coma, hypotension or hypertension, extrapyramidal symptoms, dystonia, abnormal involuntary muscle movements, agitation, seizures, dysrhythmias, ECG changes, hypothermia or hyperthermia, and autonomic nervous system dysfunction.

Treatment is symptomatic and supportive and includes maintaining vital signs, airway, stable body temperature, and fluid and electrolyte balance.

Do not induce vomiting: drug inhibits cough reflex, and aspiration may occur. Use gastric lavage, then activated charcoal and saline cathartics; dialysis does not help. Regulate body temperature as needed. Treat hypotension with I.V. fluids: *do not give epinephrine.* Treat seizures with parenteral diazepam or barbiturates; dysrhythmias with parenteral phenytoin (1 mg/kg with rate titrated to blood pressure); and extrapyramidal reactions with barbiturates, benztropine, or parenteral diphenhydramine 2 mg/kg/minute.

▶ Special considerations

• Prochlorperazine is not recommended for patients under age 2 or weighing less than 9 kg.
• Unless otherwise specified, antipsychotics are not recommended for children under age 12; be careful when using phenothiazines for nausea and vomiting, as acutely ill children (chicken pox, measles, CNS infections, dehydration) are at greatly increased risk of dystonic reactions.
• Keep patient supine for 30 to 60 minutes after dose to prevent orthostatic hypotension.
• Check vital signs regularly for decreased blood pressure (especially before and after parenteral therapy) or tachycardia; observe patient carefully for other adverse reactions.
• Check intake and output for urinary retention or constipation, which may require dosage reduction.
• Monitor bilirubin levels weekly for first 4 weeks; monitor complete blood count, ECG (for quinidine-like effects), liver and renal function studies, electrolyte levels (especially potassium) and eye examinations at baseline and periodically thereafter, especially in patients on long-term therapy.
• Observe patient for mood changes to monitor progress; benefits may not be apparent for several weeks.
• Incidence of extrapyramidal reactions is higher in children.
• Monitor for involuntary movements. Check patient receiving prolonged treatment at least once every 6 months.
• Do not withdraw drug abruptly; although physical dependence does not occur with antipsychotic drugs, rebound exacerbation of psychotic symptoms may occur, and many drug effects persist.
• Carefully follow manufacturer's instructions for reconstitution, dilution, administration, and storage of drugs; slightly discolored liquids may or may not be all right to use. Check with pharmacist.
• The liquid and injectable formulations may cause a rash after contact with skin.

• Drug may cause a pink to brown discoloration of urine.

• Prochlorperazine is associated with a high incidence of extrapyramidal effects and, in institutionalized mental patients, photosensitivity reactions; patient should avoid exposure to sunlight or heat lamps.

• Oral formulations may cause stomach upset. Administer with food or fluid.

• Dilute the concentrate in 2 to 4 oz of water. The suppository form should be stored in a cool place.

• Give I.V. dose slowly (5 mg/minute). I.M. injection may cause skin necrosis; take care to prevent extravasation. Do not administer subcutaneously.

• Administer I.M. injection deep into the upper outer quadrant of the buttock. Massaging the area after administration may prevent formation of abscesses.

• Solution for injection may be slightly discolored. Do not use if excessively discolored or if a precipitate is evident. Contact pharmacist.

• Monitor patient's blood pressure before and after parenteral administration.

• The sustained-release form should not be given to children.

• Prochlorperazine is ineffective in treating motion sickness.

• Sugarless chewing gum, hard candy, or ice chips may help relieve dry mouth.

• Protect the liquid formulation from light.

Information for parents and patient

• Explain rationale and anticipated risks and benefits of therapy, and that full therapeutic effect may not occur for several weeks.

• Patient should avoid beverages and drugs containing alcohol, and not to take any other drug (especially CNS depressants) including nonprescription products without medical approval.

• Instruct diabetic patients to monitor blood glucose levels, because drug may alter insulin needs.

• Teach parents or patient how and when to take drug, not to increase dose without medical approval, and never to discontinue drug abruptly; suggest taking full dose at bedtime if daytime sedation is troublesome.

• Advise parents to have patient lie down for 30 minutes after first dose (1 hour if I.M.) and to rise slowly from sitting or supine position to prevent orthostatic hypotension.

• Patient should avoid hazardous activities and tasks requiring mental alertness and psychomotor coordination, such as driving, until full effects of drug are established.

• Drugs are locally irritating; advise taking with milk or food to minimize GI distress. Warn that oral concentrates and solutions will irritate skin. Patient should not crush or open sustained-release products, but swallow them whole.

• Warn parents that excessive exposure to sunlight, heat lamps, or tanning beds may cause photosensitivity reactions (burn and abnormal hyperpigmentation).

• Tell parents that patient should avoid exposure to extremes of heat or cold, because of risk of hypothermia or hyperthermia induced by alteration in thermoregulatory function.

• Recommend sugarless gum, hard candy, or ice chips to relieve dry mouth.

• Explain that phenothiazines may cause pink to brown discoloration of urine.

• Explain the risks of dystonic reactions and tardive dyskinesia. Tell parents and patient to report abnormal body movements promptly.

• Tell parents to avoid spilling the liquid form. Contact with skin may cause rash and irritation.

• Tell parents to dilute the concentrate in water; explain the dropper technique of measuring dose; teach correct use of suppository.

• Urge parents to store this drug safely away from children.

• Tell parents that interactions are possible with many drugs. Patient should not take any other medication unless prescribed.

• Warn parents to report promptly if difficulty urinating, sore throat, dizziness, or fainting develop. Reassure them that most reactions can be relieved by reducing dose.

• Patient should avoid hazardous activities that require alertness until the drug's effect is established. Sedative effects subside and become tolerable in several weeks.

---

promazine hydrochloride
Prozine, Sparine

• Classification: antipsychotic, antiemetic (aliphatic phenothiazine)

How supplied
Available by prescription only
Tablets: 25 mg, 50 mg, 100 mg
Syrup: 10 mg/5 ml
Injection: 25 mg, 50 mg/ml

Indications, route, and dosage
Psychosis
Children over age 12: 10 to 25 mg P.O. or I.M. q 4 to 6 hours.
Adults: 10 to 200 mg P.O. or I.M. q 4 to 6 hours, up to 1 g daily; in acutely agitated patients, the initial I.M. or I.V. dose is 50 to 150 mg. Dose may be repeated within 5 to 10 minutes if necessary. Give I.V. dose in concentrations no greater than 25 mg/ml.

Use of doses over 1,000 mg/day has not increased therapeutic effect.

Action and kinetics
• *Antipsychotic action:* Promazine is thought to exert its antipsychotic effects by postsynaptic blockade of CNS dopamine receptors, thus inhibiting dopamine-mediated effects; antiemetic effects are attributed to dopamine receptor blockade in the medullary chemoreceptor trigger zone. Promazine has many other central and peripheral effects: it produces both alpha and ganglionic blockade and counteracts histamine- and serotonin-mediated activity. Its most prevalent side effects are antimuscarinic and sedative; it causes

---

‡May contain sulfites   ♦May contain tartrazine   ♦♦May contain benzyl alcohol

fewer extrapyramidal effects than other drugs in this class.

• *Kinetics in adults:* Promazine usually is absorbed well from the GI tract. Liquid forms have the most predictable effect, whereas tablets have erratic and variable absorption. Onset of effect ranges from ½ to 1 hour. I.M. drug is absorbed rapidly.

Promazine is distributed widely into the body, including breast milk. Peak effect occurs at 2 to 4 hours; steady-state serum level is achieved within 4 to 7 days. Drug is 91% to 99% protein-bound.

Promazine is metabolized extensively by the liver, but no active metabolites are formed.

Most of drug is excreted as metabolites in urine; some is excreted in feces via the biliary tract.

Contraindications and precautions

Promazine is contraindicated in patients with known hypersensitivity to phenothiazines and related compounds, including allergic reactions involving hepatic function; in patients with blood dyscrasias and bone marrow depression because of adverse hematologic effects; in patients with disorders accompanied by coma, CNS depression, or in patients with brain damage, because of additive CNS depression; in patients with circulatory collapse or cerebrovascular disease because of adverse effects on blood pressure; and in patients who are receiving adrenergic-blocking agents or spinal or epidural anesthetics, because of potential for excessive hypotensive response.

Promazine should be used cautiously in patients with cardiac disease (dysrhythmias, congestive heart failure, angina pectoris, valvular disease, or heart block), encephalitis, Reye's syndrome, head injury, respiratory disease, epilepsy and other seizure disorders, glaucoma, prostatic hypertrophy, urinary retention, hepatic or renal dysfunction, Parkinson's disease, pheochromocytoma, or hypocalcemia. Some oral preparations of promazine contain tartrazine; dyes may cause allergic reaction in aspirin-allergic patients.

Interactions

Concomitant use of promazine with sympathomimetics, including epinephrine, phenylephrine, phenylpropanolamine, and ephedrine (often found in nasal sprays), and with appetite suppressants may decrease their stimulatory and pressor effects.

Promazine may inhibit blood pressure response to centrally acting antihypertensive drugs, such as guanethidine, guanabenz, guanadrel, clonidine, methyldopa, and reserpine. Additive effects are likely after concomitant use of promazine with CNS depressants, including alcohol, analgesics, barbiturates, narcotics, tranquilizers, anesthetics (general, spinal or epidural), and parenteral magnesium sulfate (oversedation, respiratory depression, and hypotension); antiarrhythmic agents, quinidine, disopyramide, and procainamide (increased incidence of cardiac dysrhythmias and conduction defects); atropine and other anticholinergic drugs, including antidepressants, monoamine oxidase inhibitors, phenothiazines, antihistamines, meperidine, and antiparkinsonian agents (oversedation, paralytic ileus, visual changes,

and severe constipation); nitrates (hypotension); and metrizamide (increased risk of convulsions).

Beta-blocking agents may inhibit promazine metabolism, increasing plasma levels and toxicity.

Concomitant use with propylthiouracil increases risk of agranulocytosis; concomitant use with lithium may result in severe neurologic toxicity with an encephalitis-like syndrome, and in decreased therapeutic response to promazine.

Pharmacokinetic alterations and subsequent decreased therapeutic response to promazine may follow concomitant use with phenobarbital (enhanced renal excretion); aluminum- and magnesium-containing antacids and antidiarrheals (decreased absorption); caffeine; or heavy smoking (increased metabolism).

Promazine may antagonize the therapeutic effect of bromocriptine on prolactin secretion; it also may decrease the vasoconstricting effects of high-dose dopamine and may decrease effectiveness and increase toxicity of levodopa (by dopamine blockade). Promazine may inhibit metabolism and increase toxicity of phenytoin.

Effects on diagnostic tests

Promazine causes false-positive test results for urinary porphyrins, urobilinogen, amylase, and 5-HIAA because of darkening of urine by metabolites; it also causes false-positive urine pregnancy results in tests using human chorionic gonadotropin as the indicator.

Promazine elevates test results for liver enzymes and protein-bound iodine and causes quinidine-like effects on the ECG.

Adverse reactions

• CNS: extrapyramidal symptoms—dystonia, akathisia, torticollis, tardive dyskinesia (dose-related, long-term therapy), sedation, pseudoparkinsonism, drowsiness (frequent), neuroleptic malignant syndrome (dose-related; if untreated, fatal respiratory failure in over 10% of patients), dizziness, headache, insomnia, exacerbation of psychotic symptoms.

• CV: asystole, orthostatic hypotension, tachycardia, dizziness or fainting, dysrhythmias, ECG changes, increased anginal pain after I.M. injection.

• EENT: blurred vision, tinnitus, mydriasis, increased intraocular pressure, ocular changes (retinal pigmentary change with long-term use).

• GI: dry mouth, constipation, nausea, vomiting, anorexia, diarrhea.

• GU: urinary retention, gynecomastia, hypermenorrhea, inhibited ejaculation.

• HEMA: transient leukopenia, agranulocytosis, thrombocytopenia, anemia (within 30 to 90 days).

• Local: contact dermatitis from concentrate or injectable form, muscle necrosis from I.M. injection.

• Other: hyperprolactinemia, photosensitivity (high incidence), increased appetite or weight gain, hypersensitivity (rash, urticaria, drug fever, edema, cholestatic jaundice [in 2% to 4% of patients within first 30 days]).

After abrupt withdrawal of long-term therapy, gastritis, nausea, vomiting, dizziness, tremors, feeling of heat or cold, sweating, tachycardia, headache, or insomnia may occur.

Note: Drug should be discontinued immediately if

any of the following occurs: hypersensitivity, jaundice, agranulocytosis, neuroleptic malignant syndrome (marked hyperthermia, extrapyramidal effects, autonomic dysfunction), or severe extrapyramidal symptoms even after dosage is lowered. Drug should be discontinued 48 hours before and 24 hours after myelography using metrizamide, because of the risk of convulsions. When feasible, drug should be withdrawn slowly and gradually; many drug effects persist after withdrawal.

Overdose and treatment

CNS depression is characterized by deep, unarousable sleep and possible coma, hypotension or hypertension, extrapyramidal symptoms, abnormal involuntary muscle movements, agitation, seizures, dysrhythmias, ECG changes, hypothermia or hyperthermia, and autonomic nervous system dysfunction.

Treatment is symptomatic and supportive and includes maintaining vital signs, airway, stable body temperature, and fluid and electrolyte balance.

Do not induce vomiting: drug inhibits cough reflex, and aspiration may occur. Use gastric lavage, then activated charcoal and saline cathartics; dialysis does not help. Regulate body temperature as needed. Treat hypotension with I.V. fluids: *do not give epinephrine.* Treat seizures with parenteral diazepam or barbiturates; dysrhythmias with parenteral phenytoin (1 mg/kg with rate titrated to blood pressure); and extrapyramidal reactions with barbiturates, benztropine, or parenteral diphenhydramine 2 mg/kg/minute.

▶ Special considerations

• Promazine is not recommended for children under age 12.
• Check vital signs regularly for decreased blood pressure (especially before and after parenteral therapy) or tachycardia; observe patient carefully for other adverse reactions.
• Check intake and output for urinary retention or constipation, which may require dosage reduction.
• Monitor bilirubin levels weekly for first 4 weeks; monitor complete blood count, ECG (for quinidine-like effects), liver and renal function studies, electrolyte levels (especially potassium) and eye examinations at baseline and periodically thereafter, especially in patients on long-term therapy.
• Observe patient for mood changes to monitor progress; benefits may not be apparent for several weeks.
• Monitor for involuntary movements. Check patient receiving prolonged treatment at least once every 6 months.
• Do not withdraw drug abruptly; although physical dependence does not occur with antipsychotic drugs, rebound exacerbation of psychotic symptoms may occur, and many drug effects persist.
• Carefully follow manufacturer's instructions for reconstitution, dilution, administration, and storage of drugs; slightly discolored liquids may or may not be all right to use. Check with pharmacist.
• Liquid and injectable formulations may cause a rash after contact with skin.
• Drug may cause a pink to brown discoloration of the urine.
• Promazine is associated with a high incidence of

sedation, orthostatic hypotension, and tardive dyskinesia.
• Oral formulations may cause stomach upset. Administer with food or fluid.
• Dilute the concentrate in 2 to 4 oz of liquid, preferably water, carbonated drinks, fruit juice, tomato juice, milk, or pudding. Recommended dilution is 10 ml of liquid per 25 mg of drug.
• I.V. use is not recommended; however, if it is necessary, drug should be diluted to not more than 25 mg/ml, given slowly with special care to prevent extravasation. I.V. route should be used during surgery or for severe hiccups.
• To prevent photosensitivity reactions, patient should avoid exposure to sunlight or heat lamps.
• Administer I.M. injection deep into the upper outer quadrant of the buttock. Massaging the area after administration may prevent the formation of abscesses. I.M. injection may cause skin necrosis; take care to avoid extravasation. Monitor blood pressure before and after parenteral administration.
• Shake syrup before administration.
• Sugarless chewing gum, hard candy, or ice chips may help relieve dry mouth.
• The injection may be slightly discolored. Do not use if excessively discolored or if a precipitate is evident. Contact pharmacist.
• Protect the liquid formulation from light.

Information for parents and patient

• Explain rationale and anticipated risks and benefits of therapy, and that full therapeutic effect may not occur for several weeks.
• Teach signs and symptoms of adverse reactions and importance of reporting *any* unusual effects, especially involuntary movements.
• Tell parents that patient should avoid beverages and drugs containing alcohol, and should not take any other drug (especially CNS depressants) including nonprescription products without medical approval.
• Instruct parents of diabetic children to monitor blood glucose levels, because drug may alter insulin needs.
• Teach parents or patient how and when to take drug, not to increase dose without medical approval, and never to discontinue drug abruptly; suggest taking full dose at bedtime if daytime sedation is troublesome.
• Advise parents to have patient to lie down for 30 minutes after first dose (1 hour if I.M.) and to rise slowly from sitting or supine position to prevent orthostatic hypotension.
• Drugs are locally irritating; advise taking with milk or food to minimize GI distress. Warn that oral concentrates and solutions will irritate skin. Patient should not crush or open sustained-release products, but to swallow them whole.
• Recommend sugarless gum, hard candy, or ice chips to relieve dry mouth.
• Explain that phenothiazines may cause pink to brown discoloration of urine.
• Explain the risks of dystonic reactions and tardive dyskinesias, and the importance of reporting abnormal body movements promptly.
• Tell parents and patient to avoid spilling the liquid form. Contact with skin may cause rash and irritation.

---

‡May contain sulfites   ♦ May contain tartrazine   ♦♦ May contain benzyl alcohol

- Patient should avoid extremely hot or cold baths or exposure to temperature extremes, sunlamps, or tanning beds; drug may cause thermoregulatory changes and photosensitivity.
- Explain that patient should take drug exactly as prescribed; not to double the dose for missed doses; not to share drug with others; not to stop taking the drug suddenly, and not to take any other medications without medical approval.
- Reassure parents or patient that most adverse reactions can be alleviated by dosage reduction, but they should promptly report difficulty urinating, sore throat, dizziness, or fainting.
- Patient should avoid hazardous activities that require alertness until the drug's effect is established. Excessive sedative effects usually subside after several weeks.
- Explain which fluids are appropriate for diluting the concentrate. Explain the dropper technique of measuring dose. Tell patient to shake syrup form before administration.
- Store drug safely away from children.

promethazine hydrochloride
Anergan, Baymethazine, Ganphen, Histantil*, K-Phen, Mallergan, Pentazine, Phenameth, Phenazine, Phencen-50, Phenergan, Phenergan Fortis, Phenergan Plain, Phenoject-50, PMS Promethazine*, Prometh, Prorex, Prothazine, Prothazine Plain, Provigan, Remsed, V-Gan

- Classification: antiemetic and antivertigo agent, antihistamine, H₁-receptor antagonist, preoperative or postoperative sedative and adjunct to analgesics (phenothiazine derivative)

How supplied
Available by prescription only
Tablets: 12.5 mg, 25 mg, 50 mg
Syrup: 6.25 mg/5 ml, 10 mg/5 ml, 25 mg/5 ml
Suppositories: 12.5 mg, 25 mg, 50 mg
Injection: 25 mg/ml, 50 mg/ml

Indications, route, and dosage
Motion sickness
Children: 12.5 to 25 mg P.O., I.M., or rectally b.i.d.
Adults: 25 mg P.O. b.i.d.
Nausea
Children: 0.25 to 0.5 mg/kg I.M. or rectally q 4 to 6 hours, p.r.n.
Adults: 12.5 to 25 mg P.O., I.M., or rectally q 4 to 6 hours, p.r.n.
Rhinitis, allergy symptoms
Children: 6.25 to 12.5 mg P.O. t.i.d., or 25 mg P.O. or rectally at bedtime.
Adults: 12.5 mg P.O. before meals and at bedtime; or 25 mg P.O. at bedtime.
Sedation
Children: 12.5 to 25 mg P.O., I.M., or rectally at bedtime.

Adults: 25 to 50 mg P.O. or I.M. at bedtime or p.r.n.
Routine preoperative or postoperative sedation or as an adjunct to analgesics
Children: 12.5 to 25 mg I.M., I.V., or P.O.
Adults: 25 to 50 mg I.M., I.V., or P.O.

Actions and kinetics
- *Antiemetic and antivertigo action:* The central antimuscarinic actions of antihistamines probably are responsible for their antivertigo and antiemetic effects; promethazine also is believed to inhibit the medullary chemoreceptor trigger zone.
- *Antihistamine action:* Promethazine competes with histamine for the H₁-receptor, thereby suppressing allergic rhinitis and urticaria; drug does not prevent the release of histamine.
- *Sedative action:* CNS depressant mechanism of promethazine is unknown; phenothiazines probably cause sedation by reducing stimuli to the brain-stem reticular system.
- *Kinetics in adults:* Promethazine is well absorbed from the GI tract. Onset begins 20 minutes after oral, rectal, or I.M. administration and within 3 to 5 minutes after I.V. administration. Effects usually last 4 to 6 hours but may persist for 12 hours. Promethazine is distributed widely throughout the body; drug crosses the placenta. It is metabolized in the liver. Metabolites are excreted in urine and feces.

Contraindications and precautions
Promethazine is contraindicated in patients with known hypersensitivity to promethazine or other antihistamines or phenothiazines; during asthmatic attacks, because it thickens bronchial secretions; in acutely ill or dehydrated children, because they are at increased risk of dystonias; in patients with bone marrow depression, because it may induce blood dyscrasias; in epilepsy, because it may worsen seizure disorder; in comatose patients; and in neonates.

Like other antihistamines, promethazine has significant anticholinergic effects; it should be used with caution in patients with narrow-angle glaucoma, peptic ulcer, or pyloroduodenal obstruction or urinary bladder obstruction from narrowing of the bladder neck. It also should be used with caution in patients with cardiovascular disease or hypertension because of the risk of palpitations, tachycardia, and increased hypertension; in patients with acute or chronic respiratory dysfunction, because drug may suppress the cough reflex; in patients with hepatic dysfunction; and in children with a history of sleep apnea or a family history of sudden infant death syndrome. The relationship between these conditions and the use of promethazine has not been studied; however, a number of deaths have occurred in children who were given usual dosages of phenothiazine and antihistamines.

Antiemetic action may mask symptoms of undiagnosed diseases, drug overdose, and the ototoxic effects of aspirin — dizziness, vertigo, tinnitus — or other ototoxic drugs.

Interactions
Do not give promethazine concomitantly with epinephrine, because it may result in partial adrenergic blockade, producing further hypotension; or with MAO

inhibitors, which interfere with the detoxification of antihistamines and phenothiazines and thus prolong and intensify their sedative and anticholinergic effects. Additive CNS depression may occur when promethazine is given with other antihistamines or CNS depressants, such as alcohol, barbiturates, tranquilizers, sleeping aids, and antianxiety agents.

Effects on diagnostic tests

Promethazine should be discontinued 4 days before diagnostic skin tests to avoid preventing, reducing, or masking test response. Promethazine may cause hyperglycemia and either false-positive or false-negative pregnancy test results. It also may interfere with blood grouping in the ABO system.

Adverse reactions

• CNS: sedation, confusion, restlessness, tremors, drowsiness, extrapyramidal symptoms, dizziness, disorientation, disturbed coordination.
• CV: hypotension, hypertension.
• EENT: transient myopia, nasal congestion, oculogyric crisis.
• GI: anorexia, nausea, vomiting, constipation, dry mouth.
• GU: urinary retention.
• HEMA: leukopenia, agranulocytosis, thrombocytopenia.
• Other: photosensitivity, reversible obstructive jaundice.

Overdose and treatment

Clinical manifestations of overdose may include either CNS depression (sedation, reduced mental alertness, apnea, and cardiovascular collapse) or CNS stimulation (insomnia, hallucinations, tremors, or convulsions). Atropine-like symptoms, such as dry mouth, flushed skin, fixed and dilated pupils, and GI symptoms, are common, especially in children.

Empty stomach by gastric lavage; do not induce vomiting. Treat hypotension with vasopressors, and control seizures with diazepam or phenytoin; correct acidosis and electrolyte imbalance. Urinary acidification promotes excretion of drug. *Do not give stimulants.*

▶ Special considerations

• Use cautiously in children with respiratory dysfunction. Safety and efficacy in children under age 2 have not been established; do not give promethazine to infants under age 3 months.
• Children, especially those under age 6, may experience paradoxical hyperexcitability with restlessness, insomnia, nervousness, euphoria, tremors, and seizures.
• Drug is contraindicated during an acute asthma attack, because it may not alleviate the symptoms and because antimuscarinic effects can cause thickening of secretions.
• Monitor blood counts during long-term therapy; watch for signs of blood dyscrasias.
• Reduce GI distress by giving drug with food; give sugarless gum or candy or ice chips to relieve dry mouth; increase fluid intake (if allowed) or humidify air to decrease adverse effect of thickened secretions.

• If tolerance develops, another antihistamine may be substituted.
• Promethazine may mask ototoxicity from high doses of aspirin and other salicylates.
• Pronounced sedative effects may limit use in some ambulatory patients.
• The 50 mg/ml concentration is for I.M. use only; inject deep into large muscle mass. Do not administer drug subcutaneously; this may cause chemical irritation and necrosis. Drug may be administered I.V., in concentrations not to exceed 25 mg/ml and at a rate not to exceed 25 mg/minute; when using I.V. drip, wrap in aluminum foil to protect drug from light.
• Promethazine and meperidine (Demerol) may be mixed in the same syringe.

Information for parents and patient

• Advise parents that patient should take drug with meals or snack to prevent gastric upset and to use any of the following measures to relieve dry mouth: warm water rinses, artificial saliva, ice chips, or sugarless gum or candy. Patient should avoid overusing motuhwash, which may add to dryness (alcohol content) and destroy normal flora.
• Warn parents that patient should avoid hazardous activities requiring mental alertness until extent of CNS effects are known and should not take tranquilizers, sedatives, pain relievers, or sleeping medications without medical approval.
• Advise parents to discontinue promethazine 4 days before diagnostic skin tests to preserve accuracy of tests.
• Warn parents and patient about possible photosensitivity and teach ways to avoid it.
• When treating motion sickness, patient should take first dose 30 to 60 minutes before travel; on succeeding days, he should take dose upon arising and with evening meal.

---

proparacaine hydrochloride
Ak-Taine, Alcaine, Ophthaine Hydrochloride, Ophthetic Sterile Ophthalmic Solution

• Classification: local anesthetic

How supplied
Available by prescription only
Ophthalmic solution: 0.5%

Indications, route, and dosage
Anesthesia for tonometry, gonioscopy; suture removal from cornea; removal of corneal foreign bodies
Children and adults: Instill 1 or 2 drops of 0.5% solution in eye just before procedure.
Anesthesia for cataract extraction, glaucoma surgery
Children and adults: Instill 1 drop of 0.5% solution in eye every 5 to 10 minutes for 5 to 7 doses.

Action and kinetics
• *Anesthetic action:* Produces anesthesia by preventing initiation and transmission of impulse at the nerve cell membrane.
• *Kinetics in adults:* Onset of action is within 20 seconds of instillation. Duration of action is 15 to 20 minutes.

Contraindications and precautions
Proparacaine hydrochloride is contraindicated in patients with hypersensitivity to ester-type local anesthetics, para-aminobenzoic acid or its derivatives, or any other ingredient in the preparation. It should be used with caution in patients with cardiac disease or hyperthyroidism.

Interactions
None reported.

Effects on diagnostic tests
Proparacaine hydrochloride therapy may inhibit the growth of organisms on cultures for detection of infection.

Adverse reactions
• Eye: occasional conjunctival congestion or hemorrhage, transient pain, pupil dilation, cycloplegic effect, softening and erosion of the corneal epilthelium, hyperallergenic corneal reaction.
• Other: hypersensitivity, allergic contact dermatitis.
  Note: Drug should be discontinued if symptoms of hypersensitivity occur.

Overdose and treatment
Clinical manifestations of overdose are extremely rare with ophthalmic administration. Clinical manifestations are CNS stimulation (such as alertness, agitation), followed by depression.
  Ocular overexposure should be treated by irrigation with warm water for at least 15 minutes.

▶ Special considerations
• Proparacaine is the topical ophthalmic anesthetic of choice in diagnostic and minor surgical procedures.
• Drug is not for long-term use; may delay wound healing.
• There is no ocular condition for which the patient should treat himself with this drug. It should not be given to patient for relief of eye pain.
• Do not use discolored solution; store in tightly closed original container.
• Ophthaine brand packaging resembles that of Hemoccult in size and shape; check label carefully.

Information for parents and patient
• Warn patient not to rub or touch eye while cornea is anesthetized; this may cause corneal abrasion and greater discomfort when anesthesia wears off; advise use of a protective eye patch after procedures.
• Explain that corneal pain in abrasion is relieved only temporarily by the application of proparacaine hydrochloride.
• Tell parents and patient that local irritation or stinging may occur several hours after instillation of proparacaine.

---

propiomazine hydrochloride
Largon

• Classification: postoperative or preoperative, sedative and adjunct to analgesics (phenothiazine derivative)

How supplied
Available by prescription only
Injection: 20 mg/ml

Indications, route and dosage
Anesthesia adjunct for the relief of restlessness and apprehension, preoperatively or during surgery
Children weighing up to 27 kg: Intramuscular or intravenous, 550 mcg (0.55 mg) to 1.1 mg per kg of body weight; 0.55 to 1.1 mg/kg I.M. or I.V. alternately, adjust dosage according to age as follows:
Children age 2 to 4 years: 10 mg I.M. or I.V.
Children age 4 to 6 years: 15 mg I.M. or I.V.
Children age 6 to 12 years: 25 mg I.M. or I.V.
Preoperative
Adults: Preoperatively, 20 to 40 mg I.M. or I.V. administered with 50 mg of meperidine; during surgery with local nerve block or spinal anesthesia 10 to 20 mg I.M. or I.V. Doses may be repeated every 3 hours, if necessary.

Action and kinetics
• *Sedative action:* Propiomazine has sedative properties similar to promethazine. The mechanism of its CNS effect is unknown. Phenothiazines probably cause sedation by reducing stimuli to the brain-stem reticular system.
• *Antiemetic and antivertigo action:* The central antimuscarinic actions of antihistamines probably are responsible for their antivertigo and antimetic effects; also may inhibit the medullary chemoreceptor trigger zone.
• *Antihistamine action:* Probably competes with histamine for the H_1-receptor.
• *Kinetics in adults:* Propiomazine is probably well absorbed from parenteral sites. Peak sedative effects occur in 15 to 30 minutes after I.V. administration; in 40 to 60 minutes after I.M. administration. Peak serum concentration occurs 1 to 3 hours after I.M. administration. Like other phenothiazines, propiomazine is probably widely distributed in the body, metabolized in the liver, and excreted in the urine and bile. Duration of action is about 3 to 6 hours. It is unknown if propiomazine crosses the placenta or distributesinto breast milk.

Contraindications and precautions
Propiomazine is contraindicated in patients with known hypersensitivity to propiomazine, promethazine or other antihistamines or phenothiazides; in patients who have received large doses of CNS depressants or who are comatose; and in patients with bone marrow depression because it may induce blood dyscrasias.

Like other antihistamines, propiomazine has significant anticholinergic effects; it should be used with caution in patients with narrow-angle glaucoma, peptic ulcer, or pyloroduodenal obstruction or urinary bladder obstruction from prostatic hypertrophy or narrowing of the bladder neck. It also should be used with extreme caution in patients with hypertensive crisis, and in patients with cardiovascular disease or hypertension because of the risk of palpitations, tachycardia, and increased hypertension; in patients with acute or chronic respiratory dysfunction (especially children), because drug may suppress the cough reflex; in patients with hepatic dysfunction; and in children with a history of sleep apnea or a family history of sudden infant death syndrome—the relationship between these conditions and the use of propiomazine has not been studied; however, several deaths have occurred in children who were given usual dosages of phenothiazines and antihistamines. Propriomazine should be avoided in patients with sensitivity to sulfites because the commercial formulation contains sodium formaldehyde sulfoxylate.

Interactions

Additive or potentiated CNS depression may occur when proprimazine is given with other opiates or other analgesics and other CNS depressants such as barbiturates or other sedatives, antihistamines, tranquilizers, or alcohol. Caution is recommended and dosage of one or both agents should be reduced; dosage of barbiturates to approximately one-half of the usual dose and reduction of narcotic analgesics to approximately one-fourth to one-half of the usual dose is recommended.

Do not give propiomazine concomitantly with epinephrine, because it may result in partial adrenergic blockade, producing further hypotension, or with monoamine oxidase (MAO) inhibitors, which interfere with the detoxification of antihistamines and phenothiazines and thus prolong and intensify their sedative and anticholinergic effects. Concurrent use with mecamylamine or trimethaphan, other CNS depressants, or alcohol may potentiate the hypotensive response with increased risk of shock and cardiovascular collapse during surgery; concurrent use during titration of calcium channel blocker dosage may cause excessive hypotension; concurrent use with high dosage or rapid administration of ketamine may increase the risk of hypotension and respiratory depression.

Effects on diagnostic tests

Propiomazine may cause false-positive results of the phentolamine test; it should be withdrawn at least 24 hours, preferably 48 to 72 hours before phentolamine test.

Adverse reactions

• CNS: dizziness, drowsiness, confusion, ammnesia, restlessness, akathisia (dose related), extrapyramidal symptoms, reactivation of psychotic processes; neuroleptic malignant syndrome (NMS: hyperthermia, dehydration, cardiovascular instability; hypoxia).
• CV: transient hypotension (with rapid administration); tachycardia; cardiac arrest; hypertension.
• HEMA: blood dyscrasias.
• GI: dry mouth; hepatotoxicity; nausea, vomiting, diarrhea.
• Other: rashes, respiratory depression, altered respiratory patterns, venous irritation and thrombophlebitis (after I.V. administration), endocrine disturbances, ocular changes, hypersensitivity reactions.

Note: Propriomazine should be discontinued immediately if the patient develops fever; neuroleptic malignant syndrome can be fatal.

Overdose and treatment

Clinical effects of propiomazine may include convulsive seizures, severe extrapyramidal symptoms, and other effects ranging from mild CNS depression to profound hypotension and coma.

Treatment is symptomatic and supportive and requires general physiologic measures such as maintenance of adequate ventilation. Analeptics may cause seizures and should not be used. In the absence of seizures, early gastric lavage (with an endotracheal tube with cuff inflated in place to prevent aspiration of gastric contents) may be beneficial. Centrally acting emetics are probably of little value in the management of propiomazine overdosage. Seizures may be controlled with diazepam or barbiturates such as pentobarbital or secobarbital. Anticholinergic antiparkisonian agents may be used to treat severe extrapyramidal reactions. Severe hypotension may respond to administration of norepinephrine or phenylephrine. Epinephrine should not be used because it may lower the blood pressure further.

▶ Special considerations

• Unless otherwise specified, antipsychotics are not recommended for children under age 12; be careful when using phenothiazines for nausea and vomiting, because acutely ill children (chicken pox, measles, CNS infections, dehydration) are at greatly increased risk of dystonic reactions.
• Propiomazine may be administered I.V. or I.M. The drug should not be given subcutaneously or intraarterially. Dosages of propiomazine by either I.V. or I.M. administration are identical.
• Because I.V. administration of propiomazine may cause irritation and thrombophlebitis this drug should be injected only into a large, undamaged vein with special care to avoid extravasation. Propiomazine should not be administered intra-arterially because severe chemical irritation may cause severe arteriospasm, possibly resulting in impairment of circulation and gangrene.
• Safe use of propiomazine in the first trimester of pregnancy has not been established.
• I.V. injections should be administered slowly, as too rapid administration may cause transient hypotension.
• If NMS occurs, treatment is essentially sympomatic and supportive and may include the following: for hyperthermia, administering antipyretics (aspirin or acetaminophen), and using cooling blanket; for dehydration, restoring fluids and electrolytes; for cardiovascular instability, monitoring blood pressure and cardiac rhythm closely and administering sodium ni-

---

‡May contain sulfites   ◆May contain tartrazine   ◆◆May contain benzyl alcohol

troprusside to allow vasodilation, with subsequent heat loss from the skin in patients with less dominant muscle rigidity; for hypoxia, administering oxygen and providing mechanical ventilation if necessary; for muscle rigidity, administering dantrolene sodium (100 to 300 mg per day in divided doses; 1.25 to 1.5 mg per kg of body weight, intravenously); or administering amantadine 100 mg twice daily, or bromocriptine, 5 mg three times a day, to restore central balance of dopamine and acetylcholine at the receptor site.

• Aqueous solutions of propiomazine are incompatible with barbiturate salts and other alkaline substances.

• Check vital signs regularly for decreased blood pressure (especially before and after parenteral therapy) or tachycardia; observe patient carefully for other adverse reactions.

• Check intake and output for urinary retention or constipation, which may require dosage reduction.

• Monitor bilirubin levels weekly for first 4 weeks; monitor complete blood count, ECG (for quinidine-like effects), liver and renal function studies, electrolyte levels (especially potassium) and eye examinations at baseline and periodically thereafter, especially in patients on long-term therapy.

• Observe patient for mood changes to monitor progress; benefits may not be apparent for several weeks.

• Monitor for involuntary movements. Check patient receiving prolonged treatment at least once every 6 months.

• Do not withdraw drug abruptly; although physical dependence does not occur with antipsychotic drugs, rebound exacerbation of psychotic symptoms may occur, and many drug effects persist.

• Carefully follow manufacturer's instructions for reconstitution, dilution, administration, and storage of drugs; slightly discolored liquids may or may not be all right to use. Check with pharmacist.

Information for parents and patient

• Explain rationale and anticipated risks and benefits of therapy, and that full therapeutic effect may not occur for several weeks.

• Teach signs and symptoms of adverse reactions and importance of reporting *any* unusual effects, especially involuntary movements.

• Tell parents that patient should avoid beverages and drugs containing alcohol, and should not take any other drug (especially CNS depressants) including nonprescription products without medical approval.

• Instruct parents of diabetic children to monitor blood glucose levels, because drug may alter insulin needs.

• Teach parents or patient how and when to administer drug, not to increase dose without medical approval, and never to discontinue drug abruptly; taking full dose at bedtime may minimize daytime sedation.

• Patient should lie down for 30 minutes after first dose (1 hour if I.M.) and to rise slowly from sitting or supine position to prevent orthostatic hypotension.

• Patient should avoid hazardous activities that require mental alertness and psychomotor coordination until full effects of drug are established.

• Drugs are locally irritating; advise taking with milk or food to minimize GI distress. Warn that oral concentrates and solutions will irritate skin. Patient should not crush or open sustained-release products, but swallow them whole.

• Warn parents that excessive exposure to sunlight, heat lamps, or tanning beds may cause photosensitivity reactions (burn and abnormal hyperpigmentation).

• Patient should avoid exposure to extremes of heat or cold, because of risk of hypothermia or hyperthermia induced by alteration in thermoregulatory function.

• Recommend sugarless gum, hard candy, or ice chips to relieve dry mouth.

• Explain that phenothiazines may cause pink to brown discoloration of urine.

propranolol
Inderal, Inderal LA

• Classification: antihypertensive, antianginal, antiarrhythmic, adjunctive therapy of migraine, adjunctive therapy of myocardial infarction (beta-adrenergic blocking agent)

How supplied
Available by prescription only
Tablets: 10 mg, 20 mg, 40 mg, 60 mg, 80 mg, 90 mg
Injection: 1 mg/ml
Capsules (extended-release): 80 mg, 120 mg, 160 mg

Indications, route, and dosage
Hypertension
Children: Initially, 1 mg/kg P.O. daily, given in equally divided doses. Dosage should be titrated according to blood pressure response and patient tolerance. Maintenance dosage in children generally ranges from 1 to 5 mg/kg daily, given P.O. in two to four divided doses. Occasionally, higher dosages may be necessary.
Adults: Initially, 80 mg P.O. daily in two to four divided doses or the sustained-release form once daily. Increase at 3- to 7-day intervals to maximum dosage of 640 mg daily. Usual maintenance dosage is 160 to 480 mg daily.

Supraventricular, ventricular, and atrial dysrhythmias; tachydysrhythmias caused by excessive catecholamine action during anesthesia, hyperthyroidism, and pheochromocytoma
Children: 0.01 to 0.1 mg/kg I.V. push; may repeat q 6 to 8 hours. Maximum single dose 1 mg. Alternatively, give 0.5 to 4 mg/kg P.O. daily in divided doses q 6 to 8 hours.

Reportedly, pediatric oral dosages exceeding 4 mg/kg daily may be necessary for the management of supraventricular tachydysrhythmias. Oral propranolol hydrochloride therapy has been initiated at 1.5 to 2 mg/kg daily and titrated upward as necessary to control the dysrhythmia, up to a maximum dosage of 16 mg/kg daily given in four divided doses.
Adults: 1 to 3 mg I.V. diluted in 50 ml dextrose 5% in water or normal saline solution infused slowly, not to exceed 1 mg/minute. After 3 mg have been infused, another dose may be given in 2 minutes; subsequent

doses no sooner than q 4 hours. Usual maintenance dosage is 10 to 80 mg P.O. t.i.d. or q.i.d.

†*Prevention of frequent, severe, uncontrollable, or disabling migraine or vascular headache*
Children less than 35 kg: 10 to 20 mg P.O. t.i.d.
Children 35 kg and over: 20 to 40 mg P.O. t.i.d.
Adults: Initially, 80 mg daily in divided doses or one sustained-release capsule once daily. Usual maintenance dosage is 160 to 240 mg daily, divided t.i.d. or q.i.d.

†*To reduce mortality after myocardial infarction*
Adults: 180 to 240 mg P.O. daily in divided doses. Usually administered in three to four doses daily, beginning 5 to 21 days after infarct.

†*Adjunctive treatment of anxiety*
Adults: 10 to 80 mg P.O. 1 hour before anxiety-provoking activity.

†*Treatment of essential or familial movement tremors*
Adults: 40 mg P.O. t.i.d. or q.i.d., as tolerated and needed.

†*Adjunctive treatment of thyrotoxicosis*
Neonates: For the treatment of tachydysrhythmias with thyrotoxicosis, dosage of 2 mg/kg P.O. daily given in two to four divided doses has been used. Occasionally, higher dosages may be needed.
Adults: 10 to 40 mg P.O. t.i.d. or q.i.d., as tolerated and needed.

Treatment of tetralogy of Fallot spells
Children: 0.15 to 0.25 mg/kg I.V. slowly (maximum dose 10 mg); may repeat once. Maintenance dose is 1 to 2 mg/kg P.O. q 6 hours.

Action and kinetics
• *Antihypertensive action:* Exact mechanism of propranolol's antihypertensive effect is unknown; drug may reduce blood pressure by blocking adrenergic receptors (thus decreasing cardiac output), by decreasing sympathetic outflow from the CNS, and by suppressing renin release.
• *Antianginal action:* Propranolol decreases myocardial oxygen consumption by blocking catecholamine access to beta-adrenergic receptors, thus relieving angina.
• *Antiarrhythmic action:* Propranolol decreases heart rate and prevents exercise-induced increases in heart rate. It also decreases myocardial contractility, cardiac output, and SA and AV nodal conduction velocity.
• *Migraine prophylactic action:* The migraine-preventive effect of propranolol is thought to result from inhibition of vasodilation.
• *Myocardial infarction prophylactic action:* The exact mechanism by which propranolol decreases mortality after myocardial infarction is unknown.
• *Kinetics in adults:* Propranolol is absorbed almost completely from the GI tract. Absorption is enhanced when given with food. Peak plasma concentrations occur 60 to 90 minutes after administration of regular-release tablets. After I.V. administration, peak concentrations occur in about 1 minute, with virtually immediate onset of action. Propranolol is distributed widely throughout the body; drug is more than 90% protein-bound. Hepatic metabolism is almost total;

oral dosage form undergoes extensive first-pass metabolism. Approximately 96% to 99% of a given dose of propranolol is excreted in urine as metabolites; remainder is excreted in feces as unchanged drug and metabolites. Biological half-life is about 4 hours.

Contraindications and precautions
Propranolol is contraindicated in patients with known hypersensitivity to the drug; and in patients with overt cardiac failure, sinus bradycardia, second- or third-degree AV block, bronchial asthma, cardiogenic shock, and Raynaud's syndrome, because drug may worsen these conditions.

Propranolol should be used cautiously in patients with coronary insufficiency, because beta-adrenergic blockade may precipitate CHF; in patients with pulmonary disease; in patients with diabetes mellitus, hypoglycemia, or hyperthyroidism because propranolol may mask tachycardia (because it does not mask dizziness and sweating caused by hypoglycemia); and in patients with impaired hepatic function. Propranolol may also mask common signs of shock.

Safety and efficacy of propranolol in children have not been established; use only if potential benefit outweighs risk.

Interactions
Concomitant use with cardiac glycosides potentiates bradycardia and myocardial depressant effects of propranolol; cimetidine may decrease clearance of propranolol via inhibition of hepatic metabolism, and thus also enhance its beta-blocking effects.

Propranolol may potentiate antihypertensive effects of other antihypertensive agents, especially such catecholamine-depleting agents as reserpine.

Propranolol may antagonize beta-adrenergic stimulating effects of sympathomimetic agents such as isoproterenol and of MAO inhibitors; use with epinephrine cause severe vasoconstriction.

Atropine, tricyclic antidepressants, and other drugs with anticholinergic effects may antagonize propranolol-induced bradycardia; nonsteroidal anti-inflammatory drugs may antagonize its hypotensive effects.

High doses of propranolol may potentiate neuromuscular blocking effect of tubocurarine and related compounds.

Concomitant use with insulin can alter dosage requirements in previously stable diabetic patients.

Effects on diagnostic tests
Propranolol may elevate serum transaminase, alkaline phosphatase, and lactic dehydrogenase levels, and may elevate BUN levels in patients with severe heart disease.

Adverse reactions
• CNS: fatigue, lethargy, vivid dreams, hallucinations, *depression, weakness.*
• CV: bradycardia, *hypotension,* CHF, peripheral vascular disease.
• DERM: rash.
• GI: *nausea, vomiting,* diarrhea.
• GU: impotence.
• Metabolic: *hypoglycemia* without tachycardia.
• Other: bronchospasm, fever, arthralgia.

‡May contain sulfites   ◆May contain tartrazine   ◆◆May contain benzyl alcohol

Note: Drug should be discontinued if signs of heart failure or bronchospasm develop.

Overdose and treatment

Clinical signs of overdose include severe hypotension, bradycardia, heart failure, and bronchospasm.

After acute ingestion, induce emesis or empty stomach by gastric lavage; follow with activated charcoal to reduce absorption, and administer symptomatic and supportive care. Treat bradycardia with atropine (0.25 to 1 mg); if no response, administer isoproterenol cautiously. Treat cardiac failure with digitalis and diuretics, and hypotension with vasopressors (epinephrine is preferred). Treat bronchospasm with isoproterenol and aminophylline.

▶ Special considerations

• Check apical pulse rate daily; discontinue and reevaluate therapy if extremes occur (for example, a pulse rate below 60 beats/minute for older children; 70 to 85 for younger children; and 90 to 110 for infants).

• Monitor blood pressure, ECG, and heart rate and rhythm frequently; be alert for progression of AV block or severe bradycardia.

• Weigh patient with CHF regularly; watch for gains of more than 5 lb (2.25 kg) per week.

• Signs of hypoglycemic shock are masked; watch diabetic patients for sweating, fatigue, and hunger.

• Do not discontinue these drugs before surgery for pheochromocytoma; before any surgical procedure, notify anesthesiologist that patient is taking a beta-adrenergic blocking agent.

• Glucagon may be prescribed to reverse signs and symptoms of beta blocker overdose.

• After prolonged atrial fibrillation, restoration of normal sinus rhythm may dislodge thrombi from atrial wall, resulting in thromboembolism; anticoagulation is often advised before cardioversion.

• Propranolol also has been used to treat aggression and rage, stage fright, recurrent GI bleeding in cirrhotic patients, and menopausal symptoms.

• Propranolol should never be administered as an adjunct in the treatment of pheochromocytoma unless the patient is pre-treated with alpha-adrenergic blocking agents.

Information for parents and patient

• Explain rationale for therapy, and emphasize importance of taking drugs as prescribed, even when patient is feeling well.

• Advise parents that patient should take drug with meals because food increases absorption.

• Warn parents that patient should not discontinue drug suddenly; abrupt discontinuation can exacerbate angina or precipitate myocardial infarction.

• Explain potential adverse effects and importance of reporting any unusual effects.

• Teach parents that patient can minimize dizziness from orthostatic hypotension by taking dose at bedtime, and by rising slowly and avoiding sudden position changes.

• Advise parents to seek medical approval before giving patient nonprescription cold preparations.

propylthiouracil (PTU)
Propyl-Thyracil*

• Classification: antihyperthyroid agent (thyroid hormone antagonist)

How supplied

Available by prescription only
Tablets: 50 mg

Indications, route, and dosage
Hyperthyroidism

Children age 6 to 10: 50 to 150 mg P.O. in divided doses q 8 hours.

Children over age 10: 150 to 300 mg P.O. t.i.d. Continue until patient is euthyroid, then start maintenance dosage of 25 mg t.i.d. to 100 mg b.i.d.

Adults: 100 mg P.O. t.i.d.; up to 300 mg q 8 hours have been used in severe cases. Continue until patient is euthyroid, then start maintenance dose of 100 mg daily to t.i.d.

Preparation for thyroidectomy

Children and adults: Same dosage as for hyperthyroidism; then iodine may be added 10 days before surgery.

Thyrotoxic crisis

Children and adults: Same dosage as for hyperthyroidism, with concomitant iodine therapy and propranolol.

Action and kinetics

• *Antithyroid action:* Used to treat hyperthyroidism, PTU inhibits synthesis of thyroid hormone by interfering with the incorporation of iodine into thyroglobulin; it also inhibits the formation of iodothyronine. Besides blocking hormone synthesis, it also inhibits the peripheral deiodination of thyroxine to triiodothyronine (liothyronine). Clinical effects become evident only when the preformed hormone is depleted and circulating hormone levels decline.

As preparation for thyroidectomy, PTU inhibits synthesis of the thyroid hormone and causes a euthyroid state, reducing surgical problems than thyroidectomy; as a result, the mortality for a single-stage thyroidectomy is low. Iodide reduces the vascularity of the gland and makes it less friable.

Used in treating thyrotoxic crisis, PTU inhibits peripheral deiodination of thyroxine to triiodothyronine. Theoretically, it is preferred over methimazole in thyroid storm because of its peripheral action.

• *Kinetics in adults:* PTU is absorbed rapidly and readily (about 80%) from the GI tract. Peak levels occur at 1 to 1½ hours. It appears to be concentrated in the thyroid gland. PTU readily crosses the placenta and is distributed into breast milk. It is 75% to 80% protein-bound. PTU is metabolized rapidly in the liver. About 35% of a dose is excreted in urine. Half-life is 1 to 2 hours in patients with normal renal function and 8½ hours in anuric patients.

Contraindications and precautions

PTU is contraindicated in patients with hypersensitivity to the drug. It should be used with caution in patients receiving other agents known to cause agranulocytosis or in those with infection or hepatic dysfunction.

Interactions

Concomitant use of PTU with adrenocorticoids or adrenocorticotropic hormone may require a dosage adjustment of the steroid when thyroid status changes. Concomitant use with bone marrow depressant agents increases the risk of agranulocytosis; use with hepatotoxic agents increases the risk of hepatotoxicity; use with iodinated glycerol, lithium, or potassium iodide may potentiate hypothyroid effects.

Effects on diagnostic tests

PTU therapy alters selenomethionine (^{75}Se) levels and prothrombin time; it also alters AST (SGOT), ALT (SGPT), and lactic dehydrogenase levels, as well as liothyronine uptake.

Adverse reactions

• CNS: headache, drowsiness, vertigo, depression, paresthesias.
• DERM: rash, *urticaria*, discoloration, pruritus, lupus-like syndrome, *exfoliative dermatitis*.
• GI: diarrhea, nausea, vomiting, epigastric distress, sialadenopathy (appear to be dose-related).
• HEMA: *agranulocytosis, leukopenia, granulocytopenia, thrombocytopenia* (appear to be dose-related).
• Hepatic: *jaundice, hepatitis*.
• Renal: nephritis.
• Other: *arthralgia*, myalgia, salivary gland enlargement, loss of taste, *drug fever*, lymphadenopathy, hair loss, edema, *malaise*.
Note: Drug should be discontinued at the first sign of hepatotoxicity or if the patient develops signs of agranulocytosis, pancytopenia, hepatitis (fever, swelling of cervical lymph nodes), or exfoliative dermatitis.

Overdose and treatment

Clinical manifestations of overdose include nausea, vomiting, epigastric distress, fever, headache, arthralgia, pruritus, edema, and pancytopenia.

Treatment includes withdrawal of the drug in the presence of agranulocytosis, pancytopenia, hepatitis, fever, or exfoliative dermatitis. For depression of bone marrow, treatment may require antibiotics and transfusions of fresh whole blood. For hepatitis, treatment includes rest, adequate diet, and symptomatic support, including analgesics, gastric lavage, I.V. fluids, and mild sedation.

▶ Special considerations

• Signs and symptoms of overdose or hypothyroidism include mental depression; changes in menstrual periods; cold intolerance; constipation; dry, puffy skin; headache; listlessness; muscle aches; nausea; vomiting; weakness; fatigue; hard, nonpitting edema; and unusual weight gain.
• Watch for signs of hypothyroidism. Monitor serum levels of thyroid-stimulating hormone as a sensitive indicator of thyroid hormone levels. Dosage adjustment may be required.
• Signs and symptoms of thyrotoxicosis or inadequate thyroid suppression include diarrhea, fever, irritability, listlessness, rapid heartbeat, vomiting, and weakness.
• Treatment with PTU requires complete blood counts periodically to detect impending leukopenia, thrombocytopenia, or agranulocytosis.
• Best response occurs when drug is administered around the clock and given at the same time each day in respect to meals.
• A beta blocker, usually propranolol, commonly is given to manage the peripheral signs of hyperthyroidism, which are primarily cardiac-related (tachycardia).
• Therapy should be discontinued if patient develops severe rash or enlarged cervical lymph nodes.

Information for parents and patient

• Advise parents to call physician immediately if patient develops sore throat, fever, or mouth sores (possible signs of developing agranulocytosis, which may not be detected by periodic blood cell counts because it can develop so rapidly). Parents should also report any skin eruptions (sign of hypersensitivity).
• Suggest to parents and patient that patient take the drug with meals to reduce GI side effects.
• Warn parents to avoid giving self-prescribed cough medicines to the patient; many contain iodine.
• Instruct parents to store drug in a light-resistant container. Warn them not to store medication in the bathroom; heat and humidity may cause the drug to deteriorate.
• Advise parents to have medical review of patient's thyroid status before patient undergoes surgery (including dental surgery).
• Teach parents and patient how to recognize the signs of hyperthyroidism and hypothyroidism and what to do if they occur.

---

pseudoephedrine hydrochloride
pseudoephedrine sulfate

Afrinol, Cenafed, Decofed, Dorcol, Myfedrine, NeoFed, Novafed, PediaCare, Pseudogest, Sudafed, Sinufed

• Classification: decongestant (adrenergic)

How supplied

Available without prescription
Oral solution: 15 mg/5 ml, 30 mg/5 ml, 7.5 mg/0.8 ml
Tablets: 30 mg, 60 mg
Tablets (extended-release): 120 mg

Indications, route, and dosage
Nasal and eustachian tube decongestant

Children age 2 to 6: 15 mg P.O. q 4 to 6 hours. Maximum dosage, 60 mg/day, or 4 mg/kg or 125 mg/m² P.O. divided q.i.d.

Children age 6 to 12: Administer 30 mg P.O. q 4 to 6 hours. Maximum dosage, 120 mg daily.

Children age 12 and over and adults: 60 mg P.O. q 4 to 6 hours. Maximum dosage, 240 mg daily, or 120 mg P.O. extended-release tablet b.i.d.

Action and kinetics

• *Decongestant action:* Pseudoephedrine directly stimulates alpha-adrenergic receptors of respiratory mucosa to produce vasoconstriction; shrinkage of swollen nasal mucous membranes; reduction of tissue hyperemia, edema, and nasal congestion; an increase in airway (nasal) patency and drainage of sinus excretions; and opening of obstructed eustachian ostia. Relaxation of bronchial smooth muscle may result from direct stimulation of beta-adrenergic receptors. Mild CNS stimulation may also occur.

• *Kinetics in adults:* Nasal decongestion occurs within 30 minutes and persists 4 to 6 hours after oral dose of 60-mg tablet or oral solution. Effects persist 8 hours after 60-mg dose and up to 12 hours after 120-mg dose of extended-release form. Pseudoephedrine is widely distributed throughout the body. Drug is incompletely metabolized in liver by N-demethylation to inactive compounds. 55% to 75% of a dose is excreted unchanged in urine; remainder is excreted as unchanged drug and metabolites.

Contraindications and precautions

Pseudoephedrine is contraindicated in patients with hypersensitivity to the drug and to other sympathomimetics, severe hypertension, or severe coronary artery disease and in those taking MAO inhibitors because of the potential for severe adverse cardiovascular effects.

Administer cautiously to patients with hyperthyroidism, diabetes, ischemic heart disease, elevated intraocular pressure, or prostatic hypertrophy, because the drug may worsen these conditions.

Interactions

Concomitant use with other sympathomimetics may produce additive effects and toxicity; with reserpine, methyldopa, mecamylamine, and *Veratrum* alkaloids, may reduce their anithypertensive effects.

Beta blockers may increase pressor effects of pseudoephedrine. Tricyclic antidepressants may antagonize effects of pseudoephedrine. MAO inhibitors potentiate pressor effects of pseudoephedrine.

Effects on diagnostic tests

None reported.

Adverse reactions

• CNS: *nervousness,* excitability, *restlessness,* dizziness, weakness, insomnia, headache, drowsiness, light-headedness, fear, anxiety, tremors, hallucinations, seizures.

• CV: cardiovascular collapse, tachycardia, palpitations, dysrhythmias.

• GI: nausea, vomiting, anorexia, dry mouth.

• Other: pallor, respiratory difficulty, dysuria.

Note: Drug should be discontinued if hypersensitivity, cardiac dysrhythmias, or hypertension occurs.

Overdose and treatment

Clinical manifestations of overdose include exaggeration of common adverse reactions, particularly seizures, cardiac dysrhythmias, and nausea and vomiting.

Treatment may include an emetic and gastric lavage within 4 hours of ingestion. Charcoal is effective only if administered within 1 hour, unless extended-release form was used. If renal function is adequate, forced diuresis will increase elimination. Do not force diuresis in severe overdose. Monitor vital signs, cardiac state, and electrolyte levels. I.V. propranolol may control cardiac toxicity; I.V. diazepam may be helpful to manage delirium or convulsions; dilute potassium chloride solutions (I.V.) may be given for hypokalemia.

▶ **Special considerations**

• Extended-release preparations should not be administered to patients under age 12.

• Administer last daily dose several hours before bedtime to minimize insomnia.

• If symptoms persist longer than 5 days or fever is present, re-evaluate therapy.

• Observe patient for complaints of headache or dizziness; monitor blood pressure.

Information for parents and patient

• If patient finds swallowing medication difficult, suggest opening capsules and mixing contents with applesauce, jelly, honey, or syrup. Mixture must be swallowed without chewing.

• Drug may cause dry mouth. Suggest using ice chips or sugarless gum or candy for relief.

• Instruct parents that patient should take missed dose if remembered within 1 hour. If beyond 1 hour, patient should resume regular schedule and should not double dose.

• Caution parents that many nonprescription preparations may contain sympathomimetics, which can cause additive, hazardous reactions.

• Patient should take last dose at least 2 to 3 hours before bedtime to avoid insomnia.

• Tell parents to store drug away from heat and light (not in bathroom medicine cabinet) and safely out of reach of small children.

pyrantel pamoate
Antiminth

• Classification: anthelmintic (pyrimidine derivative)

How supplied

Available by prescription only
Oral suspension: 50 mg/ml

Indications, route, and dosage
Roundworm and pinworm infections

Children over age 2 and adults: Single dose of 11 mg/kg P.O. up to a maximum dose of 1 g. For pinworm infection, dosage should be repeated in 2 weeks.

Action and kinetics

• *Anthelmintic action:* Pyrantel causes the release of acetylcholine and inhibits cholinesterases, paralyzing the worms. It is active against *Enterobius vermicularis, Ascaris lumbricoides, Ancylostoma duodenale, Necator americanus,* and *Trichostrongylus orientalis.*

• *Kinetics in adults:* Pyrantel pamoate is absorbed poorly; peak concentrations occur in 1 to 3 hours. The small amount of absorbed drug is metabolized partially in the liver. Over 50% of an oral dose of pyrantel pamoate is excreted unchanged in feces; about 7% is excreted in urine as unchanged drug or known metabolites. It is unknown if pyrantel pamoate is excreted in urine.

Contraindications and precautions

Pryantel pamoate is contraindicated in patients with known hypersensitivity to the drug. It should be used with caution in malnourished or anemic patients and in patients with hepatic disease because it may cause transient elevations in liver function tests.

Interactions

Pyrantel pamoate antagonizes the effects of piperazine.

Effects on diagnostic tests

Pyrantel pamoate may cause transient elevations of liver function tests.

Adverse reactions

• CNS: headache, dizziness, drowsiness, insomnia.
• DERM: rashes.
• GI: *anorexia, nausea, vomiting,* gastralgia, cramps, diarrhea, tenesmus.
• Hepatic: *transient AST (SGOT) level elevation.*
• Other: fever, weakness.
  Note: Drug should be discontinued if signs of hypersensitivity or toxicity occur.

Overdose and treatment

Treatment of overdose is largely supportive, particularly of cardiovascular and respiratory functions. After recent ingestion (within 4 hours), empty stomach by induced emesis or gastric lavage. Follow with activated charcoal to decrease absorption. Osmotic cathartics may be helpful.

▶ Special considerations

• Safety and efficacy for children under age 2 have not been established.
• Shake suspension well before measuring, to ensure accurate dosage.
• Drug may be given with milk, fruit juice, or food.
• Laxatives, enemas, or dietary restrictions are unnecessary.
• Protect drug from light.
• Treat all family members.

Information for parents and patient

• Emphasize importance of washing patient's perianal area daily and changing undergarments and bedclothes daily, and of hand washing and nail cleaning after defecation and before handling, preparing, or eating food.

• Explain routes of transmission and encourage testing and, if necessary, treatment of other household members and suspected contacts.

pyrazinamide
PMS-Pyrazinamide*, Tebrazid*

• Classification: antituberculosis agent (synthetic pyrazine analogue of nicotinamide)

How supplied

Available by prescription only
Tablets: 500 mg

Indications, route, and dosage
Adjunctive treatment of tuberculosis (when primary and secondary antitubercular drugs cannot be used or have failed)

†*Children:* 15 to 30 mg/kg P.O. daily in divided doses. Maximum dosages is 2 g daily.
Adults: 20 to 35 mg/kg P.O. daily, in one or more doses. Maximum dosage is 3 g daily. Lower dosage is recommended in decreased renal function.

Action and kinetics

• *Antibiotic action:* The mechanism of action of pyrazinamide is unknown; drug may be bactericidal or bacteriostatic depending on organism susceptibility and drug concentration at infection site. Pyrazinamide is active only against *Mycobacterium tuberculosis.* Pyrazinamide is considered adjunctive in tuberculosis therapy and is given with other drugs to prevent or delay development of resistance to pyrazinamide by *M. tuberculosis.*

• *Kinetics in adults:* Pyrazinamide is absorbed well after oral administration; peak serum levels occur 2 hours after an oral dose. Pyrazinamide is distributed widely into body tissues and fluids, including lungs, liver, and CSF; drug is 50% protein-bound. It is hydrolyzed in the liver; some hydrolysis occurs in stomach. Pyrazinamide is excreted almost completely in urine by glomerular filtration. It is not known if pyrazinamide is excreted in breast milk. Elimination halflife in adults is 9 to 10 hours. Half-life is prolonged in renal and hepatic impairment.

Contraindications and precautions

Pyrazinamide is contraindicated in children with known hypersensitivity to pyrazinamide and in patients with severe hepatic disease.

Pyrazinamide should be used cautiously in patients with acute intermittent porphyria, decreased renal function, diabetes, or a history of peptic ulcer disease or gout.

Interactions

None reported.

Effects on diagnostic tests

Pyrazinamide may interfere with urine ketone determinations. The drug's systemic effects may temporarily decrease 17-ketosteroid levels; it may increase

---

‡May contain sulfites   ◆May contain tartrazine   ◆◆May contain benzyl alcohol

protein-bound iodine and urate levels and results of liver enzyme tests.

Adverse reactions
• CNS: neuromuscular blockade.
• DERM: maculopapular rash, photosensitivity (skin turns reddish brown).
• GI: anorexia, nausea, vomiting.
• GU: dysuria.
• HEMA: sideroblastic anemia, possible bleeding tendency due to thrombocytopenia.
• Hepatic: hepatitis, jaundice.
• Metabolic: interference with control in diabetes mellitus, hyperuricemia.
• Other: malaise, fever, arthralgia, porphyria.
   Note: Drug should be discontinued if patient shows signs of hypersensitivity reactions or hepatic damage.

Overdose and treatment
No specific recommendations are available. Treatment is supportive. After recent ingestion (4 hours or less), empty stomach by induced emesis or gastric lavage. Follow with activated charcoal to decrease absorption.

▶ Special considerations
• Pyrazinamide is not recommended for use in children unless essential for therapy.
• Monitor liver function, especially enzyme and bilirubin levels, and renal function, especially serum uric acid levels, before therapy and thereafter at 2- to 4-week intervals; observe patient for signs of liver damage or decreased renal function.
• In a patient with diabetes mellitus, pyrazinamide therapy may hinder stabilization of serum glucose levels.
• Pyrazinamide frequently elevates serum uric acid levels. Although usually asymptomatic, a uricosuric agent, such as probenecid or allopurinol, may be necessary.
• Combined therapy with isoniazid and rifampin may shorten duration of therapy.

Information for parents and patient
• Explain disease process and rationale for long-term therapy.
• Teach signs and symptoms of hypersensitivity and other adverse reactions, and emphasize need to report them; urge parents to report *any* unusual reactions, especially signs of gout.
• Be sure parents and patient understand how and when to take drugs. Patient should complete entire prescribed regimen, comply with instructions for around-the-clock dosage, and keep follow-up appointments.
• Tell parents and patient to keep fluid intake at 2 quarts (about 2 liters)/day; explain need for good hydration to prevent renal damage.

pyridostigmine bromide
Mestinon, Regonol

• Classification: muscle stimulant (cholinesterase inhibitor)

How supplied
Available by prescription only
Tablets: 60 mg
Tablets (timed-release): 180 mg
Syrup: 60 mg/5 ml
Injection: 5 mg/ml in 2-ml ampule or 5-ml vial

Indications, route, and dosage
Curariform antagonist postoperatively
Adults: 10 to 30 mg I.V. preceded by atropine sulfate 0.6 to 1.2 mg I.V.
Myasthenia gravis
Neonates of myasthenic mothers: 0.05 to 0.15 mg/kg I.M.
Children: 1 to 2 mg/kg P.O. q 3 to 4 hours while awake.
Children: 0.1 to .25 mg/kg I.V. with atropine or glycopyrrolate.
Adults: 60 to 180 mg P.O. b.i.d. or q.i.d. Usual dose 600 mg daily, but higher doses may be needed (up to 1,500 mg daily). Give ⅓₀ of oral dose I.M. or I.V. Dosage must be adjusted for each patient, depending on response and tolerance of adverse effects.

Action and kinetics
• *Muscle stimulant action:* Pyridostigmine blocks acetylcholine's hydrolysis by cholinesterase, resulting in acetylcholine accumulation at cholinergic synapses, increasing stimulation of cholinergic receptors at the myoneural junction.
• *Kinetics in adults:* Pyridostigmine is poorly absorbed from the GI tract. Onset of action usually occurs 30 to 45 minutes after oral administration, 2 to 5 minutes after I.V., and 15 minutes after I.M.
   Little is known about pyridostigmine's distribution; however, drug may cross the placenta, especially when administered in large doses.
   Exact metabolic fate is unknown. Duration of effect is usually 3 to 6 hours after oral dose and 2 to 3 hours after I.V. dose, depending on patient's physical and emotional status and disease severity. Pyridostigmine is not hydrolyzed by cholinesterase.
   Drug and metabolites are excreted in urine.

Contraindications and precautions
Pyridostigmine is contraindicated in patients with intestinal or urinary tract obstruction because of its stimulatory effect on smooth muscle and in patients with bradycardia, because drug may exacerbate this condition.
   Administer pyridostigmine with extreme caution to patients with bronchial asthma, because it may precipitate asthma attacks. Administer pyridostigmine cautiously to patients with epilepsy, because the drug may cause CNS stimulation; to patients with vagotonia, hyperthyroidism, or cardiac dysrhythmias.

---

because the drug may exacerbate these conditions; and to patients with peptic ulcer disease, because the drug may increase gastric acid secretion.

Interactions
Concomitant use with procainamide or quinidine may reverse pyridostigmine's cholinergic effect on muscle. Corticosteroids may decrease pyridostigmine's cholinergic effect; when corticosteroids are stopped, this effect may increase, possibly affecting muscle strength.

Concomitant use with succinylcholine may result in prolonged respiratory depression from plasma esterase inhibition, delaying succinylcholine hydrolysis. Concomitant use with ganglionic blockers, such as mecamylamine, may critically decrease blood pressure; effect is usually preceded by abdominal symptoms. Magnesium has a direct depressant effect on skeletal muscle and may antagonize pyridostigmine's beneficial effects.

Effects on diagnostic tests
None reported.

Adverse reactions
• CNS: headache (with high doses), fasciculations, convulsions.
• CV: bradycardia, hypotension (rare).
• DERM: rash, excessive sweating.
• EENT: miosis.
• GI: abdominal cramps, nausea, vomiting, diarrhea, excessive salivation.
• Other: thrombophlebitis (with I.V. administration), bronchospasm, bronchoconstriction, increased bronchial secretions, weakness, muscle cramps.

Note: Drug should be discontinued if hypersensitivity, headache, convulsions, difficulty breathing, skin rash, or paralysis occurs.

Overdose and treatment
Clinical effects of overdose include nausea, vomiting, diarrhea, blurred vision, miosis, excessive tearing, bronchospasm, increased bronchial secretions, hypotension, incoordination, excessive sweating, muscle weakness, cramps, fasciculations, paralysis, bradycardia or tachycardia, excessive salivation, and restlessness or agitation.

Support respiration; bronchial suctioning may be performed. The drug should be discontinued immediately. Atropine may be given to block pyridostigmine's muscarinic effects; however, it will not counter skeletal muscle paralysis. Avoid atropine overdose, because it may lead to bronchial plug formation.

▶ Special considerations
• Observe patients closely for cholinergic reactions, especially in parenteral forms.
• Have atropine available to reduce or reverse hypersensitivity reactions.
• Administer atropine prior to or concurrently with late doses of parenteral anticholinesterases to counteract muscarinic side effects.
• Dosage must be individualized according to severity of disease and patient response.
• Myasthenic patients may become refractory to this drug after prolonged use; however, responsiveness may be restored by reducing the dose or discontinuing the drug for a few days.
• If muscle weakness is severe, determine if this effect stems from drug toxicity or exacerbation of myasthenia gravis. A test dose of edrophonium I.V. will aggravate drug-induced weakness but will temporarily relieve weakness that results from the disease.
• Avoid giving large pyridostigmine doses to patients with decreased GI motility, because toxicity may result once motility has been restored.
• Give pyridostigmine with food or milk to reduce the risk of muscarinic adverse effects.
• Discontinue all other cholinergic drugs during pyridostigmine therapy to avoid additive toxicity.

Information for parents and patient
• When administering pyridostigmine to patient with myasthenia gravis, stress the importance to the parents and patient of taking the drug exactly as ordered, on time, and in evenly spaced doses.
• If patient is taking sustained-release tablets, explain to the parents and patient how these work and instruct the patient to take them at the same time each day and to swallow these tablets whole, rather than crushing them.
• Teach parents how to evaluate muscle strength; instruct them to observe changes in muscle strength and to report muscle cramps, rash, or fatigue.
• Tell parents to have patient take drug with food or milk to reduce adverse effects.
• Advise parents to keep daily record of dose and effects during initial phase of therapy to help identify an optimum therapeutic regimen.
• Advise parents to store drug away from children, and from direct heat and light.

---

pyridoxine hydrochloride (vitamin B₆)
Bee six, Hexa-Betalin, Pyroxine

• Classification: nutritional supplement (vitamin)

How supplied
Available by prescription only
Injection: 10-ml vial (100 mg/ml), 30-ml vial (100 mg/ml), 10-ml vial (100 mg/ml, with 1.5% benzyl alcohol), 30-ml vial (100 mg/ml, with 1.5% benzyl alcohol), 10-ml vial (100 mg/ml, with 0.5% chlorobutanol), 1-ml vial (100 mg/ml)
Tablets: 10 mg, 25 mg, 50 mg, 100 mg, 200 mg, 250 mg, 500 mg, 500 mg timed-release

Indications, route, and dosage
Dietary vitamin B₆ deficiency
Children: 100 mg P.O., I.M., or I.V. to correct deficiency, then an adequate diet with supplementary RDA doses to prevent recurrence.
Adults: 10 to 20 mg P.O., I.M., or I.V. daily for 3 weeks, then 2 to 5 mg daily as a supplement to a proper diet.

*Seizures related to vitamin B₆ deficiency or
dependency*
Children and adults: 100 mg I.M. or I.V. in single dose.
*Vitamin B₆-responsive anemias or depen-
dency syndrome (inborn errors of metabo-
lism)*
Children: 100 mg I.M. or I.V., then 2 to 10 mg I.M.
or 10 to 100 mg P.O. daily.
Adults: Up to 600 mg P.O., I.M., or I.V. daily until
symptoms subside, then 50 mg daily for life.
*Prevention of vitamin B₆ deficiency during
isoniazid therapy*
Infants: 0.1 to 0.5 mg P.O. daily.
Children: 0.5 to 1.5 mg P.O. daily.
   If neurologic symptoms develop in pediatric pa-
tients, increase dosage as necessary.
Adults: 25 to 50 mg P.O. daily.
*Treatment of vitamin B₆ deficiency secondary
to isoniazid*
Children: Titrate dosages.
Adults: 100 mg P.O. daily for 3 weeks, then 50 mg
daily.

Action and kinetics
• *Metabolic action:* Natural vitamin B₆ contained in
plant and animal foodstuffs is converted to physiologically active forms of vitamin B₆, pyridoxal phosphate and pyridoxamine phosphate. Exogenous forms
of the vitamin are metabolized in humans. Vitamin
B₆ acts as a coenzyme in protein, carbohydrate, and
fat metabolism and participates in the decarboxyl-
ation of amino acids in protein metabolism. Vitamin
B₆ also helps convert tryptophan to niacin or serotonin as well as the deamination, transamination, and
transulfuration of amino acids. Finally, vitamin B₆ is
responsible for the breakdown of glycogen to glucose-
1-phosphate in carbohydrate metabolism. The total
adult body store consists of 16 to 27 mg of pyridoxine.
The need for pyridoxine increases with the amount
of protein in the diet.
• *Kinetics in adults:* After oral administration, pyridoxine and its substituents are absorbed readily from
the GI tract. GI absorption may be diminished in patients with malabsorption syndromes or following gastric resection. Normal serum levels of pyridoxine are
30 to 80 ng/ml. Pyridoxine is stored mainly in the
liver. The total body store is approximately 16 to 27
mg. Pyridoxal and pyridoxal phosphate are the most
common forms found in the blood and are highly protein-bound. Pyridoxal crosses the placenta; fetal
plasma concentrations are five times greater than
maternal plasma concentrations. After maternal intake of 2.5 to 5.0 mg/day of pyridoxine, the concentration of the vitamin in breast milk is approximately
240 ng/ml.
   Pyridoxine is degraded to 4-pyridoxic acid in the
liver. In erythrocytes, pyridoxine is converted to pyridoxal phosphate, and pyridoxamine is converted to
pyridoxamine phosphate. The phosphorylated form of
pyridoxine is transaminated to pyridoxal and pyridoxamine, which is phosphorylated rapidly. The conversion of pyridoxine phosphate to pyridoxal phosphate
requires riboflavin.

Contraindications and precautions
Pyridoxine is contraindicated in patients with a history of pyridoxine sensitivity. Pyridoxine should not
be administered I.V. to patients with heart disease.
An inadequate diet may cause multiple vitamin deficiencies; proper nutrition is important. Pyridoxine-
dependent seizures in infants may result from the use
of large doses of pyridoxine during pregnancy.

Interactions
Pyridoxine reverses the therapeutic effects of levodopa by accelerating peripheral metabolism. Concomitant use of pyridoxine with phenobarbital or phenytoin
may cause a 50% decrease in serum concentrations
of these anticonvulsants. Isoniazid, cycloserine, penicillamine, hydralazine, and oral contraceptives may
increase pyridoxine requirements.

Effects on diagnostic tests
Pyridoxine therapy alters determinations for urobilinogen in the spot test using Ehrlich's reagent, resulting in a false-positive reaction.

Adverse reactions
• CNS: paresthesias, headache, somnolence, seizures
(with I.V. administration).
• GI: nausea.
• Local: burning or stinging at I.M. or S.C. site.
• Other: allergic reactions.

Overdose and treatment
Clinical manifestations of overdose include: ataxia
and severe sensory neuropathy after chronic consumption of high daily doses of pyridoxine (2 to 6 g).
These neurologic deficits usually resolve after pyridoxine is discontinued.

▶ Special considerations
• Safety and efficacy have not been established for
children.
• The use of large doses of pyridoxine during pregnancy has been implicated in pyridoxine-dependency
seizures in neonates.
• Prepare a dietary history. A single vitamin deficiency is unusual; lack of one vitamin often indicates
a deficiency of others.
• Initial dosing should be accompanied by EEG monitoring.
• Monitor protein intake; excessive protein intake increases pyridoxine requirements.
• The recommended daily allowance for vitamin B₆ is
0.3 to 1.6 mg in children and 1.8 to 2.2 mg in adults;
during pregnancy, dosages of 2.5 to 10 mg daily have
been recommended.
• A dosage of 25 mg/kg/day is well-tolerated. Adults
consuming 200 mg/day for 33 days and on a normal
dietary intake develop vitamin B₆ dependency.
• Do not mix with sodium bicarbonate in the same
syringe.
• Patients receiving levodopa shouldn't take pyridoxine in dosages greater than 5 mg/day.
• To treat seizures and coma from isoniazid overdose,
dosage equals dosage of isoniazid.
• Store in a tight, light-resistant container.

• Do not use injection solution if it contains precipitate. Slight darkening is acceptable.
• Dilute in dextrose 5% in water or normal saline solution.
• Pyridoxine is sometimes of value for treating nausea and vomiting during pregnancy.

Information for parents and patient
Teach the parents and patient about dietary sources of vitamin B_6, such as yeast, wheat germ, liver, whole-grain cereals, bananas, and legumes.

---

pyrimethamine
Daraprim

• Classification: antimalarial (aminopyrimidine derivative [folic acid antagonist])

How supplied
Available by prescription only
Tablets: 25 mg of pyrimethamine

Indications, route, and dosage
Malaria prophylaxis and transmission control
Children under age 4: 6.25 mg P.O. weekly. Alternatively, give 0.5 mg/kg P.O. (maximum dose 25 mg) once weekly.
Children ages 4 to 10: 12.5 mg P.O. weekly.
Children over age 10 and adults: 25 mg P.O. weekly.
    Dosage should be continued for all age-groups for at least 10 weeks after leaving endemic areas.
Acute attacks of malaria
Not recommended alone in nonimmune persons; use with faster-acting antimalarials, such as chloroquine, for 2 days to initiate transmission control and suppressive cure. For chloroquine-resistant strain, administer with sulfonamides, and possibly quinine.
Children under age 15: 12.5 mg P.O. daily for 2 days.
Children over age 15 and adults: 25 mg P.O. daily for 2 days.
Toxoplasmosis
Children: Initially, 1 mg/kg daily divided into two equal doses; after 2 to 4 days, decrease dose by one half and continue for about 1 month. Give with 100 mg sulfadiazine/kg/day divided q 6 hours.
Adults: Initially, 50 to 75 mg daily with 1 g sulfadiazine P.O. q 6 hours; after 1 to 3 weeks, decrease dose by one half and continue for 4 to 5 weeks more.

Action and kinetics
• *Antimalarial action:* Pyrimethamine inhibits the reduction of dihydrofolate to tetrahydrofolate, thereby blocking folic acid metabolism needed for survival of susceptible organisms. This mechanism is distinct from sulfonamide-induced folic acid antagonism. Chloroquine, quinine or quinacrine are preferred for acute attacks of malaria; but these drugs combined with pyramethamine may initiate suppression cure. Pyrimethamine is active against the asexual erythrocytic forms of susceptible plasmodia and against *Toxoplasma gondii*. It is usually used with a sulfonamide.

• *Kinetics in adults:* Pyrimethamine is well absorbed from the intestinal tract; peak serum concentrations occur within 2 hours. Pyrimethamine is distributed to the kidneys, liver, spleen, and lungs; it is approximately 80% bound to plasma proteins. Pyrimethamine is metabolized to several unidentified compounds. Pyrimethamine is excreted in the urine and in breast milk; elimination half-life is 2 to 6 days. Its half-life is not changed in end-stage renal disease.

Contraindications and precautions
Pyrimethamine is contraindicated in children with megaloblastic anemia from folate deficiency, because it is a folate antagonist, and in patients with known hypersensitivity to the drug. Pyrimethamine also is contraindicated in chloroquine-resistant malaria and should be used with caution after therapy with chloroquine. The drug should be used with caution in patients with glucose-6-phosphate dehydrogenase (G6PD) deficiency because it may induce hemolytic anemia.
    Initial dosage for toxoplasmosis in patients with seizure disorders should be lowered to avoid CNS toxicity.
Concomitant use with sulfadoxine is contraindicated in patients with porphyria and should be used with caution in patients with impaired hepatic or renal function, severe allergy, bronchial asthma, or G6PD deficiency.

Interactions
Pyrimethamine and sulfonamides act synergistically against some organisms, because each inhibits folic acid synthesis at a different level.
    Pyrimethamine and sulfadoxine should not be given concomitantly with other sulfonamides or with co-trimoxazole because of additive adverse effects. Concomitant use with para-aminobenzoic acid and folic acid reduce the antitoxoplasmic effects of pyrimethamine and may require higher dosage of the latter drug.

Effects on diagnostic tests
Pyrimethamine therapy may decrease white blood cell, red blood cell, and platelet counts.

Adverse reactions
• CNS: stimulation and seizures (acute toxicity), ataxia, tremors.
• DERM: rashes, erythema multiforme (Stevens-Johnson syndrome), toxic epidermal necrolysis.
• GI: anorexia, vomiting, diarrhea, atrophic glossitis, abdominal cramps.
• HEMA: agranulocytosis, aplastic anemia, megaloblastic anemia, bone marrow suppression, leukopenia, thrombocytopenia, pancytopenia.
    Note: Drug should be discontinued or dosage reduced if signs of folic acid or folinic acid deficiency develop. Parenteral folinic acid (leucovorin) may be given (up to 9 mg I.M. daily for 3 days) until blood counts are restored to normal.

Overdose and treatment
Overdose is marked by anorexia, vomiting, and CNS stimulation, including seizures. Megaloblastic ane-

---

mia, thrombocytopenia, leukopenia, glossitis, and crystalluria may also occur.

Treatment of overdose consists of gastric lavage followed by a cathartic; barbiturates may help to control seizures. Leucovorin (folinic acid) in a dosage of 3 to 9 mg daily for 3 days or longer is used to restore decreased platelet or leukocyte counts.

▶ Special considerations

• Give with meals to minimize GI distress.
• Monitor complete blood counts, including platelet counts twice a week.
• Monitor patient for signs of folate deficiency or bleeding when platelet count is low; if abnormalities appear, decrease dosage or discontinue drug. Leucovorin (folinic acid) may be prescribed to raise blood counts during reduced dosage or after drug is discontinued.
• When pyrimethamine with sulfadoxine (Fansidar) is used prophylactically, the first dose should be given 1 or 2 days before travel to an area where malaria is endemic.
• Because severe reactions may occur, pyrimethamine with sulfadoxine should be given only to patients traveling to areas where chloroquine-resistant malaria is prevalent and only if traveler will be in such areas longer than 3 weeks.

Information for parents and patient

• Teach parents how to recognize signs and symptoms of adverse blood reactions; tell parents to report them immediately. Teach emergency measures to control overt bleeding.
• Teach parents and the patient signs and symptoms of folate deficiency.
• Counsel patient and family about need to report any adverse effects and to keep follow-up medical appointments.
• Keep drug out of reach of small children.

QR

quinacrine hydrochloride
Atabrine hydrochloride

- Classification: anthelmintic, antiprotozoal, antimalarial (acridine derivative)

How supplied
Available by prescription only
Tablets: 100 mg

Indications, route, and dosage
Giardiasis
Children: 8 mg/kg P.O. daily given in three divided doses after meals for 5 days. Maximum dosage is 300 mg/day. If necessary, the dosage may be repeated in 2 weeks.
Adults: 300 mg P.O. in three divided doses for 5 to 7 days.
Tapeworm (beef, pork, and fish) infections
Children ages 5 to 10: 400 mg as a total dosage, administered in three or four divided doses, 10 minutes apart.
Children ages 11 to 14: 600 mg as a total dosage, administered in three or four divided doses, 10 minutes apart.
Children over age 14 and adults : Four doses of 200 mg given 10 minutes apart (800 mg total).
Malaria
Children over age 8 and adults: 200 mg with 1 g sodium bicarbonate q 6 hours for five doses, then 100 mg t.i.d. for 6 days.
Children ages 4 to 8: 200 mg t.i.d. for 1 day, then 100 mg q 12 hours for 6 days.
Children ages 1 to 4: 100 mg t.i.d. for 1 day, then 100 mg once daily for 6 days.
Suppression
Children: 50 mg daily for 1 to 3 months.
Adults: 100 mg daily for 1 to 3 months.

Action and kinetics
- *Antiprotozoal action:* Mechanism of action is unknown.
- *Anthelmintic and antimalarial actions:* Quinacrine intercalates into the parasite's DNA, inhibiting replication and protein synthesis. It is active against *Giardia lamblia, Diphyllobothrium latum, Dipylidium caninum, Hymenolepis diminuta, H. nana, Taenia saginata,* and *T. solium.* It also is active against asexual forms of *Plasmodium malariae, P. vivax,* and *P. falciparum.*
- Metronidazole and similar nitromidazole compounds have generally replaced quinacrine in the treatment of giardiasis because they are less toxic and more effective. Some clinicians consider quinacrine obsolete for the treatment of malaria and tapeworm.
- *Kinetics in adults:* Quinacrine is absorbed readily;

peak serum concentrations occur at 1 to 8 hours. Drug is distributed widely to tissues, especially into the pancreas, lungs, liver, spleen, bone marrow, erythrocytes, and skeletal muscle; it crosses the placenta. The drug is highly protein-bound. Quinacrine appears to be metabolized slowly.It is excreted slowly into the urine; small amounts are excreted in feces, sweat, saliva, bile, and breast milk. Half-life is 5 days.

Contraindications and precautions
Quinacrine is contraindicated in patients taking primaquine. It should be used with caution in patients with severe cardiac disease or glucose-6-phosphate dehydrogenase deficiency; in patients with severe renal disease because the drug accumulates; in patients with hepatic disease or in those taking hepatotoxic drugs, because it concentrates in the liver; in patients with psoriasis or porphyria because it may exacerbate these conditions; and in psychotic patients because it can cause psychosis. Quinacrine also should be used with caution in infants under age 1.

Interactions
Quinacrine increases primaquine's plasma concentrations to potentially toxic levels. Quinacrine may inhibit alcohol dehydrogenase. Patients should avoid alcohol ingestion during therapy with quinacrine.

Quinacrine potentiates the toxicity of antimalarial agents structurally related to primaquine and should not be used concomitantly.

Effects on diagnostic tests
Quinacrine may cause falsely elevated cortisol concentrations in urine and plasma.

Adverse reactions
- CNS: headache, dizziness, nervousness, vertigo, mood shifts, nightmares, seizures, *transient psychosis.*
- DERM: pleomorphic skin eruptions, *yellow skin,* exfoliative dermatitis, contact dermatitis.
- EENT: corneal damage with long-term therapy.
- GI: *diarrhea, anorexia, nausea, abdominal cramps, vomiting.*
- HEMA: *bone marrow depression.*
- Other: bright yellow urine.
Note: Drug should be discontinued if signs of hypersensitivity or toxicity occur.

Overdose and treatment
Clinical signs of overdose include restlessness, psychic stimulation, seizures, nausea, vomiting, abdominal cramps, diarrhea, hypotension, dysrhythmias, and yellow skin.

To treat overdose, perform gastric lavage. Symptomatic treatment may include diazepam to control initial seizures, phenytoin to control refractory seizures, and respiratory and vasopressor support as

‡May contain sulfites   ♦May contain tartrazine   ♦♦May contain benzyl alcohol

needed. After the acute phase, forced fluids and urinary acidification may help.

▶ **Special considerations**
• Use with caution in infants under age 1.
• Give quinacrine after meals with a large glass of water, tea, or fruit juice to reduce GI irritation. Honey or jam may disguise bitter taste. Concomitant sodium bicarbonate may reduce nausea and vomiting associated with large doses.
• Patient should have a bland, nonfat, semisolid diet for 24 hours before treatment and should fast after the evening meal before treatment.
• Patient should have a saline cathartic and cleansing enema before treatment to reduce amount of stool for examination; the cathartic should be repeated 1 to 2 hours after ingestion of drug, to expel worm.
• Collect all stool expelled for 48 hours after treatment; examine stool for worm's attachment organ, which will be stained yellow by drug. Worm usually passes in 4 to 10 hours after treatment.
• Patient should have regular CBCs and ophthalmoscopic examinations during prolonged treatment to detect adverse effects.
• Be alert for signs of drug-induced behavioral changes and psychosis, which may last up to 4 weeks after drug is discontinued.

Information for parents and patient
• Explain that the drug temporarily will turn skin and urine bright yellow – it is not jaundice.
• Explain that the drug turns some patients' ears, nasal cartilage, and fingernail beds a bluish gray, resembling cyanosis; it usually disappears about 2 weeks after drug is discontinued.
• Teach parents the signs and symptoms of adverse reactions. Tell parents to report them immediately.
• Advise follow-up stool examinations for 3 to 6 months to ensure elimination of worm.
• Warn parents to store drug out of reach of small children.

---

quinidine gluconate
Duraquin, Quinaglute Dura-Tabs, Quinalan, Quinate

quinidine polygalacturonate
Cardioquin

quinidine sulfate
Apo-Quinidine*, Cin-Quin, Novoquinidin, Quinidex Extentabs, Quinora

• Classification: ventricular antiarrhythmic, supraventricular antiarrhythmic, atrial antitachyarrhythmic (cinchona alkaloid)

How supplied
Available by prescription only
Tablets: 325 mg* (gluconate); 324 mg, 330 mg (ex-

tended-release, polygalacturonate); 100 mg, 200 mg, 300 mg (sulfate); 300 mg (extended-release, sulfate)
Capsules: 300 mg (sulfate)
Injection: 80 mg/ml (gluconate); 200 mg/ml (sulfate); 190 mg/ml*

Indications, route, and dosage
Atrial flutter or fibrillation
Children: Give test dose of 2 mg/kg, then 3 to 6 mg/kg P.O. q 2 to 3 hours for five doses daily.
Adults: 200 mg of quinidine sulfate or equivalent base P.O. q 2 to 3 hours for five to eight doses with subsequent daily increases until sinus rhythm is restored or toxic effects develop. Administer quinidine only after digitalization, to avoid increasing AV conduction. Maximum dosage is 3 to 4 g daily.
Paroxysmal supraventricular tachycardia
Children: Give test dose of 2 mg/kg, then 3 to 6 mg/kg P.O. q 2 to 3 hours for five doses daily.
Adults: 400 to 600 mg I.M. of gluconate q 2 to 3 hours until toxic effects develop or dysrhythmia subsides.
Premature atrial and ventricular contractions, paroxysmal atrioventricular junctional rhythm or atrial and ventricular tachycardia, maintenance of cardioversion
Children: Give test dose of 2 mg/kg, then 3 to 6 mg/kg P.O. q 2 to 3 hours for five doses daily.
Adults: Give test dose of 50 to 200 mg P.O., then monitor vital signs before beginning therapy: 200 to 400 mg of quinidine sulfate or equivalent base P.O. q 4 to 6 hours; or initially, 600 mg of quinidine gluconate I.M., then up to 400 mg q 2 hours, p.r.n.; or 800 mg of quinidine gluconate I.V. diluted in 40 ml of dextrose 5% in water, infused at 16 mg (1 ml)/minute. Alternately, give 600 mg of quinidine sulfate in extended-release form, or 324 to 648 mg of quinidine gluconate in extended-release form, q 8 to 12 hours.

Action and kinetics
• *Antiarrhythmic action:* A Class IA antiarrhythmic, quinidine depresses phase 0 of the action potential. It is considered a myocardial depressant because it decreases myocardial excitability and conduction velocity and may depress myocardial contractility. It also exerts anticholinergic activity, which may modify its direct myocardial effects. In therapeutic doses, quinidine reduces conduction velocity in the atria, ventricles, and His-Purkinje system. It helps control atrial tachydysrhythmias by prolonging the effective refractory period (ERP) and increasing the action potential duration in the atria, ventricles and His-Purkinje system. Because ERP prolongation exceeds action potential duration, tissue remains refractory even after returning to resting membrane potential (membrane-stabilizing effect). Quinidine shortens the effective refractory period of the AV node. Because quinidine's anticholinergic action also may increase AV node conductivity, digitalis should be administered for atrial tachydysrhythmias before quinidine therapy begins, to prevent ventricular tachydysrhythmias. Quinidine also suppresses automaticity in the His-Purkinje system and ectopic pacemakers, making it useful in treating ventricular premature beats. At therapeutic doses, quinidine prolongs the QRS dura-

tion and QT interval; these ECG effects may be used as an index of drug effectiveness and toxicity.

• *Kinetics in adults:* Although all quinidine salts are well absorbed from the GI tract, serum drug levels vary greatly among individuals. Onset of action of quinidine sulfate is from 1 to 3 hours. For extended-release forms, onset of action may be slightly slower but duration of effect is longer, because this drug delivery system allows longer than usual dosing intervals. Peak plasma levels occur in 3 to 4 hours for quinidine gluconate and 6 hours for quinidine polygalacturonate. Quinidine is well distributed in all tissues except the brain. It concentrates in the heart, liver, kidneys, and skeletal muscle. Distribution volume decreases in patients with CHF, possibly requiring reduction in maintenance dosage. Approximately 80% of drug is bound to plasma proteins; the unbound (active) fraction may increase in patients with hypoalbuminemia from various causes, including hepatic insufficiency. Usual therapeutic serum levels depend on assay method and ranges as follows:

—Specific assay (EMIT, HPLC, fluorescence polarization): 2 to 5 mcg/ml

—Nonspecific assay (fluorometric): 4 to 8 mcg/ml.

About 60% to 80% of drug is metabolized in the liver to two metabolites that may have some pharmacologic activity. Approximately 10% to 30% of an administered dose is excreted in the urine within 24 hours as unchanged drug. Urine acidification increases quinidine excretion; alkalinization decreases excretion. Most of an administered dose is eliminated in the urine as metabolites; elimination half-life ranges from 5 to 12 hours (usual half-life is about 6½ hours). Duration of effect ranges from 6 to 8 hours.

Contraindications and precautions

Quinidine is contraindicated in patients with complete AV block with an AV junctional or idioventricular pacemaker, because of potential for asystole; and in patients with intraventricular conduction defects (especially with prolonged QT interval or QRS duration, or digitalis toxicity manifested by dysrhythmias or AV conduction disorders), because quinidine in therapeutic concentration increases the QT interval and QRS duration through AV node and His-Purkinje effects. Further prolongation would be detrimental in these conditions; complete heart block, ventricular tachycardia, ventricular fibrillation, or asystole may result.

Quinidine is contraindicated in patients with myasthenia gravis, because the drug's anticholinergic effects may exacerbate muscle weakness; and in patients with hypersensitivity to quinidine or related compounds.

Use quinidine with caution in patients with incomplete AV block, because CHF may occur; in patients with congestive heart failure, because the drug's direct myocardial depressant effect may worsen heart failure; in patients with hypotension, because the drug causes alpha blockade, which exacerbates hypotension (especially when given I.V.); in patients with renal and hepatic dysfunction because toxic drug accumulation may result; and in patients with asthma, muscle weakness, or infection with fever, because

these conditions may mask hypersensitivity reactions to the drug.

Interactions

Concomitant use of quinidine with hypotensive agents may cause additive hypotensive effects (mainly when administered I.V.); with phenothiazines or reserpine, it may cause additive cardiac depressant effects.

Concomitant use with digoxin or digitoxin may cause increased (possibly toxic) serum digoxin levels. (Some experts recommend a 50% reduction in digoxin dosage when quinidine therapy is initiated, with subsequent monitoring of serum concentrations.)

Concomitant use with anticonvulsants (such as phenytoin and phenobarbital) increases the rate of quinidine metabolism; this leads to decreased quinidine levels. Concomitant use with coumarin may potentiate coumarin's anticoagulant effect, possibly leading to hypoprothrombinemic hemorrhage.

When used concomitantly, cholinergic agents may fail to terminate paroxysmal supraventricular tachycardia, because quinidine antagonizes cholinergics' vagal excitation effect on the atria and AV node. Also, quinidine's anticholinergic effects may negate the effects of such anticholinesterase drugs as neostigmine and pyridostigmine when these agents are used to treat myasthenia gravis.

Concomitant use with anticholinergic agents may lead to additive anticholinergic effects. Concomitant use with neuromuscular blocking agents (such as pancuronium bromide, succinylcholine chloride, tubocurarine chloride, gallium triethiodide, metocurine iodide, and decamethonium bromide) may potentiate anticholinergic effects. Use of quinidine should be avoided immediately after use of these agents; if quinidine must be used, respiratory support may be needed.

Concomitant use with thiazide diuretics, some antacids, and sodium bicarbonate may decrease quinidine elimination when urine pH increases, requiring close monitoring of therapy.

Concomitant use with rifampin may increase quinidine metabolism and decrease serum quinidine levels, possibly necessitating dosage adjustment when rifampin therapy is initiated or discontinued.

Concomitant use with nifedipine may result in decreased quinidine levels. Concomitant use with verapamil may result in significant hypotension in some patients with hypertrophic cardiomyopathy.

Concomitant use with other antiarrhythmic agents (such as amiodarone, lidocaine, phenytoin, procainamide, or propranolol) may cause additive or antagonistic cardiac effects and additive toxic effects. For example, concurrent use of quinidine and other antiarrhythmics that increase the QT interval may further prolong the QT interval and lead to Torsades de Pointes tachycardia.

Effects on diagnostic tests
None reported.

Adverse reactions
• CNS: vertigo, headache, light-headedness, confusion, restlessness, cold sweat, pallor, fainting, dementia.
• CV: premature ventricular contractions, severe hy-

---

‡May contain sulfites　　　◆May contain tartrazine　　　◆◆May contain benzyl alcohol

potension, SA and AV block, ventricular fibrillation, ventricular tachycardia, aggravated CHF, ECG changes (particularly widening QRS complex, notched P waves, widened QT interval, and ST-segment depression), Torsades de Pointes tachycardia.
• DERM: rash, petechial hemorrhage of buccal mucosa, pruritus.
• EENT: tinnitus, excessive salivation, blurred vision.
• GI: diarrhea, nausea, vomiting, anorexia, abdominal pain.
• HEMA: hemolytic anemia, thrombocytopenia, agranulocytosis.
• Hepatic: hepatotoxicity, including granulomatous hepatitis.
• Other: angioedema, acute asthmatic attack, respiratory arrest, fever, cinchonism, lupus erythematosus syndrome.

Note: Drug should be discontinued if the following problems develop: blood dyscrasias; hepatic dysfunction; renal dysfunction; syncope; cardiotoxicity, including conduction defects (25% widening of QRS complex); ventricular tachycardia or flutter; frequent premature ventricular contractions; or complete AV block.

Overdose and treatment

The most serious clinical effects of overdose include severe hypotension, ventricular dysrhythmias (including Torsades de Pointes), and seizures. QRS complexes and QT and PR intervals may be prolonged, and ataxia, anuria, respiratory distress, irritability, and hallucinations may develop. If ingestion was recent, gastric lavage, emesis, and activated charcoal may be used to decrease absorption. Urine acidification may be used to help increase quinidine elimination.

Treatment involves general supportive measures (including cardiovascular and respiratory support) with hemodynamic and ECG monitoring. Metaraminol or norepinephrine may be used to reverse hypotension (after adequate hydration has been ensured). CNS depressants should be avoided, because CNS depression may occur, possibly with seizures. Cardiac pacing may be necessary. Isoproterenol and/or ventricular pacing possibly may be used to treat Torsades de Pointes tachycardia.

I.V. infusion of ⅙ molar sodium lactate solution reduces quinidine's cardiotoxic effect. Hemodialysis, although rarely warranted, also may be effective.

▶ Special considerations

• When drug is used to treat atrial tachydysrhythmias, ventricular rate may be accelerated from drug's anticholinergic effects on AV node. This can be prevented by previous treatment with digitalis.
• Because conversion of chronic atrial fibrillation may be associated with embolism, anticoagulant should be administered before quinidine therapy begins.
• Check apical pulse rate, blood pressure, and ECG tracing before starting therapy.
• I.V. route is generally avoided because of the potential for severe hypotension; it should be used to treat acute dysrhythmias only.
• Never use discolored (brownish) quinidine solution.
• For maintenance, give only by oral or I.M. route.

Dosage requirements vary. Some patients may require drug q 4 hours, others q 6 hours. Titrate dose by both clinical response and blood levels.
• When changing administration route, alter dosage to compensate for variations in quinidine base content.
• Dosage should be decreased in patients with CHF and hepatic disease.
• Monitor ECG, especially when large doses of the drug are being administered.
• Monitor liver function tests during first 4 to 8 weeks of therapy.
• Drug may increase toxicity of digitalis derivatives. Use with caution in patients who are receiving digitalis. Monitor digoxin levels.
• GI side effects, especially diarrhea, are signs of toxicity. Check quinidine blood levels; suspect toxicity when they exceed 8 mcg/ml. GI symptoms may be minimized by giving drug with meals.
• Lidocaine may be effective in treating quinidine-induced dysrhythmias, because it increases AV conduction.
• Quinidine may cause hemolysis in patients with G6PD deficiency.
• Quinidine is hemodialyzable. Dosage adjustment may be necessary in patients undergoing dialysis.
• The amount of quinidine in the various salt forms varies as shown below:
—Gluconate: 62% quinidine (324 mg of gluconate, 250 mg sulfate)
—Polygalacturonate: 60% quinidine (275 mg polygalacturonate, 200 mg sulfate)
—Sulfate: 83% quinidine. The sulfate form is considered the standard dosage preparation.
• Quinidine gluconate is reported to be as or more active in vitro against *Plasmodium falciparum* than quinine dihydrochloride. Since the latter drug is only available through the CDC, quinidine gluconate may be useful in the treatment of severe malaria when delay of therapy may be life-threatening. The current CDC protocol involves follow-up treatment with either tetracycline or sulfadoxine and pyrimethamine.

Information for parents and patient

Instruct parent to report any skin rash, fever, unusual bleeding, bruising, ringing in ears, or visual disturbance.

---

quinine sulfate
Quinaminoph, Quinamm, Quine, Quinite

• Classification: antimalarial, skeletal muscle relaxant (cinchona alkaloid)

How supplied

Available by prescription and without prescription
Capsules: 130 mg, 195 mg, 200 mg, 260 mg, 300 mg, 325 mg
Tablets: 260 mg, 325 mg

Indications, route, and dosage
Malaria (chloroquine-resistant)
Children: 25 mg/kg/day divided into three doses for 10 days.
Adults: 650 mg P.O. q 8 hours for 10 days, with 25 mg pyrimethamine q 12 hours for 3 days and with 500 mg sulfadiazine q.i.d. for 5 days.

I.V. quinine is available from the Centers for Disease Control (CDC) for the treatment of severe malaria with coma.

Dosage in renal failure

Creatinine clearance (ml/min/ 1.73 m²)	Percent of usual dose	Interval
≥50	100	q 8 hours
10 to 50	>5	q 8 to 12 hours
<10	30 to 50	q 24 hours

Action and kinetics
• *Antimalarial action:* Quinine intercalates into DNA, disrupting the parasite's replication and transcription; it also depresses its oxygen uptake and carbohydrate metabolism. It is active against the asexual erythrocytic forms of *Plasmodium falciparum, P. malariae, P. ovale,* and *P. vivax* and is used for chloroquine-resistant malaria.
• *Skeletal muscle relaxant effects:* Quinine increases the refractory period, decreases excitability of the motor endplate, and affects calcium distribution within muscle fibers.
• *Kinetics in adults:* Quinine is absorbed almost completely; peak serum concentrations occur at 1 to 3 hours. It is distributed widely into the liver, lungs, kidneys, and spleen; CSF levels reach 2% to 5% of serum levels. Quinine is about 70% bound to plasma proteins and readily crosses the placenta. Drug is metabolized in the liver. Less than 5% of a single dose is excreted unchanged in the urine; small amounts of metabolites appear in the feces, gastric juice, bile, saliva, and breast milk. Half-life is 4 to 21 hours in healthy or convalescing persons; it is longer in patients with malaria. Urine acidification hastens elimination.

Contraindications and precautions
Quinine is contraindicated in pregnant patients and in patients with known hypersensitivity to the drug, glucose-6-phosphate dehydrogenase deficiency, optic neuritis, or tinnitus; and in patients with a history of blackwater fever or of thrombocytopenic purpura associated with previous quinine ingestion.

Quinine should be used with caution in patients with cardiac dysrhythmias and in those receiving sodium bicarbonate.

Interactions
Quinine may increase plasma levels of digoxin and digitoxin. It may potentiate the effects of neuromuscular blocking agents, and it may potentiate the action of warfarin by depressing synthesis of vitamin K–dependent clotting factors.

Concomitant use of aluminum-containing antacids may delay or decrease absorption of quinine. Concomitant use of sodium bicarbonate or acetazolamide may increase absorption of quinine by decreasing urinary excretion.

Effects on diagnostic tests
Quinine may decrease platelet and red blood cell counts. It also may cause hypoglycemia and false elevations of urinary catecholamines and may interfere with 17-hydroxycorticosteroid and 17-ketogenic steroid tests.

Adverse reactions
• CNS: severe headache, apprehension, excitement, confusion, delirium, syncope, hypothermia, seizures (with toxic doses).
• CV: hypotension, cardiovascular collapse with overdosage of rapid I.V. administration, conduction disturbances.
• DERM: rashes, pruritus.
• EENT: altered color perception, photophobia, blurred vision, night blindness, amblyopia, scotoma, diplopia, mydriasis, optic atrophy, tinnitus, impaired hearing.
• GI: epigastric distress, diarrhea, nausea, vomiting.
• GU: renal tubular damage, anuria.
• HEMA: hemolytic anemia, thrombocytopenia, agranulocytosis, hypoprothrombinemia.
• Local: thrombosis at infusion site.
• Other: asthma, flushing, fever, facial edema, dyspnea, vertigo, hypoglycemia.
Note: Drug should be discontinued if signs of hypersensitivity or toxicity occur.

Overdose and treatment
Signs of overdose include tinnitus, vertigo, headache, fever, rash, cardiovascular effects, GI distress (including vomiting), blindness, apprehension, confusion, and seizures.

Treatment includes gastric lavage followed by supportive measures, which may include fluid and electrolyte replacement, artificial respiration, and stabilization of blood pressure and renal function.

Anaphylactic reactions may require epinephrine, corticosteroids, or antihistamines. Urinary acidification may increase elimination of quinine but will also augment renal obstruction. Hemodialysis or hemoperfusion may be helpful. Vasodilator therapy or stellate blockage may relieve visual disturbances.

▶ Special considerations
• Administer quinine after meals to minimize gastric distress; do not crush tablets, as drug irritates gastric mucosa.
• Discontinue drug if signs of idiosyncrasy or toxicity occur.
• Serum concentrations of 10 mg/ml or more may confirm toxicity as the cause of tinnitus or hearing loss.
• Quinine is no longer used for acute malarial attack by *Plasmodium vivax* or for suppression of malaria from resistant organisms.
• Parenteral form may be obtained from the CDC when oral therapy is unfeasible; administer by slow infusion (over 1 hour), and monitor I.V. sites and patient for adverse effects.

---

‡May contain sulfites   ♦May contain tartrazine   ♦♦May contain benzyl alcohol

Information for parents and patient
• Teach parents about adverse reactions and the need to report these immediately—especially tinnitus and hearing impairment.
• Tell parents to avoid concomitant administration of aluminum-containing antacids because these may alter drug absorption.
• Warn parents to keep drug out of reach of small children.

---

rabies immune globulin, human (RIG)
Hyperab, Imogam Rabies Immune Globulin

• Classification: rabies prophylaxis agent (immune serum)

How supplied
Available by prescription only
Injection: 150 IU/ml in 2-ml and 10-ml vials

Indications, route, and dosage
Rabies exposure
Children and adults: 20 IU/kg at time of first dose of rabies vaccine. Use half dose to infiltrate wound area. Give remainder I.M. Don't give rabies vaccine and RIG in same syringe or at same site.

Action and kinetics
• *Postexposure rabies prophylaxis:* RIG provides passive immunity to rabies.
• *Kinetics in adults:* After slow I.M. absorption, rabies antibody appears in serum within 24 hours and peaks within 2 to 13 days. RIG probably crosses the placenta and distributes into breast milk. No information is available about metablism.

    The serum half-life for rabies antibody titer is reportedly about 24 days.

Contraindications and precautions
RIG is contraindicated in patients with known hypersensitivity to thimerosal, a component of this immune serum.

Interactions
Concomitant use of this product with corticosteroids and immunosuppressant agents may interfere with the immune response to RIG. Whenever possible, avoid using these agents during the postexposure immunization period. Because antirabies serum may partially suppress the antibody response to rabies vaccine, use only the recommended dose of antirabies vaccine. Also, RIG may interfere with the immune response to live virus vaccine and rubella virus vaccine. Do not administer live virus vaccines within 3 months after administration of RIG.

Effects on diagnostic tests
None reported.

Adverse reactions
• Local: pain, redness, and induration at injection site.
• Systemic: slight fever, headache, malaise, angioedema, nephrotic syndrome, anaphylaxis.

Overdose and treatment
No information available.

▶ Special considerations
• Obtain a thorough history of the animal bite, allergies, and reactions to immunizations.
• Epinephrine solution 1:1,000 should be available to treat allergic reactions.
• Repeated doses of RIG should not be given after rabies vaccine is started.
• Do not administer more than 0.5 ml I.M. per injection site; divide I.M. doses greater than 5 ml and administer them at different sites.
• Do not confuse this drug with rabies vaccine, which is a suspension of attenuated or killed microorganisms used to confer active immunity. These two drugs are often given together prophylactically after exposure to known or suspected rabid animals.
• Because rabies can be fatal if untreated, the use of RIG during pregnancy appears justified. No fetal risk from RIG use has been reported to date.
• Ask patient when he received his last tetanus immunization because a booster may be indicated.
• Patients previously immunized with a tissue culture-derived rabies vaccine and those who have confirmed adequate rabies antibody titers should receive only the vaccine.
• RIG has not been associated with an increased frequency of acquired immunodeficiency syndrome. The immune globulin is devoid of human immunodeficiency virus (HIV). Immune globulin recipients do not develop antibodies to HIV.
• Store between 36° to 46° F. (2° and 8° C.). Do not freeze.

Information for parents and patient
• Explain to parents and patient that the body needs about a week to develop immunity to rabies after the vaccine is administered. Therefore, patients receive RIG to provide antibodies in their blood for immediate protection against rabies.
• Reactions to antirabies serum may occur up to 12 days after this product is administered. Encourage parents and patient to report skin changes, difficulty breathing, or headache.
• Patient also may experience some local pain, swelling, and tenderness at the injection site. Recommend acetaminophen to alleviate these minor effects.

---

*Canada only   †Unlabeled clinical use   Italicized adverse reactions have been observed in children.

ranitidine
Zantac

• Classification: antiulcer agent (histamine₂-receptor antagonist)

How supplied
Available by prescription only
Tablets: 150 mg, 300 mg
Injection: 25 mg/ml

Indications, route, and dosage
Duodenal and gastric ulcer (short-term treatment); pathologic hypersecretory conditions, such as Zollinger-Ellison syndrome
†*Children:* 2 to 4 mg/kg P.O. daily in divided doses q 12 hours; or 1 to 2 mg/kg I.V. daily in divided doses q 6 to 8 hours
Adults: 150 mg P.O. b.i.d. or 300 mg h.s. Dosages up to 6.3 g daily may be prescribed in patients with Zollinger-Ellison syndrome.

Drug also may be administered parenterally: 50 mg I.V. or I.M. q 6 to 8 hours.
Maintenance therapy in duodenal ulcer
Adults: 150 mg P.O. h.s.
Gastroesophageal reflux disease (GERD)
Adults: 150 mg P.O. b.i.d.

Action and kinetics
• *Antiulcer action:* Ranitidine competitively inhibits histamine's action at H₂-receptors in gastric parietal cells. This reduces basal and nocturnal gastric acid secretion as well as that caused by histamine, food, amino acids, insulin, and pentagastrin.
• *Kinetics in adults:* Approximately 50% to 60% of an oral dose is absorbed; food does not significantly affect absorption. After I.M. injection, drug is absorbed rapidly from parenteral sites. Ranitidine is distributed to many body tissues and appears in CSF and breast milk. Drug is about 10% to 19% protein-bound. Ranitidine is metabolized in the liver and is excreted in urine and feces.

Contraindications and precautions
Ranitidine is contraindicated in patients with ranitidine allergy. Use drug cautiously in patients with impaired hepatic function; dosage adjustment may be necessary in patients with impaired renal function.

Interactions
Antacids decrease ranitidine absorption; separate drugs by at least 1 hour.

Effects on diagnostic tests
Ranitidine may cause false-positive results in urine protein tests using Multistix.

Ranitidine may increase serum creatinine, lactic dehydrogenase, alkaline phosphatase, AST (SGOT), ALT (SGPT), and total bilirubin levels. Drug may decrease WBC, RBC, and platelet counts.

Adverse reactions
• CNS: malaise, dizziness, insomnia, vertigo, reversible confusion, agitation, hallucinations.
• DERM: rash.
• GI: constipation, nausea, abdominal pain.
• HEMA (rare): reversible leukopenia, granulocytopenia, agranulocytosis, thrombocytopenia.
• Local: itching and burning at injection site.

Overdose and treatment
No cases of overdose have been reported. However, treatment would involve emesis or gastric lavage and supportive measures as needed. Hemodialysis will remove ranitidine.

▶ Special considerations
• For administration through nasogastric tube, tablets may be ground into powder to make slurry; tube should be flushed afterward to ensure drug's passage to stomach and prevent obstruction.
• When administering I.V. push, dilute to a total volume of 20 ml and inject over a period of 5 minutes. No dilution necessary when administering I.M. May also be administered by intermittent I.V. infusion. Dilute 50 mg ranitidine in 100 ml of dextrose 5% in water and infuse over 15 to 20 minutes.
• Patients with impaired renal function may require dosage adjustment.
• Dialysis removes ranitidine; administer drug after treatment.

Information for parents and patient
• Explain that patient should take drug as directed, even after pain subsides, to ensure proper healing.
• Advise patient to take a single daily dose at bedtime.
• Patient should avoid taking drug with antacids or with food or drinks (such as those containing caffeine) that stimulate gastric secretion.
• Patient should not smoke and should avoid taking aspirin and other drugs that can cause gastric irritation.
• Inform parents and patient that drug may cause drowsiness.
• Teach parents how to recognize adverse reactions that should be reported.

ribavirin
Virazole

• Classification: antiviral agent (synthetic nucleoside)

How supplied
Available by prescription only
Powder to be reconstituted for inhalation: 6 g in 100-ml glass vial

---

Indications, route, and dosage
Treatment of hospitalized infants and young children infected by respiratory syncytial virus (RSV)

Infants and young children: Usually, 1 vial is administered per treatment day. Solution in concentration of 20 mg/ml delivered via the Viratek Small Particle Aerosol Generator (SPAG-2) results in a mist with a concentration of 190 mcg/liter. Treatment is carried out for 12 to 18 hours/day for at least 3, and no more than 7, days with a flow rate of 12.5 liters of mist per minute.

Action and kinetics
• *Antiviral action:* Drug action probably involves inhibition of ribonucleic acid (RNA) and deoxyribonucleic acid (DNA) synthesis, inhibition of RNA polymerase, and interference with completion of viral polypeptide coat.
• *Kinetics in adults:* Some ribavirin is absorbed systemically. Ribavirin concentrates in bronchial secretions; plasma levels are subtherapeutic for plaque inhibition. It is metabolized to 1,2,4-triazole-3-carboxamide (deribosylated ribavirin). Most of dose is excreted renally. First phase of plasma half-life is 9½ hours; second phase has extended half-life of 40 hours (from slow drug release from red blood cell binding sites).

Contraindications and precautions
Ribavirin is contraindicated in patients who might become pregnant during therapy because of drug's potentially teratogenic or embryocidal effects.

Ribavirin should be administered with extreme caution to patients requiring ventilatory assistance because drug may precipitate in ventilatory apparatus, impairing ventilation.

Interactions
None reported.

Effects on diagnostic tests
Transient increases in serum bilirubin and liver function studies may occur.

Adverse reactions
• GI: *nausea, vomiting, poor appetite.*
• HEMA: *anemia,* reticulocytosis.
• Other: *rash, conjunctivitis, erythema at eyelids, irritability (crying), hypoactivity.*

Overdose and treatment
Unknown in humans; high doses in animals have produced GI symptoms.

▶ Special considerations
• Ribavirin aerosol is indicated only for lower respiratory tract infection caused by RSV. (Although treatment may begin before test results are available, RSV infection must eventually be confirmed.)
• Drug is most useful for infants with most severe RSV form—typically premature infants and those with underlying disorders, such as cardiopulmonary disease. (Most other infants and children with RSV

infection do not require treatment because disease is self-limiting.)
• Administer ribavirin aerosol only by SPAG-2. Do not use any other aerosol-generating device.
• To prepare drug, reconstitute solution with USP sterile water for injection or inhalation, then transfer aseptically to sterile 500-ml Erlenmeyer flask. Dilute further with sterile water to 300 ml to yield final concentration of 20 mg/ml. Solution remains stable for 24 hours at room temperature.
• Do not use bacteriostatic water (or any other water containing antimicrobial agent) to reconstitute drug.
• Discard unused solution in SPAG-2 unit before adding newly reconstituted solution. Solution should be changed at least every 24 hours.
• Monitor ventilator-dependent patients carefully because drug may precipitate in ventilatory apparatus.
• Drug therapy must be accompanied by appropriate respiratory and fluid therapy.
• Nursing staff who are or may be pregnant should not be assigned to care for children who are receiving this potentially teratogenic drug. Exclude all visitors who are or may be pregnant.

Information for parents and patient
Explain therapy to parents and patient. Have parents monitor for adverse reactions.

---

riboflavin (vitamin B₂)

• Classification: nutritional supplement (vitamin)

How supplied
Available without prescription, as appropriate
Tablets: 5 mg, 10 mg, 25 mg
Tablets (sugar-free): 50 mg, 100 mg

Indications, route, and dosage
Riboflavin deficiency or adjunct to thiamine treatment for polyneuritis or cheilosis secondary to pellagra

Children under age 12: 2 to 10 mg P.O., S.C., I.M., or I.V. daily, depending on severity.
Children age 12 and older and adults: 5 to 50 mg P.O., S.C., I.M., or I.V. daily, depending on severity. For maintenance, increase nutritional intake and supplement with vitamin B complex.

Action and kinetics
• *Metabolic action:* Riboflavin, a coenzyme, functions in the forms of flavin adenine dinucleotide (FAD) and flavin mononucleotide (FMN) and plays a vital metabolic role in numerous tissue respiration systems. FAD and FMN act as hydrogen-carrier molecules for several flavoproteins involved in intermediary metabolism. Riboflavin is also directly involved in maintaining erythrocyte integrity.

Riboflavin deficiency causes a clinical syndrome with the following symptoms: cheilosis, angular stomatitis, glossitis, keratitis, scrotal skin changes, ocular changes, and seborrheic dermatitis. In severe deficiency, normochromic, normocytic anemia and

---

neuropathy may occur. Clinical signs may become evident after 3 to 8 months of inadequate riboflavin intake. Administration of riboflavin reverses signs of deficiency. Riboflavin deficiency rarely occurs alone and is often associated with deficiency of other B vitamins and protein.

• *Kinetics in adults:* Although riboflavin is absorbed readily from the GI tract, the extent of absorption is limited. Absorption occurs at a specialized segment of the mucosa; riboflavin absorption is limited by the duration of the drug's contact with this area. Before being absorbed, riboflavin-5-phosphate is rapidly dephosphorylated in the GI lumen. GI absorption increases when the drug is administered with food and decreases when hepatitis, cirrhosis, biliary obstruction, or probenecid administration is present. FAD and FMN are distributed widely to body tissues. Free riboflavin is present in the retina. Riboflavin is stored in limited amounts in the liver, spleen, kidneys, and heart, mainly in the form of FAD. FAD and FMN are approximately 60% protein-bound in blood. Riboflavin crosses the placenta, and breast milk contains about 400 ng/ml.

Riboflavin is metabolized in the liver. After a single oral dose or I.M. administration, the biological half-life is approximately 66 to 84 minutes in healthy individuals. Riboflavin is metabolized to FMN in erythrocytes, GI mucosal cells, and the liver; FMN is converted to FAD in the liver. Approximately 9% of the drug is excreted unchanged in the urine after normal ingestion. Excretion involves renal tubular secretion and glomerular filtration. The amount renally excreted unchanged is directly proportional to the dose. Removal of riboflavin by hemodialysis is slower than by natural renal excretion.

Contraindications and precautions
None reported.

Interactions
Concomitant use of riboflavin with propantheline bromide delays the absorption rate of riboflavin but increases the total amount absorbed. If the patient is using oral contraceptives, riboflavin's dose may need to be increased.

Effects on diagnostic tests
Riboflavin therapy alters urinalysis based on spectrophotometry or color reactions. Large doses of the drug result in bright yellow urine. Riboflavin produces fluorescent substances in urine and plasma, which can falsely elevate fluorometric determinations of catecholamines and urobilinogen.

Adverse reactions
GU: bright yellow urine with high doses.

Overdose and treatment
No information available.

▶ Special considerations
• The RDA of riboflavin is 0.4 to 1.4 mg/day in children, 1.2 to 1.7 mg/day in adults, and 1.5 to 1.8 mg/day in pregnant and lactating women.

• Give the oral preparation of riboflavin with food to increase absorption.
• Obtain a dietary history because other vitamin deficiencies may coexist.

Information for parents and patient
• Inform parents and patient that riboflavin may cause a yellow discoloration of the urine.
• Teach the parents and patient about good dietary sources of riboflavin, such as liver, kidney, heart, eggs, dairy products, whole-grain cereals, and green vegetables.
• Advise storing riboflavin in a tight, light-resistant container.

---

rifampin
Rifadin, Rimactane

• Classification: antituberculosis agent, (semisynthetic rifamycin B derivative [macrocyclic antibiotic])

How supplied
Available by prescription only
Capsules: 150 mg, 300 mg
Kit: 60 capsules, 300 mg

Indications, route, and dosage
Primary treatment in pulmonary tuberculosis
Children over age 5: 10 to 20 mg/kg P.O. daily single dose 1 hour before or 2 hours after meals. Maximum dose is 600 mg daily. Concomitant administration of other effective antitubercular drugs is recommended.
Adults: 600 mg P.O. daily single dose 1 hour before or 2 hours after meals.
Asymptomatic meningococcal carriers
Infants age 3 months to 1 year: 5 mg/kg P.O. b.i.d. for 2 days.
Children age 1 to 10: 10 mg/kg P.O. b.i.d. for 2 days.
Adults: 600 mg P.O. b.i.d. for 2 days.
   Note: Reduce dosage in liver dysfunction.
Prophylaxis of Haemophilus influenzae type B
Children and adults: 20 mg/kg (up to 600 mg) once daily for 4 consecutive days.

Action and kinetics
• *Antibiotic action:* Rifampin impairs ribonucleic acid (RNA) synthesis by inhibiting deoxyribonucleic acid-dependent RNA polymerase. Rifampin may be bacteriostatic or bactericidal, depending on organism susceptibility and drug concentration at infection site.

Rifampin acts against *Mycobacterium tuberculosis, M. bovis, M. marinum, M. kansasii,* some strains of *M. fortuitum, M. avium,* and *M. intracellulare,* and many gram-positive and some gram-negative bacteria. Resistance to rifampin by *M. tuberculosis* can develop rapidly; rifampin is usually given with other antituberculosis drugs to prevent or delay resistance.

• *Kinetics in adults:* Rifampin is absorbed completely from the GI tract after oral administration; peak serum concentrations occur 1 to 4 hours after ingestion. Food delays absorption. Rifampin is distributed widely into

---

‡May contain sulfites   ♦May contain tartrazine   ♦♦May contain benzyl alcohol

body tissues and fluids, including ascitic, pleural, seminal, and cerebrospinal fluids, tears, and saliva; and into liver, prostate, lungs, and bone. Rifampin crosses the placenta; it is 84% to 91% protein-bound.

Rifampin is metabolized extensively in the liver by deacetylation. It undergoes enterohepatic circulation, and drug and metabolite are excreted primarily in bile; drug, but not metabolite, is reabsorbed. From 6% to 30% of rifampin and metabolite appear unchanged in urine in 24 hours; about 60% is excreted in feces. Some drug is excreted in breast milk. Plasma half-life in adults is 1½ to 5 hours; serum levels rise in obstructive jaundice. Dosage adjustment is not necessary for patients with renal failure.

Contraindications and precautions

Rifampin is contraindicated in children with known hypersensitivity to any rifamycin. Use rifampin with caution and at reduced dosages in patients with hepatic disease or alcoholism and in patients taking other hepatotoxic drugs.

Interactions

Concomitant use of para-aminosalicylate may decrease oral absorption of rifampin, lowering serum concentrations; administer drugs 8 to 12 hours apart. Rifampin-induced hepatic microsomal enzymes inactivate the following drugs: propranolol, metoprolol, methadone, oral sulfonylureas, corticosteroids, digitalis derivatives, oral contraceptives and anticoagulants, chloramphenicol, disopyramide, quinidine, estrogens, dapsone, cyclosporine, and clofibrate; decreased serum concentrations of those drugs require dosage adjustments. Daily use of alcohol while using rifampin may increase risk of hepatotoxicity.

Effects on diagnostic tests

Rifampin alters standard serum folate and vitamin B_{12} assays. The drug's systemic effects may cause asymptomatic elevation of liver function tests (14%) and serum uric acid and may reduce vitamin D levels.

Rifampin may cause temporary retention of sulfobromophthalein in the liver excretion test; it may also interfere with contrast material in gallbladder studies and urinalysis based on spectrophotometry.

Adverse reactions

- CNS: headache, fatigue, drowsiness, ataxia, dizziness, mental confusion, generalized numbness.
- DERM: pruritus, urticaria, rash.
- EENT: visual disturbances, conjunctivitis.
- GI: epigastric distress, anorexia, nausea, vomiting, abdominal pain, diarrhea, flatulence, sore mouth and tongue, pseudomembranous colitis.
- HEMA: thrombocytopenia, transient leukopenia, *hemolytic anemia.*
- Hepatic: serious hepatotoxicity as well as transient abnormalities in liver function tests.
- Metabolic: hyperuricemia.
- Other: flu-like syndrome, red-orange discoloration of skin, sweat, tears, feces, and urine.

Note: Drug should be discontinued if patient shows signs of hypersensitivity reactions or hepatotoxicity or if severe diarrhea indicates pseudomembranous colitis.

Overdose and treatment

Signs of overdose include lethargy, nausea, and vomiting; hepatotoxicity from massive overdose includes hepatomegaly, jaundice, elevated liver function studies and bilirubin levels, and loss of consciousness.

Treat by gastric lavage, followed by activated charcoal; if necessary, force diuresis. Perform bile drainage if hepatic dysfunction persists beyond 24 to 48 hours.

▶ Special considerations

- Safety in children under age 5 has not been established. However, drug is recommended for prophylaxis and treatment by the CDC and the American Academy of Pediatrics.
- Give drug 1 hour before or 2 hours after meals for maximum absorption; capsule contents may be mixed with food or fluid to enhance swallowing.
- Obtain specimens for culture and sensitivity testing before first dose but do not delay therapy; repeat periodically to detect drug resistance.
- Observe patient for adverse reactions and monitor hematologic, renal and liver function studies, and serum electrolytes to minimize toxicity. Watch for signs of hepatic impairment (anorexia, fatigue, malaise, jaundice, dark urine, liver tenderness).
- Increased liver enzyme activity inactivates certain drugs (especially warfarin, corticosteroids, and oral hypoglycemics), requiring dosage adjustments.
- Avoid contact with the skin.
- Almost all bacteria may develop resistance to drug—except for short term use this drug should *not* be used alone.
- Patients who cannot swallow rifampin capsules may benefit from oral suspension that can be compounded by pharmacist. It is stable for 4 weeks.

Information for parents and patient

- Explain disease process and rationale for long-term therapy.
- Teach parents signs and symptoms of hypersensitivity and other adverse reactions, and emphasize need to report *any* unusual reactions.
- Tell parents to give rifampin on an empty stomach, at least 1 hour before or 2 hours after a meal. If GI irritation occurs, patient may need to take drug with food.
- Urge parents and child to comply with prescribed regimen, not to miss doses, and not to discontinue drug without medical approval. Explain importance of follow-up appointments.
- Urge prompt reporting of any flu-like symptoms, weakness, sore throat, loss of appetite, unusual bruising, rash, itching, dark urine, clay-colored stools, or yellow discoloration of eyes or skin.
- Explain that drug turns all body fluids red-orange; advise patient of possible permanent stains on clothes and soft contact lenses.
- If appropriate, explain that oral contraceptive users should substitute other methods; rifampin inactivates such drugs and may alter menstrual patterns.

Ringer's injection

• Classification: electrolyte and fluid replenishment

How supplied
Available by prescription only
Injection: 250 ml, 500 ml, 1,000 ml

Indications, route, and dosage
Fluid and electrolyte replacement
Children and adults: Dose highly individualized according to patient's size and clinical condition, but usually 1.5 to 3 liters (2% to 6% body weight) infused I.V. over 18 to 24 hours.

Action and kinetics
• *Fluid and electrolyte replacement:* Ringer's injection replaces fluid and supplies important electrolytes: sodium 147 mEq/liter, potassium 4 mEq/liter, calcium 4.5 mEq/liter, and chloride 155.5 mEq/liter. However, clinically, the addition of potassium and calcium only slightly increases the therapeutic value of an isotonic sodium chloride solution. Neither potassium nor calcium is present in sufficient concentration in Ringer's injection to correct a deficit of these ions adequately. As with sodium chloride injection, large volumes of Ringer's injection usually cause minimal distortion of cation composition of the extracellular fluid. However, either solution may alter the acid-base balance.
• *Kinetics in adults:* Drug is given by direct I.V. infusion, and is widely distributed.There is no significant metabolism. Drug is excreted primarily in urine, with minor excretion in feces.

Contraindications and precautions
Ringer's injection is contraindicated in renal failure, except as an emergency volume expander. Use with caution in renal dysfunction, congestive heart failure, circulatory insufficiency, hypoproteinemia, or pulmonary edema.

Interactions
Several drugs, as well as packed red blood cells, are incompatible with Ringer's solution. Consult specialized references for further information.

Effects on diagnostic tests
None reported.

Adverse reactions
• CV: fluid overload.
• Other: hypernatremia, hyperkalemia, hypercalcemia, hyperchloremia.

Overdose and treatment
If overinfusion occurs, stopping infusion is usually sufficient treatment. In some cases, a loop diuretic, such as furosemide, may be necessary to increase the rate of fluid and electrolyte elimination. Dialysis may be needed in renal failure.

▶ Special considerations
Monitor for acid-base imbalance when large volume of solution is infused. Ringer's injection is a colorless, odorless solution with a salty taste and a pH between 5.0 and 7.5.

Information for parents and patient
Explain therapy and need for restraints and frequent monitoring to parents and patient.

Ringer's injection, lactated

• Classification: electrolyte and fluid replenishment (electrolyte-carbohydrate solution)

How supplied
Available by prescription only
Injection: 250 ml, 500 ml, 1,000 ml

Indications, route, and dosage
Fluid and electrolyte replacement
Children and adults: Dose highly individualized, but usually 1.5 to 3 liters (2% to 6% body weight) infused I.V. over 18 to 24 hours.

This solution approximates the contents of the blood more closely than Ringer's injection does; however, additional electrolytes may have to be added to meet the patient's needs. Specific formulations of I.V. solutions are frequently preferred to this premixed formulation. The lactate has an alkalinizing effect in the body, requiring 1 to 2 hours to be fully effective.

Action and kinetics
• *Fluid and electrolyte replacement:* Ringer's injection (lactated) replaces fluid and supplies important electrolytes: sodium 130 mEq/liter, potassium 4 mEq/liter, calcium 2.7 mEq/liter, chloride 109.7 mEq/liter, and lactate 27 mEq/liter. However, clinically, the addition of potassium and calcium only slightly increases the therapeutic value of an isotonic sodium chloride solution. Neither potassium nor calcium is present in sufficient concentration in Ringer's injection to correct a deficit of these ions. As with sodium chloride injection, large volumes of Ringer's injection usually cause minimal distortion of cation composition of the extracellular fluid. However, either solution may alter the acid-base balance.

Ringer's injection (lactated) may be used for its alkalinizing effect, because the lactate is ultimately metabolized to bicarbonate. In persons with normal cellular oxidative activity, the alkalinizing effect will be fully realized in 1 to 2 hours.
• *Kinetics in adults:* Drug is given by direct I.V. infusion. Ringer's injection is distributed widely. There is no significant metabolism. Lactate is oxidized to bicarbonate. Ringer's injection is excreted primarily in urine, with minor excretion in feces.

Contraindications and precautions
Ringer's injection (lactated) is contraindicated in patients with renal failure, except as a volume expander in hypovolemic emergencies; and in patients with lac-

tic acidosis because of the lactate content. Use cautiously in patients with renal dysfunction, congestive heart failure, circulatory insufficiency, hypoproteinemia, or pulmonary edema because of potential for fluid overload.

Interactions
Several drugs, as well as packed red blood cells, are incompatible with Ringer's solution. Consult specialized references for further information.

Effects on diagnostic tests
None reported.

Adverse reactions
• CV: fluid overload.
• Other: hypernatremia, hyperkalemia, hypercalcemia, hyperchloremia.

Overdose and treatment
If overinfusion occurs, stopping infusion is usually sufficient treatment. Dialysis may be needed in renal failure. Monitor blood acid-base balance.

▶ Special considerations
• The solution is colorless and odorless with a salty taste and a pH between 6.0 and 7.5. The absence of bicarbonate from the solution stabilizes the calcium, which may precipitate as calcium bicarbonate. It contains no antibacterial agent.
• Monitor for acid-base imbalance when large volume of solution is infused.

Information for parents and patient
Explain therapy and need for frequent monitoring and restraints to parents and patient.

scopolamine
Transderm Scōp, Transderm V∗

scopolamine hydrobromide
Isopto Hyoscine, Triptone

- Classification: antimuscarinic, antiemetic/antivertigo agent, antiparkinsonian agent, cycloplegic mydriatic (anticholinergic)

How supplied
Available without prescription
Capsules: 0.25 mg

Available by prescription only
Transdermal patch: 1.5 mg
Injection: 0.3, 0.4, 0.5, 0.6, and 1 mg/ml in 1-ml vials and ampules; 0.86 mg/ml in 0.5-ml ampules
Ophthalmic solution: 0.25%

Indications, route, and dosage
Antimuscarinic; adjunct to anesthesia
Infants age 4 to 7 months: 100 mcg I.M. or I.V.
Children age 8 months to 3 years: 150 mcg. I.M. or I.V.
Children age 3 to 8 years: 200 mcg I.M. or I.V.
Children age 8 to 12 years: 300 mcg I.M. or I.V.
Adults: 0.3 to 0.6 I.M. or I.V. as a single dose.
Prevention of nausea and vomiting associated with motion sickness
Adults: 250 to 800 mcg P.O. 1 hour before antiemetic effect is required; or one transdermal patch designed to deliver 0.5 mg/day over 3 days (72 hours), applied to the skin behind the ear at least 4 hours before the antiemetic is required.
Not recommended for children.
Postencephalitic parkinsonism and other spastic states
Infants age 4 to 7 months: 0.1 mg I.M. or S.C.
Children: 0.006 mg/kg P.O. or S.C. t.i.d. to q.i.d.; or 0.2 mg/m².
Adults: 0.5 to 1 mg P.O. t.i.d. to q.i.d.; 0.3 to 0.6 mg S.C., I.M., or I.V. (with suitable dilution) t.i.d. to q.i.d.
Cycloplegic refraction
Children: 1 drop 0.25% solution b.i.d. for 2 days before refraction.
Adults: 1 to 2 drops 0.25% solution in eye 1 hour before refraction.

Action and kinetics
- *Antimuscarinic action:* Scopolamine inhibits acetylcholine's muscarinic actions on autonomic effectors, resulting in decreased secretions and GI motility; it also blocks vagal inhibition of the sinoatrial node.
- *Antiemetic action:* Although its exact mechanism of action is unknown, scopolamine may affect neural pathways affecting the vestibular input to the CNS originating in the labyrinth of the ear, thereby inhibiting nausea and vomiting in patients with motion sickness.
- *Antiparkinsonian action:* Scopolamine blocks central cholinergic receptors, helping to balance cholinergic activity in the basal ganglia. It may also prolong dopamine's effects by blocking dopamine reuptake and storage at central receptor sites.
- *Mydriatic action:* Scopolamine competively blocks acetylcholine at cholinergic neuroeffector sites, antagonizing acetylcholine's effects on the sphincter muscle and ciliary body, thereby producing mydriasis and cycloplegia; these effects are used to produce cycloplegic refraction and pupil dilation to treat preoperative and postoperative iridocyclitis.
- *Kinetics in adults:* Scopolamine is well absorbed percutaneously from behind the ear and is well absorbed in the G.I. tract.

Scopolamine is distributed widely throughout body tissues. It crosses the placenta and probably the blood-brain barrier.

Scopolamine is probably metabolized completely in the liver; however, its exact metabolic fate is unknown.

Scopolamine is probably excreted in urine as metabolites.

Contraindications and precautions
Scopolamine is contraindicated in children with glaucoma or a tendency toward glaucoma, because drug-induced cycloplegia and mydriasis may increase intraocular pressure; and in patients with obstructive uropathy, obstructive GI tract disease, asthma, chronic pulmonary disease, myasthenia gravis, paralytic ileus, intestinal atony, or toxic megacolon, because the drug may exacerbate these conditions.

Administer scopolamine cautiously to patients with autonomic neuropathy, hyperthyroidism, coronary artery disease, congestive heart failure, hypertension, or ulcerative colitis, because the drug may exacerbate these conditions; to patients with hepatic or renal disease, because toxic accumulation may occur; to patients with cardiac dysrhythmias, because the drug may block vagal inhibition of the sinoatrial node pacemaker, worsening the dysrhythmia; to patients with hiatal hernia associated with reflux esophagitis, because this drug may decrease lower esophageal sphincter tone; to young children, because they may be more sensitive to drug effects; and to patients with known hypersensitivity to belladonna alkaloids.

Interactions
Concomitant use of scopolamine with CNS depressants (alcohol, tranquilizers, and sedative-hypnotics) may increase CNS depression.

Concurrent administration of antacids decreases oral absorption of anticholinergics. Administer scopolamine at least 1 hour before antacids.

---

‡May contain sulfites   ◆May contain tartrazine   ◆◆ May contain benzyl alcohol

Concomitant administration of drugs with anticholinergic effects may cause additive toxicity.

Decreased GI absorption of many drugs has been reported after the use of anticholinergics (for example, levodopa and ketoconazole). Conversely, slowly dissolving digoxin tablets may yield higher serum digoxin levels when administered with anticholinergics.

Use cautiously with oral potassium supplements (especially wax-matrix formulations) because the incidence of potassium-induced GI ulcerations may be increased.

Effects on diagnostic tests
None reported.

Adverse reactions
• CNS: headache, disorientation, restlessness, drowsiness, irritability, dizziness, hallucinations, memory disturbances, confusion, violent behavior, amnesia, unconsciousness, spastic extremities.
• CV: palpitations, tachycardia, paradoxical bradycardia.
• DERM: flushing, dryness, rash, erythema.
• EENT: dilated pupils; blurred vision; photophobia; cycloplegia; increased intraocular pressure; dry, itchy, or red eyes; acute narrow-angle glaucoma; ocular congestion (prolonged use).
• GI: constipation, dry mouth, dysphagia, nausea, vomiting, epigastric distress.
• GU: dysuria.
• Other: bronchial plug formation, fever, respiratory depression.
  Note: Drug should be discontinued if urinary retention, confusion, difficulty breathing, hypersensitivity, or eye pain occurs.

Overdose and treatment
Clinical effects of overdose include excitability, seizures, CNS stimulation followed by depression, and such psychotic symptoms as disorientation, confusion, hallucinations, delusions, anxiety, agitation, and restlessness. Peripheral effects include dilated, nonreactive pupils; blurred vision; flushed, hot, dry skin; dryness of mucous membranes; dysphagia; decreased or absent bowel sounds; urinary retention; hyperthermia; tachycardia; hypertension; and increased respiration.

Treatment is primarily symptomatic and supportive, as needed. Maintain patent airway. If patient is awake and alert, induce emesis (or use gastric lavage) and follow with a saline cathartic and activated charcoal to prevent further drug absorption. In severe cases, physostigmine may be administered to block scopolamine's antimuscarinic effects. Give fluids, as needed, to treat shock; diazepam to control psychotic symptoms; and pilocarpine (instilled into the eyes) to relieve mydriasis. If urinary retention develops, catheterization may be necessary. Mild symptoms will be transient and disappear after removing patch.

▶ Special considerations
• Monitor patient's vital signs, urine output, visual changes, and for signs of impending toxicity.
• Give ice chips, cool drinks, or sugarless hard candy to relieve dry mouth.

• Constipation may be relieved by stool softeners or bulk laxatives.
• Therapeutic doses may produce amnesia, drowsiness, and euphoria (desired effects for use as an adjunct to anesthesia). As necessary, reorient patient.
• Some patients may experience transient excitement or disorientation.

Ophthalmic administration
• Have patient lie down, tilt his head back, or look at ceiling to aid instillation.
• Apply pressure to the lacrimal sac for 1 minute after instillation to reduce the risk of systemic drug absorption.

Information for parents and patient
• Teach parents and patient how and when to administer drug; caution patient to take drug only as prescribed and not to add other medications except as prescribed.
• Warn patient that drug may cause dizziness, drowsiness, or blurred vision.
• Patient should avoid beverages and medications that contain alcohol, because they may cause additive CNS effects.
• Advise patient to consume plenty of fluids and dietary fiber to help avoid constipation.
• Tell parents or patient to promptly report dry mouth, blurred vision, skin rash, eye pain, any significant change in urine volume, or pain or difficulty on urination.
• Warn parents or patient that drug may cause increased sensitivity or intolerance to high temperatures, resulting in dizziness.
• Instruct parents to watch for signs of confusion and to check for rapid or pounding heartbeat and to report these effects promptly.
• Instruct parents and patient to apply pressure to bridge of nose for about 1 minute after ophthalmic instillation. Advise patient not to close eyes tightly or blink for about 1 minute after instillation.

---

secobarbital sodium
Novosecobarb*, Seconal

• Classification: sedative-hypnotic, anticonvulsant (barbiturate)
• Controlled substance schedule II (suppositories are schedule III)

How supplied
Available by prescription only
Injection: 50 mg/ml in 1-ml and 2-ml disposable syringe; 50 mg/ml in 20-ml vial
Capsules: 50 mg, 100 mg
Tablets: 100 mg
Rectal suppositories: 200 mg

Indications, route, and dosage
Preoperative sedation
Children: 50 to 100 mg P.O. or 4 to 5 mg/kg rectally 1 to 2 hours before surgery.
Adults: 200 to 300 mg P.O. 1 to 2 hours before surgery.

Insomnia
Children: 3 to 5 mg/kg I.M., not to exceed 100 mg, with no more than 5 ml injected in any one site. Or 4 to 5 mg/kg rectally.
Adults: 100 to 200 mg P.O. or I.M.
Acute psychotic agitation
Adults: Initially, 50 mg/minute I.V. up to 250 mg I.V.; additional doses given cautiously after 5 minutes if desired response is not obtained. Not to exceed 500 mg total.

Action and kinetics
• *Sedative-hypnotic action:* Secobarbital acts throughout the CNS as a nonselective depressant with a rapid onset of action and short duration of action. Particularly sensitive to this drug is the reticular activating system, which controls CNS arousal. Secobarbital decreases both presynaptic and postsynaptic membrane excitability by facilitating the action of gamma-aminobutyric acid (GABA). The exact cellular site and mechanism(s) of action are unknown.
• *Kinetics in adults:* After oral administration, 90% of secobarbital is absorbed rapidly. After rectal administration, secobarbital is nearly 100% absorbed. Peak serum concentration after oral or rectal administration occurs between 2 and 4 hours. The onset of action is rapid, occurring within 15 minutes when administered orally. Peak effects are seen 15 to 30 minutes after oral and rectal administration, 7 to 10 minutes after I.M. administration, and 1 to 3 minutes after I.V. administration. Concentrations of 1 to 5 mcg/ml are needed to produce sedation; 5 to 15 mcg/ml are needed for hypnosis. Hypnosis lasts for 1 to 4 hours after oral doses of 100 to 150 mg.

Secobarbital is distributed rapidly throughout body tissues and fluids; approximately 30% to 45% is protein-bound.

Secobarbital is oxidized in the liver to inactive metabolites. Duration of action is 3 to 4 hours.

95% of a secobarbital dose is eliminated as glucuronide conjugates and other metabolites in urine.

Contraindications and precautions
Secobarbital is contraindicated in patients with known hypersensitivity to barbiturates and in patients with bronchopneumonia, status asthmaticus, or other severe respiratory distress because of the potential for respiratory depression. Secobarbital should not be used in patients who are depressed or have suicidal ideation, because the drug can worsen depression; in patients with uncontrolled acute or chronic pain, because exacerbation of pain and paradoxical excitement can occur; and in patients with porphyria, because this drug can trigger symptoms of this disease.

Secobarbital should be used cautiously in patients who must perform hazardous tasks requiring mental alertness, because the drug causes drowsiness. Administer parenteral phenobarbital slowly and with extreme caution to patients with hypotension or severe pulmonary or cardiovascular disease because of potential adverse hemodynamic effects. Because tolerance and physical or psychological dependence may occur, prolonged use of high doses should be avoided.

Interactions
Secobarbital may add to or potentiate CNS and respiratory depressant effects of other sedative-hypnotics, antihistamines, narcotics, antidepressants, tranquilizers, and alcohol.

Secobarbital enhances the enzymatic degradation of warfarin and other oral anticoagulants; patients may require increased doses of the anticoagulant. Drug also enhances hepatic metabolism of some drugs, including digitoxin (not digoxin), corticosteroids, oral contraceptives and other estrogens, theophylline and other xanthines, and doxycycline. Secobarbital impairs the effectiveness of griseofulvin by decreasing absorption from the GI tract.

Valproic acid, phenytoin, disulfiram, and monoamine oxidase inhibitors decrease the metabolism of secobarbital and can increase its toxicity. Rifampin may decrease secobarbital levels by increasing metabolism.

Effects on diagnostic tests
Secobarbital may cause a false-positive phentolamine test. The physiologic effects of the drug may impair the absorption of cyanocobalamin ^{57}Co; it may decrease serum bilirubin concentrations in neonates, epileptic patients, and in patients with congenital nonhemolytic unconjugated hyperbilirubinemia. EEG patterns show a change in low-voltage, fast activity; changes persist for a time after discontinuation of therapy.

Adverse reactions
• CNS: drowsiness, lethargy, vertigo, headache, CNS depression, *paradoxical excitement*, confusion and agitation (especially in elderly patients), rebound insomnia, increased dreams or nightmares, possibly seizures (after acute withdrawal or reduction in dosage).
• CV: hypotension (after rapid I.V. administration), bradycardia, circulatory collapse.
• DERM: urticaria, rash, exfoliative dermatitis, Stevens-Johnson syndrome.
• EENT: miosis.
• GI: nausea, vomiting, diarrhea, constipation.
• Local: thrombophlebitis, pain and possible tissue damage at site of extravascular injection.
• Other: respiratory depression, laryngospasm, bronchospasm. Reported vitamin K deficiency and bleeding have occurred in newborns of mothers treated during pregnancy. Hyperalgesia may occur with low doses or in patients with chronic pain.
Note: Drug should be discontinued if hypersensitivity reaction, profound CNS or respiratory depression, or skin eruption occurs.

Overdose and treatment
Clinical manifestations of overdose include unsteady gait, slurred speech, sustained nystagmus, somnolence, confusion, respiratory depression, pulmonary edema, areflexia, and coma. Typical shock syndrome with tachycardia and hypotension, jaundice, hypothermia followed by fever, and oliguria may occur.

Maintain and support ventilation and pulmonary function as necessary; support cardiac function and circulation with vasopressors and I.V. fluids as needed.

‡May contain sulfites   ♦ May contain tartrazine   ♦ ♦ May contain benzyl alcohol

If patient is conscious and gag reflex is intact, induce emesis (if ingestion was recent) by administering ipecac syrup. If emesis is contraindicated, perform gastric lavage while a cuffed endotracheal tube is in place to prevent aspiration. Follow with administration of activated charcoal or saline cathartic. Measure intake and output, vital signs, and laboratory parameters; maintain body temperature. Patient should be rolled from side to side every 30 minutes to avoid pulmonary congestion.

Alkalinization of urine may be helpful in removing drug from the body; hemodialysis may be useful in severe overdose.

▶ **Special considerations**
• Premature infants are more susceptible to the depressant effects of barbiturates because of immature hepatic metabolism.
• Secobarbital may cause paradoxical excitement in children; use cautiously.
• Dosage of secobarbital must be individualized for each patient, because different rates of metabolism and enzyme induction occur.
• Assess level of consciousness before and frequently during therapy to evaluate effectiveness of drug. Monitor neurologic status for possible alterations or deteriorations. Monitor seizure character, frequency, and duration for changes. Institute seizure precautions, as necessary.
• Assess patient's sleeping patterns before and during therapy to ensure effectiveness of drug.
• Institute safety measures—side rails, assistance when out of bed, call light within reach—to prevent falls and injury.
• Anticipate possible rebound confusion and excitatory reactions in patient.
• Assess bowel elimination patterns; monitor for complaints of constipation. Advise diet high in fiber, if indicated.
• Monitor prothrombin time carefully in patients taking anticoagulants; dosage of anticoagulant may require adjustment to counteract possible interaction.
• Observe patient to prevent hoarding or self-dosing, especially in depressed or suicidal patients, or those who are or have a history of being drug-dependent.
• Abrupt discontinuation may cause withdrawal symptoms; discontinue slowly.
• Death is common with an overdose of 2 to 10 g; it may occur at much smaller doses if alcohol is also ingested.
• Use I.V. route of administration only in emergencies or when other routes are unavailable.
• Dilute secobarbital injection with sterile water for injection solution, 0.9% sodium chloride injection, or Ringer's injection. Do not use if solution is discolored or if a precipitate forms.
• Avoid I.V. administration at a rate greater than 50 mg/15 seconds to prevent hypotension and respiratory depression. Have emergency resuscitative equipment on hand.
• Administer I.M. dose deep into large muscle mass to prevent tissue injury.
• Store suppositories in refrigerator. To ensure accurate dosage, do not divide suppository.
• Secobarbital sodium injection, diluted with luke-warm tap water to a concentration of 10 to 15 mg/ml, may be administered rectally in children. A cleansing enema should be administered before secobarbital enema.
• Monitor hepatic and renal studies frequently to prevent possible toxicity.

Information for parents and patient
• Warn parents or patient to avoid concurrent use of other drugs with CNS depressant effects, such as antihistamines, analgesics, and alcohol, because they will have additive effects and result in increased drowsiness. Instruct parents to seek medical approval before giving patient any nonprescription cold or allergy preparations.
• Caution parents and patient not to increase or decrease dose or frequency without medical approval; abrupt discontinuation of medication may trigger rebound insomnia, with increased dreaming, nightmares, or seizures.
• Patient should avoid hazardous tasks that require alertness while taking secobarbital.
• Be sure parents and patient understand that secobarbital can cause physical or psychological dependence (addiction), and that these effects may be transmitted to the fetus; withdrawal symptoms can occur in neonates whose mothers took barbiturates in the third trimester.
• Instruct parents or patient to report any skin eruption or other marked adverse effect.
• Explain that a morning hangover is common after therapeutic use of barbiturates.

---

silver nitrate, silver nitrate 1%
Dey Drops Silver Nitrate

• Classification: ophthalmic antiseptic; topical cauterizing agent, heavy metal (silver compound)

How supplied
Available by prescription only
Ophthalmic solution: 1%

Indications, route, and dosage
Prevention of gonorrheal ophthalmia neonatorum
Neonates: Cleanse lids thoroughly; instill 1 drop of 1% solution into each eye.

Action and kinetics
• *Antiseptic action:* Liberated silver ions precipitate bacterial proteins, resulting in germicidal activity. Drug is effective mainly in preventing gonorrheal ophthalmia neonatorum.
• *Cauterizing action:* Denatures protein, producing a caustic or corrosive effect.
• *Kinetics in adults:* Unknown.

Contraindications and precautions
Not to be confused with topical ointment which is used to cauterize wounds in adults. Silver nitrate is contraindicated in patients with hypersensitivity to

the preparation or any of its components. For ophthalmic use, the 1% solution is considered optimal but still must be used with caution, because cauterization of the cornea and blindness may result, especially with repeated applications.

Interactions
None reported.

Effects on diagnostic tests
None reported.

Adverse reactions
• Eye: periorbital edema, temporary staining of lids and surrounding tissue, conjunctivitis (with concentrations of 1% or greater).

Overdose and treatment
Clinical manifestations of overdose are extremely rare with ophthalmic use.

Toxicity is highly dependent on the concentration of silver nitrate and extent of exposure. Oral overdose would be treated by dilution with 4 to 8 oz of water. To remove the chemical, administer sodium chloride (10 g/liter) by lavage in order to precipitate silver chloride. Activated charcoal or a cathartic can be used. Treat eye overexposure initially by irrigation with tepid water for at least 15 minutes. Treat dermal overexposure by washing with soap and water twice. Dizziness, seizures, mucous membrane irritation, nausea, vomiting, stomach ache and diarrhea, methemoglobinemia, dermatitis, rash, and hypochloremia with associated hyponatremia may occur. Treat seizures with diazepam. Depending on the extent of exposure, evaluate for methemoglobinemia; treat with methylene blue.

▶ Special considerations
• Silver nitrate is bacteriostatic, germicidal, and astringent.
• Do not use repeatedly.
• If solution stronger than 1% is accidentally used in eye, promptly irrigate with isotonic sodium chloride to prevent eye irritation.
• Instillation may be briefly delayed to allow neonate to bond with mother. Instillation at birth is required by law in most states; do not irrigate eyes after instillation. Store wax ampules away from light and heat.
• Do not use solution if it is discolored or contains a precipitate.

Information for parents and patient
• Explain that preparations may stain skin and clothing. Teach parents that silver nitrate may discolor neonate's eyelids temporarily.
• Inform parents that instillation of antiseptic at birth is required by law in most states.

silver protein, mild
Argyrol S.S.

• Classification: antiseptic (silver compound)

How supplied
Available by prescription only
Topical (ophthalmic solution): 20%

Indications, route, and dosage
Topical application for inflammation of eye, ear, nose, throat, rectum, urethra, and vagina
Children and adults: Apply p.r.n. as a 5% to 20% solution.

Action and kinetics
• *Antiseptic action:* Silver protein stains and coagulates mucus and inhibits the growth of both gram-positive and gram-negative organisms. When instilled in the eye before ophthalmic surgery, removal of stained material may reduce incidence of postoperative infection.
• *Kinetics in adults:* Unknown.

Contraindications and precautions
Silver protein is contraindicated in patients with hypersensitivity to any component of the preparation. It is not recommended for prolonged use.

Interactions
When used concomitantly with sulfacetamide, silver protein may result in precipitates.

Effects on diagnostic tests
None reported.

Adverse reactions
• DERM: argyria (permanent discoloration of skin and conjunctiva) with long-term use.
• Eye: chemical conjunctivitis.

Overdose and treatment
Clinical manifestations of ingested overdose include argyria (blue-gray discoloration of the skin, mucous membranes, and eyes), neuropathies, severe gastroenteritis, blindness. Because some silver salts may be corrosive, do not induce emesis. Sodium chloride may be administered by gastric lavage to remove the drug. Treat ocular exposure by flushing the eye for 15 minutes with warm water.

▶ Special considerations
• Store drug in amber glass bottles; protect from light.
• Do not use if drug is discolored or contains a precipitate.
• Prolonged use should be avoided.

Information for parents and patient
• Demonstrate correct application and proper storage.
• Caution parents against long-term use.

---

silver sulfadiazine
Flint SSD, Silvadene

• Classification: topical antibacterial (synthetic anti-infective)

How supplied
Available by prescription only
Cream: 1%

Indications, route, and dosage
Adjunct in the prevention and treatment of wound infection for second- and third-degree burns
Children and adults: Apply ⅟₁₆″ (16-mm) thickness of ointment to cleansed and debrided burn wound once or twice daily. Reapply if accidentally removed.

Action and kinetics
• *Antibacterial action:* Acts on bacterial cell membrane and bacterial cell wall. Silver sulfadiazine has a broad spectrum of activity, including gram-negative and gram-positive organisms.
• *Kinetics in adults:* Absorption is limited with topical use. Silver sulfadiazine is excreted in the urine.

Contraindications and precautions
Silver sulfadiazine is contraindicated in pregnant women near term and in premature infants because drug has produced kernicterus in neonates. Do not use on women of childbearing age unless benefits outweigh the possibility of fetal damage.

Silver sulfadiazine should be used cautiously in patients with known hypersensitivity to the drug. The possibility of cross-hypersensitivity with other sulfonamides should be kept in mind. It should be used cautiously in patients with impaired hepatic or renal function.

Interactions
None reported.

Effects on diagnostic tests
If used on extensive areas of body surface, systemic absorption may result in a decreased neutrophil count, indicating a reversible leukopenia.

Adverse reactions
• Local: pain, burning, rash, itching.
• Other: reversible leukopenia.
Note: Drug should be discontinued if sensitization develops.

Overdose and treatment
To treat local overapplication, discontinue drug and cleanse area thoroughly.

▶ Special considerations
• Silver sulfadiazine is contraindicated in premature infants or infants younger than age 2 months.
• Avoid contacting drug with eyes and mucous membranes.

• Apply drug with a sterile gloved hand. The burned area should be covered with cream at all times.
• Daily bathing is an aid in debridement of burn patients. Whirlpool baths are now contraindicated because they increase the risk of infection.
• Continue treatment until site is healed or is ready for skin grafting.
• Monitor for signs of fungal superinfection.
• Delayed eschar separation may result when drug is used.

Information for parents and patient
• Teach proper wound care.
• Reassure parents and patient that silver sulfadiazine does not stain the skin.

sodium benzoate and sodium phenylacetate
Ucephan

• Classification: urea cycle enzymopathy adjunct (enzyme substrate combination)

How supplied
Available by prescription only
Solution: 10 g sodium benzoate and 10 g sodium phenylacetate per 100 ml in 100-ml multiple-unit bottles.

Indications, route, and dosage
Adjunct for prevention and treatment of hyperammonemia in the chronic management of patients with urea cycle enzymopathies (UCE)
Neonates, infants, and children: 2.5 ml/kg/day (250 mg sodium benzoate and 250 mg sodium phenylacetate) in three to six equally divided doses. Total daily dosage should not exceed 100 ml (10 g each of sodium benzoate and sodium phenylacetate). Must be diluted before use.

Action and kinetics
• *Metabolic action:* Sodium benzoate and sodium phenylacetate decrease elevated blood ammonia concentrations in patients with inborn errors of ureagenesis. The mechanisms for this action are conjugation reactions involving acylation of amino acids which results in decreased ammonia formation. Benzoate and phenylacetate activate conjugation pathways which then substitute for or supplement the defective ureagenic pathway in patients with UCE, preventing the accumulation of ammonia.

The therapeutic regimens of sodium benzoate and sodium phenylacetate also include dietary manipulation and amino acid supplementation. This combined regimen has effected an 80% survival rate for UCE, which was previously almost universally fatal in the first year of life. The survival rate for each complete enzyme deficiency studied was carbamylphosphate synthetase, 75%; ornithine transcarbamylase (males), 59%; argininosuccinate synthetase, 96%. Survival in heterozygous females with partial ornithine transcarbamylase deficiency was 95%; for patients with other partial deficiencies, 86%. Early diagnosis and treatment are important in minimizing developmental disabilities. Treatment is unlikely to reverse preexisting neurologic impairment, and neurologic deterioration may continue in some patients.

• *Kinetics in adults:* Peak levels occur 1 hour after oral administration. Distribution has not been characterized. The major sites for metabolism of benzoate and phenylacetate are the liver and kidneys. Approximately 80% to 100% of the compound is excreted by the kidneys within 24 hours as metabolites.

Contraindications and precautions

Do not administer to patients with known hypersensitivities to sodium benzoate or sodium phenylacetate.

Solutions containing sodium ions should be used with great care, if at all, in patients with congestive heart failure, severe renal insufficiency, and in clinical states marked by sodium retention with edema. In patients with diminished renal function, administration of solutions containing sodium ions may result in sodium retention.

Exercise special care in calculating and preparing dosage. The solution is highly concentrated. Compound is not intended as sole therapy for UCE patients and must be combined with dietary management (low protein diet) and amino acid supplementation for best results.

Use with caution in neonates with hyperbilirubinemia, since in vitro experiments suggest that benzoate competes for bilirubin binding sites on albumin.

The benefits of treating neonatal hyperammonemic coma with this drug have not been established. The treatment of choice in neonatal hyperammonemic coma is hemodialysis. Peritoneal dialysis may be helpful if hemodialysis is not available.

Interactions

Penicillin may compete with conjugated products of sodium benzoate and sodium phenylacetate for active secretion by renal tubules.

Probenecid inhibits the renal transport of many organic compounds, including amino hippuric acid, and may affect renal excretion of the conjugation products of sodium benzoate and sodium phenylacetate.

Effects on diagnostic tests

None reported.

Adverse reactions

• GI: side effects associated with salicylates, such as nausea and vomiting, exacerbation of peptic ulcers.
• Other: mild hyperventilation and mild respiratory alkalosis.

Note: If an adverse reaction occurs, discontinue drug, evaluate the patient, and institute appropriate treatment.

Overdose and treatment

Four overdoses of sodium phenylacetate or sodium benzoate in UCE patients have been reported, two after use of an I.V. infusion. Two patients became irritable and vomited after receiving three-fold overdoses of oral sodium benzoate. Both recovered with-

out treatment 24 hours after the drug was discontinued.

Discontinue the drug and institute supportive measures for metabolic acidosis and circulatory collapse. Hemodialysis or peritoneal dialysis may be beneficial.

▶ Special considerations

• Dilute each dose in 4 to 8 ounces of infant formula or milk and administer with meals. Dilution in other beverages, especially acidic ones, may cause precipitation of the drug, depending on pH and the final concentration. Inspect the mixture for compatibility before administration.
• Because sodium phenylacetate has a lingering odor, exercise care to minimize contact with skin and clothing during mixing and administration of the drug.
• Store drug at room temperature; avoid exposing it to excessive heat.

Information for parents and patient

Explain to parents the disease process and the importance of maintaining dietary and drug therapy.

---

sodium bicarbonate
Neut, Soda Mint

• Classification: systemic and urinary alkalinizing agent, systemic hydrogen ion buffer, oral antacid

---

How supplied

Available by prescription only
Injection: 4% (2.4 mEq/5 ml), 4.2% (5 mEq/10 ml), 5% (297.5 mEq/500 ml), 7.5% (8.92 mEq/10 ml and 44.6 mEq/50 ml), 8.4% (10 mEq/10 ml and 50 mEq/50 ml)

Available without prescription
Tablets: 300 mg, 325 mg, 600 mg, 650 mg

Indications, route, and dosage
Adjunct to advanced cardiac life support

Neonates and infants to age 2: 0.5 to 1 mEq/kg I.V. bolus of a 4.2% solution. Dose may be repeated every 10 minutes depending on blood gas values. Dosage not to exceed 8 mEq/kg daily.
Children over age 2 and adults: Although no longer routinely recommended, 1 mEq/kg I.V. bolus of a 7.5% or 8.4% solution followed by 0.5 mEq/kg every 10 minutes depending on blood gas values. Further doses are based on subsequent blood gas values. If blood gas values are unavailable, use 0.5 mEq/kg q 10 minutes until spontaneous circulation returns.
Metabolic acidosis
Children and adults: Dose depends on blood CO_2 content, pH, and patient's clinical condition. Generally, 2 to 5 mEq/kg I.V. infused over 4 to 8 hours.
Urinary alkalization
Children: 1 to 10 mEq (12 to 120 mg) per kg daily.
Adults: 48 mEq (4 g) P.O. followed by 12 to 24 mEq (1 to 2 g) every 4 hours.
Antacid
Adults: 300 mg to 2 g P.O. one to four times daily.

Action and kinetics
• *Alkalizing buffering action:* Sodium bicarbonate is an alkalinizing agent that dissociates to provide bicarbonate ion. Bicarbonate in excess of that needed to buffer hydrogen ions causes systemic alkalinization and, when excreted, urinary alkalinization as well.
• *Oral antacid:* Taken orally, sodium bicarbonate neutralizes stomach acid by the above mechanism.
• *Kinetics in adults:* Sodium bicarbonate is well absorbed after oral administration as sodium ion and bicarbonate. Bicarbonate occurs naturally and is confined to the systemic circulation. There is no metabolism. Bicarbonate is filtered and reabsorbed by the kidney; less than 1% of filtered bicarbonate is excreted.

Contraindications and precautions
Sodium bicarbonate is contraindicated in patients with metabolic or respiratory alkalosis; in patients with hypochloremic alkalosis from diuretics, vomiting, or nasogastric suction; and in patients with hypocalcemia because alkalosis may produce tetany. Sodium bicarbonate should be used cautiously in patients with CHF, pulmonary disease, ascites, or other fluid-retaining states because of the large sodium load; in patients with potassium depletion because alkalosis may lower serum potassium levels, predisposing the patient to cardiac dysrhythmias; and in neonates and children under age 2 because rapid injection of hypertonic sodium may cause hypernatremia.

Interactions
If urinary alkalinization occurs, sodium bicarbonate increases half-life of quinidine, amphetamines, ephedrine, and pseudoephedrine, and it increases urinary excretion of tetracyclines and methotrexate.

Effects on diagnostic tests
Sodium bicarbonate therapy may alter serum electrolyte levels and may increase serum lactate levels.

Adverse reactions
• CNS: altered consciousness, obtundation (hypernatremia), tremors.
• CV: *fluid retention, worsening heart failure.*
• GI: *bloating and flatulence after oral use,* cramps, *nausea, vomiting.*
• GU: renal calculi.
• Metabolic: *alkalosis,* hypernatremia, hypercholemia, hyperosmolarity, *hypercapnia, hypercalcemia.*
• Local: *pain and tissue necrosis after I.V. extravasation.*
• Other: *increased vascular volume and serum osmolarity, hyperirritability, tetany, intraventricular hemorrhage.*
   Note: Drug should be discontinued if metabolic alkalosis occurs.

Overdose and treatment
Clinical signs of overdose include depressed consciousness and obtundation from hypernatremia, tetany from hypocalcemia, cardiac dysrhythmias from hypokalemia, and seizures from alkalosis. Correct fluid, electrolyte, and pH abnormalities. Monitor vital signs and fluid and electrolytes closely.

▶ Special considerations
• Avoid rapid infusion (10 ml/minute) of hypertonic solutions in children under age 2. The 4.2% solution (5 mEq/10 ml) is preferred.
• Monitor vital signs regularly; when drug is used as urinary alkalinizer, monitor urine pH.
• Avoid extravasation of I.V. solutions. Addition of calcium salts may cause precipitate; bicarbonate may inactivate catecholamines in solution (epinephrine, phenylephrine, and dopamine).
• Discourage use as an oral antacid because of hazardous excessive systemic absorption.
• Assess patient for milk-alkali syndrome if drug use is long-term.

Information for parents and patient
• Advise parents to avoid chronic use as oral antacid, and recommend nonabsorbable antacids.
• Advise parent that patient should take oral drug 1 hour before or 2 hours after enteric-coated medications, because it may cause enteric-coated products to dissolve in the stomach.

sodium chloride
Slo-Salt, Thermotab

• Classification: sodium and chloride replacement (electrolyte)

How supplied
Available by prescription only
Tablets (slow-release): 600 mg
Tablets (enteric-coated): 1 g
Injection: 0.45% sodium chloride 500 ml, 1,000 ml; 0.9% sodium chloride 50 ml, 100 ml, 150 ml, 250 ml, 500 ml, 1,000 ml; 3% sodium chloride 500 ml; 5% sodium chloride 500 ml

Indications, route, and dosage
Water and electrolyte replacement in hyponatremia from electrolyte loss or severe sodium chloride depletion
Children and adults: Calculate sodium deficit as follows: 140 mEq/L − [Na] × T.B.W. = mEq Na
   where [Na] = patient's serum sodium level;
      T.B.W. = total body water (in liters) *or*
      0.6 L/kg × body weight (kg).
      mEq Na = sodium deficit.
For severe hyponatremia (serum sodium below 120 mEq/ml), give 3% or 5% solution, with no more than 100 ml being administered over a 1-hour period.
   To correct sodium depletion of isotonic proportions, infuse 0.9% sodium chloride (2% to 6% of body weight) over 18 to 24 hours; 0.9% sodium chloride also is used as a priming fluid for hemodialysis procedures and to initiate and terminate blood transfusions. The usual oral replacement dosage of sodium chloride is 1 to 2 g t.i.d.
   Hypotonic solutions (usually 0.45% containing 77 mEq sodium and chloride per liter) are usually given with dextrose solutions for maintenance therapy for 1 to 3 days in patients unable to take fluid and nu-

---

trients orally and are administered without dextrose in the management of hyperosmolar diabetes mellitus.

Management of "heat cramps" and heat prostration from excessive perspiration during exposure to high temperatures
Adults: Give 1 g orally with a full glass of water 1 to 10 times daily. Do not exceed 4.8 g/day. A solution of 3 to 4 g of sodium chloride and 1.5 to 2 g of sodium bicarbonate per liter also is acceptable for oral use if patient cannot tolerate solid foods.

Sodium chloride solution is also used as a vehicle for drugs. The pharmacy may admix compatible drugs in sodium chloride for infusion.

Action and kinetics
• *Electrolyte replacement:* Sodium chloride solution replaces deficiencies of the sodium and chloride ions in the blood plasma.
• *Kinetics in adults:* Oral and parenteral sodium chloride are absorbed readily. Sodium chloride is distributed widely. No significant metabolism occurs. Sodium and chloride are eliminated primarily in urine, but also in the sweat, tears, and saliva.

Contraindications and precautions
The 3% and 5% sodium chloride solutions are contraindicated in the presence of elevated, normal, or only slightly decreased plasma sodium and chloride concentrations. They should be given slowly in small volumes (200 to 400 ml) because of the danger of hypervolemia caused by water flowing from the intercellular space to the hyperosmolar plasma.

Use 0.9% sodium chloride cautiously in patients with congestive heart failure (CHF), renal failure, cirrhotic and nephrotic disease, or hypoproteinemia. Use cautiously in patients receiving corticosteroids or corticotropin.

Infusion of isotonic (0.9%) sodium chloride during or immediately after surgery may result in excessive sodium retention. Infusion of a potassium-free solution may cause hypokalemia.

Pediatric patients (especially neonates) should not receive sodium chloride with benzyl alcohol as preservative (antimicrobial agent), nor should solution be used to flush I.V. catheters in neonates. Administration of sodium chloride with benzyl alcohol has caused deaths that were preceded by metabolic acidosis, CNS depression, respiratory distress progressing to gasping respiration, hypotension, renal failure, and, occasionally, seizures and intracranial hemorrhage.

Interactions
None reported.

Effects on diagnostic tests
None reported.

Adverse reactions
• CNS: irritability, restlessness, weakness, muscular twitching, headache, dizziness, obtundation with possible coma.
• CV: aggravation of CHF; hypervolemia; edema; hypertension, tachycardia, and fluid accumulation.

• HEMA: hyperosmolarity with confusion, stupor, or coma.
• Metabolic: hypernatremia and aggravation of existing acidosis with excessive infusion; severe electrolyte disturbance, loss of potassium. Excessive infusion of chloride may cause the loss of bicarbonate ions, causing acidification of the blood.
• Respiratory: pulmonary edema (if too much is given or rate of administration is too rapid); respiratory arrest.
• Other: Contaminated I.V. solutions may cause fever, infection at the infusion site, and extravasation.

Overdose and treatment
Sodium chloride overdose causes serious electrolyte disturbances. Oral ingestion of large quantities irritates the GI mucosa and may cause nausea and vomiting, diarrhea, and abdominal cramps.

Treatment of oral overdose consists of emptying the stomach, giving magnesium sulfate as a cathartic, and supportive therapy. Provide airway and ventilation if necessary. Excessive I.V. administration requires discontinuation of sodium chloride infusion.

▶ Special considerations
• Use only for correcting severe sodium deficits (sodium below 120 mEq/ml). The 3% and 5% solutions should be infused very slowly and with caution to avoid pulmonary edema. Patient should be observed constantly. Electrolyte levels should be determined frequently.
• Concentrated solutions (3.5 and 4 mEq/ml) are available for addition to parenteral nutrition solutions.
• Monitor changes in fluid balance, serum electrolyte disturbances, and acid-base imbalances.
• Monitor for hypokalemia with administration of potassium-free solutions.
• Sodium chloride 0.9% may be used in managing extreme dilution of hyponatremia and hypochloremia resulting from administration of sodium-free fluids during fluid and electrolyte therapy, and in managing extreme dilution of extracellular fluid after excessive water intake (for example, after multiple enemas).

Information for parents and patient
Explain disease process and therapy to parents or patient. Advise parents to monitor for adverse reactions.

sodium fluoride
ACT, Fluorigard, Fluorinse, Fluoritabs, Flura, Flura-Drops, Flura-Loz, Gel II, Karidium, Karigel, Karigel-N, Listermint with Fluoride, Luride, Luride Lozi-Tabs, Luride-SF Lozi-Tabs, Pediaflor, Phos-Flur, Point Two, PreviDent, Thera-Flur, Thera-Flur-N

• Classification: dental caries prophylactic (mineral)

How supplied
Available without prescription
Rinse: 0.01% (180 ml, 260 ml, 540 ml, 720 ml); 0.02% (180 ml, 300 ml, 360 ml, 480 ml)

Available by prescription only
Tablets: 0.5 mg, 1 mg (sugar-free)
Tablets (chewable): 0.25 mg (sugar-free)
Drops: 0.125 mg/drop (30 ml), 0.125 mg/drop (60 ml, sugar-free), 0.25 mg/drop (19 ml), 0.25 mg/drop (24 ml, sugar-free), 0.5 mg/ml (50 ml)
Rinse: 0.02% (250 ml, 480 ml, 500 ml), 0.09% (250 ml, 480 ml), 0.09% (480 ml, sugar-free)
Gel: 0.5% (24 g, 30 g, 60 g, 120 g, 125 g, 130 g), 0.5% sugar-free (250 g), 1.23% (480 g)
Gel drops: 0.5% (24 ml, 60 ml)

Indications, route, and dosage
Aid in the prevention of dental caries
Oral
Children to age 1: 0.25 mg daily
Children to age 3: 0.5 mg daily.
Children over age 3: 1 mg daily.
Topical rinse
Children age 6 to 12: 5 ml of 0.2% solution.
Children over age 12 and adults: 10 ml of 0.2% solution. Use once daily after thoroughly brushing teeth and rinsing mouth. Rinse around and between teeth for 1 minute, then spit out.

Action and kinetics
• *Dental caries prophylactic action:* Sodium fluoride acts systemically before tooth eruption and topically afterward by increasing tooth resistance to acid dissolution, by promoting remineralization, and by inhibiting the cariogenic microbial process. Acidulation provides greater topical fluoride uptake by dental enamel than neutral solutions. When topical fluoride is applied to hypersensitive exposed dentin, the formation of insoluble materials within the dentinal tubules blocks transmission of painful stimuli.
• *Kinetics in adults:* Sodium fluoride is absorbed readily and almost completely from the GI tract. A large amount of an oral dose may be absorbed in the stomach, and the rate of absorption may depend on the gastric pH. Oral fluoride absorption may be decreased by simultaneous ingestion of aluminum or magnesium hydroxide or calcium. Normal total plasma fluoride concentrations range from 0.14 to 0.19 mcg/ml. Sodium fluoride is stored in bones and developing teeth after absorption. Because of the storage-mobi-

lization mechanism in skeletal tissue, a constant fluoride supply may be provided. Although teeth have a small mass, they also serve as storage sites. Fluoride deposited in teeth is not released readily. Fluoride has been found in all organs and tissues with a low accumulation in noncalcified tissues. Fluoride is distributed into sweat, tears, hair, and saliva. Fluoride crosses the placenta and is distributed into breast milk. Fluoride concentrations in milk range from approximately 0.05 to 0.13 ppm and remain fairly constant. Fluoride is excreted rapidly, mainly in the feces. About 90% of fluoride is filtered by the glomerulus and reabsorbed by the renal tubules.

Contraindications and precautions
Sodium fluoride is contraindicated in patients with hypersensitivity to the fluoride ion and when the fluoride content of drinking water exceeds 0.7 ppm. Patients on a low-sodium or sodium-free diet should avoid sodium fluoride. If the fluoride content of drinking water is 0.3 ppm or more, 1-mg tablets or rinse must not be used in children under age 3. The 1-mg rinse should not be used in children under age 6 because young children cannot perform the necessary rinse correctly. Some formulations contain tartrazine, which may precipitate allergic reaction in certain individuals.

Interactions
Incompatibility of systemic fluoride with dairy foods has reportedly caused calcium fluoride formation.
Concomitant use with magnesium or aluminum hydroxide may impair the absorption of sodium fluoride.

Effects on diagnostic tests
None reported.

Adverse reactions
• CNS: headaches, weakness.
• DERM: hypersensitivity reactions, such as atopic dermatitis, eczema, and urticaria.
• GI: gastric distress.

Overdose and treatment
In children, acute ingestion of 10 to 20 mg of sodium fluoride may cause excessive salivation and GI disturbances; 500 mg may be fatal. GI disturbances include salivation, nausea, abdominal pain, vomiting, and diarrhea. CNS disturbances include CNS irritability, paresthesias, tetany, hyperactive reflexes, seizures, and respiratory or cardiac failure (from the calcium-binding effect of fluoride). Hypoglycemia and hypocalcemia are frequent laboratory findings.
By using gastric lavage with 0.15% calcium hydroxide, the fluoride may be precipitated. Administer glucose I.V. in normal saline solution; parenteral calcium administration may be indicated for tetany. Adequate urine output should be maintained.

▶ Special considerations
• Young children usually cannot perform the rinse process necessary with oral solutions.
• Because prolonged ingestion or improper techniques may result in dental fluorosis and osseous changes,

the dosage must be carefully adjusted according to the amount of fluoride ion in drinking water.
• Review dietary history with the family. A diet that includes large amounts of fish, mineral water, and tea provides approximately 5 mg/day of fluoride.
• Fluoride supplementation must be continuous from infancy to age 14 to be effective.
• Tablets can be dissolved in the mouth, chewed, swallowed whole, added to drinking water or fruit juice, or added to water in infant formula or other foods.
• Drops may be administered orally undiluted or added to fluids or food.
• Sodium fluoride may be preferred to stannous fluoride to avoid staining tooth surfaces. Neutral sodium fluoride may also be preferred to acidulated fluoride to avoid dulling of porcelain and ceramic restorations.
• Prolonged intake of drinking water containing a fluoride ion concentration of 4 to 8 ppm may result in increased density of bone mineral and fluoride osteosclerosis.
• An oral sodium fluoride dose of 40 to 65 mg/day has resulted in adverse rheumatic effects.
• Used investigationally to treat osteoporosis.

Information for parents and patient
• Patient should take sodium fluoride tablets and drops with meals. Milk and other dairy products may decrease the absorption of sodium fluoride tablets; patient should avoid simultaneous ingestion.
• Advise parents and patient that rinses and gels are most effective if used immediately after brushing or flossing and taken just before retiring to bed.
• Patient should expectorate — and not swallow — any excess liquid or gel.
• Patient should not eat, drink, or rinse his mouth for 15 to 30 minutes after application, and should use a plastic container — not glass — to dilute drops or rinse, because the fluoride interacts with glass.
• Encourage parents to notify the patient's dentist if mottling of teeth occurs.
• Advise parents to contact dentist if they move to another area. Changed water supply could cause excessive dosage of fluoride and mottled tooth enamel.
• Warn parents to treat fluoride tablets as a drug and to keep them away from children.

sodium lactate

• Classification: systemic alkalizer (alkalinizing agent)

How supplied
Available by prescription only
Injection: ⅙ molar solution
Injection, for preparations of I.V. admixtures: 2.5 mEq/ml

Indications, route, and dosage
To alkalize urine
Adults: 30 ml of a ⅙ molar solution/kg of body weight given in divided doses over 24 hours P.O.

Mild to moderate metabolic acidosis
Children and adults: Dosage is highly individualized and depends on the severity of the acidosis and the patient's age, weight, and clinical condition, and on laboratory determinants. The following formula is used to determine sodium lactate dosage for administration by I.V. infusion.

$$\text{Dose in ml of } \frac{1}{6} \text{ molar solution} = \frac{(60 - \text{plasma CO}_2)}{} \times (0.8 \times \text{body weight in lb})$$

Action and kinetics
• *Alkalizing action:* Sodium lactate is metabolized in the liver, producing bicarbonate, the primary extracellular alkalotic buffer for the body's acid-base system, and glycogen. The simultaneous removal of lactate and hydrogen ion during metabolism also produces alkalinization.
• *Kinetics in adults:* Lactate ion occurs naturally throughout the human body. It is metabolized in the liver to glycogen.

Contraindications and precautions
Sodium lactate is contraindicated in patients with lactic acidosis, which impairs lactate metabolism and prevents formation of bicarbonate; in patients with metabolic, systemic, or respiratory alkalosis; and in patients with hypernatremia because the drug may worsen these conditions.
Sodium lactate should be used cautiously in patients with CHF or other edematous or sodium-retaining states; in patients with oliguria or anuria; and in patients receiving corticosteroids or corticotropin, because of its sodium content.

Interactions
Sodium lactate is physically incompatible with sodium bicarbonate solutions.

Effects on diagnostic tests
None reported.

Adverse reactions
• CV: excess fluid retention, worsening heart failure.
• Other: metabolic alkalosis.
Note: Drug should be discontinued if adverse effects occur.

Overdose and treatment
Clinical manifestations of overdose include tetany from hypocalcemia, seizures from alkalosis, and cardiac dysrhythmias from hypokalemia. Correct fluid, electrolyte, and pH abnormalities. Monitor vital signs and fluid status closely.

▶ Special considerations
• Drug is safe to use in children; lower doses are usually indicated.
• Assess electrolyte, fluid, and acid-base status throughout infusion to prevent alkalosis.
• Monitor injection site for infiltration or extravasation or both.
• The drug should not be used to treat severe metabolic acidosis because the production of bicarbonate from lactate may take 1 to 2 hours.

---

‡May contain sulfites   ◆May contain tartrazine   ◆◆May contain benzyl alcohol

• I.V. infusion rate should not exceed 300 ml/hour.

Information for parents and patient
Explain therapy to parents and patient. Advise parents to monitor for adverse reactions.

---

sodium phosphates
(sodium phosphate and sodium biphosphate)
Fleet Phospho-Soda

• Classification: saline laxative (acid salt)

How supplied
Available without prescription
Liquid: 2.4 g sodium phosphate and 900 mg sodium biphosphate/5 ml
Enema: 160 mg/ml sodium phosphate and 60 mg/ml sodium biphosphate

Indications, route, and dosage
Constipation
Adults: 5 to 20 ml liquid P.O. with water; or 20 to 46 ml solution mixed with 4 oz cold water; or 2- to 4.5-oz enema.

Action and kinetics
• *Laxative action:* Sodium phosphate and sodium biphosphate exert an osmotic effect in the small intestine by drawing water into the intestinal lumen, producing distention that promotes peristalsis and bowel evacuation.
• *Kinetics in adults:* About 1% to 20% of sodium and phosphate is absorbed; the extent of absorption is unknown. With oral administration, action begins in 3 to 6 hours; with enema administration, in 2 to 5 minutes; with suppository administration, in 30 minutes.

Contraindications and precautions
Sodium phosphate and sodium biphosphate are contraindicated in patients with fluid and electrolyte disturbances, impaired renal function, edema, or congestive heart failure and in other patients required to limit sodium intake; and in patients with appendicitis, abdominal pain, nausea or vomiting, fecal impaction, or intestinal obstruction or perforation, because the drug may worsen the symptoms of these disorders.

Drugs should be used cautiously in patients with large hemorrhoids or anal excoriation because of the potential for irritation.

Interactions
Concomitant administration of drug with antacids may cause inactivation of both.

Effects on diagnostic tests
None reported.

Adverse reactions
• GI: abdominal cramps, nausea (rare).
• Metabolic: fluid and electrolyte disturbances (hypernatremia, hyperphosphatemia) in chronic use.
• Other: laxative dependence in long-term use.
Note: Drug should be discontinued if abdominal pain develops.

Overdose and treatment
No information available; probable clinical effects include abdominal pain and diarrhea.

▶ Special considerations
• Dilute drug with water before giving orally (add 30 ml of drug to 120 ml of water). Follow drug administration with full glass of water.
• Monitor serum electrolyte levels; when drug is given as saline laxative, up to 10% of sodium content may be absorbed.
• Drug is not routinely used to treat constipation but is commonly used to evacuate the bowel.

Information for parents and patient
• Instruct patient on how to mix the drug and on dosage schedule.
• Warn parents that frequent or prolonged use of drug may lead to laxative dependence.

---

sodium polystyrene sulfonate
Kayexalate, SPS

• Classification: cation-exchange (potassium-removing resin)

How supplied
Available by prescription only
Oral powder: 1.25 g/5 ml suspension
Rectal: 1.25 g/5 ml suspension

Indications, route, and dosage
Hyperkalemia
Neonates: 1 g/kg P.O. or rectally (q 20 minutes p.r.n.)
Children: 1 g/kg P.O. q 6 hours or q 2 to 6 hours rectally. Exchange rate: 1 mEq K per 1 g resin.
Adults: 15 g P.O. daily to q.i.d. in water or sorbitol. Alternatively, 30 to 50 g p.r.n. as a retention enema.

Action and kinetics
• *Potassium-removing action:* Sodium polystyrene sulfonate releases sodium in exchange for other cations such as potassium.
• *Kinetics in adults:* Sodium polystyrene sulfonate is not absorbed. The onset of action varies from hours to days. Drug is excreted unchanged in feces.

Contraindications and precautions
Use sodium polystyrene sulfonate cautiously in patients with renal failure and in those in whom sodium intake must be restricted. Do not administer with laxatives containing magnesium or aluminum because alkalosis may result.

Interactions
When used concomitantly, magnesium- and calcium-containing antacids are bound by the resin, possibly causing metabolic alkalosis in patients with renal impairment.

Effects on diagnostic tests
Sodium polystyrene sulfonate therapy may alter serum magnesium and calcium levels.

Adverse reactions
• GI: anorexia, *nausea, vomiting, constipation,* gastric irritation, diarrhea (with sorbitol emulsion).
• Other: *electrolyte imbalances,* ECG abnormalities, hypokalemia, sodium retention.
   Note: Drug should be discontinued if hypokalemia occurs.

Overdose and treatment
Clinical manifestations of overdose include signs and symptoms of hypokalemia (irritability, confusion, cardiac dysrhythmias, ECG changes, severe muscle weakness, and sometimes paralysis) and digitalis toxicity in digitalized patients. Drug may be discontinued or dose lowered when serum potassium level falls to the 4 to 5 mEq/liter range.

▶ Special considerations
• Adjust dosage based upon a calculation of 1 mEq of potassium bound for each 1 g of resin.
• For oral administration: mix resin only with water or sorbitol; never mix with orange juice (high K^+ content).
• Chill oral suspension to increase palatability; do not heat because that inactivates resin.
• The rectal route is recommended when vomiting, P.O. restrictions, or upper GI tract problems are present.
• For rectal administration, mix polystyrene resin only with water and sorbitol for rectal use. Do not use other vehicles (that is, mineral oil) for rectal administration, to prevent impactions. Ion exchange requires aqueous medium. Sorbitol content prevents impaction. Prepare rectal dose at room temperature. Stir emulsion gently during administration.
• Monitor serum potassium at least once daily. Watch for other signs of hypokalemia.
• Monitor for symptoms of other electrolyte deficiencies (magnesium, calcium) because drug is nonselective. Monitor serum calcium in patients receiving sodium polystyrene therapy for more than 3 days. Supplementary calcium may be needed.
• Constipation is more likely to occur when drug is given with concurrent phosphate binders (such as aluminum hydroxide).
• If hyperkalemia is severe, more drastic modalities should be added; for example, dextrose 50% with regular insulin I.V. push. Do not depend solely on polystyrene resin to lower serum potassium levels in severe hyperkalemia.

Information for parents and patient
• Instruct parents in the importance of following a prescribed low-potassium diet.
• Explain necessity of retaining enema, as appropriate to patient's age. Retention for 6 to 10 hours is ideal, but 30 to 60 minutes is acceptable.

---

sodium salicylate
Uracel

• Classification: nonnarcotic analgesic, antipyretic, anti-inflammatory (salicylate)

How supplied
Available by prescription only
Injection: 1 g/10 ml for dilution

Available without prescription
Tablets: 325 mg, 650 mg
Tablets (enteric-coated): 325 mg, 650 mg

Indications, route, and dosage
Minor pain
Children over age 12 and adults: 325 to 650 mg P.O. q 4 hours, p.r.n., or 500 mg slow I.V. infusion over 4 to 8 hours. Maximum dosage is 1 g daily.
Children age 2 to 11: 25 to 50 mg/kg or 1.5 g/m² P.O. in four or six divided doses. Dosage in children age 2 or younger must be individualized.
Rheumatoid arthritis, osteoarthritis, or other inflammatory conditions
Children: 80 to 100 mg/kg P.O. daily in divided doses.
Adults: 3.6 to 5.4 g P.O. daily in divided doses.

Action and kinetics
• *Analgesic action:* Sodium salicylate produces analgesia by an ill-defined effect on the hypothalamus (central action) and by blocking generation of pain impulses (peripheral action). The peripheral action may involve inhibition of prostaglandin synthesis.
• *Anti-inflammatory action:* The drug exerts its anti-inflammatory effect by inhibiting prostaglandin synthesis; it may also inhibit the synthesis or action of other mediators of inflammation.
• *Antipyretic action:* The drug relieves fever by acting on the hypothalamic heat-regulating center to produce peripheral vasodilation. This increases peripheral blood supply and promotes sweating, which leads to loss of heat and to cooling by evaporation.
• *Kinetics in adults:* Sodium salicylate is absorbed rapidly and completely from the GI tract. Sodium salicylate is distributed widely into most body tissues and fluids. Protein-binding is concentration-dependent, varies from 75% to 90%, and decreases as serum concentrations increase. Severe toxic side effects may occur at serum concentrations greater than 400 mcg/ml. Therapeutic blood salicylate concentrations for arthritis are 20 to 30 mg/100 ml. Sodium salicylate is hydrolyzed in the liver and metabolites are excreted in urine.

Contraindications and precautions
Sodium salicylate is contraindicated in patients with GI ulcer, GI bleeding, or known hypersensitivity to the drug or other nonsteroidal anti-inflammatory drugs (NSAIDs).

---

‡May contain sulfites   ◆May contain tartrazine   ◆ ◆ May contain benzyl alcohol

Sodium salicylate should be used cautiously in patients with renal impairment, hypoprothrombinemia, vitamin K deficiency, and bleeding disorders; and in patients with congestive heart failure (CHF) and hypertension because of the drug's sodium content.

Interactions

Concomitant use of sodium salicylate with drugs that are highly protein-bound (phenytoin, sulfonylureas, warfarin) may cause displacement of either drug, and adverse effects. Monitor therapy closely for both drugs. Concomitant use of other GI-irritating drugs (steroids, antibiotics, other NSAIDs) may potentiate the adverse GI effects of sodium salicylate. Use together with caution.

Ammonium chloride and other urine acidifiers increase sodium salicylate blood levels; monitor for sodium salicylate toxicity. Antacids in high doses, and other urine alkalizers, decrease sodium salicylate blood levels; monitor for decreased sodium salicylate effect. Corticosteroids enhance sodium salicylate elimination. Food and antacids delay and decrease absorption of sodium salicylate.

Effects on diagnostic tests

False-positive urine glucose test results may occur if the copper sulfate method is used in patients undergoing high-dose (2.4 mg/day) therapy; false-negative results may occur in these patients if the glucose oxidase method is used. Sodium salicylate may interfere with urinary vanillylmandelic acid determination or the Gerhardt test for urine aceto-acetic acid. False increases in serum uric acid may occur.

Adverse reactions

- DERM: rash, bruising.
- EENT: tinnitus and hearing loss.
- GI: nausea, vomiting, GI distress, occult bleeding.
- Local: thrombophlebitis (from I.V. use); extravasation of injection may cause sloughing of tissue.
- Other: hypersensitivity manifested by anaphylaxis or asthma, elevated liver function tests, hepatitis.
Note: Drug should be discontinued if hypersensitivity, hepatotoxicity, or salicylism occurs.

Overdose and treatment

Clinical manifestations of overdose, including respiratory alkalosis, hyperpnea, and tachypnea, are caused by increased CO_2 production and direct stimulation of the respiratory center.

To treat sodium salicylate overdose, empty stomach immediately by inducing emesis with ipecac syrup or by gastric lavage. Administer activated charcoal (most effective if given within 2 hours of ingestion) by nasogastric tube. Provide symptomatic and supportive measures (respiratory support and correction of fluid and electrolyte imbalances). Monitor laboratory parameters and vital signs closely. Alkalinization of urine may enhance excretion.

▶ Special considerations

- Each gram of sodium salicylate contains 6.25 mEq of sodium and should be avoided in sodium-restricted patients. Monitor patient for signs and symptoms of fluid retention.

- Dosage of sodium salicylate for children under age 2 must be individualized.
- Because of epidemiologic association with Reye's syndrome, the Centers for Disease Control recommend that children with chicken pox or flulike symptoms not be given salicylates.
- Do not use long-term salicylate therapy in children under age 14; safety of this use has not been established.
- Children may be more susceptible to toxic effects of salicylates. Use with caution.
- Children usually should not take salicylates more than five times or for more than 5 days.
- Use salicylates with caution in patients with a history of GI disease, increased risk of GI bleeding, or decreased renal function.
- Administer non-enteric-coated tablets with food or after meals to minimize gastric upset.
- Tablets may be chewed, broken, or crumbled and administered with food or fluids to aid swallowing.
- Patient should take drug with enough water or milk to ensure passage into stomach. Patient should sit up for 15 to 30 minutes after taking salicylates to prevent lodging of salicylate in esophagus.
- Administer antacids with salicylates, except enteric-coated forms. Separate doses of antacids and enteric-coated salicylates by 1 to 2 hours to ensure adequate absorption.
- Monitor vital signs frequently, especially temperature.
- Salicylates may mask the signs and symptoms of acute infection (fever, myalgia, erythema); carefully evaluate patients at risk for infections, such as those with diabetes.
- Monitor CBC; platelets; prothrombin times; and BUN, serum creatinine, and liver function studies periodically during salicylate therapy to detect abnormalities.
- Assess hearing function before and periodically during therapy to prevent ototoxicity.
- Assess level of pain and inflammation before initiation of therapy. Evaluate effectiveness of therapy as evidenced by relief of these symptoms.
- Assess for signs and symptoms of potential hemorrhage, such as petechiae, bruising, coffee ground vomitus, and black tarry stools.
- If fever or illness causes fluid depletion, dosage should be reduced.
- Dilute injectable formulation in 1 liter 0.9% normal saline or lactated Ringer's solution.
- Administer I.V. dose slowly over 4 to 8 hours to prevent possible thrombophlebitis.
- Check I.V. site for signs of phlebitis and extravasation.
- Monitor serum salicylate levels, especially when administering I.V., to avoid possible toxicity.
- Do not administer sodium salicylate with mineral acids or ferric salts. They are incompatible.
- Store in tightly closed container away from light. Medication turns pink when exposed to light.

Information for parents and patient

- Tell parents to have child take tablet or capsule forms of medication with enough water to ensure pas-

sage to stomach and not to lie down for 15 to 30 minutes after swallowing the drug.
• Tell parents to have patient take the medication 30 minutes before or 2 hours after meals, or with food or milk if gastric irritation occurs.
• Explain that taking the drug as directed is necessary to achieve the desired effect; 2 to 4 weeks of treatment may be needed before benefit is seen.
• Advise parents of patients on chronic salicylate therapy that follow-up laboratory tests may be necessary.
• Advise parents to avoid giving patient aspirin-containing medications without medical approval.
• Warn parents or patient that use of alcoholic beverages with salicylates may cause increased GI irritation and possibly GI bleeding.
• Instruct parents and patient to follow prescribed regimen. Caution them not to change prescribed drug regimen without medical approval.
• Patient should take a missed dose as soon as he remembers, unless it is almost time for next dose; then skip the missed dose and return to regular schedule. Patient should not to take self-prescribed drug for more than 10 consecutive days unless otherwise directed.
• Advise parents to report adverse reactions, especially bleeding or changes in hearing.

---

somatrem
Protropin

• *Classification:* human growth hormone (anterior pituitary hormone)

How supplied
Available by prescription only
Injectable lyophilized powder: 5 mg (10 IU)/vial

Indications, route, and dosage
Long-term treatment of growth failure from lack of adequate endogenous growth hormone secretion
Children (prepuberty): Up to 0.1 mg/kg I.M. three times weekly. Some clinicians consider drug equally effective if given subcutaneously and more effective if given daily in doses up to 0.05 mg/kg, not to exceed 0.3 mg/kg/week.

Action and kinetics
• *Growth-stimulating action:* Somatrem is a purified polypeptide hormone of recombinant DNA origin containing a sequence of 192 amino acids identical to the naturally occurring human growth hormone (plus methionine). Somatrem stimulates growth of linear bone, skeletal muscle, and organs and increases red blood cell mass by stimulating erythropoietin. Most actions are mediated through somatomedins (liver-synthesized hormones).
• *Kinetics in adults:* Somatrem is given by I.M. injection. Distribution is not fully understood. Approximately 90% of a dose is metabolized in the liver. Approximately 0.1% of a dose is excreted in urine

unchanged. Half-life is 20 to 30 minutes; however, tissue effects are long-lasting.

Contraindications and precautions
Somatrem is contraindicated in patients with known hypersensitivity to the drug or to benzyl alcohol, closed epiphyses (because the drug stimulates bone growth), or an intracranial lesion actively growing within the previous 12 months.
The drug's diabetogenic action requires that it be used cautiously in patients with a family history of diabetes. Untreated hypothyroidism may interfere with growth response to somatrem.

Interactions
Concomitant use of somatrem with adrenocorticoids, glucocorticoids, or corticotropin may inhibit growth response. Concomitant use of somatrem with anabolic steroids, androgens, estrogens, or thyroid hormones may accelerate epiphyseal maturation.

Effects on diagnostic tests
Somatrem therapy alters glucose tolerance test (reduced with high doses) and total protein and thyroid function tests (thyroxine-binding capacity and radioactive iodine uptake may be decreased).

Adverse reactions
• Endocrine: hypothyroidism, hyperglycemia.
• Local: pain and swelling at injection site.
• Other: antibody to growth hormone.
   Note: Drug should be discontinued if patient reaches mature adult height, patient's epiphyses close, or patient shows evidence of recurrent intracranial tumor growth.

Overdose and treatment
Clinical manifestations of overdose include gigantism in children and acromegalic features, organ enlargement, diabetes mellitus, atherosclerosis, and hypertension in patients who are not growth hormone deficient. The drug should be discontinued in such situations.

▶ Special considerations
• To prepare the solution, inject the bacteriostatic water for injection (supplied) into the vial containing the drug. Then swirl the vial with a gentle rotary motion until the contents are completely dissolved. *Do not shake the vial.*
• After reconstitution, vial solution should be clear. Do not inject if the solution is cloudy or contains any particles.
• Store reconstituted vial in refrigerator. Must be used within 7 days.
• Be sure to check the expiration date.
• Observe patient for signs of glucose intolerance.
• Monitor thyroid function tests for development of hypothyroidism.

Information for parents and patient
• Emphasize to parents the importance of regular follow-up visits.
• Advise parents to seek medical approval before administering any other medication.

---

somatropin, recombinant (human growth hormone)
Humatrope

• Classification: growth hormone (anterior pituitary hormone)

How supplied
Available by prescription only
Injection: 5 mg

Indications, route, and dosage
Growth failure in children caused by pituitary growth hormone (GH) deficiency including FH deficiency caused by cranial irradiation; growth failure associated with Turner's syndrome.
Children: Initially 0.02 to 0.04 mg (0.05 to 0.1 International Unit [IU]) per kg of body weight I.M. or S.C. every other day or three times a week.
Note: In some patients, daily dosing to reach a similar cumulative weekly dose may be more effective than every-other-day or three-times-weekly dosing.

Action and kinetics
• *Growth stimulating action:* Somatropin stimulates linear growth by affecting cartilaginous growth areas of long bones, by increasing the number and size of muscle cells, influencing the size of organs, and increasing red cell mass through erythropoietin stimulation.
• *Kinetics in adults:* Somatropin is metabolized in the liver (approximately 90%). Half life is approximately 20 minutes; however, effects are long-lasting. Approximately 0.1% of a dose is excreted in the urine as unchanged drug.

Contraindications and precautions
Use of somatropin in patients with untreated hypothyroidism may interfere with growth response to drug; adequate thyroid hormone replacement therapy is recommended. Drug requires consideration of potential risk and benefit in patient with a history of malignancy, especially of intracranial tumor, within the previous 12 months.

Interactions
Concurrent use with adrenocorticoids, glucocorticoid or corticotropin may inhibit growth response unless adrenocorticoid dosage can be reduced to about half of the maximum oral dosage. If chronic use of larger doses is required (except for short-term stress dosages), use of growth hormone should be deferred. Use with high doses of anabolic steroids, androgens, estrogens, or thyroid hormones may accelerate epiphyseal closure; however, in patients with deficiencies of these hormones, supplemental use may be necessary to allow growth response to human growth hormone.

Effects of diagnostic tests
Somatropin therapy may alter results of glucose tolerance and thyroid function tests. Serum thyroxine (T_4) concentration, radioactive iodine uptake (RAIU), and thyroxine-binding capacity may be slightly decreased.

Adverse reactions
• Local: pain and swelling at injection site (rare).
• Systemic: hypothyroidism in patients with hypopituitarism.

Overdose and treatment
None reported.

▶ Special considerations
• Patients receiving human growth hormone should be under supervision of a pediatric endocrinologist familiar with growth hormone therapy.
• Failure to grow must be documented by a subnormal growth rate. GH deficiency is usually identified by absence of response to provocative tests for the release of somatropin or by evidence of impaired spontaneous secretion of bioactivity of endogenous GH.
• Human growth hormone is ineffective in patients with closed epiphyses. Use is not usually recommended in patients with epiphyseal maturation over 15 to 16 years in males or 14 to 15 years in females. However, therapy may be useful in some older patients if epiphyses have not closed.
• Use of human growth hormone by athletes to enhance athletic performance and increase muscle size is highly controversial and is not recommended.
• A patient whose growth rate does not exceed 1″ (2.5 cm) in 6 months of treatment should be checked for the presence of antibodies or other medical problems such as hypothyroidism. Somatropin dosage may be doubled for the next 6 months up to a dosage of 0.08 mg (0.2 to 0.25 IU) per kg of body weight every other day or three times a week or its equivalent. If no response, discontinue treatment and reevaluate patient.
• Patient monitoring should include anti-growth hormone antibody determinations (with emphasis on binding capacity, if growth rate falls during therapy); bone age determinations (annually during therapy, especially in pubertal patients, receiving concurrent androgen, estrogen, or thyroid replacement, which may accelerate epiphyseal closure); growth rate determinations from stadiometer measurements (every 3 to 6 months during therapy); and regular thyroid function determinations (untreated hypothyroidism may impair response to human growth hormone).
• Prolonged use of growth hormone in patients who are not GH deficient may cause acromegaly, organ enlargement, diabetes mellitus, atherosclerosis, and hypertension.
• The dosage and schedule of administration must be individualized for each patient.
• Dosage may be increased above the recommended dosage in older hypopituitary children, especially those who have open epiphyses.
• Usually, after 2 or more years of treatment, growth rate will decrease despite continued treatment. If this occurs, the patient should be checked for antibodies,

other medical problems (such as hypothyroidism), or for poor compliance. Increased dosage of human growth hormone, or concomitant low doses of androgens or estrogens may restore the response, as long as epiphyseal maturation of 11 years or greater is present.

• Therapy should continue as long as response continues, until the patient reaches a mature adult height, or until epiphyses close.

• Recombinant somatropin, produced biosynthetically by a recombinant DNA process, has the same amino acid sequence as pituitary-derived somatropin. Somatrem, also produced by a recombinant DNA process, differs from pituitary-derived and recombinant somatropin by addition of an extra amino acid.

• Recombinant somatropin does not have the potential for contamination with viruses or other particles that may have accounted for the cases of Creutzfeldt-Jakob disease associated with human pituitary-derived somatropin administration.

• Antibodies to somatrem or to pituitary-derived somatropin may be formed in the first 3 to 6 months of treatment, but rarely cause failure to respond to therapy. Antibodies to recombinant somatropin have been detected in patients treated for 6 months or more.

• To prepare recombinant somatropin for injection, add 1.5 ml of water for injection provided by the manufacturer to the vial and swirl gently to dissolve, producing a clear solution containing 0.4 to 0.13 mg (approximately 1 to 0.33 IU) per ml (2-mg vial) or 3.3 to 1 mg (approximately 8.67 to 2.6 IU) per ml (5-mg vial). Do not shake the vial.

• After reconstitution, drug may be stored for up to 14 days in the refrigerator.

Information for parents and patient
• Explain therapy to parents and patient. Advise parents to report if pain or swelling occurs at the injection site.

---

spectinomycin hydrochloride
Trobicin

• Classification: antibiotic (aminocyclitol)

How supplied
Available by prescription only
Injection: 2-g vial with 3.2-ml diluent; 4-g vial with 6.2-ml diluent

Indications, route, and dosage
Uncomplicated gonorrhea
†*Children:* 40 mg/kg I.M. as a single dose. Usually reserved for children allergic to cephalosporins or penicillins; children over 8 may be treated with tetracycline P.O.
Adults: 2 to 4 g I.M. single dose injected deeply into upper outer quadrant of the buttocks.
Disseminated gonorrhea
Adults: 2 g I.M. b.i.d. for 3 to 7 days. Inject deeply into upper outer quadrant of the buttocks.

Action and kinetics
• *Antibacterial action:* Bacteriostatic effect results from binding of drug to 30S ribosomal subunits, thus inhibiting protein synthesis. Although drug is effective against many gram-positive and gram-negative organisms, it is used mostly against penicillin-resistant *Neisseria gonorrhoeae.*

• *Kinetics in adults:* Spectinomycin is not absorbed orally. I.M. injection results in rapid absorption; peak concentrations occur in 1 and 2 hours for 2-g and 4-g doses, respectively. Spectinomycin's distribution and metabolism are largely unknown. Most of dose is excreted unchanged in the urine. Elimination half-life ranges from 1 to 3 hours. Drug dosage is unchanged in renal failure.

Contraindications and precautions
Spectinomycin is contraindicated in patients with known hypersensitivity to the drug.

Spectinomycin should be administered cautiously to patients with strong history of drug allergies.

Interactions
None reported.

Effects on diagnostic tests
BUN, AST (SGOT), and serum alkaline phosphatase levels increase, and hemoglobin, hematocrit, and creatinine clearance levels decrease during spectinomycin therapy.

Adverse reactions
• CNS: insomnia, dizziness.
• DERM: urticaria, rash, pruritus.
• GI: nausea, vomiting.
• GU: decreased urine output.
• Local: pain at injection site.
• Other: fever, chills.

Overdose and treatment
No information available.

▶ Special considerations
• Because its safety in infants and children has not been established, drug is not first choice in treating these patients. A single dose of 40 mg/kg is recommended by the Centers for Disease Control.

• Obtain culture and sensitivity tests before starting therapy.

• Drug is usually reserved for patients with penicillin-resistant gonorrhea strains or for whom other drugs are contraindicated.

• To prepare drug, add supplied diluent to vial and shake until completely dissolved. Use reconstituted solution within 24 hours.

• Inject deep I.M. into upper outer quadrant of gluteal muscle. Give 2-g dose at single site; divide 4-g dose into two equal injections and give at two sites.

• Drug is ineffective against syphilis and may mask symptoms of incubating syphilis infection.

• Lack of response to drug usually results from reinfection.

---

‡May contain sulfites   ♦May contain tartrazine   ♦♦May contain benzyl alcohol

Information for parents and patient
• Tell parents of sexually active patient that sexual partners must be treated.
• Inform parents and patient about adverse reactions.

---

spironolactone
Aldactone

• Classification: potassium-sparing diuretic for treatment of edema and diuretic-induced hypokalemia; antihypertensive; diagnosis of primary hyperaldosteronism

---

How supplied
Available by prescription only
Tablets: 25 mg, 50 mg, 100 mg

Indications, route, and dosage
Edema
Children: Initially, 3.3 mg/kg or 60 mg/m² P.O. daily in one or more doses.
Adults: 25 to 200 mg P.O. daily in divided doses.
Detection of primary hyperaldosteronism
Children: 125 to 375 mg/m² P.O. in divided doses over 24 hours (short test). If hypokalemia and hypertension are corrected, a presumptive diagnosis of primary hyperaldosteronism is made.
Adults: 400 mg P.O. daily for 4 days (short test) or for 3 to 4 weeks (long test).

Action and kinetics
• *Diuretic and potassium-sparing action:* Spironolactone competitively inhibits aldosterone effects on the distal renal tubules, increasing sodium and water excretion and decreasing potassium excretion.

Spironolactone is used to treat edema associated with excessive aldosterone secretion, such as that associated with hepatic cirrhosis, nephrotic syndrome, and CHF. It is also used to treat diuretic-induced hypokalemia.
• *Antihypertensive action:* The mechanism of action is unknown; spironolactone may block the effect of aldosterone on arteriolar smooth muscle.
• *Diagnosis of primary hyperaldosteronism:* Spironolactone inhibits the effects of aldosterone; therefore, correction of hypokalemia and hypertension is presumptive evidence of primary hyperaldosteronism.
• *Kinetics in adults:* About 90% of spironolactone is absorbed after oral administration. Onset of action is gradual; maximum effect occurs on 3rd day of therapy. Spironolactone and its major active metabolite, canrenone, are more than 90% plasma protein-bound. Spironolactone is metabolized rapidly and extensively to canrenone; this and other metabolites are excreted primarily in urine, and a small amount is excreted in feces via the biliary tract. Half-life of canrenone is 13 to 24 hours.

Contraindications and precautions
Spironolactone is contraindicated in patients with serum potassium levels above 5.5 mEq/liter; in patients who are receiving other potassium-sparing diuretics or potassium supplements, because these drugs conserve potassium and can cause severe hyperkalemia in such patients; in patients with anuria, acute or chronic renal insufficiency, or diabetic nephropathy, because of risk of hyperkalemia; and in patients with known hypersensitivity to the drug.

Spironolactone should be used cautiously in patients with severe hepatic insufficiency because electrolyte imbalance may precipitate hepatic encephalopathy and in patients with diabetes, who are at increased risk of hyperkalemia.

Interactions
Spironolactone may potentiate the hypotensive effects of other antihypertensive agents; this may be used to therapeutic advantage.

Spironolactone increases the risk of hyperkalemia when administered with other potassium-sparing diuretics, angiotensin-converting enzyme inhibitors (captopril or enalapril), potassium supplements, potassium-containing medications (parenteral penicillin G), or salt substitutes.

Nonsteroidal anti-inflammatory agents, such as indomethacin or ibuprofen, may impair renal function and thus affect potassium excretion. Aspirin may slightly decrease the clinical response to spironolactone.

Effects on diagnostic tests
Spironolactone therapy alters fluorometric determinations of plasma and urinary 17-hydroxycorticosteroid levels and may cause false elevations on radioimmunoassay of serum digoxin.

Adverse reactions
• CNS: *headache, drowsiness.*
• DERM: urticaria, *rash.*
• GI: anorexia, *nausea, diarrhea, vomiting.*
• Metabolic: hyperkalemia, dehydration, hyponatremia, transient rise in BUN level, acidosis.
• Other: *gynecomastia* in males, breast soreness and menstrual disturbances in females.

Overdose and treatment
Clinical signs of overdose are consistent with dehydration and electrolyte disturbance.

Treatment is supportive and symptomatic. In acute ingestion, empty stomach by emesis or lavage. In severe hyperkalemia (> 6.5 mEq/liter), reduce serum potassium levels with I.V. sodium bicarbonate or glucose with insulin. A cation exchange resin, sodium polystyrene sulfonate (Kayexalate), given orally or as a retention enema, may also reduce serum potassium levels.

▶ Special considerations
• When administering spironolactone to children, crush tablets and administer them in cherry syrup as an oral suspension.
• Use drugs with caution; children are more susceptible to hyperkalemia.
• Monitor for hyperkalemia and cardiac dysrhythmias; measure serum potassium and other electrolyte levels frequently, and check for significant changes. Monitor the following at baseline and periodic inter-

---

vals: CBC, including WBC count; CO_2, BUN, and creatinine levels; and, especially, liver function studies.
• Monitor vital signs, intake and output, weight, and blood pressure daily; check patient for edema, oliguria, or lack of diuresis, which may indicate drug tolerance.
• Patient should be weighed each morning immediately after voiding and before breakfast in the same type of clothing and on the same scale; the patient's weight provides an index for therapeutic response.
• Monitor patient with hepatic disease in whom mild drug-induced acidosis may be hazardous; watch for mental confusion, lethargy, or stupor. Patients with hepatic disease are especially susceptible to diuretic-induced electrolyte imbalance; in extreme cases, coma and death can result.
• Administer spironolactone in morning to ensure that major diuresis occurs before bedtime. To prevent nocturia, do not prescribe diuretics for use after 6 p.m.
• Establish safety measures for all ambulatory patients until response to spironolactone is known; diuretic therapy may cause orthostatic hypotension, weakness, ataxia, and confusion.
• Consider possible dosage adjustments in the following circumstances: reduced dosage for patients with hepatic dysfunction and for those taking other antihypertensive agents; increased dosage in patients with renal impairment; and changes in insulin requirements in diabetic patients.
• Monitor for other signs of toxicity: lethargy, confusion, stupor, muscle twitching, increased reflexes, and convulsions (water intoxication); severe weakness, headache, abdominal pain, malaise, nausea, and vomiting (metabolic acidosis); sore throat, rash, or jaundice (blood dyscrasia from hypersensitivity); joint swelling, redness, and pain (hyperuricemia); hypotension (in patients taking other antihypertensive drugs); and hyperglycemia (in diabetic patients).
• Patient should have urinal or commode readily available.
• Give drug with meals to enhance absorption.
• Diuretic effect may be delayed 2 to 3 days if drug is used alone; maximum antihypertensive effect may be delayed 2 to 3 weeks.
• Protect drug from light.
• Adverse reactions are related to dosage levels and duration of therapy and usually disappear with withdrawal of the drug; however, gynecomastia may not.
• Spironolactone is antiandrogenic and has been used to treat hirsutism in dosages of 200 mg/day.
• Unnecessary use of spironolactone should be avoided. This drug has been shown to induce tumors in laboratory animals.

Information for parents and patient
• Explain signs and symptoms of possible adverse effects and the importance of reporting any unusual effect, especially weakness, fatigue, shortness of breath, chest or back pain, heaviness in the legs, muscle cramps, headache, dizziness, palpitations, mental confusion, nausea, vomiting, or diarrhea.
• Tell parents to watch for and to report if patient experiences increased edema or excess diuresis (more than 2% weight loss or gain) and to record weight each morning after voiding and before dressing and breakfast, using same scale.
• Teach parents and patient how to minimize dizziness from orthostatic hypotension by avoiding sudden postural changes.
• Because drug may cause dizziness, warn parents that patient should avoid hazardous activities, until response to drug is known.
• Patient should avoid potassium-rich food and potassium-containing salt substitutes or supplements, which increase the hazard of hyperkalemia.
• Patient should take drug at the same time each morning to avoid interrupted sleep from nighttime diuresis.
• Advise taking the drug with or after meals to minimize GI distress.
• Tell parents to seek medical approval before administering unprescribed drugs; many contain sodium and potassium and can cause electrolyte imbalance.
• Explain that maximal diuresis may not occur until the 3rd day of therapy and that diuresis may continue for 2 to 3 days after drug is withdrawn.
• Explain that adverse reactions usually disappear after drug is discontinued; gynecomastia, however, may persist.
• Emphasize importance of regular medical follow-up to monitor effectiveness of diuretic therapy.

stanozolol
Winstrol

• Classification: angioedema prophylactic (anabolic steroid)

How supplied
Available by prescription only
Tablets: 2 mg

Indications, route, and dosage
Prevention of hereditary angioedema
Children up to age 6: 1 mg P.O. daily administered only during an attack.
Children age 6 to 12: Up to 2 mg P.O. daily administered only during an attack.
Adults: Initially, 2 mg P.O. t.i.d.
    Dosage for continuous treatment is highly individualized.

Action and kinetics
• *Angioedema prophylactic action:* Stanozolol increases the concentration of C1 esterase inhibitor in patients with hereditary angioedema. This leads to an increased level of the C4 component of complement, which may be deficient in these patients, thus decreasing the number and severity of attacks of this disorder.
• *Kinetics in adults:* Stanozolol is metabolized by the liver. Its pharmacokinetics are otherwise poorly described.

---

‡May contain sulfites   ◆May contain tartrazine   ◆◆May contain benzyl alcohol

Contraindications and precautions

Stanozolol is contraindicated in patients with severe renal or cardiac disease, which may be worsened by the fluid and electrolyte retention this drug may cause; in patients with hepatic disease because impaired elimination may cause toxic accumulation of the drug; in male patients with breast cancer, benign prostatic hypertrophy with obstruction, or undiagnosed abnormal genital bleeding because this drug can stimulate the growth of cancerous breast or prostate tissue in males; and in pregnant or breast-feeding patients because animal studies have shown that administration of anabolic steroids during pregnancy causes masculinization of the fetus. Because of its hypercholesterolemic effects, stanozolol should be administered cautiously in patients with a history of coronary artery disease.

Interactions

In patients with diabetes, decreased blood glucose levels require adjustment of insulin dosage.

Stanozolol may potentiate the effects of warfarin-type anticoagulants, prolonging prothrombin time. Use with adrenocorticosteroids or adrenocorticotropin results in increased potential for fluid and electrolyte retention.

Effects on diagnostic tests

Stanozolol may cause abnormal results of fasting plasma glucose, glucose tolerance, and metyrapone tests. It may increase sulfobromophthalein retention. Thyroid function test results (protein-bound iodine, radioactive iodine uptake, thyroid-binding capacity) and 17-ketosteroid levels may decrease. Liver function test results, prothrombin time (especially in patients receiving anticoagulant therapy), and serum creatinine levels may be elevated. Because of this agent's anabolic activity, serum sodium, potassium, calcium, phosphate, and cholesterol levels may all rise.

Adverse reactions

• Androgenic: *in females:* deepening of voice, clitoral enlargement, changes in libido; *in males:* prepubertal—premature epiphyseal closure, priapism, phallic enlargement; postpubertal—testicular atrophy, oligospermia, decreased ejaculatory volume, impotence, gynecomastia, epididymitis.
• CNS: headache, mental depression.
• CV: edema.
• DERM: acne, oily skin, hirsutism, flushing, sweating.
• GI: gastroenteritis, nausea, vomiting, diarrhea, constipation, change in appetite, weight gain.
• GU: bladder irritability, vaginitis, menstrual irregularities.
• Hepatic: reversible jaundice, hepatotoxicity.
• Other: hypercalcemia.
  Note: Drug should be discontinued if hypercalcemia, edema, hypersensitivity reaction, priapism, or excessive sexual stimulation occurs or if virilization occurs in females.

Overdose and treatment

No information available.

▶ Special considerations

• Anabolic steroids should be used with caution in prepubertal children. Boys should be closely observed for precocious development of male sexual characteristics.
• In children, X-rays of wrist bones should establish level of bone maturation before therapy is initiated. During treatment, bone maturation may proceed more rapidly than linear growth. Intermittent dosage and periodic X-rays are recommended to monitor skeletal effects.
• Watch female patients for signs of virilization. If possible, discontinue therapy when virilization first becomes apparent because some adverse effects (deepening of voice, clitoral enlargement) are irreversible.
• Anabolic steroids do not improve athletic performance. Risks associated with their use for this purpose far outweigh any possible benefits. Proof of anabolic steroid use is grounds for disqualification in many athletic events.
• Hypercalcemia symptoms may be difficult to distinguish from symptoms of condition being treated unless anticipated and thought of as a cluster.
• Edema usually is controllable with salt restriction, diuretics, or both. Monitor weight routinely.
• Watch for symptoms of jaundice. Dosage adjustment may reverse condition. Periodic liver function tests are recommended.
• Observe patient on concomitant anticoagulant therapy for ecchymotic areas, petechiae, or abnormal bleeding. Monitor prothrombin time.
• Watch for symptoms of hypoglycemia in patients with diabetes. Change of antihypoglycemic drug dosage may be required.
• Anabolic steroids may alter many laboratory studies during therapy and for 2 to 3 weeks after therapy is stopped.
• Use with diet high in calories and protein unless contraindicated. Give small, frequent meals.
• Long-term administration is generally not recommended for children.
• Smaller doses (2 mg b.i.d.) may be used in females to minimize virilization. Routinely monitor for side effects.
• Check serum cholesterol level in cardiac patients. These patients also should be on salt-restricted diets.
• Stanozolol has been used investigationally to increase hemoglobin levels in patients with aplastic anemia.

Information for parents and patient

• Advise parents and patient to administer drug with foods or meals if it causes GI upset.
• Tell parents and female patient to report menstrual irregularities; therapy should be discontinued pending etiologic determination.

---

streptomycin sulfate

• Classification: antibiotic (aminoglycoside)

How supplied
Available by prescription only
Injection: 400 mg/ml, 500 mg/ml, 1-g vial, 5-g vial

Indications, route, and dosage
Primary and adjunctive treatment in tuberculosis
Children with normal renal function: 20 to 40 mg/kg I.M. daily in divided doses injected deeply into large muscle mass. Give concurrently with other antitubercular agents, but *not* with capreomycin, and continue until sputum specimen becomes negative.
Adults with normal renal function: 1 g I.M. daily for 2 to 3 months, then 1 g two or three times a week. Inject deeply into upper outer quadrant of buttocks.
Streptomycin sensitive systemic infections
Neonates: 20 to 30 mg/kg/day I.M., divided q 12 hours, for up to 10 days.
Children: 20 to 40 mg/kg/day I.M., divided q 8 hours, for up to 10 days.
Adults: 15 to 25 mg/kg/day I.M., divided q 12 hours for 7 to 10 days, the 1 g/dose daily.
Dosage in renal failure
Children and adults: Initial dosage is same as for those with normal renal function. Subsequent doses and frequency determined by renal function study results and blood serum concentrations; keep peak serum levels between 5 and 25 mcg/ml, and trough levels below 5 mcg/ml. Patients with a creatinine clearance > 50 ml/min usually can tolerate the drug daily; if creatinine clearance is 10 to 50 ml/min, administration interval is increased to every 24 to 72 hours. Patients with a creatinine clearance < 10 ml/min may require 72 to 96 hours between doses.

Action and kinetics
• *Antibiotic action:* Streptomycin is bactericidal; it binds directly to the 30S ribosomal subunit, thus inhibiting bacterial protein synthesis. Its spectrum of activity includes many aerobic gram-negative organisms and some aerobic gram-positive organisms. Streptomycin is generally less active against many gram-negative organisms than is tobramycin, gentamicin, amikacin, or netilmicin. Streptomycin is also active against *Mycobacterium* and *Brucella.*
• *Kinetics in adults:* Streptomycin is absorbed poorly after oral administration and usually is given parenterally; peak serum concentrations occur 1 to 2 hours after I.M. administration.
Streptomycin is distributed widely after parenteral administration; intraocular penetration is poor. CSF penetration is low, even in patients with inflamed meninges. Streptomycin crosses the placenta; it is 36% protein-bound.
Streptomycin is excreted unmetabolized, primarily in urine by glomerular filtration; small amounts may be excreted in bile and breast milk. Elimination half-

life in adults is 2 to 3 hours. In severe renal damage, half-life may extend to 110 hours.
• *Kinetics in children:* The half-life is prolonged in premature infants and neonates because of the immaturity of their renal systems.

Contraindications and precautions
Streptomycin is contraindicated in patients with known hypersensitivity to streptomycin or any other aminoglycoside.
Streptomycin should be used cautiously in neonates and other infants; in patients with decreased renal function; in patients with tinnitus, vertigo, and high-frequency hearing loss who are susceptible to ototoxicity; and in patients with dehydration, myasthenia gravis, parkinsonism, and hypocalcemia; and in elderly patients.

Interactions
Concomitant use with the following drugs may increase the hazard of nephrotoxicity, ototoxicity, and neurotoxicity: methoxyflurane, polymyxin B, vancomycin, capreomycin, cisplatin, cephalosporins, amphotericin B, and other aminoglycosides; hazard of ototoxicity is also increased during use with ethacrynic acid, furosemide, bumetanide, urea, or mannitol. Dimenhydrinate and other antiemetic and antivertigo drugs may mask streptomycin-induced ototoxicity.
Concomitant use with penicillins results in synergistic bactericidal effect against *Pseudomonas aeruginosa, Escherichia coli, Klebsiella, Citrobacter, Enterobacter, Serratia,* and *Proteus mirabilis;* however, the drugs are physically and chemically incompatible and are inactivated when mixed or given together. In vivo inactivation has been reported when aminoglycosides and penicillins are used concomitantly.
Streptomycin may potentiate neuromuscular blockade from general anesthetics or neuromuscular blocking agents such as succinylcholine and tubocurarine.

Effects on diagnostic tests
Streptomycin may cause false-positive reaction in copper sulfate test for urine glucose (Benedict's reagent or Clinitest).
Streptomycin-induced nephrotoxicity may elevate levels of blood urea nitrogen, nonprotein nitrogen, or serum creatinine levels and increase urinary excretion of casts.

Adverse reactions
• CNS: headache, lethargy, *neuromuscular blockade.*
• EENT: ototoxicity (tinnitus, vertigo, hearing loss).
• GI: diarrhea.
• GU: some nephrotoxicity (less frequent than with other aminoglycosides).
• HEMA: transient agranulocytosis.
• Local: pain, irritation, and sterile abscesses at injection site.
• Other: hypersensitivity reactions (rash, fever, urticaria, angioneurotic edema, *anaphylaxis*), bacterial and fungal superinfection.
Note: Drug should be discontinued if patient shows signs of ototoxicity, nephrotoxicity, or hypersensitiv-

ity, or if severe diarrhea indicates pseudomembranous colitis.

Overdose and treatment

Clinical signs of overdose include ototoxicity, nephrotoxicity, and neuromuscular toxicity. Remove drug by hemodialysis or peritoneal dialysis. Treatment with calcium salts or anticholinesterases reverses neuromuscular blockade.

▶ Special considerations

• Protect hands when preparing drug; drug irritates skin.
• In primary tuberculosis therapy, discontinue streptomycin when sputum test is negative.
• Because streptomycin is dialyzable, patients undergoing hemodialysis may need dosage adjustments.
• Assess patient's allergic history; do not give streptomycin to a patient with a history of hypersensitivity reactions to any aminoglycoside; monitor patient continuously for this and other adverse reactions.
• Obtain results of culture and sensitivity tests before first dose; however, therapy may begin before tests are completed. Repeat tests periodically to assess drug efficacy.
• Monitor vital signs, electrolyte levels, and renal function studies before and during therapy; be sure patient is well hydrated to minimize chemical irritation of renal tubules; watch for signs of declining renal function.
• Keep peak serum levels and trough serum levels at recommended concentrations, especially in patients with decreased renal function. Draw blood for peak level 1 hour after I.M. injection (30 minutes to 1 hour after I.V. infusion); for trough level, draw sample just before the next dose. Time and date all blood samples. Do not use heparinized tube to collect blood samples; it interferes with results.
• Evaluate patient's hearing before and during therapy; monitor for complaints of tinnitus, vertigo, or hearing loss.
• Avoid concomitant use with other ototoxic or nephrotoxic drugs.
• Usual duration of therapy is 7 to 10 days; if no response occurs in 3 to 5 days, drug should be discontinued and cultures repeated for re-evaluation of therapy.
• Closely monitor patients on long-term therapy—especially debilitated patients and others receiving immunosuppressant or radiation therapy—for possible bacterial or fungal superinfection; monitor especially for fever.
• Administer I.M. dose deep into large muscle mass (gluteal or midlateral thigh); rotate injection sites to minimize tissue injury; do not inject more than 2 g of drug per injection site. Apply ice to injection site for pain.
• Solutions should always be clear, colorless to pale yellow (in most cases, darkening indicates deterioration), and free of particles; do not give solutions containing precipitates or other foreign matter.
• Dosage alterations may be necessary in infants and children.

Information for parents and patient

• Teach parents how to recognize signs and symptoms of hypersensitivity and other adverse reactions to aminoglycosides; bacterial or fungal superinfections (especially if the child has low resistance from immunosuppressants or irradiation); urge them to report any unusual effects promptly.
• Teach parents and patients how to recognize signs of superinfection, and how to prevent it by practicing meticulous oral and anogenital hygiene. Parents of infants and toddlers should keep diaper area clean and dry and avoid using plastic pants.

sucralfate
Carafate

• Classification: antiulcer agent (pepsin inhibitor)

How supplied

Available by prescription only
Tablets: 1 g

Indications, route, and dosage
Short-term (up to 8 weeks) treatment of duodenal ulcer

Children over age 12 and adults: 1 g P.O. q.i.d. 1 hour before meals and h.s.

Action and kinetics

• *Antiulcer action:* Sucralfate has a unique mechanism of action. The drug adheres to proteins at the ulcer site, forming a protective coating against gastric acid, pepsin, and bile salts. It also inhibits pepsin, exhibits a cytoprotective effect, and forms a viscous, adhesive barrier on the surface of the intact intestinal mucosa and stomach.
• *Kinetics in adults:* Only about 3% to 5% of a dose is absorbed. Drug activity is not related to the amount absorbed. Sucralfate acts locally, at the ulcer site. Absorbed drug is distributed to many body tissues, including the liver and kidneys. It is not metabolized. About 90% of a dose is excreted in feces; absorbed drug is excreted unchanged in urine. Duration of effect is 5 hours.

Contraindications and precautions

Sucralfate is contraindicated in patients with sucralfate allergy.

Interactions

Sucralfate decreases absorption of tetracycline, phenytoin, digoxin, quinidine, cimetidine, ranitidine, theophylline, and fat-soluble vitamins A, D, E, and K.

Effects on diagnostic tests

None reported.

Adverse reactions

• CNS: dizziness, drowsiness, vertigo.
• GI: *constipation* (most common), diarrhea, nausea, dry mouth, gastric discomfort, indigestion.
• Other: rash, pruritus, back pain.

Note: Drug should be discontinued if abdominal pain develops.

Overdose and treatment
No information available.

▶ Special considerations
• Safety and effectiveness in children have not been established.
• Sucralfate may inhibit absorption of other drugs. Schedule other medications 2 hours before or after sucralfate.
• Sucralfate is poorly water-soluble. For administration by nasogastric tube, have pharmacist prepare water-sorbitol suspension of sucralfate. Alternatively, place tablet in 60-ml syringe; add 20 ml water. Let stand with tip up for about 5 minutes, occasionally shaking gently. A suspension will form that may be administered from the syringe. After administration, tube should be flushed several times to ensure that the patient receives the entire dose.
• Patients who have difficulty swallowing tablet may place it in 15 to 30 ml of water at room temperature, allow it to disintegrate, and then ingest the resulting suspension. This is particularly useful for patient with esophagitis and painful swallowing.
• Monitor patient for constipation.
• Therapy exceeding 8 weeks is not recommended.
• Some experts believe that 2 g given b.i.d. are as effective as standard regimen.
• Drug treats ulcers as effectively as histamine₂-receptor antagonists.
• Some clinicians have used sucralfate to treat stomatitis associated with chemotherapy.

Information for parents and patient
• Patient should take the drug on an empty stomach and should take sucralfate at least 1 hour before meals.
• Patient should continue taking drug as directed, even after pain begins to subside, to ensure adequate healing, but should not take drug longer than 8 weeks.
• Tell parents that they may give patient an antacid 30 minutes before or 1 hour after sucralfate.

sulfacetamide sodium
AK-Sulf Forte, AK-Sulf Ointment, Bleph-10, Cetamide, Isopto Cetamide, Sodium Sulamyd 30%, Sulamyd, Sulf-10, Sulfair, Sulfair Forte, Sulfex∗, Sulten-10

• Classification: antibiotic (sulfonamide)

How supplied
Available by prescription only
Ophthalmic solution: 10%, 15%, 30%
Ophthalmic ointment: 10%

Indications, route, and dosage
Inclusion conjunctivitis, corneal ulcers, trachoma, prophylaxis to ocular infection
Children and adults: Instill 1 or 2 drops of 10% solution into lower conjunctival sac q 2 to 3 hours during day, less often at night; or instill 1 or 2 drops of 15% solution into lower conjunctival sac q 1 to 2 hours initially, increasing interval as condition responds; or instill 1 drop of 30% solution into lower conjunctival sac q 2 hours. Instill ½" to 1" of 10% ointment into conjunctival sac q.i.d. and at bedtime. May use ointment at night along with drops during the day.

Action and kinetics
• *Antibacterial action:* Sulfonamides act by inhibiting the uptake of para-aminobenzoic acid, which is required in the synthesis of folic acid needed for bacterial growth.
• *Kinetics in adults:* Pharmacokinetics are unknown.

Contraindications and precautions
Sulfacetamide is contraindicated in patients with known or suspected sensitivity to sulfonamides or to any ingredients of the preparation. It should be used with caution to avoid overgrowth of non-susceptible organisms during prolonged therapy.

Interactions
Tetracaine or other local anesthetics that are para-aminobenzoic acid derivatives may decrease the antibacterial activity of sulfacetamide. Concomitant use of silver preparations is not recommended.

Sulfonamides are inactivated by para-aminobenzoic acid present in purulent exudates.

Effects on diagnostic tests
None reported.

Adverse reactions
• Eye: blurred vision, transient burning and stinging, hyperemia, epithelial keratitis.
• Other: hypersensitivity (including itching or burning), headache, overgrowth of nonsusceptible organisms, Stevens-Johnson syndrome (rare), sensitivity to light, systemic lupus erythematosus.
Note: Drug should be discontinued if any signs of sensitivity occur.

Overdose and treatment
No information available.

▶ Special considerations
• Drug has largely been replaced by antibiotics for treating major infections, but it is still used in minor ocular infections.
• Purulent exudate interferes with sulfacetamide action; remove as much as possible from lids before instilling sulfacetamide.

Information for parents and patient
• Instruct parents and patient in correct administration technique. Tell them to remove exudate from eye before applying the drug. Warn them not to touch tip of tube or dropper to eye or surrounding tissue.
• Explain that eye drops may burn slightly. However,

tell parents and patient to watch for signs of sensitivity, such as itching lids or constant burning, and to report these immediately.

• Advise parents and patient to wait for 10 minutes before using another eye preparation.

• Tell parents to have patient avoid sharing washcloths and towels with family members.

• Tell parents to store drug in tightly closed, light-resistant container away from heat and light; do not use discolored (dark brown) solution.

---

sulfadiazine
Microsulfon

• Classification: antibiotic (sulfonamide)

How supplied
Available by prescription only
Tablets: 500 mg

Indications, route, and dosage
Urinary tract infection
Children: Initially, 75 mg/kg or 2 g/m² P.O.; then 150 mg/kg or 4 g/m² P.O. in four to six divided doses daily. Maximum daily dosage is 6 g.
Adults: Initially, 2 to 4 g P.O.; then 500 mg to 1 g P.O. q 6 hours.
Rheumatic fever prophylaxis, as an alternative to penicillin
Children weighing less than 30 kg: 500 mg P.O. daily.
Children weighing more than 30 kg: 1 g P.O. daily.
Adjunctive treatment in toxoplasmosis
Children: 100 mg/kg P.O. in divided doses q 6 hours for 3 to 4 weeks; given with pyrimethamine 2 mg/kg daily for 3 days, then 1 mg/kg daily for 3 to 4 weeks.
Adults: 4 g P.O. in divided doses q 6 hours for 3 to 4 weeks, discontinued for 1 week; given with pyrimethamine 25 mg P.O. daily for 3 to 4 weeks.
Uncomplicated attacks of malaria
Children: 25 to 50 mg/kg P.O. q.i.d. for 5 days if combined with quinine and pyrimethamine.
Adults: 500 mg P.O. q.i.d. for 5 days.
Asymptomatic meningococcal carriers
Children age 2 to 12 months: 500 mg P.O. once daily for 2 days
Children age 1 to 12 years: 500 mg P.O. b.i.d. for 2 days
Children over age 12 and adults: 1 g P.O. for 2 days
Use only when the organism is known to be susceptible to sulfonamides. The CDC currently recommends the use of Rifampin when the organism's susceptibility is unknown.

Action and kinetics
• *Antibacterial action:* Sulfadiazine is bacteriostatic. It inhibits formation of dihydrofolic acid from para-aminobenzoic acid (PABA), thus preventing bacterial cell synthesis of essential nucleic acids. It acts synergistically with agents such as trimethoprim that block folic acid synthesis at a later stage, thus delaying or preventing bacterial resistance.
It is active against many gram-positive bacteria,

Chlamydia trachomatis, many Enterobacteriaceae, and some strains of *Toxoplasma gondii* and *Plasmodium.*
• *Kinetics in adults:* Sulfadiazine is absorbed from the GI tract after oral administration; peak serum levels occur at 2 hours.
It is distributed widely into most body tissues and fluids, including synovial, pleural, amniotic, prostatic, peritoneal, and seminal fluids; CSF penetration is poor.
Sulfadiazine crosses the placenta; it is 32% to 56% protein-bound. Sulfadiazine is metabolized partially in the liver.
Both unchanged drug and metabolites are excreted primarily in urine by glomerular filtration and, to a lesser extent, renal tubular secretion; some drug is excreted in breast milk. Urine solubility of unchanged drug increases as urine pH increases.

Contraindications and precautions
Sulfonamides are contraindicated in children with known hypersensitivity to sulfonamides or to any other drug containing sulfur (e.g., thiazides, furosemide, or oral sulfonylureas); in patients with severe renal or hepatic dysfunction, or porphyria; and in infants under age 2 months.
Administer sulfadiazine with caution to children with mild to moderate renal or hepatic impairment, urinary obstruction (because of the risk of drug accumulation), severe allergies, asthma, blood dyscrasias, or glucose-6-phosphate dehydrogenase deficiency.

Interactions
Sulfadiazine may inhibit hepatic metabolism of oral anticoagulants, displacing them from binding sites and enhancing anticoagulant effects.
Concomitant use with PABA antagonizes effects of sulfonamides; with oral hypoglycemics (sulfonylureas), enhances their hypoglycemic effects, probably by displacing sulfonylureas from protein-binding sites with either trimethoprim or pyrimethamine (folic acid antagonists with different mechanisms of action) results in synergistic antibacterial effects and delay or prevents bacterial resistance.
Concomitant use of urine acidifying agents (ammonium chloride or ascorbic acid) or methenamine decreases sulfonamide solubility, which increases risk of crystalluria.

Effects on diagnostic tests
Sulfadiazine alters urine glucose tests utilizing cupric sulfate (Benedict's reagent or Clinitest). Sulfadiazine may elevate liver function test results; it may decrease serum levels of erythrocytes, platelets, or leukocytes.

Adverse reactions
• CNS: headache, mental depression, *seizures,* hallucinations.
• DERM: erythema multiforme (Stevens-Johnson syndrome), generalized skin eruption, epidermal necrolysis, *exfoliative dermatitis,* photosensitivity, urticaria, pruritus.
• GI: nausea, vomiting, diarrhea, abdominal pain, anorexia, stomatitis.
• GU: toxic nephrosis with oliguria and anuria, crystalluria, hematuria.

• HEMA: agranulocytosis, *aplastic anemia*, megaloblastic anemia, thrombocytopenia, leukopenia, hemolytic anemia.
• Hepatic: jaundice.
• Local: irritation, extravasation.
• Other: hypersensitivity, serum sickness, drug fever, *anaphylaxis*, bacterial and fungal superinfection.

Note: Drug should be discontinued if signs of toxicity or hypersensitivity occur; if hematologic abnormalities are accompanied by sore throat, pallor, fever, jaundice, purpura, or weakness; if crystalluria is accompanied by renal colic, hematuria, oliguria, proteinuria, urinary obstruction, urolithiasis, increased BUN levels, or anuria; or if severe diarrhea indicates pseudomembranous colitis.

Overdose and treatment
Clinical signs of overdose include dizziness, drowsiness, headache, unconsciousness, anorexia, abdominal pain, nausea, and vomiting. More severe complications, including hemolytic anemia, agranulocytosis, dermatitis, acidosis, sensitivity reactions, and jaundice, may be fatal.

Treatment includes gastric lavage, if ingestion has occurred within the preceding 4 hours followed by correction of acidosis, forced fluids, and urinary alkalinization to enhance solubility and excretion. Treatment of renal failure as well as transfusion of appropriate blood products (in severe hematologic toxicity) may be required.

▶ Special considerations
• Assess patient's history of allergies; do not give sulfadiazine to any patient with a history of hypersensitivity reactions to sulfonamides or to any other drug containing sulfur (such as thiazides, furosemide, and oral sulfonylureas).
• Sulfonamides are also contraindicated in the child with severe or hepatic dysfunction or prophyria. Sulfonamides may cause kernicterus in infants, because they displace bilirubin at the binding site, cross the placenta, and are excreted in breast milk. Infants under age 2 months should receive sulfonamides only if there is no therapeutic alternative.
• Administer sulfonamides with caution to children with the following conditions: mild to moderate renal or hepatic impairment or urinary obstruction, because of the risk of drug accumulation; severe allergies; asthma; blood dyscrasias; or G6PD deficiency.
• Give sulfonamides with caution to children with fragile X chromosome associated with mental retardation, because they are vulnerable to psychomotor depression from folate depletion.
• Monitor continuously for possible hypersensitivity reactions or other untoward effects; patients with acquired immunodeficiency syndrome have a much higher incidence of adverse reactions.
• Obtain results of cultures and sensitivity tests before first dose, but therapy may begin before laboratory tests are complete; check test results periodically to assess drug efficacy. Monitor urine cultures, complete blood counts, and urinalysis before and during therapy.
• Monitor patients on long-term therapy for possible superinfection or if receiving immunosuppressants or radiation therapy.
• Sulfadazine is a less soluble sulfonamide and therefore more likely to cause crystalluria. Avoid concomitant use of urine acidifiers (check urine pH) and ensure adequate fluid intake.
• Administer with full glass (8 oz [240 ml]) of water, and ensure adequate hydration during therapy.
• Give oral sulfonamide at least 1 hour before or 2 hours after meals for maximum absorption.

Information for parents and patient
• Advise parents and patient of the need to avoid exposure to direct sunlight because of risk of photosensitivity reaction.
• Give oral sulfonamides at least 1 hour before or 2 hours after meals for maximum absorption.
• Be sure parents understand how and when to administer drugs; urge them to complete entire prescribed regimen, to comply with instructions for around-the-clock dosage, and to keep follow-up appointments.
• Teach signs and symptoms of hypersensitivity and other adverse reactions, and emphasize need to report these. Specifically urge patient to report bloody urine, difficult breathing, rash, fever, chills, or severe fatigue.
• Teach signs and symptoms of bacterial and fungal superinfection to patients and parents and if low resistance from immunosuppressants or irradiation is evident, emphasize need to report them.
• Advise patient to avoid vitamin preparations containing high doses of vitamin C during therapy.
• Teach parents and patient to prevent superinfection by practicing meticulous oral and anogenital hygiene. Parents of infants and toddlers should keep diaper area clean and dry and avoid using plastic pants.
• Explain to parents of diabetic patients that sulfonamides may increase effects of oral hypoglycemic and not to monitor urine glucose levels with Clinitest; sulfonamides alter results of tests utilizing cupric sulfate.
• Advise parents and patient to tell new dentist or physician of sulfonamide therapy.
• Teach parents to check expiration date of drug and how to store drug, and to discard unused drug.

sulfadoxine and pyrimethamine
Fansidar

• Classification: antiprotozoal; antimalarial agent (folate antagonist/sulfonamide combination)

How supplied
Available by prescription only
Tablets: 500 mg of sulfadozine and 25 mg of pyrimethamine

Indications, route, and dosage
Prophylaxis of chloroquine-resistant *Plasmodium falciparum malaria*
Infants and children ages 2 months to 4 years: ¼ tablet P.O. once q 7 days, or ½ tablet P.O. q 14 days.
Children ages 4 to 8: ½ tablet P.O. once, q 7 days, or 1 tablet once q 14 days.
Children ages 9 to 14: ¾ tablet P.O. once q 7 days, or 1½ tablet P.O. once, q 14 days.
Adults: 1 tablet P.O. once q 7 days, or 2 tablets once q 14 days.

Treatment of chloroquine-resistant *P. falciparum malaria*
Infants and children age 2 months to 4 years: ½ tablet P.O. as a single dose, alone or sequentially with quinine.
Children ages 4 to 8: 1 tablet P.O. as a single dose, alone or sequentially with quinine.
Children ages 9 to 14: 2 tablets P.O. alone or sequentially with quinine.

Action and kinetics
• *Antiprotozoal action:* Pyrimethamine and sulfadoxine act synergistically against susceptible plasmodia. Pyrimethamine is a folic acid antagonist. By binding to and reversibly inhibiting dihydrofolate reductase, it inhibits the reduction of dihydrofolic acid to tetrahydrofolic acid (folinic acid). It impairs synthesis of tetrahydrofolic acid in malarial parasites at a point immediately succeeding that where sulfonamides act.

Sulfadoxine, a structural analog of *p*-aminobenzoic acid (PABA), competively inhibits dihydrofolic acid synthesis which is necessary for the conversation of PABA to folic acid.

• *Kinetics in adults:* Sulfadoxine and pyrimethamine are well absorbed from the GI tract. After oral administration of a single tablet containing 500 mg of sulfadozine and 25 mg of pyrimethamine, peak plasma concentrations of pyrimethamine (0.13 to 0.4 μg/mL) occur within 1.5 to 8 hours; peak plasma concentrations of sulfadoxine (51 to 76 μg/mL) occur within 2.5 to 6 hours.

Pyrimethamine is distributed mainly to the kidneys, lungs, liver, and spleen and has an apparent volume of distribution of about 3 liters/kg in adults. Sulfadoxine is widely distributed in the body. Pyrimethamine is approximately 80% bound to plasma proteins. Pyrimethamine and sulfadoxine are both distributed into milk. Average plasma half-life of pyrimethamine is 111 hours (range, 54 to 148 hours); the plasma half-life of sulfadoxine is 169 hours (range is 100 to 232 hours).

Pyrimethamine and several unidentified metabolites of the drug are excreted in urine. Sulfadoxine is excreted mainly in urine.

Contraindications and precautions
Sulfadoxine and pyrimethamine is contraindicated in patients hypersensitive to either pyrimethamine or sulfonamides and in patients with megaloblastic anemia caused by folate deficiency.

Sulfadoxine and pyrimethamine should be used with caution in patients with possible folate deficiency and in patients with impaired renal or hepatic function. Use in patients with impaired renal function requires urinalysis (including microscopic examinations) and renal function tests during therapy.

Drug should be used with caution in patients with severe allergy or bronchial asthma.

Because it contains a sulfonamide, the usual precautions and contraindications of sulfonamide therapy apply, including an adequate fluid intake to prevent crystalluria.

Drug should be used with caution in patients with blood dyscrasias or megaloblastic anemia due to folate deficiency, because pyrimethamine may cause folic acid deficiency, and sulfonamides and pyrimethamine may cause blood dyscrasias; in patients with convulsive disorders, because pyrimethamine may cause CNS toxicity; in patients with glucose-6-phosphate dehydrogenase (G6PD) deficiency, because hemolytic anemia may occur; with hepatic impairment, because sulfonamides and pyrimethamine are metabolized in the liver and may cause fulminant hepatic necrosis; with porphyria, because sulfonamides may precipitate an acute attack of porphyria; and with renal function impairment because drug may worsen this condition.

Interactions
Concurrent use with *p*-aminobenzoic acid (PABA) interferes with the action of pyrimethamine. Concomitant use with other sulfonamides or with cotrimoxazole may cause additive adverse effects.

Concurrent use with aminobenzoates may antagonize the bacteriostatic effect of sulfonamides and is not recommended; with anesthetics may impair the antibacterial activity of sulfonamides; with anticoagulants (coumarin- or indandione-derivative), or anticonvulsants (hydantoin), oral antidiabetic agents or methotrexate may result in increased or prolonged effects or toxicity and may require dosage adjustments; concurrent use with bone marrow depressants may increase the leukopenic or thrombocytopenic effects and requires close observation for myelotoxic effects.

Concurrent use with oral contraceptives may result in reduced contraceptive reliability and increased incidence of breakthrough bleeding; use with other folate antagonists is not recommended because of the possibility of megaloblastic anemia; use with other hemolytics may increase the potential for toxicity; use with other hepatotoxic medications increases the incidence of hepatotoxicity and requires careful monitoring of liver functions; with methenamine or methenamine-containing medications may increase the risk of crystalluria and is not recommended; with phenylbutazone may potentiate effects of phenylbutazone because of displacement from plasma protein-binding sites; use with penicillins may interfere with the bactericidal effect of penicillins; and should not be used in the treatment of meningitis or in other situations where a rapid bactericidal effect is necessary; use with other photosensitizing drugs may cause additive photosensitivity and is not recommended; use with probenecid may decrease renal tubular secretion of sulfanamides resulting in increased and more prolonged sulfonamide serum concentrations or toxicity; use with sulfinpyrazone may displace sulfonamides from protein-binding sites and may cause decreased renal excretion and increased sulfonamide serum concentrations or toxicity and may require dosage adjustments; use with vitamin K may increase requirements for vitamin K; use with zidovudine may competitively inhibit the hepatic glucoronidation and decrease the clearance of zidovudine and should be avoided because it may potentiate the toxicity of zidovudine.

Effects on diagnostic tests
None reported.

Adverse reactions
• CNS: dizziness, headache, reversible hyperesthesia (rarely).
• DERM: skin rash, redness, blistering, peeling or loosening of skin, photosensitivity, exfoliative dermatitis, urticaria.
• EENT: change in or loss of taste; soreness, redness, swelling, burning or stinging of tongue; sore throat; difficulty in swallowing; ulcerative stomatitis, yellow eyes, goiter
• GI: diarrhea, anorexia, nausea, vomiting
• GU: hematuria, pain or burning while urinating, crystalluria
• HEMA: unusual bleeding or bruising, leukopenia, granulocytopenia, agranulocytosis, hemolysis (in patients with glucose-6-phosphate dehydrogenase [G6PD] deficiency)
• Hepatic: abnormal liver function results (e.g., elevated serum, ALT [SGPT], AST [SGOT], alkaline phosphatase, and bilirubin concentrations), jaundice, hepatomegaly, and hepatitis).
• Other: pale skin, unusual tiredness or weakness, aching of joints or muscles, fever, lower back pain, pruritis, serum sickness reactions, vasculitis (cutaneous or generalized).
  Note: Therapy should be discontinued at the first sign of skin rash; symptoms of folic acid deficiency; if a significant reduction in any formed blood element is noted; or if active bacterial or fungal infection occurs. Some clinicians recommend that sulfadoxine and pyrimethamine therapy be discontinued immediately if a hepatic reaction is suspected.

Overdose and treatment
Clinical effects of overusage of sulfadoxine and pyrimethamine may result in acute intoxication manifested by anorexia, vomiting and CNS stimulation including seizures. Megaloblastic anemia, leukopenia, thrombocytopenia, glossitis, and crystalluria may also occur.

Treatment may include emesis and gastric lavage followed by catharsis. Parenteral barbiturates should be used to control seizures. If platelet or leukocyte counts are decreased, leucovorin should be administered in a dosage of 3 to 9 mg daily for 3 days or longer. Renal and hematopoietic functions should be monitored for at least 1 month afterward.

▶ Special considerations
• Sulfadoxine and pyrimethamine combination is contraindicated in infants under 2 months of age since sulfonamides may cause kernicterus in neonates.
• Fatal reactions including erythema multiforme, Stevens-Johnson syndrome, and toxic epidermal necrol-

ysis have followed use of sulfadoxine and pyrimethamine in travelers who received the drug for prophylaxis of malaria. Because sulfonamides have also caused fatal hypersensitivity reactions, hepatocellular necrosis, agranulocytosis, aplastic anemia, and other blood dyscrasias, the CDC and most clinicians recommend sulfadoxine and pyrimethamine for prophylaxis only when the risk of chloroquine-resistant *P. falciparum* is substantial.
• During prolonged therapy with sulfadoxine and pyrimethamine, urinalysis and complete blood counts (CBCs) should be performed periodically.
• Drug may cause a change in or loss of taste; soreness, redness, swelling, buring, or stinging of the tongue; sore throat or difficulty in swallowing; and ulcers, sores, or white spots in the mouth.
• This drug's leukopenic and thrombocytopenic effects may increase the incidence of certain microbial infections, delayed healing, and gingival bleeding.
• Patients who develop leukopenia or thrombocytopenia should defer dental work until blood counts have returned to normal.
• Teach proper oral hygiene including caution in use of dental floss and toothbrushes.
• Reportedly, patients with AIDS may be at increased risk of developing severe hypersensitivity reactions to sulfadoxine and pyrimethamine, similar to the increased risk associated wtih co-trimoxazole. Such reactions (Stevens-Johnson syndrome) have been reported in some AIDS patients receiving this combination; however, it appeared to be associated with a lower risk of adverse effects than co-trimoxazole in a small group of AIDS patients and it has been used in a few patients who could not tolerate co-trimoxazole.
• Fluid intake should be sufficient to maintain adequate urine output.
• High doses of this drug may cause gastric irritation, sometimes resulting in vomiting. If this occurs, drug may be taken with food or dosage may be reduced.
• Therapy with sulfadoxine and pyrimethamine combination should be discontinued if skin rash or symptoms of folic acid or folinic acid deficiency occur. If folic acid or folinic acid deficiency occurs, folates may be administered concurrently to restore normal hematopoiesis. Folates do not impair antiprotozoal activity since protozoa are unable to utilize preformed folates. In adults, 5 to 15 mg of leucovorin (folinic acid) may be given orally, intramuscularly, or intravenously once a day for 3 days or as required; 9 mg of leucovorin may be given (folinic acid) two or three times a week. Infants may be given 1 mg of leucovorin once a day.
• Malaria prophylaxis should begin 1 to 2 weeks before the patient enters a malarious area and should continue for 4 to 6 weeks after the patient leaves the area. Starting the medication in advance allows time to substitute other antimalarials if the patient develops allergies or other adverse effects.

Information for parents and patient
• Warn parents to store pyrimethamine and sulfadoxine out of the reach of children. Accidental ingestion of pyrimethamine has been fatal.
• Warn parents that sore throat, fever, pallor, arthral-

gia, cough, shortness of breath, purpura, glossitis, or jaundice also may be an early sign of a serious adverse reaction.
• Warn parents that overdose is especially dangerous in children.
• Tell parents to give drug with plenty of water and to encourage taking several drinks of water every day, unless otherwise directed. If this drug upsets the patient's stomach or causes vomiting, it may be taken with meals or a snack.
• If patient is taking this drug to *prevent* malaria, tell parents the following: Drug therapy may be prescribed to begin 1 to 2 weeks before travel to an area where there is a chance of contracting malaria. This will help to evaluate patient's reaction to the drug. The patient should keep taking this drug while he is in the endemic area and for 4 to 6 weeks after he leaves it. It is important to keep taking the drug for the full time ordered. Parents should immediately report fever that develops during the patient's travels or within 2 months afterward.
• Advise parents that this drug works best when taken on a regular schedule without missing any doses. If the patient does miss a dose, he should take it as soon as possible unless it is almost time for the next dose; then he should skip the missed dose and resume the regular schedule. Do not double-dose.
• If patient is taking drug to *treat* malaria, advise parents and patient to take drug *exactly* as directed. If symptoms do not improve within a few days or become worse, they should notify the physician.
• Advise parents to store drug away from heat, direct light, and moisture. Heat or moisture may cause drug to deteriorate. Outdated or left-over drug should be discarded, safely out of the reach of children.
• Advise parents to report adverse reactions immediately.
• Advise parents and patient on methods they may use to prevent malaria. Because malaria is spread by mosquitoes, they should if possible, sleep under mosquito netting, wear long-sleeved shirts or blouses and long trousers to protect arms and legs, and apply mosquito repellent to uncovered areas of the skin, especially from dusk through dawn when mosquitoes are out.
• Advise parents that drug may cause dizziness. Patient should avoid hazardous activities that require mental alertness until reaction to drug is known.
• Advise parents that drug may increase the chance of certain infections, slow healing, and bleeding of the gums. The patient should be careful when using toothbrushes and dental floss. Dental work should be delayed until blood counts have returned to normal.
• Tell parents that some people who take drug may become abnormally sensitive to sunlight. Patient should avoid excessive exposure to sunlight and should avoid using a sunlamp.

sulfamethoxazole
Gamazole, Gantanol, Gantanol DS, Methanoxanol

• Classification: antibiotic (sulfonamide)

How supplied
Available by prescription only
Tablets: 500 mg, 1,000 mg
Suspension: 500 mg/5 ml

Indications, route, and dosage
Urinary tract and systemic infections
Children and infants over age 2 months: Initially, 50 to 60 mg/kg P.O., then 25 to 30 mg/kg b.i.d. Maximum dosage should not exceed 75 mg/kg daily.
Adults: Initially, 2 g P.O.; then 1 g P.O. b.i.d., up to t.i.d. for severe infections.

Action and kinetics
• *Antibacterial action:* Sulfamethoxazole is bacteriostatic. It acts by inhibiting formation of dihydrofolic acid from para-aminobenzoic acid (PABA), thus preventing bacterial cell synthesis of essential nucleic acids. It acts synergistically with agents such as trimethoprim that block folic acid synthesis at a later stage, thus delaying or preventing bacterial resistance.

Sulfamethoxazole's spectrum of action includes some gram-positive bacteria, *Chlamydia trachomatis,* many Enterobacteriaceae, and some strains of *Toxoplasma* and *Plasmodium.*
• *Kinetics in adults:* Sulfamethoxazole is absorbed from the GI tract after oral administration; and is distributed widely into most body tissues and fluids, including cerebrospinal, synovial, pleural, amniotic, prostatic, peritoneal, and seminal fluids. Sulfamethoxazole crosses the placenta; it is 50% to 70% protein-bound.

Sulfamethoxazole is metabolized partially in the liver and excreted primarily in urine by glomerular filtration and, to a lesser extent, renal tubular secretion; some drug is excreted in breast milk.

Contraindications and precautions
Sulfamethoxazole is contraindicated in children with known hypersensitivity to sulfonamides or to any other drug containing sulfur (for example, thiazides, furosemide, or oral sulfonylureas); in patients with severe renal or hepatic dysfunction, or porphyria; during pregnancy at term, and during lactation; and in infants under age 2 months.

Administer sulfonamides with caution to children with mild to moderate renal or hepatic impairment, urinary obstruction (because of the risk of drug accumulation), severe allergies, asthma, blood dyscrasias, or glucose-6-phosphate dehydrogenase deficiency.

Interactions
Sulfamethoxazole may inhibit hepatic metabolism of oral anticoagulants, displacing them from binding sites and enhancing anticoagulant effects. Concomitant use

with PABA antagonizes sulfonamide effects; with oral hypoglycemics (sulfonylureas) enhances their hypoglycemic effects, probably by displacing sulfonylureas from protein-binding sites; and with either trimethoprim or pyrimethamine (folic acid antagonists with different mechanisms of action) results in synergistic antibacterial effects and delays or prevents bacterial resistance.

Concomitant use of urine acidifying agents (ammonium chloride or ascorbic acid) decreases urine pH and sulfonamide solubility, thus increasing risk of crystalluria.

Effects on diagnostic tests

Sulfamethoxazole alters results of urine glucose tests utilizing cupric sulfate (Benedict's reagent or Clinitest).

Sulfamethoxazole may elevate liver function test results; it may decrease serum levels of erythrocytes, platelets, or leukocytes.

Adverse reactions

• CNS: headache, mental depression, seizures, hallucinations.
• DERM: erythema multiforme (Stevens-Johnson syndrome), generalized skin eruption, epidermal necrolysis, exfoliative dermatitis, photosensitivity, urticaria, pruritus.
• GI: nausea, vomiting, diarrhea, abdominal pain, anorexia, stomatitis.
• GU: toxic nephrosis with oliguria and anuria, crystalluria, hematuria.
• HEMA: agranulocytosis, aplastic anemia, megaloblastic anemia, thrombocytopenia, leukopenia, hemolytic anemia.
• Hepatic: jaundice.
• Other: hypersensitivity, serum sickness, drug fever, *anaphylaxis*, bacterial and fungal superinfection.

Note: Drug should be discontinued if signs of toxicity or hypersensitivity occur; if hematologic abnormalities are accompanied by sore throat, pallor, fever, jaundice, purpura, or weakness; if crystalluria is accompanied by renal colic, hematuria, oliguria, proteinuria, urinary obstruction, urolithiasis, increased BUN levels, or anuria; or if severe diarrhea indicates pseudomembranous colitis.

Overdose and treatment

Clinical signs of overdose include dizziness, drowsiness, headache, unconsciousness, anorexia, abdominal pain, nausea, and vomiting. More severe complications, including hemolytic anemia, agranulocytosis, dermatitis, acidosis, sensitivity reactions, and jaundice, may be fatal.

Treat by gastric lavage, if ingestion has occurred within the preceding 4 hours, followed by correction of acidosis, forced fluids, and urinary alkalinization to enhance solubility and excretion. Treatment of renal failure and transfusion of appropriate blood products (in severe hematologic toxicity) may be required.

▶ Special considerations

• Assess patient's history of allergies; do not give sulfamethoxazole to any patient with a history of hypersensitivity reactions to sulfonamides or to any

other drug containing sulfur (such as thiazides, furosemide, and oral sulfonylureas).
• Sulfonamides are also contraindicated in the child with severe or hepatic dysfunction or porphyria. Sulfonamides may cause kernicterus in infants, because they displace bilirubin at the binding site, cross the placenta, and are excreted in breast milk. Infants under age 2 months should receive sulfamethoxazole only if there is no therapeutic alternative.
• Administer sulfamethoxazole with caution to children with the following conditions: mild to moderate renal or hepatic impairment, urinary obstruction, because of the risk of drug accumulation; severe allergies; asthma; blood dyscrasias; or G6PD deficiency.
• Give sulfamethoxazole with caution to children with fragile X chromosome associated with mental retardation, because they are vulnerable to psychomotor depression from folate depletion.
• Monitor continuously for possible hypersensitivity reactions or other untoward effects; patients with acquired immunodeficiency syndrome have a much higher incidence of adverse reactions.
• Obtain results of cultures and sensitivity tests before first dose, but therapy may begin before laboratory tests are complete, check test results periodically to assess drug efficacy. Monitor urine cultures, complete blood counts, and urinalysis before and during therapy.
• Monitor patients on long-term therapy and those receiving immunosuppressants or radiation therapy for possible superinfection.

Administration

• Give oral dosage with full glass (8 oz [240 ml]) of water, and encourage increased fluid intake as appropriate for patient's weight. Patient's urine output should be at least 1,500 day.
• Tablet may be swallowed with water to facilitate passage into stomach and maximum absorption.
• Give oral sulfonamide at least 1 hour before or 2 hours after meals for maximum absorption.
• Shake oral suspension well before administering to ensure correct dosage.

Information for parents and patient

• Patient should avoid exposure to direct sunlight because of risk of photosensitivity reaction. Recommend use of a sunscreen.
• Tell parents to give sulfamethoxazole at least 1 hour before or 2 hours after meals for maximum absorption. Shake oral suspensions well before administering to ensure correct dosage.
• Tell parents to give drug with a generous amount of water and to encourage adequate intake of water; explain that tablet may be crushed and swallowed with water to ensure maximal absorption.
• Be sure parents understand how and when to administer sulfamethoxazole; urge them to complete entire prescribed regimen, to comply with instructions for around-the-clock dosage, and to keep follow-up appointments.
• Patient should avoid large doses of vitamin C which could acidify urine.
• Teach signs and symptoms of hypersensitivity and other adverse reactions, and emphasize need to report these, specifically urge patient to report bloody urine,

---

‡May contain sulfites　　　　　◆May contain tartrazine　　　　　◆ ◆May contain benzyl alcohol

difficult breathing, rash, fever, chills, or severe fatigue.

• Teach signs and symptoms of bacterial and fungal superinfection to patients and parents and if low resistance from immunosuppressants or irradiation is evident, emphasize need to report them.

• Teach parents and patient to prevent superinfection by practicing meticulous oral and anogenital hygiene. Parents of infants and toddlers should keep diaper area clean and dry and avoid using plastic pants.

• Advise parents of diabetic patients that drug may increase effects of oral hypoglycemic and not to monitor urine glucose levels with Clinitest; sulfonamides alter results of tests utilizing cupric sulfate.

• Advise patient or parents to tell new dentist or physician of sulfamethoxazole therapy.

• Teach parents to check expiration date of drug and how to store drug, and to discard unused drug.

---

sulfasalazine
Azaline, Azaline EC, Azulfidine,
Azulfidine En-tabs, S.A.S.-500,
Salazopyrin*

• Classification: antibiotic (sulfonamide)

How supplied
Available by prescription only
Tablets: 500 mg with or without enteric coating
Suspension: 250 mg/5 ml

Indications, route, and dosage
Mild to moderate ulcerative colitis, adjunctive therapy in severe ulcerative colitis
Infants over age 2 and children: Initially, 6.7 to 10 mg/kg q 4 hours, or 10 to 15 mg/kg q 6 hours, or 13.3 to 20 mg/kg q 8 hours.

Higher initial doses (up to 150 mg/kg daily divided into three to six doses) may be necessary in some patients. Maintenance dosage is 7.5 to 10 mg/kg q 6 hours.
Adults: Initially, 3 to 4 g P.O. daily in evenly divided doses. Maintenance dose is 1.5 to 2 g P.O. daily in divided doses q 6 hours. May need to start with 1 to 2 g initially, with a gradual increase in dose to minimize adverse reactions.

Action and kinetics
• *Antibacterial action:* The exact mechanism of action of sulfasalazine in ulcerative colitis is unknown; it is believed to be a pro-drug metabolized by intestinal flora in the colon. The metabolites (sulfapyridine and 5-aminosalicylic acid) appear to be the active components.
• *Kinetics in adults:* Sulfasalazine is absorbed poorly from the GI tract after oral administration; about 80% is transported to the colon where intestinal flora metabolize the drug to its active ingredients, sulfapyridine (antibacterial) and 5-aminosalicylic acid (antiinflammatory), which exert their effects locally. Sulfapyridine is absorbed from the colon, but 5-aminosalicylic acid is not.

Human data on sulfasalazine distribution are lacking. Parent drug and both metabolites cross the placenta.

Sulfasalazine is cleaved by intestinal flora in the colon. Systemically absorbed sulfasalazine is excreted chiefly in urine; some parent drug and metabolites are excreted in breast milk. Plasma half-life is about 6 to 8 hours.

Contraindications and precautions
Like all sulfonamides, sulfasalazine is contraindicated in children with known hypersensitivity to sulfonamides or to any other drug containing sulfur (for example, thiazides, furosemide, or oral sulfonylureas) in patients with known hypersensitivity to salicylates; in patients with severe renal or hepatic dysfunction, or porphyria; during pregnancy, at term, and during lactation; and in infants and children under age 2. Sulfasalazine is also contraindicated in children with intestinal or urinary tract obstructions because of the risk of local GI irritation and of crystalluria.

Administer sulfonamides with caution to children with mild to moderate renal or hepatic impairment, severe allergies, asthma, blood dyscrasias, or glucose-6-phosphate dehydrogenase deficiency.

Interactions
Sulfasalazine may inhibit hepatic metabolism of oral anticoagulants, displacing them from binding sites and enhancing anticoagulant effects.

Concomitant use with oral hypoglycemics (sulfonylureas) enhances hypoglycemic effects, probably by displacing sulfonylureas from protein-binding sites.

Sulfasalazine may reduce GI absorption of digoxin and folic acid.

Concomitant use of urine acidifying agents (ammonium chloride, ascorbic acid) decreases urine pH and sulfonamide solubility, thus increasing risk of crystalluria. Concomitant use with antibiotics that alter intestinal flora may interfere with conversion of sulfasalazine to sulfapyridine and 5-aminosalicylic acid, decreasing its effectiveness.

Concomitant use of antacids may cause premature dissolution of enteric-coated tablets (which are designed to dissolve in the intestines), thus increasing systemic absorption and hazard of toxicity.

Effects on diagnostic tests
Sulfasalazine alters results of urine glucose tests utilizing cupric sulfate (Benedict's reagent or Clinitest).

Sulfasalazine may elevate liver function test results; it may decrease serum levels of erythrocytes, platelets, or leukocytes.

Adverse reactions
• CNS: headache, mental depression, *seizures,* hallucinations, tinnitus.
• DERM: erythema multiforme (Stevens-Johnson syndrome), generalized skin eruption, *epidermal necrolysis,* exfoliative dermatitis, photosensitivity, urticaria pruritus.
• GI: nausea, vomiting, diarrhea, abdominal pain, anorexia, stomatitis.

- GU: toxic nephrosis with oliguria and anuria, crystalluria, hematuria, oligospermia, infertility.
- HEMA: agranulocytosis, aplastic anemia, megaloblastic anemia, thrombocytopenia, leukopenia, hemolytic anemia.
- Hepatic: jaundice.
- Other: hypersensitivity, serum sickness, drug fever, *anaphylaxis*, bacterial and fungal superinfection.

Note: Drug should be discontinued if signs of toxicity or hypersensitivity occur; if hematologic abnormalities are accompanied by sore throat, pallor, fever, jaundice, purpura, or weakness; if crystalluria is accompanied by renal colic, hematuria, oliguria, proteinuria, urinary obstruction, urolithiasis, increased BUN levels, or anuria; if severe diarrhea indicates pseudomembranous colitis; or if severe nausea, vomiting, or diarrhea persists.

Overdose and treatment

Clinical signs of overdose include dizziness, drowsiness, headache, unconsciousness, anorexia, abdominal pain, nausea, and vomiting. More severe complications, including hemolytic anemia, agranulocytosis, dermatitis, acidosis, sensitivity reactions, and jaundice, may be fatal.

Treat by gastric lavage, if ingestion has occurred within the preceding 4 hours, followed by correction of acidosis, forced fluids, and urinary alkalinization to enhance solubility and excretion. Treatment of renal failure and transfusion of appropriate blood products (in severe hematologic toxicity) may be required.

▶ Special considerations

- Assess patient's history of allergies; do not give sulfasalazine to any patient with a history of hypersensitivity reactions to sulfonamides or to any other drug containing sulfur (such as thiazides, furosemide, and oral sulfonylureas).
- Sulfonamides are also contraindicated in the child with severe renal or hepatic dysfunction or porphyria. Sulfonamides may cause kernicterus in infants, because they displace bilirubin at the binding site, cross the placenta, and are excreted in breast milk. Infants under age 2 months should receive sulfonamides only if there is no therapeutic alternative.
- Administer sulfasalazine with caution to children with the following conditions: mild to moderate renal or hepatic impairment, urinary obstruction, because of the risk of drug accumulation; severe allergies; asthma; blood dyscrasias; or G6PD deficiency.
- Give sulfasalazine with caution to children with fragile X chromosome associated with mental retardation, because they are vulnerable to psychomotor depression from folate depletion.
- Monitor continuously for possible hypersensitivity reactions or other untoward effects; patients with acquired immunodeficiency syndrome have a much higher incidence of adverse reactions.
- Obtain results of cultures and sensitivity tests before first dose, but therapy may begin before laboratory tests are complete; check test results periodically to assess drug efficacy. Monitor urine cultures, complete blood counts, and urinalysis before and during therapy.
- Monitor patients on long-term therapy and those who are receiving immunosuppressants or radiation therapy for possible superinfection.
- Most adverse effects from sulfasalazine involve the GI tract; minimize reactions and facilitate absorption by spacing doses evenly and administering drug after food.
- Drug colors urine orange-yellow. Patient's skin may also turn orange-yellow.
- Do not administer antacids concomitantly with enteric-coated sulfasalazine; they may alter absorption.

Administration

- Ensure adequate hydration during therapy.
- Give oral dosage with generous amount of water to facilitate passage into stomach and maximum absorption.
- Give oral sulfonamide at least 1 hour before or 2 hours after meals for maximum absorption.
- Shake oral suspensions well before administering to ensure correct dosage.

Information for parents and patient

- Tell patient that sulfasalazine normally turns urine orange-yellow. Warn patient that skin may also turn orange-yellow.
- Advise patient not to take antacids simultaneously with sulfasalazine.
- Advise patient to take drug after meals to reduce GI distress and to facilitate passage into intestines.
- Patient should avoid large doses of vitamin C which could acidify urine.
- Patient should avoid exposure to direct sunlight because of risk of photosensitivity reaction. Recommend use of sunscreen.
- Shake oral suspensions well before administering to ensure correct dosage.
- Explain that tablet may be crushed and swallowed with water to ensure maximal absorption.
- Be sure parents understand how and when to administer sulfasalazine; urge them to complete entire prescribed regimen, to comply with instructions for around-the-clock dosage, and to keep follow-up appointments.
- Teach signs and symptoms of hypersensitivity and other adverse reactions, and emphasize need to report these, specifically urge patient to report bloody urine, difficult breathing, rash, fever, chills, or severe fatigue.
- Teach signs and symptoms of bacterial and fungal superinfection to patients and parents and if low resistance from immunosuppressants or irradiation is evident, emphasize need to report them.
- Teach parents and patients to prevent superinfection by practicing meticulous oral and anogenital hygiene. Parents of infants and toddlers should keep diaper area clean and dry and avoid using plastic pants.
- Advise parents of diabetic patients not to monitor urine glucose levels with Clinitest; sulfonamides alter results of tests utilizing cupric sulfate.
- Advise patient or parents to tell new dentist or physician of sulfasalazine therapy.
- Teach parents to check expiration date of drug and how to store drug, and to discard unused drug.

---

‡May contain sulfites   ♦May contain tartrazine   ♦♦May contain benzyl alcohol

sulfisoxazole
Gantrisin, Gulfasin, Lipo Gantrisin

• Classification: antibiotic (sulfonamide)

How supplied
Available by prescription only
Tablets: 500 mg
Liquid: 500 mg/5 ml
Long-acting emulsion: 0.5 g/5 ml

Indications, route, and dosage
Urinary tract and systemic infections
Infants under 1 month of age: Except as concurrent adjunctive therapy with pyrimethamine in the treatment of congenital toxoplasmosis, use is contraindicated since sulfonamides may cause kernicterus in neonates.
Adults: Initially, 2 g P.O.; then 1 g P.O. b.i.d., up to t.i.d. for severe infections.
Systemic and urinary tract infections
Infants over age 1 month and children: Initially 75 mg/kg or 2 g/m² P.O., then 25 mg/kg or 667 mg/kg P.O. q 4 hours.
Adults: Initially, 2 g. P.O. then 1 g P.O. b.i.d. or t.i.d.
Otitis media
Infants over age 2 months and children: 37.5 mg/kg P.O. every 6 hours for 10 days, along with erythromycin ethylsuccinate 12.5 mg/kg P.O. q 6 hours.
Prophylaxis of recurrent otitis media
Infants over age 2 months and infants: 25 to 37.5 mg/kg P.O. b.i.d.
Treatment of acute pelvic inflammatory disease in prepubertal children
Children over age 1 month: 25 mg/kg P.O. q 4 hours, in combination with I.V. ceftriazone or cefurozime for at least 4 days, and preferably 2 days after the child shows substantial improvement. Oral sulfisoxazole therapy is continued for at least 14 days.
Note: The maximum dose for children should not exceed 6 g daily.

Action and kinetics
• *Antibacterial action:* Sulfisoxazole is bacteriostatic. It acts by inhibiting formation of dihydrofolic acid from para-aminobenzoic acid (PABA), thus preventing bacterial cell synthesis of essential nucleic acids. It acts synergistically with folic acid antagonists such as trimethoprim, that block folic acid synthesis at a later stage, thus delaying or preventing bacterial resistance.

Sulfisoxazole is active against some gram-positive bacteria, *Chlamydia trachomatis,* many Enterobacteriaceae, and some strains of *Toxoplasma* and *Plasmodium.*
• *Kinetics in adults:* Sulfisoxazole is absorbed readily from the GI tract after oral administration and distributed into extracellular compartments; CSF penetration is 8% to 57% in uninflamed meninges. Sulfisoxazole crosses the placenta.

Sulfisoxazole is metabolized partially in the liver and excreted primarily in urine by glomerular filtration and, to a lesser extent, renal tubular secretion; some drug is excreted in breast milk.

Contraindications and precautions
Sulfisoxazole is contraindicated in children with known hypersensitivity to sulfonamides or to any other drug containing sulfur (for example, thiazides, furosemide, or oral hypoglycemics); in patients with severe renal or hepatic dysfunction, or porphyria; during pregnancy, at term, and during lactation; and in infants under age 2 months.

Administer sulfonamides with caution to children with mild to moderate renal or hepatic impairment, urinary obstruction (because of hazard of drug accumulation), severe allergies, asthma, blood dyscrasias, or glucose-6-phosphate dehydrogenase (G-6-PD) deficiency.

Interactions
Sulfisoxazole may inhibit hepatic metabolism of oral anticoagulants, displacing them from binding sites and exaggerating anticoagulant effects. Concomitant use with PABA antagonizes effects of sulfonamides; with oral hypoglycemics (sulfonylureas) enhances hypoglycemic effects, probably by displacing sulfonylureas from protein-binding sites; with either trimethoprim or pyrimethamine (folic acid antagonists with different mechanisms of action) results in synergistic antibacterial effects and delays or prevents bacterial resistance.

Concomitant use of urine acidifying agents (ammonium chloride, ascorbic acid) decreases urine pH and sulfonamide solubility, thus increasing risk of crystalluria.

Effects on diagnostic tests
Sulfisoxazole alters results of urine glucose tests utilizing cupric sulfate (Benedict's reagent or Clinitest).

Sulfisoxazole may elevate liver function test results; it may decrease serum levels of erythrocytes, platelets, or leukocytes.

Adverse reactions
• CNS: headache, mental depression, seizures, hallucinations, kernicterus.
• DERM: erythema multiforme (Stevens-Johnson syndrome), generalized skin eruption, *epidermal necrolysis,* exfoliative dermatitis, photosensitivity, urticaria, pruritus.
• GI: nausea, vomiting, diarrhea, abdominal pain, anorexia, stomatitis.
• GU: toxic nephrosis with oliguria and anuria, crystalluria, hematuria.
• HEMA: agranulocytosis, aplastic anemia, megaloblastic anemia, thrombocytopenia, leukopenia, hemolytic anemia.
• Hepatic: jaundice.
• Other: hypersensitivity, serum sickness, drug fever, *anaphylaxis,* bacterial and fungal superinfection.
Note: Drug should be discontinued if signs of toxicity or hypersensitivity occur; if hematologic abnormalities are accompanied by sore throat, pallor, fever, jaundice, purpura, or weakness; if crystalluria is accompanied by renal colic, hematuria, oliguria, proteinuria, urinary obstruction, urolithiasis, increased

BUN levels, or anuria; or if severe diarrhea indicates pseudomembranous colitis.

Overdose and treatment

Clinical signs of overdose include dizziness, drowsiness, headache, unconsciousness, anorexia, abdominal pain, nausea, and vomiting. More severe complications, including hemolytic anemia, agranulocytosis, dermatitis, acidosis, sensitivity reactions, and jaundice, may be fatal.

Treatment requires gastric lavage, if ingestion has occurred within the preceding 4 hours, followed by correction of acidosis, and forced fluids and urinary alkalinization to enhance solubility and excretion. Treatment of renal failure and transfusion of appropriate blood products (in severe hematologic toxicity) may be required.

▶ Special considerations

• Assess patient's history of allergies; do not give sulfisoxazole to any patient with a history of hypersensitivity reactions to sulfonamides or to any other drug containing sulfur (such as thiazides, furosemide, and oral sulfonylureas).

• Sulfonamides are also contraindicated in the child with severe renal or hepatic dysfunction or porphyria. Sulfonamides may cause kernicterus in infants, because they displace bilirubin at the binding site, cross the placenta, and are excreted in breast milk. Infants under age 2 months should receive sulfonamides only if there is no therapeutic alternative.

• Administer sulfisoxazole with caution to children with the following conditions: mild to moderate renal or hepatic impairment, urinary obstruction, because of the risk of drug accumulation; severe allergies; asthma; blood dyscrasias; or G6PD deficiency.

• Give sulfisoxazole with caution to children with fragile X chromosome associated with mental retardation, because they are vulnerable to psychomotor depression from folate depletion.

• Monitor continuously for possible hypersensitivity reactions or other untoward effects; patients with acquired immunodeficiency syndrome have a much higher incidence of adverse reactions.

• Obtain results of cultures and sensitivity tests before first dose, but therapy may begin before laboratory tests are complete; check test results periodically to assess drug efficacy. Monitor urine cultures, complete blood counts, and urinalysis before and during therapy.

• Monitor patients on long-term therapy and those receiving immunosuppressants or radiation therapy for possible superinfection.

• Do not use Gantrisin suspension and Lipo-Gantrisin interchangeably; the latter is an extended-release preparation.

• Gantrisin, which offers longer stability without refrigeration than other antibiotics, is a practical choice for extended therapy.

Administration

• Give oral dosage with a generous amount of water, to facilitate passage into stomach and maximum absorption. Ensure adequate hydration during therapy. Patient's urine output should be at least 1,500 day.

• Give oral sulfonamide at least 1 hour before or 2 hours after meals for maximum absorption.

• Shake oral suspensions well before administering to ensure correct dosage.

Information for parents and patient

• Patient should avoid exposure to direct sunlight because of risk of photosensitivity reaction. Recommend use of a sunscreen.

• Give sulfisoxazole at least 1 hour before or 2 hours after meals for maximum absorption. Shake oral suspensions well before administering to ensure correct dosage.

• Patient should avoid large doses of vitamin C, which could acidify urine.

• Tell parents to give drug with a generous amount of water and to encourage adequate fluid intake. Explain that tablet may be crushed and swallowed with water to ensure maximal absorption.

• Be sure parents understand how and when to administer sulfisoxazole; urge them to complete entire prescribed regimen, to comply with instructions for around-the-clock dosage, and to keep follow-up appointments.

• Teach signs and symptoms of hypersensitivity and other adverse reactions, and emphasize need to report these, specifically urge patient to report bloody urine, difficult breathing, rash, fever, chills, or severe fatigue.

• Teach signs and symptoms of bacterial and fungal superinfection to patients and parents and if low or resistance from immunosuppressants or irradiation is evident, emphasize need to report them.

• Teach parents and patients to prevent superinfection by practicing meticulous oral and anogenital hygiene. Parents of infants and toddlers should keep diaper area clean and dry and avoid using plastic pants.

• Advise parents of diabetic patients not to monitor urine glucose levels with Clinitest; sulfonamides alter results of tests utilizing cupric sulfate.

• Advise patient or parents to tell new dentist or physician of sulfonamide therapy.

• Teach parents to check expiration date of drug and how to store drug, and to discard unused drug.

---

sutilains
Travase

• Classification: topical debriding agent (proteolytic enzyme)

How supplied

Available by prescription only
Ointment: 82,000 Casein units/g

Indications, route, and dosage

Debridement of major burns, decubitus ulcers, ulcers in peripheral vascular disease and incisional, traumatic, and pyogenic wounds

Children and adults: After cleansing and moistening wound area, apply thinly to area, extending ¼" to

---

½″ beyond area to be debrided. Cover with loose, wet dressing t.i.d. or q.i.d.

Action and kinetics
• *Proteolytic action:* Sutilains converts denatured proteins found in necrotic tissue and exudates to peptides and amino acids.
• *Kinetics in adults:* Absorption is limited with topical use.

Contraindications and precautions
Sutilains is contraindicated for use on wounds communicating with major body cavities or those containing exposed major nerves or nerve tissue; on fungating neoplastic ulcers; and in pregnant women and women of childbearing age. Sutilains should be used with caution near the eyes or mucous membranes. Avoid applying the drug to more than 10% to 15% of the burned area at one time.

Interactions
Concomitant use with detergents and anti-infectives, such as benzalkonium chloride, hexachlorophene, and nitrofurazone iron, and with metallic compounds, such as thimerosal and silver nitrate, may decrease activity of sutilains.

Effects on diagnostic tests
None reported.

Adverse reactions
• Local: pain, paresthesias, bleeding, and transient dermatitis.
  Note: Drug should be discontinued if sensitization develops or if bleeding or dermatitis occurs at wound site.

Overdose and treatment
If drug accidentally contacts eyes, flush eyes repeatedly with large amounts of normal saline solution or sterile water.

▶ Special considerations
• Maintain strict aseptic conditions when applying drug.
• Cleanse area with normal saline solution or water before applying the drug. Wound area should be well moistened before applying sutilains.
• Concomitant systemic or topical antibiotic therapy or prophylaxis may be necessary; if topical, apply sutilains first.
• Refrigerate ointment at 36.6° to 50° F. (2° to 10° C.).
• Maximal effect usually is achieved in 5 to 7 days for burns and wounds and in 8 to 12 days for decubital and peripheral vascular ulcers.

---

terbuterline sulfate
Brethine, Bricanyl

• Classification: bronchodilator (adrenergic [beta₂ agonist])

How supplied
Available by prescription only
Tablets: 2.5 mg, 5 mg
Aerosol inhaler: 200 mcg/metered spray
Injection: 1 mg/ml parenteral

Indications, route, and dosage
Relief of bronchospasm in patients with reversible obstructive airway disease
†*Children under age 12:* Initially, 0.05 mg/kg P.O. t.i.d.; maximum dosage, 5 mg daily. Or, 0.005 to 0.010 mg/kg S.C.; may be repeated q 20 minutes.
Children age 12 and over and adults: Administer 5 mg P.O. t.i.d. at 6-hour intervals. Maximum dosage, 15 mg daily. If adverse reactions occur or for children ages 12 to 15, dosage may be reduced to 2.5 mg P.O. t.i.d.; maximum, 7.5 mg daily. Alternatively, 0.25 mg S.C. may be repeated in 15 to 30 minutes; maximum, 0.5 mg q 4 hours. Alternatively, 2 inhalations q 4 to 6 hours with 1 minute elapsing between inhalations.

Action and kinetics
• *Bronchodilator action:* Terbutaline acts directly on beta₂-adrenergic receptors to relax bronchial smooth muscle, relieving bronchospasm and reducing airway resistance. Cardiac and CNS stimulation may occur with high doses.
• *Kinetics in adults:* 33% to 50% of an oral dose is absorbed through the GI tract. Onset of action occurs within 30 minutes, peaks within 2 to 3 hours, and persists for 4 to 8 hours. After S.C. injection, onset occurs within 15 minutes, peaks within 30 to 60 minutes, and persists for 1½ to 4 hours. After oral inhalation, onset of action occurs within 5 to 30 minutes, peaks within 1 to 2 hours, and persists for 3 to 4 hours.
Terbutaline is widely distributed throughout the body and partially metabolized in the liver to inactive compounds. After parenteral administration, 60% is excreted unchanged in urine, 3% in feces via bile, and the remainder in urine as metabolites. After oral administration, most of the drug is excreted as metabolites.

Contraindications and precautions
Terbutaline is contraindicated in patients with known hypersensitivity to the drug or to other sympathomimetics. It should be used with caution in patients with diabetes, hypertension, hyperthyroidism, or cardiac disease (especially when associated with dysrhythmias).

Interactions
When used concomitantly with other sympathomimetics, terbutaline may potentiate adverse cardiovascular effects of the other drugs; however, as an aerosol bronchodilator (adrenergic stimulator type), concomitant use may relieve acute bronchospasm in patients on long-term oral terbutaline therapy.
Beta blockers may antagonize bronchodilating effects of terbutaline. Use of MAO inhibitors within 14 days of terbutaline or the concomitant use of tricyclic antidepressants may potentiate terbutaline's effects on the vascular system.

Effects on diagnostic tests
None reported.

Adverse reactions
• CNS: *nervousness, tremors,* dizziness, *headache,* anxiety, restlessness, *lethargy,* vertigo, drowsiness, insomnia, *irritability.*
• CV: *increased heart rate,* palpitations, tachycardia, dysrhythmias, angina, ECG changes, *hypotension or hypertension.*
• GI: *nausea, vomiting,* digestive disorders.
• Other: bronchoconstriction, *sweating,* tinnitus, dyspnea, wheezing, unusual taste, drying or irritation of oropharynx.
Note: Drug should be discontinued if hypersensitivity or bronchoconstriction occurs.

Overdose and treatment
Clinical manifestations of overdose include exaggeration of common adverse reactions, particularly dysrhythmias, seizures, nausea, and vomiting. Treatment requires supportive measures. If patient is conscious and ingestion was recent, induce emesis and follow with gastric lavage. If patient is comatose, after endotracheal tube is in place with cuff inflated, perform gastric lavage; then administer activated charcoal to reduce drug absorption. Maintain adequate airway, provide cardiac and respiratory support, and monitor vital signs closely.

▶ Special considerations
• Monitor blood pressure, pulse, and respiratory and urinary output carefully during therapy.
• The preservative sodium bisulfite is present in many adrenergic formulations. Patients with a history of allergy to sulfites should avoid preparations that contain this preservative.
• Therapy should be administered when patient arises in morning and before meals to reduce fatigue by improving lung ventilation.
• Adrenergic inhalation may be alternated with other drug administration (steroids, other adrenergics) if

---

‡May contain sulfites   ♦May contain tartrazine   ♦♦May contain benzyl alcohol

necessary, but should not be administered simultaneously because of danger of excessive tachycardia.
• Do not use discolored or precipitated solutions.
• Protect solutions from light, freezing, and heat. Store at controlled room temperature.
• Systemic absorption can follow applications to nasal and conjunctival membranes, though infrequently. If symptoms of systemic absorption occur, patient should stop the drug.
• Prolonged or too-frequent use may cause tolerance to bronchodilating and cardiac stimulant effect. Rebound bronchospasm may follow end of drug effect.
• Protect injection solution from light. Do not use if discolored.
• Double-check dosage: oral is 2.5 mg, whereas S.C. is 0.25 mg. *Note:* A decimal error can be fatal.
• Give S.C. injection in lateral deltoid area.
• Cardiovascular effects are more likely with S.C. route and when patient has dysrhythmias. Check pulse rate and blood pressure before each dose, and monitor for any changes from baseline.
• Most adverse reactions are transient; however, tachycardia may persist for a relatively long time.
• Patient may use tablets and aerosol concomitantly. Carefully monitor patient for toxicity.
• Aerosol terbutaline produces minimal cardiac stimulation and tremors.
• Monitor neonate for hypoglycemia if the mother used terbutaline to prevent premature labor.

Information for parents and patient
• Treatment should start with first symptoms of bronchospasm.
• Dosage and recommended method of inhaling may vary with type of nebulizer and formulation used. Carefully instruct parents and patient in correct use of nebulizer and warn the patient to use lowest effective dose.
• Information and instructions are furnished with the aerosol forms of these drugs. Urge parents and patient to read them carefully and ask questions if necessary.
• Instruct patient to wait 1 full minute after initial 1 to 2 inhalations of adrenergic to be sure of necessity for another dose. Drug action should begin immediately and peak within 5 to 15 minutes.
• Teach parents and patient that a single aerosol treatment is usually enough to control an asthma attack and to call promptly if the patient requires more than three aerosol treatments in 24 hours. Explain that overuse of adrenergic bronchodilators may cause tachycardia, palpitations, headache, nausea and dizziness, loss of effectiveness, possible paradoxical reaction, and cardiac arrest.
• Tell parents to call if bronchodilator causes dizziness, chest pain, or lack of therapeutic response to usual dose.
• Tell parents that patient should avoid other adrenergic medications unless they are prescribed.
• Instruct parents and patient to avoid simultaneous administration with adrenocorticoid aerosol. Separate administration time by 15 minutes.
• Inform parents and patient that saliva and sputum may appear pink after inhalation treatment.
• Demonstrate and give parents and patient instructions on proper use of inhaler: Shake canister thoroughly to activate; place mouthpiece well into mouth, aimed at back of throat. Close lips and teeth around mouthpiece. Exhale through nose as completely as possible, then inhale through mouth slowly and deeply while actuating the nebulizer to release dose. Hold breath 10 seconds (count "1-100, 2-100, 3-100," until "10-100" is reached); remove mouthpiece, and then exhale slowly.
• Caution patient to keep spray away from eyes.
• Tell parents and patient that increased fluid intake facilitates clearing of secretions.
• Teach parents and patient how to accomplish postural drainage, to cough productively, and to clap and vibrate to promote good respiratory hygiene.
• Instruct parents and patient taking oral terbutaline on how to take pulse rate and to call if pulse varies significantly from baseline.
• Warn parents and patient not to puncture aerosol terbutaline container. Contents are under pressure. Instruct the parents and patient not to store it near heat or open flame; to expose it to temperatures above 120° F. (48.9° C.), which may burst the container; or to discard container into a fire or incinerator. Drug should be stored out of small children's reach.
• Advise parents that patient should take a missed dose within 1 hour. After 1 hour, he should omit dose and resume regular schedule; patient should not double the dose.
• Instruct the parents and patient to use terbutaline only as directed. If the drug produces no relief or his condition worsens, parents should call promptly. Excessive or prolonged use of aerosol form can lead to tolerance.
• Warn parents not to give patient nonprescription drugs without medical approval. Many cold and allergy remedies contain a sympathomimetic agent that may be harmful when combined with terbutaline.
• Tell parents and patient not to discard drug applicator. Refill units are available.

terfenadine
Seldane

• Classification: antihistamine H$_1$-receptor antagonist (butyrophenone derivative)

How supplied
Available by prescription only
Tablets: 60 mg

Indications, route, and dosage
Rhinitis, allergy symptoms
Children age 3 to 5: 15 mg P.O. b.i.d.
Children age 6 to 12: 30 to 60 mg P.O. b.i.d.
Children over age 12 and adults: 60 mg P.O. b.i.d.

Action and kinetics
• *Antihistamine action:* Antihistamines compete with histamine for histamine H$_1$-receptor sites on the smooth muscle of the bronchi, GI tract, uterus, and large blood vessels; by binding to cellular receptors, they prevent access of histamine and suppress his-

tamine-induced allergic symptoms, even though they do not prevent its release.

• *Kinetics in adults:* Terfenadine is well absorbed from the GI tract; after a 60-mg dose, action begins within 1 to 2 hours and peaks in 3 to 6 hours. Terfenadine is distributed mainly into the lungs, liver, GI tract, spleen, and bile; lower concentrations have been detected in the blood, kidneys, and heart.

Terfenadine is extensively (97%) protein-bound; it does not cross the blood-brain barrier, and it is unknown if the drug crosses the placenta or is distributed into breast milk. Plasma half-life of terfenadine is 3½ hours. Terfenadine is metabolized almost completely in the GI tract and liver (first-pass effect). Terfenadine's elimination half-life is about 16 to 23 hours. Only 1% of drug is excreted unchanged; about 60% of drug and metabolites is excreted in feces, with the remaining 40% excreted in urine.

Contraindications and precautions
Terfenadine is contraindicated in patients with known hypersensitivity to the drug. It should be used with caution in patients with asthma or other lower respiratory diseases, because its mild anticholinergic effects might aggravate these conditions.

Interactions
No significant interactions have been reported. Unlike other antihistamines, terfenadine has minimal anticholinergic activity and does not potentiate the CNS effects of alcohol, antianxiety agents, or other CNS depressants.

Effects on diagnostic tests
Terfenadine should be discontinued 2 days before using diagnostic skin tests, to prevent masking of test response.

Adverse reactions
• CNS: fatigue, dizziness, headache.
• EENT: dry mouth and throat, nasal stuffiness.
• GI: nausea, abdominal distress.

Overdose and treatment
Patients involved in the few known instances of overdose have been asymptomatic or have had mild headache, nausea, and confusion. One patient who ingested 56 tablets (3,360 mg) of Seldane developed ventricular dysrhythmia progressing to fibrillation; he responded well to defibrillation and lidocaine. Because the potential for cardiac dysrhythmias exists, continue cardiac monitoring for at least 24 hours.

Treat overdose by inducing emesis with ipecac syrup (in conscious patient), followed by activated charcoal to absorb any excess drug that may have remained in the stomach. Use gastric lavage if the patient is unconscious or if induction of vomiting fails. It is unknown if terfenadine is dialyzable.

▶ **Special considerations**
• Although its safety has not been established in children under age 12, terfenadine has been used in children age 3 to 12.
• Children, especially those under age 6, may experience paradoxical hyperexcitability with restless-

ness, insomnia, nervousness, euphoria, tremors, and seizures.
• Drug may have drying effect in patients with asthma or other lower airway disease; keep patient well hydrated.
• Terfenadine does not cause drowsiness and sedation associated with other antihistamines because it does not cross the blood-brain barrier; anticholinergic and antiserotonin effects are mild.
• Reduce GI distress by giving drug with food; give sugarless gum, sour hard candy, or ice chips to relieve dry mouth; increase fluid intake (if allowed) or humidify air to decrease adverse effect of thickened secretions.

Information for parents and patient
• Advise parents that patient should take drug with meals or snack to prevent gastric upset and use any of the following measures to relieve dry mouth; warm water rinses, artificial saliva, ice chips, or sugarless gum or candy. Patient should avoid overusing mouthwash, which may add to dryness (alcohol content) and destroy normal flora.
• Warn parents that child should avoid hazardous activities that require balance or alertness until the extent of CNS effects are known and to seek medical approval before administering tranquilizers, sedatives, pain relievers, or sleeping medications.
• Warn parents to discontinue terfenadine 2 days before diagnostic skin tests, to preserve accuracy of tests.
• Instruct parents and patient not to exceed prescribed dosage.
• Tell parents to store the drug in a tightly sealed container away from heat and direct sunlight.

testosterone
Andro 100, Andronaq-50, Histerone, Testaqua, Testoject-50, T pellets

testosterone cypionate
Andro-Cyp 100, Andro-Cyp 200, Andronate, dep Andro 100, dep Andro 200, Depo-Testosterone, Duratest, Testa-C, Testoject LA

testosterone enanthate
Andro L.A. 200, Andryl, Delatestryl, Everone, Testone L.A., Testrin-P.A.

testosterone propionate
Testex

• Classification: androgen replacement, antineoplastic (androgen)

How supplied
Available by prescription only
Testosterone
Injection (aqueous suspension): 25 mg/ml, 50 mg/ml, 100 mg/ml
Pellets (sterile) for subcutaneous implantation: 75 mg

---

‡May contain sulfites   ◆May contain tartrazine   ◆◆May contain benzyl alcohol

Testosterone cypionate (in oil)
Injection: 50 mg/ml, 100 mg/ml, 200 mg/ml
Testosterone enanthate (in oil)
Injection: 100 mg/ml, 200 mg/ml
Testosterone propionate (in oil)
Injection: 25 mg/ml, 50 mg/ml, 100 mg/ml

Indications, route, and dosage
Male hypogonadism
Testosterone or testosterone propionate
Adults: 10 to 25 mg I.M. two or three times weekly.
Testosterone cypionate or enanthate
Adults: 50 to 400 mg I.M. q 2 to 4 weeks. Then testosterone pellets (150 mg to 450 mg) S.C. q 3 to 6 months.
Delayed puberty in males
Testosterone or testosterone propionate
Adolescents: 12.5 to 25 mg I.M. two or three times weekly for up to 6 months.
Testosterone cypionate or enanthate
Adolescents: 25 to 200 mg I.M. q 2 to 4 weeks for up to 6 months.

Action and kinetics
• *Androgenic action:* Testosterone is the endogenous androgen that stimulates receptors in androgen-responsive organs and tissues to promote growth and development of male sexual organs and secondary male sexual characteristics.
• *Antineoplastic action:* Testosterone exerts inhibitory, antiestrogenic effects on hormone-responsive breast tumors and metastases.
• *Kinetics in adults:* Testosterone and its esters must be administered parenterally because they are inactivated rapidly by the liver when given orally. The onset of action of testosterone's cypionate and enanthate esters is somewhat slower than that of testosterone itself.

Testosterone is normally 98% to 99% plasma-protein bound, primarily to the testosterone-estradiol binding globulin.

Testosterone is metabolized to several 17-ketosteroids by two main pathways in the liver. A large portion of these metabolites then form glucuronide and sulfate conjugates. The plasma half-life of testosterone ranges from 10 to 100 minutes. The cypionate and enanthate esters of testosterone have longer durations of action than testosterone.

Very little unchanged testosterone appears in urine or feces. Approximately 90% of metabolized testosterone is excreted in urine in the form of sulfate and glucuronide conjugates.

Contraindications and precautions
Testosterone is contraindicated in patients with severe renal or cardiac disease, which may be worsened by the fluid and electrolyte retention caused by this drug; in patients with hepatic disease because impaired elimination of the drug may cause toxic accumulation; in male patients with prostatic or breast cancer, benign prostatic hypertrophy with obstruction, or undiagnosed abnormal genital bleeding because the drug can stimulate the growth of cancerous breast or prostate tissue; and in pregnant or breast-feeding patients because animal studies have shown that administration of androgens during pregnancy causes masculinization of the fetus.

Interactions
In patients with diabetes, decreased blood glucose levels may require adjustment of insulin dosage.

Testosterone may potentiate the effects of warfarin-type anticoagulants, prolonging prothrombin time. Concurrent administration with oxyphenbutazone may increase serum oxyphenbutazone concentrations.

Effects on diagnostic tests
Testosterone may cause abnormal results of glucose tolerance tests. Thyroid function test results (protein-bound iodine, radioactive iodine uptake, thyroid-binding capacity) and serum 17-ketosteroid levels may decrease. Liver function test results, prothrombin time (especially in patients on anticoagulant therapy), and serum creatinine levels may be elevated. Because of the anabolic activity of testosterone, increases may occur in serum sodium, potassium, calcium, phosphate, and cholesterol levels.

Adverse reactions
• Androgenic *in females:* deepening of voice, clitoral enlargement, changes in libido; *in males:* prepubertal—premature epiphyseal closure, priapism, phallic enlargement; postpubertal—testicular atrophy, oligospermia, decreased ejaculatory volume, impotence, gynecomastia, epididymitis.
• CNS: headache, anxiety, mental depression, generalized paresthesias.
• CV: edema.
• DERM: acne, oily skin, hirsutism, flushing, sweating, male pattern baldness.
• GI: gastroenteritis, nausea, vomiting, diarrhea, constipation, change in appetite, weight gain.
• GU: bladder irritability, vaginitis, menstrual irregularities.
• HEMA: polycythemia; suppression of clotting factors II, V, VII, and X.
• Hepatic: cholestatic hepatitis, jaundice.
• Local: pain at injection site, induration, irritation and sloughing with pellet implantation, postinjection furunculosis, edema.
• Other: hypercalcemia, hepatocellular cancer (with long-term use).
Note: Drug should be discontinued if hypercalcemia, edema, hypersensitivity reaction, priapism, or excessive sexual stimulation develops or if virilization occurs in females.

Overdose and treatment
No information available.

▶ Special considerations
• Children receiving androgens must be observed carefully for excessive virilization and precocious puberty. Androgen therapy may cause premature epiphyseal closure and short stature. Regular X-ray examinations of hand bones may be used to monitor skeletal maturation during therapy.
• Hypercalcemia symptoms may be difficult to distinguish from symptoms of the condition being treated unless anticipated and thought of as a cluster.

---

*Canada only †Unlabeled clinical use Italicized adverse reactions have been observed in children.

• Priapism in males indicates that dosage is excessive. Serious acute toxicities from large overdoses have not been reported.
• Yellowing of the sclera of the eyes, or of the skin, may indicate hepatic dysfunction resulting from administration of androgens.
• Androgens do not improve athletic performance, but they are abused for this purpose by some athletes. Risks associated with their use for this purpose far outweigh any possible benefits.
• Inject deeply I.M., preferably into a large muscle mass such as the upper outer quadrant of the gluteal muscle.
• Testosterone enanthate has been used to stimulate erythropoiesis.
• Testosterone pellets are administered by subcutaneous implantation. Use an injector or administer by surgical incision. The areas implanted are usually the infrascapular region or the posterior axillary line.
• Solutions of long-acting esters (enanthate and cypionate) may become cloudy if a wet needle is used to draw up the solution. This will not affect potency.
• Warming (to room temperature) and shaking vial will help redissolve crystals that have formed after storage.

Information for parents and patient

• Tell parents and patient to report GI upset, which may be caused by the drug.
• Advise patient to report too frequent or persistent penile erections.
• Advise parents and patient to report persistent GI distress, diarrhea, or the onset of jaundice.

tetanus antitoxin (TAT), equine

• Classification: tetanus antitoxin

How supplied

Available by prescription only
Injection: not less than 400 units/ml in 1,500-unit and 20,000-unit vials

Indications, route, and dosage

Indicated for tetanus prophylaxis or treatment only when human tetanus immune globulin is unavailable.
Tetanus prophylaxis
Children under 65 lb (30 kg): 1,500 units I.M. or S.C.
Children over 65 lb (30 kg) and adults: 3,000 to 5,000 units I.M. or S.C.
Tetanus treatment
Children and adults: 10,000 to 20,000 units injected into wound. Give additional 40,000 to 100,000 units I.V. Administer adsorbed tetanus toxoid at same time but at different sites and with a different syringe, because toxoid neutralization may occur.

Action and kinetics

• *Antitoxin action:* TAT neutralizes and binds toxin.
• *Kinetics in adults:* No information is available.

Contraindications and precautions

Use TAT with caution in patients allergic to equine-derived preparations.

Interactions

No significant interactions have been reported.

Effects on diagnostic tests

None reported.

Adverse reactions

• Local: pain, numbness, or skin eruptions at or near injection site.
• Systemic: joint pain, difficulty breathing, hypersensitivity, anaphylaxis, serum sickness.
Note: Drug should be discontinued if severe systemic reactions occur.

Overdose and treatment

No information available.

▶ Special considerations

• Obtain a thorough patient history of allergies, especially to horses and horse immune serum, and of previous reactions to immunizations.
• Test patient for sensitivity (against a control of normal saline solution in the other arm) before administration. Give 0.1 ml of a 1:100 dilution of antitoxin in 0.9% normal saline solution intradermally (0.05 ml of a 1:1,000 dilution in patients with a history of allergy).
• Epinephrine solution 1:1,000 should be available to treat allergic reactions.
• Use only when human tetanus immune globulin is not available.
• A preventive dose should be given to those with dirty wounds who have had three or fewer injections of tetanus toxoid and who have tetanus-prone injuries more than 24 hours old.
• Protection from TAT lasts approximately 15 days; duration of protection may be shorter in those who received a recent injection of a product derived from a horse.
• Because this product is derived from an animal source (that is, horses), patient may have anaphylactic reactions, such as rash, joint swelling or pain, fever, serum sickness, or difficulty breathing. Monitor patient closely and treat with medication, as ordered, if these effects occur.
• Store TAT between 36° and 46° F. (2° and 8° C.).

Information for parents and patient

Tell parents that the patient may experience pain, numbness, or rash at or near the injection site.

tetanus immune globulin, human (TIG)
Homo-Tet, Hyper-Tet

- Classification: tetanus prophylaxis agent (immune serum)

How supplied
Available by prescription only
Injection: 250 units per vial or syringe

Indications, route, and dosage
Tetanus exposure
Children and adults: 250 to 500 units I.M.
Tetanus treatment
Children and adults: Single doses of 3,000 to 6,000 units have been used. Optimal dosage schedules not established. Don't give at same site as toxoid.

Action and kinetics
- *Antitetanus action:* TIG provides passive immunity to tetanus. Antibodies remain at effective levels for 3 weeks or longer, which is several times the duration of antitoxin-induced antibodies. TIG protects the patient for the incubation period of most tetanus cases.
- *Kinetics in adults:* Slow. The serum half-life of TIG is approximately 28 days.

Contraindications and precautions
TIG should be used with caution in patients with known hypersensitivity to thimerosal, a component of this preparation.

Interactions
None reported.

Effects on diagnostic tests
None reported.

Adverse reactions
- Local: pain, tenderness, stiffness, and erythema at injection site.
- Systemic: slight fever, hives, angioedema, anaphylaxis.

Overdose and treatment
No information available.

▶ Special considerations
- Obtain a thorough history of injury, tetanus immunizations, last tetanus toxoid injection, allergies, and reactions to immunizations.
- Epinephrine solution 1:1,000 should be available to treat allergic reactions.
- For wound management, use TIG for prophylaxis in patients with dirty wounds if patient has had fewer than three previous tetanus toxoid injections, or if the immunization history is unknown or uncertain.
- Thoroughly cleanse and remove all foreign matter and necrotic tissue from wound.
- Immune globulin (gamma globulin) should only be given when TIG is not available.

- Do not confuse this drug with tetanus toxoid, which should be given at the same time (but at different sites) to produce active immunization.
- Administer I.M. in the deltoid muscle for adults and in the anterolateral thigh for infants and small children. Do not inject I.V.
- Tetanus risks severe morbidity and mortality in both mother and fetus if untreated. No fetal risk from the use of immune globulin has been reported to date.
- TIG has not been associated with an increased frequency of acquired immunodeficiency syndrome (AIDS). The immune globulin is devoid of human immunodeficiency virus (HIV). Immune globulin recipients do not develop antibodies to HIV.
- Store between 36° and 46° F. (2° and 8° C.). Do not freeze.

Information for parents and patient
- Explain to parents that the patient's chances of getting AIDS or hepatitis after receiving TIG are very small.
- Tell parents and patient that patient may experience some local pain, swelling, and tenderness at the injection site. Recommend acetaminophen to alleviate these minor effects.
- Encourage parents to report headache, skin changes, or difficulty breathing.

tetanus toxoid, adsorbed

tetanus toxoid, fluid

- Classification: tetanus prophylaxis agent (toxoid)

How supplied
Available by prescription only
Adsorbed toxoid
Injection: 5 to 10 Lf units of inactivated tetanus/0.5-ml dose, in 0.5-ml syringes and 5-ml vials
Fluid toxoid
Injection: 4 to 5 Lf units of inactivated tetanus/0.5-ml dose, in 0.5-ml syringes and 7.5-ml vials

Indications, route, and dosage
Primary immunization (adsorbed formulation)
Children and adults: 0.5 ml I.M. 4 to 6 weeks apart for two doses, then a third dose 1 year after the second dose. Booster dosage is 0.5 ml I.M. every 10 years.
Primary immunization (fluid formulation)
Children and adults: 0.5 ml I.M. or S.C. 4 to 8 weeks apart for three doses, then a fourth dose 6 to 12 months after the third dose. Booster dosage is 0.5 ml I.M. or S.C. every 10 years.
Tetanus prophylaxis in wound management
Children and adults: In patients with history of primary immunization and booster less than 10 years ago and a clean wound—no tetanus toxoid is required. In patients with history of primary immunization and booster more than 10 years ago and a clean wound—give 0.5 ml of adsorbed tetanus toxoid I.M. All patients with a dirty (tetanus-prone) wound and a history of primary immunization or booster more than 5 years

before should receive a booster dose of adsorbed tetanus toxoid I.U. In patients with incomplete or unknown history of immunization – give 0.5 ml adsorbed tetanus toxoid I.M. and complete primary immunization. In patients with no history of primary immunization – initiate primary immunization.

Concurrent use of tetanus immune globulin depends on primary immunization history, the type of wound (tetanus-prone), and care received for the wound. (See the "Tetanus immune globulin" entry for more information.)

Action and kinetics
• *Tetanus prophylaxis:* Tetanus toxoid promotes active immunity by inducing production of tetanus antitoxin.
• *Kinetics in adults:* Absorption is slow. Fluid formulation provides quicker booster effect. Distribution and metabolism are unknown. Excretion is unknown. Active immunity usually persists for 10 years. Adsorbed tetanus toxoid usually produces more persistent antitoxin titers than fluid tetanus toxoid.

Contraindications and precautions
Tetanus toxoid is contraindicated in patients with a history of neurologic or severe hypersensitivity reaction following a previous dose.

Interactions
Concomitant use with chloramphenicol, corticosteroids, or immunosuppressants theoretically may impair the immune response to tetanus toxoid. Avoid elective immunization under these circumstances.

Effects on diagnostic tests
None reported.

Adverse reactions
• Local: stinging, edema, erythema, pain, induration; nodule may develop and last for several weeks.
• Systemic: slight fever, chills, malaise, arthralgia, myalgia, flushing, urticaria, pruritus, tachycardia, hypotension, neurologic disorders, anaphylaxis, Arthus-like reaction.

Overdose and treatment
No information available.

▶ Special considerations
• Obtain a thorough history of allergies and reactions to immunizations.
• Epinephrine solution 1:1,000 should be available to treat allergic reactions.
• Determine tetanus immunization status and date of last tetanus immunization.
• The preferred I.M. injection site is the deltoid or midlateral thigh in adults and children and the midlateral thigh in infants.
• Preferably, tetanus immunization should be completed and maintained using multiple antigen preparations appropriate for the patient's age, such as diphtheria and tetanus toxoids (combined), or diphtheria and tetanus toxoids and pertussis vaccine.
• Shake vial vigorously to ensure a uniform suspension before withdrawing the dose.

• Do not confuse this drug with tetanus immune globulin.
• These toxoids are used to prevent, not treat, tetanus infections.
• Store at 36° to 46° F. (2° to 8° C.). Do not freeze.

Information for parents and patient
• Tell parents and patient what to expect after immunization: discomfort at the injection site and a nodule that may develop there and persist for several weeks. Patient also may develop fever, general malaise, or body aches and pains. Recommend acetaminophen to alleviate these effects.
• Instruct parents and patient not to use hot or cold compresses at the injection site because this may increase the severity of the local reaction.
• Encourage parents to report distressing adverse reactions.
• Tell parents that immunization requires a series of injections. Stress the importance of keeping scheduled appointments for subsequent doses.

---

tetracycline hydrochloride
Achromycin, Cefracycline*, Cyclopar, Medicycline*, Neo-Tetrine*, Novotetra*, Panmycin, Retet-s, Robitet, SK-Tetracycline, Sumycin, Tetracyn, Tetralean*, Tetrex, Topicycline (topical)

• Classification: antibiotic (tetracycline)

How supplied
Available by prescription only
Capsules: 250 mg, 500 mg
Tablets: 250 mg, 500 mg
Suspension: 125 mg/5 ml
Injectable: 100 mg, 250 mg, 500 mg
Topical: 2.2-mg/ml solution, 3% ointment

Indications, route, and dosage
Infections caused by sensitive organisms
Children over age 8: 6.25 to 12.5 mg/kg P.O. q 6 hours, or 12.5 or 25 mg/kg P.O. q 12 hours. Alternatively, give 5 to 8.3 mg/kg I.M. q 8 hours, or 7.5 to 12.5 mg/kg I.V. q 12 hours. Maximum daily dose is 250 mg.
Adults: 250 to 500 mg P.O. q 6 hours; 250 mg I.M. daily or 150 mg I.M. q 12 hours; or 250 to 500 mg I.V. q 8 to 12 hours (I.M. and I.V. hydrochloride salt only).
Gonorrhea
Children age 8 and older: 10 mg/kg P.O. q.i.d. for 5 days. Children under age 8 should receive spectromycin.
Adults: 500 mg P.O. q.i.d. for 7 days after penicillin, spectromycin or cephalosporin therapy.
†Early stages of Lyme disease
Children age 9 and older and adults: 250 mg P.O. q.i.d. for 10 to 20 days.

Acne
Adolescents and adults: Initially, 250 mg P.O. q 6 hours; then 125 to 500 mg P.O. daily or every other day, apply topical ointment generously to affected areas b.i.d. until skin is thoroughly wet.

Shigellosis
Adults: 2.5 g P.O. in one dose.

Superficial ocular infections and inclusion conjunctivitis
Adults and children: Instill 1 to 2 drops of ophthalmic solution in eye b.i.d., q.i.d., or more often, depending on severity of infection.

Trachoma
Children and adults: Instill 2 drops of ophthalmic solution in each eye b.i.d., t.i.d., or q.i.d. Continue for 1 to 2 months or longer, or use 1% ointment t.i.d. or q.i.d. for 30 days.

Prophylaxis of ophthalmia neonatorum
Neonates: 1 to 2 drops of ophthalmic solution into each eye shortly after delivery.

Infection prophylaxis in minor skin abrasions and treatment of superficial infections caused by susceptible organisms
Children and adults: Apply topical ointment to infected area one to five times daily.

Action and kinetics
• *Antibacterial action:* Tetracycline is bacteriostatic; it binds reversibly to ribosomal subunits, thus inhibiting bacterial protein synthesis. Its spectrum of action includes many gram-negative and gram-positive organisms, *Mycoplasma, Rickettsia, Chlamydia,* and spirochetes.

It is useful against brucellosis, glanders, mycoplasma pneumonia infections (some clinicians prefer erythromycin), leptospirosis, early stages of Lyme disease, rickettsial infections (such as Rocky Mountain spotted fever, Q fever, and typhus fever), and chlamydial infections. It is an alternative to penicillin for Neisseria gonorrhea, but because of a high level of resistance in the United States, other alternative agents should be considered.

• *Kinetics in adults:* Tetracycline is absorbed after oral administration; food and/or milk products significantly reduce oral absorption.

Tetracycline is distributed widely into body tissues and fluids, including synovial, pleural, prostatic, and seminal fluids, bronchial secretions, saliva, and aqueous humor; CSF penetration is poor. Tetracycline crosses the placenta; it is 20% to 67% protein-bound.

Tetracycline is not metabolized. It is excreted primarily unchanged in urine by glomerular filtration; plasma half-life is 6 to 12 hours in adults with normal renal function.

• *Kinetics in children:* Tetracyclines form a stable complex in bone-forming tissue and may cause permanent enamel hypoplasia or yellow-gray discoloration of teeth in children under age 8.

Contraindications and precautions
Tetracycline is contraindicated in children with known hypersensitivity to any tetracycline; in children under age 8 because of the risk of permanent discoloration of teeth, enamel defects, and retardation of bone growth; and in pregnancy.

Drug should be used cautiously in children with decreased renal function because it may elevate BUN levels and exacerbate renal dysfunction; and children apt to be exposed to direct sunlight or ultraviolet light, because of the risk of photosensitivity reactions.

Interactions
Tetracycline absorption may be decreased by antacids containing aluminum, calcium, or magnesium and laxatives containing magnesium because of chelation, and by food and dairy products, oral iron, and sodium bicarbonate.

Tetracycline may antagonize bactericidal effects of penicillin, inhibiting cell growth from bacteriostatic action; administer penicillin 2 to 3 hours before tetracycline.

Concomitant use of tetracycline increases the risk of nephrotoxicity from methoxyflurane.

Concomitant use of tetracycline necessitates lowered dosage of oral anticoagulants because of enhanced effects, and lowered dosage of digoxin because of increased bioavailability.

Effects on diagnostic tests
Tetracycline causes false-negative results in urine tests using glucose oxidase reagent (Clinistix or Tes-Tape), and false elevations in fluorometric tests for urinary catecholamines.

Tetracycline may elevate BUN levels in patients with decreased renal function.

Adverse reactions
• CNS: dizziness, headache, intracranial hypertension.
• CV: pericarditis.
• DERM: maculopapular and erythematous rashes, urticaria, photosensitivity, increased pigmentation, discolored nails and teeth. With topical use: temporary stinging or burning on application, slight yellowing of treated skin (especially in persons of fair complexion), severe dermatitis, fluorescence of treated skin under black light.
• EENT: sore throat, glossitis, dysphagia, eye itching (with ophthalmic use).
• GI: anorexia, epigastric distress, nausea, vomiting, diarrhea, stomatitis, enterocolitis, inflammatory lesions in anogenital region.
• GU: reversible nephrotoxicity (Fanconi's syndrome) with *outdated* tetracycline.
• HEMA: neutropenia, eosinophilia.
• Hepatic: hepatotoxicity with large doses given I.V.
• Metabolic: increased BUN level.
• Local: irritation after I.M. injection, thrombophlebitis.
• Other: bacterial and fungal superinfection.

   Note: Drug should be discontinued if signs of toxicity or hypersensitivity, progressive renal dysfunction, or superinfection occur; if erythema follows exposure to sunlight or ultraviolet light; or if severe diarrhea indicates pseudomembranous colitis.

Overdose and treatment
Clinical signs of overdose are usually limited to GI tract; give antacids or empty stomach by gastric lavage if ingestion occurs within the preceding 4 hours.

▶ Special considerations

• Assess child's allergic history; do not give tetracycline to any patient with a history of hypersensitivity reactions to any other tetracycline; monitor continuously for this and other adverse reactions.
• Obtain results of cultures and sensitivity tests before first dose, but do not delay therapy, check cultures periodically to assess drug efficacy.
• Monitor vital signs, electrolytes, and renal function studies before and during therapy.
• Check expiration dates. Outdated tetracycline may cause nephrotoxicity.
• Monitor for bacterial and fungal superinfection especially in debilitated children and those who are receiving immunosuppressants or radiation therapy; watch especially for oral candidiasis.
• Check patient's tongue for sign of monilia infection. Stress good oral hygiene. Stop drug if superinfection occurs. Carefully monitor patient's vital signs, especially temperature.
• Monitor for diarrhea, which may result from local irritation or superinfection.
• Children age 8 and under should not receive tetracycline unless there is no alternative. Tetracyclines can cause permanent discoloration of teeth, enamel hypoplasia and a reversible decrease in bone calcification.
• Reversible decreases in bone calcification have been reported in infants.
• Tetracycline may be administered by intracavitary instillation (chest tube) as a pleural sclerosing agent in malignant pleural effusion.

Oral administration
• Give oral tetracycline 1 hour before or 2 hours after meals for maximum absorption; do not give with food, milk or other dairy products, sodium bicarbonate, iron compounds, or antacids, which may impair absorption.
• Give water with and after oral drug to facilitate passage to stomach, because incomplete swallowing can cause severe esophageal irritation; do not administer within 1 hour of bedtime, to prevent esophageal reflux.
• Always follow manufacturer's directions for reconstitution and storage; keep product refrigerated and away from light.

Parenteral use administration
• Discard I.M. solutions after 24 hours because they deteriorate.
• Inject I.M. dose deeply into large muscle. Warn patient that it may be painful. Rotate sites. I.M. preparations in many cases contain a local anesthetic; ask patient about hypersensitivity to local anesthetics.
• For I.V. use, reconstitute 100 mg and 250 mg of powder for injection with 5 ml of sterile water; with 10 ml for 500 mg. Further dilute in dextrose 5% in 0.9% saline solution to volume appropriate for patient's weight. Refrigerate diluted solution if I.V. use and use within 24 hours.
• Do not mix tetracycline solution with any other I.V. additive; may cause drug inactivation or interaction.
• Avoid I.V. use of drug in patients with decreased renal function.
• I.V. use of tetracyclines in children with renal impairment, especially when dosage exceeds 2 g/day can cause hepatic failure.
• Monitor I.V. injection sites and rotate routinely to minimize local irritation. I.V. administration may cause severe phlebitis.
• For I.M. use, reconstitute 100 mg powder for injection with 2 ml sterile water for injection. Do not administer more than 2 ml per injection site. Concentration will be 50 mg/ml. Amount of diluent for 250 mg injection varies according to brand. Check with pharmacy or follow manufacturer's instructions.

Ophthalmic administration
• For prophylaxis of ophthalmia neonatorum, apply ointment no later than 1 hour after birth.
• Always wash hands before and after applying solution.
• Cleanse eye area of excessive exudate before application.
• Apply light finger-pressure on lacrimal sac for 1 minute after drops are instilled.
• Store in tightly closed, light-resistant container.

Topical administration
• Discontinue if no improvement or condition worsens.
• To control the rate of flow, increase or decrease pressure of applicator against skin.
• Avoid contact with eyes, nose, and mouth.
• Solution should be used within 2 months.

Information for parents and patient

• Teach signs and symptoms of adverse reactions, and emphasize need to report these promptly; urge parents to report any unusual effects.
• Teach parents of children with low resistance from immunosuppressants or irradiation how to recognize signs and symptoms of bacterial and fungal superinfection.
• Advise parents to prevent patient's direct exposure to sunlight and to use a sunscreen to help prevent photosensitivity reactions.
• Patient should take oral tetracycline with a full glass of water (to facilitate passage to the stomach), 1 hour before or 2 hours after meals for maximum absorption and not less than 1 hour before bedtime (to prevent irritation from esophageal reflux). Patient may need to take drug with food if drug causes vomiting or diarrhea.
• Emphasize that taking the drug with food, milk or other dairy products, sodium bicarbonate, or iron compounds may interfere with absorption. The patient who needs antacids should take them 3 hours after tetracycline.
• Emphasize importance of completing prescribed regimen exactly as ordered and keeping follow-up appointments.
• Teach parents and patient to prevent superinfection by practicing meticulous oral and anogenital hygiene. Parents of infants and toddlers should keep diaper area clean and dry and avoid using plastic pants.

Ophthalmic use
• Show patient how to instill ophthalmic form correctly. Warn patient not to touch tip of dropper to eye or surrounding tissue and to avoid sharing washcloths and towels with family members.
• If ophthalmic use causes signs of sensitivity, such

as itching lids or constant burning, parents should discontinue drug and call immediately.

Topical use
• Patient may continue normal use of cosmetics during topical use.
• Tell patient stinging may occur after topical use but will resolve quickly, and that drug may stain clothing.
• Explain that floating plug in bottle of topical tetracycline is an inert and harmless result of proper reconstitution of the preparation and should not be removed.
• Tell parents to check expiration dates and discard any expired drug.

---

theophylline
Aerolate, Bronkodyl, Constant-T, Elixophyllin, Quibron-T, Slo-bid, Slo-Phyllin, Somophyllin-T, Sustaire, Theobid, Theoclear, Theo-Dur, Theolair, Theophyl, Theospan-SR, Theo-24, Theovent, Uniphyl

theophylline sodium glycinate
Synophylate

• Classification: bronchodilator (xanthine derivative)

How supplied
Available by prescription only
Capsules: 50 mg, 100 mg, 200 mg, 250 mg
Capsules (extended-release): 50 mg, 60 mg, 65 mg, 75 mg, 100 mg, 125 mg, 130 mg, 200 mg, 250 mg, 260 mg, 300 mg
Elixir: 27 mg/5 ml, 50 mg/5 ml
Oral solution: 27 mg/5 ml, 53 mg/5 ml
Oral suspension: 100 mg/5 ml
Syrup: 27 mg/5 ml, 50 mg/5 ml
Tablets: 100 mg, 125 mg, 200 mg, 225 mg, 250 mg, 300 mg
Tablets (chewable): 100 mg
Tablets (extended-release): 100 mg, 200 mg, 250 mg, 300 mg, 400 mg, 500 mg
Theophylline and Dextrose 5%
Injection: 200 mg in 50 ml or 100 ml; 400 mg in 100 ml, 250 ml, 500 ml, or 1,000 ml; 800 mg in 500 ml or 1,000 ml
Theophylline sodium glycinate
Elixir: 110 mg/5 ml (equivalent to 55 mg anhydrous theophylline per 5 ml)

Indications, route, and dosage
Symptomatic relief of bronchospasm in patients not currently receiving theophylline who require rapid relief of acute symptoms
Loading dose: 6 mg/kg anhydrous theophylline, then—
Neonates and children under age 6 months: Dosage is highly individualized.
Children age 6 months to 9 years: 4 mg/kg q 4 hours for three doses; then 4 mg/kg q 6 hours.
Children age 9 to 16: 3 mg/kg q 4 hours for three doses; then 3 mg/kg q 6 hours.

Loading dose: 1 mg/kg for each 2 mcg/ml increase in theophylline concentration; then—
Premature infants (under 40 weeks' gestational age): 1 mg/kg q 12 hours.
Infants up to age 4 weeks: 1 to 2 mg/kg q 12 hours.
Infants age 4 to 8 weeks: 1 to 2 mg/kg q 8 hours.
Infants age 8 weeks to 6 months: 1 to 3 mg/kg q 6 hours.
Parenteral theophylline for patients not currently receiving theophylline
Loading dose: 4.7 mg/kg I.V. slowly; then maintenance infusion.
Children age 6 months to 9 years: 0.95 mg/kg/hour for 12 hours; then 0.79 mg/kg/hour.
Children age 9 to 16: 0.79 mg/kg/hour for 12 hours; then 0.63 mg/kg/hour.
Switch to oral theophylline as soon as patient shows adequate improvement.
Prophylaxis of bronchial asthma, bronchospasm of chronic bronchitis and emphysema
Children and adults: 16 mg/kg P.O. daily anhydrous theophylline divided q 6 or 8 hours; do not exceed 400 mg/day. Increase dose at 2- to 3-day intervals to maximum daily dose.
Children under age 9: 24 mg/kg P.O. daily in divided doses.
Children age 9 to 12: 20 mg/kg P.O. daily in divided doses.
Children age 12 to 16: 18 mg/kg P.O. daily in divided doses.
Neonatal apnea
Neonates: Loading dose 5.5 mg/kg P.O. Maintenance dose 1.1 mg/kg P.O. q 6 to 8 hours. Maintain blood level of 10 to 15 mcg/ml.
Symptomatic relief of bronchospasm in patients currently receiving theophylline
Children and adults: Each 0.5 mg/kg I.V. or P.O. (loading dose) plasma levels by 1 mcg/ml. Ideally, dose is based upon current theophylline level. In emergency situations, some clinicians recommend a 2.5 mg/kg P.O. dose of rapidly absorbed form if no obvious signs of theophylline toxicity are present.
Note: Dosage individualization is required. Use peak plasma and trough levels to estimate dose. Therapeutic range is 15 to 20 mcg/ml for bronchodilator effect, 10 to 15 mcg/ml for neonatal apnea. All doses are based upon theophylline anhydrous and lean body weight.
• Use with caution in neonates.
• Children usually require higher doses (on a mg/kg basis) than adults. Maximum recommended doses are 24 mg/kg/day in children younger than age 9; 20 mg/kg/day in children age 9 to 12; 18 mg/kg/day in children age 12 to 16; 13 mg/kg/day or 900 mg (whichever is less) in children and adults age 16 or older.

Action and kinetics
• *Bronchodilator action:* Mechanism of action is unknown. Drug may act by antagonizing adenosine receptors in the bronchi, or increasing intracellular cyclic AMP levels by inhibiting phosphodestrase, resulting in relaxation of the smooth muscle.
Drug also increases sensitivity of the medullary respiratory center to CO_2, to reduce apneic episodes.

It also prevents muscle fatigue, especially that of the diaphragm.

• *Kinetics in adults:* Drug is well absorbed. Rate and onset of action depend upon the dosage form; food may further alter rate of absorption.

Drug is distributed throughout the extracellular fluids; equilibrium between fluid and tissues occurs within an hour of an I.V. loading dose. Therapeutic plasma levels are 10 to 20 mcg/ml.

Theophylline is metabolized in the liver to inactive compounds. Half-life is 7 to 9 hours in adults, 4 to 5 hours in smokers, 20 to 30 hours in premature infants, and 3 to 5 hours in children. However, children younger than age 6 months may exhibit marked variability in theophylline metabolism.

Approximately 10% of the dose is excreted in urine unchanged. The other metabolites include 1,3 dimethyluric acid, 1 methyluric acid, and 3-methylxanthine.

Contraindications and precautions

Theophylline is contraindicated in patients with hypersensitivity to xanthines. Use cautiously in patients with compromised cardiac or circulatory function, diabetes, glaucoma, hypertension, hyperthyroidism, peptic ulcer, or gastroesophageal reflux.

Interactions

When used concomitantly, theophylline increases the excretion of lithium. Also, cimetidine, allopurinol (high dose), propranalol, erythromycin, and troleandomycin may cause an increase in serum concentrations of theophylline by decreasing the hepatic clearance. Barbiturates and phenytoin enhance hepatic metabolism of theophylline, decreasing plasma levels. Beta-adrenergic blockers exert an antagonistic pharmacologic effect.

Effects on diagnostic tests

Theophylline increases plasma free fatty acids and urinary catecholamines. Depending on assay used, theophylline levels may be falsely elevated in the presence of furosemide, phenylbutazone, probenecid, theobromine, caffeine, tea, chocolate, cola beverages, and acetaminophen.

Adverse reactions

• CNS: *irritability, restlessness,* headache, insomnia, dizziness, depression, *seizures.*
• CV: palpitations, *hypotension, sinus tachycardia, ventricular tachycardia* and other life-threatening dysrhythmias, extrasystoles, circulatory failure.
• GI: *nausea, vomiting,* epigastric pain, *loss of appetite, diarrhea.*
• Respiratory: tachypnea, respiratory arrest.
• Other: Fever, flushing, urinary retention, *hyperglycemia, muscle twitching.*

Note: Drug should be discontinued if any adverse reaction intensifies; this signals impending overdose.

Overdose and treatment

Clinical manifestations of overdose include nausea, vomiting, insomnia, irritability, tachycardia, extrasystoles, tachypnea, or tonic/clonic seizures. The onset of toxicity may be sudden and severe, seizures as the first sign. Induce emesis except in convulsing patients, then give activated charcoal (every 4 hours) and cathartics. Treat seizures with I.V. diazepam 0.1 to 0.3 mg/lg I.V. up to 10 mg; support respiratory and cardiovascular systems. Although theophylline clearance is usually rapid, charcoal hemoperfusion may be useful in severe overdose (plasma theophylline levels over 40 mcg/ml).

▶ Special considerations

• Many dosage forms and agents are available; it is important to select the form that offers maximum potential for patient compliance and minimal toxicity to the individual. Timed-release preparations may not be crushed or chewed.
• Dosage should be calculated from lean body weight, because theophylline does not distribute into fatty tissue.
• Individuals metabolize theophylline at different rates, and metabolism is influenced by many factors, including age and life-style (smoking).
• Daily dosage may need to be adjusted in patients with congestive heart failure or hepatic disease. Monitor carefully, using blood levels.
• Theophylline blood levels are used to monitor therapy.
• Do not crush extended-release tablets.
• Monitor vital signs and observe for signs and symptoms of toxicity.
• Serum theophylline measurements are recommended for patients receiving long-term therapy. Ideally, levels should be between 10 and 20 mcg/ml. Check every 6 months. If levels are less than 10 mcg/ml, increase dose by about 25% each day. If levels are 20 to 25 mcg/ml, decrease dose by about 10% each day. If levels are 25 to 30 mcg/ml, skip next dose and decrease by 25% each day. If levels are over 30 mcg/ml, skip next 2 doses and decrease by 50% each day. Repeat serum level determination.
• Drug is excreted in breast milk and may cause irritability, insomnia, or fretfulness in the breast-fed infant.

Information for parents and patient

• Instruct parents thoroughly regarding theophylline and dosage schedule; they should give a missed dose as soon as possible but should not double the dose.
• Tell parents to administer drug at regular intervals as instructed, around the clock.
• Advise parents of the adverse effects and possible signs of toxicity.
• Tell parents to restrict xanthine-containing foods and beverages. Emphasize that caffeine increases potential for adverse effects.
• Tell patient smoking reduces drug's effectiveness.
• If GI upset occurs with liquid preparations or non-sustained release forms, give with food. Some timed-release capsules (Theo-Dur Sprinkle) may be opened, and the contents sprinkled on a spoonful of soft food such as applesauce or pudding.
• Tell parents that child must swallow granules whole (without chewing) and follow with juice or water.

thiabendazole
Mintezol

• Classification: anthelmintic (benzimidazole)

How supplied
Available by prescription only
Tablets (chewable): 500 mg
Oral suspension: 500 mg/5 ml

Indications, route, and dosage
Infections with pinworm, roundworm, threadworm, whipworm, cutaneous larva migrans, and trichinosis
Children and adults: 25 mg/kg P.O. b.i.d. for 2 to 5 days. Maximum dosage is 3 g daily. If lesions persist after 2 days, repeat course.
Note: Course of therapy varies depending on organism.
Pinworm—two doses daily for 1 day; repeat in 7 days; *Roundworm, threadworm, and whipworm*—two doses daily for 2 successive days; *Trichinosis*—two doses daily for 2 to 4 successive days.

Action and kinetics
• *Anthelmintic action:* Thiabendazole kills susceptible helminths by inhibiting fumarate reductase. It is the drug of choice for *Strongyloides stercoralis* (threadworm) infections and may be useful in disseminated strongyloidiasis. It is also preferred for oral and topical therapy of *Ancylostoma braziliense, Toxocara canis,* and *T. cati.* It has shown activity in certain other nematode infections, but other agents are preferred for the treatment of ascariasis, trichuriasis, uncinariasis, and enterobiasis.
• *Kinetics in adults:* Thiabendazole is absorbed readily; peak serum concentrations occur at 1 to 2 hours. Little is known about the distribution of thiabendazole. Thiabendazole is metabolized almost completely by hydroxylation and conjugation. Approximately 90% of a thiabendazole dose is excreted in urine as metabolites within 48 hours; about 5% is excreted in feces.

Contraindications and precautions
Thiabendazole is contraindicated in patients with known hypersensitivity to the drug. It should be used with caution in patients with compromised renal or hepatic function, in patients with malnutrition or anemia, and in patients in whom vomiting would be hazardous.

Interactions
Thiabendazole may inhibit the metabolism of aminophylline; concomitant use raises theophylline levels.

Effects on diagnostic tests
Transient elevations of AST (SGOT) levels have been reported.

Adverse reactions
• CNS: impaired mental alertness, impaired physical coordination, drowsiness, giddiness, headache, dizziness.
• DERM: rash, pruritus, erythema multiforme.
• GI: anorexia, nausea, vomiting, diarrhea, epigastric distress.
• Other: lymphadenopathy, fever, flushing, chills.
   Note: Drug should be discontinued if hypersensitivity reactions occur.

Overdose and treatment
Signs of overdose may include visual disturbances and altered mental status. Treatment includes induced emesis or gastric lavage if ingested within 4 hours, followed by supportive and symptomatic treatment.

▶ Special considerations
• Give drug after meals; shake suspension well to ensure accurate dosages.
• Drug may be given with milk, fruit juice, or food.
• Laxatives, enemas, and dietary restrictions are unnecessary.
• Assess patient and review laboratory reports for signs of anemia, dehydration, or malnutrition before starting therapy.
• Monitor patient for adverse reactions, which usually occur 3 to 4 hours after drug is administered. Adverse effects are usually mild and related to dosage and duration of therapy.

Information for parents and patient
• Warn parents and patient that drug causes drowsiness or dizziness.
• Teach parents and patient the signs of hypersensitivity and to call immediately if they occur.
• Patient should wash perianal area daily and change undergarments and bedclothes daily.
• Explain routes of transmission, and encourage testing of other household members and suspected contacts.
• To help prevent reinfection, instruct parents and patient in personal hygiene, including sanitary disposal of feces and hand washing and nail cleaning after defecation and before handling, preparing, or eating food.

---

thiamine hydrochloride (vitamin B₁)
Betalin S

• Classification: nutritional supplement (B complex vitamin)

How supplied
Available by prescription only
Injection: 1-ml ampules (100 mg/ml), 1-ml vials (100 mg/ml), 2-ml vials (100 mg/ml), 10-ml vials (100 mg/ml), 30-ml vials (100 mg/ml), 30-ml vials (200 mg/ml), 30-ml vials (100 mg/ml, with 0.5% chlorobutanol)

Available without a prescription
Tablets: 5 mg, 10 mg, 25 mg, 50 mg, 100 mg, 250 mg, 500 mg
Elixir: 2.25 mg/5 ml (with alcohol 10%)

Indications, route, and dosage
Beriberi
Children: Depending on severity, 10 to 50 mg I.M. daily for several weeks with adequate dietary intake.
Adults: Depending on severity, 10 to 500 mg I.M. t.i.d. for 2 weeks, followed by dietary correction and multivitamin supplement containing 5 to 10 mg thiamine daily for 1 month.
Anemia secondary to thiamine deficiency; polyneuritis secondary to alcoholism, pregnancy, or pellagra
Children: 10 to 50 mg P.O. daily in divided doses.
Adults: 100 mg P.O. daily.
"Wet beriberi," with myocardial failure
Adults and children: 100 to 500 mg I.V. for emergency treatment.
Dietary supplement
Infants: 300 to 500 mcg (0.3 to 0.5 mg) per day P.O.
Children: 500 mcg (0.5 mg) to 1 mg per day P.O.

Action and kinetics
• *Metabolic action:* Exogenous thiamine is required for carbohydrate metabolism. Thiamine combines with adenosine triphosphate to form thiamine pyrophosphate, a coenzyme in carbohydrate metabolism and transketolation reactions. This coenzyme is also necessary in the hexose monophosphate shunt during pentose utilization. One sign of thiamine deficiency is an increase in pyruvic acid. The body's need for thiamine is greater when the carbohydrate content of the diet is high. Within 3 weeks of total absence of dietary thiamine, significant vitamin depletion can occur. Thiamine deficiency can cause beriberi.
• *Kinetics in adults:* Thiamine is absorbed readily after oral administration of small doses; after oral administration of a large dose, the total amount absorbed is limited to 8 to 15 mg. In alcoholics and in patients with cirrhosis or malabsorption, GI absorption of thiamine is decreased. When thiamine is given with meals, its GI rate of absorption decreases, but total absorption remains the same. After I.M. administration, thiamine is absorbed rapidly and completely. Thiamine is distributed widely into body tissues. When intake exceeds the minimal requirements, tissue stores become saturated. About 100 to 200 mcg/day of thiamine is distributed into the milk of breast-feeding women on a normal diet. Thiamine is metabolized in the liver. Excess thiamine is excreted in the urine. After administration of large doses (more than 10 mg), both unchanged thiamine and metabolites are excreted in urine after tissue stores become saturated.

Contraindications and precautions
Thiamine is contraindicated in patients with suspected vitamin B_1 sensitivity; an intradermal test dose is recommended before parenteral administration. Thiamine is contraindicated in patients hypersensitive to the drug or to any ingredient in thiamine preparations. In suspected thiamine deficiency, administer thiamine before a glucose load is given.

Interactions
Concomitant use of thiamine with neuromuscular blocking agents may enhance the latter's effects.
Thiamine may not be combined with alkaline solutions (such as carbonates, citrates, or bicarbonates); thiamine is unstable in neutral or alkaline solutions.

Effects on diagnostic tests
Thiamine therapy may produce false-positive results in the phosphotungstate method for determination of uric acid and in the urine spot tests with Ehrlich's reagent for urobilinogen.
Large doses of thiamine interfere with the Schack and Waxler spectrophotometric determination of serum theophylline concentrations.

Adverse reactions
• CNS: restlessness.
• CV: hypotension after rapid I.V. injection, angioneurotic edema, cyanosis.
• DERM: warmth, pruritus, urticaria, sweating.
• EENT: tightness of throat (allergic reaction).
• GI: nausea, hemorrhage, diarrhea.
• Local: pain at I.M. injection site.
• Other: anaphylactic reactions, weakness, pulmonary edema, death.

Overdose and treatment
Very large doses of thiamine administered parenterally may produce neuromuscular and ganglionic blockade and neurologic symptoms. Treatment is supportive.

▶ Special considerations
• The RDA of thiamine is 0.4 to 1.4 mg/day in children, 1.2 to 1.7 mg/day in adults, and 1.4 to 1.6 mg/day during pregnancy and lactation.
• Give intradermal skin test before I.V. thiamine administration if sensitivity is suspected, because anaphylaxis can occur. Keep epinephrine available when administering large parenteral doses.
• I.M. injection may be painful. Rotate injection sites and apply cold compresses to ease discomfort.
• Accurate dietary history is important during vitamin replacement therapy. Help patient develop a practical plan for adequate nutrition.
• Total absence of dietary thiamine can produce a deficiency state in about 3 weeks.
• Subclinical deficiency of thiamine or other B vitamins is common in patients who are poor, are chronic alcoholics, follow fad diets, or are pregnant.
• Store in light-resistant, nonmetallic container.

Information for parents and patient
Inform parents about dietary sources of thiamine, such as yeast, pork, beef, liver, whole grains, peas, and beans.

---

‡May contain sulfites　　　◆May contain tartrazine　　　◆◆May contain benzyl alcohol

---

thioguanine (6-thioguanine, 6-TG)
Lanvis*, Thioguanine Tabloid

• Classification: antineoplastic (antimetabolite [cell cycle-phase specific, S phase])

How supplied
Available by prescription only
Tablets (scored): 40 mg

Indications, route, and dosage
Dosage and indications may vary. Check current literature for recommended protocol.
Acute lymphoblastic and myelogenous leukemia, acute nonlymphocytic leukemia, chronic granulocytic leukemia
Children and adults: Initially, 2 mg/kg daily P.O. (usually calculated to nearest 20 mg) or 75 to 100 mg/m²/day P.O.; then, if no toxic effects occur, increase gradually over 3 to 4 weeks to 3 mg/kg/day. Maintenance dosage is 2 to 3 mg/kg/day P.O. or 100 mg/m²/day P.O.

Action and kinetics
• *Antineoplastic action:* Thioguanine requires conversion intracellularly to its active form to exert its cytotoxic activity. Acting as a false metabolite, thioguanine inhibits purine synthesis. Cross-resistance exists between mercaptopurine and thioguanine.
• *Kinetics in adults:* After an oral dose, the absorption of thioguanine is incomplete and variable. The average bioavailability is 30%. Thioguanine distributes well into bone marrow cells. The drug does not cross the blood-brain barrier to any appreciable extent. Thioguanine is extensively metabolized to a less active form in the liver and other tissues. Plasma concentrations of thioguanine decrease in a biphasic manner, with a half-life of 15 minutes in the initial phase and 11 hours in the terminal phase. Thioguanine is excreted in the urine, mainly as metabolites.

Contraindications and precautions
Thioguanine is contraindicated in patients with a history of resistance to previous therapy with the drug. Use with caution in renal or hepatic dysfunction because of the potential for drug accumulation.

Interactions
None reported.

Effects on diagnostic tests
Thioguanine therapy may increase blood and urine levels of uric acid.

Adverse reactions
• GI: *nausea, vomiting, stomatitis,* diarrhea, anorexia. kopenia, anemia, thrombocytopenia (occurs slowly over 2 to 4 weeks).
• Hepatic: *hepatotoxicity,* jaundice.
• Metabolic: hyperuricemia.
  Note: Drug should be discontinued if jaundice occurs.

Overdose and treatment
Clinical manifestations of overdose include myelosup pression, nausea, vomiting, malaise, hypertension, and diaphoresis.
  Treatment is usually supportive and includes trans fusion of blood components and antiemetics. Induction o emesis may be helpful if performed soon after ingestion

▶ Special considerations
• Follow all established procedures for the safe and proper handling, administration, and disposal of chemo therapy.
• Attempt to alleviate or reduce anxiety in patient an family before treatment.
• Monitor BUN, hematocrit, platelet count, ALT (SGPT) AST (SGOT), LDH, serum bilirubin, serum creatinine uric acid, total and diferential leukocyte, and others a required.
• Total daily dosage can be given at one time.
• Give dose between meals to facilitate complete absorp tion. May administer at bedtime to minimize nausea an vomiting.
• Dose modification may be required in renal or hepati dysfunction.
• Monitor serum uric acid levels. Use oral hydration t prevent uric acid nephropathy. Alkalinize urine if serur uric acid levels are elevated.
• Stop drug if hepatotoxicity or hepatic tenderness oc curs. Watch for jaundice; may reverse if drug stoppe promptly.
• Do CBC daily during induction, then weekly durin maintenance therapy.
• Drug is sometimes ordered as 6-thioguanine.
• Avoid all I.M. injections when platelet count is low.

Information for parents and patient
• Instruct patient in proper oral hygiene including cau tion when using toothbrush, dental floss, and tooth picks. Chemotherapy can increase incidence of microbia infection, delayed healing, and bleeding gums.
• Patient's dental work should be completed before ther apy whenever possible, or delayed until blood counts ar normal.
• Stress importance of keeping follow-up appointment for monitoring hematologic status.
• Teach parents and patient to check for signs of blee ing/bruising. Parents may need to restrict child's partic ipation in contact sports. Such activity is dangerou when patient's platelets are low.
• Instruct parents to monitor neutropenic patient's tem perature every 4 hours (not rectally) and to report feve cough and other signs of infection *promptly.*
• Instruct patient to clean teeth with toothettes, gauz or soft toothbrush when platelets are low. Patient shou perform frequent oral hygiene and should avoid usir commercial mouthwashes which may contain alcoh and have an irritating effect. Solutions of sodium bica bonate or hydrogen peroxide are more appropriate ri ses.
• Instruct patient to avoid foods that are spicy and e> tremely hot or cold. Topical anesthetics administere before meals (swish and spit) may relieve mouth discom fort.
• Warn patient to avoid close contact with persons wl have taken a live vaccine (polio, measles, mumps, r

---

bella) and to avoid exposure to persons with bacterial or viral infection, because chemotherapy may increase susceptibility to infection. Instruct him to report signs of infection immediately.

• Patient should not receive immunizations during therapy and for several weeks after therapy. Members of the same household should not receive live virus immunizations during the same period. Explain importance of promptly reporting susceptible patient's exposure to chicken pox.

• Emphasize the importance of continuing drug despite nausea and vomiting. Tell parents to call promptly if vomiting occurs shortly after a dose is taken.

• Premedicating with an antiemetic may prevent nausea and vomiting. If vomiting occurs, administer antiemetics p.r.n.

• Patients who have received drugs with strong emetic properties may experience anticipatory nausea and vomiting at subsequent treatments. They may benefit from treatment with an anxiolytic drug.

• Encourage adequate fluid intake to increase urine output and facilitate excretion of uric acid.

• Instruct parents or patient to recognize signs of hepatotoxicity (jaundice) and emphasize the importance of reporting them promptly.

• As appropriate explain that sexually active patients should practice contraception while taking this drug.

---

thioridazine
Mellaril-S

thioridazine hydrochloride
Apo-Thioridazine*, Mellaril, Millazine, Novoridazine*, PMS Thioridazine*

• Classification: antipsychotic (phenothiazine [piperidine derivative])

How supplied
Available by prescription only
Tablets: 10 mg, 15 mg, 25 mg, 50 mg, 100 mg, 200 mg
Syrup: 10 mg/5 ml
Oral concentrate: 30 mg/ml, 100 mg/ml (3% to 4.2% alcohol)
Suspension: 25 mg/5 ml, 100 mg/5 ml

Indications, route, and dosage
Dysthymic disorder (neurotic depression), alcohol withdrawal, behavioral problems in children
Children over age 2: 1 mg/kg daily in divided doses.
Adults: Initially, 25 mg P.O. t.i.d. Maintenance dosage is 20 to 200 mg daily.

Action and kinetics
• *Antipsychotic action:* Thioridazine is thought to exert its antipsychotic effects by postsynaptic blockade of CNS dopamine receptors, thereby inhibiting dopamine-mediated effects.

Thioridazine has many other central and peripheral effects: It produces both alpha and ganglionic blockade and counteracts histamine- and serotonin-me-

diated activity. Its most prevalent adverse reactions are antimuscarinic and sedative; it causes fewer extrapyramidal effects than other antipsychotics.

• *Kinetics in adults:* Rate and extent of absorption vary with administration route: oral tablet absorption is erratic and variable, with onset ranging from ½ to 1 hour. Oral concentrates and syrups are much more predictable.

Thioridazine is distributed widely into the body, including breast milk. Peak effects occur at 2 to 4 hours; steady-state serum level is achieved within 4 to 7 days. Drug is 91% to 99% protein-bound.

Thioridazine is metabolized extensively by the liver and forms the active metabolite mesoridazine; duration of action is 4 to 6 hours.

Most of drug is excreted as metabolites in urine; some is excreted in feces via the biliary tract.

Contraindications and precautions
Thioridazine is contraindicated in patients with known hypersensitivity to phenothiazines and related compounds, including allergic reactions involving hepatic function; in patients with blood dyscrasias or bone marrow depression (adverse hematologic effects); in patients with disorders accompanied by coma, brain damage, CNS depression, circulatory collapse, or cerebrovascular disease (additive CNS depression and adverse effects on blood pressure); and in patients receiving adrenergic-blocking agents or spinal or epidural anesthetics (excessive respiratory, cardiac, and CNS depression).

Thioridazine should be used cautiously in patients with cardiac disease (dysrhythmias, congestive heart failure, angina pectoris, valvular disease, or heart block), encephalitis, Reye's syndrome, head injury, respiratory disease, epilepsy and other seizure disorders, glaucoma, prostatic hypertrophy, urinary retention, Parkinson's disease, and pheochromocytoma, because drug may exacerbate these conditions; and in hypocalcemia, because it increases the risk of extrapyramidal reactions.

Interactions
Concomitant use of thioridazine with sympathomimetics, including epinephrine, phenylephrine, phenylpropanolamine, and ephedrine (often found in nasal sprays), and with appetite suppressants may decrease their stimulatory and pressor effects. Thioridazine may cause epinephrine reversal.

Thioridazine may inhibit blood pressure response to centrally acting antihypertensive drugs, such as guanethidine, guanabenz, guanadrel, clonidine, methyldopa, and reserpine. Additive effects are likely after concomitant use of thioridazine with CNS depressants, including alcohol, analgesics, barbiturates, narcotics, tranquilizers, anesthetics (general, spinal, or epidural), and parenteral magnesium sulfate (oversedation, respiratory depression, and hypotension); antiarrhythmic agents, including quinidine, disopyramide, and procainamide (increased incidence of cardiac dysrhythmias and conduction defects); atropine and other anticholinergic drugs, including antidepressants, MAO inhibitors, phenothiazines, antihistamines, meperidine, and antiparkinsonian agents (oversedation, paralytic ileus, visual changes, and

---

‡May contain sulfites   ◆May contain tartrazine   ◆◆May contain benzyl alcohol

severe constipation); nitrates (hypotension); and metrizamide (increased risk of convulsions).

Beta-blocking agents may inhibit thioridazine metabolism, increasing plasma levels and toxicity.

Concomitant use with propylthiouracil increases risk of agranulocytosis; concomitant use with lithium may result in severe neurologic toxicity with an encephalitis-like syndrome and in decreased therapeutic response to thioridazine.

Pharmacokinetic alterations and subsequent decreased therapeutic response to thioridazine may follow concomitant use with phenobarbital (enhanced renal excretion); aluminum- and magnesium-containing antacids and antidiarrheals (decreased absorption); caffeine; or heavy smoking (increased metabolism).

Thioridazine may antagonize therapeutic effect of bromocriptine on prolactin secretion; it also may decrease the vasoconstricting effects of high-dose dopamine and may decrease effectiveness and increase toxicity of levodopa (by dopamine blockade). Thioridazine may inhibit metabolism and increase toxicity of phenytoin.

Effects on diagnostic tests

Thioridazine causes false-positive test results for urinary porphyrins, urobilinogen, amylase, and 5-HIAA, because of darkening of urine by metabolites; it also causes false-positive urine pregnancy results in tests using human chorionic gonadotropin as the indicator.

Thioridazine elevates test results for liver enzymes and protein-bound iodine and causes quinidine-like effects on the ECG.

Adverse reactions

• CNS: extrapyramidal symptoms – dystonia, akathisia, torticollis, tardive dyskinesia (dose-related, long-term therapy), sedation (high incidence), pseudoparkinsonism, drowsiness (frequent), neuroleptic malignant syndrome (dose-related; if untreated, fatal respiratory failure in over 20% of patients), dizziness, headache, insomnia, exacerbation of psychotic symptoms.
• CV: asystole, orthostatic hypotension (high incidence), tachycardia, dizziness or fainting, dysrhythmias, ECG changes, increased anginal pain after I.M. injection.
• EENT: blurred vision, tinnitus, mydriasis, increased intraocular pressure, ocular changes (retinal pigmentary change with long-term use).
• GI: dry mouth, constipation, nausea, vomiting, anorexia, diarrhea.
• GU: urinary retention, gynecomastia, hypermenorrhea, inhibited ejaculation.
• HEMA: transient leukopenia, *agranulocytosis*, thrombocytopenia, anemia (within 30 to 90 days).
• Local: contact dermatitis from concentrate or injectable form, muscle necrosis from I.M. injection.
• Other: hyperprolactinemia, photosensitivity (high incidence), increased appetite or weight gain, hypersensitivity (rash, urticaria, drug fever, edema, cholestatic jaundice [in 2% to 4% of patients within first 30 days]).

After abrupt withdrawal of long-term therapy, gastritis, nausea, vomiting, dizziness, tremors, feeling of heat or cold, sweating, tachycardia, headache, or insomnia may occur.

Note: Drug should be discontinued if any of the following occur: hypersensitivity, jaundice, agranulocytosis, neuroleptic malignant syndrome (marked hyperthermia, extrapyramidal effects, autonomic dysfunction), or severe extrapyramidal symptoms even after dose is lowered. Drug should be discontinued 48 hours before and 24 hours after myelography using metrizamide, because of the risk of convulsions. When feasible, drug should be withdrawn slowly and gradually; many drug effects persist after withdrawal.

Overdose and treatment

CNS depression is characterized by deep, unarousable sleep and possible coma, hypotension or hypertension, extrapyramidal symptoms, abnormal involuntary muscle movements, agitation, seizures, dysrhythmias, ECG changes, hypothermia or hyperthermia, and autonomic nervous system dysfunction.

Treatment is symptomatic and supportive and includes maintaining vital signs, airway, stable body temperature, and fluid and electrolyte balance.

Do not induce vomiting: Drug inhibits cough reflex, and aspiration may occur. Use gastric lavage, then activated charcoal and saline cathartics; dialysis does not help. Regulate body temperature as needed. Treat hypotension with I.V. fluids: *do not give epinephrine.* Treat seizures with parenteral diazepam or barbiturates; dysrhythmias with parenteral phenytoin (1 mg/kg with rate titrated to blood pressure); and extrapyramidal reactions with barbiturates, benztropine, or parenteral diphenhydramine 2 mg/kg/minute.

▶ Special considerations

• Check vital signs regularly for decreased blood pressure (especially before and after parenteral therapy) or tachycardia; observe patient carefully for other adverse reactions.
• Check intake and output for urinary retention or constipation, which may require dosage reduction.
• Monitor bilirubin levels weekly for first 4 weeks; monitor complete blood count, ECG (for quinidine-like effects), liver and renal function studies, electrolyte levels (especially potassium) and eye examinations at baseline and periodically thereafter, especially in patients on long-term therapy.
• Observe patient for mood changes to monitor progress; benefits may not be apparent for several weeks.
• Do not withdraw drug abruptly; although physical dependence does not occur with antipsychotic drugs, rebound exacerbation of psychotic symptoms may occur, and many drug effects persist.
• Carefully follow manufacturer's instructions for reconstitution, dilution, administration, and storage of drugs; slightly discolored liquids may or may not be all right to use. Check with pharmacist.
• Liquid and injectable formulations may cause a rash if skin contact occurs.
• Drug causes pink to brown discoloration of patient's urine.
• Thioridazine is associated with a high incidence of sedation, anticholinergic effects, orthostatic hypotension, and photosensitivity reactions.

---

*Canada only   †Unlabeled clinical use   Italicized adverse reactions have been observed in children

• Oral formulations may cause stomach upset. Administer with food or fluid.
• Check patient regularly for abnormal body movements (at least once every 6 months).
• Concentrate must be diluted in 2 to 4 oz of liquid, preferably water, carbonated drinks, fruit juice, tomato juice, milk, or pudding.
• Sugarless chewing gum, hard candy, or ice chips may help alleviate dry mouth.
• Protect liquid formulation from light.

Information for parents and patient
• Explain rationale and anticipated risks and benefits of therapy, and that full therapeutic effect may not occur for several weeks.
• Patient should avoid beverages and medications containing alcohol, and not take any other drug (especially CNS depressants) including nonprescription products without medical approval.
• Instruct parents of diabetic patients to monitor blood glucose levels, because drug may alter insulin needs.
• Teach parents or patient how and when to take drug, not to increase dose without medical approval, and never to discontinue drug abruptly; suggest taking full dose at bedtime if daytime sedation is troublesome.
• Advise parents to have patient lie down for 30 minutes after first dose (1 hour if I.M.) and to rise slowly from sitting or supine position to prevent orthostatic hypotension.
• Drugs are locally irritating; advise taking with milk or food to minimize GI distress. Warn that oral concentrates and solutions will irritate skin. Patient should not crush or open sustained-release products, but swallow them whole.
• Warn parents that excessive exposure to sunlight, heat lamps, or tanning beds may cause photosensitivity reactions (burn and abnormal hyperpigmentation); and that patient should avoid exposure to extremes of heat or cold, because of risk of hypothermia or hyperthermia induced by alteration in thermoregulatory function.
• Recommend sugarless gum, hard candy, or ice chips to relieve dry mouth.
• Explain that phenothiazines may cause pink to brown discoloration of urine.
• Explain the risks of dystonic reactions and tardive dyskinesia, and tell parents to report any abnormal body movements.
• Warn parents that spilling the liquid on the skin may cause rash and irritation.
• Explain that many drug interactions are possible. Patient should not take any other medication unless prescribed.
• Tell parents to call the physician promptly if patient develops difficulty urinating, sore throat, dizziness or fainting.
• Patient should avoid hazardous activities that require alertness until the drug's effect is established. Excessive sedation usually subsides after several weeks.
• Explain which fluids are appropriate for diluting the concentrate and the dropper technique of measuring dose.
• Store drug safely away from children.

thiotepa

• Classification: antineoplastic (alkylating agent [cell cycle-phase nonspecific])

How supplied
Available by prescription only
Injection: 15-mg vials

Indications, route, and dosage
Dosage and indications may vary. Check current literature for recommended protocol.
Breast, lung, and ovarian cancer; Hodgkin's disease; lymphomas
Children age 12 and over and adults: 0.2 mg/kg I.V. daily for 5 days, repeated q 2 to 4 weeks; or 0.3 to 0.4 mg/kg I.V. q 1 to 4 weeks.
Bladder tumor
Children age 12 and over and adults: 30 to 60 ml of a 1 mg/ml solution (thiotepa in distilled water) instilled in bladder once weekly for 4 weeks.
Neoplastic effusions
Children age 12 and over and adults: 0.6 to 0.8 mg/kg intracavity or intratumor q 1 to 4 weeks. Maintenance dosage is 0.07 to 0.8 mg/kg q 1 to 4 weeks.

Action and kinetics
• *Antineoplastic action:* Thiotepa exerts its cytotoxic activity as an alkylating agent, cross-linking strands of DNA and RNA and inhibiting protein synthesis, resulting in cell death.
• *Kinetics in adults:* The absorption of thiotepa across the GI tract is incomplete. Absorption from the bladder is variable, ranging from 10% to 100% of an instilled dose. Absorption is increased by certain pathologic conditions. Intramuscular and pleural membrane absorption of thiotepa is also variable. Thiotepa crosses the blood-brain barrier. Thiotepa is metabolized extensively in the liver; thiotepa and its metabolites are excreted in urine.

Contraindications and precautions
Thiotepa is contraindicated in patients with a history of hypersensitivity to the drug and in patients with preexisting hepatic, renal, or bone marrow impairment, because of the potential for additive toxicity.

Interactions
When used concomitantly, thiotepa may cause prolonged respirations and apnea in patients receiving succinylcholine. Thiotepa appears to inhibit the activity of pseudocholinesterase, the enzyme that deactivates succinylcholine. Use succinylcholine with extreme caution in patients receiving thiotepa.

Effects on diagnostic tests
Thiotepa therapy may increase blood and urine levels of uric acid and decrease plasma pseudocholinesterase concentrations.

---

‡May contain sulfites   ◆May contain tartrazine   ◆◆May contain benzyl alcohol

Adverse reactions
- CNS: dizziness.
- DERM: hives, rash.
- GI: *nausea, vomiting,* anorexia.
- GU: *interference with spermatogenesis, menstrual dysfunction.*
- HEMA: *bone marrow depression* (dose-limiting), leukopenia (begins within 5 to 30 days), thrombocytopenia, neutropenia, anemia.
- Metabolic: hyperuricemia.
- Local: *intense pain at administration site.*
- Other: headache, fever, tightness of throat, *pulmonary infiltrates and fibrosis.*

  Note: Drug should be discontinued if leukocyte or platelet count drops rapidly.

Overdose and treatment
Clinical manifestations of overdose include nausea, vomiting, and precipitation of uric acid in the renal tubules.

Treatment is usually supportive and includes transfusion of blood components, antiemetics, hydration, and allopurinol.

▶ Special considerations
- Follow established procedures for safe handling, administration, and disposal.
- Vital signs and patency of catheter or I.V. line throughout administration should be monitored.
- Treat extravasation promptly.
- Monitor BUN, hematocrit, platelet count, ALT (SGPT), AST (SGOT), LDH, serum bilirubin, serum creatinine, uric acid total and differential leukocyte.
- To reconstitute drug, use 1.5 ml of sterile water for injection to yield a concentration of 10 mg/ml. The solution is clear to slightly opaque.
- A 1 mg/ml solution is considered isotonic.
- Premedicating with an antiemetic may prevent nausea and vomiting. If vomiting occurs, administer antiemetics p.r.n.
- Patients who have received drugs with strong emetic properties may experience anticipatory nausea and vomiting at subsequent treatments. They may benefit from treatment with an anxiolytic drug.
- Use only sterile water for injection to reconstitute. Refrigerated solution is stable 5 days.
- Refrigerate dry powder; protect from light.
- Drug can be given by all parenteral routes, including direct injection into the tumor.
- Stop drug or decrease dosage if WBC count falls below 4,000/mm³ or if platelet count falls below 150,000/mm³.
- Drug may be mixed with procaine 2% or epinephrine 1:1,000, or both, for local use.
- Drug may be further diluted to larger volumes with normal saline solution, dextrose 5% in water, or lactated Ringer's solution for administration by I.V. infusion, intracavitary injection, or perfusion therapy.
- Withhold fluids for 8 to 10 hours before bladder instillation. Instill 60 ml of drug into bladder by catheter; ask patient to retain solution for 2 hours. Volume may be reduced to 30 ml if discomfort is too great. Reposition patient every 15 minutes for maximum area contact.
- To prevent hyperuricemia with resulting uric acid

nephropathy, allopurinol may be given; keep patient well hydrated. Monitor uric acid.
- Monitor CBC weekly for at least 3 weeks after last dose. Warn patient to report even mild infections.
- Use cautiously in bone marrow depression and renal or hepatic dysfunction.
- Avoid all I.M. injections when platelet count is low. Watch closely for signs of bleeding. Instruct patient to avoid nonprescription products containing aspirin.
- Toxicity may be delayed and prolonged because drug binds to tissues and stays in body several hours.
- GU adverse reactions are reversible in 6 to 8 months.

Information for parents and patient
- Advise parents to have patient avoid exposure to persons with bacterial or viral infections because chemotherapy can increase susceptibilty to infection. Parents should watch for and report any signs of infection promptly.
- Patient should avoid contact with persons who have received live virus immunizations (polio, measles/mumps/rubella). Explain importance of promptly reporting susceptible patient's exposure to chicken pox.
- Instruct parents to monitor neutropenic patient's temperature every 4 hours (not rectally) and to report fever, cough and other signs of infection *promptly.*
- Patient should complete dental work before therapy whenever possible, or delay it until blood counts are normal.
- Inform parents or patient that drug may cause headache and fever.
- Warn parents that patient may bruise easily because of drug's effect on blood count. Tell them to report any unusual bruising or bleeding promptly.
- Teach parents and patient to check for signs of bleeding and bruising. Parents may need to restrict child's participation in contact sports. Such activity is dangerous when patient's platelets are low.
- Stress importance of keeping follow-up appointments for monitoring hematologic status.
- Instruct patient to clean teeth with toothettes, gauze, or soft toothbrush when platelets are low. Patient should perform frequent oral hygiene and should avoid using commercial mouthwashes which may contain alcohol and have an irritating effect. Solutions of sodium bicarbonate or hydrogen peroxide are more appropriate rinses.
- Instruct patient to avoid foods that are spicy and extremely hot or cold. Topical anesthetics administered before meals (swish and spit) may relieve mouth discomfort.
- Advise parents that immunizations should be avoided if possible during therapy.
- Advise parents to encourage patient to drink plenty of fluids to facilitate the excretion of uric acid.
- If appropriate, explain that drug may cause menstrual irregularities, but sexually active patient should continue contraception during therapy with this drug.

thyroglobulin
Proloid

• Classification: thyroid hormone

How supplied
Available by prescription only
Tablets: 32 mg, 65 mg, 100 mg, 130 mg, 200 mg

Indications, route, and dosage
Cretinism and juvenile hypothyroidism
Children age 1 to 4 months: Initially, 15 to 30 mg P.O. daily, increased at 2-week intervals. Usual maintenance dosage is 30 to 45 mg P.O. daily.
Children age 4 to 12 months: 60 to 80 mg P.O. daily.
Children over age 1: Dosage may approach adult dosage (60 to 180 mg P.O. daily), depending on response.

Action and kinetics
• *Thyrotropic action:* Thyroglobulin affects protein and carbohydrate metabolism, promotes gluconeogenesis, increases the utilization and mobilization of glycogen stores, stimulates protein synthesis, and regulates cell growth and differentiation. The major effect of thyroglobulin is to increase the metabolic rate of tissue.
• *Kinetics in adults:* Thyroglobulin is absorbed from the GI tract. Distribution is not fully understood. It is highly protein-bound.

Contraindications and precautions
Thyroglobulin is contraindicated in patients with hypersensitivity to beef or pork and in patients with thyrotoxicosis, acute myocardial infarction, and uncorrected adrenal insufficiency because thyroid hormones increase tissue metabolic demands. Thyroglobulin is also contraindicated for treating obesity because it is ineffective and can cause life-threatening adverse reactions.

Thyroglobulin should be used cautiously in patients with angina or other cardiovascular disease because of the risk of increased metabolic demands; in patients with diabetes mellitus because of reduced glucose tolerance; in patients with malabsorption states; and in patients with long-standing hypothyroidism or myxedema because these patients may be more sensitive to the effects of thyroid hormones.

Interactions
Concomitant use of thyroglobulin with an adrenocorticoid or corticotropin changes thyroid status and may require dosage changes of thyroid, adrenocorticoid, or corticotropin. Concomitant use with an anticoagulant may alter the anticoagulant's effects, requiring an increase in thyroglobulin dosage. Concomitant use with tricyclic antidepressants or sympathomimetics may increase the effects of these medications or of thyroglobulin, possibly leading to coronary insufficiency or cardiac dysrhythmias.

Use with insulin may affect the dosage requirements of these agents. Estrogens, which increase serum thyroxine-binding globulin levels, raise thyroid hormone requirements. Hepatic enzyme inducers (such as phenytoin) may increase hepatic degradation of levothyroxine and raise dosage requirements of levothyroxine. Concomitant use with somatrem may accelerate epiphyseal maturation. I.V. phenytoin may release free thyroid. Cholestyramine or colestipol may impair absorption.

Effects on diagnostic tests
Thyroglobulin alters ^{131}I thyroid uptake, protein-bound iodine levels, and liothyronine uptake.

Adverse reactions
• CNS: nervousness, insomnia, tremors.
• CV: tachycardia, palpitations, dysrhythmias, angina pectoris, hypertension, elevated pulse pressure, cardiac arrest.
• GI: change in appetite, nausea, diarrhea.
• Other: headache, leg cramps, weight loss, sweating, heat intolerance, allergic skin reactions, fever, menstrual irregularities.
Note: Drug should be discontinued if patient develops signs of allergic reaction or hyperthyroidism.

Overdose and treatment
Clinical manifestations of overdose include signs and symptoms of hyperthyroidism, including weight loss, increased appetite, palpitations, nervousness, diarrhea, abdominal cramps, sweating, tachycardia, increased pulse and blood pressure, angina, cardiac dysrhythmias, tremors, headache, insomnia, heat intolerance, fever, and menstrual irregularities.

Overdose treatment requires reduction of GI absorption and efforts to counteract central and peripheral effects, primarily sympathetic activity. Use gastric lavage or induce emesis (follow with activated charcoal, up to 4 hours after ingestion). If the patient is comatose or is having seizures, inflate cuff on endotracheal tube to prevent aspiration. Treatment may include oxygen and artificial ventilation to support respiration. It should also include appropriate measures to treat CHF and control fever, hypoglycemia, and fluid loss. Propranolol may be used to combat many of the effects of increased sympathetic activity. Thyroid therapy should be withdrawn gradually over 2 to 6 days, then resumed at a lower dose.

▶ Special considerations
• During first few months of therapy, children may suffer partial hair loss. Reassure child and parents that this is temporary.
• Drug dosage varies widely among patients. Treatment should start at the lowest level, titrating to higher doses according to patient's symptoms and laboratory data, until euthyroid state is reached.
• Monitor prothrombin time; patients taking anticoagulants usually require lower doses.
• Monitor for signs of overdosage or hyperthyroidism, including changes in menstrual periods, coldness, constipation, dry puffy skin, headache, listlessness, muscle aches, nausea, vomiting, weakness, fatigue, and unusual weight gain.
• Signs of thyrotoxicosis or inadequate dosage therapy include diarrhea, fever, irritability, listlessness, rapid heartbeat, vomiting, and weakness.

- Variable hormonal content of commercial preparations may produce fluctuations of liothyronine and levothyroxine.
- Monitor patient's pulse rate and blood pressure.
- A.M. administration helps to prevent insomnia.

Information for parents and patient
- Advise parents and patient to report headache, diarrhea, nervousness, excessive sweating, heat intolerance, chest pain, increased pulse rate, or palpitations.
- Patient should take daily dose at the same time each day, preferably in the morning to avoid insomnia.
- Tell patient not to store medication in warm, humid areas, such as the bathroom, to prevent deterioration of the drug.

thyroid USP (desiccated)
Armour Thyroid, Dathroid, Delcoid, S-P-T, Thermoloid, Thyrar, Thyrocrine, Thyroid Strong, Thyro-teric

- Classification: thyroid hormone

How supplied
Available by prescription only
Tablets: 16 mg, 32 mg, 65 mg, 98 mg, 130 mg, 195 mg, 260 mg, 325 mg
Tablets (enteric-coated): 32 mg, 65 mg, 130 mg
Tablets (bovine origin): 32 mg, 65 mg, 130 mg
Capsules (porcine origin): 65 mg, 130 mg, 195 mg, 325 mg
Strong tablets (50% stronger than thyroid USP, and containing 0.3% iodine): 32 mg, 65 mg, 130 mg, 195 mg

Indications, route, and dosage
Cretinism and juvenile hypothyroidism
Children age 1 to 4 months: Initially, 15 to 30 mg P.O. daily, increased at 2-week intervals. Usual maintenance dosage is 30 to 45 mg P.O. daily.
Children age 4 to 12 months: 30 to 60 mg P.O. daily.
Children over age 1: Dosage may approach adult dosage (60 to 180 mg daily), depending on response.
Adult hypothyroidism
Adults: Initially, 60 mg P.O. daily, increased by 60 mg q 30 days until desired response is achieved. Usual maintenance dosage is 60 to 180 mg P.O. daily as a single dose.

Action and kinetics
- *Thyrotropic action:* Thyroid USP affects protein and carbohydrate metabolism, promotes gluconeogenesis, increases the utilization and mobilization of glycogen stores, stimulates protein synthesis, and regulates cell growth and differentiation. The major effect of thyroid is to increase the metabolic rate of tissue.
- *Kinetics in adults:* Thyroid USP is absorbed from the GI tract. Distribution is not fully understood. Thyroid USP is highly protein-bound. Metabolism and excretion are also not fully understood.

Contraindications and precautions
Thyroid USP is contraindicated in patients with hypersensitivity to beef or pork and in those with thyrotoxicosis, acute myocardial infarction, or uncorrected adrenal insufficiency (thyroid increases tissue metabolic demands). Thyroid USP also is contraindicated for treating obesity because it is ineffective and can cause life-threatening adverse reactions.

Thyroid USP should be used cautiously in patients with angina or other cardiovascular disease because of the risk of increased metabolic demands; in patients with diabetes mellitus because of reduced glucose tolerance; in patients with malabsorption states; and in patients with chronic hypothyroidism or myxedema because these patients may be more sensitive to the effects of thyroid.

Interactions
Concomitant use of thyroid USP with adrenocorticoids or corticotropin causes changes in thyroid status, and changes in thyroid dosages may require adrenocorticoid or corticotropin dosage changes as well. Concomitant use with anticoagulants may alter anticoagulant effect; an increased thyroid USP dosage may necessitate a lower anticoagulant dose.

Use with tricyclic antidepressants or sympathomimetics may increase the effects of these medications or of thyroid USP, possibly leading to coronary insufficiency or cardiac dysrhythmias. Use with insulin may affect dosage requirements of insulin. Estrogens, which increase serum thyroxine-binding globulin levels, raise thyroid USP requirements.

Hepatic enzyme inducers (for example, phenytoin) may increase hepatic degradation of levothyroxine, causing increased dosage requirements of levothyroxine. Concomitant use with somatrem may accelerate epiphyseal maturation. I.V. phenytoin may release free thyroid from thyroglobulin. Cholestyramine and colestipol may decrease absorption.

Effects on diagnostic tests
Thyroid USP therapy alters ^{131}I thyroid uptake, protein-bound iodine levels, and liothyronine uptake.

Adverse reactions
- CNS: nervousness, insomnia, tremors.
- CV: tachycardia, palpitations, dysrhythmias, angina pectoris, hypertension, widened pulse pressure, cardiac arrest.
- GI: change in appetite, nausea, diarrhea.
- Other: headache, leg cramps, weight loss, sweating, heat intolerance, allergic skin reactions, fever, menstrual irregularities.
Note: Drug should be discontinued if patient develops allergic reaction or signs of hyperthyroidism.

Overdose and treatment
Clinical manifestations of overdose include signs and symptoms of hyperthyroidism, including weight loss, increased appetite, palpitations, nervousness, diarrhea, abdominal cramps, sweating, tachycardia, increased pulse and blood pressure, angina, cardiac dysrhythmias, tremors, headache, insomnia, heat intolerance, fever, and menstrual irregularities.
Treatment requires reduction of GI absorption and

efforts to counteract central and peripheral effects, primarily sympathetic activity. Use gastric lavage or induce emesis (followed with activated charcoal, if less than 4 hours after ingestion). If the patient is comatose or is having seizures, inflate cuff on endotracheal tube to prevent aspiration. Treatment may include oxygen and artificial ventilation to support respiration. It also should include appropriate measures to treat CHF and control fever, hypoglycemia, and fluid loss. Propranolol may be used to combat many of the effects of increased sympathetic activity. Thyroid USP therapy should be withdrawn gradually over 2 to 6 days, then resumed at a lower dosage.

▶ **Special considerations**
• During first few months of therapy, children may suffer partial hair loss. Reassure child and parents that this is temporary.
• Drug dosage varies widely among patients. Treatment should start at the lowest level, titrating to higher doses according to patient's symptoms and laboratory data, until euthyroid state is reached.
• Drug should be administered at the same time each day. A.M. administration helps prevent insomnia.
• Monitor pulse rate and blood pressure.
• Monitor prothrombin time; patients taking anticoagulants usually require lower doses.
• Monitor for signs of inadequate dosage or hypothyroidism, including changes in menstrual periods, coldness, constipation, dry puffy skin, headache, listlessness, muscle aches, nausea, vomiting, weakness, fatigue, and unusual weight gain.
• Signs of thyrotoxicosis or overdosage include diarrhea, fever, irritability, listlessness, rapid heartbeat, vomiting, and weakness.
• Commercial preparations from different manufacturers may have variable hormonal content and produce fluctuating liothyronine and levothyroxine levels. Do not change brands after the patient is stabilized.
• In children, sleeping pulse rate and basal morning temperature are guides to treatment.
• Enteric-coated tablets give unreliable absorption.

Information for parents and patient
• Encourage patient to take daily dose at the same time each day, preferably in the morning to avoid insomnia.
• Advise parents to call if patient experiences headache, diarrhea, nervousness, excessive sweating, heat intolerance, chest pain, increased pulse rate, or palpitations.
• Tell parents not to store this medication in warm, humid areas, such as the bathroom, to prevent deterioration of the drug.

thyrotropin (thyroid-stimulating hormone, or TSH)
Thytropar

• Classification: thyrotropic hormone (anterior pituitary hormone)

How supplied
Available by prescription only
Powder for injection: 10 units (IU)/vial

Indications, route, and dosage
Diagnosis of thyroid cancer remnant with ^{131}I after surgery
Children and adults: 10 units I.M. or S.C. for 3 to 7 days.
Differential diagnosis of primary and secondary hypothyroidism
Children and adults: 10 units I.M. or S.C. for 1 to 3 days.
In protein-bound iodine or ^{131}I uptake determinations for differential diagnosis of subclinical hypothyroidism or low thyroid reserve
Children and adults: 10 units I.M. or S.C.
Therapy for thyroid carcinoma (local or metastatic) with [131]I
Children and adults: 10 units I.M. or S.C. for 3 to 8 days.
To determine thyroid status of patient receiving thyroid
Children and adults: 10 units I.M. or S.C. for 1 to 3 days.

Action and kinetics
• *Thyrotropic action:* Thyrotropin produces increased uptake of iodine by the thyroid and increased formation and release of thyroid hormone.
• *Kinetics in adults:* Onset of effect occurs within minutes after injection. Drug is concentrated primarily in the thyroid gland. Metabolism and excretion are not fully understood.

Contraindications and precautions
Thyrotropin is contraindicated in patients with hypersensitivity to the drug, recent myocardial infarction, or untreated Addison's disease.

Drug should be used cautiously in patients with angina, hypertension, or heart failure, because of the risk of sudden metabolic demands; and in patients with adrenocortical insufficiency or hypopituitarism, because thyrotropin administration can provoke acute adrenocortical crisis.

Interactions
None reported.

Effects on diagnostic tests
Thyrotropin therapy alters ^{131}I thyroid uptake.

‡May contain sulfites   ◆May contain tartrazine   ◆◆May contain benzyl alcohol

Adverse reactions

- CNS: headache, fainting.
- CV: tachycardia, atrial fibrillation, angina pectoris, CHF, hypotension.
- GI: nausea, vomiting.
- GU: urinary frequency.
- Other: thyroid hyperplasia (large doses), fever, menstrual irregularities, *allergic reactions* (postinjection flare, urticaria, anaphylaxis, wheezing, tightness of throat).

Note: Drug should be discontinued if hypersensitivity reaction occurs.

Overdose and treatment

Clinical manifestations of overdose include headache, irritability, nervousness, sweating, tachycardia, increased GI motility, and menstrual irregularities. Angina or CHF may be aggravated. Shock may develop.

Treatment includes administering propranolol (or another beta blocker) to treat adrenergic effects of hyperthyroidism. Recommended adult dosage of propranolol is 1 mg/dose over at least 1 minute, repeated every 2 to 5 minutes (to a maximum of 5 mg). Dosage in children is 0.01 to 0.1 mg/kg over 10 minutes (to a maximum of 1 mg). Monitor blood pressure and cardiac function. Exchange transfusions may be beneficial in acute overdose. Diuresis and dialysis are not effective.

▶ Special considerations

- During first few months of therapy, children may suffer partial hair loss. Reassure child and parents that this is temporary.
- Drug dosage varies widely among patients. Treatment should start at the lowest level, titrating to higher doses according to patient's symptoms and laboratory data, until euthyroid state is reached.
- Drug should be administered at the same time each day. A.M. administration helps prevent insomnia.
- Monitor pulse rate and blood pressure.
- Monitor prothrombin time; patients taking anticoagulants usually require lower doses.
- Monitor for signs of overdosage or hypothyroidism, including changes in menstrual periods, coldness, constipation, dry puffy skin, headache, listlessness, muscle aches, nausea, vomiting, weakness, fatigue, and unusual weight gain.
- Signs of thyrotoxicosis or inadequate dosage therapy include diarrhea, fever, irritability, listlessness, rapid heartbeat, vomiting, and weakness.
- Allergic reactions are common in patients who have previously received thyrotropin.
- Thyrotropin may cause thyroid hyperplasia.
- Three-day dosage schedule may be used in longstanding pituitary myxedema or with prolonged use of thyroid medication.

Information for parents and patient

Warn patient to call immediately if he experiences itching, redness, or swelling at the injection site; skin rash; tightness of throat or wheezing; chest pain; irritability; nervousness; rapid heartbeat; shortness of breath; or unusual sweating.

ticarcillin disodium
Ticar

- Classification: antibiotic (extended-spectrum penicillin, alpha-carboxypenicillin)

How supplied

Available by prescription only
Injection: 1 g, 3 g, 6 g
Pharmacy bulk package: 20 g, 30 g
I.V. infusion: 3 g

Indications, route, and dosage
Serious infections caused by susceptible organisms

Neonates age 0 to 7 days weighing ≤ *2,000 g:* 150 mg/kg/day I.V. or I.M., divided q 12 hours.
Neonates age 0 to 7 days weighing > *2,000 g:* 225 mg/kg/day I.V. or I.M., divided q 8 hours.
Neonates age 7 days to 4 weeks weighing ≤ *2,000 g:* 225 mg/kg/day I.V. or I.M., divided q 8 hours.
Neonates age 7 days to 4 weeks weighing > *2,000 g:* 300 mg/kg/day I.V. or I.M., divided q 6 hours.
Infants and children: 200 to 400 mg/kg/day I.V. or I.M., divided q 4 to 6 hours.
Children under 40 kg: 200 to 300 mg/kg I.V. or I.M. daily, divided into doses given q 4 to 6 hours.
Adults: 200 to 300 mg/kg I.V. or I.M. daily, divided into doses given q 3, 4, or 6 hours.
Dosage in renal failure

Creatinine clearance (ml/min/1.73 m²)	Dosage in adults
> 60	3 g I.V. q 4 hours
30 to 60	2 g I.V. q 4 hours
10 to 30	2 g I.V. q 8 hours
< 10 with hepatic failure	2 g I.V. q 24 hours or 1g I.V. q 12 hours
Patients on hemodialysis	2 g I.V. q 12 hours with 3 g I.V. after each treatment
Patients on peritoneal dialysis	3 g I.V. q 12 hours

Action and kinetics

- *Antibiotic action:* Ticarcillin is bactericidal; it adheres to bacterial penicillin-binding proteins, thus inhibiting bacterial cell wall synthesis. Extended-spectrum penicillins are more resistant to inactivation by certain beta-lactamases, especially those produced by gram-negative organisms, but are still liable to inactivation by certain others.

Ticarcillin's spectrum of activity includes many gram-negative aerobic and anaerobic bacilli, many gram-positive and gram-negative aerobic cocci, and some gram-positive aerobic and anaerobic bacilli. Ticarcillin may be effective against some strains of carbenicillin-resistant gram-negative bacilli.

It is often more active (by weight) against *Pseudomonas aeruginosa* than is carbenicillin. Its primary use is in combination with an aminoglycoside to treat *P. aeruginosa* infections.

When ticarcilin is used alone, resistance develops rapidly. It is almost always used with other antibiotics (such as aminoglycosides).

• *Kinetics in adults:* Peak plasma concentrations occur 30 to 75 minutes after an I.M. dose.

Ticarcillin disodium is distributed widely. It penetrates minimally into CSF with uninflamed meninges. Ticarcillin crosses the placenta; it is 45% to 65% protein-bound.

About 13% of a dose is metabolized by hydrolysis to inactive compounds.

Ticarcillin is excreted primarily (80% to 93%) in urine by renal tubular secretion and glomerular filteration; it is also excreted in bile and in breast milk. Elimination half-life in adults is about 1 hour; in severe renal impairment, half-life is extended to about 3 hours. Ticarcillin sodium is removed by hemodialysis but not by peritoneal dialysis.

Contraindications and precautions
Ticarcillin is contraindicated in patients with known hypersensitivity to any other penicillin or to cephalosporins.

Ticarcillin should be used cautiously in patients with renal impairment because it is excreted in urine; decreased dosage is required in moderate to severe renal failure. Use cautiously in patients with bleeding tendencies, hypokalemia, or sodium restriction.

Interactions
Concomitant use with aminoglycoside antibiotics results in synergistic bactericidal effects against *Pseudomonas aeruginosa, Escherichia coli, Klebsiella, Citrobacter, Enterobacter, Serratia,* and *Proteus mirabilis.* However, the drugs are physically and chemically incompatible and are inactivated when mixed or given together.

Concomitant use of ticarcillin (and other extended-spectrum penicillins) with clavulanic acid also produces a synergistic bactericidal effect against certain beta-lactamase-producing bacteria.

Probenecid blocks renal tubular secretion of ticarcillin, raising ticarcillin's serum concentrations.

Large doses of penicillins may interfere with renal tubular secretion of methotrexate, thus delaying elimination and elevating serum concentrations of methotrexate.

Effects on diagnostic tests
Ticarcillin alters tests for urinary or serum proteins; it interferes with turbidimetric methods that use sulfosalicylic acid, trichloroacetic acid, acetic acid, or nitric acid. Ticarcillin does not interfere with tests using bromophenol blue (Albustix, Albutest, Multi-Stix).

Ticarcillin may falsely decrease serum aminoglycoside concentrations. Systemic effects of ticarcillin may cause positive Coombs' test, hypokalemia and hypernatremia, and may prolong prothrombin times (PTs); it may also cause transient elevations in liver function studies and transient reductions in red blood cell, white blood cell, and platelet counts.

Adverse reactions
• CNS: neuromuscular irritability, seizures.
• GI: nausea, diarrhea, vomiting, pseudomembranous colitis.
• GU: acute interstitial nephritis.
• HEMA: leukopenia, neutropenia, eosinophilia, thrombocytopenia, hemolytic anemia, bleeding at high doses.
• Metabolic: hypokalemia.
• Local: pain at injection site, vein irritation, phlebitis.
• Other: hypersensitivity reactions, (rash, pruritus, urticaria, chills, fever, edema, anaphylaxis), bacterial and fungal superinfection.

Note: Drug should be discontinued if immediate hypersensitivity reactions occur, if bleeding complications occur, or if severe diarrhea occurs, as this may indicate pseudomembranous colitis.

Overdose and treatment
Clinical signs of overdose include neuromuscular hypersensitivity or seizures resulting from CNS irritation by high drug concentrations. Ticarcillin can be removed by hemodialysis.

▶ Special considerations
• Ticarcillin contains 5.2 mEq of sodium per gram of drug. Use with caution in patients who require sodium restriction.
• Ticarcillin reconstituted for I.M. use with bacteriostatic water for injection containing benzyl alcohol should not be used in neonates because of toxicity.
• Assess patient's history of allergies; do not give ticarcillin to any patient with a history of hypersensitivity reactions to either penicillins or cephalosporins. Try to ascertain whether previous reactions were true hypersensitivity reactions or another reaction, such as GI distress, which the patient has interpreted as allergy.
• Keep in mind that a negative history for penicillin hypersensitivity does not preclude future allergic reactions; monitor patient continuously for possible allergic reactions or other untoward effects.
• In patients with renal impairment, dosage should be reduced if creatinine clearance is below 10 ml/minute.
• Assess level of consciousness, neurologic status, and renal function when high doses are used, because excessive blood levels can cause CNS toxicity.
• Obtain results of cultures and sensitivity tests before first dose; however, therapy may begin before test results are complete. Repeat tests periodically to assess drug efficacy.
• Monitor vital signs, electrolytes, and renal function studies; monitor body weight for fluid retention with extended-spectrum penicillins for possible hypokalemia or hypermatremia.
• Coagulation abnormalities, even frank bleeding, can follow high doses, especially of extended-spectrum penicillins; monitor prothrombin times and platelet counts, and assess patient for signs of occult or frank bleeding.
• Monitor patients on long-term therapy for possible

superinfection, especially debilitated patients and others receiving immunosuppressants or radiation therapy; monitor closely, especially for fever.
• Ticarcillin is almost always used with another antibiotic, such as an aminoglycoside, in life-threatening situations.
• Monitor intake, output, and weight; monitor serum electrolytes to prevent hypokalemia and hypernatremia.
• Monitor neurologic status. High concentrations may cause seizures.
• Check complete blood count, differential, PT, and partial thromboplastin time. Drug may cause thrombocytopenia or later platelet aggregation. Watch for signs of bleeding.
• Because ticarcillin is dialyzable, patients undergoing hemodialysis may need dosage adjustments.

Parenteral administration
• Give penicillins at least 1 hour before giving bacteriostatic antibiotics (tetracyclines, erythromycins, and chloramphenicol); these drugs inhibit bacterial cell growth, decreasing rate of penicillin uptake by bacterial cell walls.
• Always consult manufacturer's directions for reconstitution, dilution, and storage of drugs; check expiration dates.
• Do not add or mix other drugs with I.V. infusions—particularly aminoglycosides, which will be inactivated if mixed with penicillins; they are chemically and physically incompatible. If other drugs must be given I.V., temporarily stop infusion of primary drug.
• Infuse I.V. drug continuously or intermittently (over 30 minutes) and assess I.V. site frequently to prevent infiltration or phlebitis; rotate infusion site q 48 hours; intermittent I.V. infusion may be diluted in sterile water, 0.9% sodium chloride, dextrose 5% in water, dextrose 5% in water and half normal saline, or lactated Ringer's solution. Lower volumes of diluent may be used, provided that final concentration of solution does not exceed 100 mg/ml.
• Solutions should always be clear, colorless to pale yellow, and free of particles; do not give solutions containing precipitates or other foreign matter.

Information for parents and patient
• Teach signs and symptoms of hypersensitivity and other adverse reactions, and emphasize need to report any unusual reactions.
• Teach signs and symptoms of bacterial and fungal superinfection to parents and patient, especially for debilitated patients and others with low resistance from immunosuppressants or irradiation; emphasize need to report signs of infection.
• Teach parents and patients how to prevent superinfection by practicing meticulous oral and anogenital hygiene. Parents of infants and toddlers should keep diaper area clean and dry and avoid using plastic pants.

---

ticarcillin disodium/clavulanate potassium
Timentin

• Classification: antibiotic (extended-spectrum penicillin, beta-lactamase inhibitor)

How supplied
Available by prescription only
Injection: 3 g ticarcillin and 100 mg clavulanic acid

Indications, route, and dosage
Infections of the lower respiratory tract, urinary tract, bones and joints, skin and skin structure, and septicemia when caused by susceptible organisms
†*Children 15 months to age 12:* 207 to 310 mg/kg (based on ticarcillin component) I.V. daily in divided doses every 4 to 6 hours.
Adults: 3.1 g (contains 3 g ticarcillin and 0.1 g clavulanate potassium) diluted in 50 to 100 ml dextrose 5% and water, sodium chloride, or lactated Ringer's injection and administered by I.V. infusion over 30 minutes q 4 to 6 hours.

Dosage in renal failure
Loading dose: 3.1 g (3 g ticarcillin with 100 mg clavulanate)

Creatinine clearance (ml/min/1.73 m²)	Dosage in adults
> 60	3.1 g I.V. q 4 hours
30 to 60	2 g I.V. q 4 hours
10 to 30	2 g I.V. q 8 hours
< 10	2 g I.V. q 12 hours
< 10 with hepatic failure	2 g I.V. q 24 hours
Patients on hemodialysis	2 g I.V. every 12 hours, then 3.1 g after treatment
Patients on peritoneal dialysis	3.1 g I.V. q 12 hours

Action and kinetics
• *Antibiotic action:* Ticarcillin is bactericidal; it adheres to bacterial penicillin-binding proteins, thus inhibiting bacterial cell wall synthesis. Extended-spectrum penicillins are more resistant to inactivation by certain beta-lactamases, especially those produced by gram-negative organisms, but are still liable to inactivation by certain others.
Clavulanic acid has only weak antibacterial activity and does not affect the action of ticarcillin. However, clavulanic acid has a beta-lactam ring and is structurally similar to penicillin and cephalosporins; it binds irreversibly with certain beta-lactamases, preventing inactivation of ticarcillin and broadening its bactericidal spectrum.
Ticarcillin's spectrum of activity includes many gram-negative aerobic and anaerobic bacilli, many gram-positive and gram-negative aerobic cocci, and

---

some gram-positive aerobic and anaerobic bacilli. The combination of ticarcillin and clavulanate potassium is also effective against many beta-lactamase-producing strains, including *Staphylococcus aureus, Hemophilus influenzae, Neisseria gonorrhoeae, Escherichia coli, Klebsiella, Providencia,* and *Bacteroides fragilis,* but not *Pseudomonas aeruginosa.*

• *Kinetics in adults:* Ticarcillin disodium/clavulanate potassium is only administered intravenously; peak plasma concentration occurs immediately after infusion is complete.

Ticarcillin disodium is distributed widely. It penetrates minimally into CSF with uninflamed meninges; clavulanic acid penetrates into pleural fluid, lungs, and peritoneal fluid.

Ticarcillin sodium achieves high concentrations in urine. Protein-binding is 45% to 65% for ticarcillin and 22% to 30% for clavulanic acid; both cross the placenta.

About 13% of a ticarcillin dose is metabolized by hydrolysis to inactive compounds; clavulanic acid is thought to undergo extensive metabolism, but its fate is as yet unknown.

Ticarcillin is excreted primarily (83% to 90%) in urine by renal tubular secretion and glomerular filtration; it is also excreted in bile and in breast milk. Clavulanate's metabolites are excreted in urine by glomerular filtration and in breast milk. Elimination half-life of ticarcillin in adults is about 1 hour and that of clavulanate is about 1 hour; in severe renal impairment, ticarcillin's half-life is extended to about 3 hours and that of clavulanate to about 4½ hours. Both drugs are removed by hemodialysis but only slightly by peritoneal dialysis.

Contraindications and precautions

Ticarcillin/clavulanate potassium is contraindicated in patients with known hypersensitivity to any other penicillin or to cephalosporins.

Ticarcillin/clavulanate potassium should be used with caution in patients with renal impairment because it is excreted in urine; decreased dosage is required in moderate to severe renal failure.

Interactions

Concomitant use of ticarcillin and clavulanate potassium with aminoglycoside antibiotics results in synergistic bactericidal effects against *Pseudomonas aeruginosa, Escherichia coli, Klebsiella, Citrobacter, Enterobacter, Serratia,* and *Proteus mirabilis.* However, the drugs are physically and chemically incompatible and are inactivated when mixed or given together. In vivo inactivation has been reported when aminoglycosides and extended-spectrum penicillins are used concomitantly.

Probenecid blocks tubular secretion of ticarcillin, raising its serum concentration; it has no effect on clavulanate.

Large doses of penicillin may interfere with renal tubular secretion of methotrexate, thus delaying elimination and elevating serum concentrations of methotrexate.

Effects on diagnostic tests

Ticarcillin/clavulanate potassium alters tests for urinary or serum proteins; it interferes with turbidimetric methods that use sulfosalicylic acid, trichloroacetic acid, acetic acid, or nitric acid. Ticarcillin/clavulanate potassium does not interfere with tests using bromophenol blue (Albustix, Albutest, MultiStix). Ticarcillin/clavulanate potassium may falsely decrease serum aminoglycoside concentration.

Systemic effects of ticarcillin/clavulanate potassium may cause positive Coombs' test, hypokalemia, and hypernatremia and may prolong prothrombin times; it may also cause transient elevations in liver function studies and transient reductions in red blood cell, white blood cell, and platelet counts.

Adverse reactions

• CNS: neuromuscular irritability, seizures.
• GI: nausea, diarrhea, vomiting, pseudomembranous colitis.
• HEMA: leukopenia, neutropenia, eosinophilia, thrombocytopenia, hemolytic anemia, bleeding at high doses.
• Metabolic: hypokalemia.
• Local: pain at injection site, vein irritation, phlebitis.
• Other: hypersensitivity reactions (rash, pruritus, urticaria, chills, fever, edema, anaphylaxis), bacterial and fungal superinfection.

Note: Drug should be discontinued if immediate hypersensitivity reactions occur, if bleeding complications occur, or if severe diarrhea occurs, as this may indicate pseudomembranous colitis.

Overdose and treatment

Clinical signs of overdose include neuromuscular hypersensitivity or seizures; ticarcillin and clavulanate potassium can be removed by hemodialysis.

▶ Special considerations

• Ticarcillin contains 5.2 mEq of sodium per gram of drug. Use with caution in patients with sodium restriction.

• Assess patient's history of allergies; do not give drug to any patient with a history of hypersensitivity reactions to either penicillins or cephalosporins. Try to determine whether previous reactions were true hypersensitivity reactions or another reaction, such as GI distress, which the patient has interpreted as allergy.

• Ticarcillin/clavulanate potassium is almost always used with another antibiotic, such as an aminoglycoside, in life-threatening situations.

• Keep in mind that a negative history for penicillin hypersensitivity does not preclude future allergic reactions; monitor patient continuously for possible allergic reactions or other untoward effects.

• In patients with renal impairment, dosage should be reduced if creatinine clearance is below 10 ml/minute.

• Assess level of consciousness, neurologic status, and renal function when high doses are used, because excessive blood levels can cause CNS toxicity.

• Obtain results of cultures and sensitivity tests before first dose; however, therapy may begin before test

---

‡May contain sulfites   ◆May contain tartrazine   ◆◆May contain benzyl alcohol

results are complete. Repeat tests periodically to assess drug efficacy.

• Monitor vital signs, electrolytes, and renal function studies; monitor body weight for fluid retention with extended-spectrum penicillins for possible hypokalemia or hypernatremia.

• Coagulation abnormalities, even frank bleeding, can follow high doses, especially of extended-spectrum penicillins; monitor prothrombin times and platelet counts, and assess patient for signs of occult or frank bleeding.

• Monitor patients on long-term therapy for possible superinfection, especially debilitated patients and others receiving immunosuppressants or radiation therapy; monitor closely, especially for fever.

• Monitor intake, output, weight and serum electrolytes. Observe for signs of hypernatremia and hypokalemia.

• Monitor neurologic status. High blood levels may cause seizures.

• Because ticarcillin/clavulanate potassium is dialyzable, patients undergoing hemodialysis may need dosage adjustments.

• Check complete blood count, PT, and partial thromboplastin time. Drug may cause thrombocytopenia and alter platelet aggregation. Watch for signs of bleeding.

Oral and parenteral administration

• Give penicillins at least 1 hour before giving bacteriostatic antibiotics (tetracyclines, erythromycins, and chloramphenicol); these drugs inhibit bacterial cell growth, decreasing rate of penicillin uptake by bacterial cell walls.

• Always consult manufacturer's directions for reconstitution, dilution, and storage of drugs; check expiration dates.

• Do not add or mix other drugs with I.V. infusions — particularly aminoglycosides, which will be inactivated if mixed with penicillins; they are chemically and physically incompatible. If other drugs must be given I.V., temporarily stop infusion of primary drug.

• Infuse I.V. drug continuously or intermittently (over 30 minutes) and assess I.V. site frequently to prevent infiltration or phlebitis; rotate infusion site q 48 hours; intermittent I.V. infusion may be diluted in sterile water, 0.9% sodium chloride, dextrose 5% in water, dextrose 5% in water and half normal saline, or lactated Ringer's solution to volumes appropriate for the patient's weight.

• Solutions should always be clear, colorless to pale yellow, and free of particles; do not give solutions containing precipitates or other foreign matter.

Information for parents and patient

• Teach signs and symptoms of hypersensitivity and other adverse reactions, and emphasize need to report any unusual reactions.

• Teach signs and symptoms of bacterial and fungal superinfection to parents and patients, especially for debilitated patients and others with low resistance from immunosuppressants or irradiation; emphasize need to report signs of infection.

tobramycin sulfate
Nebcin, Nebcin Pediatric

• Classification: antibiotic (aminoglycoside)

How supplied

Available by prescription only
Injection: 40 mg/ml, 10 mg/ml (pediatric)
Ophthalmic solution: 0.3%
Ophthalmic ointment: 0.3%

Indications, route, and dosage

Serious infections caused by sensitive Escherichia coli, Proteus, Klebsiella, Enterobacter, Serratia, Staphylococcus aureus, Pseudomonas, Citrobacter, and Providencia

Premature infants < 34 weeks' gestation and those with renal or hepatic impairment: 2 to 2.5 mg/kg I.M. or I.V. q 18 to 24 hours.

Neonates age 1 to 7 days: 2 to 2.5 mg/kg I.M. or I.V. q 12 hours. For I.V. use, dilute in 50 to 100 ml normal saline solution or dextrose 5% in water for adults and in less volume for children. Infuse over 20 to 60 minutes.

Neonates age 8 days or older: 2 to 2.5 mg/kg I.M. or I.V. q 8 hours.

Children and adults with normal renal function: 3 mg/ kg I.M. or I.V. daily, divided q 8 hours. Up to 5 mg/ kg I.M. or I.V. daily, divided q 6 to 8 hours for life-threatening infections.

Patients with impaired renal function: Initial dosage is same as for those with normal renal function. Subsequent doses and frequency determined by renal function study results and blood levels; keep peak serum concentrations between 4 and 10 mcg/ml, and trough serum concentrations between 1 and 2 mcg/ ml.

Treatment of external ocular infection caused by susceptible gram-negative bacteria

Children and adults: In mild to moderate infections, instill 1 or 2 drops into affected eye q 4 hours. In severe infections, instill 2 drops into the affected eye hourly.

Acute exacerbation of cystic fibrosis

Children: 6 to 10 mg/kg/day divided q 6 to 8 hours.

Dosage in renal failure

Several methods have been used to calculate tobramycin dosage in renal failure.

After a 1 mg/kg loading dose, adjust subsequent dosage by reducing doses administered at 8-hour intervals or by prolonging the interval between normal doses. Both of these methods are useful when serum levels of tobramycin cannot be measured directly. They are based on either creatinine clearance (preferred) or serum creatinine because these values correlate with the half-life of tobramycin.

To calculate reduced dosage for 8-hour intervals, use available nomograms; or, if the patient's steady state serum creatinine values are known, divide the normally recommended dose by the patient's serum creatinine value. To determine frequency in hours for normal dosage (if creatinine clearance rate is no available), divide the normal dose by the patient's serum creatinine value. Dosage schedules derived from either method require careful clinical and laboratory observations of the patient and should be adjusted as appropriate. These methods of calculation may be misleading in elderly patients and those with severe wasting; neither should be used when dialysis is performed.

Hemodialysis removes 50% of a dose in 6 hours. In anephric patients maintained by dialysis, 1.5 to 2 mg/kg after each dialysis usually maintains therapeutic, nontoxic serum levels. Patients receiving peritoneal dialysis twice a week should receive a 1.5 to 2mg/kg loading dose followed by 1 mg/kg every 3 days. Those receiving dialysis every 2 days should receive a 1.5 mg/kg loading dose after the first dialysis and 0.75 mg/kg after each subsequent dialysis.

Action and kinetics

• *Antibiotic action:* Tobramycin is bactericidal; it binds directly to the 30S ribosomal subunit, thereby inhibiting bacterial protein synthesis. Its spectrum of activity includes many aerobic gram-negative organisms, including most strains of *Pseudomonas aeruginosa* and some aerobic gram-positive organisms. Tobramycin may act against some bacterial strains resistant to other aminoglycosides; many strains resistant to tobramycin are susceptible to amikacin, gentamicin, or netilmicin.

• *Kinetics in adults:* Tobramycin is absorbed poorly after oral administration and usually is given parenterally; peak serum concentrations occur 30 to 90 minutes after I.M. administration.

Tobramycin is distributed widely after parenteral administration; intraocular penetration is poor. CSF penetration is low, even in patients with inflamed meninges. Protein binding is minimal. Tobramycin crosses the placenta.

Tobramycin is excreted unmetabolized, primarily in urine by glomerular filteration; small amounts may be excreted in bile and breast milk. Elimination half-life in adults is 2 to 3 hours. In severe renal damage, half-life may extend to 24 to 60 hours.

• *Kinetics in children:* Plasma elimination half-life is reported to be 4.6 hours in full-term infants, and 8.7 hours in low birth weight infants.

Contraindications and precautions

Tobramycin is contraindicated in patients with known hypersensitivity to tobramycin or any other aminoglycoside.

Tobramycin should be used cautiously in neonates and other infants; in patients with decreased renal function; in patients with tinnitus, vertigo, and high-frequency hearing loss who are susceptible to ototoxicity; in patients with dehydration, myasthenia gravis, parkinsonism, and hypocalcemia; and in elderly patients.

Interactions

Concomitant use with the following drugs may increase the hazard of nephrotoxicity, ototoxicity, and neurotoxicity: methoxyflurane, polymyxin B, vancomycin, capreomycin, cisplatin, cephalosporins, amphotericin B, and other aminoglycosides; hazard of

ototoxicity is also increased during use with ethacrynic acid, furosemide, bumetanide, urea, or mannitol. Dimenhydrinate and other antiemetic and antivertigo drugs may mask tobramycin-induced ototoxicity.

Concomitant use with penicillin results in a synergistic bactericidal effect against *P. aeruginosa, E. coli, Klebsiella, Citrobacter, Enterobacter, Serratia,* and *Proteus mirabilis.* However, the drugs are physically and chemically incompatible and are inactivated when mixed or given together. In vivo inactivation has been reported when aminoglycosides and penicillins are used concomitantly.

Tobramycin may potentiate neuromuscular blockade from general anesthetics or neuromuscular blocking agents such as succinylcholine and tubocurarine.

Effects on diagnostic tests

Tobramycin may elevate BUN, nonprotein nitrogen, or serum creatinine levels and increase urinary excretion of casts.

Adverse reactions

• CNS: *headache, lethargy, neuromuscular blockade with respiratory depression.*
• EENT: *ototoxicity (tinnitus, vertigo, hearing loss);* with ophthalmic use, *burning or stinging on instillation, lid itching or lid swelling.*
• GI: *diarrhea, nausea, vomiting.*
• GU: *nephrotoxicity* (cells or casts in the urine, oliguria, proteinuria, decreased creatinine clearance, increased BUN, serum creatinine, and nonprotein nitrogen levels).
• HEMA: *anemia, agranuloytopenia.*
• Hepatic: increased AST (SGOT), ALT (SGPT).
• Other: *hypersensitivity reactions (eosinophilia, fever, rash, urticaria, pruritus),* bacterial or fungal superinfection.

Note: Drug should be discontinued if signs of ototoxicity, nephrotoxicity, or hypersensitivity occur.

Overdose and treatment

Clinical signs of overdose include ototoxicity, nephrotoxicity, and neuromuscular toxicity. Remove drug by hemodialysis or peritoneal dialysis. Treatment with calcium salts or anticholinesterases reverses neuromuscular blockade.

▶ Special considerations

• Some studies suggest tobramycin may be less nephrotoxic than gentamicin.
• Tobramycin is inactive against chlamydia, fungi, viruses, and most anaerobic bacteria.
• The half-life of aminoglycosides is prolonged in neonates and premature infants because of immaturity of their renal systems; dosage alterations may be necessary in infants and children.
• Tobramycin has been administered intrathecally and intraventricularly. Many clinicians prefer intraventricular administration to ensure adequate CSF levels in the treatment of ventriculitis.
• Discontinue ophthalmic use if keratitis, erythema, lacrimation, edema, or lid itching occurs.
• Assess patient's allergic history; do not give tobramycin to a patient with a history of hypersensitivity

reactions to any aminoglycoside; monitor patient continuously for this and other adverse reactions.
• Obtain results of culture and sensitivity tests before first dose; however, therapy may begin before tests are completed. Repeat tests periodically to assess drug efficacy.
• Monitor vital signs, electrolyte levels, and renal function studies before and during therapy; be sure patient is well hydrated to minimize chemical irritation of renal tubules; watch for signs of declining renal function.
• Because tobramycin is dialyzable, patients undergoing hemodialysis may need dosage adjustments.
• Keep peak serum levels and trough serum levels at recommended concentrations, especially in patients with decreased renal function. Draw blood for peak level 1 to 2 hours after I.M. injection (30 minutes to 1 hour after I.V. infusion); for trough level, draw sample just before the next dose. Time and date all blood samples. Do not use heparinized tube to collect blood samples; it interferes with results.
• Evaluate patient's hearing before and during therapy; monitor for complaints of tinnitus, vertigo, or hearing loss.
• Avoid concomitant use with other ototoxic or nephrotoxic drugs.
• Usual duration of therapy is 7 to 10 days; if no response occurs in 3 to 5 days, drug should be discontinued and cultures repeated for reevaluation of therapy.
• Closely monitor patients on long-term therapy—especially debilitated patients and others receiving immunosuppressant or radiation therapy—for possible bacterial or fungal superinfection; monitor especially for fever.

Parenteral administration
• Consult manufacturer's directions for reconstitution, dilution, and storage of drugs; check expiration dates.
• Administer I.M. dose deep into large muscle mass (gluteal or midlateral thigh); rotate injection sites to minimize tissue injury; do not inject more than 2 g of drug per injection site. Apply ice to injection site for pain.
• Do not add or mix other drugs with I.V. infusions—particularly penicillins, which will inactivate aminoglycosides; the two groups are chemically and physically incompatible. If other drugs must be given I.V., temporarily stop infusion of primary drug.
• Too-rapid I.V. administration may cause neuromuscular blockade. Infuse I.V. drug continuously or intermittently over 30 to 60 minutes for adults, 20 to 60 minutes for infants; dilution volume for children is determined individually.
• Solutions should always be clear, colorless to pale yellow (in most cases, darkening indicates deterioration), and free of particles; do not give solutions containing precipitates or other foreign matter.

Information for parents and patient
• Teach parents how to recognize signs and symptoms of hypersensitivity; bacterial or fungal superinfections (especially if the child has low resistance from immunosuppressants or irradiation); and other adverse reactions to aminoglycosides, urge them to report *any* unusual effects promptly.

• Teach parents and patients to prevent superinfection by practicing meticulous oral and anogenital hygiene. Parents of infants and toddlers should keep diaper area clean and dry and avoid using plastic pants.
• Be sure parents understand how and when to administer drug; urge them to complete entire prescribed regimen, to comply with instructions for around-the-clock dosage, and to keep follow-up appointments.

---

tolazoline hydrochloride
Priscoline

• Classification: antihypertensive (peripheral vasodilator, alpha-adrenergic blocking agent)

How supplied
Available by prescription only
Injection: 25 mg/ml in 10-ml vials

Indications, route, and dosage
Persistant pulmonary vasoconstriction and hypertension of the newborn (persistent fetal circulation)
Neonates: Initially, 1 to 2 mg/kg I.V. via an upper body vein over 10 minutes, followed by an I.V. infusion of 1 to 2 mg/kg/hour.

Action and kinetics
• *Antihypertensive action:* Tolazoline, by direct relaxation of vascular smooth muscle, causes peripheral vasodilation and decreased peripheral resistance. Tolazoline inhibits responses to adrenergic stimuli by competitively blocking alpha-adrenergic receptors; however, at usual doses, this effect is relatively transient and incomplete.
• *Kinetics in adults:* Tolazoline is absorbed rapidly and almost completely after parenteral administration. Tolazoline concentrates primarily in kidneys and liver. It is excreted in urine, primarily as unchanged drug; half-life is 3 to 10 hours in neonates.

Contraindications and precautions
Tolazoline is contraindicated in patients with known hypersensitivity to the drug and in patients with known or suspected coronary artery disease or after a cerebrovascular accident.
Tolazoline should be used cautiously in patients with gastritis or peptic ulcer disease because the drug can stimulate gastric secretion; and in patients with mitral stenosis because the drug can increase or decrease pulmonary artery pressure and total pulmonary resistance. Tolazoline may activate stress ulcers.

Interactions
Tolazoline may cause a disulfiram-type reaction after alcohol ingestion because of the accumulation of acetaldehyde.
Concomitant use with epinephrine or norepinephrine may cause "epinephrine reversal"—a paradoxical decrease in blood pressure followed by exaggerated rebound hypertension.

Effects on diagnostic tests
None reported.

Adverse reactions
• CV: *hypotension, tachycardia,* dysrhythmias, pulmonary hemorrhage, marked hypertension, shock.
• DERM: *flushing,* increased pilomotor activity.
• GI: nausea, vomiting, diarrhea, hepatitis, *abdominal distention, increased secretion, GI bleeding, gastric perforation.*
• GU: *oliguria, hematuria.*
• HEMA: *thrombocytopenia,* agranulocytosis, *bone marrow suppression.*
• Other: headache, dizziness, sweating, *hyponatremia.*

Overdose and treatment
Clinical manifestations of overdose include flushing, hypotension, and shock.

Treat overdose symptomatically and supportively; if vasopressor is necessary, use ephedrine, which has both central and peripheral actions. Avoid epinephrine or norepinephrine because epinephrine reversal may occur from the alpha-blocking effects of tolazoline.

▶ Special considerations
• Drug is indicated for neonatal hypertension and pulmonary vasoconstriction.
• Pretreatment of infants with antacids may prevent GI bleeding.
• Keeping patient warm increases drug's effect.
• Monitor blood pH for acidosis, which may reduce drug's effect. Obtain blood gases before and during drug use.
• Continuously monitor patient's blood pressure during therapy.
• Test stool and gastric aspirate for occult blood.
• When administering drug, keep in mind the following. Filter drug when drawing it up; drug may be diluted with normal saline solution, dextrose 5% in water, or dextrose 10% in water; solution is good for 24 hours; I.V. infusion should be administered through the branches of superior vena cava (scalp or upper limb vessels if possible); titrate increased and decreased doses.
• Consider administration of Maalox for tolazoline-induced gastric hemorrhage.
• Tolazoline has been used in adults as a provocative test for glaucoma; intra-arterially to improve vascular visualization during angiography; as a diagnostic agent to distinguish between vasospastic or obstructive components of occlusive peripheral vascular disease; and as adjunctive treatment of peripheral vascular disorders.

Information for parents and patient
Explain treatment required.

tolmetin sodium
Tolectin, Tolectin DS

• Classification: nonnarcotic analgesic, antipyretic (nonsteroidal anti-inflammatory)

How supplied
Available by prescription only
Tablets: 200 mg
Capsules: 400 mg

Indications, route, and dosage
Rheumatoid arthritis and osteoarthritis, juvenile rheumatoid arthritis
Children age 2 or older: 15 to 30 mg/kg/day in three or four divided doses.
Adults: 400 mg P.O. t.i.d. or q.i.d. Maximum dosage is 2 g/day.

Action and kinetics
• *Anti-inflammatory, analgesic, and antipyretic actions:* Mechanisms of action are unknown; the drug is thought to inhibit prostaglandin synthesis.
• *Kinetics in adults:* Drug is absorbed rapidly from the GI tract. Tolmetin is highly protein-bound and is metabolized in the liver. Tolmetin is excreted in urine.

Contraindications and precautions
Tolmetin is contraindicated in patients with known hypersensitivity to tolmetin or zomepirac, or in patients in whom aspirin or other nonsteroidal anti-inflammatory drugs (NSAIDs) induce symptoms of asthma, urticaria, or rhinitis.

Tolmetin should be used cautiously in patients with a history of GI bleeding or GI ulcer because the drug may irritate the GI tract; in patients with renal disease because the drug may be nephrotoxic; or in patients with cardiac disease because it may cause peripheral edema, sodium retention, and hypertension.

Patients with known "triad" symptoms (aspirin hypersensitivity, rhinitis/nasal polyps, and asthma) are at high risk of cross-sensitivity to tolmetin with precipitation of bronchospasm.

The signs and symptoms of acute infection (fever, myalgias, erythema) may be masked by the use of tolmetin. Evaluate patients with high infection risk (such as those with diabetes) carefully.

Interactions
When used concomitantly, anticoagulants and thrombolytic drugs may be potentiated by the platelet-inhibiting effect of tolmetin. Concomitant use of tolmetin with highly protein-bound drugs (for example, phenytoin, sulfonylureas, warfarin) may cause displacement of either drug and adverse effects. Monitor therapy closely for both drugs. Concomitant use with other GI-irritating drugs (such as steroids, antibiotics, NSAIDs) may potentiate the adverse GI effects of tolmetin. Use together with caution.

Antacids and food delay and decrease the absorption of tolmetin. NSAIDs are known to decrease renal clearance of lithium carbonate, thus increasing lithium serum levels and risks of adverse effects. Concomitant use of tolmetin and aspirin may decrease plasma levels of tolmetin.

Effects on diagnostic tests

Tolmetin falsely elevates results of urinary protein assays (pseudoproteinuria) in tests using sulfusalicylic acid (not reagent strips like Albustix or Unistix). The physiologic effects of the drug may result in an increased bleeding time; increased BUN, serum potassium, and serum transaminase levels; and decreased hemoglobin and hematocrit levels.

Adverse reactions
• CNS: headache, drowsiness, dizziness.
• CV: hypertension, congestive heart failure (CHF).
• DERM: pruritus, rash, urticaria.
• EENT: tinnitus, visual disturbances.
• GI: *epigastric distress*, nausea, occult blood loss, diarrhea, constipation, *GI bleeding.*
• GU: nephrotoxicity, hematuria, urinary tract infection, pseudoproteinuria.
• HEMA: prolonged bleeding time, leukopenia, hemolytic anemia.
• Other: sodium retention, edema, hepatotoxicity.
   Note: Drug should be discontinued if hypersensitivity or signs and symptoms of hepatic or renal toxicity occur.

Overdose and treatment

Clinical manifestations of overdose include dizziness, drowsiness, mental confusion, lethargy.

   To treat tolmetin overdose, empty stomach immediately by inducing emesis or by gastric lavage followed by administration of activated charcoal. Provide symptomatic and supportive measures (respiratory support and correction of fluid and electrolyte imbalances). Monitor laboratory parameters and vital signs closely. Alkalinization of urine via sodium bicarbonate ingestion may enhance renal excretion of tolmetin.

▶ Special considerations
• The safe use of tolmetin in children under age 2 has not been established.
• Use drug cautiously in patients with a history of GI disease, increased risk of GI bleeding, or decreased renal function.
• Patients with known "triad" symptoms (aspirin hypersensitivity, rhinitis/nasal polyps, and asthma) are at high risk of bronchospasm.
• Drug may mask the signs and symptoms of acute infection (fever, myalgia, erythema); carefully evaluate patients at high risk for infection (for example, those with diabetes).
• Administer drug with a full 9-oz glass of water to ensure adequate passage into stomach. Have patient sit up for 15 to 30 minutes after taking the drug to prevent lodging of the drug in the esophagus.
• Tablets may be crushed and mixed with food or fluids to aid swallowing, and with antacids to minimize gastric upset.
• Assess level of pain and inflammation before start of therapy. Evaluate patient for relief or reduction of these symptoms.
• Monitor for signs and symptoms of bleeding.
• Monitor ophthalmic and auditory function before and periodically during therapy to prevent toxicity.
• Monitor CBC, platelets, prothrombin times, and hepatic and renal function studies periodically to detect abnormalities.
• Patients who do not respond to one NSAID may respond to another NSAID.
• Use of an NSAID with an opioid analgesic has an additive effect. Use of lower doses of the opioid analgesic may be possible.
• Assess cardiopulmonary status closely. Tolmetin may cause sodium retention. Monitor vital signs closely, especially heart rate and blood pressure.
• Assess renal function periodically during therapy; monitor intake and output and daily weight.
• Monitor for presence and amount of edema.
• Therapeutic effect usually occurs within a few days to 1 week of therapy but may take as long as 6 weeks. Evaluate patient's response to drug as evidenced by relief of symptoms.

Information for parents and patient
• Patient should take medication with enough water to ensure passage to the stomach 30 minutes before or 2 hours after meals, or with food or milk if gastric irritation occurs.
• Explain that taking the drug as directed is necessary to achieve the desired effect. Up to 6 weeks of treatment may be needed before benefit is seen.
• Advise parents of patients on chronic therapy that follow-up laboratory tests may be necessary.
• Warn parent and patient that use of alcoholic beverages while taking drug therapy may cause increased GI irritation and, possibly GI bleeding.
• Advise parents to avoid giving child nonprescription medications unless medically approved. Warn them not to give patient sodium bicarbonate, which may decrease effectiveness of drug.
• Advise parents to report any signs of edema; encourage routine check of blood pressure.
• Instruct parents to check patient's weight and to report any significant gain of 3 pounds or more within 1 week.
• Instruct parents in safety measures to prevent injury.

---

tretinoin
Retin-A

• Classification: antiacne agent (vitamin A derivative)

How supplied
Available by prescription only
Cream: 0.025%, 0.05%, 0.1%
Gel: 0.025%, 0.01%
Solution: 0.05%

Indications, route, and dosage
Acne vulgaris (especially grades I, II, and III)
Children and adults: Cleanse affected area and lightly apply solution once daily at bedtime or as directed.

Action and kinetics
• *Antiacne action:* Mechanism of action of tretinoin has not been determined; however, it appears that tretinoin acts as a follicular epithelium irritant, preventing horny cells from sticking together and inhibiting the formation of additional comedones.
• *Kinetics in adults:* Absorption is limited with topical use. A minimal amount is excreted in the urine.

Contraindications and precautions
Tretinoin is contraindicated in patients with known hypersensitivity to vitamin A/retinoic acid. It should be used cautiously in patients with eczema. Avoid contact of drug with eyes, mouth, angles of the nose, mucous membranes, or open wounds. Use of topical preparations containing high concentrations of alcohol, menthol, spices, or lime should be avoided, as they may cause skin irritation. Avoid use of medicated cosmetics on treated skin.

Interactions
Concomitant use with sulfur, resorcinol, benzoyl peroxide, or salicylic acid should be undertaken with caution because of the possibility of interactions.

Effects on diagnostic tests
None reported.

Adverse reactions
• Local: peeling, erythema, blisters, crusting, hyperpigmentation and hypopigmentation, contact dermatitis.
Note: Drug should be discontinued if sensitization or extreme redness and blistering of skin occurs.

Overdose and treatment
No information available. Discontinue use and rinse area thoroughly.

▶ Special considerations
• Make sure that patient knows how to use medication and is aware of time required for clinical effect; therapeutic effect normally occurs in 2 to 3 weeks but may take 6 weeks or more. Relapses generally occur within 3 to 6 weeks of stopping medication.
• Patients who cannot or will not minimize sun exposure should not use this medication.

Information for parents and patient
• Advise sparing application to thoroughly clean, dry skin, which minimizes irritation; to wash face with mild soap no more than once or twice a day. Stress importance of thorough removal of dirt and make up before application and of hand washing after each use, but warn against use of strong, medicated, or perfumed cosmetics, soaps, or skin cleansers.
• Explain that application of the drug may cause a temporary feeling of warmth. If discomfort occurs, tell patient to decrease amount, but not to discontinue medication.

• Because of potential for severe irritation and peeling, patient should use low concentrations initially. If tolerated, higher concentrations may then be used.
• Stress that initial exacerbation of inflammatory lesions is common and that redness and scaling (usually occurring in 7 to 10 days) are normal skin responses; these disappear when medication is decreased or discontinued.
• If severe local irritation develops, patient should stop drug temporarily and readjust dosage when irritation or inflammation subsides.
• Caution parents to keep patient's exposure to sunlight or ultraviolet rays to a minimum and, if sunburned, to delay therapy until sunburn fades. Patient who cannot avoid exposure to sunlight should use #15 or higher sunscreen and protective clothing.

---

triamcinolone
Systemic: Aristocort, Kenacort, Ledercort*

triamcinolone acetonide
Systemic: Kenalog, Kenalone, Triam-A

Oral inhalant: Azmacort

Topical: Adcortyl*, Adcortyl in Orabase*, Aristocort, Flutex, Kenalog, Kenalog in Orabase, Triacet, Triaderm*, Trianide*

triamcinolone diacetate
Systemic: Amcort, Aristocort, Aristocort Forte, Aristocort Intralesional, Articulose LA, Cenocort Forte, Cinalone, Kenacort, Triam-Forte, Triamolone, Tristoject

triamcinolone hexacetonide
Systemic: Aristospan Intra-articular, Aristospan Intralesional

• Classification: anti-inflammatory, immunosuppressant (glucocorticoid)

How supplied
Available by prescription only
Triamcinolone
Tablets: 1 mg, 2 mg, 4 mg, 8 mg
Syrup: 2 mg/ml, 4 mg/ml
Triamcinolone acetonide
Cream, ointment: 0.025%, 0.1%, 0.5%
Lotion: 0.025%, 0.1%
Aerosol: 0.015%, 0.2 mg/2-second spray
Oral inhalation aerosol: 100 mcg/metered spray, 240 doses/inhaler
Injection: 10 mg/ml, 40 mg/ml suspension
Triamcinolone diacetate
Injection: 25 mg/ml, 40 mg/ml suspension
Triamcinolone hexacetonide
Injection: 5 mg/ml, 20 mg/ml suspension

---

‡May contain sulfites   ◆May contain tartrazine   ◆◆May contain benzyl alcohol

Indications, route, and dosage
Adrenal insufficiency
Triamcinolone
Children: 117 mcg/kg or 3.3 mg/m² P.O. daily, in a single dose or divided.
Adults: 4 to 12 mg P.O. daily, in a single dose or divided.

Severe inflammation or immunosuppression
Triamcinolone
Children: 416 mcg to 1.7 mg/kg or 12.5 to 50 mg/m² P.O. daily, in a single dose or divided.
Adults: 4 to 60 mg P.O. daily, in a single dose or divided.

Triamcinolone acetonide
Children over age 6: 40 mg I.M. q 4 weeks; or 2.5 to 15 mg intra-articularly as needed.
Adults: 40 to 80 mg I.M. q 4 weeks; or 2.5 to 15 mg intra-articularly; or up to 1 mg intralesionally as needed.

Triamcinolone diacetate
Children over age 6: 40 mg I.M. once a week.
Adults: 40 mg I.M. once a week; or 3 to 40 mg intra-articularly, intrasynovially, or intralesionally q 1 to 8 weeks.

Triamcinolone hexacetonide
Adults: 2 to 20 mg intra-articularly q 3 to 4 weeks as needed; or up to 0.5 mg intralesionally per square inch of skin.

Steroid-dependent asthma
Triamcinolone acetonide
Children age 6 to 12: 1 or 2 inhalations t.i.d. to q.i.d. Maximum dosage is 12 inhalations daily.
Adults: 2 inhalations t.i.d. to q.i.d. Maximum dosage is 16 inhalations daily.

Inflammation of corticosteroid-responsive dermatoses
Triamcinolone acetonide
Children: Apply 0.025% cream, ointment, lotion or 0.015% aerosol sparingly to affected areas once or twice daily.

Apply 0.1 or 0.5% ointment, cream or lotion once a day.
Adults: Apply cream, ointment, or lotion sparingly b.i.d to q.i.d. Apply aerosol by spraying affected area for about 2 seconds from a distance of 3″ to 6″ (7.5 to 15 cm) t.i.d. or q.i.d. Apply paste to oral lesions by pressing a small amount into lesion without rubbing until thin film develops. Apply two or three times daily after meals and at bedtime.

Action and kinetics
• *Anti-inflammatory action:* Triamcinolone stimulates the synthesis of enzymes needed to decrease the inflammatory response. It suppresses the immune system by reducing activity and volume of the lymphatic system, thus producing lymphocytopenia (primarily of T-lymphocytes), decreases immunoglobulin and complement concentrations, decreases passage of immune complexes through basement membranes, and possibly depresses reactivity of tissue to antigen-antibody interactions.

Triamcinolone is an intermediate-acting glucocorticoid. The addition of a fluorine group in the molecule increases the anti-inflammatory activity, which is five times more potent than an equal weight of hydrocor-

tisone. It has essentially no mineralocorticoid activity.

Triamcinolone may be administered orally. The diacetate and acetonide salts may be administered by I.M., intra-articular, intrasynovial, intralesional or sublesional, and soft-tissue injection. The diacetate suspension is slightly soluble, providing a prompt onset of action and a longer duration of effect (1 to 2 weeks). Triamcinolone acetonide is relatively insoluble and slowly absorbed. Its extended duration of action lasts for several weeks. Triamcinolone hexacetonide is relatively insoluble, is absorbed slowly, and has a prolonged action of 3 to 4 weeks. Do not administer any of the parenteral suspensions intravenously.

Triamcinolone acetonide is used as an oral inhalant to treat bronchial asthma in patients who require corticosteroids to control symptoms.
• *Kinetics in adults:* Triamcinolone is absorbed readily after oral administration. After oral and I.V. administration, peak effects occur in about 1 to 2 hours. The suspensions for injection have variable onset and duration of action, depending on whether they are injected into an intra-articular space or a muscle, and on the blood supply to that muscle.

Systemic absorption from the lungs is similar to that observed from oral administration. Peak levels are attained in 1 to 2 hours. After oral inhalation, 10% to 25% of the drug is distributed to the lungs. The remainder is swallowed or deposited within the mouth. Triamcinolone is metabolized mainly by the liver. Some drug that reaches the lungs may be metabolized locally.

After topical application, absorption depends on the potency of the preparation, the amount applied, and the skin at the application site. It ranges from about 1% in areas with a thick stratum corneum (such as the palms, soles, elbows, and knees) to as high as 36% in areas of the thinnest stratum corneum (face, eyelids, and genitals). Absorption increases in areas of skin damage, inflammation, or occlusion. After topical application, triamcinolone is distributed throughout the local skin layer and metabolized primarily in the skin. A small amount is absorbed, especially through the oral mucosa.

Triamcinolone is removed rapidly from the blood and distributed to muscle, liver, skin, intestines, and kidneys. Triamcinolone is extensively bound to plasma proteins (transcortin and albumin). Only the unbound portion is active. Adrenocorticoids are distributed into breast milk and through the placenta.

Triamcinolone is metabolized in the liver to inactive glucuronide and sulfate metabolites. The inactive metabolites and small amounts of unmetabolized drug are excreted by the kidneys. Insignificant quantities of drug are also excreted in feces. The biologic half-life of triamcinolone is 18 to 36 hours.

Contraindications and precautions
Triamcinolone is contraindicated in patients with hypersensitivity to ingredients of adrenocorticoid preparations and in patients with systemic fungal infections (except in adrenal insufficiency). Patients receiving triamcinolone should not be given live virus

vaccines because triamcinolone suppresses the immune response.

Triamcinolone should be used with extreme caution in patients with GI ulceration, renal disease, hypertension, osteoporosis, diabetes mellitus, thromboembolic disorders, seizures, myasthenia gravis, CHF, tuberculosis, hypoalbuminemia, hypothyroidism, cirrhosis of the liver, emotional instability, psychotic tendencies, hyperlipidemias, glaucoma, or cataracts because the drug may exacerbate these conditions.

Because adrenocorticoids increase susceptibility to and mask symptoms of infection, triamcinolone should not be used (except in life-threatening situations) in patients with viral infections or bacterial infections not controlled by anti-infective agents.

Triamcinolone inhalant is contraindicated in patients with acute status asthmaticus or a hypersensitivity to any component of the preparation.

Drug should be used with caution in patients receiving systemic corticosteroids because of increased risk of hypothalamic-pituitary-adrenal axis suppression; when substituting inhalant for oral systemic therapy (because withdrawal symptoms may occur); and in patients with tuberculosis, healing nasal septal ulcers, oral or nasal surgery or trauma, or bacterial, fungal, or viral respiratory infection.

Topical use of triamcinolone is contraindicated in patients who are hypersensitive to any component of the preparation. It should be used cautiously in patients with viral, fungal, or tubercular skin lesions. It should also be used with extreme caution in patients with impaired circulation because the drug may increase the risk of skin ulceration.

Interactions
When used concomitantly, triamcinolone rarely may decrease the effects of oral anticoagulants.

Glucocorticoids increase the metabolism of isoniazid and salicylates; cause hyperglycemia, requiring dosage adjustment of insulin in diabetic patients; and may enhance hypokalemia associated with diuretic or amphotericin B therapy. The hypokalemia may increase the risk of toxicity in patients concurrently receiving digitalis glycosides.

Barbiturates, phenytoin, and rifampin may cause decreased corticosteroid effects because of increased hepatic metabolism. Cholestyramine, colestipol, and antacids decrease triamcinolone's effect by adsorbing the corticosteroid, decreasing the amount absorbed.

Concomitant use with estrogens may reduce the metabolism of triamcinolone by increasing the concentration of transcortin. The half-life of the corticosteroid is then prolonged because of increased protein-binding. Concomitant administration of ulcerogenic drugs, such as nonsteroidal anti-inflammatory agents, may increase the risk of GI ulceration.

Effects on diagnostic tests
Triamcinolone suppresses reactions to skin tests; causes false-negative results in the nitroblue tetrazolium test for systemic bacterial infections; decreases ^{131}I uptake and protein-bound iodine concentrations in thyroid function tests; may increase glucose and cholesterol levels; may decrease serum potassium, calcium, thyroxine, and triiodothyronine levels; and may increase urine glucose and calcium levels.

Adverse reactions
When administered in high doses or for prolonged therapy, triamcinolone suppresses release of adrenocorticotropic hormone (ACTH) from the pituitary gland; in turn, the adrenal cortex stops secreting endogenous corticosteroids. The degree and duration of hypothalamic-pituitary-adrenal (HPA) axis suppression produced by the drugs is highly variable among patients and depends on the dose, frequency, and time of administration, and duration of glucocorticoid therapy.
- CNS: euphoria, insomnia, headache, psychotic behavior, *pseudotumor cerebri*, mental changes, nervousness, restlessness, *psychoses*.
- CV: CHF, *hypertension*, edema.
- DERM: delayed healing, *acne*, skin eruptions, striae, burning, itching, irritation, dryness, folliculitis, hypertrichosis, acneiform eruptions, hypopigmentation, perioral dermatitis, allergic contact dermatitis, maceration, secondary infection, atrophy, miliaria.
- EENT: *cataracts*, glaucoma, thrush, rash, dry mouth, hoarseness, irritation of mouth or throat, dysgeusia.
- GI: *peptic ulcer*, irritation, increased appetite.
- Immune: immunosuppression, *increased susceptibility to infection*, fungal overgrowth of nose, mouth, or throat.
- Metabolic: *hypokalemia*, sodium retention, fluid retention, weight gain, hyperglycemia, *osteoporosis*, growth suppression in children, *glycosuria*.
- Musculoskeletal: muscle atrophy, weakness, *myopathy*.
- Other: pancreatitis, *hirsutism*, *cushingoid symptoms*, withdrawal syndrome (nausea, fatigue, anorexia, dyspnea, hypotension, hypoglycemia, myalgia, arthralgia, fever, dizziness, and fainting), *ecchymoses*. Sudden withdrawal may exacerbate the underlying disease or may be fatal. Acute adrenal insufficiency may occur with increased stress (infection, surgery, trauma) or abrupt withdrawal after long-term therapy.

Note: Topical use should be discontinued if local irritation, infection, systemic absorption, or hypersensitivity reaction occurs. Inhalant should be discontinued if no improvement is evident after 3 weeks or if an oral infection develops.

Overdose and treatment
Acute ingestion, even in massive doses, is rarely a clinical problem. Toxic signs and symptoms rarely occur if the drug is used for less than 3 weeks, even at large doses. However, chronic use causes adverse physiologic effects, including suppression of the HPA axis, cushingoid appearance, muscle weakness, and osteoporosis.

▶ Special considerations
- Chronic use of adrenocorticoids or corticotropin in children and adolescents may delay growth and maturation.
- If possible, avoid long-term administration of pharmacologic dosages of glucocorticoids in children because these drugs may retard bone growth.

---

‡May contain sulfites   ◆May contain tartrazine   ◆◆May contain benzyl alcohol

Manifestations of adrenal suppression in children include retardation of linear growth, delayed weight gain, low plasma cortisol concentrations, and lack of response to corticotropin stimulation. In children who require prolonged therapy, closely monitor growth and development. Alternate-day therapy is recommended to minimize growth suppression.
• Establish baseline blood pressure, fluid intake and output, weight, and electrolyte status. Watch for any sudden patient weight gain, edema, change in blood pressure, or change in electrolyte status.
• During times of physiologic stress (trauma, surgery, infection), the patient may require additional steroids and may experience signs of steroid withdrawal; patients who were previously steroid-dependent may need systemic corticosteroids to prevent adrenal insufficiency.
• After long-term therapy, the drug should be reduced gradually. Rapid reduction may cause withdrawal symptoms.
• Be aware of the patient's psychological history and watch for any behavioral changes.
• Observe for signs of infection or delayed wound healing.
• Acute withdrawal of drug may result in fever, myalgia, arthralgia, malaise, hypotension, or hypoglycemia shock.

Topical administration
• The 0.5% cream and ointment are recommended only for dermatoses refractory to treatment with lower concentrations.
• Children may show greater susceptibility to topical corticosteroid-induced HPA axis suppression and Cushing's syndrome than mature patients because of a higher ratio of skin surface area to body weight. HPA axis suppression, Cushing's syndrome, and intracranial hypertension have been reported in children receiving topical corticosteroids. Signs of adrenal suppression in children include linear growth retardation, delayed weight gain, low plasma cortisol levels, and absence of response to ACTH stimulation. Signs of intracranial hypertension include bulging fontanels, headaches, and bilateral papilledema.
• Topical administration to children should be limited to the lowest effective amount. Chronic corticosteroid therapy may interfere with growth and development.
• Discontinue if the patient develops signs of systemic absorption (including Cushing's syndrome, hyperglycemia, or glucosuria), skin irritation or ulceration, hypersensitivity, or infection. (If antifungals or antibiotics are being used with corticosteroids and the infection does not respond immediately, corticosteroids should be stopped until infection is controlled).
• Monitor patient response. Observe area of inflammation and elicit patient comments concerning pruritus. Inspect skin for infection, striae, and atrophy. Skin atrophy is common and may be clinically significant within 3 to 4 weeks of treatment with high-potency preparations; it also occurs more readily at sites where percutaneous absorption is high.
• Do not apply occlusive dressings over topical steroids because this may lead to secondary infection, maceration, atrophy, striae, or miliaria caused by increasing steroid penetration and potency.

Inhalant administration
• In children, systemic corticosteroid therapy may be successfully substituted with nasal or oral inhalant corticosteroid therapy, thus reducing the risk of adverse systemic effects. However, the risk of HPA axis suppression and Cushing's syndrome still exists, particularly if excessive dosages are used.
• The therapeutic effects of intranasal inhalants, unlike those of sympathomimetic decongestants, are not immediate. Full therapeutic benefit requires regular use and is usually evident within a few days, although a few patients may require up to 3 weeks of therapy for maximum benefit.
• Use of nasal or oral inhalation therapy may occasionally allow a patient to discontinue systemic corticosteroid therapy. Systemic therapy should be discontinued by gradually tapering the dosage while carefully observing the patient for signs of adrenal insufficiency (joint pain, lassitude, depression).
• After the desired clinical effect is obtained, maintenance dose should be reduced to the smallest amount necessary to control symptoms.
• The drug should be discontinued if the patient develops signs of systemic absorption (including Cushing's syndrome, hyperglycemia, or glucosuria), mucosal irritation or ulceration, hypersensitivity, or infection. (If antifungals or antibiotics are being used with corticosteroids and the infection does not respond immediately, discontinue corticosteroids until the infection is controlled.)

Information for parents and patient
• Be sure that parents and patient understand the need to take the adrenocorticosteroid as prescribed. Give instructions on what to do if a dose is inadvertently missed.
• Warn the parents and patient not to discontinue the drug abruptly.
• Inform the parents and patient of the possible therapeutic and adverse effects of the drug, so that they may report any complications as soon as possible.
• Advise the parents that the patient should wear a Medic Alert bracelet or necklace indicating the need for supplemental adrenocorticoids during times of stress.

For patients using a nasal inhaler
• Instruct patient to use only as directed. Inform him that full therapeutic effect is not immediate but requires regular use of inhaler.
• Encourage patient with blocked nasal passages to use an oral decongestant ½ hour before intranasal corticosteroid adminsitration to ensure adequate penetration. Advise patient to clear nasal passages of secretions before using the inhaler.
• Advise patient to read manufacturer's instructions and demonstrate use of inhaler. Assist patient until proper use of inhaler is demonstrated.
• Instruct patient to clean inhaler according to manufacturer's instructions.

For patients using an oral inhaler
• Instruct patient to use only as directed.
• Advise patient receiving bronchodilators by inhalation to use the bronchodilator before the corticosteroid inhalant to enhance penetration of the corticosteroid into the bronchial tree. Patient shoul

wait several minutes to allow time for the broncho-dilator to relax the smooth muscle.

• Ask patient to read manufacturer's instructions and demonstrate use of inhaler. Assist patient until proper use of inhaler is demonstrated.

• Instruct patient to hold breath for a few seconds to enhance placement and action of the drug and to wait 1 minute before taking subsequent puffs of medication.

• Tell patient to rinse mouth with water after using the inhaler to decrease the chance of oral fungal infections. Tell him to check nasal and oral mucous membranes frequently for signs of fungal infection.

• Warn asthma patients not to increase use of corticosteroid inhaler during a severe asthma attack, but to call for adjustment of therapy, possibly by adding a systemic steroid.

For patients using either type of inhaler

• Tell patient to report decreased response; an adjustment in dosage or discontinuation of the drug may be necessary.

• Instruct patient to observe for adverse effects, and if fever or local irritation develops, to discontinue use and report the effect promptly.

Method for applying topical preparations

Instruct parents and patient in application of the drug. Tell them the following:

• Wash your hands before and after applying the drug.

• Gently cleanse the area of application. Washing or soaking the area before application may increase drug penetration.

• Apply sparingly in a light film; rub in lightly. Avoid contact with patient's eyes, unless using an ophthalmic product.

• Avoid prolonged application in areas near the eyes, genitals, rectum, on the face, and in skin folds. High-potency topical corticosteroids are more likely to cause striae in these areas because of their higher rates of absorption.

• Monitor patient response. Observe area of inflammation and elicit patient comments concerning pruritus. Inspect skin for infection, striae, and atrophy. Skin atrophy is common and may be clinically significant within 3 to 4 weeks of treatment with high-potency preparations; it also occurs more readily at sites where percutaneous absorption is high.

• Do not apply occlusive dressings over topical steroids because this may lead to secondary infection, maceration, atrophy, striae, or miliaria caused by increasing steroid penetration and potency.

• To use with an occlusive dressing: apply cream, then cover with a thin, pliable, noninflammable plastic film; seal to adjacent unaffected skin with hypoallergenic tape. Minimize adverse reactions by using occlusive dressing intermittently. Do not leave it in place longer than 16 hours each day.

• For patients with eczematous dermatitis who may develop irritation from adhesive material, hold dressings in place with gauze, elastic bandages, stockings, or stockinette.

• Warn patient not to use nonprescription topical preparations other than those specifically recommended.

• Advise parents not to use tight-fitting diapers or plastic pants on a child being treated in the diaper area, since such garments may serve as occlusive dressings.

trichlormethiazide
Aquazide, Diurese, Metahydrin, Naqua, Trichlorex*

• Classification: diuretic, antihypertensive (thiazide)

How supplied
Available by prescription only
Tablets: 2 mg, 4 mg

Indications, route, and dosage
Edema
Children over age 6 months: 0.07 mg/kg or 2 mg/m² P.O. daily or in two divided doses.
Adults: 1 to 4 mg P.O. daily or in two divided doses.
Hypertension
Children over age 6 months: 0.07 mg/kg or 2 mg/m² P.O. daily or in two divided doses.
Adults: 2 to 4 mg P.O. daily.

Action and kinetics
• *Diuretic action:* Trichlormethiazide increases urinary excretion of sodium and water by inhibiting sodium reabsorption in the cortical diluting tubule of the nephron, thereby relieving edema.

• *Antihypertensive action:* The exact mechanism of trichlormethiazide's antihypertensive effect is unknown; it may result from direct arteriolar vasodilation. Trichlormethiazide also reduces total body sodium and total peripheral resistance.

• *Kinetics in adults:* Trichlormethiazide is absorbed from the GI tract after oral administration. Limited data are available on other pharmacokinetic parameters; the drug appears to be primarily excreted unchanged in urine.

Contraindications and precautions
Trichlormethiazide is contraindicated in patients with anuria and in those with known hypersensitivity to the drug or to other sulfonamide derivatives. Trichlormethiazide should be used cautiously in patients with severe renal disease, because it may decrease glomerular filtration rate and precipitate azotemia; in patients with impaired hepatic function or liver disease, because electrolyte alterations may induce hepatic coma; and in patients taking digoxin, because hypokalemia may predispose them to digitalis toxicity.

Metahydrin and Trichlorex contain tartrazine, which may cause allergic reactions, including bronchospasm, in asthmatic and aspirin-sensitive patients.

Interactions
Trichlormethiazide potentiates the hypotensive effects of most other antihypertensive drugs; this may be used to therapeutic advantage.

Trichlormethiazide may potentiate hyperglycemic, hypotensive, and hyperuricemic effects of diazoxide, and its hyperglycemic effect may increase insulin requirements in diabetic patients.

Trichlormethiazide may reduce renal clearance of

lithium, elevating serum lithium levels, and may necessitate reduction in lithium dosage by 50%.

Trichlormethiazide turns urine slightly more alkaline and may decrease urinary excretion of some amines, such as amphetamine and quinidine; alkaline urine also may decrease therapeutic efficacy of methenamine compounds, such as methenamine mandelate.

Cholestyramine and colestipol may bind trichlormethiazide, preventing its absorption; give drugs 1 hour apart.

Effects on diagnostic tests

Trichlormethiazide therapy may alter serum electrolyte levels and may increase serum urate, glucose, cholesterol, and triglyceride levels. It also may interfere with tests for parathyroid function and should be discontinued before such tests.

Adverse reactions

- CV: volume depletion and dehydration, orthostatic hypotension, hypercholesterolemia, hypertriglyceridemia.
- DERM: dermatitis, photosensitivity, rash.
- GI: anorexia, nausea, pancreatitis.
- HEMA: aplastic anemia, agranulocytosis, leukopenia, thrombocytopenia.
- Hepatic: hepatic encephalopathy.
- Metabolic: asymptomatic hyperuricemia; gout; hyperglycemia and impairment of glucose tolerance; fluid and electrolyte imbalances, including dilutional hyponatremia and hypochloremia, hypercalcemia, and hypokalemia; metabolic alkalosis.
- Other: hypersensitivity reactions, such as pneumonitis and vasculitis.

Note: Drug should be discontinued if rising BUN and serum creatinine levels indicate renal impairment or if patient shows signs of impending coma.

Overdose and treatment

Clinical signs of overdose include GI irritation and hypermotility, diuresis, and lethargy, which may progress to coma.

Treatment is mainly supportive; monitor and assist respiratory, cardiovascular, and renal function as indicated. Monitor fluid and electrolyte balance. For recent ingestion (within 4 hours), induce vomiting with ipecac in conscious patient; otherwise, use gastric lavage to avoid aspiration. Do not give cathartics; these promote additional loss of fluids and electrolytes.

▶ Special considerations

- Monitor weight and serum electrolyte levels regularly.
- Monitor serum potassium levels; encourage high-potassium diet. Foods rich in potassium include citrus fruits, tomatoes, bananas, dates, and apricots. Watch for signs of hypokalemia (for example, muscle weakness or cramps). Patients also taking digitalis have an increased risk of digitalis toxicity from the potassium-depleting effect of the drug.
- Trichlormethiazide may be used with potassium-sparing diuretics to attenuate potassium loss.

- Check insulin requirements in patients with diabetes.
- Monitor serum creatinine and BUN levels regularly. Drug is not as effective if these levels are more than twice normal.
- Monitor blood uric acid levels.
- A.M. administration is recommended to prevent nocturia.
- Antihypertensive effects persist for approximately 1 week after discontinuation of the drug.
- Instruct parents to observe for and to report any joint swelling, pain, or redness; these signs may indicate hyperuricemia.

Information for parents and patient

- Explain rationale of therapy and diuretic effects of drug.
- Advise parents to watch for and promptly report signs of electrolyte imbalance: weakness, fatigue, muscle cramps, paresthesias, confusion, nausea, vomiting, diarrhea, headache, dizziness, and palpitations.
- Tell parents to report any increased edema or weight or excess diuresis (more than a 2% weight loss or gain) and to record child's weight each morning after voiding and before breakfast on the same scale and wearing the same type of clothing.
- Advise parents to give drug with food to minimize gastric irritation; to encourage child to eat potassium-rich foods, such as citrus fruits, potatoes, dates, raisins, and bananas; and to restrict child's access to salt and high-sodium foods, such as lunch meat, smoked meats, and processed cheeses. Inform parents that low-sodium formulas are available for infants.
- Tell parents to seek medical approval before giving patient nonprescription drugs; many contain sodium and potassium and can cause electrolyte imbalances.
- Explain photosensitivity reactions. In thiazide-related photosensitivity, ultraviolet radiation alters drug structure, causing allergic reactions in some persons; such reactions occur 10 days to 2 weeks after initial sun exposure.
- Warn parents to supervise the child's activities closely to prevent falls and other injuries that may result from dizziness, especially at beginning of therapy.
- Caution patient to change position slowly, especially when rising to upright position, to prevent dizziness from orthostatic hypotension.
- Advise parents to watch closely for chest, back, or leg pain, or shortness of breath, and to call immediately if they occur.
- Advise parents to administer drug only as prescribed and at the same time each day, to prevent nighttime diuresis and interrupted sleep.
- Emphasize importance of regular medical follow-up to monitor effectiveness of diuretic therapy.

trientine hydrochloride
Cuprid

• Classification: heavy metal antagonist (chelating agent)

How supplied
Available by prescription only
Capsules: 250 mg

Indications, route, and dosage
Wilson's disease in patients who are intolerant of penicillamine
Children under age 12: 500 to 750 mg in doses divided b.i.d. to q.i.d. Maximum dosage is 1,500 mg daily.
Adults: 750 to 1,250 mg in doses divided b.i.d. to q.i.d. Maximum dosage is 2 g daily.

Action and kinetics
• *Chelating action:* Trientine forms a soluble complex with free serum copper that is renally excreted, removing excess copper.
• *Kinetics in adults:* Trientine is well absorbed after oral administration. Drug is excreted in urine as unchanged drug or a trientine-copper complex.

Contraindications and precautions
Trientine is contraindicated in patients with known or suspected hypersensitivity to the drug; it is not intended for use in patients with rheumatoid arthritis, biliary cirrhosis, or cystinuria.

Drug should be used with caution in patients who have or are at risk for iron deficiency, because trientine also chelates iron; and in patients with idiopathic or penicillamine-induced systemic lupus erythematosus (SLE), because trientine may reactivate the disease.

Interactions
Concomitant ingestion of trientine with mineral supplements, especially iron, reduces absorption of the drug.

Effects on diagnostic tests
None reported.

Adverse reactions
• DERM: dermatitis.
• EENT: bronchitis, asthma.
• Other: SLE, iron deficiency anemia.
Note: Drug should be discontinued if SLE or hypersensitivity occurs.

Overdose and treatment
Data on effects of overdose are unavailable. Treat symptomatically.

▶ Special considerations
• Safety and efficacy in children have not been established; drug should be used with caution.
• Drug is designed for use only in patients unable to tolerate penicillamine, which remains the standard therapy for Wilson's disease.

• Daily dosage may be increased if clinical response is inadequate or free serum copper level remains above 20 mcg/dl.
• Observe patient for any signs or symptoms of hypersensitivity, such as asthma, fever, or skin eruptions; monitor all patients for iron deficiency anemia.
• For optimal therapeutic effect, give drug 1 hour before or 2 hours after meals and at least 1 hour apart from any other drug, food, or milk.

Information for parents and patient
• Explain disease process and rationale for therapy, stress importance of compliance with low-copper diet and follow-up visits.
• Tell parents and patient how and when to take drug; especially advise patient to swallow capsule whole (do not open or chew), and to drink full glass (8 oz) of water with each dose.
• Advise parents to check for fever nightly for the first month of treatment and to report any signs, such as fever or skin eruption.
• Explain that trientine causes contact dermatitis; after accidental contact, flood exposed area with water promptly.

trifluoperazine hydrochloride
Apo-Trifluoperazine∗, Novoflurazine∗, Solazine∗, Stelazine, Suprazine, Terfluzine∗

• Classification: antipsychotic, antiemetic (phenothiazine [piperazine derivative])

How supplied
Available by prescription only
Tablets (regular and film-coated): 1 mg, 2 mg, 5 mg, 10 mg
Oral concentrate: 10 mg/ml
Injection: 2 mg/ml

Indications, route, and dosage
Anxiety states
Adults: 1 to 2 mg P.O. b.i.d.
Schizophrenia and other psychotic disorders
Children age 6 to 12 (hospitalized or under close supervision): 1 mg P.O. daily or b.i.d.; may increase gradually to 15 mg daily.
Adults: For outpatients, 1 to 2 mg P.O. b.i.d., increased as needed. For hospitalized patients, 2 to 5 mg P.O. b.i.d.; may increase gradually to 40 mg daily. For I.M. injection, 1 to 2 mg q 4 to 6 hours, p.r.n.

Action and kinetics
• *Antipsychotic action:* Trifluoperazine is thought to exert its antipsychotic effects by postsynaptic blockade of CNS dopamine receptors, thereby inhibiting dopamine-mediated effects; antiemetic effects are attributed to opamine receptor blockade in the medullary chemoreceptor trigger zone. Trifluoperazine has many other central and peripheral effects; it produces alpha and ganglionic blockade and counteracts histamine- and serotonin-mediated activity. Its most

prevalent adverse reactions are extrapyramidal; it has less sedative and autonomic activity than aliphatic phenothiazines.

• *Kinetics in adults:* Rate and extent of absorption vary with route of administration: oral tablet absorption is erratic and variable, with onset of action ranging from ½ to 1 hour; oral concentrate absorption is much more predictable. I.M. drug is absorbed rapidly.

Trifluoperazine is distributed widely in the body, including breast milk. Drug is 91% to 99% protein-bound. Peak effect occurs in 2 to 4 hours; steady-state serum levels are achieved within 4 to 7 days.

Trifluoperazine is metabolized extensively by the liver, but no active metabolites are formed; duration of action is about 4 to 6 hours.

Most of drug is excreted in urine via the kidneys; some is excreted in feces via the biliary tract.

Contraindications and precautions

Trifluoperazine is contraindicated in patients with known hypersensitivity to phenothiazines and related compounds, including allergic reactions involving hepatic function; in patients with blood dyscrasias and bone marrow depression (adverse hematologic effects); in patients with disorders accompanied by coma, brain damage, CNS depression, circulatory collapse, or cerebrovascular disease (additive CNS depression and adverse blood pressure effects); and in patients taking adrenergic-blocking agents or spinal or epidural anesthetics (excessive respiratory, cardiac, and CNS depression).

Trifluoperazine should be used with caution in patients with cardiac disease (dysrhythmias, congestive heart failure, angina pectoris, valvular disease, or heart block); encephalitis; Reye's syndrome; head injury; respiratory disease; epilepsy and other seizure disorders; glaucoma; prostatic hypertrophy; urinary retention; Parkinson's disease and pheochromocytoma, because it may exacerbate these conditions; in patients with hypocalcemia because it increases the risk of extrapyramidal reactions; and in patients with hepatic or renal dysfunction (diminished metabolism and excretion cause the drug to accumulate).

Interactions

Concomitant use of trifluoperazine with sympathomimetics, including epinephrine, phenylephrine, phenylpropanolamine, and ephedrine (often found in nasal sprays), and appetite suppressants may decrease their stimulatory and pressor effects. Use epinephrine as a pressor agent in patients taking trifluoperazine may result in epinephrine reversal or further lowering of blood pressure.

Trifluoperazine may inhibit blood pressure response to centrally acting antihypertensive drugs, such as guanethidine, guanabenz, guanadrel, clonidine, methyldopa, and reserpine. Additive effects are likely after concomitant use of trifluoperazine with CNS depressants, including alcohol, analgesics, barbiturates, narcotics, tranquilizers, anesthetics (general, spinal, epidural), and parenteral magnesium sulfate (oversedation, respiratory depression, and hypotension); antiarrhythmic agents, quinidine, disopyramide, and procainamide (increased incidence of cardiac dysrhythmias and conduction defects); atropine and other anticholinergic drugs, including antidepressants, monoamine oxidase inhibitors, phenothiazines, antihistamines, meperidine, and antiparkinsonian agents (oversedation, paralytic ileus, visual changes, and severe constipation); nitrates (hypotension); and metrizamide (increased risk of convulsions).

Beta-blocking agents may inhibit trifluoperazine metabolism, increasing plasma levels and toxicity.

Concomitant use of trifluoperazine with propylthiouracil increases risk of agranulocytosis; concomitant use with lithium may result in severe neurologic toxicity with an encephalitis-like syndrome and in decreased therapeutic response to trifluoperazine.

Pharmacokinetic alterations and subsequent decreased therapeutic response to trifluoperazine may follow concomitant use with phenobarbital (enhanced renal excretion), aluminum and magnesium-containing antacids and antidiarrheals (decreased absorption), caffeine, and heavy smoking (increased metabolism).

Trifluoperazine may antagonize therapeutic effect of bromocriptine on prolactin secretion; it also may decrease the vasoconstricting effects of high-dose dopamine and may decrease effectiveness and increase toxicity of levodopa (by dopamine blockade). Trifluoperazine may inhibit metabolism and increase toxicity of phenytoin.

Effects on diagnostic tests

Trifluoperazine causes false-positive test results for urine porphyrins, urobilinogen, amylase, and 5-HIAA levels from darkening of urine by metabolites; it also causes false-positive urine pregnancy results in tests using human chorionic gonadotropin as the indicator.

Trifluoperazine elevates tests for liver function and protein-bound iodine and causes quinidine-like effects on the ECG.

Adverse reactions

• CNS: extrapyramidal symptoms (dystonia, akathisia, torticollis, tardive dyskinesia, sedation (low incidence), pseudoparkinsonism, drowsiness (frequent), neuroleptic malignant syndrome (dose-related; fatal respiratory failure in over 10% of patients if untreated), dizziness, headache, insomnia, exacerbation of psychotic symptoms.

• CV: asystole, orthostatic hypotension, tachycardia, dizziness or fainting, dysrhythmias, ECG changes, increased anginal pain after I.M. injection.

• EENT: blurred vision, tinnitus, mydriasis, increased intraocular pressure, ocular changes (retinal pigmentary change with long-term use).

• GI: dry mouth, constipation, nausea, vomiting, anorexia, diarrhea.

• GU: urinary retention, gynecomastia, hypermenorrhea, inhibited ejaculation.

• HEMA: transient leukopenia, agranulocytosis, thrombocytopenia, anemia (within 30 to 90 days).

• Local: contact dermatitis from concentrate or injection, muscle necrosis from I.M. injection.

• Other: hyperprolactinemia, photosensitivity, increased appetite or weight gain, hypersensitivity (rash, urticaria, drug fever, edema, cholestatic jaundice [2% to 4% in first 30 days]).

After abrupt withdrawal of long-term therapy, gastritis, nausea, vomiting, dizziness, tremors, feeling of heat or cold, sweating, tachycardia, headache, or insomnia may occur.

Note: Drug should be discontinued immediately if any of the following occur: hypersensitivity, jaundice, agranulocytosis, neuroleptic malignant syndrome (marked hyperthermia, extrapyramidal effects, autonomic dysfunction), severe extrapyramidal symptoms even after dosage is lowered. Drug should be discontinued 48 hours before and 24 hours after myelography using metrizamide, because of risk of convulsions. When feasible, drug should be withdrawn slowly and gradually; many drug effects persist after withdrawal.

Overdose and treatment

CNS depression is characterized by deep, unarousable sleep and possible coma, hypotension or hypertension, extrapyramidal symptoms, dystonia, abnormal involuntary muscle movements, agitation, seizures, dysrhythmias, ECG changes, hypothermia or hyperthermia, and autonomic nervous system dysfunction.

Treatment is symptomatic and supportive and includes maintaining vital signs, airway, stable body temperature, and fluid and electrolyte balance.

Do not induce vomiting: Drug inhibits cough reflex, and aspiration may occur. Use gastric lavage, then activated charcoal and saline cathartics; dialysis is usually ineffective. Regulate body temperature as needed. Treat hypotension with I.V. fluids: *Do not give epinephrine.* Treat seizures with parenteral diazepam or barbiturates; dysrhythmias with parenteral phenytoin (1 mg/kg with rate titrated to blood pressure); extrapyramidal reactions with barbiturates, benztropin, or parenteral diphenhydramine 2 mg/kg/minute.

▶ Special considerations

• Drug is not recommended for children under age 6.
• Check vital signs regularly for decreased blood pressure (especially before and after parenteral therapy) or tachycardia; observe patient carefully for other adverse reactions.
• Check intake and output for urinary retention or constipation, which may require dosage reduction.
• Monitor bilirubin levels weekly for first 4 weeks; monitor complete blood count, ECG (for quinidine-like effects), liver and renal function studies, electrolyte levels (especially potassium) and eye examinations at baseline and periodically thereafter, especially in patients on long-term therapy.
• Observe patient for mood changes to monitor progress; benefits may not be apparent for several weeks.
• Do not withdraw drug abruptly; although physical dependence does not occur with antipsychotic drugs, rebound exacerbation of psychotic symptoms may occur, and many drug effects persist.
• Carefully follow manufacturer's instructions for reconstitution, dilution, administration, and storage of drugs.
• When drug is given for anxiety, do not exceed 6 mg daily for longer than 12 weeks. However, some clinicians recommend against use of this drug for anything but psychosis.

• Administer I.M. injection deep in the upper outer quadrant of the buttock. Massaging the area after administration may prevent formation of abscesses. I.M. injection may cause skin necrosis; do not extravasate.
• Solution for injection may be slightly discolored. Do not use if excessively discolored or a precipitate is evident. Contact pharmacist.
• Shake concentrate before administration.
• Chewing sugarless gum, hard candy, or ice chips may help relieve dry mouth.
• Worsening anginal pain has been reported in patients receiving trifluoperazine; however, ECG reactions are less frequent with this drug than with other phenothiazines.
• Liquid and injectable formulations may cause a rash after contact with skin.
• Drug may cause pink to brown discoloration of urine.
• Trifluoperazine is associated with a high incidence of extrapyramidal symptoms and photosensitivity reactions. Monitor for involuntary movements. Check patient receiving prolonged treatment at least once every 6 months. Patient should avoid exposure to sunlight or heat lamps.
• Oral formulations may cause stomach upset. Administer with food or fluid.
• Concentrate must be diluted in 2 to 4 oz of liquid, preferably water, carbonated drinks, fruit juice, tomato juice, milk, or pudding.
• Protect the liquid formulation from light.

Information for parents and patient

• Explain rationale and anticipated risks and benefits of therapy, and that full therapeutic effect may not occur for several weeks.
• Patient should avoid beverages and drugs containing alcohol, and not take any other drug (especially CNS depressants) including nonprescription products without medical approval.
• Instruct parents of diabetic children to monitor blood glucose levels, because drug may alter insulin needs.
• Teach parents or patient how and when to take drug, not to increase dose without medical approval, and never to discontinue drug abruptly; suggest taking full dose at bedtime if daytime sedation is troublesome.
• Advise parents to have patient lie down for 30 minutes after first dose (1 hour if I.M.) and to rise slowly from sitting or supine position to prevent orthostatic hypotension.
• Drugs are locally irritating; advise taking with milk or food to minimize GI distress. Warn that oral concentrates and solutions will irritate skin. Patient should not crush or open sustained-release products, but swallow them whole.
• Warn parents that excessive exposure to sunlight, heat lamps, or tanning beds may cause photosensitivity reactions (burn and abnormal hyperpigmentation).
• Patient should avoid exposure to extremes of heat or cold, because of risk of hypothermia or hyperthermia induced by alteration in thermoregulatory function.
• Recommend sugarless gum, hard candy, or ice chips to relieve dry mouth.

• Explain that phenothiazines may cause pink to brown discoloration of urine.
• Explain the risks of dystonic reactions, akathisia, and tardive dyskinesia, and tell parents to report abnormal body movements.
• Explain that many drug interactions are possible. Patient should not take any other medication unless prescribed.
• Tell parents that many adverse reactions may be alleviated by dosage reduction. However, parents should report if patient experiences difficulty urinating, sore throat, dizziness, or fainting.
• Patient should avoid hazardous activities that require alertness until the effect of the drug is established. Sedative effects usually subside in several weeks.
• Advise parents to store medication safely away from children.

---

triflupromazine hydrochloride
Vesprin

• Classification: antipsychotic, antiemetic (aliphatic phenothiazine)

How supplied
Available by prescription only
Injection: 10 mg, 20 mg/ml

Indications, route, and dosage
Psychotic disorders
Children over age 2½: 0.2 to 0.25 mg/kg I.M. in divided doses. Maximum dosage is 10 mg daily.
Adults: 60 to 150 mg I.M. in two or three divided doses.

Nausea and vomiting
Children: 0.2 mg/kg to 0.25 mg/kg I.M. up to maximum of 10 mg daily.
Adults: 1 mg I.V.; may be repeated up to a maximum of 3 mg daily; or 5 to 15 mg I.M. daily up to maximum of 60 mg daily.
Note: I.V. form is not recommended for use in children.

Action and kinetics
• *Antipsychotic and antiemetic actions:* Triflupromazine is thought to exert its antipsychotic effects by postsynaptic blockade of CNS dopamine receptors, thereby inhibiting dopamine-mediated effects; antiemetic effects are attributed to dopamine receptor blockade in the medullary chemoreceptor trigger zone. Triflupromazine has many other central and peripheral effects; it produces alpha and ganglionic blockade and counteracts histamine- and serotonin-mediated activity. Its most prominent adverse reactions are antimuscarinic and sedative; it causes fewer extrapyramidal effects than other antipsychotics.
• *Kinetics in adults:* I.M. drug is absorbed rapidly. Triflupromazine is distributed widely into the body, including breast milk. Steady-state serum level is achieved within 4 to 7 days. Drug is 91% to 99% protein-bound. Triflupromazine is metabolized exten-

sively by the liver and forms 10 to 12 metabolites. Majority of drug is excreted as metabolites in urine; some drug is excreted in feces via the biliary tract.

Contraindications and precautions
Triflupromazine is contraindicated in patients with known hypersensitivity to phenothiazines and related compounds, including allergic reactions involving hepatic function; in patients with blood dyscrasias and bone marrow depression (adverse hematologic effects); in patients with disorders accompanied by coma, brain damage, CNS depression (additive CNS depression), circulatory collapse, or cerebrovascular disease (adverse effects on blood pressure); and in patients taking adrenergic-blocking agents or spinal or epidural anesthetics (excessive respiratory, cardiac, and CNS depression).

Triflupromazine should be used cautiously in patients with cardiac disease (dysrhythmias, congestive heart failure, angina pectoris, valvular disease, or heart block); encephalitis; Reye's syndrome; head injury; respiratory disease; epilepsy and other seizure disorders; glaucoma; prostatic hypertrophy; urinary retention; hepatic or renal dysfunction; Parkinson's disease and pheochromocytoma, because it may worsen these conditions; and in patients with hypocalcemia because it increases the risk of extrapyramidal reactions. Drug therapy for uncomplicated nausea and vomiting in children should be avoided to prevent masking symptoms of serious underlying illness such as Reye's syndrome.

Interactions
Concomitant use of triflupromazine with sympathomimetics, including epinephrine, phenylephrine, phenylpropanolamine, and ephedrine (often found in nasal sprays) and with appetite suppressants may decrease their stimulatory and pressor effects. Triflupromazine may cause epinephrine reversal.

Triflupromazine may inhibit blood pressure response to centrally acting antihypertensive drugs, such as guanethidine, guanabenz, guanadrel, clonidine, methyldopa, and reserpine. Additive effects are likely after concomitant use of triflupromazine with CNS depressants (including alcohol, analgesics, barbiturates, narcotics, tranquilizers, and general, spinal, and epidural anesthetics) and parenteral magnesium sulfate (oversedation, respiratory depression, and hypotension); antiarrhythmic agents, quinidine, disopyramide, and procainamide (increased incidence of cardiac dysrhythmias and conduction defects); atropine and other anticholinergic drugs, including antidepressants, monoamine oxidase inhibitors, phenothiazines, antihistamines, meperidine, and antiparkinsonian agents (oversedation, paralytic ileus, visual changes, and severe constipation); nitrates (hypotension); and metrizamide (increased risk of convulsions).

Beta-blocking agents may inhibit triflupromazine metabolism, increasing plasma levels and toxicity.

Concomitant use of triflupromazine with propylthiouracil increases risk of agranulocytosis; concomitant use with lithium may result in severe neurologic toxicity with an encephalitis-like syndrome and in decreased therapeutic response to triflupromazine.

---

*Canada only   †Unlabeled clinical use   Italicized adverse reactions have been observed in children.

Pharmacokinetic alterations and subsequent decreased therapeutic response to triflupromazine may follow concomitant use with phenobarbital (enhanced renal excretion); aluminum- and magnesium-containing antacids and antidiarrheals (decreased absorption); caffeine; and heavy smoking (increased metabolism).

Triflupromazine may antagonize therapeutic effect of bromocriptine on prolactin secretion; it also may decrease the vasoconstricting effects of high-dose dopamine and may decrease effectiveness and increase toxicity of levodopa (by dopamine blockade). Triflupromazine may inhibit metabolism and increase toxicity of phenytoin.

Effects on diagnostic tests
Triflupromazine causes false-positive test results for urine porphyrins, urobilinogen, amylase, and 5-HIAA from darkening of urine by metabolites; it also causes false-positive urine pregnancy results in tests using human chorionic gonadotropin as the indicator.

Triflupromazine elevates levels for liver function tests and protein-bound iodine and causes quinidine-like ECG effects.

Adverse reactions
• CNS: extrapyramidal symptoms, including dystonia, akathisia, torticollis, tardive dyskinesia, sedation (high incidence), pseudoparkinsonism, drowsiness (frequent), neuroleptic malignant syndrome (dose-related; if untreated, fatal respiratory failure in over 10% of patients), dizziness, headache, insomnia, decreased libido, and exacerbation of psychotic symptoms.
• CV: asystole, orthostatic hypotension, tachycardia, dizziness and fainting, dysrhythmias, ECG changes, increased anginal pain after I.M. injection.
• EENT: blurred vision, tinnitus, mydriasis, increased intraocular pressure, ocular changes (retinal pigmentary change with long-term use).
• GI: dry mouth, constipation, nausea, vomiting, anorexia, diarrhea.
• GU: urinary retention, gynecomastia, hypermenorrhea, inhibited ejaculation.
• HEMA: transient leukopenia, agranulocytosis, thrombocytopenia, anemia (within 30 to 90 days).
• Local: contact dermatitis from concentrate or injectable form, muscle necrosis from I.M. injection.
• Other: hyperprolactinemia, photosensitivity, increased appetite and weight gain, hypersensitivity (rash, urticaria, drug fever, edema, cholestatic jaundice [in 2% to 4% of patients within first 30 days]).

After abrupt withdrawal of long-term therapy, gastritis, nausea, vomiting, dizziness, tremors, feeling of heat or cold, sweating, tachycardia, headache, and insomnia may occur.

Note: Drug should be discontinued if any of the following occur: hypersensitivity, jaundice, agranulocytosis; neuroleptic malignant syndrome (marked hyperthermia, extrapyramidal effects, autonomic dysfunction); severe extrapyramidal symptoms even after dosage is lowered. Drug should be discontinued 48 hours before and 24 hours after myelography using metrizamide, because of risk of convulsions. When feasible, drug should be withdrawn slowly and gradually; many drug effects persist after withdrawal.

Overdose and treatment
CNS depression is characterized by deep, unarousable sleep and possible coma, hypotension or hypertension, extrapyramidal symptoms, abnormal involuntary muscle movements, agitation, seizures, dysrhythmias, ECG changes, hypothermia or hyperthermia, and autonomic nervous system dysfunction.

Treatment is symptomatic and supportive, including maintenance of vital signs and airway, stable body temperature, and fluid and electrolyte balance.

Do not induce vomiting—drug inhibits cough reflex, and aspiration may occur. Use gastric lavage, then activated charcoal and saline cathartics; dialysis does not help. Regulate body temperature as needed. Treat hypotension with I.V. fluids—*do not give epinephrine*. Treat seizures with parenteral diazepam or barbiturates; dysrhythmias with parenteral phenytoin (1 mg/kg with rate titrated to blood pressure); extrapyramidal reactions with barbiturates, benztropin, or parenteral diphenhydramine 2 mg/kg/minute.

▶ Special considerations
• Drug is not recommended for patients under age 2½.
• Unless otherwise specified, antipsychotics are not recommended for children under age 12; be careful when using phenothiazines for nausea and vomiting, as acutely ill children (chicken pox, measles, CNS infections, dehydration) are at greatly increased risk of dystonic reactions.
• Check vital signs regularly for decreased blood pressure (especially before and after parenteral therapy) or tachycardia; observe patient carefully for other adverse reactions.
• Carefully follow manufacturer's instructions for reconstitution, dilution, administration, and storage of drugs.
• Administer drug I.M. deep in the upper outer quadrant of the buttock. Massaging the area after administration may prevent formation of abscesses. I.M. injection may cause skin necrosis; monitor to prevent extravasation.
• Check intake and output for urinary retention or constipation, which may require dosage reduction.
• Monitor bilirubin levels weekly for first 4 weeks; monitor complete blood count, ECG (for quinidine-like effects), liver and renal function studies, electrolyte levels (especially potassium) and eye examinations at baseline and periodically thereafter, especially in patients on long-term therapy.
• Observe patient for mood changes to monitor progress; benefits may not be apparent for several weeks.
• Do not withdraw drug abruptly; although physical dependence does not occur with antipsychotic drugs, rebound exacerbation of psychotic symptoms may occur, and many drug effects persist.
• Drug may cause a rash after contact with skin.
• Drug may cause pink to brown discoloration of urine.
• Triflupromazine is associated with a high incidence of sedation, orthostatic hypotension, and photosensitivity reaction. Blood pressure should be checked

before and after parenteral administration. Patient should avoid exposure to sunlight or heat lamps.
• Monitor patient regularly for abnormal movements (at least once every 6 months).
• Solution for injection may be slightly discolored. Do not use if excessively discolored or a precipitate is evident. Contact pharmacist.
• Sugarless chewing gum, hard candy, or ice chips may help relieve dry mouth.

Information for parents and patient
• Explain rationale and anticipated risks and benefits of therapy, and that full therapeutic effect may not occur for several weeks.
• Patient should avoid beverages and drugs containing alcohol, and not take any other drug (especially CNS depressants) including nonprescription products without medical approval.
• Instruct parents of diabetic children to monitor blood glucose levels, because drug may alter insulin needs.
• Teach parents or patient how and when to take drug, not to increase dose without medical approval, and never to discontinue drug abruptly; suggest giving full dose at bedtime if daytime sedation is troublesome.
• Explain that many drug interactions are possible. Patient should not take any other medication without medical approval.
• Patient should lie down for 30 minutes after first dose (1 hour if I.M.) and rise slowly from sitting or supine position to prevent orthostatic hypotension.
• Patient should avoid hazardous activities that require mental alertness and psychomotor coordination, until full effects of drug are established; emphasize that sedative effects subside after several weeks.
• Excessive exposure to sunlight, heat lamps, or tanning beds may cause photosensitivity reactions (burn and abnormal hyperpigmentation).
• Patient should avoid exposure to extremes of heat or cold, because of risk of hypothermia or hyperthermia induced by alteration in thermoregulatory function.
• Recommend sugarless gum, hard candy, or ice chips to relieve dry mouth.
• Explain that phenothiazines may cause pink to brown discoloration of urine.
• Explain the risks of dystonic reactions and tardive dyskinesia, and tell parents to report abnormal body movements.

trimeprazine tartrate
Panectyl*, Temaril

• Classification: antipruritic (phenothiazine-derivative antihistamine)

How supplied
Available by prescription only
Tablets: 2.5 mg
Spansule capsules (sustained-release): 5 mg
Syrup: 2.5 mg/5 ml (5.7% alcohol)

Indications, route, and dosage
Pruritus
Children age 6 months to 2 years: 1.25 mg P.O. at bedtime or t.i.d., p.r.n.
Children age 3 to 5: 2.5 mg P.O. at bedtime or t.i.d., p.r.n.
Children age 6 to 11: One Spansule capsule (5 mg) daily. Spansule capsules are not recommended for children under age 6.
Children age 12 and older and adults: 2.5 mg P.O. q.i.d.; or (timed-release) 5 mg P.O. q 12 hours.

Action and kinetics
• *Antipruritic action:* Antihistamines compete for histamine H_1-receptor sites by binding to cellular receptors; they prevent access of histamine and suppress histamine-induced allergic symptoms, even though they do not prevent its release.
• *Kinetics in adults:* Absorption, distribution, metabolism, and excretion have not been reported.

Contraindications and precautions
Trimeprazine is contraindicated in patients with known hypersensitivity to trimeprazine or to phenothiazines; during acute asthma attacks, because it thickens bronchial secretions; in acutely ill or dehydrated children, because they are at increased risk of developing dystonias; in patients with bone marrow depression, because the drug may exacerbate this syndrome; in patients with epilepsy, because the drug may increase the incidence of seizures; and in comatose patients and newborns.
    It also should be used with caution in children with a history of sleep apnea or a family history of sudden infant death syndrome. The relationship between these conditions and trimeprazine has not been studied; however, death has occurred in children given usual doses of phenothiazine antihistamines.
    Because of its significant anticholinergic activity, trimeprazine should be used with caution in patients with narrow-angle glaucoma; in those with pyloroduodenal obstruction or urinary bladder obstruction from narrowing of the bladder neck; in patients with cardiovascular disease or hypertension, because of the hazard of palpitations and tachycardia; and in patients with acute or chronic respiratory dysfunction (especially children), because trimeprazine may suppress the cough reflex.

Interactions
MAO inhibitors interfere with the detoxification of antihistamines and phenothiazines and thus prolong and intensify their central depressant and anticholinergic effects; added sedation and CNS depression may occur when trimeprazine is used concomitantly with other CNS depressants, including alcohol, barbiturates, tranquilizers, sleeping aids, and antianxiety agents.
    Phenothiazines potentiate the CNS depressant and analgesic effect of narcotics; the phenothiazine activity of trimeprazine is potentiated by oral contraceptives, progesterone, reserpine, and nylidrin hydrochloride.
    Do not give epinephrine to reverse trimeprazine-

induced hypotension; partial adrenergic blockade may cause further hypotension.

Effects on diagnostic tests

Trimeprazine should be discontinued 4 days before diagnostic skin tests, to avoid preventing, reducing, or masking positive test response. Trimeprazine may cause false-positive or false-negative urine pregnancy test results.

Adverse reactions

• CNS: drowsiness, dizziness, confusion, headache, restlessness, tremors, irritability, insomnia, extrapyramidal symptoms (especially at high doses), muscular weakness, disturbed coordination, increased appetite, paradoxical excitation.
• CV: postural hypotension, reflex tachycardia, palpitations, ECG changes.
• DERM: urticaria, rash, photosensitivity, systemic lupus erythematosus-like syndrome.
• GI: anorexia, nausea, vomiting, constipation, dry mouth and throat.
• GU: urinary frequency, urinary retention, gynecomastia.
• HEMA: agranulocytosis, leukopenia.
• Metabolic: hyperprolactinemia.
• Respiratory: chest tightness, wheezing, thickened bronchial secretions.
• Long-term therapy: skin hyperpigmentation; ocular changes, including corneal opacities and impaired vision.

Overdose and treatment

Clinical manifestations of overdose may include either CNS depression (sedation, reduced mental alertness, apnea, and cardiovascular collapse) or CNS stimulation (insomnia, hallucinations, tremors, or convulsions). Anticholinergic symptoms, such as dry mouth, flushed skin, fixed and dilated pupils, and GI symptoms, are common, especially in children. The manufacturer warns against inducing emesis, because dystonic reaction of head and neck may result in aspiration of vomitus. Use gastric lavage followed by activated charcoal. Treat hypotension with vasopressors, and control seizures with diazepam or phenytoin I.V. *Do not give stimulants.*

▶ Special considerations

• Drug is contraindicated for use in neonates; infants and children under age 6 may experience paradoxical hyperexcitability.
• Children, especially those under age 6, may experience paradoxical hyperexcitability with restlessness, insomnia, nervousness, euphoria, tremors, and seizures.
• Drug is contraindicated during an acute asthma attack, because it may not alleviate the symptoms and because antimuscarinic effects can cause thickening of secretions.
• Monitor blood counts during long-term therapy; watch for signs of blood dyscrasias.
• Reduce GI distress by giving drug with food; give sugarless gum or candy or ice chips to relieve dry mouth; increase fluid intake (if allowed) or humidify air to decrease adverse effect of thickened secretions.

Information for parents and patient

• Warn parents and patient about risk of photosensitivity; recommend sunscreen, and advise patient to report skin reactions immediately.
• Instruct parents to store drug in a tightly closed container away from direct sunlight and heat.
• Advise parents that patient should take drug with meals or snack to prevent gastric upset and to use any of the following measures to relieve dry mouth: warm water rinses, artificial saliva, ice chips, or sugarless gum or candy. Patient should avoid overusing mouthwash, which may add to dryness (alcohol content) and destroy normal flora.
• Warn parents that patient should avoid hazardous activities requiring mental alertness until extent of CNS effects are known and should not take tranquilizers, sedatives, pain relievers, or sleeping medications without medical approval.
• Advise parents to discontinue trimeprazine 4 days before diagnostic skin tests, to preserve accuracy of tests.

trimethadione
Tridione

• Classification: anticonvulsant (oxazolidinedione derivative)

How supplied

Available by prescription only
Capsules: 150 mg, 300 mg
Solution: 40 mg/ml

Indications, route, and dosage
Refractory absence (petit mal) seizures

Children: 20 to 50 mg/kg P.O. daily, divided q 6 to 8 hours. Usual maintenance dosage is 40 mg/kg or 1 g/m² P.O. daily in divided doses t.i.d. or q.i.d., not to exceed 900 mg/day.
Adults: Initially, 300 mg P.O. t.i.d.; may increase by 300 mg weekly, up to 600 mg P.O. q.i.d.

Action and kinetics

• *Anticonvulsant action:* Trimethadione raises the threshold for cortical seizures but does not modify the seizure pattern. It decreases projection of focal activity and reduces both repetitive spinal cord transmission and spike-and-wave patterns of absence (petit mal) seizures.
• *Kinetics in adults:* Trimethadione is well and rapidly absorbed from the GI tract. Peak plasma concentrations occur in 30 minutes to 2 hours. Trimethadione is distributed widely throughout the body; protein-binding is insignificant. Drug is metabolized in the liver to an active metabolite and is excreted slowly in urine.

Contraindications and precautions

Trimethadione is contraindicated in patients with known hypersensitivity to oxazolidinedione derivatives and in patients with renal or hepatic dysfunction. It should be used with caution in patients with severe

‡May contain sulfites   ♦May contain tartrazine   ♦♦May contain benzyl alcohol

blood dyscrasias, acute intermittent porphyria, or diseases of the retina or optic nerve.

Trimethadione is highly teratogenic and is contraindicated during pregnancy.

Interactions
Concomitant use of trimethadione and mephenytoin or phenacemide may result in a high incidence of toxicity; such combinations should be avoided.

Effects on diagnostic tests
Trimethadione may elevate liver function test results.

Adverse reactions
• CNS: drowsiness, fatigue, malaise, insomnia, dizziness, headache, paresthesias, irritability.
• CV: hypertension, hypotension.
• DERM: acneiform and morbilliform rash, exfoliative dermatitis, erythema multiforme, petechiae, alopecia.
• EENT: hemeralopia, diplopia, photophobia, epistaxis, retinal hemorrhage.
• GI: nausea, vomiting, anorexia, abdominal pain, bleeding gums.
• GU: nephrosis, albuminuria, vaginal bleeding.
• HEMA: neutropenia, leukopenia, eosinophilia, thrombocytopenia, pancytopenia, agranulocytosis, hypoplastic and aplastic anemia.
• Hepatic: abnormal liver function test results.
• Other: lymphadenopathy.
Note: Drug should be discontinued if signs of hypersensitivity, any rash (even acneiform), or unusual skin lesions occur; if scotomata occur; if neutrophil count falls to or below 2,500/mm³; if any of the following signs of blood dyscrasia occur: joint pain, fever, sore throat, or unusual bleeding or bruising; if patient has persistent or increasing albuminuria; if jaundice or other signs of hepatic dysfunction occur; or if syndromes resembling systemic lupus erythematosus, malignant lymphoma, or myasthenia gravis occur.

Overdose and treatment
Symptoms of overdose include nausea, drowsiness, ataxia, and visual disturbances; coma may follow massive overdose. Treat overdose by immediate gastric lavage or emesis, with supportive measures. Monitor vital signs and fluid and electrolyte balance carefully. Alkalinization of urine may hasten renal excretion. Monitor blood counts and hepatic and renal function after recovery. Contact local or regional poison control center for more information.

▶ Special considerations
• Trimethadione should not be withdrawn abruptly; this can precipitate absence seizures.
• Monitor CBCs and liver enzyme levels periodically during therapy.

Information for parents and patient
• Advise parents that follow-up laboratory tests are essential.
• Explain incidence of teratogenesis to parents of adolescents and emphasize importance of reporting suspected pregnancy immediately.
• Patients should avoid ingesting alcoholic beverages.

• Tell parents to have patient take drug with food or milk if GI upset occurs.
• Advise parents to have patient wear a Medic Alert bracelet or necklace indicating medication use and epilepsy.
• Explain that the drug may cause sensitivity to bright light. Sunscreens and protective clothing may be necessary.
• Warn that the drug may cause drowsiness or blurred vision. Advise parents that patient should avoid hazardous activities that require mental alertness until response to drug is determined.
• Advise parents to report the following: visual disturbances, excessive drowsiness, dizziness, sore throat, fever, unusual bleeding or bruising, or skin rash.
• Inform parents and patient that hemeralopia (day blindness) may be relieved by wearing dark glasses.

---

trimethobenzamide hydrochloride
Tegamide, T-Gen, Ticon, Tigan, Tiject-20

• Classification: antiemetic (ethanolamine-related antihistamine)

How supplied
Available by prescription only
Capsules: 100 mg, 250 mg
Suppositories: 100 mg, 200 mg
Injection: 100 mg/ml

Indications, route, and dosage
Nausea and vomiting (treatment)
Children under 13.6 kg: 100 mg rectally t.i.d. or q.i.d.
Children 13.6 to 45 kg: 100 to 200 mg P.O. or rectally t.i.d. or q.i.d.
Adults: 250 mg P.O. t.i.d. or q.i.d.; or 200 mg I.M. or rectally t.i.d. or q.i.d.

Action and kinetics
• *Antiemetic action:* Trimethobenzamide is a weak antihistamine with limited antiemetic properties. Its exact mechanism of action is unknown. Drug effect may occur in the brain's chemoreceptor trigger zone; however, the drug apparently does not inhibit direct impulses to the vomiting center.
• *Kinetics in adults:* Approximately 60% of an oral dose is absorbed. After oral administration, action begins in 10 to 40 minutes; after I.M. administration in 15 to 35 minutes. Distribution is unknown. Approximately 50% to 70% of a dose is metabolized, probably in the liver. Drug is excreted in urine and feces. After oral administration, duration of effect is 3 to 4 hours; after I.M. administration, 2 to 3 hours.

Contraindications and precautions
Trimethobenzamide is contraindicated in patients with hypersensitivity to this drug, benzocaine, or other local anesthetics. The injectable form is contraindicated in children; suppositories are contraindicated

in neonates and premature infants. Some clinicians consider the use of centrally acting antiemetics a contributing factor in the development of Reye's syndrome.

Trimethobenzamide should be used cautiously in patients with acute febrile illness, encephalitis, Reye's syndrome, encephalopathy, gastroenteritis, dehydration, or electrolyte imbalance, because the drug may mask the symptoms of these conditions.

Antiemetic effect may mask signs of overdose of toxic agents, intestinal obstruction, brain tumor, or other conditions. Antiemetics should not be the sole therapy. They should be used with restoration of fluid and electrolyte balance and relief of the underlying disease.

Interactions
Alcohol and other CNS depressants, including tricyclic antidepressants, antihypertensives, phenothiazines, and belladonna alkaloids, may increase trimethobenzamide toxicity.

Effects on diagnostic tests
None reported.

Adverse reactions
• CNS: *drowsiness, dizziness* (at high doses), headache, seizures, depression, opisthotonos, coma, *confusion, extrapyramidal symptoms*.
• CV: hypotension.
• GI: diarrhea, hepatotoxicity, jaundice, exacerbation of preexisting nausea (at high doses).
• Other: hypersensitivity reactions; parkinson-like symptoms; pain, burning, stinging, erythema, and swelling at injection site; muscle cramps.
Note: Drug should be discontinued if CNS or hypersensitivity reactions occur.

Overdose and treatment
Signs and symptoms of overdose may include severe neurologic reactions, such as opisthotonos, seizures, coma, and extrapyramidal reactions. Discontinue the drug and provide supportive care.

▶ Special considerations
• Injectable form not recommended for use in children.
• Record frequency and volume of vomiting; observe patient for signs and symptoms of dehydration.
• Drug may be less effective against severe vomiting than other agents.
• Drug has little or no value in treating motion sickness.

Information for parents and patient
• Warn parents that patient should avoid hazardous activities that require alertness, because drug may cause drowsiness, and should avoid consuming alcohol to prevent additive sedations.
• Instruct parents or patient to monitor amount of emesis, to observe for signs of dehydration, and report persistent vomiting.
• If appropriate, instruct parents in correct administration and storage of suppositories.

---

tripelennamine citrate
PBZ

tripelennamine hydrochloride
PBZ, PBZ-SR, Pelamine

• Classification: antihistamine H_1-receptor antagonist (ethylenediamine-derivative)

How supplied
Available with or without prescription
Tablets: 25 mg, 50 mg tripelennamine hydrochloride
Tablets (extended-release): 50 mg, 100 mg tripelennamine hydrochloride
Elixir: 37.5 mg/5 ml tripelennamine citrate; 37.5 mg tripelennamine citrate equal 25 mg tripelennamine hydrochloride
Topical cream: 2%

Indications, route, and dosage
Rhinitis, allergy symptoms, allergic reactions to blood or plasma, adjunct to epinephrine in anaphylaxis
Infants and children: 5 mg/kg or 150 mg/m² daily in four to six divided doses. Do not use timed-release tablets in children.
Adults: 25 to 50 mg P.O. q 4 to 6 hours; or (timed-release) 50 to 100 mg P.O. b.i.d. or t.i.d. Maximum dosage is 600 mg daily.
Pruritus, minor burns, insect bites, sunburn, skin irritations
Children and adults: Apply topical cream t.i.d. or q.i.d.
  Drug dosages are based on tripelennamine hydrochloride (tablets only); dosage of tripelennamine citrate (elixir only) is about 1½ times that of tripelennamine hydrochloride; 5 mg tripelennamine hydrochloride equals 7.5 mg tripelennamine citrate.

Action and kinetics
• *Antihistamine action:* Tripelennamine competes with histamine for the H_1-receptor, thereby ameliorating histamine effects in target tissues; drug does not prevent the release of histamine.
• *Kinetics in adults:* Tripelennamine is well absorbed; distribution, metabolism, and excretion have not been reported.

Contraindications and precautions
Tripelennamine is contraindicated in patients with known hypersensitivity to this drug or antihistamines with a similar chemical structure, such as pyrilamine; in neonates and other infants, because young children may be more susceptible to the toxic effects of antihistamines; during asthma attacks, because it thickens bronchial secretions; and in patients who have taken MAO inhibitors within the preceding 2 weeks.

Because of significant anticholinergic effects, tripelennamine should be used with caution in patients with narrow-angle glaucoma; in those with pyloroduodenal obstruction or urinary bladder obstruction from narrowing of the bladder neck; and in patients

---

◦ May contain sulfites   ◆ May contain tartrazine   ◆◆ May contain benzyl alcohol

with cardiovascular disease or hypertension, because drug may cause palpitations.

Safe use in neonates and premature infants is not established. Other infants and children under age 6 may experience paradoxical hyperexcitability.

Interactions

MAO inhibitors interfere with the detoxification of antihistamines and phenothiazines, and thus prolong and intensify their central depressant and anticholinergic effects; additive CNS depression and sedation may occur when tripelennamine is administered with other CNS depressants, such as alcohol, barbiturates, tranquilizers, sleeping aids, or antianxiety agents.

Effects on diagnostic tests

Tripelennamine should be discontinued 4 days before diagnostic skin tests, to avoid preventing, reducing, or masking test response.

Adverse reactions

• CNS: drowsiness, dizziness, confusion, vertigo, tinnitus, fatigue, disturbed coordination, paresthesias, euphoria, nervousness, restlessness, tremors, irritability, insomnia.
• CV: mild hypertension, hypotension, palpitations, chest tightness.
• DERM: rash, urticaria, photosensitivity.
• EENT: diplopia, blurred vision, dry nose and throat.
• GI: anorexia, diarrhea, constipation, nausea, vomiting.
• GU: urinary frequency or retention.
• HEMA: leukopenia, agranulocytosis, hemolytic anemia.
• Respiratory: thickened bronchial secretions.
• Topical: sensitization.

Overdose and treatment

Clinical manifestations of overdose may include either CNS depression (sedation, reduced mental alertness, apnea, and cardiovascular collapse) or CNS stimulation (insomnia, hallucinations, tremors, or seizures). Anticholinergic symptoms, such as dry mouth, flushed skin, fixed and dilated pupils, and GI symptoms, are common, especially in children; children also may experience fever, excitement, ataxia, and athetosis.

Treat overdose by inducing emesis with ipecac syrup (in conscious patient), followed by activated charcoal to reduce further drug absorption. Use gastric lavage if patient is unconscious or ipecac fails. Treat hypotension with vasopressors, and control seizures with diazepam, phenytoin, or short-acting barbiturates. *Do not give stimulants.*

▶ Special considerations

• Be alert to change in drug dosage when substituting elixir for tablets, or vice versa.
• Give extended-release tablets whole; do not crush.
• Drug is contraindicated during an acute asthma attack, because it may not alleviate the symptoms and because antimuscarinic effects can cause thickening secretions.
• Children, especially those under age 6, may experience paradoxical hyperexcitability with restless-

ness, insomnia, nervousness, euphoria, tremors, and seizures.
• Reduce GI distress by giving drug with food; give sugarless gum or candy or ice chips to relieve dry mouth; increase fluid intake (if appropriate) or humidify air to decrease adverse effect of thickened secretions.

Information for parents and patient

• Advise patient to take drug with meals or snack to prevent gastric upset and to use any of the following measures to relieve dry mouth: warm water rinses, artificial saliva, ice chips, or sugarless gum or candy. Patient should avoid overusing mouthwash, which may add to dryness (alcohol content) and destroy normal flora.
• Warn parents that child should avoid hazardous activities that require balance or alertness until extent of CNS effects are known. Advise them to seek medical approval before administering tranquilizers, sedatives, pain relievers, or sleeping medications.
• Warn parents to discontinue tripelennamine 4 days before diagnostic skin tests, to preserve accuracy of tests.

---

triprolidine hydrochloride
Actidil, Myidyl

• Classification: antihistamine derivative

How supplied

Available with or without prescription
Tablets: 2.5 mg
Syrup: 1.25 mg/5 ml

Indications, route, and dosage
Colds and allergy symptoms

Children age 4 months to 1 year: 0.3 mg every 6 to 8 hours; maximum daily dosage is 1.25 mg.
Children age 2 to 3: 0.6 mg every 6 to 8 hours; maximum daily dosage is 2.5 mg.
Children age 4 to 5: 0.9 mg q 6 to 8 hours; maximum daily dosage is 3.75 mg.
Children age 6 to 11: 1.25 mg q 4 to 6 hours; maximum daily dosage is 5 mg.
Children age 12 and older and adults: 2.5 mg P.O. 4 to 6 hours; maximum daily dosage is 10 mg.

Action and kinetics

• *Antihistamine action:* Antihistamines compete with histamine for histamine H_1-receptor sites on the smooth muscle of the bronchi, GI tract, uterus, and large blood vessels; by binding to cellular receptors they prevent access of histamine and suppress histamine-induced allergic symptoms, even though they do not prevent its release.
• *Kinetics in adults:* Triprolidine is well absorbed from the GI tract; it has a rapid onset of action, with peak effects occurring in about 3½ hours, and a duration of about 12 hours. Triprolidine's distribution is not fully known; drug is distributed to the lungs, spleen,

---

and kidneys. Drug is metabolized by the liver; half-life is about 2 to 6 hours.

Contraindications and precautions

Triprolidine is contraindicated in patients with known hypersensitivity to this drug or other antihistamines with similar chemical structures (brompheniramine, chlorpheniramine, and dexchlorpheniramine); during asthma attacks, because triprolidine thickens bronchial secretions; and in patients who have taken MAO inhibitors within the previous 2 weeks.

Triprolidine should be used with caution in patients with narrow-angle glaucoma; in those with pyloro-duodenal obstruction or urinary bladder obstruction from narrowing of the bladder neck, because of their marked anticholinergic effects; in patients with cardiovascular disease, hypertension, or hyperthyroidism, because of the risk of palpitations and tachycardia; and in patients with renal disease, diabetes, bronchial asthma, urinary retention, or stenosing peptic ulcers.

Drug is not indicated for use in premature or newborn infants; infants and children under age 6 may experience paradoxical hyperexcitability.

Interactions

MAO inhibitors interfere with the detoxification of antihistamines and thus prolong and intensify their central depressant and anticholinergic effects; added CNS depression may occur when triprolidine is given concomitantly with other CNS depressants, such as alcohol, barbiturates, tranquilizers, sleeping aids, and antianxiety agents.

Triprolidine may diminish the effects of sulfonylureas and may partially counteract the anticoagulant effects of heparin.

Effects on diagnostic tests

Discontinue triprolidine 4 days before diagnostic skin tests; antihistamines can prevent, reduce, or mask positive skin response to the tests.

Adverse reactions

- CNS: drowsiness, dizziness, restlessness, insomnia, stimulation.
- DERM: urticaria, rash.
- EENT: dry nose and throat.
- GI: anorexia, diarrhea, constipation, nausea, vomiting, dry mouth.
- GU: urinary frequency or retention.
- Respiratory: thick bronchial secretions.

Overdose and treatment

Clinical manifestations of overdose may include either CNS depression (sedation, reduced mental alertness, apnea, and cardiovascular collapse) or CNS stimulation (insomnia, hallucinations, tremors, or seizures). Anticholinergic symptoms, such as dry mouth, flushed skin, fixed and dilated pupils, and GI symptoms, are common, especially in children.

Treat overdose by inducing emesis with ipecac syrup (in conscious patient), followed by activated charcoal to reduce further drug absorption. Use gastric lavage if patient is unconscious or ipecac fails. Treat hypotension with vasopressors, and control seizures with diazepam or phenytoin. *Do not give stimulants.*

▶ Special considerations

- Triprolidine has a low incidence of drowsiness.
- Drug is contraindicated during an acute asthma attack, because it may not alleviate the symptoms and because antimuscarinic effects can cause thickening secretions.
- Children, especially those under age 6, may experience paradoxical hyperexcitability with restlessness, insomnia, nervousness, euphoria, tremors, and seizures.
- Monitor blood counts during long-term therapy; watch for signs of blood dyscrasias.
- Reduce GI distress by giving drug with food; give sugarless gum, sour hard candy, or ice chips to relieve dry mouth; increase fluid intake (if allowed) or humidify air to decrease adverse effect of thickened secretions.

Information for parents and patient

- Advise patient to take drug with meals or snack to prevent gastric upset and to use any of the following measures to relieve dry mouth: warm water rinses, artificial saliva, ice chips, or sugarless gum or candy. Patient should avoid overusing mouthwash, which may add to dryness (alcohol content) and destroy normal flora.
- Warn parents that child should avoid hazardous activities that require balance or alertness until extent of CNS effects are known.
- Advise them to seek medical approval before administering tranquilizers, sedatives, pain relievers, or sleeping medications.
- Warn parents to discontinue tripelennamine 4 days before diagnostic skin tests, to preserve accuracy of tests.

tromethamine
Tham, Tham-E

- Classification: systemic alkalinizer (sodium-free organic amine)

How supplied

Available by prescription only
Injection: 36 g, 36 mg/ml (18 g/500 ml)

Indications, route, and dosage
Correction of metabolic acidosis (associated with cardiac bypass surgery or with cardiac arrest)

Dosage depends on base deficit. Calculate as follows:

$$
\begin{array}{l}
\text{ml of 0.3 molar} \\
\text{tromethamine} \\
\text{solution required} \\
\text{(without electro-} \\
\text{lytes)}
\end{array} =
\begin{array}{l}
\text{body} \\
\text{weight} \\
\text{in kg}
\end{array} \times
\begin{array}{l}
\text{base} \\
\text{deficit in} \\
\text{mEq/liter} \\
\times 1.1.
\end{array}
$$

Total dosage should be administered over at least 1 hour and should not exceed 500 mg/kg for an adult.

---

‡May contain sulfites   ◆May contain tartrazine   ◆◆May contain benzyl alcohol

The usual dose of a 0.3 molar solution (3.6 to 10.8 g of tromethamine) may be administered into a large peripheral vein. If the chest is open, 55 to 165 ml of a 0.3 molar solution (2 to 6 g of tromethamine) has also been injected into the ventricular cavity (*not into the cardiac muscle*).

For systemic acidosis during cardiac bypass surgery, the usual single dose of a 0.3 molar solution is 9 ml/kg (324 mg/kg of tromethamine) or about 500 ml (18 g of tromethamine) for most adults.

To titrate the excess acidity of stored blood used to prime the pump oxygenator during cardiac bypass surgery
Add 14 to 70 ml of 0.3 molar solution to each 500 ml of blood, depending on the pH of the blood.

Action and kinetics
• *Systemic alkalizing action:* Tromethamine, as a weak base, acts as a proton acceptor to prevent or correct acidosis; drug reduces hydrogen ion concentration. It also acts as a weak osmotic diuretic, increasing the flow of alkaline urine.
• *Kinetics in adults:* Absorption is immediate because tromethamine is available for I.V. use only. At pH of 7.4, about 25% of drug is un-ionized; this portion may enter cells to neutralize acidic ions of intracellular fluid. There is no metabolism. Tromethamine is excreted renally as the bicarbonate salt.

Contraindications and precautions
Tromethamine is contraindicated in patients with uremia or anuria, because of renal excretion; in patients with chronic respiratory acidosis, because it decreases serum carbon dioxide levels and may cause respiratory failure; in pregnant patients; or when used longer than 24 hours, except in life-threatening emergencies.

Drug should be used with caution in neonates and other infants, and in patients with renal disease and poor urine output, because drug may accumulate in patients with decreased renal function.

Interactions
Concomitant use with other respiratory or CNS depressants may cause cumulative respiratory depression.

Effects on diagnostic tests
Tromethamine alters serum electrolyte levels. Transient decreases in blood glucose concentrations may occur.

Adverse reactions
• CNS: *respiratory depression.*
• Local: *tissue irritation,* chemical phlebitis, venospasm, I.V. thrombophlebitis.
• Other: *hypoglycemia,* severe hepatic necrosis in newborns and infants (with 1.2 molar solution), hydropic degeneration of hepatic and renal tubular cells (with a 1.5 molar solution), *hyperkalemia, increased coagulation time.*
Note: Drug should be discontinued if signs of hypersensitivity, severe hypoglycemia, or respiratory depression occur, or if infusion extravasates.

Overdose and treatment
Clinical signs of overdose include respiratory or systemic alkalosis, cardiac dysrhythmias secondary to hypokalemia, respiratory depression, and hypoglycemia. Discontinue drug and correct pH; use decreased ventilation and systemic acidifiers if necessary. Treat hypokalemia cautiously with potassium (serum potassium levels will rise with correction of alkalosis), and hypoglycemia with I.V. glucose as needed.

▶ Special considerations
• Drug should be used with caution in pediatric patients; severe hepatic necrosis has occurred in infants and neonates after administration of a 1.2 molar solution through the umbilical vein.
• Monitor vital signs, blood pH levels, carbon dioxide tension, and bicarbonate, glucose, and electrolyte levels before, during, and after infusion.
• Tromethamine should be administered by slow I.V. into the largest antecubital vein or via a large needle, indwelling catheter, or pump-oxygenator. Infusion site should be checked frequently to avoid extravasation of solution and prevent tissue damage. If extravasation occurs, aspirate as much fluid as possible. Infiltrating area with 1% procaine hydrochloride to which hyaluronidase has been added may aid in extravasation and venospasm. Local injection of phentolamine can be used to reverse venospasm.

---

tropicamide
Mydriacyl

• Classification: cycloplegic, mydriatic (anticholinergic agent)

How supplied
Available by prescription only
Ophthalmic solution: 0.5%, 1%

Indications, route, and dosage
Cycloplegic refractions
Children and adults: Instill 1 or 2 drops of 0.5% or 1% solution in each eye; repeat in 5 minutes.
Fundus examinations
Children and adults: Instill 1 or 2 drops of 0.5% or 1% solution in each eye 15 to 20 minutes before examination. May be repeated in 30 minutes.

Action and kinetics
• *Mydriatic action:* Anticholinergic action prevents the sphincter muscle of the iris and the muscle of the ciliary body from responding to cholinergic stimulation, producing pupillary dilation (mydriasis) and paralysis of accommodation (cycloplegia).
• *Kinetics in adults:* Peak effect usually occurs in 20 to 40 minutes. Recovery from cycloplegic and mydriatic effects usually occurs in about 6 hours.

Contraindications and precautions
Tropicamide is contraindicated in patients with narrow-angle glaucoma and in patients hypersensitive

---

any component of the preparation. Drug should be used with caution in patients in whom increased intraocular pressure may occur; and in children, because of increased risk of cardiovascular and CNS effects.

Interactions
None significant.

Effects on diagnostic tests
None reported.

Adverse reactions
• CNS: ataxia, *behavorial disturbances in children.*
• DERM: dryness, flushing.
• ENT: nose and throat dryness.
• Eye: transient stinging, increased intraocular pressure, blurred vision, photophobia.
• Other: fever, *cardiopulmonary collapse.*
   Note: Drug should be discontinued if behavioral disturbances occur.

Overdose and treatment
Clinical manifestations of overdose include dry, flushed skin; dry mouth; dilated pupils; delirium; hallucination; tachycardia; and decreased bowel sounds. Treat accidental ingestion with emesis or activated charcoal. Use physostigmine to antagonize tropicamide's anticholinergic activity in severe toxicity and propranolol to treat symptomatic tachydysrhythmias unresponsive to physostigmine.

▶ Special considerations
Infants and small children may be especially susceptible to CNS disturbances from systemic absorption. Psychotic reactions, behavioral disturbances, and cardiopulmonary collapse have been reported in children.

Tropicamide is the shortest-acting cycloplegic, but its mydriatic effect is greater than its cycloplegic effect.

Apply finger pressure to patient's lacrimal sac for 1 to 2 minutes after instillation to avoid systemic absorption of drug.

Information for parents and patient
Advise patient to protect eyes from bright illumination for comfort.

Instruct parents and patient to wait 5 minutes before using another eye preparation.

---

tuberculosis skin test antigens

tuberculin purified protein derivative (PPD)
Aplisol, PPD-Stabilized Solution (Mantoux), Tubersol

tuberculin cutaneous multiple-puncture device
Aplitest, Mono-Vacc Test (Old Tuberculin), Sclavo-Test (PPD), Tine Test (Old Tuberculin)

• Classification: diagnostic skin test antigen (*Mycobacterium tuberculosis* and *Mycobacterium bovis* antigen)

How supplied
Available by prescription only
Tuberculin PPD
Injection (intradermal): 1 tuberculin unit/0.1 ml, 5 tuberculin units/0.1 ml, 250 tuberculin units/0.1 ml
Tuberculin cutaneous multiple-puncture device
Test: 25 devices/pack

Indications, route, and dosage
Diagnosis of tuberculosis; evaluation of immunocompetence in patients with cancer or malnutrition
Children and adults: Intradermal injection of 5 tuberculin units/0.1 ml.

A single-use, multiple-puncture device is used for determining tuberculin sensitivity. All multiple-puncture tests are equivalent to or more potent than 5 tuberculin units of PPD (Mantoux).
Children and adults: Apply the unit firmly and without any twisting to the upper one-third of the forearm for approximately 3 seconds; this will ensure stabilizing the dried tuberculin B in the tissue lymph. Exert enough pressure to ensure that all four tines have entered the skin of the test area and a circular depression is visible.

Action and kinetics
• *Diagnosis of tuberculosis:* Administration to a patient with a natural infection with *M. tuberculosis* usually results in sensitivity to tuberculin and a delayed hypersensitivity reaction (after administration of old tuberculin or PPD). The cell-mediated immune reaction to tuberculin in tuberculin-sensitive individuals, which results mainly from cellular infiltrates of the skin's dermis, usually causes local edema.
• *Diagnosis of immunocompetence in patients with cancer or malnutrition:* PPD is given intradermally with three or more antigens to detect anergy, the absence of an immune response to the test. The reaction may not be evident. Injection into a site subject to excessive exposure to sunlight may cause a false-negative reaction.
• *Kinetics in adults:* When PPD is injected intradermally, or a multiple-puncture device is used, a delayed hypersensitivity reaction is evident in 5 to 6 hours

and peaks in 48 to 72 hours. Injection must be given intradermally or by skin puncture; a subcutaneous injection invalidates the test.

Contraindications and precautions

Severe reactions from tuberculin PPD are rare and usually result from extreme sensitivity to the tuberculin.

Inadvertent subcutaneous administration of PPD may result in a febrile reaction in highly sensitized patients. Old tubercular lesions are not activated by administration of PPD.

Interactions

When PPD antigen is used 4 to 6 weeks after immunization with live or inactivated viral vaccines, the reaction to tuberculin may be suppressed. False-negative reactions may also occur if test is used in patients receiving systemic corticosteroids or aminocaproic acid.

Topical alcohol theoretically may inactivate the PPD antigen and invalidate the test.

Effects on diagnostic tests

None reported.

Adverse reactions

• Local: pain, pruritus, vesiculation, ulceration, necrosis may occur in some tuberculin-sensitive patients.
• Other: hypersensitivity (immediate reaction may occur at the test site in the form of a wheal or flare that lasts less than a day; this should not interfere with the PPD test reading at 48 to 72 hours), anaphylaxis, Arthus reaction.

Overdose and treatment

No information available.

▶ Special considerations

Tuberculin PPD
• Obtain a history of allergies and previous skin test reactions before administration of the test.
• Epinephrine 1:1,000 should be available to treat rare anaphylactic reaction.
• Intradermal injection should produce a "bleb" 6 to 10 mm in diameter on skin. If bleb does not appear, retest at a site at least 5 cm from the initial site.
• Read test in 48 to 72 hours. An induration of 10 mm or greater is a significant reaction in patients who are not suspected to have tuberculosis and who have not been exposed to active tuberculosis. An induration of 5 mm or greater is significant in patients suspected to have tuberculosis or who have recently been exposed to active tuberculosis. A reaction of 2 mm or greater may be considered significant in infants or children. The amount of induration at the site, not the erythema, determines the significance of the reaction.

For either test, keep a record of the administration technique, manufacturer and tuberculin lot number, date and location of administration, date test is read, and the size of the induration in millimeters.

Multiple-puncture device

• Obtain history of allergies, especially to acacia (contained in the Tine Test as stabilizer), and reactions to skin tests.
• Report all known cases of tuberculosis to appropriate public health agency.
• Reaction may be depressed in patients with malnutrition, immunosuppression, or miliary tuberculosis.
• Interpretation: Read test at 48 to 72 hours. Measure the size of the largest induration in millimeters. A large reaction may cause the area around the puncture site to be indistinguishable.
Positive reaction: If vesiculation is present, the test may be interpreted as positive if induration is greater than 2 mm, but consider further diagnostic procedures.
Negative reaction: Induration is less than 2 mm. There is no reason to retest the patient unless the person is a contact of a patient with tuberculosis or there is clinical evidence of the disease.
Diagnosis of tuberculosis: PPD administration to a patient with a natural infection with *Mycobacterium tuberculosis* usually results in sensitivity to tuberculin and a delayed hypersensitivity reaction after administration of old tuberculin or PPD. The cell-mediated immune reaction to tuberculin in tuberculin-sensitive individuals is seen as erythema and induration, which mainly results from cellular infiltrates of the skin's dermis; usually causes local edema.
Diagnosis of immunocompetence in patients with such conditions as cancer or malnutrition: PPD is given intradermally with three or more antigens (such as Multitest CMI) to detect anergy.
• No evidence to date of adverse effects to fetus. Benefits of test are thought to outweigh the potential risk to the fetus.

Information for parents and patient

• Advise parents to report any unusual side effects. Explain that the induration will disappear in a few days.
• Reinforce the benefits of treatment if test is positive for tuberculosis.

UVW

uracil mustard

Classification: antineoplastic (alkylating agent [cell cycle-phase nonspecific])

How supplied
Available by prescription only
Capsules: 1 mg

Indications, route, and dosage
Dosage and indications may vary. Check current literature for recommended protocol.

Chronic lymphocytic and myelocytic leukemia; Hodgkin's disease; non-Hodgkin's lymphomas of the histiocytic and lymphocytic types; reticulum cell sarcoma; lymphomas; mycosis fungoides; polycythemia vera; ovarian, cervical, and lung cancer
Children: 0.3 mg/kg P.O. weekly for 4 weeks.
Adults: 1 to 2 mg P.O. daily for 3 months or until desired response or toxicity occurs; maintenance dosage is 1 mg daily for 3 out of 4 weeks until optimum response or relapse occurs. Alternatively, 3 to 5 mg P.O. for 7 days, not to exceed total dose of 0.5 mg/kg, followed by 1 mg daily until response occurs, then 1 mg daily 3 out of 4 weeks; or 0.15 mg/kg P.O. once weekly for 4 weeks.
Thrombocytosis
Adults: 1 to 2 mg P.O. daily for 14 days.

Action and kinetics
Antineoplastic action: Uracil mustard exerts its cytotoxic activity by cross-linking strands of DNA, interfering with DNA and RNA replication and disrupting normal nucleic acid function, resulting in cell death.

Kinetics in adults: In animal studies, uracil mustard is absorbed quickly but incompletely after oral administration. Distribution and metabolism are unknown. In studies using dogs, elimination of uracil mustard from the plasma is rapid, with no drug detected 2 hours after administration. Less than 1% of a dose is excreted unchanged in urine.

Contraindications and precautions
Uracil mustard is contraindicated in patients with a history of hypersensitivity to tartrazine, a dye contained in the capsules. The incidence of hypersensitivity is low, but it seems to occur frequently in patients allergic to aspirin.

Drug should be used cautiously in patients whose bone marrow shows infiltration with malignant cells, because hematopoietic toxicity may be increased.

Interactions
None reported.

Effects on diagnostic tests
Uracil mustard therapy may increase blood and urine uric acid levels.

Adverse reactions
• CNS: irritability, nervousness, mental cloudiness, depression.
• DERM: pruritus, dermatitis, hyperpigmentation.
• GI: nausea, vomiting, diarrhea, epigastric distress, abdominal pain, anorexia.
• HEMA: bone-marrow depression (dose-limiting), thrombocytopenia, leukopenia, anemia.
• Metabolic: hyperuricemia.
• Other: alopecia (rare).

Overdose and treatment
Clinical manifestations of overdose include myelosuppression, nausea, and vomiting.

Treatment is usually supportive and includes antiemetics and transfusion of blood components.

▶ Special considerations
• Attempt to alleviate or reduce anxiety in parents and patient before treatment.
• Monitor BUN, hematocrit, platelet count, ALT (SGPT), AST (SGOT), LDH, serum bilirubin, serum creatinine, uric acid total and differential leukocyte.
• Give at bedtime to reduce nausea.
• Drug is usually not administered until 2 or 3 weeks after the maximum effect of previous drugs is reached or until radiation effects are evident.
• Watch for signs of ecchymoses, easy bruising, and petechiae.
• To prevent hyperuricemia and resulting uric acid nephropathy, allopurinol can be given; keep patient hydrated. Monitor uric acid levels.
• Monitor platelet count regularly. Perform a CBC one to two times weekly for 4 weeks, then 4 weeks after stopping drug.
• Avoid all I.M. injections when platelet count is below 100,000/mm³.
• Anticoagulants should be used cautiously. Watch closely for signs of bleeding. Instruct patient to avoid nonprescription products containing aspirin.
• Dose modification may be required in severe thrombocytopenia, aplastic anemia or leukopenia, or acute leukemia.
• Uracil mustard capsules contain tartrazine, a dye which may cause allergic reactions in certain individuals, especially these sensitive to aspirin.

Information for parents and patient
• Stress importance of keeping follow-up appointments for monitoring hematologic status.
• Instruct parents to monitor neutropenic patient's temperature every 4 hours (not rectally) and to report fever, cough, and other signs of infection *promptly.*
• Advise parents to avoid patient's exposure to per-

---

sons with bacterial or viral infections because chemotherapy can increase susceptibility to infection.
• Advise parents that immunizations should be avoided if possible during therapy.
• Patient should avoid contact with persons who have received live-virus immunizations (polio, measles/mumps/rubella). Explain importance of promptly reporting susceptible patient's exposure to chicken pox.
• Warn parents that patients may bruise easily because of drug's effect on blood count.
• Teach parents and patient to check for signs of bleeding and bruising. Parents may need to restrict child's participation in contact sports. Such activity is dangerous when patient's platelets are low.
• Instruct patient to clean teeth with toothettes, gauze, or soft toothbrush when platelets are low.
• Advise parents that patient should complete dental work before therapy whenever possible, or delay it until blood counts are normal.
• Emphasize the importance of continuing the drug despite nausea and vomiting. Tell parents to call immediately if vomiting occurs shortly after taking a dose.
• Advise parents to encourage patient to drink plenty of fluids to increase urine output and facilitate excretion of uric acid. Patient should void frequently.

---

urea (carbamide)
Ureaphil

• Classification: osmotic diuretic (carbonic acid salt)

How supplied
Available by prescription only
Injectable: 40-g vial

Indications, route, and dosage
Reduction of intracranial or intraocular pressure
Children under age 2: As little as 0.1 g/kg by slow I.V. infusion may be effective.
Children over age 2: 0.5 to 1.5 g/kg or 35 g/m² daily by slow I.V. infusion.
Adults: 1 to 1.5 g/kg as a 30% solution given by slow I.V. infusion over 1 to 2½ hours.
Maximum daily adult dosage is 120 g. To prepare 135 ml of 30% solution, mix contents of a 40-g vial of urea with 105 ml of dextrose 5% or 10% in water or with 10% invert sugar in water. Each ml of 30% solution provides 300 mg of urea.
†*Diuresis*
Children: 800 mg/kg or 25 g/m² P.O. daily, divided q 8 hours.
Adults: 20 g P.O. two to five times daily.

Action and kinetics
• *Diuretic action:* Urea elevates plasma osmolality, enhancing the flow of water into extracellular fluid, such as blood, and reducing intracranial and intraocular pressure.
• *Kinetics in adults:* I.V. urea produces diuresis and maximal reduction of intraocular and intracranial

pressure within 1 to 2 hours; even though drug is administered I.V., it is hydrolyzed and absorbed from the GI tract. Urea distributes into intracellular and extracellular fluid, including lymph, bile, and cerebrospinal fluid. Drug is hydrolyzed in the GI tract by bacterial uridase; it is excreted by the kidneys.

Contraindications and precautions
Urea is contraindicated in patients with severely impaired renal function, because it is excreted in urine; marked dehydration follows volume depletion and liver failure.

Interactions
Urea may enhance renal excretion of lithium and lower serum lithium levels.

Effects on diagnostic tests
Urea therapy alters electrolyte balance.

Adverse reactions
• CNS: headache.
• CV: tachycardia, CHF, pulmonary edema.
• GI: nausea, vomiting.
• Metabolic: sodium and potassium depletion.
• Local: irritation or necrotic sloughing may occur with extravasation.
Note: Drug should be discontinued if BUN level rises above 75 mg/dl or if diuresis does not occur within 1 to 2 hours.

Overdose and treatment
Clinical signs of overdose include polyuria, cellular dehydration, hypotension, and cardiovascular collapse. Discontinue infusion and institute supportive measures.

▶ Special considerations
• Monitor I.V. infusion carefully for inflammation at the infusion site.
• Patient should have frequent mouth care or fluids as appropriate to relieve thirst.
• In patients with urethral catheter, an hourly urometer collection bag should be used to facilitate accurate measurement of urine output. For the patient who is not catheterized, a urine collection bag should be in place. Diapers should be weighed.
• Avoid rapid I.V. infusion, which may cause hemolysis or increased capillary bleeding. Also avoid extravasation, which may cause reactions ranging from mild irritation to necrosis.
• Do not administer through the same infusion line as blood.
• Do not infuse into leg veins; this may cause phlebitis or thrombosis.
• Watch for hyponatremia or hypokalemia (muscle weakness, lethargy); such signs may indicate electrolyte depletion before serum levels are reduced.
• Maintain adequate hydration; monitor fluid and electrolyte balance.
• In renal disease, monitor BUN levels frequently.
• Indwelling urethral catheter should be used in comatose patients to ensure bladder emptying. Use of an hourly urometer collection bag facilitates accurate measurement of urine output.

• If satisfactory diuresis does not occur in 6 to 12 hours, urea should be discontinued and renal function re-evaluated.

• Use only freshly reconstituted urea for I.V. infusion; solution turns to ammonia when left standing. Use within minutes of reconstitution.

• Urea has been used orally on an investigational basis for migraine prophylaxis, acute sickle-cell crisis prevention, and the correction of syndrome of inappropriate antidiuretic hormone (SIADH).

• Mix oral medication with carbonated beverages, jelly, or jam to disguise unpleasant flavor.

Information for parents and patient
• The patient may feel thirsty or experience mouth dryness. Emphasize importance of drinking only the amount of fluids provided, as ordered.

• With initial doses, patient should change position slowly, especially when rising to an upright position, to prevent dizziness from orthostatic hypotension.

• Instruct parents to watch patient for chest, back, or leg pain or shortness of breath, and to report these effects immediately.

---

valproic acid
Depakene

divalproex sodium
Depakote

• Classification: anticonvulsant (carboxylic acid derivative)

How supplied
Available by prescription only
Valproic acid
Capsules: 250 mg
Syrup: 250 mg/ml
Divalproex sodium
Tablets (enteric-coated): 125 mg, 250 mg, 500 mg

Indications, route, and dosage
Simple and complex absence seizures (petit mal) and mixed seizure types; investigationally in major motor (tonic-clonic) seizures
Children and adults: Initially, 15 mg/kg P.O. daily, divided b.i.d. or t.i.d.; may increase by 5 to 10 mg/kg daily at weekly intervals up to a maximum of 60 mg/kg daily, divided b.i.d. or t.i.d. B.i.d. dosage is recommended for the enteric-coated tablets.

Note: Dosages of divalproex sodium (Depakote) are expressed as valproic acid.

Action and kinetics
• *Anticonvulsant action:* Valproic acid's mechanism of action is unknown; effects may be from increased brain levels of gamma-aminobutyric acid (GABA), an inhibitory transmitter. Valproic acid also may decrease GABA's enzymatic catabolism. Onset of therapeutic effects may require a week or more. Valproic acid may be used with other anticonvulsants.

• *Kinetics in adults:* Valproate sodium and divalproex sodium quickly convert to valproic acid after administration of oral dose; peak plasma concentrations occur in 1 to 4 hours (with uncoated tablets) and 3 to 5 hours (with enteric-coated tablets); bioavailability of drug is same for both dosage forms.

Valproic acid is distributed rapidly throughout the body; drug is 80% to 95% protein-bound.

Valproic acid is metabolized by the liver.

Valproic acid is excreted in urine; some drug is excreted in feces and exhaled air. Breast milk levels are 1% to 10% of serum levels.

Contraindications and precautions
Valproic acid is contraindicated in patients with known hypersensitivity to valproic acid and in patients with a history of hepatic disease because valproic acid may be hepatotoxic. It should be used with caution in patients taking oral anticoagulants or multiple anticonvulsants. Patients with congenital metabolic or seizure disorders with mental retardation, especially in children under age 2, appear to be at increased risk of adverse effects.

Interactions
Valproic acid may potentiate effects of monoamine oxidase (MAO) inhibitors and other CNS antidepressants and of oral anticoagulants. Besides additive sedative effects, valproic acid increases serum levels of primidone and phenobarbital; such combinations may cause excessive somnolence and require careful monitoring. Concomitant use with clonazepam may cause absence seizures and should be avoided.

Effects on diagnostic tests
Valproic acid may cause false-positive test results for urinary ketones; it also may cause abnormalities in liver function test results.

Adverse reactions
Because drug usually is used with other anticonvulsants, the adverse reactions reported may not be caused by valproic acid alone.
• CNS: *sedation,* emotional upset, depression, psychosis, *aggression, hyperactivity,* behavioral deterioration, muscle weakness, tremors, ataxia, headache, hallucinations.
• EENT: stomatitis, hypersalivation, nystagmus, diplopia, scotomata.
• GI: nausea, vomiting, indigestion, diarrhea, abdominal cramps, constipation, increased appetite and weight gain, anorexia, pancreatitis. *Note:* Lower incidence of GI effects occurs with divalproex.
• HEMA: inhibited platelet aggregation, thrombocytopenia, increased bleeding time.
• Hepatic: enzyme level elevations, toxic hepatitis.
• Metabolic: elevated serum ammonia levels.
• Other: alopecia, enuresis, curling or waving hair.
Note: Drug should be discontinued if signs of hypersensitivity, hepatic dysfunction (markedly elevated liver enzyme levels or jaundice), or coagulation abnormalities (bruising or hemorrhage) occur.

Overdose and treatment
Symptoms of overdose include somnolence and coma. Treat overdose supportively: Maintain adequate urine

---

‡May contain sulfites   ◆May contain tartrazine   ◆◆May contain benzyl alcohol

output, and monitor vital signs and fluid and electrolyte balance carefully. Naloxone reverses CNS and respiratory depression but also may reverse anticonvulsant effects of valproic acid. Valproic acid is not dialyzable.

▶ **Special considerations**
- Valproic acid is not recommended for use in children under age 2; this age-group is at highest risk of adverse effects. Reportedly, hyperexcitability and aggressiveness have occurred in a few children.
- Patient should have review of liver function, platelet counts, and prothrombin times at baseline and at monthly intervals—especially during first 6 months.
- Therapeutic range is not well established, but most patients respond to serum levels of 50 to 100 mcg/ml. Some patients may require higher levels.
- Drug should not be withdrawn abruptly.
- Tremors may indicate need for dosage reduction.
- Administer drug with food to minimize GI irritation. Enteric-coated formulation may be better tolerated.

Information for parents and patient
- Patient may take drug with food to avoid GI upset.
- Advise parents and patient not to discontinue drug suddenly, not to alter dosage without medical approval, and to consult pharmacist before changing brand or using generic drug because therapeutic effect may change.
- Patient should swallow tablets whole to avoid local mucosal irritation and, if necessary, take with food but not with carbonated beverages because tablet may dissolve before swallowing, causing irritation and unpleasant taste.
- Patient should avoid ingestion of alcohol, which may decrease drug's effectiveness and may increase CNS adverse effects.
- Patient should avoid hazardous activities that require mental alertness until degree of CNS sedative effect is determined. Drug may cause drowsiness and dizziness.
- Teach parents and patient signs and symptoms of hypersensitivity and adverse effects, and the need to report them.
- Encourage parents to have child wear a Medic Alert bracelet or necklace, listing drug taken and seizure disorders.

---

vancomycin
Lyphocin, Vancor, Vancoted, Vanocin

- Classification: antibiotic (glycopeptide)

How supplied
Available by prescription only
Powder for oral solution: 1-g, 10-g bottles
Powder for injection: 500-mg, 1-g vials

Indications, route, and dosage
Severe staphylococcal infections when other antibiotics are ineffective or contraindicated
Neonates age 0 to 7 days weighing < 1,000 g: 10 mg/kg I.V. q 24 hours.
Neonates age 0 to 7 days weighing 1,000 to 2,000 g: 10 mg/kg I.V. q 18 hours.
Neonates age 0 to 7 days and weighing > 2,000 g: 10 mg/kg I.V. q 12 hours.
Infants > 7 days weighing < 1,000 g: 10 mg/kg I.V. q 18 hours.
Infants > 7 days weighing 1,000 to 2,000 g: 10 mg/kg I.V. q 12 hours.
Infants > 7 days weighing > 2,000 g: 10 mg/kg I.V. q 8 hours.
Older infants and children: 30 to 45 mg/kg I.V. daily divided q 8 hours.
Adults: 40 mg/kg/day I.V. in divided doses q 6 hours, not to exceed 2 g daily.
Endocarditis prophylaxis in penicillin-sensitive patients undergoing dental instrumentation procedures
Children under 27 kg: 20 mg/kg I.V. 1 hour before procedure. Dose may be repeated in 8 to 12 hours in high-risk patients.
Children over 27 kg and adults: 1 g I.V. 1 hour before procedure. Dose may be repeated in 8 to 12 hours in high-risk patients.
Endocarditis prophylaxis in penicillin-sensitive patients undergoing GI, GU, or biliary tract surgery
Children under 27 kg: 20 mg/kg I.V. 1 hour before procedure, with 2 mg/kg gentamicin I.V. or I.M. 30 minutes to 1 hour before procedure. Dose may be repeated in 8 to 12 hours.
Children over 27 kg and adults: 1 g I.V. 1 hour before procedure, with gentamicin 1.5 mg/kg I.V. or I.M. 30 minutes to 1 hour before procedure. Dose may be repeated in 8 to 12 hours.
Antibiotic associated pseudomembraneous and staphyloccal enterocolitis
Children: 10 mg/kg P.O. q 6 hours. Do not exceed 2 g/day.
Adults: 125 to 500 mg P.O. q 6 hours for 7 to 10 days.
Dosage in renal failure
Dosage and/or frequency of administration should be modified according to degree of renal impairment, severity of infection, and susceptibility of the causative organism. Dosage should be based upon serum concentrations of drug.

The recommended initial dose is 15 mg/kg. Subsequent doses should be adjusted as needed. Some clinicians use the following schedule:

Serum creatinine level	Dosage in adults
< 1.5 mg/100 ml	1 g q 12 hr
1.5 to 5 mg/100 ml	1 g q 3 to 6 days
> 5 mg/100 ml	1 g q 10 to 14 days

Action and kinetics
- *Antibacterial action:* Vancomycin hinders cell-wall synthesis by blocking glycopeptide polymerization. It

---

spectrum of activity includes many gram-positive organisms, including those resistant to other antibiotics. It is useful for *Staphylococcus epidermidis* and methicillin-resistant *S. aureus*. It is also useful for penicillin-resistant *S. pneumococcus.*

• *Kinetics in adults:* Minimal systemic absorption occurs when vancomycin is administered orally. (However, drug may accumulate in patients with colitis or renal failure.)

Vancomycin is distributed widely in body fluids, including pericardial, pleural, ascitic, synovial, and placental fluid. It will achieve therapeutic levels in CSF in patients with inflamed meninges. Predicted serum levels are 18 to 26 mcg/ml; suggested therapeutic levels are usually 15 to 30 mcg/ml at peak; preinfusion troughs are 5 to 10 mcg/ml. Trough levels have not been correlated with clinical effect. Vancomycin's metabolism is unknown.

When administered parenterally, vancomycin is excreted renally, mainly by filtration. When administered orally, drug is excreted in feces. In patients with normal renal function, plasma half-life is 6 hours; in patients with creatinine clearance ranging from 10 to 30 ml/minute, plasma half-life is about 32 hours; if creatinine clearance is below 10 ml/minute, plasma half-life is 146 hours.

Contraindications and precautions

Vancomycin is contraindicated in patients with known hypersensitivity to the drug.

Vancomycin should be administered cautiously to patients with hearing loss because of its ototoxic effects (especially at high serum levels), and to patients with renal impairment because of its nephrotoxic effects.

Interactions

When used concomitantly, vancomycin may have additive nephrotoxic effects with other nephrotoxic drugs such as aminoglycosides, polymyxin B, colistin, amphotericin B, capreomycin, methoxyflurane, and cisplatin.

Effects on diagnostic tests

Blood urea nitrogen (BUN) and serum creatinine levels may increase, and neutropenia and eosinophilia may occur during vancomycin therapy.

Adverse reactions

• CNS: neurotoxicity.
• DERM: rash.
• EENT: tinnitus, deafness, *ototoxicity.*
• GI: *nausea and vomiting.*
• GU: *nephrotoxicity.*
• HEMA: neutropenia, eosinophilia.
• Local: *phlebitis, pain at I.V. site.*
• Other: *anaphylaxis; fever; chills; hypotension; flushing; rash on face, neck, trunk, and upper extremities (from overly rapid infusion).*

Note: Drug should be discontinued if hypersensitivity develops. Do not confuse hypersensitivity with maculopapular rash.

Overdose and treatment

No information available.

▶ Special considerations

• Obtain culture and sensitivity tests before starting therapy (unless drug is being used for prophylaxis). Mycobacteria and fungi are highly resistent to vancomycin.

• To prepare drug for oral administration, reconstitute as directed in manufacturer's instructions. Reconstituted solution remains stable for 2 weeks when refrigerated.

• To prepare drug for I.V. injection, reconstitute 500-mg or 1-g vial with 10 ml of sterile water for injection, to yield 50 mg/ml or 100 mg/ml, respectively. Withdraw desired dose and further dilute to appropriate volume with normal saline solution or dextrose 5% in water. Infuse over at least 60 minutes to avoid adverse effects related to rapid infusion rate. Reconstituted solution remains stable for 96 hours when refrigerated.

• Do not give I.M. because drug is highly irritating. Monitor for patency during infusion.

• Monitor blood counts and BUN, serum creatinine, AST (SGOT), ALT (SGPT), and drug levels.

• If patient develops maculopapular rash on face, neck, trunk, and upper extremities, slow infusion rate. Premedication with Benadryl before infusion may prevent this reaction.

• If patient has preexisting auditory dysfunction or requires prolonged therapy, auditory function tests may be indicated before and during therapy.

• Hemodialysis and peritoneal dialysis remove only minimal drug amounts. Patients receiving these treatments require usual dose only once every 5 to 7 days.

• Monitor renal function closely. Renal function studies may be required before and during therapy.

Information for parents and patient

• If patient is receiving drug orally, remind parents to have patient continue taking it as directed, even if he feels better.

• Advise parents not to administer antidiarrheal agents concomitantly with drug except as prescribed.

• Instruct parent to watch for signs of ringing in the ears or deafness and to report it promptly.

varicella-zoster immune globulin (VZIG)

• Classification: varicella-zoster prophylaxis agent (immune serum)

How supplied

Available by prescription only
Injection: 10% to 18% solution of the globulin fraction of human plasma containing 125 units of varicella-zoster virus antibody (volume is about 1.25 ml)

☆May contain sulfites   ◆May contain tartrazine   ◆◆May contain benzyl alcohol

Indications, route, and dosage
Passive immunization of susceptible patients, primarily immunocompromised patients and children exposed in utero, after exposure to varicella (chicken pox or herpes zoster)
Children and adults: 125 units per 10 kg of body weight I.M., to a maximum of 625 units. Higher doses may be needed in immunocompromised adults.

Action and kinetics
• *Postexposure prophylaxis:* This agent provides passive immunity to varicella-zoster virus.
• *Kinetics in adults:* After I.M. absorption, the persistence of antibodies is unknown, but protection should last at least 3 weeks. Protection is sufficient to prevent or lessen the severity of varicella infections.

Contraindications and precautions
VZIG should be used with caution in patients with known hypersensitivity to thimerosal, a component of this immune serum.

Interactions
Concomitant use of VZIG with corticosteroids or immunosuppressants may interfere with the immune response to this immune globulin. Whenever possible, avoid using these agents during the postexposure immunization period.

Also, VZIG may interfere with the immune response to live-virus vaccines (for example, those for measles, mumps, and rubella). Do not administer live-virus vaccines within 3 months after administering VZIG. If it becomes necessary to administer VZIG and a live-virus vaccine concomitantly, confirm seroconversion with follow-up serologic testing.

Effects on diagnostic tests
None reported.

Adverse reactions
• Local: discomfort and rash at injection site.
• Systemic: gastrointestinal distress, malaise, headache, respiratory distress, anaphylaxis, angioneurotic edema.

Overdose and treatment
No information available.

▶ Special considerations
• Obtain a thorough history of allergies and reactions to immunizations.
• Epinephrine solution 1:1,000 should be available to treat allergic reactions.
• VZIG is recommended primarily for immunodeficient patients under age 15 and certain infants exposed in utero, although use in other patients (especially immunocompromised patients of any age, normal adults, pregnant women, and premature and full-term infants) should be considered on a case-by-case basis.
• Administer only by deep I.M. injection. Never administer I.V. Use the anterolateral thigh in infants and small children; the deltoid or anterolateral thigh in older children and adults; and the upper outer quadrant of the gluteal muscle in adults receiving large doses.

• For maximum benefit, administer VZIG within 96 hours of presumed exposure.
• Store unopened vials between 36° and 46° F. (2° and 8° C.). Do not freeze.

Information for parents and patient
• Explain to parents that patient's chances of getting AIDS or hepatitis from VZIG are very small.
• Tell parents that patient may experience some local pain, swelling, and tenderness at the injection site. Recommend acetaminophen to alleviate these minor effects.
• Encourage parents to report severe reactions.

---

vasopressin (antidiuretic hormone [ADH])
Pitressin

vasopressin tannate
Pitressin Tannate in Oil

• Classification: antidiuretic hormone, peristaltic stimulant, hemostatic agent (posterior pituitary hormone)

How supplied
Available by prescription only
Vasopressin
Injection: 0.5-ml and 1-ml ampules, 20 units/ml
Vasopressin tannate
Injection: 1-ml ampules, 5 units/ml

Indications, route, and dosage
Nonnephrogenic, nonpsychogenic diabetes insipidus
Children: 2.5 to 10 units I.M. or S.C. b.i.d. to q.i.d., p.r.n.; or intranasally (spray or cotton balls) in individualized doses. For chronic therapy, inject 1.25 to 2.5 units of Pitressin Tannate in Oil suspension I.M. or S.C. q 2 to 3 days.
Adults: 5 to 10 units I.M. or S.C. b.i.d. to q.i.d., p.r.n.; or intranasally (spray or cotton balls) in individualized doses, based on response. For chronic therapy, inject 2.5 to 5 units of Pitressin Tannate in Oil suspension I.M. or S.C. q 2 to 3 days.
Postoperative abdominal distention
Children: Dosage is highly individualized. Reduce adult dosage proportionately.
Adults: 5 units (aqueous) I.M. initially, then q 3 to 4 hours, increasing dosage to 10 units, if needed.

Action and kinetics
• *Antidiuretic action:* Vasopressin is used as an antidiuretic to control or prevent signs and complications of neurogenic diabetes insipidus. Acting primarily at the renal tubular level, vasopressin increases cyclic 3′,5′-adenosine monophosphate, which increases water permeability at the renal tubule and collecting duct, resulting in increased urine osmolality and decreased urinary flow rate.
• *Peristaltic stimulant action:* Used to treat postoperative abdominal distention and to facilitate abdom

---

inal radiographic procedures, vasopressin induces peristalsis by directly stimulating contraction of smooth muscle in the GI tract.

• *Hemostatic action:* In patients with GI hemorrhage, vasopressin administered I.V. or intra-arterially into the superior mesenteric artery controls bleeding of esophageal varices by directly stimulating vasoconstriction of capillaries and small arterioles.

• *Kinetics in adults:* Vasopressin is destroyed by trypsin in the GI tract and must be administered intranasally or parenterally. Absorption of vasopressin tannate in oil after I.M. or S.C. administration may be erratic. Vasopressin tannate in oil is absorbed more slowly than the aqueous preparation after I.M. administration. Vasopressin is distributed throughout the extracellular fluid, with no evidence of protein-binding. Most of a dose is destroyed rapidly in the liver and kidneys. Approximately 5% of an S.C. dose of aqueous vasopressin is excreted unchanged in urine after 4 hours. Duration of action after I.M. administration of vasopressin tannate in oil is 24 to 72 hours; after I.M. or S.C. administration of the aqueous form, 2 to 8 hours. Half-life is 10 to 20 minutes.

Contraindications and precautions
Vasopressin is contraindicated in patients with chronic nephritis accompanied by nitrogen retention or hypersensitivity to the drug.

It should be used with caution in patients with seizure disorders, migraines, asthma, or heart failure, because rapid addition of extracellular water may be hazardous; and in those with vascular disease, angina pectoris, or coronary thrombosis, because large doses may precipitate myocardial infarction. Preoperative and postoperative polyuric patients may have considerably reduced hormone requirements.

Interactions
Concomitant use of vasopressin with carbamazepine, chlorpropamide, or clofibrate may potentiate vasopressin's antidiuretic effect; use with demeclocycline, lithium, norepinephrine, epinephrine, heparin, or alcohol may decrease antidiuretic effect.

Effects on diagnostic tests
None reported.

Adverse reactions
• CNS: tremors, dizziness, headache.
• CV: angina in patients with vascular disease, vasoconstriction. Large doses may cause hypertension, ECG changes. With intra-arterial infusion: bradycardia, cardiac dysrhythmias, pulmonary edema.
• DERM: circumoral pallor.
• GI: abdominal cramps, nausea, vomiting, diarrhea, intestinal hyperactivity.
• GU: uterine cramps, anuria.
• Other: water intoxication (drowsiness, listlessness, headache, confusion, weight gain), hypersensitivity reactions (urticaria, angioneurotic edema, bronchoconstriction, fever, rash, wheezing, dyspnea, anaphylaxis), sweating.
Note: Drug should be discontinued if signs or symptoms of anaphylaxis, hypersensitivity, or water intoxication occur.

Overdose and treatment
Clinical manifestations of overdose include drowsiness, listlessness, headache, confusion, anuria, and weight gain (water intoxication). Treatment requires water restriction and temporary withdrawal of vasopressin until polyuria occurs. Severe water intoxication may require osmotic diuresis with mannitol, hypertonic dextrose, or urea, either alone or with furosemide.

▶ Special considerations
• Children show increased sensitivity to the effects of vasopressin. Use with caution.
• Establish baseline vital signs and intake and output ratio at the initiation of therapy.
• Monitor patient's blood pressure twice daily. Watch for excessively elevated blood pressure or lack of response to drug, which may be indicated by hypotension. Also monitor fluid intake and output and daily weights.
• Adjust fluid intake to reduce risk of water intoxication and sodium depletion, especially in young patients.
• Question the patient with abdominal distention about passage of flatus and stool.
• A rectal tube will facilitate gas expulsion after vasopressin injection.
• Observe for signs of early water intoxication (drowsiness, listlessness, headache, confusion, and weight gain) to prevent seizures, coma, and death.
• Overdose may cause oxytocic or vasopressor activity. If patient develops uterine cramps, increased GI activity, fluid retention, or hypertension, withhold drug until effects subside. Furosemide may be used if fluid retention is excessive.
• Some patients may have difficulty measuring and inhaling drug into nostrils. Teach patient correct method of administration.
• Never inject vasopressin tannate in oil I.V.
• Never inject during first stage of labor; this may cause ruptured uterus.
• Overhydration is more likely to occur with long-acting tannate oil suspension than with aqueous vasopressin solution.
• Use extreme caution to avoid extravasation because of the risk of necrosis and gangrene.
• Place vasopressin tannate in oil ampule in warm water for 10 to 15 minutes. Remove and *shake thoroughly* to ensure a uniform suspension before drawing up dose. Poor response may be from inadequate shaking.

Information for parents and patient
• Teach parents and patient correct administration method. Some patients may have difficulty measuring and inhaling drug into nostrils.
• Instruct parents or patient using vasopressin tannate in oil to always warm the ampule in his hands and shake it vigorously before drawing the solution into the needle to allow uniform mixture of drug. Encourage rotation of injection sites.
• Patient should drink one or two glasses of water with each dose of vasopressin. This reduces the adverse reactions of unusual paleness, nausea, abdominal cramps, and vomiting.

‡May contain sulfites   ◆May contain tartrazine   ◆◆May contain benzyl alcohol

- Teach parents and patient how to maintain a fluid intake and output record.
- Show parents and patient how to check the expiration date.
- Tell parents to call immediately if any of the following signs or symptoms occur: chest pain, confusion, fever, hives, skin rash, headache, problems with urination, seizures, weight gain, unusual drowsiness, wheezing, trouble with breathing, or swelling of face, hands, feet, or mouth.

verapamil hydrochloride
Calan, Isoptin

- Classification: antianginal, antihypertensive, antiarrhythmic (calcium channel blocker)

How supplied
Available by prescription only
Tablets: 80 mg, 120 mg; 240 mg (extended-release)
Injection: 2.5 mg/ml

Indications, route, and dosage
Supraventricular tachydysrhythmias
Children under age 1: 0.1 to 0.2 mg/kg (0.75 to 2 mg) as I.V. bolus over 2 minutes. Dose may be repeated in 30 minutes if no response occurs.
Children age 1 to 15: 0.1 to 0.3 mg/kg (2 to 5 mg) as I.V. bolus over 2 minutes. Dose should not exceed 5 mg. Dose may be repeated in 30 minutes if no response occurs (should not exceed 10 mg).
Adults: 0.075 to 0.15 mg/kg (5 to 10 mg) I.V. push over 2 minutes. If no response occurs, give a second dose of 10 mg (0.15 mg/kg) 15 to 30 minutes after the initial dose.
Note: Use in infants is associated with severe adverse reactions and is not recommended by pediatric cardiologists.
Prevention of recurrent paroxysmal supraventricular tachycardia
Adults: 240 to 480 mg P.O. daily in three to four divided doses.
Control of ventricular rate in digitalized patients with chronic atrial flutter and/or fibrillation
Adults: 240 to 320 mg P.O. daily in three to four divided doses.
Hypertension
Adults: Usual starting dose is 80 mg P.O. t.i.d., or one 240-mg sustained-release tablet or capsule P.O. daily in the morning. Dosage may be increased at weekly intervals. For patients taking sustained-release product, dosage may be increased in 120-mg increments, with second dose added in the evening.

Action and kinetics
- *Antianginal action:* Verapamil manages unstable and chronic stable angina by reducing afterload, both at rest and with exercise, thereby decreasing oxygen consumption. It also decreases myocardial oxygen demand and cardiac work by exerting a negative inotropic effect, reducing heart rate, relieving coronary artery spasm (via coronary artery vasodilation), and dilating peripheral vessels. The net result of these effects is relief of angina-related ischemia and pain. In patients with Prinzmetal's variant angina, verapamil inhibits coronary artery spasm, resulting in increased myocardial oxygen delivery.
- *Antihypertensive action:* Verapamil reduces blood pressure mainly by dilating peripheral vessels. Its negative inotropic effect blocks reflex mechanisms that lead to increased blood pressure.
- *Antiarrhythmic action:* Verapamil's combined effects on the SA and AV nodes help manage dysrhythmias. The drug's primary effect is on the AV node; slowed conduction reduces the ventricular rate in atrial tachydysrhythmias and blocks reentry paths in paroxysmal supraventricular dysrhythmias.
- *Kinetics in adults:* Verapamil is absorbed rapidly and completely from the GI tract after oral administration; however, only about 20% to 35% of the drug reaches systemic circulation because of first-pass effect. When administered orally, peak effects occur within 1 to 2 hours with conventional tablets and within 4 to 8 hours with sustained-release preparations. When administered I.V., effects occur within minutes after injection and usually persist about 30 to 60 minutes (although they may last up to 6 hours). Steady-state distribution volume in healthy adults ranges from about 4.5 to 7 liters/kg but may increase to 12 liters, kg in patients with hepatic cirrhosis. Approximately 90% of circulating drug is bound to plasma proteins. Verapamil is metabolized in the liver and is excreted in the urine as unchanged drug and active metabolites. Elimination half-life is normally 6 to 12 hours and increases to as much as 16 hours in patients with hepatic cirrhosis. In infants, elimination half-life may be 5 to 7 hours.

Contraindications and precautions
Verapamil is contraindicated in patients with severe hypotension (systolic blood pressure below 90 mm Hg or cardiogenic shock, because of the drug's hypotensive effect; in patients with second- or third-degree AV block or sick sinus syndrome (unless a functioning artificial ventricular pacemaker is in place), because of the drug's effects on the cardiac conduction system; in patients with severe left ventricular dysfunction (indicated by pulmonary wedge pressure above 20 mm Hg and left ventricular ejection fraction below 20%) unless heart failure results from supraventricular tachycardia, because the drug may worsen the condition; in patients with ventricular dysfunction or AV abnormalities who are receiving beta-adrenergic blockers, because of the drug's negative inotropic effect and inhibition of the cardiac conduction system and in patients with known hypersensitivity to the drug.

All verapamil forms should be used with caution in patients with moderately severe ventricular dysfunction or heart failure, because the drug may precipitate or worsen the condition; in patients with hypertrophic cardiomyopathy, because the drug may cause serious and sometimes fatal adverse cardiovascular effects (such as pulmonary edema, hypotension, heart block, or sinus arrest); in patients with hepatic or renal impairment, because the drug may accumulate (generally, the dose should be reduced and the patient carefully monitored); in patients with sick sinus syndrome or atrial flutter or fibrillation with an accessory bypass tract (such as Wolff-Parkinson-White or Lown-Ganong-Levine syndrome), because the drug may precipitate life-threatening adverse effects (for example, ventricular fibrillation or cardiac arrest); in patients with wide-complex ventricular tachycardia, because the drug may cause marked hemodynamic deterioration and ventricular fibrillation; and in patients receiving the drug I.V., because of possible adverse hemodynamic effects (hypotension) and adverse ECG effects (such as bradycardia and heart block).

Interactions

Concomitant use of verapamil with beta blockers may cause additive effects leading to CHF, conduction disturbances, dysrhythmias, and hypotension, especially if high beta-blocker doses are used, if the drugs are administered I.V., or if the patient has moderately severe to severe CHF, severe cardiomyopathy, or recent myocardial infarction.

Concomitant use of oral verapamil with digoxin may increase serum digoxin concentration by 50% to 75% during the 1st week of therapy. Concomitant use with antihypertensives may lead to combined antihypertensive effects, resulting in clinically significant hypotension. Concomitant use with drugs that attenuate alpha-adrenergic response (such as prazosin and methyldopa) may cause excessive blood pressure reduction. Concomitant use with disopyramide may cause combined negative inotropic effects; with quinidine to treat hypertrophic cardiomyopathy, may cause excessive hypotension; with carbamazepine, may cause increased serum carbamazepine levels and subsequent toxicity; with rifampin, may substantially reduce verapamil's oral bioavailability.

Effects on diagnostic tests

None reported.

Adverse reactions

CNS: dizziness, headache, fatigue.
CV: *transient hypotension, heart failure, bradycardia,* AV block, ventricular asystole, peripheral edema, *pnea.*
GI: constipation, nausea (primarily with oral form).
Hepatic: elevated liver enzyme levels.
Note: Drug should be discontinued if systolic presure falls below 90 mm Hg, if heart failure worsens, or if dysrhythmias, hemodynamically significant bradycardia, or second- or third-degree heart block occur.

Overdose and treatment

Clinical effects of overdose are primarily extensions of adverse reactions. Heart block, asystole, and hypotension are the most serious reactions and require immediate attention.

Treatment may include administering I.V. isoproterenol, norepinephrine, epinephrine, atropine, or calcium gluconate in usual doses. Adequate hydration should be ensured.

In patients with hypertrophic cardiomyopathy, alpha-adrenergic agents, including methoxamine, phenylephrine, and metaraminol, should be used to maintain blood pressure. (Isoproterenol and norepinephrine should be avoided.) Inotropic agents, including dobutamine and dopamine, may be used if necessary.

If severe conduction disturbances, such as heart block and asystole, occur with hypotension that does not respond to drug therapy, cardiac pacing should be initiated immediately, with cardiopulmonary resuscitation measures as indicated.

In patients with Wolff-Parkinson-White or Lown-Ganong-Levine syndrome and a rapid ventricular rate caused by hemodynamically significant antegrade conduction, synchronized cardioversion may be used. Lidocaine and/or procainamide may be used as adjuncts.

▶ **Special considerations**

• Currently, only the I.V. form is indicated for use in pediatric patients to treat supraventricular tachydysrhythmias.
• Because administration of verapamil to infants younger than age 1 has been associated with severe and fatal adverse reactions, many pediatric cardiologists consider such use contraindicated.
• Use of verapamil in patient receiving carbamazepine may require a 40% to 50% reduction in carbamazepine dosage. Monitor patient closely for signs of toxicity.
• Reduce dosage in patients with renal or hepatic impairment.
• Monitor cardiac rate and rhythm and blood pressure carefully when initiating therapy or increasing dose.
• Total serum calcium concentrations are not affected by calcium channel blocking agents.
• If patient is receiving I.V. verapamil, monitor ECG continuously.
• If verapamil is added to therapy of patient receiving digoxin, digoxin dose should be reduced by half with subsequent monitoring of serum drug levels.
• During long-term combination therapy involving verapamil and digoxin, monitor ECG periodically to observe for AV block and bradycardia, because of drugs' possible additive effects on the AV node.
• Obtain periodic liver function tests.
• Patients with severely compromised cardiac function and those receiving beta blockers should receive lower verapamil doses. Monitor these patients closely.
• Discontinue disopyramide 48 hours before starting verapamil therapy and do not reinstitute until 24 hours after verapamil has been discontinued.

Information for parents and patient

• Urge parents and patient to report signs of CHF, such as swelling of hands and feet or shortness of breath.
• Advise parents of patient who is receiving nitrate therapy while verapamil dose is being titrated to have patient comply with prescribed therapy.
• Tell parents not to abruptly discontinue the drug; gradual dosage reduction may be necessary.
• Patient who misses a dose should take the dose as soon as possible, but not if almost time for next dose. Warn against taking a double dose.

vidarabine monohydrate (adenosine arabinoside)
Vira-A

- Classification: antiviral agent (purine nucleoside)

How supplied
Available by prescription only
Concentrate for I.V. infusion: 200 mg/ml in 5-ml vial (equivalent to 187.4 mg vidarabine)
Ophthalmic ointment: 3% in 3.5-g tube (equivalent to 2.8% vidarabine)

Indications, route, and dosage
Herpes simplex virus encephalitis
Neonates: 15 to 30 mg/kg as a single daily dose.
Children and adults: 15 mg/kg daily for 10 days. Slowly infuse the total daily dosage by I.V. infusion at a constant rate over a 12- to 24-hour period. Avoid rapid or bolus injection.
Herpes zoster in immunocompromised patient
Infants and children: 10 to 30 mg/kg daily.
Adults: 10 mg/kg I.V. daily for 5 days at constant rate over 12 to 24 hours/day.
Acute keratoconjunctivitis and recurrent epithelial keratitis caused by herpes simplex virus Types I and II
Children and adults: Administer ½" (1.3 cm) of ointment into lower conjunctival sac five times daily at 3-hour intervals.
Dosage in renal failure
Children and adults: Dosage should be reduced by at least 25% in patients with creatinine clearance < 10 ml/min.

Action and kinetics
- *Antiviral action:* Vidarabine is an adenosine analog. Its exact mechanism of action is unknown; presumably it involves inhibition of DNA polymerase and viral replication by incorporation into viral DNA.
- *Kinetics in adults:* Vidarabine is absorbed poorly when administered orally, I.M., or S.C. I.V. administration results in rapid deamination to the active metabolite, arabinosyl-hypoxanthine. Vidarabine and arabinosyl-hypoxanthine are distributed widely in body tissues and fluids. CSF concentration equals about 30% of serum levels. Parent compound is 20% to 30% plasma protein-bound; arabinosyl-hypoxanthine is 1% to 3% plasma protein-bound.

Vidarabine is metabolized into the active metabolite arabinosyl-hypoxanthine. Both parent compound and active metabolite are excreted primarily by the kidneys. Half-lives of parent compound and active metabolite are 1½ and 3½ hours, respectively.

Contraindications and precautions
Vidarabine is contraindicated in patients with known hypersensitivity to the drug.

Vidarabine should be administered cautiously to patients with hepatic or renal dysfunction because they may be more susceptible to dose-related adverse effects, and to patients with restricted fluid intake because they may not tolerate the large fluid volumes needed for drug administration.

Interactions
When used concomitantly, vidarabine may inhibit theophylline metabolism, increasing the risk of theophylline toxicity. Concomitant use with allopurinol may inhibit vidarabine metabolism, causing tremors, anemia, nausea, pain, or pruritus.

Effects on diagnostic tests
AST (SGOT) and serum bilirubin levels may increase and leukocyte, platelet, reticulocyte, hemoglobin, and hematocrit values may decrease during vidarabine therapy.

Adverse reactions
- CNS: tremors, dizziness, hallucinations, confusion, psychosis, ataxia, coma (especially in patients in renal failure).
- DERM: pruritus, rash.
- EENT (with ophthalmic application): lacrimation, foreign body sensation, conjunctival injection, burning, irritation, superficial keratitis, pain, photophobia, punctal occlusion, sensitivity.
- GI: anorexia, nausea, vomiting, diarrhea.
- HEMA: anemia, neutropenia, thrombocytopenia.
- Hepatic: elevated AST (SGOT) and bilirubin levels.
- Local: pain at injection site.
- Other: weight loss.

Overdose and treatment
Clinical effects of overdose may reflect fluid overload and potential risk of heart failure caused by volume of fluid needed to administer drug. Carefully monitor renal, hepatic, and hematologic status in patient who received excessive dose.

▶ Special considerations
- Drug proves effective only if patient has at least minimal immunocompetence.
- Definitive diagnosis of herpes simplex conjunctivitis should be made before administration of ophthalmic form.
- Drug reduces mortality from herpes simplex encephalitis from 70% to 28%. However, no evidence suggests that drug is effective against encephalitis caused by other viruses.
- Do not give I.M. or S.C. because drug is poorly and unreliably absorbed by these routes.
- To prepare I.V. infusion, shake vial well to achieve uniform suspension before transferring to I.V. solution container. Examine vial for uniformity. Use at least 1 liter for every 450 mg of drug (every milligram requires at least 2.22 ml of I.V. fluid). Infuse drug via continuous drip over 12 to 24 hours. Avoid rapid or bolus injection. Use I.V. in-line filter (0.45 microns or smaller).
- To facilitate dissolution, warm solution to 95° to 104° F. (35° to 40° C.). Once in solution, vidarabine remains stable at room temperature for 48 hours. Do not refrigerate diluted solution.
- Any crystalloid solution may be used to prepare I.V. drug. Do not use biological (blood) or colloidal (albumin) fluids.

If patient is receiving drug concomitantly with theophylline, monitor serum theophylline levels and observe for signs and symptoms of theophylline toxicity. Monitor hepatic and hematologic status during therapy.

Information for parents and patient

Warn parents and patient receiving ophthalmic ointment not to exceed recommended frequency or duration of therapy. Instruct them to wash hands before and after applying ointment, and warn them against allowing tip of tube to touch eye or surrounding area.

Advise parents that patient should wear sunglasses if photosensitivity occurs.

Advise patient to store ophthalmic ointment in tightly sealed, light-resistant container.

vinblastine sulfate (VLB)
Velban, Velbe*

Classification: antineoplastic (vinca alkaloid [cell cycle-phase specific, M phase])

How supplied
Available by prescription only
Injection: 10-mg vials (lyophilized powder), 10 mg/10 ml vials

Indications, route, and dosage
Dosage and indications may vary. Check current literature for recommended protocol.

Breast or testicular cancer, Hodgkin's and non-Hodgkin's lymphomas, choriocarcinoma, lymphosarcoma, †neuroblastoma, lung cancer, mycosis fungoides, histiocytosis, head and neck carcinoma, renal carcinoma, ovarian germ cell tumors, Kaposi's sarcoma
Children: 2.5 mg/m² I.V. as a single dose every week, increased weekly in increments of 1.25 mg/m² to a maximum of 7.5 mg/m². Dose should not be repeated if WBC count falls below 4,000/mm³.
Adults: 0.1 mg/kg or 3.7 mg/m² I.V. weekly or q 2 weeks. May be increased in weekly increments of 50 mcg/kg or 1.8 to 1.9 mg/m² to maximum dose of 0.5 mg/kg or 18.5 mg/m² I.V. weekly, according to response. Dose should not be repeated if WBC count falls below 4,000/mm³.

Action and kinetics
Antineoplastic action: Vinblastine exerts its cytotoxic activity by arresting the cell cycle in the metaphase portion of cell division, resulting in a blockade of mitosis. The drug also inhibits DNA-dependent RNA synthesis and interferes with amino acid metabolism, inhibiting purine synthesis.
Kinetics in adults: Vinblastine is absorbed unpredictably across the GI tract after oral administration, which is why it must be given I.V.

Vinblastine is distributed widely into body tissues. The drug crosses the blood-brain barrier but does not achieve therapeutic concentrations in the CSF.

Vinblastine is metabolized partially in the liver to an active metabolite and is excreted primarily in bile as unchanged drug. A smaller portion is excreted in urine. The plasma elimination of vinblastine is described as triphasic, with half-lives of 35 minutes, 53 minutes, and 19 hours for the alpha, beta, and terminal phases, respectively.

Contraindications and precautions
Vinblastine is contraindicated in patients with severe leukopenia or bacterial infections because treatment with myelosuppressive drugs such as vinblastine causes an increased frequency of infections. Instruct patients to report any symptoms of sore throat and fever and of unusual bruising or bleeding. Leukocyte, erythrocyte, and platelet counts, and hemoglobin should be monitored weekly during therapy. Vinblastine can impair fertility. Aspermia has occurred after treatment with vinblastine.

Interactions
Concomitant use of vinblastine increases the effect of methotrexate by increasing cellular uptake of methotrexate. This interaction allows a lower dose of methotrexate, reducing the potential for methotrexate toxicity.

Effects on diagnostic tests
Vinblastine therapy may increase blood and urine concentrations of uric acid.

Adverse reactions
• CNS: depression, paresthesias, peripheral neuropathy and neuritis, numbness, *loss of deep tendon reflexes, muscle pain* and weakness.
• DERM: dermatitis, vesiculation.
• EENT: pharyngitis.
• GI: *nausea, vomiting, stomatitis,* ulcer, bleeding, constipation, *paralytic ileus, anorexia, weight loss, abdominal pain.*
• GU: oligospermia, aspermia, urinary retention.
• HEMA: *bone marrow depression* (dose-limiting), leukopenia (nadir on days 4 to 10 and lasts another 7 to 14 days), thrombocytopenia.
• Local: *irritation, phlebitis, cellulitis, necrosis if I.V. extravasates.*
• Other: acute bronchospasm, reversible alopecia in 5% to 10% of patients, pain in tumor site, low fever, *jaw pain, inappropriate ADH secretion.*

Note: Drug should be discontinued if patient develops stomatitis.

Overdose and treatment
Clinical manifestations of overdose include stomatitis, ileus, mental depression, paresthesias, loss of deep reflexes, permanent CNS damage, and myelosuppression.

Treatment is usually supportive and includes transfusion of blood components and appropriate symptomatic therapy.

▶ Special considerations
• To reconstitute drug, use 10 ml of preserved normal saline injection to yield a concentration of 1 mg/ml.
• Drug may be administered by I.V. push injection over

1 minute into the tubing of a freely flowing I.V. infusion.

• Dilution into larger volume is not recommended for infusion into peripheral veins. This method increases risk of extravasation. Drug may be administered as an I.V. infusion through a central venous catheter.

• Drug is a vesicant. Treat extravasation promptly according to institutional policy.

• Take special care to avoid extravasation. Treatment of extravasation includes liberal injection of hyaluronidase into the site, followed by warm compresses to minimize the spread of the reaction. Prepare hyaluronidase by adding 3 ml of normal saline injection to the 150-unit vial.

• Give an antiemetic before administering drug, to reduce nausea.

• Do not administer more frequently than every 7 days to allow review of effect on leukocytes before administration of next dose. Leukopenia may develop. Monitor CBC.

• Reduced dosage may be required in patients with liver disease.

• After administering, monitor for life-threatening acute bronchospasm. This reaction is most likely to occur in a patient who is also receiving mitomycin.

• Prevent uric acid nephropathy with generous oral fluid intake and administration of allopurinol.

• Give laxatives as needed. Stool softeners may be used prophylactically.

• Drug is less neurotoxic than vincristine.

Information for parents and patient

• Stress importance of keeping follow-up appointments for monitoring hematologic status.

• Teach parents and patient to check for signs of bleeding and bruising. Parents may need to restrict child's participation in contact sports. Such activity is dangerous when patient's platelets are low.

• Instruct parents to monitor neutropenic patient's temperature every 4 hours (not rectally) and to report fever, cough, and other signs of infection *promptly*.

• Patient should avoid contact with persons who have received live-virus immunizations (polio, measles/mumps/rubella). Explain importance of promptly reporting susceptible patient's exposure to chicken pox.

• Instruct patient to clean teeth with toothettes, gauze, or soft toothbrush when platelets are low. Patient should perform frequent oral hygiene and should avoid using commercial mouthwashes which may contain alcohol and have an irritating effect. Solutions of sodium bicarbonate or hydrogen peroxide are more appropriate rinses.

• Instruct patient to avoid foods that are spicy and extremely hot or cold. Topical anesthetics administered before meals (swish and spit) may relieve mouth discomfort.

• Advise the parents to encourage the patient to drink plenty of fluids to increase urine output and facilitate excretion of uric acid.

• Explain that therapeutic response is not immediate. Adequate trial is 12 weeks.

• Reassure parents and patient that hair should grow back after treatment has ended.

vincristine sulfate
Oncovin, Vincasar

• Classification: antineoplastic (vinca alkaloid [cell cycle-phase specific, M phase])

How supplied
Available by prescription only
Injection: 1 mg/1 ml, 2 mg/2 ml, 5 mg/5 ml multiple-dose vials; 1 mg/1 ml, 2 mg/2 ml preservative-free vials

Indications, route, and dosage
Dosage and indications may vary. Check current literature for recommended protocol.
Acute lymphoblastic and other leukemias; Hodgkin's disease; lymphosarcoma; †reticulum cell, †osteogenic, and †other sarcomas; neuroblastoma; rhabdomyosarcoma; Wilms' tumor; †lung and breast cancer
Children 10 kg and less or with a body surface area $< 1 m^2$: Initate therapy at 0.05 mg/kg once weekly.
Children over 10 kg or with a body surface area $> 1 m^2$: 2 mg/m² I.V. weekly.
Adults: 10 to 30 mcg/kg I.V. or 0.4 to 1.4 mg/m² I.V. weekly.
Maximum single dose (adults and children) is 2 mg.

Action and kinetics
• *Antineoplastic action:* Vincristine exerts its cytotoxic activity by arresting the cell cycle in the metaphase portion of cell division, resulting in a blockade of mitosis. The drug also inhibits DNA-dependent RNA synthesis and interferes with amino acid metabolites inhibiting purine synthesis.

• *Kinetics in adults:* Vincristine is absorbed unpredictably across the GI tract after oral administration and therefore must be given I.V.
Vincristine is rapidly and widely distributed into body tissues and is bound to erythrocytes and platelets. The drug crosses the blood-brain barrier but does not achieve therapeutic concentrations in the cerebrospinal fluid.
Vincristine is extensively metabolized in the liver and its metabolites are primarily excreted into bile. A smaller portion is eliminated through the kidneys. The plasma elimination of vincristine is described as triphasic, with half-lives of about 4 minutes, 2¼ hours, and 85 hours for the distribution, second, and terminal phases, respectively.

Contraindications and precautions
Vincristine is contraindicated in patients with the demyelinating form of Charcot-Marie-Tooth syndrome because of the drug's neurotoxic effects.
Treatment with myelosuppressive drugs such as vincristine causes an increased frequency of infections. Patient should call if sore throat or fever develops. Use with caution in patients with preexisting neuromuscular disease, closely monitoring for neurotoxicity. Leukocyte count and hemoglobin should

be checked before each dose. Use cautiously in patients with jaundice or hepatic dysfunction.

Interactions
Concomitant use of vincristine increases the therapeutic effect of methotrexate. This interaction may be used to therapeutic advantage; it allows a lower dose of methotrexate, reducing the potential for methotrexate toxicity. Concomitant use with other neurotoxic drugs increases neurotoxicity through an additive effect.

Effects on diagnostic tests
Vincristine therapy may increase blood and urine concentrations of uric acid and serum potassium.

Adverse reactions
• CNS: neurotoxicity (dose-limiting), *peripheral neuropathy*, sensory loss, deep tendon reflex loss, paresthesias, wristdrop and footdrop, ataxia, cranial nerve palsies (headache, jaw pain, hoarseness, vocal cord paralysis, visual disturbances), muscle weakness and cramps, depression, agitation, insomnia; some neurotoxicities may be permanent.
• EENT: diplopia, optic and extraocular neuropathy, ptosis.
• GI: *constipation*, cramps, *paralytic ileus*, nausea, vomiting, anorexia, stomatitis, weight loss, dysphagia.
• GU: urinary retention.
• HEMA: *bone marrow depression*, rapidly reversible mild anemia and leukopenia.
• Local: *severe local reaction when extravasated*, phlebitis, cellulitis.
• Other: acute bronchospasm, *reversible alopecia* (in up to 71% of patients), *jaw pain, inappropriate ADH secretion, hepatic damage.*

Overdose and treatment
Clinical manifestations of overdose include alopecia, myelosuppression, paresthesias, neuritic pain, motor difficulties, loss of deep tendon reflexes, nausea, vomiting, and ileus.

Treatment is usually supportive and includes transfusion of blood components, antiemetics, enemas for ileus, phenobarbital for convulsions, and other appropriate symptomatic therapy. Administration of calcium leucovorin at a dosage of 15 mg I.V. q 3 hours for 24 hours, then q 6 hours for 48 hours may help protect cells from the toxic effects of vincristine.

▶ Special considerations
• Drug may be administered by I.V. push injection over 1 minute into the tubing of a freely flowing I.V. infusion.
• Dilution into larger volumes is not recommended for infusion into peripheral veins; this method increases risk of extravasation. Drug may be administered as an I.V. infusion through a central venous catheter.
• Drug is a vesicant. Avoid placement of I.V. site at or near a joint that may be immobilized if extravasation occurs. During I.V. administration, monitor continuously for extravasation. If it occurs, stop infusion, remove I.V., and treat promptly according to institutional policy.

• Do not administer more than 2 mg per week.
• After administering, monitor for life-threatening bronchospasm reaction. It is most likely to occur in a patient who is also receiving mitomycin.
• Because of potential for neurotoxicity, do not give drug more than once a week. Children are more resistant to neurotoxicity than adults. Neurotoxicity is dose-related and usually reversible; reduce dose if symptoms of neurotoxicity develop.
• Monitor for neurotoxicity by checking for depression of Achilles tendon reflex, numbness, tingling, footdrop or wristdrop, difficulty in walking, ataxia, and slapping gait. Also check ability to walk on heels. Patient should have support during walking.
• Prevent uric acid nephropathy with generous oral fluid intake and administration of allopurinol. Alkalinization of urine may be required if serum uric acid concentration is increased.
• Monitor CBC before therapy and weekly before each dose.
• Monitor bowel function. Patient should have stool softener, laxative, or water before dosing. Constipation may be an early sign of neurotoxicity.
• Patients with obstructive jaundice or liver disease should receive a reduced dosage.
• Vials of 5 mg are for multiple-dose use only. Do not administer entire vial to patient as single dose. Do not store drug in plastic syringes. Protect drug from light.
• Drug may cause inappropriate ADH secretion. Treatment requires fluid restriction and a loop diuretic.

Information for parents and patient
• Stress importance of keeping follow-up appointments for monitoring hematologic status.
• Instruct parents to monitor neutropenic patient's temperature every 4 hours (not rectally) and to report fever, cough, and other signs of infection *promptly.*
• Patient should avoid contact with persons who have received live-virus immunizations (polio, measles/mumps/rubella). Explain importance of promptly reporting susceptible patient's exposure to chicken pox.
• Teach parents and patient to check for signs of bleeding and bruising. Parents may need to restrict child's participation in contact sports. Such activity is dangerous when patient's platelets are low.
• Instruct patient to clean teeth with toothettes, gauze, or soft toothbrush when platelets are low.
• Instruct parents to report signs of neuropathy promptly (weakness, jaw pain, numbness, slapping gait, walking on toes, constipation).
• Sexually active patients should continue contraception while taking this drug.
• Patient should take a stool softener to prevent constipation. Tell parents to call if patient develops constipation or stomach pain.
• Advise parents to encourage the child to drink plenty of fluids to increase urine output and facilitate excretion of uric acid.
• Assure parents and patient that hair growth should resume after treatment is discontinued.

vindesine sulfate
Eldisine*

- Classification: antineoplastic (vinca alkaloid [cell cycle-phase specific, M phase])

How supplied
Available only through investigational protocols
Injection: 5-mg, 10-mg ampules

Indications, route, and dosage
Dosage and indications may vary. Check current literature for recommended protocol.
†*Acute lymphoblastic leukemia, breast cancer, malignant melanoma, lymphosarcoma, non-small-cell lung carcinoma*
Children: 4 mg/m² I.V. route q 7 to 10 days, or 2 mg/m²/day for 2 days, followed by 5 to 7 days without the drug.
Adults: 3 to 4 mg/m² I.V. q 7 to 14 days, or continuous I.V. infusion 1.2 to 1.5 mg/m² daily for 5 days q 3 weeks.

Action and kinetics
- *Antineoplastic action:* Vindesine exerts its cytotoxic activity by arresting the cell cycle in the metaphase portion of cell division, resulting in a blockade of mitosis. The drug also inhibits DNA-dependent RNA synthesis and interferes with amino acid metabolism, inhibiting purine synthesis.
- *Kinetics in adults:* Vindesine is absorbed unpredictably across the GI tract after oral administration and therefore must be administered I.V.

Vindesine is widely distributed into body tissues. The drug crosses the blood-brain barrier but does not achieve therapeutic concentrations in the cerebrospinal fluid. Extensive tissue-binding occurs.

Vindesine is partially metabolized in the liver to an active metabolite and is excreted primarily in bile as unchanged drug. A smaller portion is eliminated in urine. The plasma elimination of vindesine has been described as triphasic, with half-lives of 3 minutes, 100 minutes, and greater than 20 hours for the distribution, second, and terminal phases, respectively.

Contraindications and precautions
Vindesine is contraindicated in patients with severe leukopenia or bacterial infections because treatment with myelosuppressive drugs such as vindesine causes an increased frequency of infections. Patients should promptly report sore throat and fever and any unusual bleeding or bruising. Leukocyte and platelet counts should be monitored frequently during therapy.

Do not administer with other vinca alkaloids because of increased potential for cumulative neurotoxicity.

Interactions
Compatibility with other drugs has not been determined. Avoid concomitant use.

Effects on diagnostic tests
Vindesine therapy may increase blood and urine concentrations of uric acid.

Adverse reactions
- CNS: paresthesias, decreased deep tendon reflex, muscle weakness.
- GI: constipation, abdominal cramping, nausea, vomiting.
- HEMA: bone marrow depression (dose-limiting), leukopenia, thrombocytopenia.
- Local: phlebitis, necrosis on extravasation.
- Other: acute bronchospasm, reversible alopecia, jaw pain, fever with continuous infusions.

Overdose and treatment
Clinical manifestations of overdose include ileus, mental depression, paresthesias, loss of deep tendon reflexes, stomatitis, nausea, vomiting, and myelosuppression. Treatment is generally supportive and includes transfusion of blood components, antiemetics, enemas for the ileus, and other appropriate symptomatic therapy.

▶ Special considerations
- To reconstitute, use 10 ml of normal saline injection to yield a concentration of 1 mg/ml.
- Drug may be administered by I.V. push injection over 1 minute into the tubing of a freely flowing I.V. infusion.
- Do not give as a continuous infusion unless patient has a central I.V. line.
- When reconstituted with the 10-ml diluent provided or normal saline solution, the drug is stable for 30 days under refrigeration.
- Dosage should be adjusted in patients with impaired hepatic function.
- After administering, monitor for life-threatening acute bronchospasm reaction. It is most likely to occur in a patient who is also receiving mitomycin.
- Monitor CBC.
- Because drug is a painful vesicant, give 10-ml normal saline solution flush before drug to test vein patency and 10-ml normal saline solution flush to remove any remaining drug from tubing after drug is given.
- Take special care to avoid extravasation. Treatment of extravasation includes liberal injection of hyaluronidase into the site, followed by warm compresses to minimize the spread of the reaction. Prepare hyaluronidase by adding 3 ml of normal saline injection to the 150-unit vial.
- Neuropathy may be assessed by recording patient signatures before each course of therapy and observing for deterioration of handwriting.
- Assess for depression of Achilles tendon reflex, foot drop or wristdrop, or slapping gait (late signs of neurotoxicity).
- To prevent paralytic ileus, encourage patient to force fluids, increase ambulation, and use stool softeners.
- Prevent uric acid nephropathy with generous oral fluid intake and administration of allopurinol.

Information for parents and patient
- Stress importance of keeping follow-up appointments for monitoring hematologic status.

• Teach parents and patient to check for signs of bleeding and bruising. Parents may need to restrict child's participation in contact sports. Such activity is dangerous when patient's platelets are low.
• Instruct parents to monitor neutropenic patient's temperature every 4 hours (not rectally) and to report fever, cough, and other signs of infection *promptly*.
• Patient should avoid contact with persons with bacterial or viral infections or who have received live-virus immunizations (polio, measles/mumps/rubella). Explain importance of promptly reporting susceptible patient's exposure to chicken pox.
• Instruct patient to clean teeth with toothettes, gauze, or soft toothbrush when platelets are low.
• Advise parents to encourage the patient to drink plenty of fluids to increase urine output and facilitate excretion of uric acid.
• Instruct parents and patient to report any signs of neurotoxicity: numbness and tingling of extremities, jaw pain, constipation (may be early sign of neurotoxicity).
• Reassure parents and patient that hair should grow back after treatment has ended.

---

vitamin A
Aquasol A

• Classification: nutritional supplement (fat-soluble vitamin)

How supplied
Available by prescription only
Tablets: 10,000 IU
Capsules: 25,000 IU, 50,000 IU
Injection: 2-ml vials (50,000 IU/ml with 0.5% chlorobutanol, polysorbate 80, butylated hydroxyanisol, and butylated hydroxytoluene)

Available without prescription, as appropriate
Drops: 30 ml with dropper (50,000 IU/0.1 ml)
Capsules: 10,000 IU

Indications, route, and dosage
Severe vitamin A deficiency with xerophthalmia
Children over age 8 and adults: 500,000 IU P.O. daily for 3 days, then 50,000 IU P.O. daily for 14 days, then maintenance dosage of 10,000 to 20,000 IU P.O. daily for 2 months, followed by adequate dietary nutrition and recommended daily allowance (RDA) of vitamin A.

Severe vitamin A deficiency
Infants under age 1: 7,500 to 15,000 IU I.M. daily for 10 days.
Children ages 1 to 8: 17,500 to 35,000 IU I.M. daily for 10 days.
Children over age 8 and adults: 100,000 IU P.O. or I.M. daily for 3 days, then 50,000 IU P.O. daily for 14 days, then maintenance dosage of 10,000 to 20,000 IU P.O. daily for 2 months, followed by adequate dietary nutrition and RDA vitamin A.

Maintenance only
Children under age 4: 10,000 IU I.M. daily for 2 months, then adequate dietary nutrition and RDA of vitamin A.
Children ages 4 to 8: 15,000 IU I.M. daily for 2 months, then adequate dietary nutrition and RDA of vitamin A.

Note: The RDA for vitamin A is as follows:

Infants		
birth to 6 months	420 RE	2,100 IU
ages 6 to 12 months	400 RE	2,000 IU
Children		
ages 1 to 3	400 RE	2,000 IU
ages 4 to 6	500 RE	2,500 IU
ages 7 to 10	700 RE	3,300 IU
ages 11 and over (males)	1,000 RE	5,000 IU
ages 11 and over (females)	800 RE	4,000 IU
RE = retinol equivalents		

Action and kinetics
• *Metabolic action:* One IU of vitamin A is equivalent to 0.3 mcg of retinol or 0.6 mcg of beta-carotene. Beta-carotene, or provitamin A, yields retinol after absorption from the intestinal tract.

Retinol's combination with opsin, the red pigment in the retina, helps form rhodopsin, which is necessary for visual adaptation to darkness. Vitamin A prevents growth retardation and preserves the integrity of the epithelial cells. Vitamin A deficiency is characterized by nyctalopia (night blindness), keratomalacia (necrosis of the cornea), keratinization and drying of the skin, low resistance to infection, growth retardation, bone thickening, diminished cortical steroid production, and fetal malformations.
• *Kinetics in adults:* In normal doses, vitamin A is absorbed readily and completely if fat absorption is normal. Larger doses, or regular doses in patients with fat malabsorption, low protein intake, or hepatic or pancreatic disease, may be absorbed incompletely. Because vitamin A is fat-soluble, absorption requires bile salts, pancreatic lipase, and dietary fat. Vitamin A is stored (primarily as palmitate) in Kupffer's cells of the liver. Normal adult liver stores are sufficient to provide vitamin A requirements for 2 years. Lesser amounts of retinyl palmitate are stored in the kidneys, lungs, adrenal glands, retinas, and intraperitoneal fat. Vitamin A circulates bound to a specific alpha$_1$ protein, retinol-binding protein (RBP). Blood level assays may not reflect liver storage of vitamin A because serum levels depend partly on circulating RBP. Liver storage should be adequate before discontinuing therapy. Vitamin A is distributed into breast milk. It does not readily cross the placenta. Vitamin A is metabolized in the liver. Retinol (fat-soluble) is conjugated with glucuronic acid and then further metabolized to retinal and retinoic acid. Retinoic acid is excreted in feces via biliary elimination. Retinal, retinoic acid, and other water-soluble metabolites are excreted in

---

‡May contain sulfites ◆May contain tartrazine ◆◆May contain benzyl alcohol

urine and feces. Normally, no unchanged retinol is excreted in urine, except in patients with pneumonia or chronic nephritis.

Contraindications and precautions

Vitamin A is contraindicated in patients with hypervitaminosis A and in those with sensitivity to vitamin A or other ingredients in commercially available preparations. Intravenous use is contraindicated because it may cause fatal anaphylaxis.

Vitamin A intake from fortified foods, dietary supplements, self-prescribed drugs, and prescription drug sources should be evaluated. Prolonged administration of dosages that exceed 25,000 IU/day requires close supervision.

The efficacy of large systemic doses of vitamin A in treating acne has not been established; this use should be avoided because of the potential for toxicity. Topical vitamin A acid (tretinoin) is useful in treating acne.

Interactions

Concomitant use of vitamin A with oral contraceptives significantly increases the vitamin's plasma levels. Prolonged use of mineral oil may interfere with the intestinal absorption of vitamin A. Concomitant use with cholestyramine may decrease the absorption of vitamin A by decreasing bile acids and preventing the micellar phase in the GI lumen. Daily vitamin A supplements have been recommended during long-term cholestyramine therapy. Use with neomycin may decrease vitamin A absorption. Large doses of vitamin A may interfere with the hypoprothrombinemic effect of warfarin. Because of the potential for additive adverse effects, patients receiving retinoids (such as etretinate or isotretinoin) should avoid concomitant use of vitamin A.

Effects on diagnostic tests

Vitamin A therapy may falsely increase serum cholesterol level readings by interfering with the Zlatkis-Zak reaction. Vitamin A has also been reported to falsely elevate bilirubin determinations.

Adverse reactions

Adverse reactions are usually seen only with toxicity (hypervitaminosis A).
• CNS: irritability, headache, increased intracranial pressure, fatigue, lethargy, malaise.
• DERM: alopecia; drying, cracking, scaling skin; pruritus; lip fissures; massive desquamation; increased pigmentation.
• EENT: miosis, papilledema, exophthalmos.
• GI: anorexia, epigastric pain, diarrhea, vomiting.
• GU: hypomenorrhea.
• HEMA: hypoplastic anemia, leukopenia.
• Hepatic: jaundice, hepatomegaly.
• Metabolic: hypercalcemia.
• Other: night sweating; skeletal — slow growth, decalcification of bone, fractures, hyperostosis, painful periostitis, premature closure of epiphyses, migratory arthralgia, cortical thickening over the radius and tibia, bulging fontanelles, splenomegaly. Fatal anaphylaxis has been reported after I.V. use.

Overdose and treatment

In acute toxicity, increased intracranial pressure develops within 8 to 12 hours; cutaneous desquamation follows in a few days. Toxicity can follow a single dose of 25,000 IU/kg, which in infants would represent about 75,000 IU and in adults over 2 million IU.

Chronic toxicity results from administration of 4,000 IU/kg for 6 to 15 months. In infants (age 3 to 6 months) this would represent about 18,500 IU/day for 1 to 3 months; in adults, 1 million IU/day for 3 days, 50,000 IU/day for more than 18 months, or 500,000 IU/day for 2 months.

To treat toxicity, discontinue vitamin A administration if hypercalcemia persists, and administer I.V. normal saline solution, prednisone, and calcitonin, if indicated. Perform liver function tests to detect possible liver damage.

▶ Special considerations

• Safety of amounts exceeding 6,000 IU/day during pregnancy is not known.
• In any dietary deficiency, suspect multiple vitamin deficiency.
• Give vitamin A concurrently with bile salts to patients with malabsorption caused by inadequate bile secretion.
• Vitamin A given by I.V. push is contraindicated because it can cause anaphylaxis and death.
• Use special water-miscible form of vitamin A when adding to large parenteral volumes.
• Excessive amounts, particularly in neonates, may be toxic.

Information for parents and patient

• Explain that patient must avoid prolonged use of mineral oil while taking this drug because mineral oil reduces vitamin A absorption in the intestine.
• Tell parents not to exceed recommended dosage.
• Tell parents to report promptly any symptoms of overdose (nausea, vomiting, anorexia, malaise, drying or cracking of skin or lips, irritability, headache, or loss of hair) and to discontinue the drug immediately when such symptoms occur.
• Patient should consume adequate protein, vitamin E, and zinc, which, along with bile, are necessary for vitamin A absorption.
• Tell parents to store vitamin A in a tight, light-resistant container.
• Advise parents to teach children that vitamins cannot be taken indiscriminately and that megadoses should be avoided.
• Liquid preparations may be mixed with fruit juice or cereal.

vitamin E (alpha tocopherol)
Aquasol E, CEN-E, E-Ferol, E-Ferol
Succinate, Eprolin Gelseals, Epsilan-
M, E-Vital, Pheryl-E 400, Tocopher-
Caps, Vita-Plus E, Viterra E

• Classification: nutritional supplement (vitamin)

How available
Available without prescription, as appropriate
Oral solution: 50 IU/ml
Capsules: 50 IU, 100 IU, 200 IU, 400 IU, 600 IU, 1,000 IU
Tablets: 100 IU, 200 IU, 400 IU, 500 IU, 600 IU, 1,000 IU
Tablets (chewable): 100 IU, 200 IU, 400 IU

Indications, route, and dosage
Vitamin E deficiency in premature infants and in patients with impaired fat absorption
Children: 1 mg equivalent/0.6 g of dietary unsaturated fat P.O. or I.M. daily.
Adults: Depending on severity, 60 to 75 IU P.O. or I.M. daily. Maximum dosage is 300 IU/day.
  Note: The usual recommended daily allowance (RDA) in infants up to age 1 year is 4 to 6 IU; in children age 1 to 10, 7 to 10 IU.

Action and kinetics
• *Nutritional action:* As a dietary supplement, the exact biochemical mechanism is unclear, although it is believed to act as an antioxidant. Vitamin E protects cell membranes, vitamin A, vitamin C (ascorbic acid), and polyunsaturated fatty acids from oxidation. It also may act as a cofactor in enzyme systems, and some evidence exists that it decreases platelet aggregation.
• *Kinetics in adults:* GI absorption depends on the presence of bile. Only 20% to 60% of the vitamin obtained from dietary sources is absorbed. As dosage increases, the fraction of vitamin E absorbed decreases. Vitamin E is distributed to all tissues and is stored in adipose tissue. It is metabolized in the liver by glucuronidation and excreted primarily in bile. Some enterohepatic circulation may occur. Small amounts of the metabolites are excreted in urine.

Contraindications and precautions
Vitamin E is usually nontoxic. A complex and potentially fatal syndrome has occurred in several premature infants who received I.V. therapy with vitamin E; however, this form of the drug is no longer available.

Interactions
Concomitant use of vitamin E with mineral oil, colestipol, cholestyramine, or sucralfate may increase vitamin E requirements.
  Vitamin E may have anti-vitamin K effects; patients receiving oral anticoagulants may be at risk for hemorrhage after large doses of vitamin E.

Effects on diagnostic tests
None reported.

Adverse reactions
None reported.

Overdose and treatment
Clinical manifestations of overdose include a possible increase in blood pressure. Treatment is generally supportive.

▶ Special considerations
• Give concurrently with bile salts if patient has malabsorption caused by lack of bile.
• Investigational uses of vitamin E include prevention of retrolental fibroplasia and bronchopulmonary dysplasia in neonates.
• Vitamin E may be labeled in milligrams of vitamin E activity. The conversion is 1 unit equals 1.0 mg of alpha-tocopherol acetate or 0.6 mg of alpha-tocopherol.
• Premature infants may experience anemia secondary to deficient vitamin E.

Information for parents and patient
• Inform parents and patient about dietary sources of vitamin E, such as vegetable oil, green leafy vegetables, nuts, wheat germ, eggs, meat, liver, dairy products, and cereals.
• Tell parents to store vitamin E in a tight, light-resistant container.
• Liquid vitamins may be mixed with food or juice.
• Advise the parents not to refer to vitamins or other drugs as candy and to teach children that vitamins and other drugs cannot be taken indiscriminately.

---

vitamin K derivatives

menadiol sodium diphosphate
Synkayvite

phytonadione
AquaMEPHYTON, Konakion, Mephyton

• Classification: blood coagulation modifier (vitamin K)

How supplied
All products available by prescription only
Menadiol sodium diphosphate
Tablets: 5 mg
Injection: 5 mg/ml, 10 mg/ml, 37.5 mg/ml
Phytonadione
Tablets: 5 mg
Injection (aqueous colloidal solution): 2 mg/ml, 10 mg/ml
Injection (aqueous dispersion): 2 mg/ml, 10 mg/ml

---

‡May contain sulfites   ◆May contain tartrazine   ◆◆May contain benzyl alcohol

Indications, route, and dosage

Hypoprothrombinemia secondary to vitamin K malabsorption or drug therapy, or when oral administration is desired and bile secretion is inadequate

Adults: 5 to 10 mg menadiol sodium diphosphate or phytonadione P.O. daily or 5 to 15 mg menadiol sodium diphosphate I.M. once or twice daily, or titrated to patient's requirements.

Hypoprothrombinemia secondary to vitamin K malabsorption, drug therapy, or excess vitamin A

Infants: 2 mg P.O. or parenterally. I.V. injection rate for children and infants should not exceed 3 mg/m²/minute or a total of 5 mg.

Children: 5 to 10 mg P.O. or parenterally.

Adults: 2 to 25 mg phytonadione P.O. or parenterally, repeated and increased up to 50 mg, if necessary.

Hypoprothrombinemia secondary to effect of oral anticoagulants

Adults: 2.5 to 10 mg phytonadione P.O., S.C., or I.M., based on prothrombin time, repeated, if necessary, 12 to 48 hours after oral dose or 6 to 8 hours after parenteral dose. In emergency, give 10 to 50 mg slow I.V., rate not to exceed 1 mg/minute, repeated every 6 to 8 hours, as needed.

Prevention of hemorrhagic disease in neonates

Neonates: 0.5 to 1 mg phytonadione S.C. or I.M. immediately after birth, repeated in 6 to 8 hours, if needed, especially if mother received oral anticoagulants or long-term anticonvulsant therapy during pregnancy.

Differentiation between hepatocellular disease or biliary obstruction as source of hypoprothrombinemia

Children and adults: 10 mg phytonadione I.M. or S.C.

Prevention of hypoprothrombinemia related to vitamin K deficiency in long-term parenteral nutrition

Children: 2 to 5 mg S.C. or I.M. weekly.

Adults: 5 to 10 mg phytonadione S.C. or I.M. weekly.

Prevention of hypoprothrombinemia in infants receiving less than 0.1 mg/liter vitamin K in breast milk or milk substitutes

Infants: 1 mg phytonadione S.C. or I.M. monthly.

Action and kinetics

• *Coagulation modifying action:* Vitamin K is a lipid-soluble vitamin that promotes hepatic formation of active prothrombin and several other coagulation factors.

Phytonadione (vitamin K_1) is a synthetic form of vitamin K, and is also lipid-soluble; menadiol sodium diphosphate (vitamin K_4) is a water-soluble derivative converted in the body to menadione (vitamin K_3), which has activity similar to naturally occurring vitamin K.

Vitamin K does not counteract the action of heparin.

• *Kinetics in adults:* Phytonadione requires the presence of bile salts for GI tract absorption; menadiol sodium diphosphate can be absorbed in the absence of bile salts. Once absorbed, vitamin K enters the blood directly. Onset of action after I.V. injection is more rapid, but of shorter duration, than that occurring after S.C. or I.M. injection.

Vitamin K concentrates in the liver. Action of parenteral phytonadione begins in 1 to 2 hours; hemorrhage is usually controlled within 3 to 6 hours, and normal prothrombin levels are achieved in 12 to 14 hours. Oral phytonadione begins to act within 6 to 10 hours; parenteral menadiol sodium diphosphate begins to act in 8 to 24 hours. Vitamin K is metabolized rapidly by the liver; little tissue accumulation occurs. Data are limited. High concentrations occur in feces; however, intestinal bacteria can synthesize vitamin K.

Contraindications and precautions

Vitamin K is contraindicated in patients hypersensitive to any of its analogues; and during the last few weeks of pregnancy or labor, because menadiol sodium diphosphate has caused toxic reactions in neonates. Menadiol sodium diphosphate is contraindicated in infants.

Administer vitamin K cautiously to patients with impaired hepatic function, because large doses may further decrease hepatic function. Menadiol sodium diphosphate may induce erythrocyte hemolysis in patients with glucose-6-phosphate dehydrogenase deficiency.

Interactions

Broad-spectrum antibiotics (especially cefoperazone, moxalactam, cefamandole, and cefotetan) may interfere with the actions of vitamin K, producing hypoprothrombinemia.

Mineral oil inhibits absorption of oral vitamin K; give drugs at well-spaced intervals, and monitor result.

Vitamin K antagonizes the effects of oral anticoagulants; patients receiving these agents should take vitamin K *only* for severe hypoprothrombinemia.

Effects on diagnostic tests

Phytonadione can falsely elevate urine steroid levels.

Adverse reactions

• CNS: headache, dizziness, *convulsive movements.*
• CV: transient hypotension after I.V. administration, rapid weak pulse, cardiac dysrhythmias.
• DERM: allergic rash, pruritus, urticaria, eruptions on repeated injections, sweating, flushing, erythema.
• GI: nausea, vomiting.
• Local: pain, swelling, hematoma at injection site.
• Other: bronchospasm, dyspnea, cramplike pain, anaphylaxis and anaphylactoid reactions (usually after rapid I.V. administration).
• Neonates: hyperbilirubinemia, *fatal kernicterus, severe hemolytic anemia.*

Note: Drug should be discontinued if allergic or severe CNS reactions appear.

Overdose and treatment

Excessive doses of vitamin K may cause hepatic dysfunction in adults; in neonates and premature infants, large doses may cause hemolytic anemia, kernicterus, and death. Treatment is supportive.

▶ Special considerations
• In prophylaxis and treatment of hemorrhagic disease of the newborn, phytonadione has a greater margin of safety than menadiol sodium diphosphate.
• Check product information for approved routes of administration.
• Administration of menadiol sodium diphosphate I.V. push should not exceed rate of 1 mg/minute.
• If severity of condition warrants I.V. infusion, mix with normal saline, dextrose 5% in water, or dextrose 5% in normal saline solution. Monitor for flushing, weakness, tachycardia, and hypotension; shock may follow.
• Monitor prothrombin time to determine effectiveness.
• Monitor patient response, and watch for adverse effects; failure to respond to vitamin K may indicate coagulation defects or irreversible hepatic damage.
• Excessive use of vitamin K may temporarily defeat oral anticoagulant therapy; higher doses of oral anticoagulant or interim use of heparin may be required.
• Phytonadione for hemorrhagic disease in infants causes fewer adverse reactions than do other vitamin K analogues; phytonadione is the vitamin K analogue of choice to treat an oral anticoagulant overdose.
• Patients receiving phytonadione who have bile deficiency require concomitant use of bile salts to ensure adequate absorption.

Information for parents and patient
• For patients receiving oral form, explain rationale for drug therapy; stress importance of complying with medical regimen and keeping follow-up appointments. Tell patient to take a missed dose as soon as possible, but not if it is almost time for next dose, and to report missed doses.
• Warn parents that patient should avoid taking nonprescription products containing aspirin, other salicylates, or drugs that may interact with the anticoagulant, causing an increase or decrease in the drug's action, and to seek medical approval before stopping or starting any other medication.
• Advise parents that patient should not substantially alter daily intake of leafy green vegetables (asparagus, broccoli, cabbage, lettuce, turnip greens, spinach, or watercress) or of fish, pork or beef liver, green tea, or tomatoes; these foods contain vitamin K, and widely varying daily intake may alter anticoagulant effect.
• Parents should inform every new physician and dentist that patient is taking this drug.

---

warfarin sodium
Coumadin, Panwarfin, Sofarin

• Classification: anticoagulant (coumadin derivative)

How supplied
Available by prescription only
Tablets: 2 mg, 2.5 mg, 5 mg, 7.5 mg, 10 mg
Injection: 50 mg/vial

Indications, route, and dosage
Venous thrombosis; pulmonary embolism; embolism associated with mitral valve disease and atrial fibrillation
Children and adults: 10 to 15 mg for 2 to 5 days until desired prothrombin time (PT) is reached. Maintenance dose is based on PT but is usually 2 to 10 mg P.O. daily.

Action and kinetics
• *Anticoagulant action:* Warfarin inhibits vitamin K-dependent activation of clotting factors II, VII, IX, and X, which are formed in the liver; it has no direct effect on established thrombi and cannot reverse ischemic tissue damage. However, warfarin may prevent additional clot formation, extension of formed clots, and secondary complications of thrombosis.
• *Kinetics in adults:* Warfarin is rapidly and completely absorbed from the GI tract. Drug is highly bound to plasma protein, especially albumin; it crosses placenta but does not appear to accumulate in breast milk. Warfarin is hydroxylated by liver into inactive metabolites. Metabolites are reabsorbed from bile and excreted in urine. Half-life of parent drug is 1 to 3 days. Because therapeutic effect is relatively more dependent on clotting factor depletion (factor X has half-life of 40 hours), PT will not peak for 1½ to 3 days despite use of a loading dose. Duration of action is 2 to 5 days—more closely reflecting drug's half-life.

Contraindications and precautions
Warfarin is contraindicated in patients with bleeding or hemorrhagic tendencies caused by open wounds, visceral cancer, GI ulcers, severe hepatic or renal disease, severe or uncontrolled hypertension (diastolic pressure over 110 mm Hg), subacute bacterial endocarditis, or vitamin K deficiency; or after recent brain, eye, or spinal cord surgery, because excessive bleeding can occur.
    Administer warfarin cautiously to patients with diverticulitis, colitis, mild to moderate hypertension, or mild to moderate hepatic or renal disease; during lactation; to patients with any drainage tubes; in conjunction with regional or lumbar block anesthesia; or to patients with any condition that increases risk of hemorrhage.

Interactions
Oral anticoagulants interact with many drugs; thus, any change in drug regimen, including use of nonprescription compounds, requires careful monitoring. The most significant interactions follow.
    Concomitant use with amiodarone, anabolic steroids, chloramphenicol, metronidazole, cimetidine, clofibrate, dextrothyroxine and other thyroid preparations, salicylates, streptokinase, urokinase, disulfiram, or sulfonamides markedly increases warfarin's anticoagulant effect; *avoid concomitant use.*
    Concomitant use with ethacrynic acid, indomethacin, mefenamic acid, phenylbutazone, or sulfinpyrazone increases warfarin's anticoagulant effect and causes severe GI irritation (may be ulcerogenic); *avoid concomitant use when possible.*
    Concomitant use with allopurinol, moxalactam, ce-

---

foperazone, cefamandole, cefotetan, danazol, diflunisal, erythromycin, glucagon, heparin, miconazole, quinidine, sulindac, or vitamin E increases warfarin's anticoagulant effects. Monitor carefully.

Concomitant use with glutethimide or rifampin causes decreased anticoagulant effect of major significance and should be avoided. Barbiturates may inhibit anticoagulant effect for several weeks after barbiturate withdrawal, and fatal hemorrhage can occur after cessation of barbiturate effect; if barbiturates are withdrawn, reduce anticoagulant dose.

Concomitant use with carbamazepine, oral contraceptives, corticosteroids, ethchlorvynol, griseofulvin, and vitamin K may cause decreased anticoagulant effect; monitor carefully. Cholestyramine decreases warfarin's anticoagulant effect when used close together; administer 6 hours after warfarin.

Concomitant use with chloral hydrate may increase or decrease warfarin's anticoagulant effect; monitor therapy carefully and avoid when possible. Acute alcohol intoxication increases warfarin's anticoagulant effect; chronic alcohol abuse decreases anticoagulant effect but may predispose to bleeding problems.

Effects on diagnostic tests

Warfarin prolongs both PT and partial thromboplastin time; it may enhance uric acid excretion, elevate serum transaminase levels, increase lactic dehydrogenase activity, and cause false-negative serum theophylline levels.

Adverse reactions

• DERM: dermatitis, urticaria, rash, necrosis, petechiae, *alopecia*, ecchymoses.
• GI: paralytic ileus and intestinal obstruction (caused by hemorrhage), diarrhea, vomiting, cramps, nausea, melena, hematemesis.
• GU: excessive uterine bleeding.
• HEMA: hemorrhage with high dosage, leukopenia.
• Other: fever, hemoptysis, burning sensation of feet.
   Note: Drug should be discontinued if patient shows any sign of bleeding or allergic tendencies, or shows signs of necrosis of the skin or other tissues.

Overdose and treatment

Clinical manifestations of overdose vary with severity and may include internal or external bleeding or skin necrosis of fat-rich areas, but most common sign is hematuria. Excessive prolongation of PT or minor bleeding mandates withdrawal of therapy; withholding one or two doses may be adequate in some cases. Treatment to control bleeding may include oral or I.V. phytonadione (vitamin K_1) and, in severe hemorrhage, fresh frozen plasma or whole blood. Use of phytonadione may interfere with subsequent oral anticoagulant therapy.

▶ Special considerations

• Infants, especially neonates, may be more susceptible to anticoagulants because of vitamin K deficiency.
• Obtain PT before initiation of drug and daily during initial therapy for dosage adjustment; follow hospital policy for anticoagulant administration.
• Dosage is determined by PT; therapy usually aims to maintain PT at 1.5 to 2 times normal. Numerical PT values depend on procedure and reagents used in the individual laboratory.
• During maintenance, check PT as often as twice a week or as infrequently as every 6 weeks, depending on PT and patient's reliability and clinical status.
• Because of delayed onset of action, heparin is commonly given during the first few days of treatment. Do not check PT within 5 hours of intermittent heparin use; however, PT may be checked at any time during continuous heparinization.
• Use caution when adding or stopping any drug in patients taking anticoagulants; some drugs alter clotting time, and the combination may cause either hemorrhage or rethrombosis.
• Avoid I.M. injections during therapy, because they will cause hematomas.
• Be prepared for emergency blood replacement.
• Check patient regularly for bleeding gums, bruises on arms or legs, petechiae, nosebleeds, hemoptysis, melena, hematuria, or hematemesis, which indicate increased bleeding; for sudden lumbar pain, which may signal retroperitoneal hemorrhage; and for fever and rash, which may signal other severe complications.

Information for parents and patient

• Explain disease process and rationale for drug therapy; stress importance of complying with recommended amount and timing of dosage, and of keeping follow-up appointments.
• Stress importance of taking a missed dose as soon as possible. If the missed dose is not remembered until the next day, the patient should not take it; doubling the dose can cause bleeding. Tell parents to report any missed doses.
• Patient should carry a card that identifies him as a potential bleeder and should inform any other physicians or dentists who may be treating him.
• Tell parents and patient to watch for bruising and other signs of increased bleeding and to call immediately if these or other complications occur; heavier-than-usual menses may require dosage adjustment.
• Patient should avoid nonprescription products containing aspirin, other salicylates, or other drugs that may change anticoagulant action unless they have been approved by the patient's physician.
• Explain that PT is increased by fever, long periods of hot weather, malnutrition, and diarrhea.
• Tell parents and patient that drug may turn alkaline urine red-orange.
• Patient should not substantially alter daily intake of leafy green vegetables (asparagus, broccoli, cabbage, lettuce, turnip greens, spinach, watercress) or of fish, pork or beef liver, green tea, or tomatoes; these foods contain vitamin K and widely varying daily intake may alter anticoagulant effect.
• Explain that smoking may increase dosage requirement because of changes in metabolism; light to moderate alcohol intake does not significantly alter PT.
• Patient should take special precautions against cuts and bruises; for example, patient should use a soft toothbrush to prevent gum irritation.

---

zidovudine (AZT)
Retrovir

• Classification: antiviral (thymidine analogue)

How supplied
Available by prescription only through special distribution program
Capsules: 100 mg

Indications, route, and dosage
Symptomatic human immunodeficiency virus (HIV), acquired immunodeficiency syndrome (AIDS), or advanced AIDS-related complex (ARC)
†*Children:* Optimal dosage schedule has not been established. Some trials have used 100 to 120 mg/m² P.O. q 6 hours.
Adults: 200 mg P.O. q 4 hours.

Action and kinetics
• *Antiviral action:* Zidovudine is converted intracellularly to an active triphosphate compound that inhibits reverse transcriptase (an enzyme essential for retroviral DNA synthesis), thereby inhibiting viral replication. When used in vitro, the drug inhibits certain other viruses and bacteria; however, this has undetermined clinical significance.
• *Kinetics in adults:* Zidovudine is absorbed rapidly from the GI tract. Average systemic bioavailability is 65% of dose (drug undergoes first-pass metabolism). Preliminary data reveal good CSF penetration. Approximately 36% of zidovudine dose is plasma protein-bound. Zidovudine is metabolized rapidly to an inactive compound. Parent drug and metabolite are excreted by glomerular filtration and tubular secretion in the kidneys. Urine recovery of parent drug and metabolite is 14% and 74%, respectively. Elimination half-lives of these compounds equal 1 hour.
• *Kinetics in chldren:* Pharmacokinetics is similar to that in adults.

Contraindications and precautions
Zidovudine should be administered with extreme caution to patients with compromised bone marrow function. Significant anemia may occur after 2 to 6 weeks of therapy, possibly necessitating dosage adjustment, drug discontinuation, or transfusions.

Interactions
When used concomitantly with drugs that are nephrotoxic or that affect bone marrow function or formation of bone marrow elements (such as dapsone, pentamidine, amphotericin B, flucytosine, vincristine, vinblastine, doxorubicin, and interferon), zidovudine may increase the risk of drug toxicity. Concomitant use with probenecid may impair elimination of zidovudine. Concomitant use with acetaminophen may increase the risk of granulocytopenia.

Effects on diagnostic tests
Zidovudine may cause depression of formed elements (erythrocytes, leukocytes, and platelets) in peripheral blood.

Adverse reactions
• CNS: headache, malaise, dizziness, paresthesia.
• GI: nausea, vomiting, anorexia.
• HEMA: anemia, granulocytopenia, thrombocytopenia.
• Other: myalgia.
Note: Temporarily discontinue zidovudine if marked anemia (hemoglobin level below 7.5 mg/dl or reduction by more than 25% of baseline value) or granulocytopenia (granulocyte count less than 750/mm³ or reduction by more than 50% of baseline value) occurs.

Overdose and treatment
No information available.

▶ Special considerations
• The optimum duration of treatment, as well as the dosage for optimum effectiveness and minimum toxicity, is not yet known.
• Monitor complete blood count and platelet count at least every 2 weeks. Dosage may be discontinued or reduced if hematologic toxicity occurs.
• Observe patient for signs and symptoms of opportunistic infection (including pneumonia, meningitis, and sepsis).

Information for parents and patient
• Teach parents and patient about disease, ways to prevent disease transmission, rationale for drug therapy, and drug's limitations.
• Explain that drug does not cure HIV infection or AIDS but may reduce morbidity resulting from opportunistic infections and thus prolong the patient's life.
• Teach parents or patient about proper drug administration. When the drug must be taken every 4 hours around the clock, explain the importance of maintaining an adequate blood level and suggest ways to avoid missing doses, such as the use of alarm clocks.
• Because zidovudine frequently causes a low red blood cell count, advise parents that patient may need blood transfusions during treatment.
• Inform patient about the importance of follow-up medical visits to evaluate for adverse effects and to monitor clinical status.
• Instruct parents and patient how to recognize adverse drug effects and to report these immediately.
• Warn parents that patient should not to take any other drugs for AIDS (especially from the "street") without medical approval.

---

*Canada only   †Unlabeled clinical use   Italicized adverse reactions have been observed in children.

DRUGS AVAILABLE WITHOUT PRESCRIPTION

DRUG	INDICATION AND DOSAGE	SPECIAL CONSIDERATIONS

Cough and cold drugs

dextromethorphan hydrobromide
Nonnarcotic antitussive

Nonproductive cough
Children age 2 to 5: 2.5 to 5 mg P.O. q 4 hours, or 7.5 mg q 6 to 8 hours; or 15 mg of sustained-action liquid b.i.d. Maximum dosage is 30 mg daily.
Children age 6 to 11: 5 to 10 mg P.O. q 4 hours, or 15 mg q 6 to 8 hours; or 30 mg of controlled-release liquid b.i.d. Maximum dosage is 60 mg daily.
Children age 12 and older and adults: 10 to 20 mg P.O. q 4 hours, or 30 mg q 6 to 8 hours. Or 60 mg of controlled-release liquid b.i.d. Maximum dosage is 120 mg daily.

● Syrup, tablets, and lozenges are not recommended for children under age 2. Sustained-action liquid may be used in children under age 2, but dosage must be individualized.
● Dextromethorphan is contraindicated in patients with known hypersensitivity to this drug, and in patients who have taken MAO inhibitors within the preceding 2 weeks.
● Dextromethorphan should be used with caution in patients with asthma and other respiratory conditions in which thick secretions are present, because this drug may impair mobilization of secretions.
● May cause drowsiness, dizziness, or nausea.
● Treatment is intended to relieve intensity and frequency of coughing without abolishing the protective cough reflex.
● Tell parents to call if cough persists more than 7 days.

guaifenesin
Expectorant

Excessive bronchial secretions
Children under age 2: Individualize dosage. For self-medication, the recommended dosage is half the usual dosage.
Children age 2 to 5: 50 to 100 mg P.O. q 4 hours; maximum dosage is 600 mg daily.
Children age 6 to 11: 100 to 200 mg P.O. q 4 hours; maximum dosage is 1.2 g daily.
Children age 12 and older and adults: 200 to 400 mg P.O. q 4 hours; maximum dosage is 2.4 g daily.

● Individualize dosage for children under age 2.
● May cause drowsiness. Excessive doses may cause nausea and vomiting.
● Taking drug with water helps liquefy secretions
● Instruct patients to call if cough persists for more than 1 week, if cough recurs, or if cough is accompanied by fever, skin rash, or persistent headache.

terpin hydrate
Expectorant

Excessive bronchial secretions
Children age 1 to 4: 1.25 ml of elixir P.O. t.i.d. to q.i.d.
Children age 5 to 9: 2.5 ml of elixir P.O. t.i.d. to q.i.d.
Children age 10 to 12: 5 ml of elixir P.O. b.i.d.
Children over age 12 and adults: 5 to 10 ml of elixir P.O. q 4 to 6 hours. Not to exceed 8 teaspoons daily.

● Drug contains 43% alcohol. It is contraindicated in patients with peptic ulcer. It is not recommended in children under age 12 because of its high alcohol content. It should be used with caution in patients taking other CNS depressants and during pregnancy; alcohol crosses the placental barrier and may cause congenital anomalies.
● May cause sedation, nausea, and vomiting.
● Taking drug with 8 oz (240 ml) of water helps liquefy secretions.
● Taking drug with food prevents epigastric distress.

Miscellaneous GI drugs

bisacodyl, bisacodyl tannex
Laxative (stimulant)

Constipation; surgery or bowel examination
Children up to age 3: ½ of suppository (5 mg).
Children over age 3: 5 mg P.O., or one suppository (10 mg); alternatively, may give half the contents of microenema.

● Do not give bisacodyl tannex to children under age 12.
● Bisacodyl is contraindicated in patients with fluid and electrolyte disturbances, appendicitis, any abdominal condition necessitating immediate surgery, ulcerative colitis, rectal fissures, ulcerated hemor-

DRUGS AVAILABLE WITHOUT PRESCRIPTION (continued)

DRUG	INDICATION AND DOSAGE	SPECIAL CONSIDERATIONS
Miscellaneous GI drugs (continued)		
bisacodyl, bisacodyl tannex Laxative (stimulant) (continued)	*Adults:* 10 to 15 mg P.O. in evening or before breakfast. Up to 30 mg may be used for thorough evacuation needed for examinations or surgery. Alternatively, give one suppository (10 mg), p.r.n., or contents of one retention enema.	rhoids, fecal impaction, and intestinal obstruction, because the drug may exacerbate these conditions. ● Bisacodyl tannex should not be used if multiple enemas are to be administered, because significant absorption of tannic acid may result in hepatotoxicity. ● May cause nausea, vomiting, abdominal cramps, diarrhea (with high doses); rectal burning (with suppositories). ● Drug should be discontinued if severe abdominal pain or laxative dependence occurs. ● Advise parents that patient should not take drug within 1 hour of antacids or milk.
bismuth subgallate, bismuth subsalicylate Antidiarrheal	**Mild nonspecific diarrhea** *Children age 3 to 6:* ⅓ of tablet or 5 ml of suspension P.O. *Children age 6 to 9:* ⅔ of tablet or 10 ml of suspension P.O. *Children age 9 to 12:* 1 tablet or 15 ml of suspension P.O. May repeat q ½ to 1 hour p.r.n.; not to exceed eight doses in 24 hours. *Adults:* 1 to 2 tablets chewed or swallowed whole t.i.d. (subgallate), or 30 ml of suspension or 2 tablets q ½ to 1 hour up to a maximum of eight doses and for no longer than 2 days (subsalicylate).	● May increase risk of aspirin toxicity if taken concurrently. ● May cause temporary tongue and stool darkening and fecal impaction in infants and debilitated patients. ● If patient is also receiving tetracycline, administer bismuth at least 1 hour apart; to avoid decreased drug absorption, dosages or schedules of other medications may require adjustment. ● Shake suspension well before using to ensure correct dosage. ● Tell parents to report persistent diarrhea.
calcium carbonate Antacid	**Excessive gastric acidity** *Children:* 5 to 15 ml P.O. q 3 to 6 hours or 1 to 3 hours after meals and h.s. **To prevent GI bleeding in critical illness** *Infants:* 2 to 5 ml P.O. q 1 to 2 hours. *Children:* 5 to 15 ml P.O. q 1 to 2 hours. *Adults:* 1 or 2 tablets, four to six times daily, chewed well and taken with water; or 1 g of suspension (5 ml of most products) 1 hour after meals and h.s.	● Administer ½ to 1 hour after meals and h.s. ● Do not administer with milk or other foods high in vitamin D. Can cause milk-alkali syndrome (headache, confusion, distaste for food, nausea, vomiting, hypercalcemia, hypercalciuria, calcinosis, hypophosphatemia). ● May cause enteric-coated tablets to be released prematurely in stomach. Calcium carbonate and any enteric-coated tablet should be taken 1 hour apart. ● Monitor bowel function. Manage constipation with laxatives or stool softeners. ● Monitor serum and urine calcium levels, especially in mild renal impairment and with long-term use. Observe patient for symptoms of hypercalcemia (nausea, vomiting, headache, mental confusion, anorexia).
calcium polycarbophil Laxative and antidiarrheal	**Constipation** *Children age 3 to 6:* 500 mg P.O. b.i.d. as required. Maximum dosage is 1.5 g in 24-hour period. *Children age 6 to 12:* 500 mg P.O. t.i.d. as required. Maximum dosage is 3 g in 24-hour period.	● Patient must chew tablets before swallowing; administer tablets with 8 oz (240 ml) of fluid. Administer less fluid for antidiarrheal effect. ● Do not give drug as an antidiarrheal if patient has high fever. ● Warn parents not to give pa-

(continued)

DRUGS AVAILABLE WITHOUT PRESCRIPTION (continued)

DRUG	INDICATION AND DOSAGE	SPECIAL CONSIDERATIONS

Miscellaneous GI drugs (continued)

DRUG	INDICATION AND DOSAGE	SPECIAL CONSIDERATIONS
calcium poly-carbophil Laxative and antidiarrheal (continued)	*Adults:* 1 g P.O. q.i.d. as required. Maximum dosage is 6 g in 24-hour period. **Acute nonspecific diarrhea associated with irritable bowel syndrome** *Children age 3 to 6:* 500 mg P.O. b.i.d. as required. Maximum dosage is 1.5 g in 24-hour period. *Children age 6 to 12:* 500 mg P.O. t.i.d. as required. Maximum dosage is 3 g in 24-hour period. *Adults:* 1 g P.O. q.i.d. as required. Maximum dosage is 6 g in 24-hour period. For severe diarrhea, may repeat dose q ½ hour; do not exceed maximum daily dosage.	tient more than 12 tablets in 24-hour period (6 tablets for child age 6 to 12; 3 tablets for child age 3 to 6) and to give for length of time prescribed. • If patient is taking drug as laxative, advise parents to call promptly and discontinue drug if constipation persists after 1 week or if fever, nausea, vomiting, or abdominal pain occurs. • Tell parents that patient may take smaller, more frequent doses at regular intervals throughout the day to ease abdominal discomfort or fullness.
cascara sagrada Laxative (stimulant)	**Acute constipation; bowel examination** *Children under age 2:* One-quarter of adult dose. *Children age 2 to 12:* One-half of adult dose. *Adults:* 1 tablet P.O. h.s., 1 ml of fluid extract daily, or 5 ml of aromatic fluid extract daily.	• Not a drug of choice for children. • Cascara is contraindicated in patients with fluid and electrolyte disturbances; appendicitis; nausea, vomiting, or abdominal pain; any abdominal condition necessitating immediate surgery; fecal impaction; rectal bleeding; or intestinal obstruction, because the drug may exacerbate these conditons. • May cause abdominal cramps. • Drug should be discontinued if abdominal pain occurs. • Fluid extract preparation is five times as potent as aromatic fluid extract. • Aromatic fluid extract tastes better than fluid extract. • Drug may color urine reddish pink or brown, depending on urine pH.
castor oil Laxative (stimulant)	**Bowel examination or surgery; acute constipation** *Infants:* Up to 4 ml P.O. Increased dose produces no greater effect. *Children under age 2:* 1.25 to 7.5 ml P.O. *Children age 2 and older:* 5 to 15 ml P.O. *Adults:* 15 to 60 ml of liquid P.O. or 2 to 4 capsules P.O.	• Not recommended for routine use in constipation. Castor oil is contraindicated in patients with fluid or electrolyte disturbances, because it may worsen the imbalance; in patients with appendicitis, acute surgical abdomen, fecal impaction, intestinal obstruction, or intestinal perforation, because excessive intestinal stimulation may exacerbate symptoms of these disorders; and in patients with hypersensitivity to castor beans. • Discontinue drug if abdominal pain occurs. • Do not administer drug h.s. because of rapid onset of action. • Drug is most effective when taken on an empty stomach; shake well. • Observe patient for signs and symptoms of dehydration. • Flavored preparations are available. Suggest that parents chill drug or give it with juice or carbonated beverage for improved palatability. • Reassure parents and patient that after response to drug, patient may not need to move bowels again for 1 or 2 days.

DRUGS AVAILABLE WITHOUT PRESCRIPTION (continued)

DRUG	INDICATION AND DOSAGE	SPECIAL CONSIDERATIONS

Miscellaneous GI drugs (continued)

cyclizine hydro-chloride
Antiemetic and anti-vertigo agent

Motion sickness (prophylaxis and treatment)
Children age 6 to 12: 25 mg P.O. q 4 to 6 hours p.r.n. to a maximum of 75 mg daily.
Adults: 50 mg P.O. ½ hour before travel, then q 4 to 6 hours p.r.n. to maximum of 200 mg daily.

● Cyclizine is contraindicated in children with known hypersensitivity to drug or other antiemetic antihistamines with a similar chemical structure, such as buclizine, meclizine, or dimenhydrinate.
● Cylizine should be used with caution in patients with narrow-angle glaucoma, asthma, or GI or GU obstruction, because of its anticholinergic effects. Drug may mask signs of intestinal obstruction or brain tumor. Drug is not indicated for use in children under age 6; they may experience paradoxical hyperexcitability.
● Instruct patients who are taking drug for motion sickness to position themselves in places of minimal motion, to avoid excessive intake of food or drink, and to avoid reading while in motion.
● Advise patients to take drug with meals or snack to prevent gastric upset and to use any of the following measures to relieve dry mouth: warm water rinses, artificial saliva, ice chips, or sugarless gum or candy. Patient should avoid overusing mouthwash, which may add to dryness (alcohol content) and destroy normal flora.
● Warn parents that child should avoid hazardous activities that require balance or alertness until extent of CNS effects are known. Tell them to seek medical approval before administering tranquilizers, sedatives, pain relievers, or sleeping medications.

docusate calcium, docusate potassium, docusate sodium
Laxative (emollient)

Constipation
Docusate sodium
Children under age 3: 10 to 40 mg P.O. daily.
Children age 3 to 6: 20 to 60 mg P.O. daily.
Children age 6 to 12: 40 to 120 mg P.O. daily.
Children age 12 and over and adults: 50 to 300 mg P.O. daily until bowel movements are normal. Alternatively, add 50 to 100 mg to saline or oil retention enema to treat fecal impaction.
Docusate calcium or docusate potassium
Older children and adults: 240 mg P.O. daily until bowel movements are normal.
  Higher doses are for initial therapy. Adjust dose to individual response. Usual dosage in children and adults with minimal needs is 50 to 150 mg (docusate calcium) P.O. daily.

● Docusate salts are contraindicated in patients receiving mineral oil because they may increase absorption to dangerous levels.
● May cause throat irritation, bitter taste, mild abdominal cramping, and diarrhea.
● Discontinue if severe abdominal cramping occurs.
● Liquid (but not syrup) may be diluted in juice or other flavored liquid to improve taste.
● Avoid using docusate sodium in sodium-restricted patients.
● Docusate salts are available in combination with casanthranol (Peri-Colace), danthron (Dorbantyl), senna (Senokot, Gentlax), and phenolphthalein (Ex-Lax, Feen-a-Mint, Correctol).
● Docusate salts are less likely than other laxatives to cause laxative dependence; however, their effectiveness may decrease with long-term use.

(continued)

DRUGS AVAILABLE WITHOUT PRESCRIPTION (continued)

DRUG	INDICATION AND DOSAGE	SPECIAL CONSIDERATIONS

Miscellaneous GI drugs (continued)

DRUG	INDICATION AND DOSAGE	SPECIAL CONSIDERATIONS
glycerin Laxative (osmotic)	**Constipation** *Children under age 6:* 1 to 1.5 g as a suppository or 2 to 5 ml as an enema. *Children age 6 and older and adults:* 3 g as a suppository or 5 to 15 ml as an enema.	• May cause rectal discomfort or local hyperemia. • Store in tightly closed container.
kaolin and pectin mixtures Antidiarrheal	**Mild nonspecific diarrhea** *Children age 3 to 5:* 15 ml of concentrate; or 15 to 30 ml of regular-strength suspension P.O. after each bowel movement. *Children age 6 to 11:* 30 ml of concentrate; or 30 to 60 ml of regular-strength suspension P.O. after each bowel movement. *Children age 12 and older:* 45 ml of concentrate; or 60 ml of regular-strength suspension P.O. after each bowel movement. *Adults:* 45 to 90 ml of concentrate; or 60 to 120 ml of regular-strength suspension P.O. after each bowel movement.	• May cause constipation, intestinal obstruction, and fecal impaction or ulceration in infants and debilitated patients; after chronic use, drug absorbs nutrients. • Kaolin/pectin should be discontinued and therapy re-evaluated if diarrhea persists for more than 48 hours or if fever develops. • Give kaolin/pectin at least 2 hours before or 3 to 4 hours after antibiotic. • Contraindicated in patients with bowel obstruction.
magaldrate (aluminum-magnesium complex) Antacid	**Excessive gastric acidity** *Children age 6 and older and adults:* 540 to 1,080 mg of suspension P.O. between meals and h.s. with water; 480 to 960 mg in tablet form P.O. with water between meals and h.s.; or 1 to 2 chewable tablets (chewed before swallowing) between meals and h.s.	• May cause mild diarrhea or constipation, unusual fatigue, or weight loss. • Shake suspension well; give with small amounts of water or fruit juice. • Give drug at least 1 hour apart from enteric-coated medications or other oral medications. • Chewable tablets contain sugar. • Most formulations contain less than 0.5 mg of sodium per tablet (or 5 ml of liquid). • Warn parents that patient should not take more than 18 teaspoonfuls or 20 tablets in a 24-hour period.
magnesium citrate Laxative (hyperosmotic)	**Constipation; therapeutic bowel evacuation** *Children age 2 to 5:* 2.7 to 6.25 g P.O. daily as a single dose or in divided doses. *Children age 6 to 11:* 5.5 to 12.5 g P.O. daily as a single dose or in divided doses. *Children age 12 and older and adults:* 11 to 25 g P.O. daily as a single dose or in divided doses.	• Contraindicated in appendicitis and intestinal obstruction because drug may exacerbate condition. Also contraindicated in diabetes mellitus because preparation contains of large amounts of glucose, galactose, and sucrose. • May cause abdominal cramps, diarrhea, and gas formation. • Advise patient to take dose with 8 oz (240 ml) glass of water. Or may mix with fruit juice or citrus-flavored carbonated beverage to disguise unpleasant taste. • Evacuation usually occurs within 3 hours.
magnesium hydroxide (milk of magnesia, magnesia magma) Antacid, antiulcer agent, and laxative	**Bowel evacuation before surgery** *Children over age 6 and adults:* 10 to 20 ml concentrated milk of magnesia P.O., or 15 to 60 ml milk of magnesia P.O. **Constipation** *Children age 2 to 6:* 5 to 15 ml P.O. *Children age 6 to 12:* 15 to 30 ml P.O.	• Use of magnesium hydroxide as an antacid in children requires a well-established diagnosis. • May cause diarrhea, abdominal cramps, dehydration, or fluid and electrolyte imbalances. • Drug should be discontinued if patient develops signs or symptoms of hypermagnesemia, such as hypotension, respiratory depres-

DRUGS AVAILABLE WITHOUT PRESCRIPTION *(continued)*

DRUG	INDICATION AND DOSAGE	SPECIAL CONSIDERATIONS

Miscellaneous GI drugs *(continued)*

DRUG	INDICATION AND DOSAGE	SPECIAL CONSIDERATIONS
magnesium hydroxide (milk of magnesia, magnesia magma) Antacid, antiulcer agent, and laxative *(continued)*	*Adults:* 30 to 60 ml P.O., usually h.s. **Excessive gastric acidity** *Children:* 2.5 to 5 ml P.O. as needed. *Adults:* 5 to 15 ml P.O. as needed.	sion, narcosis, ECG changes, muscle weakness, sedation, or confusion. • Give drug at least 1 hour apart from enteric-coated medications; shake suspension well. • Contraindicated in abdominal pain, ileostomy, colostomy, nausea, vomiting, fecal impaction, intestinal obstruction, intestinal perforation, and renal failure.
methylcellulose Laxative (bulk)	**Chronic constipation** *Children:* 5 to 10 ml P.O. mixed in milk or cereal one or two times daily. *Adults:* 5 to 20 ml of liquid P.O. t.i.d. with a glass of water; 15 ml of syrup P.O. morning and evening; or 1 tablespoon of powder in 8 oz (240 ml) of water, one to three times daily. **Chronic diarrhea** *Children over age 12 and adults:* One tablespoon powder in 80 ml (approximately 3 oz) of water, one to three times daily.	• Methylcellulose is contraindicated in patients with abdominal pain, acute surgical abdomen, or intestinal obstruction or perforation, because the drug may exacerbate these conditions. • May cause abdominal cramps, diarrhea, nausea, vomiting, or intestinal obstruction (if chewed or taken dry). • Drug should be discontinued if abdominal pain occurs. • When used as a laxative, encourage fluid intake. • Drug may absorb oral medications; schedule at least 1 hour apart from all other drugs. • Bulk laxatives most closely mimic natural bowel function and do not promote laxative dependence. • Explain that the drug's full effect may not occur for 2 to 3 days.
mineral oil Laxative (emollient)	**Constipation; bowel examination or surgery** *Children:* 5 to 15 ml P.O. h.s., or 1- to 2-oz enema. *Adults:* 15 to 30 ml P.O. h.s., or 4-oz enema.	• Mineral oil is contraindicated in patients with fluid and electrolyte disturbances, appendicitis, acute surgical abdomen, fecal impaction, or intestinal obstruction or perforation, because the drug may exacerbate these conditions. • The enema form is contraindicated in children under age 2 because of potential for adverse effects. • Oral forms should be avoided in children under age 4 because of the risk of oil droplet aspiration. • Repeated use is not recommended in pregnant patients; drug may cause hypoprothrombinemia and hemorrhagic disease of the neonate. • May cause nausea, vomiting and diarrhea, abdominal cramps, and anal itching. • Drug should be discontinued if abdominal pain occurs. • Avoid administering drug to patients lying flat because aspiration of drug may cause pneumonitis. • Do not give drug with food because this may delay gastric emptying, delaying drug action and increasing aspiration risk. Separate by at last 2 hours. • To improve taste, give emulsion and suspension with fruit juice or carbonated beverages.

(continued)

DRUGS AVAILABLE WITHOUT PRESCRIPTION (continued)

DRUG	INDICATION AND DOSAGE	SPECIAL CONSIDERATIONS
Miscellaneous GI drugs (continued)		
mineral oil Laxative (emollient) (continued)		• Cleansing enema should be given ½ to 1 hour after retention enema. • Reduce or divide dose or use emulsified drug form to avoid leakage through anal sphincter. • Mineral oil may impair absorption of fat-soluble vitamins (A, D, E, and K).
psyllium Laxative (bulk)	**Constipation; irritable bowel syndrome** *Children over age 6:* 1 level teaspoon or 1 packet in ½ glass of liquid P.O., one to three times daily *Adults:* 1 to 2 rounded teaspoons in full glass of liquid, one to three times daily; followed by second glass of liquid or 1 packet dissolved in water P.O., one to three times daily.	• Psyllium is contraindicated in patients with abdominal pain, fecal impaction, or intestinal obstruction or ulceration, because the drug may worsen these conditions. • Effervescent powder should be used with caution in sodium-restricted and patients because of the drug's high sodium content. Sugar-free preparations should be used with caution in patients who must restrict phenylalanine intake; these products may contain aspartame, which the GI tract metabolizes to phenylalanine. • Before administering drug, add water or juice and stir for a few seconds to improves drug's taste. Have patient drink mixture immediately to prevent it from congealing, then have him drink another glass of fluid. Patient should never swallow drug in dry form. • Separate administration of psyllium and oral anticoagulants, digitalis glycosides, and salicylates by at least 2 hours. • Drug may reduce appetite if administered before meals. • Psyllium and other bulk laxatives most closely mimic natural bowel function and do not cause laxative dependence; they are especially useful for patients with postpartum constipation or diverticular disease, for debilitated patients, for irritable bowel syndrome, and for chronic laxative users. • Give diabetic patients a sugar- and sodium-free psyllium product.
senna Laxative (stimulant)	**Acute constipation; bowel examination** *Infants age 1 month to 1 year:* 1.25 to 2.5 ml of syrup h.s. *Children age 1 to 5:* 2.5 to 5 ml of syrup h.s. *Children age 5 to 15:* 5 to 10 ml of syrup h.s. *Children under 60 lb (27 kg):* Follow manufacturer's recommendation. *Children over 60 lb (27 kg):* 1 tablet, ½ teaspoon of granules dissolved in water, or ½ suppository h.s.	• Senna is contraindicated in patients with fluid and electrolyte disturbances, appendicitis, abdominal pain, nausea or vomiting, fecal impaction, or intestinal obstruction or perforation, because the drug may worsen these conditions. • May cause nausea, vomiting, diarrhea, abdominal cramps, yellow or yellow-green cast in feces, red-pink discoloration in alkaline urine, or yellow-brown color in acidic urine. • Drug should be discontinued if abdominal pain develops.

DRUGS AVAILABLE WITHOUT PRESCRIPTION *(continued)*

DRUG	INDICATION AND DOSAGE	SPECIAL CONSIDERATIONS
Miscellaneous GI drugs *(continued)*		
senna Laxative (stimulant) *(continued)*	*Adults:* Usual dose is two tablets, 1 teaspoon of granules dissolved in water, or 10 to 15 ml of syrup h.s.; not to exceed 4 tablets b.i.d., 2 teaspoons of granules b.i.d., or 10 to 15 ml of syrup h.s.	● Warn parents and patient that drug may turn urine pink, red, violet, or brown depending on urinary pH.
simethicone Antiflatulent	**Functional gastric bloating** *Children over age 12 and adults:* 40 to 125 mg after each meal and h.s.	● Simethicone is not recommended for infant colic; it has limited use in children. ● Tell parents that patient should chew tablets thoroughly or shake suspension well before using.
Otics and optics		
acetic acid Antibacterial and antifungal	**External ear canal infection** *Children and adults:* 4 to 6 drops into ear canal t.i.d. or q.i.d.; or insert saturated wick for first 24 hours, then continue with instillations. **Prophylaxis of swimmer's ear** *Children and adults:* 2 drops in each ear b.i.d.	● May cause urticaria, irritation or itching, or overgrowth of nonsusceptible organisms. ● Drug should be discontinued if severe irritation or sensitivity develops. ● Avoid contact with eyes and mucous membranes. ● Apply to freshly cleansed area free of other medications. ● Topical application is especially useful for treating superficial gram-negative infections. ● Use aseptic technique to prevent infection.
artificial tears Demulcent	**Insufficient tear production** *Children and adults:* Instill 1 to 2 drops in eye t.i.d., q.i.d., or p.r.n.	● May cause pain on instillation, blurred vision (especially with Lacrisert), or crust formation on eyelids and eyelashes (with high-viscosity products). ● Drug should be discontinued if eye pain, change in vision, or continued redness or irritation of the eye occurs, or if the condition worsens or is not relieved within 72 hours. ● If accidentally swallowed, may cause hypotension, shock, restlessness, weakness, seizures, nausea, vomiting, diarrhea, oliguria, hypothermia, hyperthermia, or erythematous rash. ● Can be used as often as desired. There are no known toxic effects unless patient is allergic to the preservative or is sensitive to boric acid found in some preparations. ● Do not instill when contact lens is in place unless the product is specifically designed for use with contact lenses. ● Patient's eyelids should be kept clean. Some products cause gummy deposit to form on the lids. ● Lacrisert rod should be inserted with special applicator included in the package.

(continued)

DRUGS AVAILABLE WITHOUT PRESCRIPTION (continued)

DRUG	INDICATION AND DOSAGE	SPECIAL CONSIDERATIONS

Otics and optics (continued)

DRUG	INDICATION AND DOSAGE	SPECIAL CONSIDERATIONS
carbamide peroxide Cerumolytic and topical anesthetic	**Impacted cerumen; gum, mouth, or lip irritation** *Children and adults:* 5 to 10 drops of otic solution into ear canal b.i.d. for 3 to 4 days. **Inflammation or irritation of lips, mouth, or gums** *Children:* Apply undiluted gel to affected area (massage into area with finger or swab) q.i.d. *Adults:* Apply several drops undiluted solution to affected area or place 10 drops on tongue (mix with saliva, swish for 1 to 3 minutes, and expectorate) after meals and h.s.	● Carbamide peroxide is contraindicated in patients with ear drainage or discharge, ear pain, irritation or rash in the ear, dizziness, injured or perforated eardrum, or hypersensitivity to any component of the preparation. ● Use with caution in children under age 12. ● Do not use to treat swimmer's ear or itching of the ear canal, or if patient has a perforated eardrum. ● Irrigation of ear may be necessary to aid removal of cerumen. ● Tip of dropper should not touch ear or ear canal. ● Remove cerumen remaining after instillation by using a soft rubber-bulb otic syringe to gently irrigate the ear canal with warm water. ● Tell patient or parents to call if imflammation or irritation persists. ● Warn parents or patient not to use for more than 4 consecutive days and to avoid contact with eyes. ● Instruct patient to keep solution in ear for at least 15 minutes by tilting head sideways or putting cotton in ear.
naphazoline hydrochloride Decongestant and vasoconstrictor	**Ocular congestion, irritation, itching** *Adults:* Instill 1 to 2 drops in eye q 3 to 4 hours. **Nasal congestion** *Children over age 12 and adults:* Apply 1 or 2 drops or sprays to nasal mucosa, p.r.n. Do not use more than q 3 hours (drops) or q 4 to 6 hours (spray).	● Use in infants and children may result in CNS depression, leading to coma and marked reduction in body temperature. ● Naphazoline is the most widely used ocular decongestant. ● Do not shake container. ● Advise parents to report blurred vision, eye pain, or lid swelling. ● Advise parents and patient using ophthalmic solution that photophobia may follow pupil dilation; tell parents to report this effect promptly. ● Tell parents to call if nasal congestion persists after 5 days of using nasal solution. Warn them not to exceed recommended dosage; rebound nasal congestion and conjunctivitis may follow frequent or prolonged use. ● May cause headache; dizziness; nervousness; coma; hypertension; cardiovascular collapse; transient burning, stinging, dryness, or ulceration of nasal mucosa; anosmia; sneezing; transient stinging of eye; pupillary dilation; irritation; hyperemia; increased or decreased intraocular pressure; nausea; weakness; nasal congestion; or sweating. ● Drug should be discontinued if systemic symptoms occur.

DRUGS AVAILABLE WITHOUT PRESCRIPTION *(continued)*

DRUG	INDICATION AND DOSAGE	SPECIAL CONSIDERATIONS
Otics and optics *(continued)*		
tetrahydrozoline hydrochloride Decongestant and vasoconstrictor	**Nasal congestion** *Children age 2 to 6:* Apply 2 or 3 drops of 0.05% solution to nasal mucosa q 4 to 6 hours, p.r.n. *Children over age 6 and adults:* Apply 2 to 4 drops of 0.1% solution or spray to nasal musosa q 4 to 6 hours, p.r.n. **Conjuctival congestion** *Adults:* 1 or 2 drops in each eye b.i.d. or t.i.d.	• The 0.1% nasal solution is contraindicated in children under age 6. All use is contraindicated in children under age 2. • Excessive use may cause rebound effect. • Drug should not be used for more than 5 days. • Advise parents and patient not to exceed recommended dosage, and to use only when needed. • Tell patient to remove contact lenses before using. • May cause drowsiness; CNS depression; dizziness; headache; insomnia tremor; seizures; anxiety; hallucinations; weakness; prolonged psychosis; insomnia; hypertension; palpitations; sweating; dysrhythmias; transient burning, stinging, or dryness of mucosa; sneezing; rebound nasal congestion with excessive or long-term use; blurred vision; pupillary dilation; irritation; tearing; or photophobia. • Drug should be discontinued if symptoms of systemic absorption occur. • Contraindicated in narrow-angle glaucoma.
triethanolamine polypeptide oleate-condensate Ceruminolytic	**Impacted cerumen** *Children and adults:* Fill ear canal with solution, and insert cotton plug. After 15 to 30 minutes, flush ear with warm water. Do not expose ear canal to solution for more than 30 minutes.	• To determine allergic potential, do patch test: Place 1 drop of drug on inner forearm, then cover with small bandage; check in 24 hours. If any reaction (redness, swelling) occurs, do not use drug. • Moisten cotton plug with medication before insertion. • May cause dermatitis, ranging from mild redness and itching of the external ear canal to a severe reaction involving the external ear and surrounding tissue (generally lasts 2 to 10 days), as well as erythema and pruritus. • Drug should be discontinued if dermatitis reaction occurs.
xylometazoline hydrochloride Decongestant and vasoconstrictor	**Nasal congestion** *Children under age 12:* Apply 2 or 3 drops or 1 spray of 0.05% solution to nasal mucosa q 8 to 10 hours. *Children over age 12 and adults:* Apply 2 or 3 drops or 2 sprays of 0.1% solution to nasal mucosa q 8 to 10 hours.	• Children may be prone to greater systemic absorption, with resultant increase in adverse reactions. • Tell patient to report insomnia, dizziness, weakness, tremors, or irregular heartbeat. • May cause headache; drowsiness; dizziness; insomnia; tremors; psychological disturbances; seizures; CNS depression; weakness; hallucinations; prolonged psychosis; blurred vision; ocular irritation; tearing; photophobia; rebound nasal congestion or irritation with excessive or long-term use; transient burning, stinging, dryness, or ulceration of nasal mucosa; sneezing; dysuria; orofacial dystonia; pallor; or sweating.

(continued)

DRUGS AVAILABLE WITHOUT PRESCRIPTION (continued)

DRUG	INDICATION AND DOSAGE	SPECIAL CONSIDERATIONS
Otics and optics (continued)		
xylometazoline hydrochloride Decongestant and vasoconstrictor (continued)		● Drug should be discontinued if symptoms of systemic toxicity occur. ● Contraindicated in narrow-angle glaucoma.
Topicals		
benzocaine Local anesthetic	**Dental pain or dental procedures** Children and adults: Apply topical jelly (10% or 20%) or dental paste to area p.r.n. **Pruritic dermatoses, pruritus, or other irritations** Adults: Apply topical solution (20%) to affected area p.r.n.	● Excessive use may cause methemoglobinemia in infants. Do not use in children under age 1. ● Use with antibiotic to treat underlying cause of pain; using alone may mask more serious condition. ● Tell parents to call if child's pain lasts longer than 48 hours, if burning or itching occurs, or if the condition persists. ● To minimize risk of biting trauma, patient should not eat or chew gum after application to oral mucosa. ● Patient should not eat for 1 hour after application to oral mucosa because swallowing may be impaired, increasing the risk of aspiration. ● May cause urticaria and edema. ● Drug should be discontinued if symptoms of hypersensitivity occur.
ciclopirox olamine Antifungal	**Tinea pedis, tinea cruris, and tinea corporis; cutaneous candidiasis; tinea versicolor** Children over age 10 and adults: Massage gently into the affected and surrounding areas b.i.d., in the morning and evening.	● Safety and efficacy in children under age 10 have not been established. ● Advise parents that patient should use drug for full treatment period even if symptoms have improved. Parents should call if no improvement occurs in 4 weeks. ● Tell parents and patient to avoid occlusive wrapping or dressing. ● Advise parents and patient to wash hands thoroughly after applying drug to avoid contacting eyes with the medication. ● If sensitivity or chemical irritation occurs, parents should discontinue treatment and call promptly. ● Inform patient with tinea versicolor that hypopigmentation from the disease will not resolve immediately.
dibucaine Local anesthetic	**Pain and itching associated with abrasions, sunburn, minor burns, hemorrhoids, and other minor skin conditions** Children and adults: Apply to affected areas. For hemorrhoids, insert ointment into rectum using a rectal applicator in the morning, evening, and after each bowel movement.	● Use dibucaine topically only, for short periods. ● Dosage should be adjusted to patient's age, size, and physical condition. ● Advise parents and patient to call if condition worsens or if symptoms persist for more than 7 days after use. ● Caution parents to apply drug sparingly to minimize adverse effects. ● May cause urticaria, edema, burning or stinging, tenderness, irritation, inflammation, contact dermatitis, or cutaneous lesions. ● Drug should be discontinued if sensitization occurs or if condition worsens.

DRUGS AVAILABLE WITHOUT PRESCRIPTION (continued)

DRUG	INDICATION AND DOSAGE	SPECIAL CONSIDERATIONS

Topicals (continued)

pyrethrins with piperonyl butoxide
Pediculocide

Pediculosis
Children and adults: Apply gel, solution, or shampoo to the hair and scalp or skin; repeat once in 7 to 10 days. Do not apply more than twice within 24 hours.

● Pyrethrins and piperonyl butoxide combination applied topically in recommended dosage rarely causes systemic toxicity.
● When pyrethrins are injected or inhaled, they can cause nausea, vomiting, muscle paralysis, and even death; however, severe pyrethrin poisoning is rare.
● Piperonyl butoxide has been reported to cause nausea, vomiting, diarrhea, depression, and hemorrhagic enteritis when large amounts are ingested orally.
● First treatment with pyrethrins and piperonyl butoxide is often successful, but treatment should be repeated in 7 to 10 days to kill any newly hatched lice. The drug should not be used more than twice within 24 hours.
● All contaminated clothing and bed linen should be machine-washed in hot water and dried in a hot dryer for at least 20 minutes or should be dry-cleaned after treatment to avoid reinfestation or transmission of pediculosis.
● Pyrethrins with piperonyl butoxide should not be administered orally or be inhaled. Preparations containing the drugs should not be used near the eyes or allowed to come in contact with mucous membranes. If contact with an eye occurs, the affected eye should be rinsed thoroughly with water. Shampoo containers should be shaken before using.
● For the treatment of pediculosis, enough gel, shampoo, or solution should be applied to cover the affected hairy and adjacent areas, taking care to avoid contact with the eyes, eyelashes, mucous membranes, and urethral meatus. After 10 minutes, the hair is then washed thoroughly (with soap or plain shampoo and water if a solution or gel of the drug is applied, or with water if a shampoo of the drug is applied), dried with a clean towel, and combed with a fine-tooth comb to remove any remaining nit shells.
● Pyrethrins with piperonyl butoxide should not be applied to acutely inflamed skin or raw, weeping surfaces.

Vitamins

Multivitamins

Nutritional supplement
Children and adults: 1 tablet or capsule P.O. daily.

● Make sure children understand vitamins are not candy.
● Children's formulations differ from adult preparation.
● Vitamins do not replace a well-balanced diet.

CALCULATING BODY SURFACE AREA IN CHILDREN

In a child of average size, find weight and corresponding surface area on the boxed scale to the left. Or use the nomogram to the right.

Lay a straightedge on the correct height and weight points for the child, then read the intersecting point on the surface area scale.

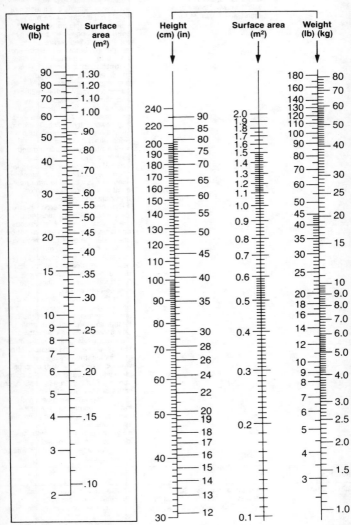

FOR CHILDREN OF NORMAL HEIGHT AND WEIGHT

NOMOGRAM

Reprinted with permission from *Nelson Textbook of Pediatrics*, W.B. Saunders Co., 1987.

TABLE OF EQUIVALENTS

Frequently used equivalents in the metric system

Metric Weight		*Metric Volume*	
1 gram (g)	= 0.001 kilogram (kg or Kg)	1 liter (L)	= 0.001 kiloliter (kl or Kl)
	= 0.01 hectogram (hg or Hg)		= 0.01 hectoliter (hl or Hl)
	= 0.1 decagram (dag or Dg)		= 0.1 decaliter (dal or Dl)
	= 10 decigrams (dg)		= 10 deciliters (dl)
	= 100 centigrams (cg)		= 100 centiliters (cl)
	= 1,000 milligrams (mg)		= 1,000 milliliters (ml)*

Frequently used equivalents in the apothecary system

Apothecary Weight		*Apothecary Volume*	
20 grains (gr)	= 1 scruple (Э)	60 minims (♍)†	= 1 fluidram (f ʒ)
3 scruples	= 1 dram (ʒ)	8 fluidrams	= 1 fluidounce (f ʒ)
8 drams	= 1 ounce (ʒ)	16 fluidounces	= 1 pint (pt)
12 ounces	= 1 pound (℔)	2 pints	= 1 quart (qt)
		4 quarts	= 1 gallon (gal)

Approximate metric and apothecary weight equivalents

Metric	*Apothecary*	*Metric*	*Apothecary*
1 gram (g)	= 15 grains	0.05 g (50 mg)	= ¾ grain
0.6 g (600 mg)	= 10 grains	0.03 g (30 mg)	= ½ grain
0.5 g (500 mg)	= 7½ grains	0.015 g (15 mg)	= ¼ grain
0.3 g (300 mg)	= 5 grains	0.001 g (1 mg)	= 1/60 grain
0.2 g (200 mg)	= 3 grains	0.6 mg	= 1/100 grain
0.1 g (100 mg)	= 1½ grains	0.5 mg	= 1/120 grain
0.06 g (60 mg)	= 1 grain	0.4 mg	= 1/150 grain

Approximate household, apothecary, and metric volume equivalents

Household	*Apothecary*	*Metric*
1 teaspoon (t or tsp)	= 1 fluidram (f ʒ)	= 4 or 5 ml‡
1 tablespoon (T or tbs)	= ½ fluidounce (f ʒ)	= 15 ml
2 tablespoons	= 1 fluidounce	= 30 ml
1 measuring cupful	= 8 fluidounces	= 240 ml
1 pint (pt)	= 16 fluidounces	= 473 ml
1 quart (qt)	= 32 fluidounces	= 946 ml
1 gallon (gal)	= 128 fluidounces	= 3,785 ml

*1 ml = 1 cubic centimeter (cc); however, ml is the preferred measurement term today.

†A minim is *almost equal* to a drop. When a drug is prescribed in minims, it is best to measure it in minims. The minim is measured with a minim glass; a drop, with a medicine dropper.

‡Although the fluidram is approximately 4 ml, in prescriptions it is considered equivalent to the teaspoon (which is 5 ml).

PEDIATRIC RECOMMENDATIONS FOR ANESTHETIC DRUGS

DRUG AND INDICATION	DOSAGE	SPECIAL CONSIDERATIONS

Halogenated inhalation anesthetics

Enflurane, halothane, isoflurane
Induction and maintenance of general anesthesia

Expressed in terms of minimal alveolar concentration (MAC)

• These agents are administered only by personnel trained to manage administration of anesthesia and related adverse reactions. They are often used with I.V. induction agents.
• Postoperatively, observe patient for cardiac dysrhythmias, hypotension, respiratory depression, and emergence delirium. Psychomotor impairment may persist for 24 hours or more.

halothane: 0.75%

• Halothane will sensitize the myocardium to catecholamines. Subsequent exposure to epinephrine may result in dysrhythmias.
• Hepatitis has been associated with halothane. It may result from hypersensitivity or from accumulation of toxic metabolites.

enflurane: 1.68%

• Because of its cardiovascular depressant effects, enflurane must be used with extreme caution in patients receiving beta blockers; rarely, it may cause CNS excitation or seizures.
• Enflurane has been associated with renal damage in patients with compromised renal function.

isoflurane: 1.15%

• Isoflurane does not have the cardiac depressant effects of enflurane or halothane, but it may depress respiration.

I.V. agents

Atracurium besylate
Adjunct to general anesthesia, to facilitate endotracheal intubation, and to provide skeletal muscle relaxation during surgery or mechanical ventilation

Dose depends on anesthetic used, individual needs, and response. Doses are representative and must be adjusted.
Children ages 1 month to 2 years: Initially, 0.3 to 0.4 mg/kg by I.V. bolus when under halothane anesthesia. Frequent maintenance doses may be needed.
Children over age 2: Initially, 0.4 to 0.5 mg/kg by I.V. bolus. Maintenance dose of 0.08 to 0.10 mg/kg within 20 to 45 minutes of initial dose should be administered during prolonged surgical procedures. Maintenance doses may be administered q 12 to 25 minutes in patients receiving balanced anesthesia.

• Safety and efficacy have not been established for children under age 1 month.
• Reduce dose and administration rate in patients in whom histamine release may be hazardous.
• Prior administration of succinylcholine does not prolong action of atracurium, but it quickens onset and may deepen neuromuscular blockade.
• Atracurium has little or no effect on heart rate and will not counteract or reverse the bradycardia caused by anesthetics or vagal stimulation. Pretreatment with anticholinergics (atropine or glycopyrrolate) is advised.
• If bradycardia occurs during atracurium administration, treat by administration of I.V. atropine.
• Alkaline solutions, such as barbiturates, should not be admixed in the same syringe or given through the same needle with atracurium.
• Peripheral nerve stimulator may be used to detect residual paralysis during recovery and to avoid atracurium overdose.
• Atracurium should be used only if endotracheal intubation, administration of oxygen under positive pressure, artificial respiration, and assisted or controlled ventilation are immediately available.
• To evaluate patient for recovery from neuromuscular blocking effect, observe for ability to breathe, to cough, to protrude tongue, to keep eyes open, to lift head keeping mouth closed, and to show adequate strength of handgrip. Assess for adequate negative inspiratory force (-25 cm H_2O).

PEDIATRIC RECOMMENDATIONS FOR ANESTHETIC DRUGS *(continued)*

DRUG AND INDICATION	DOSAGE	SPECIAL CONSIDERATIONS

I.V. agents *(continued)*

DRUG AND INDICATION	DOSAGE	SPECIAL CONSIDERATIONS
Atracurium besylate *(continued)*		• Until head and neck muscles recover from blockade effects, patient may find speech difficult. • If indicated, assess need for pain medication or sedation. Drug does not affect consciousness or relieve pain. • May cause hypotension, tachycardia, flushing, erythema, pruritus, urticaria, rash, hypothermia, increased pulmonary function impairment, respiratory depression, wheezing, increased bronchial secretions, and bronchospasm.
Fentanyl citrate Adjunct to anesthesia and post-operative analgesia	*Children ages 2 to 12:* 1 to 2 mcg/kg I.V.	• Safe use in children under age 2 has not been established. • Administer with extreme caution to patients with head injury, increased intracranial pressure, seizures, asthma, chronic obstructive pulmonary disease, severe hepatic or renal disease, acute abdominal conditions, cardiac dysrhythmias, hypovolemia, or psychiatric disorders, and to debilitated patients. Reduced doses may be necessary. • Consider possible interactions with other drugs the patient is taking. • Keep resuscitative equipment and a narcotic antagonist (naloxone) available. Be prepared to provide support of ventilation and gastric lavage. • I.V. administration should be given by slow injection, preferably in diluted solution. Rapid I.V. injection increases the incidence of adverse effects. • Parenteral injections should be given cautiously to patients who are chilled, hypovolemic, or in shock, because decreased perfusion may lead to accumulation of the drug and toxic effects. Rotate injection sites to avoid induration. • Before administration, visually inspect all parenteral products for particulate matter and discoloration. • A regular dosage schedule (rather than p.r.n.) is preferred to alleviate the symptoms and anxiety that accompany pain. • The duration of respiratory depression may be longer than the analgesic effect. Monitor the patient closely with repeated dosing. • With chronic administration, evaluate the patient's respiratory status before each dose. Because severe respiratory depression may occur (especially with accumulation from chronic dosing), watch for respiratory rate below the patient's baseline level. Evaluate the patient for restlessness, which may be a sign of compensatory response to hypoxia. • Opiates or agonist-antagonists may cause orthostatic hypotension in ambulatory patients. Have the patient sit or lie down to relieve dizziness or fainting. • Because opiates depress respiration when they are used postoperatively, encourage patient turning, coughing, and deep breathing to avoid atelectases.

(continued)

PEDIATRIC RECOMMENDATIONS FOR ANESTHETIC DRUGS (continued)

DRUG AND INDICATION	DOSAGE	SPECIAL CONSIDERATIONS

I.V. agents (continued)

Fentanyl citrate (continued)

- Observe patient for delayed onset of respiratory depression. The high lipid solubility of fentanyl may contribute to this potential adverse effect.
- Monitor patient's heart rate. Fentanyl may cause bradycardia. Pretreatment with an anticholinergic (such as atropine or glycopyrrolate) may minimize this effect.
- High doses can produce muscle rigidity. This effect can be reversed by naloxone.
- Explain that constipation may result from taking an opiate. Suggest measures to increase dietary fiber content, or recommend a stool softener.
- If patient's condition allows, instruct patient to breathe deeply, cough, and change position every 2 hours to avoid respiratory complications.
- Patient should void at least every 4 hours to avoid urinary retention.
- May cause sedation, euphoria, insomnia, agitation, confusion, headache, tremors, convulsions, dysphoria, miosis, seizures, dizziness, bradycardia, palpitations, chest wall rigidity, hypertension, hypotension, syncope, edema, shock, cardiopulmonary arrest, flushing, rash, pruritus, pain at injection site, diaphoresis, dry mouth, anorexia, biliary spasms (colic), ileus, nausea, vomiting, constipation, urinary retention or hesitancy, apnea, respiratory depression, skeletal muscle rigidity, and blurred vision.

Ketamine hydrochloride
Induction and maintenance of general anesthesia

Children: 1 to 4.5 mg/kg I.V. over 60 seconds or 6.5 to 13 mg/kg I.M. To maintain anesthesia, repeat in increments of half to full initial dose.

- Keep verbal, tactile, and visual stimulation to a minimum during induction and recovery. Emergence reactions (including dreams, visual imagery, hallucinations, and delirium) occur in 12% of patients and may occur for up to 24 hours postoperatively. They may be reduced by using lower dosage of ketamine with I.V. diazepam and can be treated with short- or ultrashort-acting barbiturates. Incidence is lower in patients under age 15 and when drug is given I.M.
- Dissociative and hallucinatory side effects have led to drug abuse.
- Barbiturates are incompatible in the same syringe.
- Warn parents that patient should avoid tasks requiring motor coordination and mental alertness for 24 hours after anesthesia.
- May cause tonic-clonic movements, respiratory depression, apnea (if administered too rapidly), hallucinations, confusion, excitement, dreamlike states, irrational behavior, psychic abnormalities, hypertension, tachycardia, hypotension and bradycardia if used with halothane, dysrhythmias, transient erythema, measles-like rash, diplopia, nystagmus, laryngospasm, mild anorexia, nausea, vomiting, or excessive salivation.
- Ketamine is a preferred agent when thiopental is contraindicated, as in patients with porphyrin or barbiturate allergy, severe asthma, airway irritability, or hypotensive hypovolemic states with cardiovascular instability.

PEDIATRIC RECOMMENDATIONS FOR ANESTHETIC DRUGS *(continued)*

DRUG AND INDICATION	DOSAGE	SPECIAL CONSIDERATIONS

I.V. agents *(continued)*

Ketamine hydrochloride *(continued)*

● Some clinicians advocate combined use with a benzodiazepine sedative, such as midazolam or diazepam, to minimize post-operative adverse reactions, such as emergence delirium, prolonged hallucinations, and nightmares.

Methohexital sodium
Induction and maintenance of general anesthesia for short procedures, such as electroconvulsive therapy or cardioversion

Children: For induction, 1% solution I.V., given at rate of 1 ml/5 seconds (dose varies from 50 to 120 mg).
For maintenance, intermittent I.V. injection of 20 to 40 mg (2 to 4 ml of 1% solution) or continuous I.V. infusion of 3 ml of 0.2% solution infused at rate of 1 drop/second.

● Avoid extravasation or intra-arterial injection because of possible tissue necrosis and gangrene.
● Drug is physically incompatible with lactated Ringer's solution; with acidic solutions, such as atropine, metocurine, and succinylcholine; and with silicone. Avoid contact with rubber stoppers or parts of syringes that have been treated with silicone.
● May cause skeletal muscle hyperactivity, anxiety, restlessness, headache, emergence delirium, transient hypotension, tachycardia, circulatory depression, peripheral vascular collapse, pain, swelling, ulceration and necrosis on extravasation, abdominal pain, nausea, vomiting, excessive salivation, respiratory depression, apnea, laryngospasm, bronchospasm, hiccups, thrombophlebitis and pain at injection site, and injury to adjacent nerves.
● Drug should be discontinued if peripheral vascular collapse, respiratory arrest, or hypersensitivity reaction occurs.

Pancuronium bromide
Adjunct to anesthesia to induce skeletal muscle relaxation, facilitate intubation and ventilation, and weaken muscle contractions in induced convulsions

Dose depends on anesthetic used, individual needs, and response. Doses are representative and must be adjusted.
Dosage for neonates under age 1 month must be carefully individualized.
Neonates: Initial (test) dose is 0.02 mg/kg. Maintenance dose is 0.03 to 0.09 mg/kg.
Children over age 1 month: Initially, 0.04 to 0.1 mg/kg I.V.; then 0.01 mg/kg q 30 to 60 minutes if needed.

● Monitor baseline electrolyte levels, intake and output, and vital signs, especially heart rate and respiration.
● Administration requires direct medical supervision, with emergency respiratory support available.
● If using succinylcholine, allow its effects to subside before administering pancuronium.
● Store drug in refrigerator and not in plastic container or syringes. Plastic syringes may be used to administer dose.
● Do not mix in same syringe or give through same needle with barbiturates or other alkaline solutions.
● Use fresh solution only.
● Neostigmine, edrophonium, or pyridostigmine may be used to reverse effects.
● Dosage should be reduced when ether or other inhalation anesthetic that enhances neuromuscular blockade is used.
● Large doses may increase frequency and severity of tachycardia.
● Drug does not relieve pain or affect consciousness; be sure to assess need for analgesic or sedative.
● May cause elevated pulse rate, especially after high doses or when administered in combination with ketamine; slight elevation in blood pressure (dose-related); burning sensation along vein (rare); excessive salivation and sweating (particularly in children); transient rash; wheezing; prolonged dose-related apnea; and residual muscular weakness.
● Drug should be discontinued if hypersensitivity or cardiovascular collapse occurs.

(continued)

PEDIATRIC RECOMMENDATIONS FOR ANESTHETIC DRUGS (continued)

DRUG AND INDICATION	DOSAGE	SPECIAL CONSIDERATIONS
I.V. agents (continued)		
Succinylcholine chloride To induce skeletal muscle relaxation; facilitate intubation, ventilation, or orthopedic manipulations; and lessen muscle contractions in induced convulsions	Dosage depends on the anesthetic used, patient's needs, and response. Doses are representative and must be adjusted. Paralysis is induced after inducing hypnosis with thiopental or other appropriate agent. *Children:* Initial dose is 1 to 2 mg/kg I.V. or 2.5 to 4 mg/kg I.M. Maintenance dose is 0.3 to 0.6 mg/kg I.V. at intervals of 5 to 10 minutes.	● Administration requires direct medical supervision by trained anesthesia personnel. ● Usually administered I.V., succinylcholine may be administered I.M. if suitable vein is inaccessible. Give deep I.M., preferably high into the deltoid muscle. ● Duration of action is prolonged to 20 minutes with continuous I.V infusion or when given with hexafluorenium bromide. ● Repeated fractional doses of succinylcholine alone are not advised; they may cause reduced response or prolonged apnea. ● Monitor baseline electrolyte determination and vital signs (check respiration every 5 to 10 minutes during infusion). ● Keep airway clear. Have emergency respiratory support (endotracheal equipment, ventilator, oxygen, atropine, neostigmine) on hand. ● Store injectable form in refrigerator. Store powder form at room temperature and keep tightly closed. Use immediately after reconstitution. ● Do not mix with alkaline solutions (thiopental, sodium bicarbonate, barbiturates). ● Tachyphylaxis may occur. ● Reassure parents and patient that postoperative stiffness is normal and will soon subside. Monitor for residual muscle weakness. ● May cause transient bradycardia, tachycardia, hypertension, hypotension, dysrhythmias, sinus arrest, increased intraocular pressure, prolonged respiratory depression, apnea, wheezing or troubled breathing, malignant hyperthermia, muscle fasciculation, postoperative muscle pain, myoglobinemia, excessive salivation, myoglobinuria, rash, and tachyphylaxis (after repeated doses). ● With large doses or prolonged administration of repeated doses, the patient may experience a prolonged "phase II" block (paralysis) that is not pharmacologically reversible.
Thiopental sodium General anesthetic	*Children and adults:* Dosage must be individualized; most physicians use 2 to 3 mg/kg I.V. as an induction dose, followed by 1 mg/kg I.V. as a maintenance dose. Maximum dose is 1 g/ 50 lb (22.7 kg) of body weight, or 1 to 1.5 g for children weighing 75 lb (34 kg) or more and 3 to 4 g for adults weighing 200 lb (90 kg) or more.	● Solutions of succinylcholine, tubocurarine, or atropine should not be mixed with thiopental but can be given to the patient concomitantly. ● Use cautiously in pediatric patients. ● May cause anxiety, restlessness, retrograde amnesia, prolonged somnolence, hypotension, tachycardia, peripheral vascular collapse, myocardial depression, dysrhythmias, nausea and vomiting, respiratory depression, apnea, laryngospasm, bronchospasm, and pain, swelling, ulceration, and necrosis on extravasation (unlikely at concentrations under 2.5%).

PEDIATRIC RECOMMENDATIONS FOR ANESTHETIC DRUGS (continued)

DRUG AND INDICATION	DOSAGE	SPECIAL CONSIDERATIONS

I.V. agents (continued)

Tubocurarine chloride
Adjunct to general anesthesia to induce skeletal muscle relaxation, facilitate intubation, and reduce fractures and dislocations

Dose depends on anesthetic used, individual needs, and response. Doses listed are representative and must be adjusted. Dosage may be calculated on the basis of 0.165 mg/kg.

Initial dose is 6 to 9 mg I.V. followed by 3 to 4.5 mg in 3 to 5 minutes if needed. Additional doses of 3 mg may be given if needed during prolonged anesthesia.
To assist with mechanical ventilation
Initial dose is 0.0165 mg/kg I.V. (average 1 mg), then adjust subsequent doses to patient's responses.

- The margin of safety between therapeutic dose and dose causing respiratory paralysis is small.
- Monitor respirations closely for early signs of paralysis.
- Allow effects of succinylcholine to subside before giving tubocurarine.
- Measure and record intake and output.
- Use only fresh solution. Discard if discolored.
- Do not mix in same syrange with barbiturates or other alkaline solutions.
- Assess baseline tests of renal function and serum electrolyte levels before drug administration. Electrolyte imbalance (particularly potassium and magnesium) can potentiate drug's effects.
- I.V. administration requires direct medical supervision. Drug should be given I.V. slowly over 60 to 90 seconds or I.M. by deep injection in deltoid muscle. Tubocurarine is usually administered by I.V. injection, but if patient's veins are inaccessible, drug may be given I.M. in same dosage as given I.V.
- Keep airway clear. Have emergency respiratory support equipment on hand. Be prepared for endotracheal intubation, suction, or assisted or controlled respiration with oxygen administration. Have atropine and the antagonists neostigmine or edrophonium (cholinesterase inhibitors) available. A nerve stimulator may be used to evaluate recovery from neuromuscular blockade.
- Muscle paralysis follows drug administration in sequence: jaw muscles, levator eyelid muscles and other muscles of head and neck, limbs, intercostals and diaphragm, abdomen, and trunk. Facial and diaphragm muscles recover first, then legs, arms, shoulder girdle, trunk, larynx, hands, feet, and pharynx. Muscle function is usually restored within 90 minutes. Patient may find speech difficult until muscles of head and neck recover.
- Monitor blood pressure, vital signs, and airway until patient recovers from drug effects.
- After neuromuscular blockade dissipates, watch for residual muscle weakness.
- Renal dysfunction prolongs drug action. Peristaltic action may be suppressed. Check for bowel sounds.
- Drug does not affect consciousness or relieve pain; assess patient's need for analgesic or sedative.
- May cause hypotension, increased salivation, decreased GI motility and tone, wheezing or troubled breathing, bronchospasm, respiratory depression to point of apnea, hypersensitivity, and residual muscle weakness.

(continued)

PEDIATRIC RECOMMENDATIONS FOR ANESTHETIC DRUGS (continued)

DRUG AND INDICATION	DOSAGE	SPECIAL CONSIDERATIONS

I.V. agents (continued)

Vecuronium bromide
Adjunct to anesthesia, to facilitate intubation, and to provide skeletal muscle relaxation during surgery or mechanical ventilation

Dose depends on anesthetic used, individual needs, and response. Doses are representative and must be adjusted.
Children ages 1 to 9: Dosage is individualized. Higher initial doses and more frequent maintenance doses may be needed in children ages 1 to 9 as compared to adults. *Children age 10 and over and adults:* Initially, 0.08 to 0.10 mg/kg I.V. bolus. Higher initial doses (up to 0.3 mg/kg) may be used for rapid onset. Maintenance doses of 0.010 to 0.015 mg/kg within 25 to 40 minutes of initial dose should be administered during prolonged surgical procedures. Maintenance doses may be given q 12 to 15 minutes in patients receiving balanced anesthetic.
   Safety and efficacy have not been established in infants under age 7 weeks. Infants ages 7 weeks to 1 year are more sensitive to neuromuscular blocking effects; less frequent administration may be necessary.

• Administer by rapid I.V. injection or I.V. infusion. Do not give I.M.
• Reconstitute using 5 ml of sterile water for injection (provided by manufacturer) to produce a solution containing 2 mg/ml.
• Do not mix in same syringe or give through same needle as barbiturates or other alkaline solutions.
• Protect solution from light.
• After reconstitution, solution should be stored in refrigerator or at room temperature not exceeding 86° F. (30° C.). Do not use if discolored. Discard unused portion after 24 hours.
• Have emergency respiratory support equipment immediately available.
• Assess baseline serum electrolyte levels, acid-base balance, and renal and hepatic function before administration.
• Peripheral nerve stimulator may be used to identify residual paralysis during recovery and is especially useful during administration to high-risk patients.
• After procedure, monitor vital signs at least every 15 minutes until patient is stable, then every 1/2 hour for the next 2 hours. Monitor airway and pattern of respirations until patient has recovered from drug effects. Anticipate problems with ventilation in obese patients and those with myasthenia gravis or other neuromuscular disease.
• Evaluate recovery from neuromuscular blockade by checking strength of handgrip and ability to breathe naturally, to take deep breaths and cough, to keep eyes open, and to lift head keeping mouth closed.
• Drug does not relieve pain or affect consciousness; if indicated, assess need for analgesic or sedative.
• May cause minimal and transient cardiovascular effects; skeletal muscle weakness or paralysis; respiratory insufficiency; respiratory paralysis; prolonged, dose-related apnea; and malignant hyperthermia.

RECOMMENDATIONS FOR PEDIATRIC IMMUNIZATION

The following charts provide a list of vaccines available in the United States, summarize the recommended schedule for active immunization of infants and children, and describe current requirements for reporting adverse reactions to immunization. These recommendations are derived from the 1989 revision of The General Recommendations on Immunization from The Centers for Disease Control (CDC) Advisory Committee of Immunization Practices.

VACCINE	TYPE	ROUTE AND COMMENT
BCG (bacillus of Calmette and Guérin)	Live bacteria	Intradermal or subcutaneous
Cholera	Inactivated bacteria	Subcutaneous or intradermal The intradermal dose is lower.
DTP (diphtheria, tetanus, pertussis)	Toxoids and inactivated bacteria	Intramuscular
Haemophilus influenzae b —Polysaccharide (HbPV)	Bacterial polysaccharide	Subcutaneous or intramuscular Route depends on the manufacturer; consult package insert for specific recommendation.
—Conjugate (HbCV)	Polysaccharide conjugated to protein	Intramuscular
HB (hepatitis B)	Inactive viral antigen	Intramuscular
Influenza	Inactivated virus or viral components	Intramuscular
IPV (inactivated poliovirus vaccine)	Inactivated viruses of all three serotypes	Subcutaneous
Measles	Live virus	Subcutaneous
Meningococcal	Bacterial polysaccharides of serotypes A/C/Y/W-135	Subcutaneous
MMR (measles, mumps, rubella)	Live viruses	Subcutaneous
Mumps	Live virus	Subcutaneous
OPV (oral poliovirus vaccine)	Live viruses of all three serotypes	Oral
Plague	Inactivated bacteria	Intramuscular
Pneumococcal	Bacterial polysaccharides of 23 pneumococcal types	Intramuscular or subcutaneous
Rabies	Inactivated virus	Subcutaneous or intradermal Intradermal dose is lower and used only for preexposure vaccination.
Rubella	Live virus	Subcutaneous
Td or DT (T = tetanus, D or d = diphtheria)	Inactivated toxins (toxoids)	Intramuscular DT = tetanus and diphtheria toxoids for use in children < age 7. Td = tetanus and diphtheria toxoids for use in persons ≥ age 7. Td contains the same amount of tetanus toxoids as DTP or DT but a reduced dose of diphtheria toxoid.
Tetanus	Inactivated toxin (toxoid)	Intramuscular Preparations with adjuvants should be given intramuscularly.
Typhoid	Inactivated bacteria	Subcutaneous Boosters may be given intradermally unless acetone-killed and dried vaccine is used.
Yellow fever	Live virus	Subcutaneous

(continued)

Recommended schedule for active immunization of normal infants and children

RECOMMENDED AGE*	VACCINE	COMMENTS
2 months	DTP#1, OPV#1	OPV and DTP can be given earlier in areas of high endemicity. DTP may be used up to the seventh birthday. The first dose can be given at age 6 weeks and the second and third doses given 4 to 8 weeks after the preceding dose.
4 months	DTP#2, OPV#2	6-week to 2-month interval desired between OPV doses.
6 months	DTP#3	An additional dose of OPV at this time is optional in areas with a high risk of poliovirus exposure.
15 months	MMR, DTP#4, OPV#3	Completion of primary series of DTP and OPV provided at least 6 months have elapsed since DTP#3 or, if fewer than 3 doses of DTP have been received, at least 6 weeks since the last previous dose of DTP or OVP. MMR vaccine should not be delayed to allow simultaneous administration with DTP and OPV. Administering MMR at age 15 months and DTP#4 and OPV#3 at age 18 months continues to be an acceptable alternative. Counties that report five or more cases of measles among preschool children during each of the last 5 years should implement a routine two-dose measles vaccination schedule for preschoolers. The first dose should be administered at age 9 months or the first health-care contact thereafter. Infants vaccinated before their first birthday should receive a second dose at about age 15 months. Single-antigen measles vaccine should be used for children < age 1 year and MMR for children vaccinated on or after their first birthday. If resources do not allow a routine two-dose schedule, an acceptable alternative is to lower the routine age for MMR vaccination to 12 months.
18 months	HbCV	Conjugate preferred over polysaccharide vaccines. Children < age 5 previously vaccinated with polysaccharide vaccine between the ages of 18 and 23 months should be revaccinated with a single dose of conjugated vaccine if at least 2 months have elapsed since they received the polysaccharide vaccine. If HbCV is not available, an acceptable alternative is to give *Haemophilus influenzae* b polysaccharide vaccine (HbPV) at age ≥ 24 months. Children at high risk for Haemophilus influenzae type b disease where conjugate vaccine is not available may be vaccinated with HbPV at age 18 months and revaccinated at 24 months.
4 to 6 years	DTP#5, OPV#4	At or before school entry up to the seventh birthday.
14 to 16 years	Td	Repeat every 10 years throughout life. Toxoids, Adsorbed (for use in persons ≥ age 7) contains the same amount of tetanus toxoid as DTP or DT but a reduced dose of diphtheria toxoid.

*These recommended ages should not be construed as absolute; for example, 2-month vaccines can be given at 6 to 10 weeks. However, MMR should not be given to children < age 12 months. If exposure to measles disease is considered likely, then children age 6 through 11 months may be immunized with single-antigen measles vaccine. These children should be reimmunized with MMR at approximately age 15 months.

For all products used, consult the manufacturers' package enclosures for instructions regarding storage, handling, dosage, and administration. Immunobiologics prepared by different manufacturers can vary, and those of the same manufacturer can change from time to time. The package inserts are useful references for specific products, but they may not be consistent with current Advisory Committee of Immunization Practices and American Academy of Pediatrics immunization schedules.

Recommended immunization schedule for infants and children up to the seventh birthday who were not immunized in early infancy*

TIMING	VACCINE	COMMENTS
First visit	DTP#1, OPV#1, MMR if child is ≥ age 15 months, and HbCV if child is ≤ age 18 months	DTP, OPV, and MMR should be administered simultaneously to children ≥ age 15 months, if appropriate. DTP, OPV, MMR, and HbCV may be given simultaneously to children ages 18 months to 5 years. DTP can be used up to the seventh birthday. If HbCV is not available, an acceptable alternative is to give Haemophilus influenzae b polysaccharide vaccine (HbPV) at age 24 months. If HbCV is unavailable and if the child is at high risk for *Haemophilus influenzae* type b disease, HbPV may be given at age 18 months with a second dose at 24 months. Children < age 5 who were previously vaccinated with HbPV between ages 18 and 23 months should be revaccinated with a single dose of HbCV at least 2 months after the initial dose of HbPV. Either HbCV or HbPV can be administered up to the fifth birthday. However, they are not generally recommended for persons ≥ age 5.
2 months after DTP#1, OPV#1	DTP#2, OPV#2	The second and third doses of DTP can be given 4 to 8 weeks after the preceding dose.
2 months after DTP#2	DTP#3	An additional dose of OPV at this time is optional in areas with high risk of poliovirus exposure.
6 to 12 months after DTP#3	DTP#4, OPV#3	
Preschoolers (4 to 6 years)	DTP#5, OPV#4	Preferably at or before school entry. The preschool doses are not necessary if the fourth dose of DTP and third dose of OPV are administered after the fourth birthday.
14 to 16 years	Td	Repeat every 10 years throughout life. Tetanus and Diphtheria Toxoids, Adsorbed (for use in persons ≥ age 7) contains the same dose of tetanus toxoid as DTP or DT and a reduced dose of diphtheria toxoid.

*If initiated in the first year of life, give DTP#1, 2, and 3 and OPV#1 and 2 according to this schedule; give MMR when the child reaches age 15 months.

Recommended immunization schedule for persons over age 7 who were not immunized in early infancy

TIMING	VACCINE	COMMENTS
First visit	Td#1, OPV#1, and MMR*	The DTP doses given to children < age 7 who remain incompletely immunized at ≥ age 7 should be counted as prior exposure to tetanus and diphtheria toxoids (for example, a child who previously received two doses of DTP needs only one dose of Td to complete a primary series for tetanus and diphtheria). OPV is not routinely recommended for persons ≥ age 18. When polio vaccine is to be given to persons ≥ age 18, inactivated poliovirus vaccine (IPV) is preferred.
2 months after Td#1, OPV#1	Td#2, OPV#2	OPV may be given as soon as 6 weeks after OPV#1.
6 to 12 months after Td#2, OPV#2	Td#3, OPV#3	OPV#3 may be given as soon as 6 weeks after OPV#2.
10 years after Td#3	Td	Repeat every 10 years throughout life.

*Persons born before 1957 can generally be considered immune to measles and mumps and need not be immunized. Because medical personnel are at higher risk for acquiring measles than the general population, medical facilities may wish to consider requiring proof of measles immunity for employees born before 1957. Rubella vaccine can be given to persons of any age, particularly to nonpregnant women of childbearing age. MMR can be used because administration of vaccine to persons already immune is not deleterious.

(continued)

Guidelines for spacing live and killed antigen administration

ANTIGEN COMBINATION	RECOMMENDED MINIMUM INTERVAL BETWEEN DOSES
≥ 2 killed antigens	None. May be given simultaneously or at any interval between doses. If possible, vaccines associated with local or systemic side effects (cholera, typhoid, plague vaccines) should be given on separate occasions to avoid accentuated reactions.
Killed and live antigens	None. May be given simultaneously or at any interval between doses except cholera vaccine with yellow fever vaccine. If time permits, these antigens should not be administered simultaneously, and at least 3 weeks should elapse between administration of yellow fever vaccine and cholera vaccine. If the vaccines must be given simultaneously or within a 3-week interval, the antibody response may not be optimal.
≥ 2 live antigens	4-week minimum interval if not administered simultaneously.

Recommendations for routine immunization of HIV-infected children and adults

| | HIV INFECTION | |
VACCINE	KNOWN ASYMPTOMATIC	SYMPTOMATIC
DTP	yes	yes
HbCV	yes	yes
Influenza	no	yes
IPV	yes	yes
MMR	yes	yes
OPV	no	no
Pneumococcal	no	yes

Recommendations for immunization of HIV-infected children have been controversial. However, the Advisory Committee of Immunization Practice of the CDC has offered the following recommendations. If the decision to vaccinate is made, symptomatic HIV-infected children should receive MMR vaccine at 15 months, the age currently recommended for vaccination of children without HIV infection and for those with asymptomatic HIV infection. When there is an increased risk of exposure to measles, such as during an outbreak, these children should receive vaccination at younger ages. At such times, infants ages 6 to 11 months should receive monovalent measles vaccine and should be revaccinated with MMR at ages 12 months or older. Children ages 12 to 14 months should receive MMR and do not need revaccination.

The use of high-dose intravenous immune globin (IGIV) administered at regular intervals is being studied to determine whether it will prevent a variety of infections in HIV-infected children. Consider that MMR vaccine may be ineffective if administered to a child who has received IGIV during the preceding 3 months.

Immune globulin (IG) can be used to prevent or modify measles infection in HIV-infected children if administered within 6 days of exposure. IG is indicated for measles-susceptible household contacts of children with asymptomatic HIV infection, particularly for those under age 1, and for measles-susceptible pregnant women. In contrast, exposed symptomatic HIV-infected patients should receive IG prophylaxis regardless of vaccination status. Intramuscular IG may not be necessary if a patient with HIV infection is receiving 100 to 400 mg/kg IGIV at regular intervals and received the last dose within 3 weeks of exposure of measles.

Requirements for reporting adverse reactions to immunization

The National Vaccine Injury Compensation Program established by the National Childhood Vaccine Injury Act of 1986 requires physicians and other health-care providers who administer vaccines to maintain permanent immunization records and to report certain adverse events to the U.S. Department of Health and Human Services. These recording and reporting requirements took effect on March 21, 1988. Reportable reactions include those listed below and those specified in the manufacturer's vaccine package insert as contraindications to further doses of that vaccine.

The appropriate method of reporting depends on the source of funds used to purchase the vaccine. Adverse events that follow administration of vaccines purchased with public (federal, state, or local government) funds must be reported by the administering health-care provider to the appropriate local, county, or state health department. Subsequently, the state health department completes and submits the correct forms to CDC. Reportable adverse events that follow administration of vaccines purchased with private funds are reported by the health-care provider directly to the Food and Drug Administration (FDA).

Reportable adverse events after vaccination

VACCINE AND TOXOID	EVENT	INTERVAL FROM VACCINATION
DTP, polio, DTP-polio combined	Anaphylaxis or anaphylactic shock	24 hours
	Encephalopathy (or encephalitis)*	7 days
	Shock-collapse or hypotonic-hyporesponsive collapse†	7 days
	Residual seizure disorder‡	Variable
	Any acute complication or sequela (including death) of above events	No time limit
	Events described in manufacturer's package insert as contraindications to additional doses of vaccine	See package insert
IPV	Anaphylaxis or anaphylactic shock	24 hours
	Any acute complication or sequela (including death) of above event	No time limit
	Events described in manufacturer's package insert as contraindications to additional doses of vaccine	See package insert
MMR; DT, Td, tetanus toxoid	Anaphylaxis or anaphylactic shock	24 hours
	Encephalopathy (or encephalitis)*	15 days for MMR vaccines; 7 days for DT, Td, and tetanus toxoids
	Residual seizure disorder‡	Variable
	Any acute complication or sequela (including death) of above events	No time limit
	Events described in manufacturer's package insert as contraindications to additional doses of vaccine	See package insert
OPV	Paralytic poliomyelitis	
	— in a non-immunodeficient recipient	30 days
	— in an immunodeficient recipient	6 months
	— in a vaccine-associated community case	No time limit
	Any acute complication or sequela (including death) of above events	No time limit
	Events described in manufacturer's package insert as contraindications to additional doses of vaccine	See package insert

*Encephalopathy means any significant acquired abnormality of, injury to, or impairment of brain function, including focal and diffuse neurologic signs, increased intracranial pressure, or changes in level of consciousness lasting at least 6 hours, with or without convulsions. The neurologic signs and symptoms of encephalopathy may be temporary with complete recovery, or they may result in various degress of permanent impairment. Signs and symptoms (such as high-pitched and unusual screaming, persistent unconsolable crying, and bulging fontanels) are compatible with an encephalopathy, but are not themselves conclusive evidence of encephalopathy. Encephalopathy usually can be documented by slow wave activity on an EEG.

†Shock-collapse or hypotonic-hyporesponsive collapse may be evidenced by such signs or symptoms as decrease in or loss of muscle tone, paralysis (partial or complete), hemiplegia, hemiparesis, loss of color or turning pale white or blue, unresponsiveness to environmental stimuli, depression of or loss of consciousness, prolonged sleeping with difficulty arousing, or cardiovascular or respiratory arrest.

‡Residual seizure disorder may be considered to have occurred if no other seizure or convulsion unaccompanied by fever or accompanied by a fever of less than 102° F. preceded the first seizure or convulsion after administration of the vaccine; in the case of MMR vaccines, if the first seizure occurred within 15 days after vaccination; or in the case of any other vaccine, if the first seizure occurred within 3 days after vaccination, and if two or more seizures without fever or with fever below 102° F. occurred within 1 year after vaccination.

The terms seizure and convulsion include grand mal, petit mal, absence, myoclonic, tonic-clonic, and focal motor seizures and signs.

IDENTIFYING THE UNKNOWN POISON

Poisoning is the fourth most common cause of death in children. Approximately 80% of accidental poisonings occur in children under age 5, who ingest soaps, detergents, plants, vitamins, and their parents' medications. Such ingestions commonly include salicylates, alkaline corrosives, acetaminophen, iron, petroleum products, antihistamines, tricyclic antidepressants, benzodiazepines, barbiturates, pesticides, and opiates. The following symptoms and signs may help identify the unknown poison.

SIGN OR SYMPTOM	SUSPECTED POISON
Agitation, delirium	Alcohol, atropine, amphetamines, aniline dyes, antihistamines, arsenic, barbiturates, belladonna alkaloids, benzene, camphor, cocaine, DDT, digitalis, lead, LSD, marijuana, phencyclidine (PCP), theophylline, tricyclics
Alopecia	Arsenic, boric acid, cancer chemotherapeutic agents, lead, radioactive agents, thallium, vitamin A
Anemia	Lead, naphthalene and other potentially hemolytic agents, snake venom
Ataxia (choreiform); ataxia (tremors)	Heavy metals Lithium
Bradycardia	Barbiturates, beta blockers, digitalis, lead, muscarine-containing mushrooms, opiates, organophosphates, quinidine, quinine
Breath odor, alcoholic	Alcohol, chloral hydrate, phenols
Breath odor, bitter almond	Cyanides
Breath odor, garlic	Arsenic, organophosphates, phosphorus
Breath odor, pears	Chloral hydrate
Breath odor, pine	Pine oil
Breath odor, sweet	Acetone, chloroform, ether
Breath odor, violets	Turpentine
Breath odor, wintergreen	Methyl salicylate
Burns	Boric acid, corrosives, thallium
Coma, obtundation	Hypnotics, sedatives, general anesthetics: alcohols, anesthetics, aniline derivatives, anticonvulsants, atropine, barbiturates, benzene, bromides, carbon dioxide, carbon monoxide, chloral hydrate, chloroform, cyanide, ethers, hypnotics, insulin, lead, mushrooms, nicotine, opiates, organophosphates, paraldehyde, phencyclidine (PCP), salicylates, scopolamine
Cyanosis	Anesthetics (locals), nitrates, nitrites, phenocetin, sulfonamides
Dry mouth	Atropine, anticholinergics, antihistamines, belladonna alkaloids, botulinus toxin, narcotics, sympathomimetics
Dysphagia	Arsenic, camphor, caustics, botulinus toxin, iodine
Dyspnea	Carbon dioxide, carbon monoxide, cyanides, volatile organic solvents (such as benzene), snake venoms
Dysrhythmias	Amphetamines, digitalis, narcotics, phenothiazines, solvents, theophylline, tricyclic antidepressants
Fever	Alcohols, antihistamines, atropine, belladonna alkaloids, camphor, food poisoning, phenothiazines, quinine, salicylates, theophylline
GI symptoms: Abdominal pain, diarrhea, nausea	Arsenic, boric acid, botulinus toxin, cocaine, corrosives, digitalis, fluorides, food poisoning, lead, mercury, methanol, mushrooms, naphthalene, nicotine, opiates, organophosphates, phosphorus, salicylates, snake bites, spider bites, thallium, theophylline

IDENTIFYING THE UNKNOWN POISON *(continued)*

SIGN OR SYMPTOM	SUSPECTED POISON
Headache	Anilines, benzene, caffeine, carbon monoxide, lead, organophosphates
Hematemesis	Arsenic, caustics, fluoride, iron, phosphorus, salicylates, theophylline, warfarin
Hematuria/hemoglobinuria	Arsenic, cyclophosphamide, mercury, naphthalene, and other potential hemolytic oxidizers
Hemorrhage	Thallium, warfarin
Hypertension	Amphetamines, cortisone, lead, nicotine, sympathomimetics
Hypotension	Chloral hydrate, iron, phenothiazines, sympatholytics, tricyclic antidepressants
Methemoglobinemia	Anilines, nitrates, nitrites
Muscle spasms	Atropine, camphor, fluorides, lead, phencyclidine (PCP), phenothiazines, spider and scorpion bites, strychnine
Nystagmus	Barbiturates, phencyclidine (PCP), phenytoin, primidone, sedatives, tricyclic antidepressants
Paresthesias, weakness, paralysis	Alcohols, arsenics, botulinus toxin, curare, carbon monoxide, cyanide, fluorides, lead, mercury nicotine, organophosphates, thallium
Proteinuria	Arsenic, mercury, phosphorus
Ptosis	Botulinus toxin, phenytoin
Pupils, constricted	Barbiturates, chloral hydrate, ethanol, opiates, organophosphates, parasympathomimetics, phencyclidine (PCP), phenothiazines, sympatholytics
Pupils, dilated	Alcohols, amphetamines, antihistamines, atropine, belladonna alkaloids, benzene, botulinus toxin, camphor, carbon monoxide, cocaine, cyanide, ephedrine, LSD, meperidine, mescaline, parasympatholytics, sympathomimetics, thallium, tricyclics
Respiratory depression	Alcohols, barbiturates, cyanides, benzodiazepines, carbon monoxide, fluorides, opiates, organophosphates, phenothiazines, snake venom
Salivation	Arsenic, bismuth, caustics, cholinergics, fluoride, mercury, muscarine-containing mushrooms, nicotine, organophosphates, phencyclidine (PCP), salicylates
Seizures	Alcohol, amphetamines, antihistamines, arsenic, atropine, barbiturate withdrawal, belladonna alkaloids, boric acid, caffeine, camphor, cocaine, cyanides, digitalis, fluoride, hydrocarbons, lead, mercury, mushrooms, narcotics, nicotine, organophosphates, phenothiazines, phencyclidine (PCP), phenytoin, propoxyphene, salicylates, strychnine, thallium, theophylline, tricyclic antidepressants
Shock	Acids, alkalis, endotoxins, food poisoning, iron, leads, opiates
Skin, flushed	Alcohol, anticholinergics, antihistamines, atropine, boric acid, carbon monoxide, phenothiazines, snake bites, sympathomimetics
Skin, hot, dry	Atropine, belladonna alkaloids, botulinus toxin, sympathomimetics
Skin color, cyanotic, brown, or blue (without respiratory depression or shock)	Carbon dioxide, chlorate, ergot, ethylene glycol, iron, nitrites, nitrobenzene, nitrates, and other drugs and chemicals

(continued)

IDENTIFYING THE UNKNOWN POISON *(continued)*

SIGN OR SYMPTOM	SUSPECTED POISON
Skin color, pink	Boric acid, carbon monoxide, cyanides
Skin color, red-orange	Rifampin
Skin color, yellow	Hepatotoxic agents (chlorinated compounds, such as carbon tetrachloride, heavy metals, mushrooms, and many drugs), agents that cause hemolytic anemia (anilines, fava beans, many drugs), quinacrine, vitamin A
Strabismus	Botulinus toxin, thallium
Sweating	Cholinergics, nicotine, organophosphates, phencyclidine (PCP)
Tachycardia	Amphetamines, atropine, cocaine, caffeine, sympathomimetics, theophylline
Tachypnea, hyperpnea	Amphetamines, atropine, belladonna alkaloids, camphor, carbon monoxide, caustics, cocaine, cyanides, hydrocarbons, salicylates, snake venoms, strychnine, talc
Tinnitus	Aminoglycosides, camphor, diuretics, methanol, nicotine, quinidine, quinine, salicylates
Twitching, facial	Lead, mercury

ANTIDOTES TO POISONING OR ENVENOMATION

The chart below summarizes the pediatric uses, dosages, and other considerations for selected antidotes. For more information, contact your local poison information center.

TYPE OF POISONING OR VENOM	ANTIDOTE	PEDIATRIC CONSIDERATIONS
Acetaminophen toxicity	**acetylcysteine (Airbron*, Muco-myst, Mucosol, Parvolex*)** *Children:* Initially, 140 mg/kg P.O., followed by 70 mg/kg q 4 hours for 17 doses (a total of 1,330 mg/kg) or until acetaminophen assay reveals nontoxic level. Alternatively, may be administered I.V.: Loading dose is 150 mg/kg I.V. in 200 ml D_5W over 15 minutes, followed by 50 mg/kg I.V. in 500 ml D_5W over 4 hours, followed by 100 mg/kg I.V. in 100 ml D_5W over 16 hours.	● When used orally for acetaminophen overdose, dilute with cola, fruit juice, or water to a 5% concentration and administer within 1 hour.
Acute oral overdose or poisoning when emesis is desirable (non-corrosive substance; non-obtunded patient)	**apomorphine** *Children:* 0.07 to 0.1 mg/kg or 3 mg/m^2 S.C. or I.M. followed by oral administration of water.	● Onset of emesis occurs in 1 to 2 minutes in children. Emetic action can be induced earlier by gently bouncing the child. If vomiting does not occur, gastric lavage should be performed. *Never repeat dose.* ● To prepare drug, dissolve tablet in 1 to 2 ml of normal saline solution or sterile water for injection. Filter before administering. Protect solution from light and air; do not use discolored solution (green or brown). ● Administer water after giving dose. Emetic action is increased if dose is followed immediately by water. ● Keep narcotic antagonist, such as naloxone, available to reverse apomorphine's effects, if necessary. ● Apomorphine is contraindicated in unconscious patients and those with poisoning caused by alkalis, corrosives, or petroleum distillates; in patients with narcosis resulting from opiates, barbiturates, or other CNS depressants; in severely inebriated patients or those with narcotic sensitivity or a depressed gag reflex because of the risk of aspiration pneumonia; in patients who are in shock because drug may cause circulatory failure; and in patients with strychnine poisoning or seizures because of the potential for aspiration and loss of airway.
Acute oral overdose or poisoning when emesis is desirable (non-corrosive substance; non-obtunded patient)	**ipecac syrup** *Children under age 1:* 5 to 10 ml P.O. followed by 100 to 200 ml of water or clear liquid. *Children age 1 to 2:* 15 ml P.O. followed by about 200 ml of water or clear liquid. *Children over age 12:* 30 ml P.O. followed by 200 to 300 ml of water or clear liquid. May repeat dose once after 20 minutes, if necessary.	● Administer ipecac syrup *before* giving activated charcoal, not after. Follow dose with 1 or 2 glasses of water. If vomiting does not occur after second dose, give activated charcoal to adsorb both ipecac syrup and ingested poison. Follow with gastric lavage. ● Ipecac syrup usually empties the stomach completely within 30 minutes (in over 90% of patients); average emptying time is 20 minutes.

*Canada only

(continued)

ANTIDOTES TO POISONING OR ENVENOMATION *(continued)*

TYPE OF POISONING OR VENOM	ANTIDOTE	PEDIATRIC CONSIDERATIONS
	ipecac syrup *(continued)*	• Be careful not to confuse ipecac syrup with ipecac fluid extract, which is rarely used but is 14 times more potent. Never store these two drugs together—the wrong drug could cause death. • In antiemetic toxicity, ipecac syrup is usually effective if less than 1 hour has passed since ingestion of antiemetic. • Advise parents to keep ipecac syrup at home at all times but to keep it out of children's reach.
Anticholinesterase insecticide	**atropine sulfate** *Children:* 2 mg I.M. or I.V. repeated every 20 to 30 minutes until muscarinic symptoms disappear. Severe cases may require up to 6 mg I.M. or I.V. q 1 hour.	• Monitor patient's vital signs, urine output, and visual changes. • Give ice chips, cool drinks, or hard candy to relieve dry mouth. • Constipation may be relieved by stool softeners or bulk laxatives. • Observe for tachycardia if patient has cardiac disorder. • With I.V. administration, drug may cause paradoxical initial bradycardia, which usually disappears within 2 minutes. • Monitor patient's fluid intake and output; drug causes urinary retention and hesitancy. If possible, patient should void before taking drug. • High doses may cause hyperpyrexia, urinary retention, and CNS effects, including hallucinations and confusion (anticholinergic delirium). Other anticholinergic drugs may increase vagal blockage.
Anticoagulant (oral); hypoprothrombinemia due to oral anticoagulants	**vitamin K derivatives:** **menadiol sodium diphosphate, phytonadione (AquaMEPHYTON, Konakion, Mephyton)** *Children:* 5 to 10 mg P.O. per day (phytonadione or menadiol tablets) *Infants:* 1 to 2 mg I.M. or S.C. (phytonadione) *Children:* 5 to 10 mg I.M. or S.C. (phytonadione) *Children:* 5 to 10 mg I.M. or S.C. one or two times a day (menadiol)	• Monitor prothrombin time to determine effectiveness. • Monitor patient response, and watch for adverse effects; failure to respond to vitamin K may indicate coagulation defects or irreversible hepatic damage.
Arsenic, gold, mercury, or lead	**dimercaprol (BAL in Oil)** *Severe arsenic or gold poisoning* *Children:* 3 mg/kg deep I.M. every 4 hours for 2 days, then q.i.d. on 3rd day; then b.i.d. for 10 days. *Mild arsenic or gold poisoning* *Children:* 2.5 mg/kg deep I.M. q.i.d. for 2 days, then b.i.d. on 3rd day; then once daily for 10 days. *Severe gold dermatitis* *Children:* 2.5 mg/kg deep I.M. every 4 hours for 2 days, then b.i.d. for 7 days. *Gold-induced thrombocytopenia* *Children:* 100 mg deep I.M. b.i.d. for 15 days.	• Fever is common, usually appearing after the second or third dose, and may persist throughout therapy. Acrodynia in infants and children has been treated with 3 mg/kg of dimercaprol I.M. every 4 hours for 2 days, then every 6 hours for 1 day, followed by every 12 hours for 7 to 8 days. • Treat patient as soon as possible after poisoning for optimal therapeutic effect; administer drug by deep I.M. injection only. • Monitor vital signs and intake and output during therapy, and keep urine alkaline to prevent renal failure.

ANTIDOTES TO POISONING OR ENVENOMATION *(continued)*		
TYPE OF POISONING OR VENOM	**ANTIDOTE**	**PEDIATRIC CONSIDERATIONS**
	dimercaprol (BAL in Oil) *(continued)* **Mercury poisoning** *Children:* Initially, 5 mg/kg deep I.M., then 2.5 mg/kg daily or b.i.d. for 10 days. **Acute lead encephalopathy or blood lead level greater than 100 mcg/dl** *Children:* 4 mg/kg deep I.M. injection, then give simultaneously with edetate calcium disodium (250 mg/m²) every 4 hours for 5 days. Use separate injection sites.	• Adverse effects of dimercaprol are usually mild and transient and occur in about one half of patients who receive an I.M. dose of 5 mg/kg. In patients who receive doses in excess of 5 mg/kg, adverse effects usually occur within 30 minutes after injection and subside in 1 to 6 hours. • Drug has strong garlic odor. Advise parents and patient that drug may cause a bad taste in the mouth and/or bad breath; a burning sensation of the lips, mouth, throat, eyes, and penis; and toothache.
Antimony, arsenic, aspirin, atropine, barbiturates, camphor, cardiac glycosides, cocaine, glutethimide, ipecac, malathion, morphine, poisonous mushrooms, opium, oxalic acid, parathion, phenol, phenothiazines, potassium permanganate, propoxyphene, quinine, strychnine, sulfonamides, or tricyclic antidepressants	**activated charcoal (Actidose-Aqua, Arm-a-char, Charcoaide, Charcocaps, Insta-char, Liquid-Antidose)** *Children:* 5 to 10 times estimated weight of drug or chemical ingested. Minimum dose is 30 g in 250 ml water to make a slurry. Give orally, preferably within 30 minutes of ingestion. Larger doses are necessary if food is in the stomach. Activated charcoal may be given 30 g q 6 hours for 1 to 2 days (gastric dialysis) to enhance removal of some drugs.	• Do not give activated charcoal to a semiconscious or unconscious patient. • Because activated charcoal absorbs and inactivates syrup of ipecac, give only after emesis is complete. • Activated charcoal is most effective when used within 30 minutes of toxin ingestion; a cathartic is commonly administered with or after activated charcoal to speed removal of the toxin-charcoal complex. • Do not give in ice cream, milk, or sherbet; dairy products reduce drug's absorptive capacity. • Powder form is most effective. Mix with tap water to form consistancy of thick syrup. A small amount of fruit juice or flavoring may be added to make mixture more palatable.
Black widow spider bite	**black widow spider (Latrodectus mactans) antivenin** *Children:* 2.5 ml (1 vial) I.M. in anterolateral thigh or deltoid muscle. If symptoms do not subside in 1 to 3 hours, an equal dose may be repeated. Antivenin also may be given I.V. in 10 to 50 ml of normal saline solution over 15 minutes (the preferred route for severe cases, such as patients in shock or those under age 12).	• Immobilize patient immediately. Splint the bitten limb to prevent spread of venom. • Obtain a thorough patient history of allergies, especially to horses and horse immune serum, and previous reactions to immunizations. • Test patient for sensitivity (against a control of normal saline solution in opposing extremity) before giving antivenin. Give 0.2 ml of the 1:10 dilution of horse serum intradermally. Read results after 5 to 30 minutes. *Positive reaction:* wheal with or without pseudopodia and surrounding erythema. If skin sensitivity test is positive, consider a conjunctival test and desensitization schedule. • Early use of antivenin is recommended for best results. • Apply tourniquet above site of I.M. injection if systemic reaction to antivenin occurs. • Epinephrine solution 1:1,000 should be available to treat allergic reactions.

(continued)

ANTIDOTES TO POISONING OR ENVENOMATION *(continued)*

TYPE OF POISONING OR VENOM	ANTIDOTE	PEDIATRIC CONSIDERATIONS
	black widow spider *(Latrodectus mactans)* antivenin *(continued)*	• Black widow spider venom is neurotoxic and may cause ascending motor convulsions. Watch patient carefully for 2 to 3 days for signs of neurotoxicity. • A black widow spider bite induces painful muscle spasms. Patient may need analgesia and prolonged warm baths. • Administer a 10-ml injection of 10% calcium gluconate to control muscle pain p.r.n. • Vital signs should be checked every 30 minutes for 1 to 3 hours.
Botulism	**botulism antitoxin, trivalent (ABE) equine** *Children:* 2 vials I.V. Dilute antitoxin 1:10 in dextrose 5% or 10% in water or normal saline solution before giving. Give first 10 ml of dilution over 5 minutes; after 15 minutes, rate may be increased.	• Drug is available through state health department or state epidemiologist. • Obtain a thorough patient history of allergies, especially to horses and horse immune serum, and previous reactions to immunizations. • Epinephrine solution 1:1,000 should be available to treat allergic reactions. • This product is derived from horses immunized with *Clostridium botulinum* toxin. Therefore, test patient for sensitivity (against a control of normal saline solution in opposing extremity) before giving it. Read results after 5 to 30 minutes. *Positive reaction:* wheal with or without pseudopodia and surrounding erythema. If skin sensitivity test is positive, desensitization is required. • Earliest possible use of antitoxin is recommended for best results. • Monitor vital signs every 30 minutes until patient's condition improves. • Assess for neurotoxicity, respiratory depression, and change in comfort level. • Warn parents and patient that delayed adverse effects may occur 5 to 13 days after the acute phase of botulism. Urge them to report any allergic reactions or other unusual symptoms.
Coral snake bite (Eastern and Texas)	**North American coral snake *(Micrurus fulvius)* antivenin** *Children:* 3 to 5 vials slow I.V. through running I.V. of normal saline solution. Give first 1 to 2 ml over 3 to 5 minutes, and watch for signs of allergic reaction. If no signs develop, continue injection. Up to 10 vials may be needed. Not effective for Sonoran or Arizona coral snake bites.	• Splint bitten limb to prevent spread of venom. • Obtain a thorough patient history of allergies, especially to horses and horse immune serum, and of previous reactions to immunizations. • Before administering antivenin, a skin test for sensitivity to equine serum should be performed, because this product is derived from horses immunized with Eastern coral snake venom. For an intradermal test, use a 1:10 dilution of the antivenin serum in normal-saline solution.

ANTIDOTES TO POISONING OR ENVENOMATION *(continued)*

TYPE OF POISONING OR VENOM	ANTIDOTE	PEDIATRIC CONSIDERATIONS
	North American coral snake (Micrurus fulvius) antivenin *(continued)*	• Epinephrine solution 1:1,000 should be available to treat allergic reactions. • Venom is neurotoxic and may rapidly cause respiratory paralysis and death. Monitor patient carefully for 24 hours. Be ready to take supportive measures, such as mechanical ventilation. • Avoid use of narcotic analgesics and other drugs that produce sedation or respiratory depression. • Monitor patient closely over the next 24 hours for reactions to both the snake bite and the antivenin.

Crotalid (pit viper) bites, including those from rattlesnakes, copperheads, and cottonmouth moccasins	**crotaline (Crotalidae) antivenin, polyvalent**
	Children: The following initial doses (given I.M., S.C., or I.V.) are recommended (based on level of envenomation): minimal—2 to 4 vials; moderate—5 to 9 vials; severe—10 to 15 or more vials.
	    Subsequent dosages are based on the patient's response: 10 ml q 30 minutes to 2 hours, as needed, may be given. If bite is in an extremity, inject part of the initial dose at various sites around the limb above the swelling; do not inject in finger or toe.
	    The smaller the patient, the larger the initial dose. The amount of antivenin given to a child is not based on weight. Children may require a larger dose than adults.
	    Note: I.V. route is preferred and is mandatory if shock is present. When given I.M., crotaline antivenin may not reach maximum blood levels until about 8 hours after administration.
		• Immobolize patient immediately. Splint the bitten extremity.
		• Obtain a thorough patient history of allergies, especially to horses and horse immune serum, and previous reactions to immunizations.
		• Early use of antivenin (within 4 hours of the bite) is recommended for best results.
		• This product is derived from horses immunized with *Crotalidae* venom. Therefore, test patient for sensitivity (against a control of normal saline solution in opposing extremity) before giving it. Give 0.02 to 0.03 ml of the 1:10 dilution of horse serum (provided) intradermally. Read results after 5 to 30 minutes.
		    Positive reaction: wheal with or without pseudopodia and surrounding erythema. If sensitivity test is positive, follow desensitization schedule.
		• Epinephrine solution 1:1,000 should be available to treat allergic reactions.
		• Monitor circumference of bitten area before and after antivenin administration.
		• Type and cross-match as soon as possible because hemolysis from venom prevents accurate cross matching.
		• Monitor intake and urine output.
		• Watch patient carefully for delayed allergic reactions or relapse.
		• Monitor vital signs frequently (q 30 minutes) until symptoms subside (usually in 1 to 3 hours). Also monitor hemoglobin, hematocrit, CBC with differential, platelets, coagulation studies, bleeding time, chemistry panel, and urinalysis.
		• Monitor for hypersensitivity, shock, anaphylaxis, and serum sickness (marked by malaise, fever, nausea, vomiting, urticaria, lymphadenopathy, edema, arthralgia, muscle weakness, and peripheral neuritis, which may occur 5 to 24 days after administration).

(continued)

ANTIDOTES TO POISONING OR ENVENOMATION *(continued)*

TYPE OF POISONING OR VENOM	ANTIDOTE	PEDIATRIC CONSIDERATIONS
Cyanide	**amyl nitrite** **†*Adjunct treatment of cyanide poisoning*** *Children:* 0.3 ml by inhalation for 15 to 30 seconds; repeat every 60 seconds until sodium nitrite I.V. infusion and sodium thiosulfate I.V. infusion are available.	● Cyanide poisoning is usually treated in three steps: 1, amyl nitrite inhalation; 2, sodium nitrite I.V. infusion (0.33 ml/kg in children); 3, sodium thiosulfate I.V. infusion (1.65 ml/kg in children). ● Keep patient sitting or lying down during and immediately after inhalation. Crush ampule (has a woven gauze covering) between fingers, and hold to patient's nose for inhalation. ● Monitor for orthostatic hypotension; do not allow patient to make rapid postural changes while inhaling drug. ● Amyl nitrite is highly flammable; keep away from open flame and extinguish all cigarettes before use.
Cyanide	**methylene blue** ***Cyanide poisoning and methemoglobinemia*** *Children:* 1 to 2 mg/kg of 1% sterile solution by slow I.V. infusion. Dose may be repeated in 1 hour if necessary.	● Monitor hemoglobin concentration for evidence of anemia, which may result from accelerated erythrocyte destruction. ● Monitor fluid intake and output. Maintain intake of at least 2,000 ml daily. ● Advise parents and patient that drug turns urine and stool blue-green. Skin stains may be removed with hypochlorite solutions.
Digoxin or digitoxin	**digoxin immune FAB (ovine)** *Children:* Administered I.V. over 30 minutes or as a bolus if cardiac arrest is imminent. Dosage varies according to the amount of drug to be neutralized; average dose is 10 vials (400 mg). However, if toxicity resulted from acute digoxin ingestion, and neither a serum digoxin level nor an estimated ingestion amount is known, 20 vials (800 mg) should be administered. Alternatively, calculate dosage if ingested glycoside dosage is known: For digoxin tablets, oral solution, and I.M. injection: $$\text{dose (mg)} = \frac{\dfrac{\text{dose ingested (mg)} \times 0.8}{0.6}} {} \times 40$$ For digitoxin tablets, digoxin capsules, and I.V digitoxin and digoxin: $$\text{dose (mg)} = \frac{\text{dose ingested (mg)}}{0.6} \times 40$$ When steady state serum glycosides levels are known: $$\text{dose (mg)} = \frac{\text{serum digoxin concentration (ng/ml)} \times \text{body wt (kg)}}{100} \times 40$$ $$\text{dose (mg)} = \frac{\text{serum digitoxin concentration (ng/ml)} \times \text{body wt (kg)}}{1000} \times 40$$	● Monitor for volume overload in small children. ● Very small doses may require diluting the reconstituted solution with 36 ml of sterile saline for injection to produce a 1 mg/ml solution. ● Infants may require smaller doses; the manufacturer recommends reconstituting as directed and administering with a tuberculin syringe. ● Give I.V. using a 0.22-micron filter needle over 30 minutes or as a bolus injection when cardiac arrest is imminent. Dose depends on amount of digoxin to be neutralized. Each 40-mg vial binds approximately 0.6 mg of digoxin or digitoxin. ● Reconstitute vial with 4 ml of sterile water for injection, mix gently, and use immediately. May be stored in refrigerator up to 4 hours. ● Measure serum digoxin or digitoxin levels before giving antidote, because serum concentrations may be difficult to interpret after therapy with antidote. ● Closely monitor temperature, blood pressure, ECG, and potassium concentration before, during, and after administration of antidote.

†Unlabeled use

ANTIDOTES TO POISONING OR ENVENOMATION *(continued)*

TYPE OF POISONING OR VENOM	ANTIDOTE	PEDIATRIC CONSIDERATIONS
	digoxin immune FAB (ovine) *(continued)*	• Potassium levels must be checked repeatedly, because severe digitalis intoxication can cause life-threatening hyperkalemia, and reversal by digoxin immune FAB may lead to rapid hypokalemia.
Heavy metals (copper, iron, mercury, lead)	**penicillamine** *Children:* 30 to 40 mg/kg or 600 to 750 mg/m³ P.O. daily for 1 to 6 months.	• Check for possible iron deficiency resulting from chronic use. • Prescribe drug to be taken 1 hour before or 2 hours after meals or other medications to facilitate absorption. • Perform urinalyses and CBC including differential blood count every 2 weeks for 4 to 6 months, then monthly; check kidney and liver function, usually every 6 months; observe for fever or allergic reactions (rash, joint pains, easy bruising); and check routinely for proteinuria. Handle patient carefully to avoid skin damage. • About one third of patients receiving penicillamine experience an allergic reaction. Monitor for allergic signs and symptoms.
Heparin overdose	**protamine sulfate** *Children:* Dosage is based on venous blood coagulation studies, usually 1 mg for each 90 units of heparin derived from lung tissue or 1 mg for each 115 units of heparin derived from intestinal mucosa. Give by slow I.V. injection over 1 to 3 minutes. Maximum dosage is 50 mg in any 10-minute period.	• Check for possible fish allergy. • Do not mix protamine with any other medication. • Reconstitute powder by adding 5 ml sterile water to 50-mg vial (25 ml to 250-mg vial); discard unused solution. • Slow I.V. administration (over 1 to 3 minutes) decreases adverse effects; have antishock equipment available. • Monitor patient continually, and check vital signs frequently; blood pressure may fall suddenly. • Dosage is based upon blood coagulation studies, as well as on route of administration of heparin and time elapsed since heparin was administered. • Advise parents and patient that patient may experience transitory flushing or feel warm after I.V. administration.
Iron (acute intoxication; chronic overload after multiple transfusions)	**deferoxamine mesylate** *Acute iron intoxication* *Children:* 1 g I.M. or I.V. followed by 500 mg I.M. or I.V. every 4 hours for two doses; then 500 mg I.M. or I.V. every 4 to 12 hours if needed. I.V. infusion rate should not exceed 15 mg/kg hourly. Do not exceed 6 g in 24 hours. *Chronic iron overload resulting from multiple transfusions* *Children:* 500 mg to 1 g I.M. daily and 3 g slow I.V. infusion in separate solution along with each unit of blood transfused. I.V. infusion rate should not exceed 15 mg/kg hourly. Alternatively, give 1 to 2 g by subcutaneous infusion over 8 to 24 hours.	• Use I.M. route for acute iron intoxication, if patient's not in shock. If patient is in shock, administer I.V. *slowly;* avoid S.C. route. • Observe for and be prepared to treat hypersensitivity reactions; monitor renal, visual, and hearing function throughout therapy. • Advise parents that ophthalmic and, possibly, audiometric examinations are needed every 3 to 6 months during continuous therapy; stress importance of reporting any changes in patient's vision or hearing. • Explain that drug may turn urine red. *(continued)*

ANTIDOTES TO POISONING OR ENVENOMATION (continued)

TYPE OF POISONING OR VENOM	ANTIDOTE	PEDIATRIC CONSIDERATIONS
Lead poisoning by radioactive and nuclear fusion products and other heavy metals except mercury, gold, or arsenic poisoning	**edetate calcium disodium** *Symptomatic lead poisoning without encephalopathy and blood lead concentrations less than 100 mcg/dl* Children: 1 g/m² I.V. or I.M. daily in divided doses for 3 to 5 days. *Severe lead poisoning with symptoms of encephalopathy and/or blood lead concentrations greater than 100 mcg/dl* Children: 250 mg/m² deep I.M. injection or continuous I.V. infusion 4 hours after injection of 4 mg/kg of dimercaprol and then at 4-hour intervals thereafter, usually for 5 days (1.5 g/m² daily).	• I.M. route is recommended for children. • Add 1% procaine before I.M. injection to decrease pain at site. • Avoid rapid and large-volume I.V. infusions in patients with lead encephalopathy. • Hydrate patient before giving drug to ensure adequate urine flow; monitor renal status frequently. • Monitor intake and output, urinalysis, BUN levels, and ECG throughout therapy. • For I.V. infusion, dilute drug with dextrose 5% solution or normal saline solution; administer one half the daily dose over at least a 1 hour in asymptomatic patients, 2 hours in symptomatic patients. The second daily infusion should be given 6 or more hours after the first infusion. If administered as a single dose, infuse over 12 to 24 hours. • If drug is administered as a continuous I.V. infusion, interrupt infusion for at least 1 hour before a blood lead concentration to avoid a falsely elevated value.
Opiate overdose, opiate-induced respiratory depression	**naloxone hydrochloride** *Postoperative narcotic depression* Children: 0.01 mg/kg dose I.M., I.V., or S.C., repeated q 2 to 3 minutes p.r.n. If initial dose does not result in clinical improvement, up to 10 times this dose (0.1 mg/kg) may be needed to be effective. *Neonatal opiate depression (asphyxia neonatorum)* Neonates: 0.01 mg/kg I.V. into umbilical vein repeated q 2 to 3 minutes for three doses. Concentration for use in neonates and children is 0.02 mg/ml.	• Naloxone should be administered cautiously to narcotic addicts, including newborns of women with narcotic dependence, in whom it may produce an acute abstinence syndrome. • Administer with extreme caution to children. Adult concentration (0.4 mg/ml) may be diluted by mixing 0.5 ml with 9.5 ml sterile water or saline solution for injection to make neonatal concentration (0.02 mg/ml). • Keep resuscitative equipment available. Be prepared to provide supported ventilation and gastric lavage. • Because naloxone's duration of activity is shorter than that of most narcotics, vigilance and repeated doses are usually necessary to manage an acute narcotic overdose in a nonaddicted patient. • Avoid relying on the drug too much; do not neglect airway, breathing, and circulation. Maintain adequate respiratory and cardiovascular status at all times. Respiratory "overshoot" may occur; monitor for respiratory rate higher than before respiratory depression. Respiratory rate increases in 1 to 2 minutes, and effect lasts 1 to 4 hours. • Naloxone is not effective in treating respiratory depression caused by non-opioid drugs.

ANTIDOTES TO POISONING OR ENVENOMATION *(continued)*

TYPE OF POISONING OR VENOM	ANTIDOTE	PEDIATRIC CONSIDERATIONS
	naloxone hydrochloride *(continued)*	● Naloxone may be administered by continuous I.V. infusion, which is often necessary to control the adverse effects of epidurally administered morphine. ● Naloxone improves circulation in refractory shock, and has been used by some researchers to relieve certain kinds of chronic constipation. ● Monitor for bleeding. Naloxone has been associated with abnormal coagulation test results.
Organophosphate pesticides	**pralidoxime chloride (2-PAM chloride, pyridine-2-aldoxime methochloride)** *Children:* 20 to 40 mg/kg I.V. infusion over 30 to 60 minutes. Pralidoxime chloride is most effective when administered within 24 hours of exposure. It should be administered with atropine.	● Institute treatment of organophosphate poisoning without waiting for laboratory test results. Draw blood for RBC and cholinesterase levels before giving pralidoxime. Begin pralidoxime and atropine therapy simultaneously. Repeat dosage if signs of toxicity reappear. Maintain some degree of atropinism for at least 48 hours. ● Treatment is most effective when started within the first 24 hours, preferably within a few hours after poisoning. Even severe poisoning may be reversed if drug is given within 48 hours. Monitor effect of therapy by ECG because of possible heart block due to the anticholinesterase. Continued absorption of the anticholinesterase from the lower bowel causes recurring toxic exposure that may require additional doses of pralidoxime q 3 to 8 hours, or over several days. ● After dermal exposure, the patient's clothing should be removed and hair and skin should be washed with sodium bicarbonate, soap, water, or alcohol as soon as possible. While cleaning the patient, caregiver should wear gloves and protective garb to avoid contamination. Patient may need a second washing. ● Subconjunctival injection is currently an unapproved method of administration but has been used to reverse adverse ocular effects resulting from systemic overdose or splashing into the eye. ● Reconstitute pralidoxime with 20 ml of sterile water for injection to provide a solution containing 50 mg/ml. For I.V. infusion, dilute calculated dose to a volume of 100 ml with normal saline injection. Use within a few hours. ● Pralidoxime usually is administered by I.V. infusion over 15 to 30 minutes. Rapid administration has produced tachycardia, laryngospasm, muscle rigidity, and transient neuromuscular blockade. Hypertension may also occur, related to dose and rate of infusion;

(continued)

ANTIDOTES TO POISONING OR ENVENOMATION *(continued)*

TYPE OF POISONING OR VENOM	ANTIDOTE	PEDIATRIC CONSIDERATIONS
	pralidoxime chloride (2-PAM chloride, pyridine-2-aldoxime methochloride) *(continued)*	it may be reversed by discontinuing the infusion, slowing the rate of infusion, or infusing 5 mg of phentolamine. Closely monitor blood pressure. ● In patients with pulmonary edema, if I.V. infusion is not practical, or a more rapid effect is needed, pralidoxime may be given by slow I.V. injection over at least 5 minutes; it may also be given I.M. or S.C.
Rabies exposure	**antirabies serum** *Children:* 40 units/kg at time of first dose of rabies vaccine. Use half dose to infiltrate wound area. Give remainder I.M. Don't give rabies vaccine and antirabies serum in same syringe or at same time. For wounds on mucous membranes, the entire dose should be administered I.M. This serum should be administered to a patient only once.	● Epinephrine solution 1:1,000 should be available to treat allergic reactions. ● Perform a sensitivity test before giving I.M. dose. Dilute antirabies serum to 1:100 or 1:1,000 with normal saline solution for injection. Inject intradermally 0.1 ml of 1:100 dilution (or 0.05 ml of 1:1,000 dilution in patient with a history of allergy) on inner forearm. Inject other arm with 0.1 ml of normal saline solution intradermally as a control. Read within 30 minutes. *Positive reaction:* wheal of 10 mm or more and erythematous flare of 20 x 20 mm. For patients hypersensitive to horse serum, use human rabies immune globulin instead. ● Equine antirabies serum is used primarily only when human rabies immune globulin is unavailable. ● Explain to parents and patient that the body takes approximately 1 week to develop immunity to rabies after the vaccine is given. Patient is receiving antirabies serum to provide antibodies for immediate protection against rabies. ● Tell parents and patient that reactions to antirabies serum may develop up to 12 days after administration and are related to the product's source, namely horses. Have patient immediately report skin changes, difficulty breathing, headache, swollen lymph nodes, or joint pain. ● Tell parents and patient that acetaminophen may relieve headache, joint pain, or other minor discomfort after injection of antirabies serum.
Tricyclic antidepressants, anticholinergics	**physostigmine salicylate, physostigmine sulfate** *Children:* Not more than 0.5 mg I.V. over at least 1 minute. Dosage may be repeated at 5- to 10-minute intervals to a maximum of 2 mg if no adverse cholinergic signs are present.	● Observe patient closely for cholinergic reactions, especially with parenteral forms. ● Have atropine available to reduce or reverse hypersensitivity reactions. ● Administer atropine before or with large doses of parenteral anticholinesterases to counteract muscarinic adverse effects.

ndex

i refers to an illustration; t refers to a table.